Biotechnology Entrepreneurship

Leading, Managing and Commercializing Innovative Technologies

Biotechnology Entrepreneurship

Leading, Managing and Commercializing Innovative Technologies

Second Edition

Edited by

Craig Shimasaki, PhD, MBA
CEO, BioSource Consulting Group and Moleculera Labs, Oklahoma City, OK, United States

ELSEVIER

ACADEMIC PRESS
An imprint of Elsevier

Academic Press is an imprint of Elsevier
125 London Wall, London EC2Y 5AS, United Kingdom
525 B Street, Suite 1650, San Diego, CA 92101, United States
50 Hampshire Street, 5th Floor, Cambridge, MA 02139, United States
The Boulevard, Langford Lane, Kidlington, Oxford OX5 1GB, United Kingdom

Notices
Knowledge and best practice in this field are constantly changing. As new research and experience broaden our understanding, changes in research methods, professional practices, or medical treatment may become necessary.

Practitioners and researchers must always rely on their own experience and knowledge in evaluating and using any information, methods, compounds, or experiments described herein. In using such information or methods they should be mindful of their own safety and the safety of others, including parties for whom they have a professional responsibility.

To the fullest extent of the law, neither the Publisher nor the authors, contributors, or editors, assume any liability for any injury and/or damage to persons or property as a matter of products liability, negligence or otherwise, or from any use or operation of any methods, products, instructions, or ideas contained in the material herein.

British Library Cataloguing-in-Publication Data
A catalogue record for this book is available from the British Library

Library of Congress Cataloging-in-Publication Data
A catalog record for this book is available from the Library of Congress

ISBN: 978-0-12-815585-1

For Information on all Academic Press publications
visit our website at https://www.elsevier.com/books-and-journals

Publisher: Wolff Andre Gerhard
Acquisitions Editor: Mary Preap
Editorial Project Manager: Sandra Harron
Production Project Manager: Kiruthika Govindaraju
Cover Designer: Matthew Limbert

Typeset by MPS Limited, Chennai, India

Dedication

I dedicate this second edition of *Biotechnology Entrepreneurship* to my mother who passed away on March 23, 2018. She and my father had recently celebrated their 65th wedding anniversary and I was there to truly understand how a lifelong relationship of love, dedication, and perseverance gives purpose and meaning to life. My mother exemplified many characteristics that in some way she passed on to me either by association, osmosis or just by me being convinced that those were "normal." Some of the things I learned included (1) perseverance, even in the most troubled times, (2) to always keep your life in perspective, (3) a belief that circumstances will always improve, but realizing that I influence the outcome, (4) to appreciate people for their inherent value, not for what they can do for me, (5) having a desire to impact others with a vision greater than I can accomplish alone. Finally, that a successful life includes harmonious relationships and a growing relationship with God, so that your labor is not in vain.

This book is also dedicated to the biotechnology entrepreneurs who are diligently working to develop effective vaccines, rapid diagnostics and innovative treatments in the fight against the recent coronovirus, SARS-CoV2. These individuals bring the passion and talent that will help them creatively solve life-altering medical problems, and build upon what past generations have accomplished in this field. The purpose and mission of this book is to impart guidance, insight, practical assistance, and inspiration such that they can experience greater successes than our previous generations. If I have been a part of helping you to navigate toward this goal, then these writings have been well worth the time and effort to pen.

Contents

List of Contributors

Chris Allen, MS, Director, Capital Projects, Paragon Bioservices Inc., Baltimore, MD, United States

Jack M. Anthony, Founder and Former Principal, BioMentorz, Inc., Healdsburg, CA, United States

Norman W. Baylor, PhD, President & CEO, Biologics Consulting Group, Inc., Alexandria, VA, United States

John F. Beeler, PhD, Translational Medicine, Bristol-Myers Squibb, Cambridge, MA, United States

Dave Boclair, Director, Operational Excellence, Paragon Bioservices Inc., Baltimore, MD, United States

Arthur A. Boni, PhD, John R. Thorne Distinguished Career Professor of Entrepreneurship, Emeritus, Tepper School of Business at Carnegie Mellon University, Pittsburgh, PA, United States

Craig C. Bradley, JD, Much Shelist, P.C., Chicago, IL, United States

Lowell W. Busenitz, PhD, MBA, Price College of Business, Center for Entrepreneurship, University of Oklahoma, Norman, OK, United States

Mark Byrne, MS, President, PriMedicus Development, Loveland, OH, United States; Chief Executive Officer, ProteoSense, Columbus, OH, United States

Robert J. Calcaterra, DSc, Founder, St. Louis Arch Angels; Co-founder and Managing Director, Exeteur Group, LLC; StartUp Partners International, LLC, St. Louis, MO, United States

John Conner, MS, Chief Manufacturing Officer, Paragon Bioservices, Inc., Baltimore, MD, United States

Gerry J. Elman, MS, JD, Elman Technology Law, P.C., Media, PA, United States

Steven M. Ferguson, CLP, Special Advisor, Office of Technology Transfer, National Institutes of Health, Rockville, MD, United States

François Ferré, PhD, ALMA Life Sciences LLC, San Diego, CA, United States

Toby Freedman, PhD, President, Synapsis Search Biotech Recruiting, Portola Valley, CA, United States

Susan Garfield, DrPH, Global Advisory Principal and Life Sciences Sector Commercial Lead, EY, Cambridge, MA, United States

The Honorable James C. Greenwood, President & CEO, Biotechnology Innovation Organization (BIO), Washington, DC, United States

Neal Gutterson, PhD, Corteva Agrisciences, Johnston, Iowa, United States

Philip Haworth, PhD, Principal, BioMentorz, Inc., Santa Fe, NM, United States

Gail H. Javitt, JD, MPH, Epstein Becker Green, PC, United States

Uma S. Kaundinya, PhD, CLP, Vice-President, Corporate Development, Goldfinch Bio, Cambridge, MA, United States

Donald R. Kirsch, PhD, Harvard Extension School, Cambridge, MA, United States

Konstantin S. Kostov, PhD, Cantina Angels, Chicago, IL, United States; Life Science Angels, Sunnyvale, CA, United States

Joan E. Kureczka, MSEM, Senior Vice President and Stacey Shackford, Director, Social Media. Bioscribe, Inc., California

Lynn Johnson Langer, PhD, MBA, Executive Dean of Academic Programs, Foundation for Advanced Education in the Sciences at the National Institutes of Health, Bethesda, MD, United States

Maria Lopez, Vice President, Quality and Regulatory Affairs, SIWA Biotech Corp., Oklahoma City, OK, United States

Lara V. Marks, D.Phil Oxon, FRSB, Honorary Research Associate, Department of Science and Technology Studies, University College London and Managing editor of www.whatisbiotechnology.org, London, United Kingdom

Magda Marquet, PhD, ALMA Life Sciences LLC, San Diego, CA, United States

Gayle M. Mills, MBA, Principal, BioMentorz, Inc., Santa Fe, NM, United States

Bill Minshall, MS, Owner, ASL Consulting, Ocala, FL, United States

Jay Peterson, Manager, Manufacturing, Cytovance Biologics Inc., Oklahoma City, OK, United States

Rabi Prusti, PhD, Executive Director, Quality Control, Cytovance Biologics Inc., Oklahoma City, OK, United States

David Sahner, MD, Chief Medical and Chief Scientific Officer, EigenMed, Inc., Santa Rosa, CA, United States; Consultant to Biotechnology, Data Science, and Venture Capital companies, Santa Cruz, CA, United States

Stephen M. Sammut, MA, MBA, DBA, Health Care Management, Wharton School, University of Pennsylvania, Philadelphia, PA, United States

Alaap B. Shah, JD, MPH, Epstein Becker Green, PC, United States

Craig Shimasaki, PhD, MBA, CEO, BioSource Consulting Group and Moleculera Labs, Oklahoma City, OK, United States

David C. Spellmeyer, PhD, Adjunct Associate Professor, Department of Pharmaceutical Chemistry, University of California, San Francisco and Principal, Interlaken Associates, LLC, San Francisco, CA, United States; Principal, Interlaken Associates, LLC, Oakland, CA, United States

Henri A. Termeer, MBA, Former CEO, Genzyme Corporation, Cambridge, MA, United States

Donna-Bea Tillman, PhD, Team Lead, Devices, Biologics Consulting Group, Inc., Alexandria, VA, United States

Gergana Todorova, PhD, Mihaylo College of Business and Economics, California State University, Fullerton, CA, United States

Tom D. Walker, MBA, CEO and President, Rev1 Ventures, Inc., Columbus, OH, United States

Robert E. Wanerman, JD, MPH, Partner at Epstein Becker Green, P.C., Washington, DC, United States

Laurie R. Weingart, PhD, Richard M. and Margaret S. Cyert Professor of Organizational Behavior and Theory, Tepper School of Business at Carnegie Mellon University, Pittsburgh, PA, United States

Gladys B. White, PhD, Adjunct Professor of Liberal Studies, Georgetown University, Washington, DC, United States

Don Wuchterl, Senior Vice President, Technical Operations and Quality, Audentes Therapeutics, San Francisco, CA, United States

Jay Z. Zhang, MS, JD, Shuwen Biotech Co. Ltd., Deqing, P.R. China; China Jiliang University Law School, Hangzhou, P.R. China

Jimmy Zhimin Zhang, PhD, MBA, Founder, Chairman and CEO, AccuGen Therapeutics, Inc., San Francisco, CA, United States; Venture Partner, Lilly Asia Ventures (LAV), Shanghai, P.R. China

Foreword to the Second Edition

I'd like to share with you why this book you are holding is a valuable and essential resource for you.

As a physics graduate student who had transplanted himself to the Cell Biology Department of the New York University School of Medicine in the mid-1970s to work on a doctoral project in structural biology, I was rather oblivious to the scientific significance of the seminal Cohen–Boyer publication that arguably sets the stage for the advent of the biotechnology industry. What was unmistakable was the excitement of the biologists in the lab any time they referred to it, and that left an indelible impression on my memory.

Fast forward to October 1980. I had just defended my PhD thesis, maybe even learned some biology in the interim, but that was of no value in comprehending the next event that captured the imagination of scientists in the lab—the IPO of Genentech! The difference was that this time I decided to take action. I was going to become a part of this new and exciting undertaking, and the role I chose for myself was borne out of my personal experience. I surmised that this new and emerging industry, this marriage of science and business, would require people to explain business to the scientists, and science to the business people. With that simple thought as my mission statement, starting from October 1980, I embarked on a lifelong embrace with biotechnology, first as one of the Wall Street's earlier crop of biotech analysts, then an investment banker, and longer term, a company founder, investor, advisor, and board member. In fact, it has mattered little in what capacity I was to be involved with the industry, all that mattered was that I could find myself at this extraordinary intersection of science, medicine, business, and finance that almost magically has been able to generate truly breakthrough medicines over the last four decades.

Since the global financial crisis of 2008, capital markets for biotech companies have been improving steadily and the IPO market has come back with unprecedented breadth and intensity. Particularly in the 2013–18 period, we have seen more capital raised (about $27.2 billion) in IPOs than the total amount raised from 1979 to 2012 (about $23.8 billion). During the same time, more than 300 companies have gone public, which, given the rate of disappearance of older companies through acquisition, bankruptcy, or refocus away from biotech, at the close of 2018 more than half of the publicly trading companies in this sector had their IPOs during the past 6 years. Not all CEOs are first-time CEOs but, clearly, we have a great number of new faces staffing the management teams of these companies, most of whom have only experienced the generous stock market environment of the past few years.

I will close with a short story that makes my point even more succinct. Recently, during a strategic consulting assignment for a young biotech company, a pair of professionals from a notable management consulting firm asked to have a telephonic interview with me to solicit some insights and recommendations. Both individuals sounded quite bright but also quite young. At one point during the conversation, I offered an opinion regarding which drug discovery and development projects were suitable for young companies by retelling a story, as I have done many times, that I had heard from the late, legendary leader George Rathmann of Amgen. George had told me, and all others who cared to listen, that for a young company, the only suitable projects are those that would allow you to analyze the clinical data "on the back of an envelope." He would then go on and say, "After seeing a few patients on erythropoietin have their hematocrit go up, we knew he had a drug." He was taking an extreme position, but he was trying to make a point. As I told the story, I paused for a moment. Even though we were on the phone, I could sense puzzlement on the other end of the line. So I asked, "Do you know who George Rathmann was?" First silence, and then came their answer, "No."

While I am not suggesting that history repeats itself in a precise fashion, I am suggesting that ignoring history and the lessons that seasoned professionals can teach us could be catastrophic.

I have recited this lengthy personal discourse to stress the fact that I have witnessed first-hand much of what has transpired in the biotechnology industry since the early 1980s. Seeing the flawed ways by which the past is brought into the present led me to coin a phrase—*in business, history often is ignored, revised, or misinterpreted*. I find this problem particularly acute in our sector. The occasional academic analyses that are generated lack the real-world point of view that only seasoned practitioners can provide. On the other hand, most seasoned practitioners typically are not very good at, or interested in, producing analytical treatises. As a result, there is scant literary works and professional resources that provide a robust historical and practical overview of the inner workings of the biotechnology industry. Without such literary resources, the next generation cannot rely on much more than personal experience and/or industry folklore when they are confronted with challenges and are seeking guidance from past experience.

This book is a rare and comprehensive practical resource, written by experienced practitioners and thoughtful biotechnology industry leaders dealing with topics that are relevant to research and business executives in this amazing industry. It has the right mix of tactical and strategic insights. It will be an invaluable companion to current entrepreneurs, academic training programs, service providers, and to those who are just trying to make sense out of the ever-evolving challenges confronting them in this industry. This book provides a systematic way to communicate to the current generation of leaders the hard-learned lessons from the past. Read, enjoy, and learn the real history and practical guidance from those who came before you.

Dr. Stelios Papadopoulos is Chairman of the Board of Directors of Biogen Inc., Exelixis Inc., and Regulus Therapeutics Inc. He is a cofounder of Exelixis Inc. as well as cofounder and former Chairman of Anadys Pharmaceuticals Inc. (acquired by Hoffman—La Roche in 2011) and Cellzome Inc. (acquired by GlaxoSmithKline in 2012). In the not-for-profit sector, Dr. Papadopoulos is a cofounder and Chairman of Fondation Santé (www.fondationsante.org)*, a member of the Board of Visitors of Duke Health, and a member of the Global Advisory Board of the Duke Institute for Health Innovation.*

Dr. Stelios Papadopoulos was formerly Vice Chairman of Cowen & Co., LLC, where as an investment banker, he focused on the biotech and pharma sectors. Prior to joining Cowen, he spent 13 years as an investment banker at PaineWebber, Incorporated where he was most recently Chairman of PaineWebber Development Corp., a PaineWebber subsidiary focusing on biotechnology. He joined PaineWebber in 1987 from Drexel Burnham Lambert where he was an analyst in the Equity Research Department covering the biotechnology industry. Prior to Drexel, he was the biotechnology analyst of Donaldson, Lufkin & Jenrette. For his work as an equity analyst, he was elected in the Institutional Investor 1987 All America Research Team. He has also received multiple honors and awards for his work in the biopharma industry as a company founder, advisor, and financier.

Before coming to Wall Street, Dr. Papadopoulos was on the faculty of the Department of Cell Biology at New York University School of Medicine. He maintains his affiliation with NYU as an Adjunct Associate Professor of Cell Biology. Dr. Papadopoulos holds graduate degrees from New York University (MS in physics, PhD in biophysics, and MBA in finance).

Stelios Papadopoulos, PhD

Foreword to the First Edition

Among the fascinating aspects of biotechnology is the fact that this endeavor did not exist when the pioneers of the industry were growing up. Back in the day, it was not a career choice in high school or college—there were no courses you could take, no majors or minors you could elect to prepare you for what was to come. And I would be willing to bet that when asked what they wanted to be when they grew up, *no one* answered "a biotechnology entrepreneur."

With a scant background in biology, then short careers in law, national security affairs, and politics, I was "adopted" by the biotech village in 1993, when the Biotechnology Industry Organization (BIO) was first formed. Associating with those pioneer scientists, CEOs, and financial gurus has been the best part of my professional life. Put simply, their risk-taking behavior in uncharted territory, resilience, and dedication to helping others remain both inspirational and instructive.

When BIO was established 20 years ago, our infant industry was struggling to apply new molecular and genetic understanding to drug discovery, was running into financial and regulatory walls, and was attempting to adapt to proposals for comprehensive health-care reform. Plus we encountered controversies over patents, cloning (remember Dolly?), NIH funding, GMOs, among others. Do these sound familiar?

Now, finally, we have this textbook, which serves as a roadmap and operating manual to guide the next generation of biotech entrepreneurs. The chapters that follow cover the waterfront—the whole constellation of issues you'll confront, the hardest nuts you'll have to crack. The authors of these chapters share their experience generously and forthrightly in a fashion that characterizes the best mentors of any industry, especially biotech.

Philosopher George Santayana's most famous reflection is often cited but too rarely heeded. Allow me to remind you that he said, "Those who do not learn from history are condemned to repeat it." Trust me, it's worth learning from the biotech pioneers who have authored the chapters that follow. Having been there, done that, they can help you avoid many of the pitfalls that remain particular to this endeavor. They have made their mistakes, and for the most part have learned from them. What follows is high-value, even inspirational guidance.

Read on and go forth, but this will not be the end of the story. A confident prediction: biotechnology will transform the 21st century well beyond what chemistry and physics accomplished earlier. There is much further uncharted territory. Those are the chapters you will write.

Carl Feldbaum grew up in Philadelphia, graduated from Princeton University with a BA in Biology and a JD from the University of Pennsylvania Law School. He served as an Assistant District Attorney in his hometown, then as a prosecutor on the Watergate Special Prosecution Force in Washington, DC. He later served as Inspector General for Defense Intelligence in the Pentagon, president of Palomar Corporation, a national security think tank, and as chief-of-staff to US Senator Arlen Specter. In 1993 he helped found the Biotechnology Industry Organization and served as its president for 12 years until his "retirement" in 2005. In 2001 he was elected to the Biotechnology Hall of Fame. Carl now serves on several public and nonprofit biotech boards of directors.

Carl B. Feldbaum, JD

Preface to the Second Edition

This unique resource contains the collective experiences and seasoned advice from pioneers and leaders in the biotechnology industry who worked and served in it for many decades. You are about to read their insights, guidance, and best practices acquired through the tough lessons they have learned. There is an old saying, "Learn from the mistakes of others because you will never live long enough to make them all yourself." History and experience are our greatest teachers, but without a chronicling of these lessons learned, others are destined to "learn" these same lessons anew. This book was conceived for that very reason—to share vital lessons learned that will help you to become more successful than your predecessors.

Seasoned biotechnology entrepreneurial leaders are our scarcest resource and yet they are *the* most critical factor in predicting the future success of a biotechnology company. Products are produced by companies, and companies are started and guided by entrepreneurial leaders and managers. Therefore it is essential to produce entrepreneurial leaders, managers, and team members who are knowledgeable, better equipped, and have the business acumen necessary to make wise decisions for building successful biotechnology companies. These individuals make choices each day that affect the likelihood of success or failure for their organization and for the life-changing products develop. Because of this, it is equally important that we continue to develop wise leaders and managers who will shepherd the next generation of biotechnology companies.

What is contained within these pages?

In this book, you will find a wealth of information and inspiration giving guidance for achieving success in this exciting, yet challenging industry. You will find this to be a practical guidebook that was born out of lessons these leaders have learned. You will hear first-hand accounts of early biotechnology company founders, confirming that starting and growing a biotechnology company is not a prescriptive endeavor. You will also hear from veteran industry professionals in diverse segments of our industry sharing their insights and the critical information you need to know for operating in this industry. Topics in this book include: what is a biotechnology entrepreneur and what are the characteristics that make them successful; building great teams; how to evaluate a product idea; legally establishing your company; how to grow biotechnology clusters in your region; strategies for licensing and protecting intellectual property; understanding motivation of investors; best sources of capital for different stages of development; understanding the product approval processes; reimbursement strategies; forming biotechnology partnerships; drug, diagnostics, and bioagriculture development simplified; biomanufacturing; public relations strategies to get the word out; and careers in the life science industry and even bioethics.

Why did I write this book?

The goal I envisioned when starting to write and recruit contributors for the first edition of *Biotechnology Entrepreneurship* was to teach, train, and inspire future biotechnology leaders and team members, so they could be more successful in translating basic research discoveries into commercial products that would impact the world. I was fortunate to have started my career at Genentech in the early 1980s and witnessed first-hand the exciting opportunities and the unforeseen challenges of developing biotechnology products. However, even with that experience, I did not feel adequately prepared for the deluge of decisions that accompanied starting, managing, and leading a biotechnology company. As years went by, I recognized familiar overarching issues that arose in each successive company, and these issues were similar to those other entrepreneurs faced as they started and grew their companies. There was a myriad of reoccurring practical issues to deal with each day working to build a biotechnology company, helping other start-ups I cofounded, or mentoring scientists, physicians, and postdocs in the companies they desired to start. Another reason I wanted to write this book was to capture the inspiration, and memorialize the stories of the pioneers and leaders in our industry. I realized that many of the founding pioneers who paved the way for us to follow were passing away, along with the knowledge they acquired navigating their entrepreneurial journey. Rob Swanson of Genentech, George Rathman of Amgen, and more recently Henri

Termeer of Genzyme. My goal was to have a practical book that covered the key elements that entrepreneurs, leaders, and managers of biotechnology companies could gain insights from and use tools that would help them become successful.

Why a second edition?

As one would expect, biotechnology discoveries are rapidly advancing, such as CRISPR-Cas9 and the potential for its endless applications, artificial intelligence, and the myriad of applications in pharmaceutical and biotech product development. There is an urgent need to rapidly advance technology and speed applications to combat some of the most devastating diseases such as HIV, Ebola, SARS, MERS and the more recent Coronavirus (SARS-Cov-2). This second edition is expansive and updated, keeping the same tenets and purpose to teach, train, and inspire leaders and managers in the biotechnology industry. New chapters have been added covering: mentors and why you need them for success; how to apply the Business Model Canvas when developing your business model; understanding biases and how investors make decisions; the financial ramifications of raising capital and what you need to know about term sheets; commercial development of medical devices; artificial intelligence and applications in biotech and pharma, and updated chapters.

There are relatively few books dedicated to teaching, training, and guiding new leaders and managers of biotechnology enterprises. There are even fewer written materials that comprehensively capture the experiences and knowledge from seasoned experts in the business of biotechnology, explaining the fundamental issues that students, practitioners, and future managers of biotechnology companies would need to know to be proficient in this industry. This resource is intended to be a practical aid for practitioners, supporters, and students of the biotechnology industry. Although this book is titled *Biotechnology Entrepreneurship*, these writings are not only for individuals who start companies but also for those who desire to work in these early stage organizations. This book was also written for the many professionals who support the biotechnology industry, government officials and community leaders who want to grow biotechnology clusters in their region, and individuals who want to be employed within this diverse industry.

The biotechnology industry is key to the transformation of longer life through diagnostics, therapeutics, and genetic information, and for improving our health and food supply through bioagriculture and health-care IT, while advancing discoveries through research tools and reagents. Biotechnology has transformative power to impact the lives of millions of individuals. A few decades ago, who would have thought we could use the word "cure" as it relates to hepatitis C? The biotechnology industry and biotechnology entrepreneurship subject matter is vast and expanding with new knowledge and discoveries occurring almost daily, and it is a formidable task to comprehensively compile all this material. It would be presumptuous to believe that this is an exhaustive treatment to everyone's satisfaction of all the information contained within this vast and expanding industry. However, this book aspires to be a major step toward compiling the essential parts and pieces necessary for biotechnology leaders, managers, and entrepreneurs to be informed of the key elements necessary to build, manage, and grow successful biotechnology enterprises.

Because biotechnology companies are a melding of both science and business, leaders and managers must be skilled at managing the risk of scientific uncertainty and business. However, you cannot manage the risks that you do not know. Our goal has been to teach, train, and inspire you to be more successful in this rewarding and challenging industry. If we have accomplished that in any way, I will have considered this work a success.

Companies in our industry fail for various reasons, whereas the differentiating factor in those that are successful is the experience of the team. So how can individuals who are relatively new to entrepreneurship improve their success? By gleaning from the advice of those who have experience—which is the purpose of this book. I would greatly appreciate any feedback about the contents of this book, and any suggestions on how we may improve its value to you. You may send any comments to me at cs@biosourceconsulting.com.

I wish you the best of success in all your entrepreneurial endeavors!

Craig Shimasaki, PhD, MBA
Co-founder, President & CEO, Moleculera Labs, Oklahoma City, OK, United States,
Founder, President & CEO, BioSource Consulting Group, Oklahoma City, OK, United States
March 17, 2020

Preface to the First Edition

This is not just a book, but a compilation of experiences, advice, and lessons learned from biotechnology pioneers and leaders who have worked and served in this industry for many decades. There is an old saying, "Learn from the mistakes of others because you will never live long enough to make them all yourself." We have all made a few of these ourselves, and experience is one of our greatest teachers. But without a recounting of lessons learned by others, we are destined to "relearn" these same lessons anew. What you are about to read are insights, guidance, and advice from veterans in this industry, sharing best practices in starting, managing, and leading biotechnology companies.

The biotechnology industry diligently pursues better, faster, and more effective methods of translating ideas into needed commercial products. Products are produced by companies, and companies are started and managed by entrepreneurial leaders. Therefore it is vital to "produce" more effective entrepreneurial leaders and managers who are knowledgeable, better equipped, and have the acumen necessary to make wise decisions for building successful biotechnology companies. Seasoned entrepreneurial leaders are one of our scarcest resources and yet they are *the* most critical factor in predicting the future success of a company. Leaders and managers make decisions each day that affect the likelihood of success or failure for their organization and for the products they are developing. I believe that it is equally, if not more, important to develop knowledgeable and wise leaders who will shepherd the next generation of biotechnology companies.

The idea for this book came about primarily from two realizations. The first one was the recognition of my own inner frustrations while toiling through an inefficient, trial-and-error learning process as a serial entrepreneur of three biotechnology companies. I was fortunate to have started my career at Genentech in the early 1980s, and I witnessed first-hand the exciting opportunities and the unforeseen challenges of developing biotechnology products. However, even with that experience, I did not feel adequately prepared for the deluge of decisions that accompanied starting, managing, and leading a biotechnology company. As years went by, I recognized familiar overarching issues that arose at each successive company, and these issues were similar to those other entrepreneurs faced as they started and grew their companies.

The second realization came while listening to successful entrepreneurs and talented professionals who shared nuggets of wisdom and insight about their experiences and journey. Inspiration came while listening to fireside chats with Henri Termeer, former Chairman, CEO, and President of Genzyme, who shared his experiences and gave us his insightful admonitions. More ideas came while hearing talks from seasoned industry professionals about how to strengthen intellectual property protection, pragmatic regulatory guidance, sensible market strategies, and practical fundraising advice. Then there was the realization that many of our early biotechnology pioneers were no longer with us. Sadly, there are relatively few books dedicated to teaching, training, and guiding new leaders and managers of biotechnology enterprises, and I found no written materials that comprehensively captured all of this knowledge.

My desire was to assemble a comprehensive work written by seasoned experts in the business of biotechnology, explaining the fundamental issues that students, practitioners, and future managers of biotechnology companies would need to know to be proficient in this industry. These writings are not only for them but also for the many professionals who support the biotechnology industry, government, and community leaders who are working to grow biotechnology clusters in their region, including individuals who want to be employed within this diverse industry.

In this book, you will find a wealth of information and inspiration that provide the next generation of biotechnology entrepreneurs an improved chance of achieving success in this exciting, yet challenging, industry. You will find this to be a guidebook to help entrepreneurial leaders, managers, practitioners, and industry supporters gain "experience" through the lessons these individuals have learned. Within these covers, you will hear first-hand accounts of early founders of biotechnology companies, confirming that starting and growing biotechnology companies are not a prescriptive endeavor. You will also hear from veteran entrepreneurs and industry professionals sharing insights about what they learned over many years in this industry. Topics, such as what is a biotechnology entrepreneur and what are the characteristics that make them successful; how to assess a technology product idea; growing biotechnology clusters in a region; licensing and protecting intellectual property strategies; what are the best sources of capital at different stages of development, angel capital, venture capital; product approval processes; reimbursement strategies; biotechnology partnerships; drug, diagnostics, and bioagriculture development processes; biomanufacturing; and careers in the life science industry and even bioethics.

The biotechnology industry and biotechnology entrepreneurship subject matter is vast and expanding with new knowledge and discoveries occurring almost daily and it is a formidable task to compile this subject matter. Yet, it would be presumptuous to believe that this is an exhaustive treatment of all the information in this vast industry to everyone's satisfaction. However, this book aspires to be a major step toward compiling the essential parts and pieces necessary for biotechnology leaders, managers, and entrepreneurs to be informed of the key elements necessary to build and manage successful biotechnology companies.

Biotechnology companies are a melding of both science and business and, therefore, successful leaders are skilled risk managers of a scientific uncertainty business. However, one cannot manage the risks that they do not know. Our purpose and goal is to teach, train, and inspire current and future biotechnology entrepreneurs, leaders, and managers to be more successful in this rewarding and challenging industry. If we have accomplished that in any way, I will have considered this work a success.

I would greatly appreciate any feedback about this book and I solicit any suggestions on how we may improve its value to you. You may send any comments to me at cs@biosourceconsulting.com.

Craig Shimasaki, PhD, MBA

Co-founder, President & CEO, Moleculera Labs, Oklahoma City, OK, United States,

Founder, President & CEO, BioSource Consulting Group, Oklahoma City, OK, United States

Acknowledgments

I am immensely grateful to each of my colleagues and contributors to the second edition of *Biotechnology Entrepreneurship*. Each of them possesses decades of experience and are successful in their own right. I am thankful that in the midst of their demanding workload, they have unselfishly shared their knowledge, wisdom, and encouragement throughout these pages. They are fervent supporters of the biotechnology industry and they all want to see you succeed.

I wish to thank Mary Preap, Acquisitions Editor of Elsevier, who recognized the need for a second edition, Sandra Harron and Anna Dubnow, Editorial Project Managers of this book, and Production Manager Kiruthika Govindaraju, each have been tremendously helpful in bringing this book to completion.

I especially appreciate and thank my wife Verna who tirelessly read and assisted me in editing the seemingly endless revisions to many of the chapters in this book. And most importantly, I acknowledge and give thanks to God, who makes all things that seem impossible—possible!

Section I

Understanding Biotechnology Entrepreneurship

Chapter 1

What is Biotechnology Entrepreneurship?

Craig Shimasaki, PhD, MBA

CEO, BioSource Consulting Group and Moleculera Labs, Oklahoma City, OK, United States

Chapter Outline

My working definition of "biotechnology entrepreneurship" is the sum of all the activities performed through a team of individuals, working together over time, to build an enterprise that creates and commercializes life-changing products through the melding of scientific and business disciplines. It is through these integrated activities that a biotechnology enterprise creates, develops, and ultimately commercializes transformative products. Some of the most amazing life-saving treatments, medical devices, advanced fuels, and efficient crops, have been conceived and developed through biotechnology enterprises. In this chapter, I will outline the unique aspects of entrepreneurship in the biotechnology industry and contrast that with other industries, discuss the biotechnology entrepreneur's background and characteristics, and the factors that should influence their decisions. We will also discuss the concept of "intrapreneurship" in large companies, which refers to entrepreneurial activity for product innovation within an existing fully-sustainable enterprise.

The Significance of the Biotechnology Entrepreneur

A single individual can successfully manage and complete a research project, whereas it requires a company to create, develop, and commercialize a biotechnology product. All companies need a capable and skilled entrepreneurial leader in order to have any hope of becoming successful; therefore without the entrepreneur, there is no company. For example, without a Rob Swanson and Herb Boyer, there is no Genentech; without an Ivor Royston and Howard Birndorf, there is also no Hybritech (not to mention the numerous companies that their employees subsequently birthed in the San Diego area). Yes, diverse teams of people are essential to the success of any organization. However, without the leadership, vision, and the driving force of an entrepreneur, biotechnology products will never be brought into existence.

Biotechnology entrepreneurs are the backbone of the biotech industry and the source of its future innovation.

Biotechnology Entrepreneurship. DOI: https://doi.org/10.1016/B978-0-12-815585-1.00001-2

Without them, there would be no biotechnology industry. Biotech entrepreneurs are leaders with vision and passion that drives them to pursue their goals, with the belief that their product or service will ultimately impact the well-being of multitudes. Biotechnology entrepreneurs start companies for various reasons. Universally, they believe that their product or service can better diagnose, treat, cure, feed, or fuel millions of people. Most biotech entrepreneurs start companies with a heavy dose of altruism, and most often, this is the driving force that propels their work and efforts forward. Without a doubt, biotechnology entrepreneurs believe that financial rewards may await them. However, it is important to realize that these individuals are not *principally* driven by aspirations of financial prosperity, as there are much easier and faster career paths for making a comfortable living. However, these individuals are motivated to prove that their discovery or invention can one day become a commercial product that will be useful to the masses. This selfless motivation is an asset to the entrepreneur, especially when they encounter challenging financial circumstances and they still press forward without giving up or quitting. Unfortunately, this altruistic motivation may also become a detriment, particularly when sound financial and business decisions must be made. Biotechnology entrepreneurship can best be described as a lengthy and challenging journey along a circuitous path toward a satisfying and rewarding destination. Seasoned and thoroughly-equipped entrepreneurs have a less-challenging journey than their counterparts who possess minimal experience. This is because the path to commercialization is not always prescriptive, and there awaits many decisions along the way that can lead to either trouble or ultimate success. As we will discuss in more detail, most founders of biotechnology companies are typically scientists, physicians, engineers, or individuals with technical knowledge in a specialized discipline. Another group of biotechnology founders are individuals with business, finance, or venture capital backgrounds, who then co-found a company with the scientific inventors. I'll discuss the advantages and shortcomings typically inherent in both these scenarios and share how these can be overcome.

The Integration of Two Distinctly Different Disciplines

Biotechnology entrepreneurship is based upon the integration of two distinctly different disciplines—science and business. Managing the complexities of this intertwined cross-discipline enterprise can take new entrepreneurs by surprise. First-time entrepreneurs in a scientific field often unknowingly embrace the belief that the ability to complete scientific research is equivalent to product-development success. Soon afterwards they learn that there is a vast difference between completing a *scientific project* and building a *scientific company* that commercializes a biotechnology product. When you include the need to make practical, strategic business and financial decisions into this mix (which is not a typical skill set most scientists possess), leading a biotechnology company can be quite challenging for the inexperienced. Throughout this book, we endeavor to equip biotechnology entrepreneurs and leadership teams with the practical and experiential knowledge, along with a few sage words of advice, to help them become successful.

The term *entrepreneur* as defined by the *Merriam-Webster dictionary* is "*one who organizes, manages, and assumes the risk of the business or enterprise.*" In other words, the entrepreneur is the owner and manager of the *business risks*. However, in a biotechnology enterprise, the entrepreneur is also the owner and manager of the *scientific risks*. This duplicity of roles requires an individual who understands both sets of risks and how they influence each other. This is because decisions made in one area impact the corresponding area, and scientific issues are often inextricably tied to business issues. For example, let's say that your latest laboratory experiment reveals an unforeseen requirement to modify your company's planned molecular therapeutic target and therefore the team needs to modify the screening assays used to select the best target molecule. This, in turn, alters the original allotted time to reach your planned development milestone. Consequently, this results in a requirement for more capital than originally planned in order to sustain the organization through this period. Without the necessary capital to continue development, a company will cease to exist. Creating a successful biotechnology enterprise requires careful integration and management of *both* the business and the scientific issues, not to mention the myriad of other start-up issues an entrepreneur faces along the path of bringing a product to market. When a biotechnology company is created, you must meld biology with business and therefore you create a business of uncertainty. As the entrepreneur and leadership team reduces the uncertainty risk, the company value increases. Therefore the biotech entrepreneur must become a successful risk manager (Fig. 1.1).

Biotechnology Entrepreneurship Versus General Entrepreneurship

All entrepreneurs are endowed with a special set of talents and abilities, but more importantly, they possess a unique perspective on how they view the world around them. When others see problems, entrepreneurs visualize a myriad of solutions. When others spot roadblocks, entrepreneurs picture untapped opportunity. When others

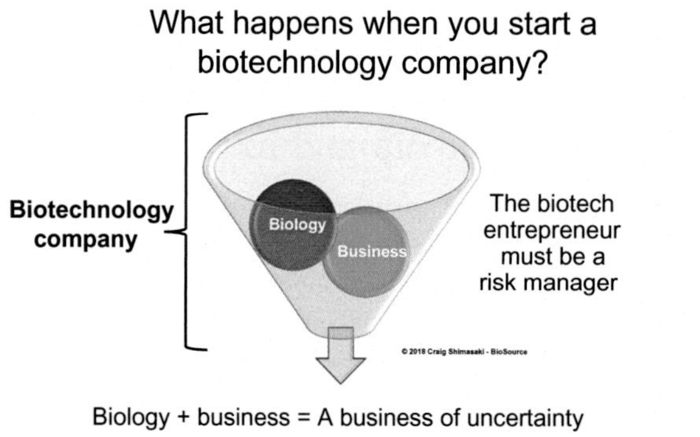
What happens when you start a biotechnology company?
Biotechnology company
Biology
Business
The biotech entrepreneur must be a risk manager
© 2018 Craig Shimasaki - BioSource
Biology + business = A business of uncertainty

FIGURE 1.1 Combining biology and business results in a business of uncertainty.

encounter challenges and are overcome by cynicism and despondency, entrepreneurs sense motivation rising within them to overcome. I believe that most individuals possess some underlying capabilities for entrepreneurial success. However, for these individuals who do not become entrepreneurs, certain life events and outcomes, coupled with their belief about the future, have altered their sight. As if wearing a green-tinted, grease-smudged pair of glasses, their eyesight is tainted by the misleading and hazy view of circumstances and a belief about their inability to change them. Sometimes entrepreneurs may be accused of inaccurately seeing the world through rose-colored glasses. However, those who have a vision of "*what could be*" achieve far more than those who believe "*they cannot.*" All good entrepreneurs should work to gain a balanced view of the real challenges yet not lose sight of their aspirational goals.

There are similarities between biotechnology entrepreneurship and consumer product entrepreneurship activities. Both require a competitive idea, a driving passion for their work, the ability to recruit and lead an experienced team, raising capital to support the endeavor through to commercialization, and a dogged perseverance to overcome roadblocks encountered along the way. However, the differences between the paths of a biotechnology product and a consumer product are greater than their similarities. Biotechnology endeavors come with unique challenges that other entrepreneurial endeavors do not face. These include the requirement for enormous amounts of capital to make product-development progress, lengthy product-development timeframes that can span over a decade, and stiffer regulatory approval requirements for products to reach commercialization. Biotechnology products include the complexity of medical insurance reimbursement and multiple customers in that the individual who orders the product does not use the product, and the individual who uses the product does not pay for the product. Biotech products also have an inherent scientific uncertainty that frequently is not fully appreciated until unexpected, but critical biological problems are encountered during development.

Time and Money Differences Between Biotechnology Products and Other Products

Every entrepreneurial enterprise requires capital to develop a product and reach commercialization. However, biotechnology endeavors require orders-of-magnitude more capital and take much longer to develop than most other enterprises. Companies that develop Internet applications or consumer-oriented products may often be able to reach commercialization with several hundred thousand dollars in capital and a couple of years in development before releasing a commercial product. Biotechnology enterprises require tens of millions, to hundreds of millions of dollars and many years, possibly a decade or more before these products have an *opportunity* to reach the market. Because of the enormous capital required to develop a product in the biotechnology industry, maximizing your company's attractiveness to investors and industry partners is vital during the growth of your organization. No matter how great a product idea or technology concept may be, without continued and uninterrupted funding, it is nearly impossible for any biotechnology product to reach commercialization. Therefore capital planning and the entrepreneur's ability to raise capital are vital prerequisites for the growth and development of a company in this industry. The biotech entrepreneur must have a working understanding of the total capital required to reach each value-enhancing milestone in order to remain attractive to subsequent investors. Funding gaps are not unusual for a development-stage company; however, it is incumbent upon the leader to be sure that these short-term and temporary funding gaps do not cause the demise of the company. In Chapter 10: *Understanding Biotechnology Product Sectors*, we discuss in more detail, the cost estimates and timeframes required for the development of various biotechnology products.

Regulatory Requirements

In addition to the cost and timeframe differences, the biotechnology industry is regulated by strict governmental requirements that must be met before marketing any biotech product. Regulatory agencies, such as the Food and Drug Administration (FDA) in the United States, the Medicines and Healthcare Products Regulatory Agency in the United Kingdom, and the European Medicines Agency in Europe, to name a few, each require extensive preclinical and human clinical testing to prove that your biotechnology product is safe and effective before it can be commercialized. Just meeting these regulatory requirements may take several years and millions of dollars. As technology and scientific methods advance and become more sophisticated, regulatory requirements also shift to keep pace with new discoveries that uncover the effects of biomedical and genetic products on human health. Since biotechnology products require numerous years of development, it would not be unusual to have regulatory requirements modified or changed between the time your product development starts and when your product is fully developed and ready for regulatory approval. The regulatory requirements differ for agricultural products, medical devices, laboratory tests, therapeutics, and biologics. Understanding the specific requirements for your product approval is critical to raising capital and commercialization success. Chapter 30: *Regulatory Approval and Compliances for Biotechnology Products*, is devoted to this subject.

The Biological Uncertainty Factor

One inherent factor within all biotechnology product-development plans is "biological uncertainty." Each biotechnology product idea carries a finite amount of biological uncertainty with it, which is not fully known until the product is developed and finally tested in the laboratory, in the field, and in animals or in humans. For medical devices and diagnostics, this biological uncertainty factor is not fully appreciated until the device or diagnostic test is validated in a large enough population of living beings, whether in animals or tested in large numbers of human clinical specimens. For therapeutics and biologics, this biological uncertainty may erroneously be presumed to be minimized by having positive preclinical, Phase 1 and Phase 2 testing results, only to discover that in Phase 3, the product is not effective in larger populations of humans. For agricultural biotechnology products, this biological uncertainty may be hidden in the plant or animal species, manifesting through an unknown effect of a gene-trait, or its effect on the downstream food chain or the eco-environment. Although it is impossible for an entrepreneurial team to eliminate this biological uncertainty, creative managers will find ways to adapt their product within the confines of these biologic uncertainties to ultimately produce a product that has great value to a target group of people. Biological uncertainty plays another role when the cause of a disease or disorder which a product is targeting may not be fully understood. This is the case with many disorders such as Alzheimer's, cancer, mental illnesses, and a host of other diseases and disorders. To add more intricacy to product development, scientific discoveries are still revealing the complex interaction of our biology and the environment, such as the microbiota interaction and the prevention or predisposition to many diseases. This inherent biological uncertainty is a risk factor that must be managed by the entrepreneur in order to successfully bring any biotechnology product to market.

Entrepreneurship and Intrapreneurship

It is possible that many individuals reading this chapter may not intend to start a biotechnology company on their own. In my example, although I never intended to start a biotechnology company, my interest and desire was to translate scientific discoveries into life-changing commercial products. Because of that interest, it led me to cofound nine biotech companies, and, for three of them, I become the CEO. Therefore even though you may not intend to start a company, one thing is for certain—you will likely work for one. Much of what we discuss in this book references an "entrepreneur;" however, the entire content of this chapter as well as this book is directly applicable to *all* managers and leaders within any biotechnology organization. For future career advancement, it is imperative for individuals to learn what it means to operate as a biotechnology *intrapreneur* irrespective of their position within an organization. So, what is an intrapreneur? An intrapreneur is someone who can operate like an entrepreneur but within a larger organization and in a smaller context. Intrapreneurs have similar characteristics that entrepreneurs have but they are confined within the boundaries of their organization or their departmental functions. Intrapreneurs are those who operate in a less-restrictive corporate environment, are given a budget or are requested to provide a budget, and have a project or product innovative idea to carry out and explore. The intrapreneur is protected from many of the downsides that an entrepreneur faces, such as the consequences of not finding capital, and failure of the product-development project, as these do not have the personal costs because the organization absorbs these losses and failures. A good intrapreneur approaches problems and makes decisions as if they were solely responsible for the outcome, and they operate as if the consequences impact them personally. An intrapreneur works to complete not only the tasks and responsibilities assigned to them, but they also observe the functions around them to be sure that those are executed properly, as they understand these can impact their own work and outcome. Great intrapreneurs know that their career advancement is determined in part by how they creatively solve problems and manage responsibilities that their company entrusts to them.

If you are not interested in being an entrepreneur or intrapreneur there are a multitude of other career opportunities for life science professionals, beyond what most individuals realize. For those who want to learn more about various career options available to individuals with scientific backgrounds, see *Chapter 40*: *Diverse Career Opportunities in the Biotechnology and Life Sciences*

Industry, which reviews the diversity of careers for new graduates or for current biotechnology professionals seeking a variety of job functions within the life science industry.

The Biotechnology Entrepreneur, Manager, and Leader

Entrepreneurial leaders typically possess a variety of skill sets and well-defined characteristics that have been studied and taught in most business schools. A set of these is outlined in *Chapter 4, Seven Characteristics of Successful Biotechnology Leaders*. Below, I list 13 biotechnology entrepreneurial characteristics, 10 of them I believe are essential to entrepreneurs in any industry. Although we will not take the time to elaborate on these general entrepreneurial characteristics, I would encourage you to reflect on the extent to which these operate within you. If you have uncertainty about any particular character trait, often by studying about them, you will find that it is easier to emulate them and can find many good books devoted to them.

Essential Entrepreneurial Characteristics in any Industry

1. A driving passion for your work
2. The ability to communicate your vision and inspire others to follow
3. Humility and the desire to learn
4. Accepting responsibility and ownership for problems
5. Perseverance in the face of adversity
6. An ability to raise money and manage it well
7. Understanding the purpose and principles of negotiation
8. Acquiring characteristics of wise leadership and skilled management
9. Embracing worthy core values
10. Utilizing creativity and imagination to solve problems

The biotechnology entrepreneur must also have honed an additional set of skills that I believe are crucial for success within this industry. Several of these characteristics are unique to this industry. Biotech entrepreneurs need to be particularly good at these three skills because of the enormous development costs, lengthy development time, and requirement of a myriad of disciplines to develop a biotechnology product. These additional skills are the ones that help leaders achieve great commercial outcomes. Unfortunately, these characteristics tend to be the ones that new leaders often struggle with the most. I'd like to elaborate on a few of the general entrepreneurial characteristics and two of the key biotechnology entrepreneur-specific characteristics in the following.

Essential Biotechnology Entrepreneurial Characteristics

1. Awareness of the unknown–unknowns
2. A multidiscipline translator: improving your ability to speak and understand the language of business and science
3. Understanding and navigating the complexity and interdependency between scientific and business decisions

Essential Biotechnology Entrepreneurial Characteristics

Awareness of the Unknown–Unknowns

The term *unknown–unknowns* may sound like circular reasoning, but it points out that there are issues that we don't even realize that we don't understand. This is the source of frequent peril during the development stage of many biotechnology companies. Its negative consequences have been painfully felt at some time or other in most all biotech enterprises. During their journey, a biotechnology entrepreneur will generally encounter two types of unknowns. The first we call the *known–unknowns*. These are issues and matters that you understand are important, but you also recognize that there is a gap in your knowledge in this particular area. All of us have experienced the feeling of having limited knowledge in an unfamiliar area, whether it be accounting, finance, regulatory laws, human resources, or a particular area of chemistry, biology, or physics. Although you may wish you possessed a working knowledge in that particular area, you recognize your knowledge gap and can hire consultants or solicit the advice of experts in that field. In other words, you are aware of what you don't know. *Known–unknowns* refer to having full recognition and awareness of limited information in an area that is critical to the company's future success, and that you are also aware that you do not have enough knowledge to make rational decisions about how to proceed. There is safety in this awareness because entrepreneur leaders can then seek the advice of experts in these fields and proceed with caution.

Then, there are the *unknown–unknowns*. This situation occurs when you do not possess knowledge about an area critical to the company, *and* you do not recognize your knowledge gap, but you proceed anyway. In other words, these are the things you do not know, that you do not know. In one consumer example of the unknown–unknowns, remember the market launch of "New Coke" by Coca-Cola. On April 23, 1985, the Coca-Cola Company announced a change to its nearly century-old secret formula by removing the original Coca-Cola from store shelves and replacing it with New Coke. This move was a major failure for the company. The fans of Coke were so angry they launched grassroots campaigns across the country to force Coca-Cola to bring back the original Coke. Interestingly, a poll showed that *only* 13% of soda drinkers liked the New Coke and that most consumers did not like it. Seventy-seven days later, the president of Coke announced the return of "Coca-Cola Classic," the original formula. This is an example of an unknown—unknown which should not have been. (Alternatively, some conspiracists believe that this was a planned marketing ploy, meaning they believed Coca-Cola was smarter than most people thought.) This is a familiar example of an organization thinking they understood something, but in reality, they did not. The major difference between an unknown—unknown for the Coca-Cola Company and a start-up biotechnology company is that the former has a large bank account and plentiful resources to recover from their mistake, whereas a young biotech company generally has one chance at commercialization success. Missteps for a development-stage biotechnology company can cost millions of dollars and ultimately jeopardize their future existence, whereas for large, well-established pharmaceutical companies, they can withstand multiple clinical trial failures and still survive to develop other products.

For Aviron, the biotechnology company that developed the FluMist influenza nasal vaccine in the late 1990s, their unknown—unknown occurred when the commercial vaccine they submitted to the FDA was not produced by the same manufacturing process and facility that was used to produce the product for their Phase 3 clinical trials. It appears that the company did not recognize this was an issue until after submitting their product license application to the FDA on June 30, 1998. This unknown—unknown required that the company confirm the clinical equivalence of their product produced at their new facility by the new process, and compare it to the process for the product manufactured at their former facility and used in their Phase 3 clinical study. The company successfully completed an additional 225-patient bridging study in Australia from December 1998 to March 1999. The results demonstrated that the new material produced at their new facility had similar immunogenicity and safety and tolerability profiles as the material produced at their previous facility (Aviron SEC S-3 Filing 2000, 2000). The company responded to the issue and announced on August 7, 2000 the hiring of a V.P. of Regulatory Affairs and a V.P. of Manufacturing. However, the impact of this unknown—unknown was a delay in the FDA approval, additional capital consumed, additional clinical testing, and a reduction in investor confidence. Fortunately for Aviron, they recovered and ultimately received FDA approval for their vaccine, and they were acquired in 2001 by MedImmune for $1.5 billion. Unfortunately, most unknown—unknowns in the biotechnology industry do not result in recovery and ultimate success such as this.

The unknown—unknowns are challenging to recognize because by definition you don't know what *you don't know*. A quote attributed to Socrates is, "*The more I learn, the more I learn how little I know.*" One good way to avoid this pitfall is to always seek counsel and advice from experienced individuals in your field before embarking on what you are wanting to do. Often, because of the need to accomplish many things quickly, we move forward with a limited understanding of the issues, only to find out later there are unforeseen consequences. This can especially be true when planning and preparing for regulatory approvals and clearances for biotechnology and bioagricultural products. Remember that regulations are constantly changing, and without current regulatory knowledge and experience, it is extremely difficult to successfully satisfy all the requirements for regulatory approval. Wise entrepreneurs surround themselves with many experienced and seasoned professionals they trust. These individuals may include other entrepreneurs, professionals in different fields, and experienced board members who bring expertise that the entrepreneur does not possess. Also, don't be afraid to ask questions. Seek plenty of advice and guidance when planning, and before proceeding. Cultivate relationships with others who have led and managed successful companies (see *Chapter 8: Building Human Relationship Networks*). When you are given any advice, it is also worth noting that sometimes guidance can be, in reality, a personal preference rather than a strict requirement. Understand that everyone will have their own opinion and you don't have to follow the advice of all people. However, there is safety in the counsel of many wise individuals.

Before we leave this topic, it is important to understand the difference between *The Goal* and *A Method*. There are a myriad of issues that a biotechnology entrepreneur must manage and navigate through when building a biotechnology company and developing a successful product. The *goal* rarely changes, whereas there are many *methods* to achieve your goal. Often, the advice from others is their preferred *method* to reach your stated *goal*. Recognize that even your own belief about how (*method*) to reach your goal can also be an opinion. Listen to the advice of others as you may formulate an even better method that you did not previously consider. Remember, methods vary, but never lose sight of your goal.

Be a Multidiscipline Translator: Improve your Ability to Speak and Understand the Language of Business and Science

All science and technology-based companies experience a normal tension that rises at the interface of the technical and business/marketing functions. A good portion of this tension exists because of the absence of individuals who are multidiscipline translators of both the science and business goals of the organization. A development-stage biotechnology company usually starts with a small team of people, so it is imperative that someone within that team has the ability to communicate both the scientific and business goals of the company. A multidiscipline translator is someone who not only understands the business, financial, marketing, and corporate issues but also understands the technical and scientific issues—and speaks both languages well enough for individuals in these respective fields to understand.

Biotechnology companies are most often founded by someone with a technical background, such as a scientist, physician, or engineer. These individuals are very proficient and accomplished within their specific technical discipline. All too often, the business aspects, such as financing, marketing, and legal issues, are not familiar to these individuals; or worse, they have no interest in learning or understanding them. Scientists are trained to be analytical and are good at questioning theories and suppositions. They are great researchers because they have been trained to be skeptical of information they don't understand until reproducible evidence is documented. Also, scientists naturally detect interpretation errors, and most scientists can quickly spot inconsistencies and problems within assumptions. These characteristics are ideal for making new discoveries, but they are ineffective communication tools when speaking to potential investors, businesspersons, and marketing people about your company's purpose and mission. It is important for scientists leading an entrepreneurial organization to learn the thinking process of businesspersons.

Reticence to learning something in another field or discipline becomes problematic for individuals in a young entrepreneurial organization as there is much to accomplish with seemingly limited resources. Although the team may be accomplishing great work scientifically, the unaddressed business, market, and financial problems can greatly reduce the interest from potential investors or partners. For instance, if the technology a company is working on is exciting and cutting-edge, but the target market they are addressing is relatively small and uninteresting, there will be limited investor interest. As such, the likelihood of raising large amounts of capital from sophisticated investors will also be limited.

When the founder is a businessperson rather than a scientist, they may lean toward operating in an artificially conceived environment in which the technology can deliver anything the market wants, when technically that may be impossible. If the businessperson founder does not understand the scientific limitations and the resulting implications it has on their product, there will be a disconnect between product development and marketing aspirations for the company. In this situation, the company may be promising future market benefits for a product that the technology cannot deliver. Sadly, when prototype or clinical testing begins, there may be great disappointment, and sometimes, failure. This reinforces the importance of being able to clearly communicate both the business and the science in a way that individuals in both disciplines can unambiguously understand.

All entrepreneurs, whether a businessperson, scientist, or engineer, should speak to their counterparts in the vocabulary of the listener. At the very least, all entrepreneurs should communicate with the assumption that the listener has little or no prior understanding of their subject matter, particularly their specialized terminology. It is not a requirement that all entrepreneurs need to memorize a business and scientific lexicon. However, proficiency and skill are required in order to convey precise meaning so the listener understands what is communicated and not confused by the jargon. For instance, when a scientist is communicating to a businessperson or investor about the benefits of their technology, instead of going headlong into a discourse about how "allelic-variation in single nucleotide polymorphisms and its haplotype chromosomal loci contributes to disease predisposition," they can just say, *"changes in the DNA of genes increase a person's likelihood of getting a disease."* The word "bacteria" works well for *Bacteroides melaninogenicus.* For the businessperson, their challenge is to translate business concepts and define their terminology so it is understandable to scientists and engineers. If a scientist asks the businessperson, *"how do we determine how much our company is worth,"* don't proceed to talk about risk-adjusted discounts to future cash flows and future earnings, but rather explain concepts through analogies such as housing prices, where the value is based upon what a willing buyer will pay at any point of time, then explain any other factors used for estimating the value. To the degree that the technical individuals understand the business and marketing objectives, to that same degree these trained problem-solving individuals can help to keep product development on track and meet the company's business objectives and market expectations.

Learn to simplify all terminology that may be commonplace in your specialty, particularly when communicating the value and significance of what you are doing to others. Use words that have meaning to the listener. Entrepreneurs should practice translating into the language of the listener and use analogies when describing complex scientific concepts or biological processes. Remember, verbal communication is simply a method of faithfully transferring thoughts and ideas from one person to another. If the listener cannot comprehend what you are verbally communicating, they certainly will not know if your thoughts are worthy of consideration. Multidiscipline translators learn to *think* about the issues encountered in other disciplines. Just as a bilingual individual will tell you that they became fluent only when they began to *think* in that language, so it is with the biotechnology entrepreneur, they must think about the issues critical to both the science and the business. Scientists should practice thinking about the business issues, and businesspersons should spend time thinking about the issues in the science, and each should frequently ask questions of the other to be sure that their understanding is consistent with the facts. Businesspersons and scientists approach problems differently and each can benefit from the thoughts and solutions offered by the other. Also, it is helpful to learn to understand the thinking process rather than just accepting an end-result or conclusion. I have seen from personal experience that by sharing a scientific issue in a way that a nonscientist can understand, great ideas have been offered though a listener who was not knowledgeable in that technical field. Don't be afraid to share issues with individuals whom you trust, even though they are trained in other disciplines or other fields. They may surprise you with good ideas and solutions. At the very least, you will have practiced simplifying the issues and concepts in a way that is understandable to others. You may even find that in doing this you solve your own problem by simplifying the issue. As we will discuss in the financing chapters, this is an essential skill that will prove valuable when raising capital.

Understanding the Purpose and Principles of Negotiation

Frequently, the term *negotiation* conjures up an image of two parties sitting on opposite sides of a table emotionally arguing the terms of an agreement or price of an asset. The connotation is arm-twisting and demanding which are believed to be associated with "negotiation." The general perception is that back-and-forth bantering is required until one party gets the upper hand and pressures the other party to succumb to their demands. These types of negotiations do occur, but this image should not reflect the majority of negotiations a biotech entrepreneur experiences, as these outcomes do not lend themselves to future collaborative relationships. It may be true that when negotiating the value of your company with investors, it may sometimes resemble the above description; however, even then, it is best not to allow negotiations to deteriorate to a verbal arm-wrestling match with the other party. The purpose of negotiation is to exchange something of value to one party, for something of different but equal value to another party. Before you begin negotiating, think about what you will be promising or giving up and be sure you are:

- Balancing obligations made to different entities (investors, regulators, partners, and customers).
- Balancing your limited time and resources.
- Securing *buy in* from those that hold or influence these resources.

Standard negotiation training seminars focus on techniques and the *dos* and *don'ts* of negotiation. However, negotiation is not just about technique, but rather understanding what is of importance to one party in order to exchange something that is equally important to the other. Negotiation is about reaching agreeable compromise where each party receives enough value to come to an agreement. Frequently, in negotiations, one party states that *everything* is important to them, and therefore there is limited compromise toward mutual agreement. In reality, every party has a hierarchy of importance for each of the terms or conditions in an agreement. The entrepreneur must learn to quickly find out what is of the highest value to the other party, and in exchange be sure to receive what is of the most value to them.

A better connotation for negotiation is the idea of a journey along an unfamiliar road navigating detours and roadblocks to ultimately arrive at your destination. Just as in this example, we sometimes say that we negotiated our way around these obstacles. When we say we negotiated, we mean that we figured out how to get past or go around obstacles in our path until we reached our goal. Great biotechnology entrepreneurs learn to be good negotiators in this sense, and they wisely negotiate as they traverse the obstacle-laden path toward product development and commercialization.

Acquiring Characteristics of Wise Leadership and Skilled Management

As a society, we are trained to value intellect and knowledge. Truly, without knowledge, we make few technological advances. However, there is an important distinction between knowledge and wisdom. Wisdom is knowing when to apply a certain portion of knowledge to a specific situation at a particular time. You may know individuals who are filled with knowledge because they talk to you authoritatively on almost any subject. However, sometimes you may find that wisdom escapes these individuals and they don't often make great leaders. We all have a certain degree of expectation of wisdom from our leaders. We follow leaders because we believe they know where they are going, we trust their judgment, and they inspire us by their vision and mission for the companies they lead.

We can train ourselves to increase our wisdom just as we can train ourselves to gain knowledge. Often learning to increase in wisdom has to do with closing our mouth more often, and listening carefully in order to understand the communicated thoughts and ideas of others. I did not say listen to the *words of others* because as we discussed above, verbal communication, or words, are just a surrogate for transmitting thoughts, ideas, concepts, and beliefs from one person to another. When we learn to readily grasp with fidelity the communicated thoughts, ideas, concepts, and beliefs of others, we can make better judgments and decisions about the best direction to take. Wisdom increases when we uncover truthful information that we did not previously know, which comes by careful listening, and it serves as a solid basis for our subsequent actions.

To become a successful entrepreneur, you must increase your leadership wisdom because a single person alone cannot accomplish what a committed group of individuals can accomplish collectively. Cohesive and united entrepreneurial teams can accomplish some of the most amazing things that larger, disorganized groups never achieve. Often, the most significant difference between these two groups is that one of them has a leader with wisdom, and a team who trusts their leader. There are many pitfalls to avoid in a development-stage biotechnology company. You will increase your likelihood of avoiding these pitfalls by increasing your leadership wisdom and by teaching your team to embody this same characteristic. There is also a difference between leadership and management. Peter Drucker, one of the most influential persons on management, said, "*Management is doing things right; leadership is doing the right things.*" The entrepreneurial leader must do both, and know the different between doing things right (executing a plan) and doing the right things (possessing the right plan).

Embracing Worthy Core Values

Each one of us possess a set of internal core values whether we recognize them or not. Our core values are the sum total of the guiding principles upon which we operate and make decisions. Sometimes these core values are worthy and good, and sometimes they can be damaging and negative. Entrepreneurs who have built strong and successful companies have been guided by worthy core values and their team exemplifies and mirrors those values. The leader's core values are the compass by which an organization will be directed. For example, a team member with the core value of *respect for others and a desire to complete a job well*, will not leave work undone simply because they put in their time. This individual will do whatever it takes to finish the job well, and they do so not because they are told to, but because their values guide their actions. They have respect for others and do not want to leave an unfinished job for someone else to complete. Conversely, an employee with self-centered core values will only do what they are told, not put in any additional effort, and believe that their responsibility ends when the clock hits 5:00 p.m.

Great leaders espouse worthy core values. Any individual can be a leader, but having good core values determines the extent of their success in the long term. It could be argued, based upon the strictest definition, that Fidel Castro was an effective *leader* because leadership is often defined as the ability to pull together resources and effectively execute a plan that others follow. Few people think of Castro as a good leader because many of his actions were based on unethical core values. Therefore, the qualification for a good leader must be placed in the context of having worthy core values. The leader's core values are the compass by which the organization will be directed, and these become the guiding principles for the culture of the company. For more insight into the connection between the leader's core values and the company culture, read *Chapter 35: Company* Growth *Stages and the Value of Corporate* Culture. Be sure to examine your own core values and that of your leader because these are the guiding principles one reaches down into when faced with difficult decisions. Foundational to a good leader is their core values. There are great books about leadership and core values that may be helpful for biotech entrepreneurs. I recommend Jim Collins' book entitled *Good to Great* as a place to start [1]. Another easy book to read on core values is *Life's Greatest Lessons: 20 Things that Matter* written by Hal Urban [2].

Utilizing Creativity and Imagination to Solve Problem

Creativity is not just an important attribute for artists and musicians; it is essential for the success of every biotechnology entrepreneur. Creativity is not limited to artistic expression but is also necessary for arriving at great solutions that are not obvious from the circumstances. Albert Einstein once stated, "*Imagination is more important than knowledge. For knowledge is limited to all we now know and understand...*" Creativity and imagination allow one to see things others do not see while in the midst of difficult circumstances.

Creativity and imagination were used to establish each of the great architectural structures we see today. The Eiffel Tower was just a grand idea that existed in the mind of two engineers, Maurice Koechlin and Émile Nouguier, many years before the first steel girder was ever set in place. Even after the imagined structure was drawn on paper, Gustave Eiffel and his two engineers encountered seemingly insurmountable challenges, and they had many reasons to quit. There was great opposition to the building of this unique tower, and criticism abounded, claiming it would cost too much, the design

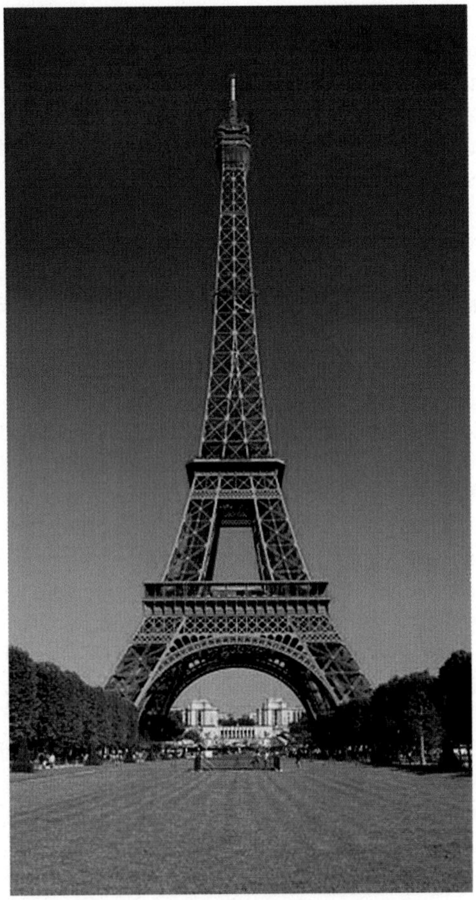

FIGURE 1.2 The Eiffel Tower: created by a vision that has become one of the most recognized architectural structures in the world.

could not support its weight, and the land where it was to be erected was not solid (see Fig. 1.2). However, through creativity and imagination, the founding team was able to overcome all these obstacles, including public opposition. As a result, the Eiffel Tower has become one of the most recognized structures in the world today. Never underestimate the value of creativity and imagination. Creative and imaginative entrepreneurs accomplish great things when coupled with having leadership wisdom.

Four Backgrounds of Biotechnology Entrepreneurs

The typical biotechnology entrepreneur who starts an enterprise usually has one of the following four background types. Although individuals from any background can start a biotechnology company—as long as they have the ideas, skills, and motivation, the odds for success are heavily weighed against anyone who is not from one of these categories. Each background comes with its own strengths and weaknesses. The four most common backgrounds of biotechnology entrepreneurs include the following:

1. The *scientist/physician/bioengineer* who comes from an academic institution (university, research foundation, or nonprofit research institute).
2. The *scientist/physician/bioengineer* who comes from the life science industry such as another biotechnology company.
3. The *businessperson*, such as a former executive in the life science, pharmaceutical, or venture capital industry, who is not a scientist/physician/bioengineer.
4. A *core group of individuals* that spun off from another life science organization within the industry.

Most biotech entrepreneurs and founders can be classified into one of these four categories and their backgrounds often influence the time required to raise capital (see Fig. 1.3).

Being the Entrepreneur for a Season

Because most early stage biotechnology companies are founded by scientists, it is worthwhile to address the issue of how to be a biotechnology entrepreneur when you don't want to lead a company. If you are a professor at a university or research institution and you simply want the opportunity to see your research become a commercial biotechnology product, you do not necessarily need to leave your day job and become the CEO. In fact, it may be ill-advised to become the CEO if you have no previous business experience. An academic scientist without prior business experience functioning as a CEO can be an impediment to a company raising money because investors bet on experienced people—not just technologies alone. Although there are examples of scientists leading successful biotech companies, unfortunately, stereotyping of scientists can and do occur. As a general rule, the more practical business experience you possess, the more confidence investors will have in your ability to successfully lead a company.

If you are an academic professor and want to remain in your position, you can still assist in starting and forming your new company and help develop the technology, and even participate in its value creation without leaving your position. If you are considering leaving your academic position, you still don't have to run the entire organization unless that is your desire. There are several ways to participate in the entrepreneurial process without shouldering the full responsibility for the entire organization. There are valuable roles you can assume which still provide the opportunity to participate in the entrepreneurial process and better equip yourself for a subsequent entrepreneurial opportunity.

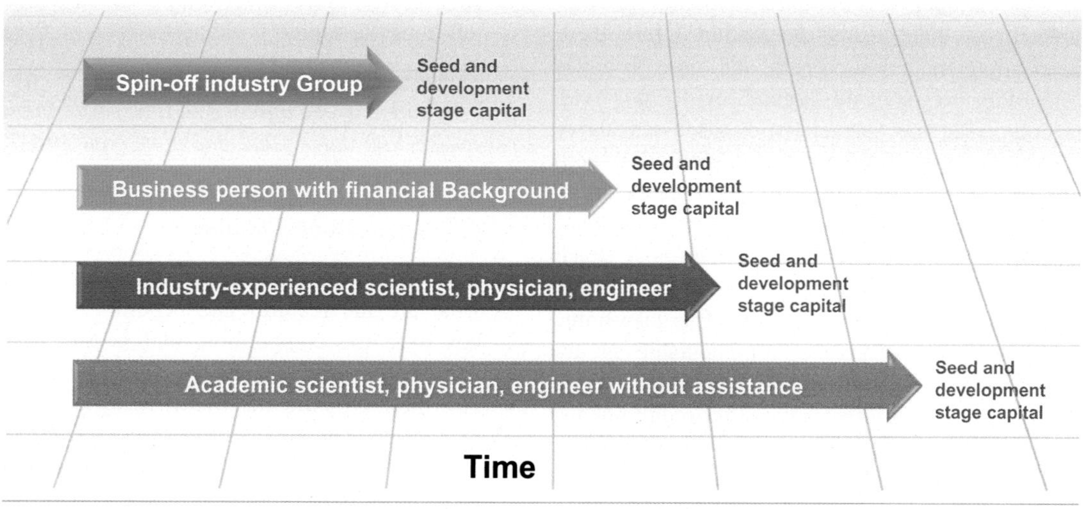

FIGURE 1.3 Backgrounds of biotechnology entrepreneurs and the impact on time typically required to raise capital. *Adapted with permission from Shimasaki, C. "The Business of Bioscience: What Goes Into Making a Biotechnology Product." Springer; 2009.*

It is important to first decide your time commitment to the new entity. Are you interested in full-time participation or only part-time? Do you only want to participate in this new venture as a consultant on an *as-needed basis*? Would you like to start on an *as-needed* basis yet have the opportunity to later participate full-time? Identify your time commitment interest first because it will help in selecting your entrepreneurial options. If you are contemplating starting a biotechnology company but are not interested in leading the organization, here are some ways you can participate.

1. Take the position of *Chief Scientific Officer or Vice President of R&D.* Participate by leading the technology development but have someone else shoulder the business and financing responsibilities of the organization.
2. Participate as a *Scientific Advisory Board Member* and assist in the overall direction and in solving problems during the technology development.
3. Participate as *Scientific Consultant* and assist on an as-needed basis.

If you are a professor with minimal business experience, you may want to consider some of these supportive roles in your new venture rather than taking responsibility for the entire organization. This way, you can learn by participating as a member of the team rather than being solely responsible for the outcome of the company. By doing this, you will gain valuable experience that can be applied to your next opportunity. You can later lead with more confidence because you will then understand the start-up process and the many issues you may face. In the beginning, regardless of your long-term interest, you will be heavily involved in establishing the company and must be willing to commit a large portion of your time during this phase. Afterward, you can then return to your academic research or medical practice while contributing in an alternate role as described above. As a founder of the company, you will most likely be involved in securing seed funding for your new venture which may come in the form of grants and/or seed capital funding from angel investors. During this time, you must identify and recruit an experienced CEO or a former entrepreneur who can give you guidance on how to move the technology forward. Initially, the founding entrepreneur is the key driving force behind the company. By participating in one these supporting roles, it will better prepare you for subsequent start-up options where you may want to assume the leadership role. However, just because you are not leading the organization does not mean you cannot participate in shaping its future.

Driving Forces Behind a Biotech Entrepreneur's Decisions

All entrepreneurs are presented with choices each day. The choices one makes can be analogous to a person deciding which path to travel along toward a desired location. Each decision, made over time, will advance you along a particular path that makes it easier or more difficult to arrive at your ultimate destination. For instance, if one lives in San Francisco and desires to travel to a final destination in New York City, there are literally hundreds of routes one can take to get there. Some paths may permit an individual to arrive faster and more economically than others, but as long as the traveler heads east and north, all travelers will eventually reach New York City. However, each time the traveler takes a south or westward step, that path will ultimately separate the individual further from their desired destination. Often, there are obstacles along one's desired path, and these obstacles require creativity to navigate around or to go over. Persistently applying the characteristics discussed above (creativity, imagination, wisdom, negotiation) will help the entrepreneur consistently move in the right direction. However, if you consistently yield to follow the path of least resistance, you will never reach your goal. Each decision and choice an entrepreneur makes plots a route toward a destination—intended or not. The take-home message is that biotechnology entrepreneurship is not forged by any single prescriptive path, even though there are facets of biotechnology that have strict requirements. The particular path you take, and the choices you make, may be different from that of another entrepreneur. However, the desired destination does not change. This analogy is another way of explaining the difference between a method and the goal. Different paths are analogous to utilizing different methods, but the goal always remains the same. All biotechnology entrepreneurs will have the best opportunity to arrive at their ultimate destination if they consistently find creative ways to navigate around and overcome obstacles within their path.

As illustrated in Fig. 1.4, there are influences that must be considered as a biotech entrepreneur makes decisions. All decisions made during the growth of a company are knowingly or unknowingly impacted by these forces. I have included a few general comments to elaborate on these forces to give an example of how decisions in these areas can impact your company's future success.

***Capital needs and timing*:**

- How much capital do you need to make enough product-development progress to reach your next value-enhancing milestone and increase your company's value?

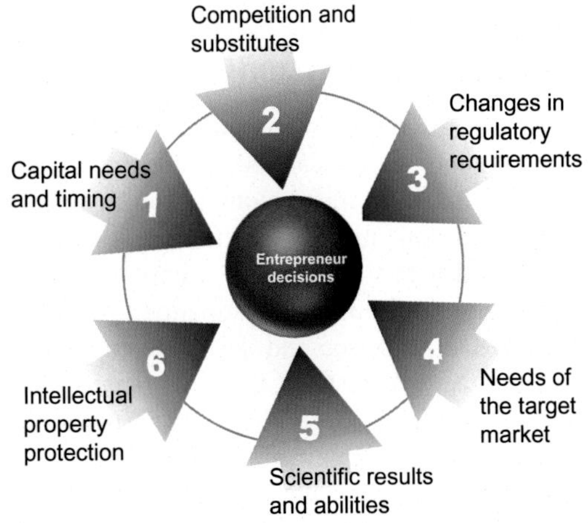

FIGURE 1.4 Forces that influence a biotech entrepreneur's decisions.

- How much capital is remaining and how much time is left until the capital is exhausted?

Summary: Decisions made on when to raise capital and the amount of capital you raise, will impact all the resources you have, and the time you are allotted to accomplish your goals.

***Competition and substitutes*:**

- What are the strengths of the existing competition, and what are the features and benefits that your product has over the competition, and is this of significant value?
- Are there existing substitutes being used comfortably and can the switching hurdles can be overcome?
- Can your product provide enough value for users to switch?

Summary: The quality of competitive products and the likelihood of new competitors will impact the interest from investors. This sets the bar for the quality, features, and benefits that are required for your product to be successful.

***Changes in regulatory requirements*:**

- What are the current and future regulations that could impact your product approval; is there any precedent for your product or technology that would make regulatory approval highly likely and less risky?
- Will you be able to provide enough supporting data to demonstrate safety and efficacy of your product or service to obtain regulatory approval?

Summary: The decisions made on regulatory issues impact the time it takes to reach commercialization or the likelihood of reaching commercialization.

***Needs of the target market*:**

- Have you chosen the best target market that has the greatest need for your product or service?
- Is there an educational or awareness requirement that can be managed easily so that those in this target market will readily adopt and utilize your product?

Summary: The target market you have selected for your product will impact the interest from investors and the likelihood of success once the product is commercialized.

***Scientific results and capabilities*:**

- Is there enough scientific evidence to support the likelihood that your future product would work and provide value to the target market selected?
- Do you possess, or can you retain, recruit, and hire, the key individuals that have the capability to make

your product perform in the manner required to provide significant value to your target market?

Summary: Your decisions on scientific direction and your ability to recruit personnel will impact the quality of the research and development, and ultimately the likelihood of reaching your product development goals.

***Intellectual property protection*:**

- Is there a path for patent coverage to protect the product features you want in your commercialized product and will this support continued investor interest?
- Can you fence your technology with broad intellectual property protection such that it would be increasingly difficult for others to come up with an equivalent competitive product?

Summary: Your decisions on the intellectual property protection strategy will impact your ability to attract investors and sustain your product value during commercialization.

Each of these forces influence in some way an entrepreneur's decisions, and these have the ability to impact many facets of your business. For instance, decisions made in choosing your target market impact the likelihood of interest from investors, whereas your ability to attract funding impacts your ability to recruit and retain the best technical staff and resources. Product development decisions affect the likelihood of securing regulatory approval, whereas the ability to obtain regulatory approval impacts investor interest. Be aware of the effect of various decisions on other aspects of your company both now and in the future.

Learning from "Failure"

Sadly, there are many company failures within the biotechnology industry. These occur for various reasons: running out of capital before reaching the next milestone, faulty product ideas, failed clinical trials, choosing the wrong target market, your biological premise did not prove to be the pathway for disease, and a host of others. The Small Business Administration tells us that approximately 50% of companies in all industries fail within the first five years. Knowing the complexity of biological discoveries, the large capital requirements and rigorous federal regulations, it would not be surprising if the biotechnology industry has at least the same, if not a greater percentage of failures compared to other industries (see Fig. 1.5).

Failure is a fact in any industry, not just biotechnology. However, the opportunity for success is what drives entrepreneurs and companies. The impact of biotechnology products on the life and well-being of our world is tremendous. The entrepreneurial team's motivation is to seek more cures, better treatments, advanced fuels, improved crops, and safer foods. It is important for the biotech entrepreneur to understand there are failures, but not to presume they are doomed to such a fate before they

Number of years since starting	Year																					
	1994	1995	1996	1997	1998	1999	2000	2001	2002	2003	2004	2005	2006	2007	2008	2009	2010	2011	2012	2013	2014	2015
1	100.0	100.0	100.0	100.0	100.0	100.0	100.0	100.0	100.0	100.0	100.0	100.0	100.0	100.0	100.0	100.0	100.0	100.0	100.0	100.0	100.0	100.0
2	79.6	78.8	78.2	78.5	80.1	79.1	78.4	75.7	78.4	79.3	78.9	80.1	78.3	77.3	75.2	76.7	78.6	79.4	79.2	79.6	79.9	–
3	68.1	67.9	66.9	68.3	68.5	67.0	66.0	64.7	67.4	68.4	69.1	68.7	66.3	64.0	63.3	66.4	68.6	69.3	68.7	69.3	–	–
4	60.6	59.8	59.7	60.2	59.6	58.5	58.2	57.6	60.0	61.4	61.2	60.2	56.7	55.5	56.5	59.9	61.6	61.9	61.5	–	–	–
5	54.3	54.1	53.4	53.0	53.0	52.7	52.8	52.3	54.8	55.3	54.5	52.6	49.8	50.2	51.7	54.8	56.0	56.3	–	–	–	–
6	49.6	48.8	48.1	47.6	48.1	48.2	48.2	48.1	50.1	50.0	48.4	46.8	45.4	46.4	47.8	50.1	51.4	–	–	–	–	–
7	45.2	44.4	43.9	43.7	44.4	44.4	44.7	44.2	45.9	44.8	43.7	43.2	42.3	43.1	44.2	46.3	–	–	–	–	–	–
8	41.5	40.7	40.5	40.5	41.2	41.4	41.6	40.9	41.8	40.9	40.5	40.5	39.6	40.1	41.1	–	–	–	–	–	–	–
9	38.3	38.0	37.8	37.7	38.7	38.6	38.6	37.4	38.4	38.1	38.2	38.2	37.1	37.5	–	–	–	–	–	–	–	–
10	35.7	35.7	35.4	35.6	36.2	36.1	35.5	34.5	36.1	36.0	36.1	35.9	34.9	–	–	–	–	–	–	–	–	–
11	33.6	33.4	33.4	33.5	34.0	33.2	32.9	32.4	34.2	34.2	34.0	33.8	–	–	–	–	–	–	–	–	–	–
12	31.8	31.6	31.5	31.5	31.5	31.0	31.2	30.9	32.5	32.3	32.1	–	–	–	–	–	–	–	–	–	–	–
13	30.3	29.9	29.7	29.3	29.5	29.4	29.8	29.5	30.8	30.8	–	–	–	–	–	–	–	–	–	–	–	–
14	28.7	28.4	28.0	27.6	28.1	28.2	28.6	28.1	29.4	–	–	–	–	–	–	–	–	–	–	–	–	–
15	27.2	26.6	26.3	26.2	26.9	27.0	27.3	26.8	–	–	–	–	–	–	–	–	–	–	–	–	–	–
16	25.5	25.1	25.1	25.1	25.7	25.8	26.3	–	–	–	–	–	–	–	–	–	–	–	–	–	–	–
17	24.1	24.0	24.1	24.1	24.7	24.8	–	–	–	–	–	–	–	–	–	–	–	–	–	–	–	–
18	23.0	23.0	23.1	23.2	23.6	–	–	–	–	–	–	–	–	–	–	–	–	–	–	–	–	–
19	22.0	22.2	22.2	22.2	–	–	–	–	–	–	–	–	–	–	–	–	–	–	–	–	–	–
20	21.2	21.3	21.3	–	–	–	–	–	–	–	–	–	–	–	–	–	–	–	–	–	–	–
21	20.3	20.4	–	–	–	–	–	–	–	–	–	–	–	–	–	–	–	–	–	–	–	–
22	19.5	–	–	–	–	–	–	–	–	–	–	–	–	–	–	–	–	–	–	–	–	–

Note: Dashes indicate not applicable.

FIGURE 1.5 Survival rates for businesses started in the United States
Survival rates for businesses in percent, from 1994 to 2015, by year started and the number of years since starting.

get started. The correct definition of *failure* is *an unsuccessful company* or an *unsuccessful product*. However, failure sometimes incorrectly carries a meaning for the entrepreneur beyond that. Often, failure may incorrectly be perceived as *a way of life*, or *an individual*. The biotechnology entrepreneur must remember that failure is simply an *event* that occurred at a particular point in time. Sometimes failure can be the most valuable learning experience and teaching resource for life—if the individual recognizes it. Thomas Edison understood that what others call *failure* is really a lack of perseverance. His belief was evident when he replied to a question about his numerous unsuccessful attempts to find the perfect filament for the light bulb by saying, "*I never failed once, it just happened to be a 2000-step process.*" For the biotech entrepreneur, this is an important distinction to remember when building a business. There are times when you may find yourself in an unfamiliar situation that is extremely challenging and has grave consequences. You may even experience a failure or two along the way. For some, the natural human instinct is to draw back and retreat which shows up in various ways such as avoiding decisions, apathy, shirking responsibilities, and limited communication with your team. During these times, you need the input from other entrepreneurs who have been in these situations before and have picked themselves up, dusted themselves off and started again. Realize that this is just a step in the process of success, and learn rather than lament. A helpful quote by Hagan, "*If you think for too long about a missed opportunity, chances are you will miss the next one too*" [3]. The world is in need of what you have to offer. Remember, that without the driving force of the entrepreneur there will be no life-saving products, no advancements in diagnostic technology, no treatments for rare diseases, no improvements in agricultural foods or crops, or breakthroughs that would benefit humankind.

Summary

If you are contemplating starting a biotechnology company and you have a product idea in mind, you will be best served by carefully reading the rest of this book. If your background is a scientist, physician, or engineer, your objective will be to sharpen your business skills and gain understanding of the norms of business and navigate with help through this process. If your background is in business, your objective will be to practice understanding and communicating with the scientists about the technical capabilities until you understand its market advantages and limitations, and can translate it into a business advantage. *Biotechnology entrepreneurship* is an amalgam of the diverse activities essential to building a successful biotechnology company. The biotechnology entrepreneur is a company builder, a product developer, and a risk manager. They are the key source of motivation, the driver of vision, and the forward momentum of the organization. Without them, the company would not exist. There are certain characteristics vital to all entrepreneurs and some that are essential to those in the biotechnology industry. When an introspective entrepreneur evaluates their weaknesses, then purposes to find help from counterparts and mentors, they can avoid the unknown–unknowns. Biotech entrepreneurs face a myriad of challenges to their product development and company success, and the entrepreneurial path can be likened to a journey toward a destination filled with roadblocks and detours along the way. There is no single prescriptive roadmap that all entrepreneurs must take, but there are guidelines that will help you navigate around these obstacles to your ultimate destination. Each decision an entrepreneur makes is influenced by the numerous forces described within this chapter. When risks are properly managed, and wise decisions are made, your entrepreneurial endeavor will lead to some of the most rewarding life-long experiences of your career.

References

[1] Collins, J., 2001. Good to Great: Why Some Companies Make the Leap and Others Don't. New York: Collins Business.

[2] Urban, H., 2003. Life's Greatest Lessons: 20 Things that Matter. 4th ed. New York: Fireside.

[3] Hagan S. [S.l.] Language of Influence and Personal Power. KPT Pub LLC; 2018.

Chapter 2

A Biotechnology Entrepreneur's Legacy - Henri A. Termeer's Story and his Advice to Entrepreneurs

Henri A. Termeer, MBA
Former CEO, Genzyme Corporation, Cambridge, MA, United States

Chapter Outline

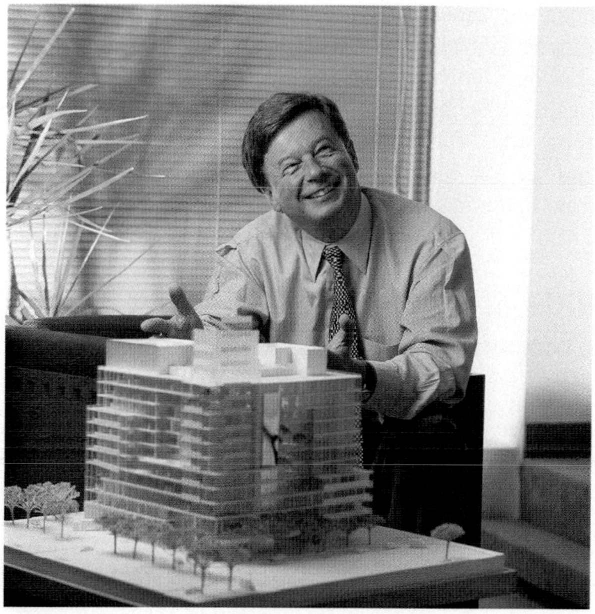

FIGURE 2.1 Henri A. Termeer.

Henri A. Termeer served as one of the longest tenured entrepreneurial CEO of any company in the biotechnology industry. His innovative approaches, achievements, and successes transposed Genzyme from a fledgling start-up to an international biopharmaceutical company with more than $4.5 billion in revenue annually. Termeer was a compassionate, caring, and generous individual with a driving passion to find innovative ways of bringing new therapies for rare diseases to those who so desperately need them. Genzyme remains the world's leading developer and manufacturer of orphan drugs. In February 2011, Genzyme was acquired by the Paris-based pharmaceutical company, Sanofi, for more than $20 billion. That transaction was the second largest sale of a biotechnology company in history, following only Roche's acquisition of Genentech in 2009. Henri passed away on May 12, 2017 at age 71, in his Marblehead home in Massachusetts.

Biotechnology Entrepreneurship. DOI: https://doi.org/10.1016/B978-0-12-815585-1.00002-4

There is an age-old question about whether entrepreneurs are "made" or "born." The theory is, if you are not born an entrepreneur, you cannot learn to become one. I am not certain about the correct answer to this frequently asked question; however, I believe that regardless of whether or not you are "born" an entrepreneur, you still must "learn" to be a good one if you want to be successful.

For me, while growing up, I had a natural interest in entrepreneurship and I seemed to gravitate toward entrepreneurial activities. I followed my natural interests with passion, and through this process, I learned entrepreneurial skills in the areas I enjoyed. I grew up in the Netherlands and studied economics at the Erasmus University in Rotterdam. Even while I was studying economics, I was simultaneously involved in activities that allowed me to learn about the early commercialization process of companies. Throughout my formal education years, I continued to follow my interests, even when it meant leaving my home in Holland to study in England. From a very young age, I always had a sense within myself that one day I would be an entrepreneur and be involved in starting a business on my own.

Path to Entrepreneurship

My educational and early career years were characterized by following my passions and being involved in things that were exciting to me, especially entrepreneurial activities. Because of my interest in the commercialization process of companies, I decided to pursue an MBA, so I moved to Virginia to attend the Darden School of Business. While at Darden in the early 1970s, Baxter (then Baxter Travenol Laboratories) approached me with an offer for an exciting opportunity within their organization after my graduation in 1973. During their recruitment process, Baxter described themselves as a fast-growing healthcare company. At that time, they were a small-to-medium-sized company with about \$200–\$300 million in revenue. Baxter told me that they needed someone to become a General Manager in Europe who spoke European languages and understood their culture. This opportunity really interested me, coupled with the possibility that one day I could return to Europe to run one of their companies there.

After graduating, I joined Baxter, and it was at that time that I was first introduced to the medical world. Baxter was headquartered in Chicago, so I moved there from Virginia. After 3 years of training and grooming, I was sent to Europe as a General Manager to run Travenol GmbH in Germany. This was a great experience for me as I was only 29 then, and yet had complete responsibility for all the operations and success of this company's products. Travenol was a premier company and had world-class clinical research and treatment programs for hemophilia. It was a wonderful learning experience and opportunity as I had the freedom to develop and grow an organization in Germany, and I had the latitude to expand and manage the market for these products. In 1979 I returned to the United States where I was stationed in Los Angeles as the Executive Vice President of Baxter's new Biological Division, with responsibility for all global research and development, marketing, and regulatory affairs.

In the early 1980s, Baxter was engaged in the beginning stages of the new biotechnology industry, and we were producing Factor VIII, blood-clotting proteins, and other blood products. Our source of starting material was plasma, which we obtained by extraction from human blood. At that time, we were just learning how to replace plasma extraction with newer biotechnology methods of production for our products. During this time, several early biotech companies such as Genentech, Genetics Institute, Genex, and Hybritech had already formed, and I had the opportunity to negotiate deals on behalf of Baxter with these young biotechnology companies. Throughout these activities, I acquired valuable knowledge about the emerging world of biotechnology, which was still in its infancy. This was a very exciting phase for me, and I had a strong intuition that the possibilities were great for developing unique and novel products through biotechnology.

Interestingly, Baxter had also acquired a reputation as a company with great entrepreneurial instincts, where young people were given the chance to do something great. As a result, many Baxter alums were sought after and became instrumental in starting and growing many biotechnology companies, such as Genetics Institute, Hybritech, and Integrated Genetics (IG). One reason for this concentration of biotech leaders from Baxter was that fledgling biotechnology companies desperately needed experienced management, and they looked for leaders in existing companies that had a good reputation. Harvard Business School published a book by Monica Higgins about the "Baxter Boys" [1] that chronicled the large number of biotechnology entrepreneurs that emerged from that company.

Risks of Joining a Biotechnology Company

In 1983, while at Baxter, I was approached by venture capitalists at Oak Ventures who invited me to become involved in the beginnings of Genzyme, a small biologics company, they recently seeded with capital in Boston. After carefully considering the opportunity, I decided to make the move. I gave up what was a relatively comfortable role at Baxter, after having worked there for 10 years, leaving a stable corporation for a new start-up in the emerging industry of biotechnology. Many others may have thought this move to be tenuous; however, I did not consider this to be as big a risk as others might have. I had the distinct advantage in that Baxter produced human proteins, not through genetic engineering but through extraction of human plasma. Because of this experience, I was keenly aware of the medical significance of producing human proteins, and I also understood the risks and problems of acquiring them from human sources. Fortunately, protein-production risks had already been a part of my life for some time, so I felt very comfortable with my decision to move to a start-up company that would ultimately focus on orphan diseases. My thought process was that the first human-protein product at Baxter, Factor VIII, was extracted from plasma and could have been thought of in some way as an orphan-type disease also. When I compared all the product development and manufacturing risks we experienced at Baxter, such as the HIV and hepatitis contamination risks, the risk of not finding enough plasma, the difficulties of storing plasma, and the product development and manufacturing risks, then moving to Genzyme did not seem to be an enormous leap to me.

There were also other reasons that convinced me to start from a clean slate at Genzyme. We had access to eight very enthusiastic full professors—seven from MIT and one from Harvard. We also decided to look for support from the top-tier group of venture capitalists to support our activities. Even though many others may have viewed this career move as risky, I was not tentative in my decision at all because I did not feel that the risks were enormous. In fact it was quite the opposite; I saw that an alternative way of producing human-derived proteins as very attractive, and to me, this was the "Holy Grail" kind-of-world.

Genzyme in the Early Days

Developing and growing a biotechnology company has never been easy, which was especially so in the early 1980s when there were no successful biotechnology business models to follow. When I started at Genzyme, there was nothing much, just a few very impressive scientists and the beginnings of a business infrastructure (Fig. 2.2). However, we had the latitude and freedom to chart our own course and build something special. I reached out to other companies and became involved in discussions with biotechnology companies that were ahead of us, such as Genetics Institute, Hybritech, Genentech, and others; we were much impressed by their knowledge of the subject.

During the early days of Genzyme, we sold a few diagnostic enzymes, having quite less income; but in reality, we had no real sustainable capital. In addition, we had no real cash reserves to speak of, so I spent a disproportionate amount of my time in the early years raising

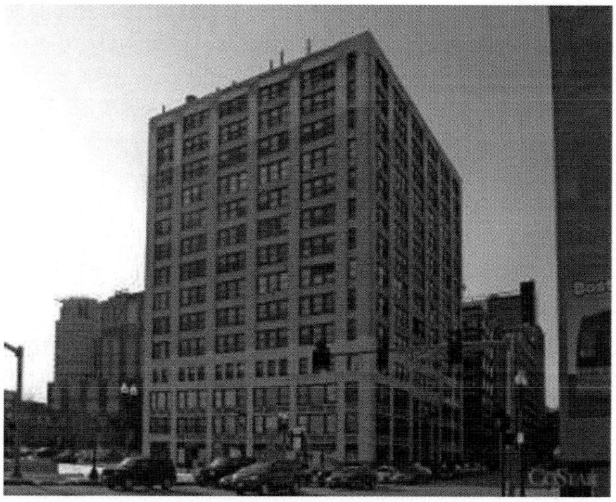

FIGURE 2.2 Early Genzyme office location. 75 Kneeland Street, Boston, MA. *From LoopNet.*

money. I raised money any way I could. Because biotechnology was new, I even had to find new ways to raise money, along with creating cost-effective ways to get things done. During the first 2 years, we raised just enough money to sustain ourselves for the following year, and we obtained two or three very small equity rounds. In the beginning, I thought I would go to pharmaceutical companies to secure our capital. After doing this, I realized that this was a very costly route because pharmaceutical companies were not really interested in us as a company; they wanted to acquire our products and, of course, I wanted to keep our products for our company. Later, we decided to raise money through selling equity. We tried many different routes to accomplish that, until we eventually went out with our IPO in 1986 and raised more than $28 million. That capital reserve became the financial basis for us to accomplish all the rest of the activities at Genzyme.

The Importance of Understanding Business and Finance

For a scientist without any financial experience or business background, starting a company can be very challenging. If you do not understand how financial systems operate, or what the company financial goals are, or you do not understand what are reasonable terms to ask for during negotiations, you will feel extremely uncomfortable. In order to be successful, an entrepreneur must have confidence in both business and finance. Biotech entrepreneurs do not necessarily need to be accountants or financial analysts, but they do need to understand what is appropriate for a financial deal structure, including the best approach for all aspects of accounting and financing of the company, understanding the impact on the company when giving up equity, the cost of capital, and the burn-rate risk to the company. Unfortunately, the consequences of raising capital and capital planning are often enormously underestimated, or even ignored by young biotechnology companies and their entrepreneurs.

Raising Capital

The single most important value creator for a biotechnology company is sustainability. You not only need to conduct great science but also need to have a time continuum long enough to research the problem and complete the work so you can make it successful. The length of time you have to do this is ultimately determined by your financial strength. In order for biotechnology companies to raise capital, they must give up something in return. It is critical to recognize what you are willing to give up because it may prove to be very costly to the company. Obviously, the best asset a biotechnology company has is their first product which creates their equity value. Unfortunately, young biotechnology companies often give up their best asset in order to raise the capital they need. I believe that a better approach is to use your second-best asset rather than giving up your most important asset. Another way of saying this in simple English is as follows: Don't give up your "first-born." Or at the very least, if you must give it up, do it in such a way that the deal is so good for the company and shareholders that it cannot be refused. Young biotechnology companies are tempted to become shortsighted because they easily become focused on raising just enough money for the next day. On top of that, the asset they use to raise the money is the one that is the most advanced and the one with the greatest value to the company.

Young companies often presume that they must relinquish their first product in order to raise capital, and then they can create a follow-on second product. However, what they do not appreciate is the enormous uncertainty and risks involved in creating a second product, not to mention the enormous amount of time and money required to accomplish that goal. Often companies end up being completely unsustainable because their first product has been "mortgaged" so to speak, and later they find themselves still in need of capital. It is important for the leader to recognize what it took for the first product to reach that stage of development and create its existing value. The flaw is that people presume that they can easily develop a second successful product, which is an unrealistic assumption because you do not always know whether or not you can discover or accomplish that goal. Moreover, most likely these steps often take 5, 10, or 15 years. I would venture to say that if you conducted a study on the thousands of companies that have had a relatively short life, often, almost all of them have some kind of collaboration early with a major company, and then they are unable to create a successful follow-on product. The truth is that the entrepreneur really does not know whether the company can create and successfully develop a second product. Unfortunately, that is why many start-up companies have limited existence.

There are, of course, different strategies of building a biotechnology company. Some entrepreneurs may just want to develop one product and find an exit for themselves. If your purpose and goal is to simply begin development for a short period of time and have an early exit, then that is a different objective. However, if you want to build sustainability into your company and grow a strong business, do not give up your "first-born," give up your "second-born" instead. From the beginning at Genzyme, we intended to establish a sustainable business with revenues generated by our own products, and we sought to retain full rights to them. There are different beliefs on how to build a sustainable biotechnology company, but this is how we approached it at Genzyme.

Managing the Uncertainty of Biotechnology

It is not uncommon for young leaders to look for and follow tried-and-true methods of success. However, building a biotechnology company and developing biotechnology products do not have straightforward prescriptive paths. Every biotechnology company's path to success is in some way different from each other. I believe that any leader who does not recognize the enormous uncertainty of product development and the need to constantly learn and adapt should not be in this business. In order to be successful in this industry, one must always be circumspect and never lose sight of the ultimate purpose and mission of the company; otherwise, you may simply follow the path of least resistance. Successful entrepreneurs understand the principle of "hedging your bets." They plan for alternatives and think about "What would happen if this approach fails?" However, please do not take this as an endorsement for pessimism. You need to identify alternatives without losing the energy necessary to motivate your team and provide your idea or approach with the best possible opportunity for success. Managing the risks in the biotechnology industry is an important responsibility of the biotechnology entrepreneur. We know that the odds of picking successes are very small because even pharmaceutical companies with billions of dollars of R&D money cannot pick successes at a predicable rate. Big Pharma has a lot of experience, a lot of money, and yet they still often fail in their product development. They fail at trying to select what can be done better by thousands of smaller companies. Remember, you do not overcome this type of risk, you simply live with it and manage it. As an entrepreneur, you are destined to fail if you believe that biotechnology product development is *not* a risky business. Biotechnology is inherently a risky business; however, it is still enormously exciting and you can succeed at if you learn to adapt to and have well-thought-out alternative plans.

Core Values

One of the most important things for an entrepreneur is to develop and establish a foundational purpose for the company. At Genzyme, we created a very purpose-driven culture that came with important breakthroughs as we developed and began to understand unique medical solutions; this purpose was larger than any single individual. When you work toward an important purpose, everyone gains a sense of urgency. Although this may seem strange, it is not about *me* just having some fun. It is about *us* making progress; it is about working together as a cohesive team and seeing needs in other areas of the company not necessarily assigned to you. The leader is the key to spreading these shared core values. If the leader does not possess good core values, good core values will not be emulated by employees. It is vital for the leader to create a culture of cooperation, shared values and responsibility, and the passion to meet unmet medical needs for patients.

Integrating the Science and Business

I am a firm believer in having every stakeholder participate in examining what we did as a company, including the scientists, the business people, the receptionist, and even the person in the warehouse. This shared responsibility created a collective sense of purpose, because we were all aligned to one goal. I made sure that our scientists never had separation between what they were thinking and doing, and what the business people were thinking and doing. We were an integrated company, and we kept it that way. As we grew in size, we naturally became quite diversified, but we still created ways for scientists and product development individuals to stay closely connected, even after our products reached the market. One cannot forget that there is always a certain amount of inherent natural tension created between the business and the science. But there is less tension if you do not allow separation between these disciplines. Companies naturally grow in size and diversification; however, it is more problematic to allow separation between functions within companies. When employees feel engaged, it is more enjoyable for everyone within the company. When everyone feels connected, they experience an enormous sense of value being able to do something special for patients, especially when employees are involved throughout the entire project.

Earlier in the development of any project, when the product is making its way through the process to become a lead compound for a particular disease, we brought patients into the company. We exposed our scientists to the patient and the patient's environment and the patient advocacy organization, if one existed. Whenever there was an important meeting for that particular disease, we did not just have the marketing people sitting in the room to discuss this, we included the scientists. Even after the product reached the clinic, we included the basic scientists and asked them to listen and make judgments about the progress; I encouraged our scientists to become involved in all these activities. As one can imagine, there were some scientists who preferred not to be involved in marketing discussions, and I accepted that. However, I would still invite scientists who were interested, to get close to the project and experience the entire process, because I understood the value of having collective interaction and participation from all disciplines. If an idea did not work or it just failed outright, it became a disappointment to the entire team. But they experienced this responsibility in a practical manner together as a team. If a project or idea did not work out, each team member learned something valuable, which allowed them to creatively think about alternative options to make it successful. Unless an individual is close to a project, it is very difficult for them to have the necessary motivation and understanding to attempt something new. Human nature is such that you do not learn much from an experience if you are not close to it. This is how I dealt with integrating the business and the science, for good or bad—there is no perfect formula.

The Value of a Business Background and Experience

Building and growing a biotechnology company is a combination of business and science. Successful entrepreneurs understand the important aspects of each discipline. I came into this industry as a businessman and had gained many years of training at a very successful health sciences company. I had previously run several different large businesses at Baxter, including R&D at the divisional or country level and at the sales and marketing and manufacturing level. By the time I started with Genzyme, my business background was fairly extensive and as a result, I was able to utilize my business experiences. Consequently, as the company grew, I did not need to second guess my experiences and did not have a feeling that I would outgrow my ability to manage this business. I also made sure that the composition of the Board of Directors kept increasing in experience by bringing different people onto the board over time. Also, when we hired new employees, I made sure that people came with the right experience. We also did a lot of things that allowed people to continue their education. I knew we would experience growing pains, so we had regular meetings to try to identify how we could become a billion-dollar company and still be a company where all of us wanted to work. As we grew, we added different business units, but we set up a system where we never really lost touch with people, and we allowed them to stay engaged with what the company as a whole was doing. We grew as new people came in, and a large company has a different feel than a smaller young one. However, our turnover was always very small—we had a very low turnover rate for a biotech company. We tried to be wise with regards to compensation, and we gave incentive compensation with options to everyone no matter what level they were in the company. Spanning almost three decades that I was there, Genzyme continued to retain an environment where people appreciated belonging, and up to the time I left, we had approximately 12,500 full-time employees. If you are the CEO of a start-up biotechnology company, your responsibility is to bring out good ideas from your team, inspire them, and provide the overarching vision that guides them to success.

One big flaw that can occur is when young entrepreneurs receive a lot of enthusiastic early financial and moral support from investors. As the company quickly develops, the support that was there in the beginning is no longer there later in the same way. Because of this, some entrepreneurs are surprised when suddenly they receive critical questions from these same investors, and the entrepreneur has no answers. Entrepreneurs must expect hard questions because that is the only way an investor can stay in touch with the company and its progress. Successful entrepreneurs are not easily discouraged because they have broad shoulders and accept responsibility and feel in charge. If you do not feel in charge because strong investors seem to be the ones in charge, you need to ask yourself the question "can I overcome this issue?" If you become too irritated by having hard questions asked of you, you will not succeed. Always remember that the questions will never stop, especially when more development obstacles come. If this bothers you, you may not be the right person, or you may not be ready to lead a company.

Driven from Within

There is no formula for building a company and developing a biotechnology product, nor is it something you simply fill in the blanks to succeed. Every entrepreneur must have an internal navigation system and a high degree of self-motivation. I absolutely believe that you cannot be successful without being driven from within yourself. You have to feel it. It requires total sensitivity 24/7. You live it. You think it. You must follow your instincts all the time because there are no universal predictable ways for success in this industry. Entrepreneurs must have these instincts and be connected with what is inside of them. If entrepreneurs need to wait for instruction from a board member as to what they can say, or be told what to do, they are in a problematic position. Investors and board members will want to tell you what to do because that is their business and it is their money. However, you should not wait for this to occur; you need to take your own cues and take the initiative before others begin telling you what to do. Yes, you can and should receive guidance from mentors and other entrepreneurs. You can, and should, bring other experienced people into your shop and listen to all the best advice and experience they have. Brainstorming can be very constructive; however, you must not sit back and wait for problems to occur before you do something. You should always take the initiative to actively lead your company from within. The entrepreneur must understand that he or she is the leader. You must take the initiative. It is a lonesome job in many ways because at the end of the day you cannot blame anyone else. Therefore having self-confidence is important for entrepreneurs because their own instincts are critical to navigating through the challenges of building a company.

In Touch with Events Outside the Company

All entrepreneurs need to be able to work effectively with the world outside of the company's four walls. I believe that this is *the* most decisive factor in facilitating your company's success. For instance, what do you need to do about reimbursement? What do you need to do about certain FDA regulations? What regulatory action needs to occur in order to get your product approved? What impact does the pricing for your product have? What is the impact of competition around the world? These are some of the things the CEO has to think about and have a feel for, even at the time of start-up. These outside issues must become a part of the entrepreneur's overall plan.

Biotech CEOs also need to be engaged with individuals outside of their company. Leaders need to become engaged in important meetings at the Biotechnology Innovation Organization; they need to have colleagues they can talk to and exchange thoughts with. The entrepreneur needs to understand that these different elements of the outside world ultimately determine the economic success of the company. Recognize that the events which occur outside the company impact the inside success. Successful entrepreneurs become part of that outside world on a continuous basis.

Good Fortune and Success

Occasionally, good things happen to companies, such that when they look back at an event, they can say "that was a fortunate break!" The entrepreneur must not forget that the opposite situation can also happen. Fortunate breaks occur when you create an environment that has ample opportunity and foresight to capture them; in other words, create a big umbrella. Companies that do not plan for contingencies or alternate events rarely have a chance to take advantage of fortunate breaks. It is probably true that in almost every instance of great success in companies, there were some fortunate series of events that catapulted them to succeed. Entrepreneurs need to know that they can increase their chances of "fortunate breaks" by incorporating foresight and planning for alternative events and being prepared to take advantage of opportunities happening outside their company.

Closing Advice

My advice to biotech entrepreneurs is "*make a difference!*" Work to create solutions for patients and help them with physical limitations improves their life. We cannot afford *not* to come up with better treatments for diseases. As a society, this is where we should spend our best energy, use our best people, and focus on our best efforts. Supporters of the biotechnology industry believe this is worth it. As a biotech entrepreneur, you can bring value and make a difference for these people. Look for a place to make a difference. Learn to do which is important and operate by a different set of criteria than others.

I believe that one of the greatest characteristics to become a successful entrepreneur is that you must be very humble. Everything of great worth requires the help of other people. Don't limit yourself to your own resources. While you do this, live and operate with passion. Passion is what makes us who we are. Passion translates into a need to do something about a difficult situation. Successful entrepreneurs also have a vision. Learn to see things that others do not. What you can visualize, you can carry forward. Ideas are simply an opportunity. Once you have the proof-of-concept, you have a responsibility to take it forward. As you move things forward, learn to take calculated risks. The ability to pioneer something, and go places that no one else has ever been, is unique. Almost anyone can do things that are predictable. Remember, most initiatives will fail, but if you have the courage to take things forward and can identify alternatives, you can make your ultimate goal successful. I wish each of you the very best of success in your endeavors!

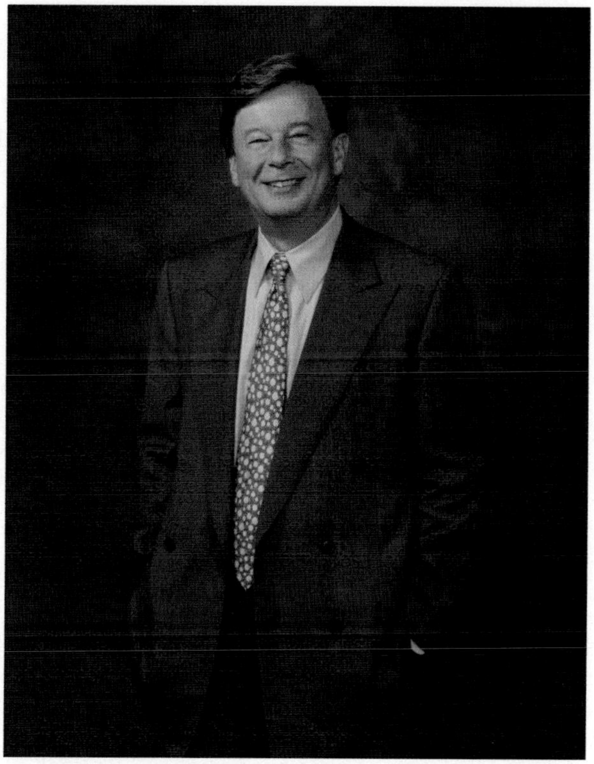

FIGURE 2.3 Henri A. Termeer: A biotech pioneer who will be dearly missed (February 28, 1946–May 12, 2017).

Reference

[1] Higgins MC. How the Baxter boys built the biotech industry. Career imprints: creating leaders across an industry. San Francisco, CA: Jossey-Bass; 2005.

A Tribute to Henri A. Termeer

by Stelios Papadopoulos, PhD

The Henri Termeer I Knew

Most people knew Henri Termeer, the biotech industry pioneer, the wise leader of Genzyme, and the mentor of young entrepreneurs. I knew him too. I also knew Henri, the visionary and the fighter.

Shortly after the June 1986 IPO of Genzyme, I decided to visit the company in my capacity as a Wall Street biotech analyst. Sandwiched between the high-profile Genetics Institute IPO and the Cytogen hot deal, Genzyme had attracted a lot of attention albeit without the obligatory exciting projects in recombinant DNA technology. Instead, the prospectus described a variety of apparently disconnected businesses and research programs. Among them, was a manufacturing contract to supply the NIH with glucocerebrocidase to be used by researchers at the NIH in clinical trials for Gaucher disease. That inconspicuous component of the early business of Genzyme ultimately led to the billion-dollar Ceredase–Cerezyme franchise and the real genesis of the orphan drug business.

In those days, Genzyme was in an old building on 75 Kneeland Street, not exactly a high-rent district of Boston. The ancient cast iron radiators hissed, and the bathroom windows did not close, but nothing seemed to take Henri away from his focus—describing his vision of how he was going to build a great company but without waiting for the science to deliver at some indeterminate point in the future. All along the way, he would be trying to graft money-making businesses onto the company, all aiming toward creating a diversified health-care product company. It was not as if the concept was terribly novel. It was straightforward but also quite risky. Except that Henri, with his conviction and enthusiasm, made you believe that he could do it. It was almost as if he possessed a collection of secret passwords that would get him out of whatever business jams he would encounter along the way. Wall Street signed up on the vision and stayed with Henri for a very long time. I was fascinated. And once I switched from equity research to investment banking the following year, I started working with Genzyme as one of their investment bankers.

Our first big idea was to merge Genzyme with another local biotech company, Integrated Genetics (IG). IG would bring biology, particularly recombinant DNA expertise, along with a variety of therapeutic protein programs, protein production capability, and a diagnostics initiative to complement Genzyme's chemistry and its other businesses. In 1987 the IG board did not find the terms of the proposed merger attractive enough to do the deal. However, after a couple of disappointments, they reconsidered, and the merger finally took place in the summer of 1989. For the rest of the year, we proceeded to raise capital through the sale of equity and by structuring a Research & Development Limited Partnership (R&DLP) to fund the clinical development of hyaluronic acid for a variety of applications.

The moment of truth and a turning point for the company came a year later. In the summer of 1989 a new financing vehicle had been introduced in biotech designed to facilitate the funding of product development without burdening the company's financial statements with the expenses associated with R&D. The first such structure, Tocor, sponsored by Centocor, was used to finance the development of several products. If Centocor were to choose to reclaim ownership of the programs from Tocor, it would have to compensate the holders of Tocor shares with a stream of royalties. Alternatively, Centocor could decide to exercise its option anytime during the first 5 years and buy back the shares of Tocor at preagreed upon prices. With some notable differences, this instrument resembled an R&DLP except that it was organized as a public corporation, and its shares were freely trading in the market.

In the summer of 1990 when Henri had to make a choice of what financial structure to use for the purpose of funding development of six different research programs, he opted for the Tocor structure rather than the conventional R&DLP. Except that he was astute enough to realize that the presence of royalties in the individual product buybacks was an unnatural legacy from the R&DLP structure and demanded that we devise a novel structure without royalties. Our initial reaction was to disagree, until we realized that Henri had a deeper intuitive understanding of our investment banking business than we did. So we created the final version of the financial structure that became the model that was copied many times after that. That was Neozyme, and the structure came to be known as Special Purpose Accelerated Research Corporation.

Devising the financial structure for Neozyme and writing the prospectus was the easy part. Selling the deal turned out to be next to impossible. The preliminary prospectus was filed with the SEC on August 13, 1990 less than 2 weeks after the Iraqi invasion in Kuwait. As time went on, the occupation of Kuwait appeared irreversible unless the United States were to mount an invasion. In the fall of 1990 the financial markets came to a grinding halt. It was against that sentiment that we were trying to generate enthusiasm for the Neozyme offering.

As the market resistance, or better yet the lack of interest, was becoming more pronounced, Henri became more determined. He was focused and passionate as he offered compelling arguments to anyone who would agree to hear the story. Behind his determination was his long-term vision for the company. Henri expected the approval of Ceredase early the following year and had correctly anticipated that the product launch would become all-consuming for the young company. Now was the time to lay the foundation and protect the investment in the diverse programs that would represent distinct pillars of the diversified health-care products company he wanted to build. The six programs in Neozyme were, indeed, in diverse areas: a cancer diagnostic and therapeutic product, a cholesterol diagnostic, pharmaceutical intermediates, a wound-repair product, devices and reagents for prenatal testing, and protein replacement as a cystic fibrosis treatment.

Finally, more than 2 months later, we launched the transaction, and after we had sweetened the terms, we scraped barely enough orders to put a deal together. The evening we priced the deal, we sat exhausted on the floor of a small office off the trading floor. In the next morning the market took a double take astonished at the news of the deal, because no financing had been priced on Wall Street for more than a week.

Henri had concluded that these programs represented substantial future options for Genzyme, and he felt that it was imperative to get them off the ground well ahead of the impending launch of Ceredase. He had the vision, the foresight, and the passion to get the deal done.

Henri was a visionary and he was a fighter.

Stelios Papadopoulos, PhD, is a former biotech analyst and investment banker. He is currently the Chairman of the Board of Biogen, Exelixis and Regulus Therapeutics.

A Tribute to Henri A. Termeer

by Peter Wirth, JD

Empathy, Generosity, Discipline, and Engagement: Reflections on the Life of Henri Termeer

As I reread Henri's advice to biotech entrepreneurs for the umpteenth time, many of the themes are familiar to me. Henri's focus on making a difference through some combination of passion, humility, vision, and calculated risk-taking captures the essence of his worldview and his management style. In fact, they are stated here with a clarity and succinctness that Henri seldom resorted to in real life. And yet, even as this chapter can serve as a sort of catechism for entrepreneurship, it does not fully capture what made Henri so special to so many people.

I have been thinking a lot about that question since Henri's untimely death in May 2017 and have come to believe that Henri's defining characteristic was his natural, instinctive ability to empathize and genuinely engage with people. Whether he was talking to a patient about their desperate need for access to an effective drug to treat an illness that affected only 1 person in 40,000, or sitting down in the Genzyme cafeteria with a group of unsuspecting young MBAs for an impromptu review of their latest corporate development project, or calmly talking to a first-time CEO through some mystifying and terrifying confrontation with her/his board of directors, Henri was unselfconsciously but intensely present with that individual. You had the feeling, at that moment in time, that you were the most important person in Henri's life, and that feeling somehow left you with a sense of comfort, confidence, and renewed optimism.

In addition to his world-class *Menschengefühl*, Henri embodied the lessons that Clayton Christensen teaches in his marvelous book, *How Will You Measure Your Life*. In a nutshell, Christensen points out that most of us talk about what is important to us (family, friends, and service to community) but then allocate our time in a completely different manner (mostly to work). Henri walked the walk, not only was he deeply immersed in leading Genzyme, but also he somehow managed to spend a full measure of time on the many other things that mattered most to him: his family, the many people inside and outside Genzyme that he mentored, the patients Genzyme served, and all the civic, cultural, and educational institutions where he served as an advisor and board member.

So what mattered most to Henri? I think his family came first. Henri led an incredibly busy professional life. Getting his attention during the day was nearly impossible. And yet I could always catch him before 6:00 a.m. He would be in the car, being driven to work, and on the phone with our European offices or getting ready for his jam-packed day. He always made time to talk between calls. Good luck getting his attention after 6:00 p.m. or on weekends. That was time reserved for his wife Belinda, his children, Adriana and Nicholas, and Woody, the family dog. Nothing except the direst emergency could intrude on that time.

Of course, Henri cared deeply about Genzyme and all the people who worked there, from the C-level executives to the maintenance crew that took care of Genzyme Centre, our environmental friendly but somewhat temperamental corporate headquarters. Within Genzyme, Henri was admired not only for his special genius as a leader who could take our company where no one had ventured before, but also he was in equal measure loved for his extraordinary empathy for each person that he took on that journey. Everyone at Genzyme felt that they had a special relationship with Henri, such that they mattered to him as a person. Hardly anyone ever left Genzyme for a "better opportunity"; our employee turnover rate was one of the lowest in our industry. And although he did not make a fuss about it, Henri was deeply committed to redefining gender stereotypes. He went out of his way to give women an equal chance at career advancement by assigning them P&L responsibility or other leadership roles. As a result, Genzyme produced more female CEOs than any other company that I know of: Mara Aspinall, Gail Maderis, Ann Merrifield, Paula Regan, Paula Soteropoulos, Alison Lawton, and Alicia Secor each benefited from Henri's mentorship and inspiration and went on to lead their own companies.

Patients were also extraordinarily important to Henri. One of the most difficult periods in his career was when we were unable to supply Cerezyme to Gaucher patients because of the failure of our Allston Landing manufacturing plant. Although he felt the pain of this failure in a very personal way, Henri was unequivocal that our limited supply of drug be allocated on the basis of medical need rather than ability to pay, with patients on free drug programs receiving equal priority to those whose treatment costs were fully reimbursed. Henri was also committed to connecting "our" patients with alternative sources of supply offered by our competitors. Many of those patients repaid Henri's loyalty by returning to Cerezyme treatment after we overcame our supply issues.

One key lesson we learned from Henri was that companies had to do well financially in order to create a sustainable ability to do good. Cerezyme, and its predecessor Ceredase, were extremely expensive drugs. They established the paradigm for the ultraorphan drug industry. Over the years, Genzyme was strongly criticized for these high drug prices. Yet Henri understood that only by charging high prices could we bring these life-altering drugs to all patients who could benefit. Genzyme had two prices for its ultraorphan drugs: a universally applicable commercial price, and free. By treating all patients who could benefit regardless of ability to pay, Henri gained the moral authority to insist that health-care systems that could afford to pay for these drugs do so. Only by generating "pharmaceutical margins" could Genzyme afford the investments in research and provide support and patient outreach that made our drugs available globally regardless of ability to pay. I believe that patients ultimately understood that their interest in access to effective therapies was completely aligned with Genzyme's financial discipline and business objectives.

Beyond Genzyme, Henri was a true Renaissance man. Yes, he was a giant in our industry, and yes he did pioneer the ultraorphan disease business model that underpins much of the industry today. But Henri was also deeply committed to serving the community in which he lived. Whether it was as a Director of the Massachusetts General Hospital or the Boston Ballet, on the Executive Committee of the Massachusetts Institute of Technology or as Chairman of the Federal Reserve Bank of Boston or BIO, Henri made enormous contributions to every institution that he was involved with. Engagement with the community was an essential part of Henri's life.

I feel extremely fortunate that Henri was an important part of my life for so many years. Of course, I will miss his kindness, wisdom, optimism, and commitment to making the world a better place. But his legacy and spirit will nurture and inspire many of us for years to come, so he really is not entirely gone from our lives. If there is any message we should take from Henri's example, it would be that we should spend our time on the people and things that matter most to us, that we should be fully present in all of our personal interactions, and that as a result we will lead happier and more productive lives, and the world will indeed become a better place.

Peter Wirth serves on the board of directors of a number of public and private biotechnology companies and is a venture partner with Quan Capital Management, a global venture capital company. While at Genzyme, he was Executive Vice President, Legal and Corporate Development, Chief Risk Officer, and Corporate Secretary.

Chapter 3

A Biotechnology Entrepreneur's Story: From Start-Up to International Contract Development and Manufacturing Organization

Magda Marquet, PhD and François Ferré, PhD
ALMA Life Sciences LLC, San Diego, CA, United States

Chapter Outline

Often the lives of entrepreneurs have varied and unusual beginnings. I (François) grew up on a farm near Poitiers, France, with four siblings and spent my youth with a close connection to nature. My father, Roger, a farmer as well as a wine maker, was passionate about medicine in his youth, but unfortunately couldn't fulfill his dream due to his obligation to uphold our family farm. My father made sure that none of his sons would ever consider farming by giving them the worst jobs on the farm during their summer vacations. It worked! All three boys ended up in the medical field. My mom, Jacqueline, was also dedicated to helping me find my passion. My fascination with the miracle, that is life, naturally gravitated me towards studying biochemistry. I completed my Masters in Toulouse and then went into the new field of molecular oncology at The Pasteur Institute in Lille. My thesis advisor, Dr. Dominique Stehelin, had just returned from San Francisco where he was a postdoctoral fellow at the laboratory of Dr. Bishop and Dr. Varmus who later shared the Nobel Prize in Medicine for their work on retroviral oncogenes. Dominique communicated his enthusiasm for the burgeoning field of oncogenes and for the unmatched research opportunities across the Atlantic.

I (Magda) grew up in Andorra, one of the smallest countries in the world, nested between France and Spain in the Pyrenees mountains. The youngest of three children, I spent my childhood hiking in the summer, skiing in the winter, and socializing with tourists in the small hotel my parents owned. At the age of 15, I went to France to attend high school where I thought about future careers I could practice in my tiny country. Needless to say, biotechnology was not on my list of future careers as the field didn't even exist at the time. Every Sunday, I called my family from a phone booth. One particular Sunday, my whole life flipped upside down, and without knowing it, my future career path was determined. On that fateful day, I found out that my mother had been hospitalized with advanced breast cancer. This news completely shattered me. As a teenager in a foreign country, I felt very alone, scared, and unequipped to deal with this family crisis. My mother had always been an example for me and, along with my father, had always told me that I could choose to be whatever I wanted to be in life. Not every girl at the time was fortunate enough to hear this empowering message, and this gave me the strong belief that I could accomplish anything. Eventually, I chose the field of biochemical engineering. I was determined to build a career in the burgeoning field of biotechnology with the intention of making a difference in health care.

Biotechnology Entrepreneurship. DOI: https://doi.org/10.1016/B978-0-12-815585-1.00003-6

While I was a Ph.D. student at INSA/University of Toulouse, my thesis advisor invited me to meet with a collaborator. This is how I met Francois. We were very fortunate to become life partners and to share a common passion for health care.

The genesis of Althea Technologies

A year before turning 40, we started playing around with the idea of starting our own business. At the time, we were only scientists with big dreams and zero business experience. We felt we had already accomplished some of our dreams by getting married and moving to San Diego, California, from Europe in the mid-1980s where we started building strong career paths in biotechnology and a family with two wonderful sons in the 1990s. Just before the millennium, we clearly got the entrepreneurial bug as we were becoming more eager to start a new business together without a precise idea of what we would be working on. We both had relevant experience and were fascinated by the emerging field of gene therapy. We quickly realized that we had developed skills in that highly technical space that could form the basis of a credible venture. Magda was at Vical, a pioneering company in the fields of gene therapy, and was very involved in the development efforts surrounding DNA vaccines. So much so that she was an integral part of the first team to approach the FDA on the development of a DNA vaccine. François was at The Immune Response Corporation working with the late Dr. Jonas Salk on a therapeutic AIDS vaccine and had developed new methods to quantify minute amounts of gene/gene products in tissues such as blood. To say the least, we were both involved in some very exciting and pioneering scientific endeavors. Not only that but we were both big believers in the promises of gene therapy. So, the idea was born. Now what?

Our first hurdle was to overcome the negative comments directed at us for starting a company together. As soon as we shared our ideas with our friends, they said, "Why would you do that? A husband and wife venture? Seriously? You have good jobs. Why take the risk? Maybe one should start the company and the other one joins later." Despite the pushback, we were adamant that it had to be the two of us. We both knew that moving down the path of starting a business would require a lot of energy and demand us to keep a very positive attitude specifically to counter the naysayers. We had to admit that their arguments were pretty compelling because even if we could overcome the negative connotation of starting a business with a spouse, we were heading for some pretty strong headwinds. We did not have any intellectual property, which was a serious handicap in attracting sophisticated investors in the biotechnology industry. Another major obstacle for us was our lack of business and financial experience. We never read a business plan, let alone contemplated writing one, neither did we have any idea of what a revenue forecast looked like. That being said, we were truly committed to our dreams so we forged ahead anyway. We realized that an integral part of entrepreneurship is taking calculated risks coupled with having plenty of perseverance in spite of what others have to say.

A couple of breakthroughs cemented our destiny. We were basically two scientists pursuing a dream, but we had enough common sense to realize that selling the story on our own would be very difficult, if not impossible. Over the years, we were lucky to be able to develop great relationships with our two bosses—Magda with the CEO of Vical, Dr. Alain Schreiber, and François with the CEO of The Immune Response Corporation, Jim Glavin. François and Jim became great friends through playing tennis together. By late May of 1997, we felt that our business ideas were mature enough to share with a few key people. After a riveting tennis match, François, who was still working for The Immune Response Corporation, mustered the courage to approach Jim with our new business concept. To our great fortune, Jim responded enthusiastically. Better yet, he flat out said that once we had a business plan and were truly committed to the venture, he would be happy to help by being our first investor. Next thing we knew, Jim joined our board, and so did Dr. Alain Schreiber. Alain also decided to invest in our new venture and brought in other investors. Shortly after, we met a very successful bioentrepreneur, Richard Chan, who decided to invest and join our Board to help raise additional capital.

We felt really blessed to have the support of these mentors who trusted us as scientists, and also knew that we would need a lot of help on the business side. So that's how it all got started, and we honestly think that they gave us the needed credibility to fundraise our new business venture.

We learned later on that one key factor to our success was to attract the right investors and people aligned with our vision to be on our Board of Directors. In addition to Jim, Alain, and Richard, we had the good fortune of being able to convince Tim Wollaeger to invest and join our Board. At the time, Tim was a very successful venture capitalist in San Diego who had built a reputation of being a maverick. So, when Martha Demski, the CFO of Vical and Magda's colleague, proposed to introduce us to Tim, we were quite intimidated. Realizing what a big step that was for us, Martha very kindly offered to coach us before the meeting. It couldn't have gone better. Tim, being a very intuitive person, makes decisions very quickly based on how he feels. Obviously, it is hard to tell what he saw in us but midway through the meeting, he stood up and declared—"Honestly, I do not fully understand the science but I like you guys, checked up on your reputation around town, and can say confidently that I'm in and would like to join your Board." We were both completely shocked and elated. What a guy! We later learned from him that he trusted us because he viewed us as big dreamers with fire in our belly. With his knowledge and experience in building successful companies, Tim proved to be a great addition to the team. He'd been there before. In his experience, Tim knew that over the course of a company's lifespan, you will experience lots of ups and downs, and you need to have the right attitude, investors, and board members to get you through it. He was really a key contributor to the success of our company.

We called the company Althea Technologies. We stumbled upon it while looking at names in a flower book and immediately connected with althea since it means "healing" in Greek. We felt it was just perfect for a company whose main focus was to help develop new treatments for patients using gene therapy (Fig. 3.1).

The First Year

It is common knowledge that most new ventures don't make it through the first year. Not so common is the fear that we wouldn't make it through the first day, and yet it was exactly how we felt on the very first day of Althea. For good measure, we started the company on April Fool's day, so we knew we had an out: "just kidding." In all seriousness, we were in real trouble. We had managed to raise $2 million, which was no small feat in the spring of 1998 when all the rage was about dot.com ventures. Although we had a decent business plan, we had no idea how to get started. The most daunting realizations were that we were responsible for other people's money and that we were racing against time. One of the best pieces of advice we received later on when we were contemplating starting a different venture was to make sure that you triple the money needed and double the time required in your business plan. It will not guarantee success but will surely help you sleep better at night. So, we had a sleepless night but we made it through the first day...

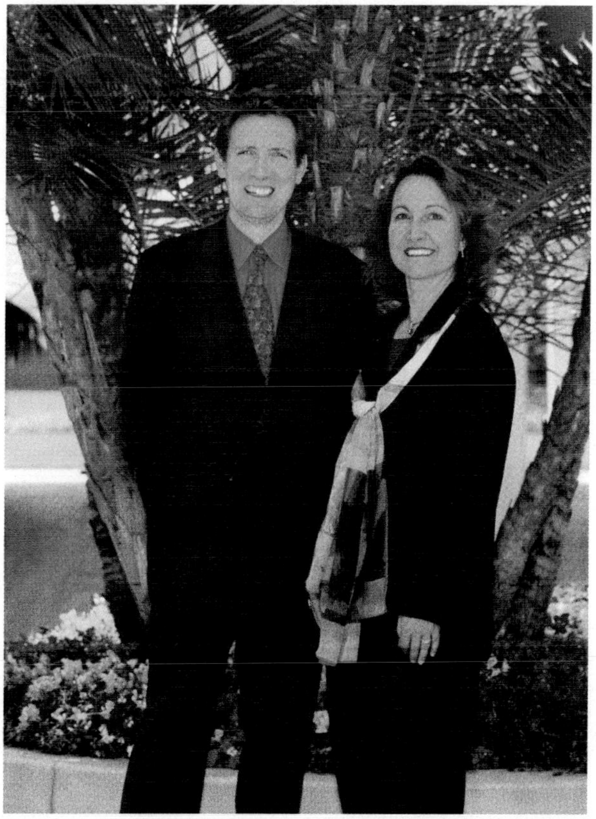

FIGURE 3.1 Dr Magda Marquet and Dr François Ferré during the early days of Althea Technologies.

We were blessed to be able to hire great people from the start. Intuitively, we knew that we needed employees who would be self-starters and versatile in their roles. In essence, we gravitated toward hiring "intrapreneurs," people who were willing and capable of wearing multiple hats to drive innovation within the company. Our business strategy was based on the development of two verticals: one pertaining to the development of molecular tests, our service business; the other one focusing on the development of research products such as DNA extraction kits, our product business. We reasoned, and it was fully highlighted in our business plan, that by developing improved molecular methods for our service business, we could channel these improvements into new molecular kits for our product business. It seemed logical and our investors liked the concept. However, as we mentioned before, start-ups are all about time and money. It turned out that we hadn't raised enough money to carry both business verticals simultaneously. In the spring of 1999, less than a year into the venture, we reached a turning point as the company was bleeding cash too fast with too little to show for in terms of product development. Fortunately, we had a little traction in the service business, so we were still hopeful that we would be able to make it through this rough patch. The board agreed with us, so we focused all our efforts in the service arena and became a contract research organization (CRO). By the fall of 1999, we had enough momentum in our molecular testing business to raise additional funding. We made it through the first year!

Reinventing the Company—Again

After the first year, we felt really good about Althea's potential for growth. Although there were numerous established and successful CROs serving the biotech and pharmaceutical industries at the time, very few players were focusing on the emerging field of gene therapy. Due to the fact that this new research and clinical area required highly specialized skills, we were able to become pioneers in developing these very precise molecular tools. Everything was smooth sailing until one day, an event completely out of our control had a major impact on the future of the company. In September 1999, the field of gene therapy got hit with a major human tragedy in the death of 18-year-old Jesse Gelsinger. He was the first person publicly identified as having died in a clinical trial for gene therapy. This tragedy pretty much destroyed this nascent field of clinical investigation, because it was so unexpected, and also, because of Jesse's dad who became a very effective crusader against gene therapy, wanting to halt all clinical development and pushing for more basic research. His efforts resulted in a major deceleration in clinical development for many years and impacted the field in a huge way—but who can blame him? We had made such a strong investment in serving this specific clinical space that for a while, the future of the company looked rather bleak. For one thing, we had to reinvent ourselves fast and furious. We had a few contracts ongoing, so those were still running their course, but we needed to pivot fast. Our Board was very concerned and unsure of what direction to take moving forward. We had one thing going for us—we hired very resourceful and bright people. With their help, we redirected the energy and focus of the company toward developing new tools to further advance the *research* side of the gene therapy field, which was still relatively strong, and to address new clinical development markets such as biologics. The Board was skeptical at first but agreed to run with the new strategy; hence we were able to pivot effectively. Less than a year later, Althea had its first profitable quarter.

Our Own Trademark: Co-CEOs

When the company was on solid grounds with steady growth and profitability, we approached the Board with a new request. At the time, François was CEO and Magda was President and COO. We decided to become co-CEOs, because it was important for us to have parity. We felt strongly that it would make us more effective leaders of the organization. The Board was not convinced and challenged us on the concept. The first objection was of course—*who's going to be the boss?* The second objection was in a similar vein—*nobody does that!*—and the third one—*if parity matters to you, why not create an Office for the President?* That last objection was a gift to us as it undermined the first objection, and the second objection could be rapidly dismissed as well since there were already several companies out there with co-CEOs at the helm. In fact, those companies were doing extremely well. Although the sample size of companies run by co-CEOs was way too small to drive any meaningful conclusion, we could still point to the fact that they did not collapse under the weight of this type of leadership. In the end, the board didn't like the decision, but we were able to convince them since we picked that fight at the right time as things were going really well within the company. On top of that, they already knew that once we had made up our minds about something, we could be quite persistent. By 2000, we officially became co-CEOs of Althea. To this day, we believe that this was a great move for the company. At the time, Althea had two very separate lines of business, and we each had our own. By having the same title, we immediately informed the teams that these business branches were of equal value to the company (which was absolutely true at the time), and therefore we were able to minimize the internal tensions that inevitably arise when growing two very different sides of a company. We believe it also had a very positive impact on the company culture as we were strongly signaling that as far as advancing your career goes, gender was a nonissue at Althea.

Building a Great Culture

We set out to create a very entrepreneurial culture based on trust and a can-do attitude where people would be rewarded for taking risks, being creative, and reinventing themselves. We also built a culture of celebration and fun. The fascinating thing about creating a great culture is that it is truly an evolutionary process. We have already mentioned the importance of hiring the right people, but what does it really mean for the organization? We learned over the years that the people who thrive in the early days of start-up life are not necessarily the ones who do well in a more mature organization. We were blessed from day 1 with some extraordinary employees who embraced the start-up life to the fullest (Fig. 3.2). They were highly technical people working around the clock, even on weekends. They were "star" employees who worked tirelessly and made a huge difference for the company. We loved them like family and appreciated everything they did for Althea. As the company grew, some of them had difficulty adapting to a more structured environment which inevitably came with a maturing enterprise. They were also very demanding of our time since we used to give it to them more freely when we were a small team. How does one manage such a dynamic? That's what building a great culture is all about. We were strong believers in personal growth and quickly realized that one of our top priorities as leaders of the organization was to catalyze the personal growth of key employees. We read many books on the subject, attended seminars, and even hired a coach. We wanted to make sure that everyone coming to work at

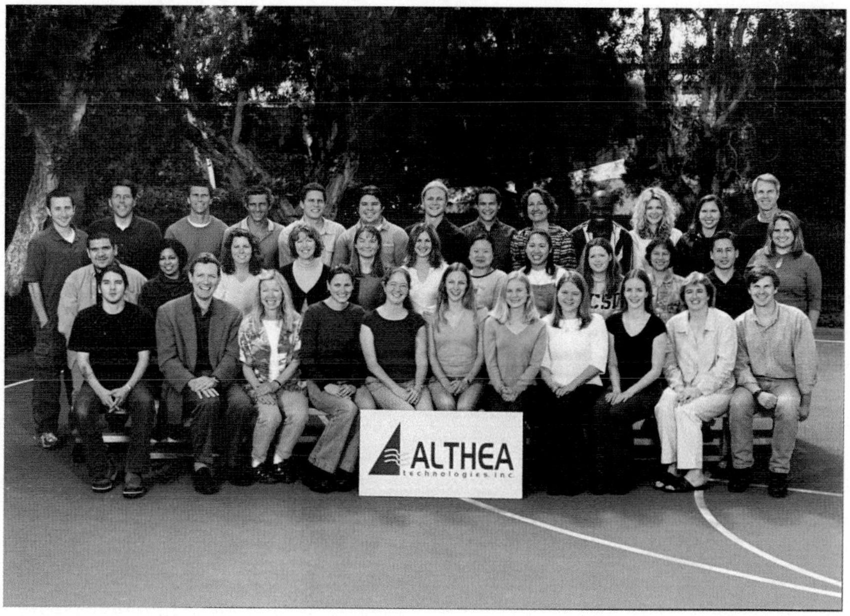

FIGURE 3.2 Althea Technologies team in the early days, circa 2000.

Althea had an opportunity to grow, to learn new skills, and to express themselves, and in doing so, helped deliver further value to the company. The results were truly astonishing. Most of our "star" employees evolved to become leaders with their tremendous "can-do" attitude intact, but also tempered by the realization that their own success was directly linked to their respective team's success. Althea rapidly became known in the industry as a company with a great culture where employees were rewarded for their creative ideas. It became known as a place where people worked hard, but also had a lot of fun playing hard together. Althea had truly developed a culture of celebration. It came to a point where pretty much anything became an excuse to celebrate. When the French national soccer team won its first game in the 1998 World Cup, champagne was flowing freely for lunch. In the early days, we celebrated every small purchase order by chanting in the hallways: "a PO a day keeps the VCs away!" We are very strong believers in celebrating the small things in life as well as the milestones, which naturally extended to our corporate life.

Accelerating the Growth of the Company

In 2002 the company was doing well. However, it became more apparent that with the on-going lines of business, it was going to be challenging to get to an accelerated phase. As a venture driven business, this was of course a real concern, as entrepreneurs and companies are rewarded on growth. We had a hunch that we should shift the company more aggressively toward the contract manufacturing organization (CMO) aspect of the business instead of being solely a CRO. One of the key impediments was linked to the fact that building a CMO business was incredibly capital intensive due to the need for costly equipment and strong customer support on the regulatory side. Since no one on the team had run a CMO business before, the Board was not very keen on raising a significant amount of money to try our hands at it. It also didn't help that they just survived a near-death experience the year before. So, what to do? Again, it is all about who you are able to bring on the bus. One of our key players who joined Althea in the first year was Rick Hancock. Rick was François' colleague at the Immune Response Corporation and had consulted for Magda when she was at Vical. Rick was a wizard in manufacturing very complex therapeutic products such as HIV vaccines. He had a true knack for making something out of nothing and had been a real asset in our ability to pivot our business strategy early on. So, when he came to us with an idea for a new line of business, we paid attention. Rick had been at the forefront of our CMO business and, in that capacity, had been talking to many customers. He noticed that a number of smaller companies struggled with getting their clinical products in a final form for use in clinical settings. This activity is called fill/finish and consists of sterilely producing the final formulation of a drug product in vials or syringes. Due to the small size of their clinical lots, our customers had a hard time finding a CMO to help them. With very limited market research and Rick's promise that he could start with little capital, we went to the Board to pitch this new line of business as our next growth opportunity. It worked. To this day, we are not sure why they liked it, but they did. It turned out that our hunch and Rick's magic led to what is today the biggest line of business for the company.

Turning a Challenge Into an Opportunity

The biotech industry is not immune to the financial conditions in the market as 2009 was a very tough year for Althea. We were still trying to recover from the 2008 financial crash that disproportionally affected our biotech customers' ability to raise and spend money on new therapeutics. In fact, the fourth quarter of 2008 was the scariest time at Althea as the phones went literally silent from October through December. By the end of 2009, we had regained some momentum, but then some really bad news hit us at the last Board meeting of the year. Our CFO announced that our main customer Altus Pharmaceuticals was unable to raise additional capital and just filed for bankruptcy protection. This was truly a double-blow since we not only lost a partner who had just signed a major multiyear contract with us, but one who also owed us a very substantial amount of money with no capacity to pay. The Board was in complete shock and was scrambling to come up with the appropriate answer to this new crisis. The beauty of facing the abyss a couple of times previously is that it forces one to somehow trust that the right answer does not have to come from some kind of rational thinking and may in fact come from a crazy idea that comes out of nowhere. Now remember, Althea was already struggling financially before the Altus news. Yet toward the end of the Board meeting and after ample deliberations, François blurted out: "Why don't we try to buy them?" Complete silence—at first glance, it made absolutely no sense, but as the stunned Board started to contemplate the possibilities, it dawned on some of us, including François, that this idea may in fact have merit. Altus had developed a very interesting proprietary technology platform for the delivery of biological molecules which could potentially be of value to some of our customers. Although there were no immediate financial rewards to contemplate, owning this technology could boost Althea's perceived value and therefore attract new venture capital. The Board decided to go for it, and in the spring of 2010, Althea acquired Altus Pharmaceuticals. As we went through the acquisition process, we learned that some of the companies that licensed the Altus technology were getting great results in clinical trials. This was exciting news, because it meant that some financial rewards in the form of licensing milestones could potentially come our way sooner than expected, and that is exactly what ended up happening. Intuition is a powerful tool that should not be overlooked; sometimes the craziest idea leads to a "lucky break."

Orchestrating a Successful Exit—New Beginning with Ajinomoto

By 2012, the company was in an accelerated growth phase; thus we had to decide how to fuel it. It turned out that it was destiny when in the spring of 2012, at the International BIO Convention, Magda was introduced by a colleague to Dr. Shiragami of Ajinomoto. Dr. Shiragami was focused on licensing a new expression system (Corinex) based on corynebacteria, the very microorganism that Magda worked on days and nights decades ago when she was a PhD student in Toulouse, France. Magda was fully aware that Ajinomoto's success over the last century was based in large part on the production of amino acids by corynebacteria. Needless to say, this serendipitous encounter was followed by many more fruitful discussions about the merits of collaborating around the Corinex platform. In August, the board decided to hire an investment banking firm to help us find a strategic partner to acquire the company. Although Ajinomoto had no intention of acquiring Althea at the time and mostly wanted to collaborate on technology development, the trust that Dr. Shiragami and Magda had established was key in Ajinomoto's decision to throw its hat in the ring. This led to the acquisition of Althea Technologies by the Ajinomoto group just a few months later in the spring of 2013. As founders of Althea, we could not have dreamed of a better outcome. Not only were the financial rewards for all stakeholders of Althea significant, but equally important was that Ajinomoto committed to build upon the foundation we had created, honored our vision, and offered every single employee of Althea a path for growth. It is common knowledge that most company integrations are disastrous. Fortunately, this wasn't the case for us. Five years later, despite the fact that there were huge differences in both company's size, culture, and business focus, the acquisition of Althea by Ajinomoto continues to be a great success, and we are tremendously grateful for it.

Final Words

As we further reflect on our experiences as entrepreneurs and creators of a successful life science company, a few key messages come to mind. We believe that the first and perhaps most important characteristic of a successful entrepreneur has to be perseverance. Building a company from scratch is a marathon, not a sprint. Let us further define perseverance in the context of successful entrepreneurship. We believe that it has to be connected somehow to the upmost conviction on the part of entrepreneurs that they will not be denied the right to realize their dreams. In the early stages of a company, so many things can go wrong and will go wrong that entrepreneurs have to develop some potent personal tools to resist the temptation to give up all together. For us, one of those tools was the wonderful quote from Helen Keller: "Life is either a daring adventure or nothing at all." When we were fund-raising, the quote was posted everywhere in our home office, by the fax machine (yes, such a dreadful instrument did exist not so long ago), and taped to our computer screen or on the wall just above it. It was inescapable. When the rejections came through the phone line, we found great solace reading it aloud. Later on, it became our rallying cry when the tough got tougher at Althea.

Perseverance is very different from stubbornness. When facing the wall, it is not about trying to plough through it, as all too often the wall will prevail. It is about humbly recognizing one's limits, genuinely asking for help with the deep conviction that a solution does exist somewhere, and being able to spot it when it shows up. That's when the miracles happen. With that in mind, entrepreneurs benefit immensely from developing an open mind and a capacity to stay centered. In most cases, this requires a substantial amount of work as the world of an entrepreneur is notoriously chaotic. We recognized early on a need for balance in our lives and decided to use the tool of meditation to get us out of the busy work. This provided some significant stress release and helped us refocus our mind. We believe to this day that it fundamentally contributed to our overall success as biotech entrepreneurs.

Magda Marquet and Francois Ferré are San Diego life sciences entrepreneurs. After founding Althea Technologies in 1998 and leading it to a successful exit 15 years later, they used a significant portion of the proceeds to start an investment fund, Alma Life Sciences, to help entrepreneurs build innovative companies. They also cofounded AltheaDx, a precision medicine company with a leading pharmacogenomics test in the areas of depression and anxiety. Both of them play a vital role in building the San Diego entrepreneurial ecosystem by their involvement and support of local organizations, universities, and research institutions. They have been recognized throughout their careers with prestigious awards such as the Regional Ernst and Young Entrepreneur of the Year Award in Life Sciences and the CONNECT Entrepreneur Hall of Fame. Magda and Francois have two sons, Alex (30) and Max (26). When they are not involved in biotech, you can find Francois on a tennis court or Magda in a yoga studio.

Chapter 4

Seven Characteristics of Successful Biotechnology Leaders

Lynn Johnson Langer, PhD, MBA

Executive Dean of Academic Programs, Foundation for Advanced Education in the Sciences at the National Institutes of Health, Bethesda, MD, United States

Chapter Outline

Leaders of biopharmaceutical companies face significantly different challenges and experience different life practices compared to the leaders of other businesses [1–3]. These differences include the manner in which biopharmaceutical leaders have to continuously adapt and learn for their companies to be successful and the communication challenges that emanate from the different cultural worlds of scientists and businesspeople, for example, the different styles of social interaction and definitions of success. A more subtle, but perhaps even more compelling, difference exists as well: leaders of biopharmaceutical organizations must balance the enormous financial pressures, development timeline concerns, and the urgency of saving human lives, against the need to carefully create and thoughtfully manage a company for long-term success. The biopharmaceutical industry is unique in this regard. Due to extreme product development costs, there is very little middle ground in this industry in which organizations can grow slowly and organically. At specific growth milestones the organization must commit to success by investing in the infrastructure, staff, talent, and resources that are required to make it through the development, clinical trials, regulatory approval, and into the commercial production. Biotechnology product development can cost up to $1 billion or more for a single commercialized therapy.

Most biopharmaceutical organizations are founded by scientists. Generally, prior experience of scientists/founders tends to come from the research laboratory, and leading a biopharmaceutical organization is very different from leading or managing a research laboratory or even other types of business. Leading a research laboratory occurs within an atmosphere of similarly trained staff members in scientific research where definitions of success are determined by the peers rather than the market approval and commercialization of drugs that lead to curing disease. Hence, the leadership demands in a research laboratory may not change over time, or at least not as rapidly as they do in a developing biopharmaceutical company. The skills required in a leader of biopharmaceutical companies are also different from other non-bioscience businesses. Biopharmaceutical companies must be market and revenue driven, as a result, the leaders too are expected to deal with complex and time-consuming regulatory factors and pressures as well as with the ethics of testing products in human subjects in order to find cures for the diseases due to which human lives are at stake. These differences between biopharmaceutical and academic organizations can frustrate a highly successful and respected scientist who has become accustomed to doing things in his or her own way. These managers are

Biotechnology Entrepreneurship. DOI: https://doi.org/10.1016/B978-0-12-815585-1.00004-8

often only accustomed to the style of leadership needed to run a successful laboratory.

In 2017 Gritzo, Fusfeld, and Carpenter published research regarding attributes for R&D managers necessary to become successful leaders. They discovered that successful R&D leaders are good at asking relevant questions and engaging in "deep listening, critical to that work." They are quick to understand and master new technical information and are often seen as more creative. When R&D managers ultimately rise to an executive level, they frequently offer "more novel ideas and foster a climate of experimentation better than nonbusiness units."

Unfortunately, R&D leaders do not necessarily manage individuals as effectively as non-R&D leaders. They often do not deal well with incompetence and with resistant employees. Interestingly, these researchers found that for those R&D managers who were promoted to higher managerial positions were perceived as being good at "offering constructive feedback, praising performance, and effectively resolving conflict" [4]. Conversely, R&D managers are "often seen as arrogant, not acting fairly and lacking work/life balance compared to non-R&D managers" [4].

There are businesspeople who start biotechnology companies and are not trained as scientists; these managers may not struggle with the same issues that scientist leaders do. However, nonscientist businesspeople will have different issues related to understanding the capabilities and limitations of the technology and its development time. This chapter briefly describes the leadership pitfalls that scientists can find themselves in and discusses about the ways they can be overcome and lead to success. Business leaders coming from other industries must also learn to adapt to the changing organizational needs, but scientist/founders in the biopharmaceutical industry must change themselves in more dramatic and fundamental ways. The successful leader must evolve from a scientist, to a scientific leader, to a scientific *and* business leader. Hence, not only must the leader of a biopharmaceutical company deal with the organizational chaos that frequently occurs in highly dynamic organizations, or what Vaill [5] calls permanent whitewater, but the successful biopharmaceutical leader must also learn to change how he or she perceives the very nature of collegial relationships, how professional success is defined, and how the creative urge must be contained. Moreover, this continuous learning and adaptation must be carried out in a context in which the lead time to fully develop a product is much longer than in any other industry. This puts an additional strain on the leader because of the extraordinarily high risk of failure and the enormous financial costs involved. The scientist/founder, who may have seldom experienced personal or professional failure, finds him or herself in a situation where failure is common in business.

As the scientist leader often enters the industry with a strong and even primary desire to help humanity by finding cures for illnesses, as well as a desire to be financially successful, they are also motivated differently than other business leaders, including those in other science and technology-driven industries and in those companies with strong ethical concerns. A business leader's appropriate concern may be with how his or her company impacts the environment, acts in a socially responsible manner, or treats employees, which is very different than an immediate concern for human life and death. The combination of these different personal motivations, and potentially a scientist's ego, make leading a biopharmaceutical organization more complex than leading other organizations. This complexity is exacerbated by the highly regulated environment in which biopharmaceutical organizations operate as well as the very nature of how these companies evolve and operate.

The biopharmaceutical industry requires a controlled and sustained focus on preclinical testing and clinical trials over long periods of time. However, traits that make many scientists successful in the lab may have the opposite effect when leading a biopharmaceutical organization. A scientists' ability to be highly creative in a scientific endeavor may cause them to be too thorough, analytical, and creative when running a business. This can slow down the process toward success. Scientific leaders may be so accustomed to coming up with novel solutions in their research that they may not realize that business solutions may already exist. Such a focus on creativity can engender a level of ambiguity in an organization that must work in a highly regulated environment. In such an environment the creative urges of the scientist must often be subsumed under the company's managerial needs for producing an approved medical product or service that is marketable. This is not to say that scientist/founders' creativity is not useful in running their companies, but in some cases, their creativity may prevent them from seeing solutions and providing the kind of sustained focus needed for success.

The underlying desire of many life scientists to help humanity when starting a company means dealing with complex communication issues, stringent regulatory requirements, and often overwhelming financial considerations, which makes leading a biopharmaceutical company truly different from leading other types of organizations. To be successful in creating and leading biopharmaceutical companies, the leader must continuously adapt and learn. The scientists may have an advantage here, for by nature, they tend to be curious and innately interested in learning. Due to personal, financial, and organizational complexities of the biopharmaceutical business, only those few who are capable of continuous adaptation and learning are likely to be successful.

Success and Failure

While no single leadership practice will guarantee success, one of the most important factors required is that the leader must be adaptable and able to lead effectively in a highly dynamic environment. Different styles of leadership are needed at different points in the company's evolution, often simultaneously. Leading a start-up, for example, requires a different approach than leading a company with hundreds or thousands of employees. In addition, as the company grows, the leader needs to consistently articulate his or her vision. The leader also needs to be a strategic decision maker and be flexible enough to allow the strategic vision to adjust to the culture as well as the environment. The leader needs to be able to communicate effectively and create an organization where communication flows efficiently at all levels. The leader also needs to recognize that clear cultural differences exist between functional groups, and the leader must not give in to the common temptation among both the scientists and the businesspeople to downplay the importance of these differences.

Organizational leaders need to empower their employees at all levels to make strategic decisions; but at the same time, the leader needs to know which decisions must be retained as his or her sole responsibility. The nature of leading biopharmaceutical organizations requires leaders who are able to adapt their style and create learning organizations. There is no middle ground in this industry for slow, organic organizational growth, and the leader must adapt quickly and use different styles of leadership almost simultaneously. The leaders of biopharmaceutical organizations face enormous financial pressures and must balance these with the urgency of saving human lives. The biopharmaceutical industry is unique in this regard.

Success or failure of the venture may result from the fact that most companies are founded by the scientists who may have little experience or training in how to successfully create and lead a biotechnology company from start-up through commercialization but this does not mean that scientist leaders cannot be successful in the biotechnology industry. The classic examples of successful organizations started and run by scientist/founders include Genentech, Amgen, and Genzyme. The biotech industry is older than 40 years, and there have been some blockbuster examples of success. These companies continually adapted and grew from the early start-up companies to multibillion dollar organizations. Yet because of the high entry barriers and high cost of biotech product development, many biotech start-ups failed. To bring a biopharmaceutical product from the research bench to the consumer is estimated ranging from $648 million to $2.7 billion when the cost of failed drugs is included [6]. Biotech leaders can ensure success by modifying their behavior and being open to change and adaptation. Over half of all biotechnology firms are founded by scientists, yet for every start-up biotech firm that succeeds, 15–20 of them fail, and 8 out of 10 drugs fail in clinical trials [7–9]. Yet, with much can be done to improve the likelihood of success.

Requirements for Achieving Success: Organizational Growth

Once R&D managers advance through the ranks, they may struggle in their relationships with upper management and do not perform as well as non-R&D managers. "This can be a problem because of the importance of alignment between senior management and non-R&D managers" [4]. Effective management of the senior manager relationships is critical to success, and unless R&D managers are able to learn to develop these skills, they are likely to be less successful.

In the 1970s, Greiner [10] argued that organizations go through five stages of growth that cause a significant change in leadership requirements and structure of the organization. These include a need for creative leaders at the outset of the company and more directive leaders when the company grows out of the early start-up phase. Greiner states that leaders need to learn to delegate, then coordinate, and finally collaborate as companies grow large. However, Greiner's findings do not go far enough to describe the needs of the biopharmaceutical organization, and many of these traits are required to function in a more organic or constructivist way than a linear progression of requirements. Biotech companies evolve differently than other organizations due to the regulated nature of the biopharmaceutical industry. They reach the key crisis points that result in the requirement of major changes in leadership and structure. For example, early-stage biopharmaceutical organizations with scientist/founders can initially be highly collaborative and entrepreneurial, but as the company grows, the decision-making styles and processes of communication must also change. This need for change is particularly true as biopharmaceutical organizations begin clinical testing of their drug products on humans. As organizations move into the clinical testing phase, the leader now needs to work within a more stringent regulatory environment such as the United States Food and Drug Administration (FDA) (USFDA)–regulated framework. Prior to human testing, the company is typically research focused, and a collaborative style is expected and accepted. However, once a protocol for testing on humans has been established, changes can only be made within regulatory approval requirements such as the USFDA and the European Medicines Agency (EMA) approval. Drug development companies require a decisive leader capable of delegating responsibility to expert senior executives in various, but interrelated, functional areas. At this point in the developmental process of the organization, decisions need to be made by the leader, which cannot be easily changed due to the greater regulatory oversight.

The step to human clinical trials moves the biopharmaceutical company from a research orientation to a more operational or product development orientation. The regulatory bodies, such as the USFDA, the EMA, and, the SFDA (State FDA) in China, oversee and regulate all testing preformed on humans and require substantial documentation. Maturing organizations need focused decision-making from their scientist/founders regarding testing on humans, but there also continues to be a need for collaborative leadership in other aspects of the organization. This is one of the paradoxes of leadership in the biopharmaceutical companies. Collaborative leadership continues to be critical in the areas such as marketing, manufacturing, and the regulatory department as they work together to plan the launch of a new product. This paradoxical challenge involves dealing with the complexity of simultaneously being both a directive and collaborative leader. Biopharmaceutical organizations experience ever-changing leadership needs within the context of "permanent whitewater" [5]. The essence of leaders who are learners and learning organizations is the ability to adapt and adjust as a complex and uncertain environment evolves. This evolution is not a linear process but one that continuously circles back on itself while continuously moving forward.

Further, successful leaders recognize the requirement of different styles of leadership and decision-making within different functional areas of the organization. Researchers, for example, may prefer a collaborative style of decision-making, whereas clinical and regulatory staff may prefer a more focused, decisive style. It is not unusual for the scientists in general to have a highly collaborative management style because they are trained to collaborate and seek the opinion of others. This style of leadership may work well in the early stages of the organization. However, once a company advances its research to the product developmental stage and begins preclinical and clinical trials, a new style of management is often needed. As the product moves from pure R&D to a regulatory environment that requires stringent oversight for testing on human subjects, the organization's managerial framework tends to become more rigid. For example, a chief medical officer (CMO) at a biopharmaceutical organization cannot accept changes in decisions related to clinical trials, or with commercialization of the product that may conflict or cause confusion with the regulatory requirements of getting a product through the critical USFDA approval process. Midstream shifts in business strategy, which may involve multiple organizational functions, can be tolerated early on, but not later when the drug begins to be tested on humans. For example, shifts in how, or to whom, the product may be marketed can no longer easily be dealt with as a collaborative decision once a product reaches a certain point. Such midstream changes are notoriously difficult to manage once a product moves out of R&D. Leaders of organizations with products in clinical trials need to trust and, in some circumstances, even defer to the opinion of the CMO or other experienced senior leaders. If the CEO is unable to trust or delegate some decisions to senior executives, a conflict may arise, and company executives may become frustrated. This requirement does not mean that the CEO must give up all control but there must be staff in place that can be trusted to make the correct decision. There is a need for directive leadership by the CMO and collaborative leadership by the CEO. There is also the reality of the distribution and marketing systems, political and other realities, all of which require a fluid style of leadership by the CEO, which enables him or her to be effective with the organization as a whole. Ultimately, when viewed from this perspective, the leadership is paradoxical. The leader must be simultaneously tough and directive while, at the same time, being collaborative and compassionate, consistent and predictable, and adaptable and open to creativity and dissent.

Business leaders understand that scientists are frequently motivated by factors other than money, such as peer recognition, job satisfaction, environment, or scientific challenges. Scientists, on the other hand, need to understand that without a business focus, their discoveries may never be fully developed. Although each group may think that they fully grasp these differences, their behavior and actions suggest that they have not always understood how these differences can adversely affect an organization. Training and continuous learning is needed at all levels of the organization to help communicate across the cultural divides between science and business and to help ensure an increase in effective cross-departmental communication. Training and continuous learning should focus on the fact that while both groups generally share similar goals for the organization, there is a need to view the company as a whole, with a system's view of the company. Without such a holistic systems perspective, it will be difficult for the company to meet its goals and succeed.

While there are a number of requirements that are important for achieving success for newly emerging biopharmaceutical organizations, these requirements center on the leader's ability to continuously learn and adapt to various organizational growth stages and organizational needs. Before a scientist even begins to establish a new organization, it is very important for him or her to have a realistic understanding of the evolving requirements involved in starting and running a biopharmaceutical company. A perception that the initial managerial, commercial, and scientific requirements will remain static may cause scientists to found organizations that will be at risk of failure as they grow beyond their initial stages. Due to the dynamic nature of this industry, scientist/founders need to learn how to suppress their ego and even be willing to give up complete control over the organization. As the company grows from its initial founding, it is very difficult for the scientist/founders to know all the aspects involved in running a vital organization, and they need to surround themselves with experienced people whose opinions they can trust and to whom they can delegate responsibilities. In addition, running a successful company will require scientist/founders to create an organization with high levels of communication and a culture of learning for all the employees.

Seven Factors for Success

After conducting research on successful biopharmaceutical companies and their leaders, we find that there are at least seven factors that are strong indicators of success. The most important lesson is that these may be predictable practices that can be learned by leaders to increase the likelihood of success.

Be Adaptable

The dynamic nature of leading biopharmaceutical organizations requires the leaders to be able to continuously adapt to their style and create learning organizations. The most crucial factor leading to success is that the leader must be adaptable to lead effectively in this highly dynamic environment. This proves to be a paradox for many leaders who find that their style though successful in some situations may not be good for other situations.

Be Authentic

The leader needs to be true to themselves and their personal value system. The leader should take the time to be reflective and better understand their personal motivations. When the leader does this, they are able to better understand how they want to proceed in difficult and unclear situations; if the leader aligns their thinking with words and actions, they will remain true to their authentic selves. By knowing what they stand for before difficult situations arise, the leader is able to act with integrity. According to Amita Shukla, author of Enduring Edge [11], "such integrity gives them the courage of their convictions to speak their mind, even when difficult. They earn respect, not through the authority of titles, but through the embodiment of universal virtues and values. Their intentions are always focused on the greater good."

Articulate Vision

Communication of the essence and culture of the organization needs to be carried out under the guiding principles created through the leadership of the scientist/founder. These principles need to be articulated and embedded within the culture so that it will continue even in the absence of the leader. The company may not need to have an articulated mission statement to be successful, but a common understanding of the vision and goals of the organization is critical. Articulating the vision of the organization can be communicated directly by the leader when the company is small, but as it grows, other means of ensuring that employees at all levels understand the culture and mission of the company must be established. Slogans on the walls are only valuable if they reflect a genuine culture of what the company is in business for. If the business does not continually reinforce slogans with its actions and tangible evidence of its vision, culture, and value, then it may come across as disingenuous.

The leader needs to consistently articulate his or her vision throughout the organization. Especially during the change, everyone in the organization should have a firm idea of the vision. If the company is small, this can be done informally by discussing with employees, but as the company grows, the leader needs to take additional steps to ensure that communication increases and that too in multiple ways. The leader needs to set an optimistic tone about the vision for the future and how the company can achieve this vision.

Strategic Decision Maker

Often, the scientist/founders face difficulty relinquishing control and trusting the judgment of others. If the leader can understand that the success of the organization depends on his or her ability to make strategic decisions that almost necessarily require input from others who have had prior success, then the leader may be more likely to accept advice from others. The leader needs to be flexible enough to allow the strategic vision adjust to the culture and the environment. The leader needs to be seen as a decision maker but also allow others in the organization to determine how individual goals will be met. Leaders need to surround themselves with experts to help them guide in subject areas in which they themselves have limited experience. One way they can do this is by taking advice from an executive coach who has experience working with other leaders within the industry. Having a confidential coach with whom the leader may discuss concerns and fears may allow the leader to test ideas before implementing them within the organization. Another way is through establishing mentoring relationships with successful entrepreneurs who are willing to share their experiences and give guidance to others. Another step the leaders can take is to have access to executive consultants who have prior experience in successful biopharmaceutical organizations. While the leader needs to be decisive, he or she also needs to understand when to accept the guidance of others and when to defer to other's expertise.

Part of strategic decision-making requires the leaders not only to be caring toward their employees but also be careful not to become too emotionally attached to them, nor should they come to think of themselves as a parent who is responsible for the general well-being of the people they oversee. Such an attitude can make it difficult to fire the employees who no longer contribute to the organization, but who may feel like part of the family. The CEO needs to be passionate, embody the mission of the company, and have concern for employees; at the same time, they must be detached enough to make non-emotional decisions that are in the best interest of the company. This is an example of the paradoxical nature of leadership in the biopharmaceutical industry.

Communication

The leader needs to be able to communicate effectively and create an organization where communication flows efficiently at all levels. Effective communication is crucial at all stages of the company, but many times as the company grows in number, the informal communication style of the small start-up leaves workers feeling left out of the loop. The leader must ensure that processes are in place to disseminate information in multiple ways. Group meetings are obvious choices, but new ways to communicate are always evolving from social networking to company functions. The main point is that communication must be frequent and ongoing.

As companies evolve and change, so must their leaders. This adaptation requires the leaders to ensure that communication processes are in place as these changes transform the organization over time. There will always be a need for high-level, regular communication to decrease fear and increase trust and synergy among employees. However, as the company evolves, informal communication becomes less effective, and more formal processes need to be established. The organization's leadership must adapt to these changing requirements. As the leader learns to delegate more, some employees may begin to feel that they are losing responsibility and worry that they are being left out of the process. New forms of communication are required so that those who are left out of some decision processes do not become fearful, confused, or insecure. For the company to be successful the CEO needs to make sure increased levels and methods of communication are in place. These processes do not need to include direct communication from the CEO to all employees, but employees need to feel that the voice and values of the leader are communicated. If the leader is not able to adapt to the leadership style required in the next phase, either the organization will flounder, or the leader may be replaced. Electronic communication common to employees under 30, such as text messaging and videoconferencing, may help in communication. As the under 30-year-old generation moves to the leadership positions, these newer forms of communication will come to a commonplace along with yet-to-be-invented forms of communication and social media.

As companies become global and geographically and culturally dispersed, communication issues can become an even greater concern. Geographic distance can increase the need for more communication to help prevent fear and mistrust. This communication can be accomplished in several ways but it must be consistent, expected, and carried out at all levels of the organization. Increased communication will promote trust and better working relationships both intra- and interdepartmentally, and across boundaries. Although face-to-face meetings are encouraged, with such vast distances between groups within the same organizations, electronic communication will become even more important. New technologies that use videoconferencing and other forms of communication between people across distances are increasingly required to build successful organizations. More traditional examples of processes that increase levels of communication might include establishing regular formal meetings, or emails that explain higher level decisions and changes. In addition, the leader needs to create an environment that encourages informal meetings and a company-wide culture of knowledge sharing.

Recognize and Use a Diverse Set of Opinions

The leader needs to recognize that clear cultural differences exist between functional groups. The biotechnology industry is increasingly global, and obvious cultural differences exist across ethnic boundaries. The leader needs to be sure to reach out to all groups and whenever possible visit all company locations. In addition, more subtle cultural differences occur between groups such as scientists, regulators, and business administrators. Personality differences can often be better understood through psychometric instruments.

The leader must not give in to the common temptation among both scientists and businesspeople to downplay the importance of these differences. For example, personality tests don't show the cultural nuances between a scientist researcher and someone in marketing and finance. Boundaries exist between functional areas, and a culture of respect must be evidenced through the leader's behaviors and actions. Better understanding of styles and norms between groups can lead to a company culture where differences are not just tolerated but respected for the important functional work that must be done to keep the company thriving and successful.

The evidence is overwhelming that increased diversity and increased number of women on company boards of directors increases a company's bottom line in terms of return on equity, return on sales, and return on invested capital [12–15]. Diversity also improves a board's decision-making, enhances the company's image, and delivers better environmental, social, and governance performance [16]. One study from the University of Leeds in the United Kingdom shows that having at least one woman on a board significantly decreased a company's chance of going out of business [16a]. Catalyst reports linked performance and gender balance on the board and found that Fortune 500 companies with three or more women on the board gain a significant performance advantage over those with the fewest and showed an increase of 73% return on sales, 83% return on equity, and a 112% return on invested capital [17,18].

While gender diversity is critical, experts pointed out that board diversity should not just include increased numbers of women on boards but more diversity in thought overall, rather than focusing on diversity of gender, race, and geography. Having women on a board doesn't mean that their worldview is different. Boards need to consider cognitive diversity to stimulate a level of collaborative challenge.

Empower and Develop Employees

Organizational leaders need to empower their employees at all levels to make strategic decisions; but at the same time, the leader needs to know which decisions must be retained as his or her sole responsibility. Some decisions are for the leader alone to make. Other decisions should be made at the functional level, often down to the individual. Participatory leaders can sometimes be seen as wishy-washy, or unable to decide. These leaders need to learn when to let go of a decision and let other managers within the organization decide but also know when to make high-level decisions alone. Workers need to trust that their leader can guide the organization through the often chaotic environment. Overall controls need to be in place so that when strategic decisions are made and articulated, the functional groups that carry out the decision have the leeway to determine their specific goals and how they will be met.

Successful biopharmaceutical companies, such as all the successful organizations, develop and reinforce a culture that empowers employees and enables them to feel a sense of opportunity and the belief that they are part of a long-term venture. Within the company, programs should be arranged to train younger executives in order to cultivate new potential leaders in the company. The culture within the organization needs to instill a sense of opportunity and belief that their organization will be a long-term, valuable venture.

First biotech company

The biotechnology industry is generally considered to have started with the first use of recombinant DNA techniques to make proteins, pioneered by geneticist, Stanley Cohen, and biochemist, Herbert Boyer, in the early 1970s. By 1976, Boyer, along with venture capitalist, Robert Swanson, founded Genentech, the first biotechnology organization and one of the most successful. The company grew to over 800 employees by 1985 and now has almost 15,000 and is consistently named a top 100 company to work for by Fortune for over 20 years. In 2009 Genentech became a subsidiary of Roche. Since its founding, Genentech has consistently maintained its entrepreneurial culture and adapted quickly to changing circumstances. Product development is boundaryless, and cross-functional teams are assembled for each new product. These teams consist of scientists, relevant business areas, and key stakeholders that are empowered to make decisions. Genentech also maintains a strong focus on its core mission, and the company regularly rejects even promising projects that are outside their expertise. The mission is clearly articulated, and the strategic vision is regularly communicated.

Largest biotech company

Amgen is one of the largest biotechnology companies in the world and consistently receives top rankings for such metrics as top 100 for best large employers by Forbes, in 2018, and it ranked number six by Fortune for World's Most Admired Company (Company Website, 2018). Amgen makes drugs to combat anemia, arthritis, and cancer. In 2003 over half of Amgen's spending was on R&D. Gordon Binder, president and CEO from 1988 until 2000, discussing Amgen's success stated that "among the key ingredients [to success] are teamwork, risk-taking and the pursuit of excellence" [19]. Binder was clearly a strategic decision maker who created a culture where all levels of employees are treated the same and where risk-taking is encouraged. "Every time we took a risk, it paid off. And when we didn't, it hurt us," Binder believes work should be fun and not stressful. He feels that as long as working at Amgen is not stressful, the company would be successful. Another key element to Amgen's success, according to Binder, is that "The people who do the work should help plan the work. The enthusiasm this creates for people who make the plan

(Continued)

(Continued)

more than makes up for the time it takes to come up with that plan."

Successful scientist/entrepreneur

An example of a successful scientist/entrepreneur founder is the late Frank Baldino, who founded and ran Cephalon from its beginning in 1987 until his death in 2010. Under the leadership of Baldino, the company grew to become one of the top-ten largest publicly traded biotechnology companies in the United States with annual revenues of approximately $2 billion having more than 3000 employees. The strength of the organization came from its charismatic leader and chief strategist, Dr. Frank Baldino. Baldino was only in his early 30s and had no prior business experience when he founded the company. Early on, he brought together a team of young scientists who were groomed and experienced from their work at various pharmaceutical organizations to become the senior executive team. Baldino was an excellent communicator who not only set the strategic vision for the company but also trusted his team to make decisions for their departments. Baldino was also exceptionally adaptable as he led the company from a small start-up to a successful biopharmaceutical company.

In the early 2000s the company sponsored internal research to determine the key ingredients for its own success. They discovered that their success stemmed from "CEO credibility, a senior team that manages expectations and implements strategy, and the availability of funds to execute the strategy and market drugs" [20].

In addition to being adaptable, a number of important attributes are required for establishing a learning organization that deals with the paradoxical nature of successfully leading biopharmaceutical companies. The leader needs to be authentic to themselves and their personal values. Second, they need to know what they stand for and why. Third, the leader should be a visionary manager who is able to consistently articulate his or her vision throughout the organization. Fourth, the leader needs to be a strategic decision maker and be flexible enough to allow the strategic vision to adjust to the culture and the environment. Fifth, the leader needs to be able to communicate effectively and create an organization where communication flows efficiently at all levels. Such communication can be extremely difficult in fast-growing organizations where effective communication is needed across cultural, geographic, or functional boundaries. Sixth, the leader needs to recognize that clear cultural differences exist between functional groups and should incorporate diversity. The leader must not give in to the common temptation among both scientists and businesspeople to downplay the importance of these differences. Within the organization, cultural differences need to be respected, whether they are between people from different countries or people with different functional backgrounds, such as science and business. Finally, organizational leader needs to empower their employees at all levels to make strategic decisions; but at the same time, the leader needs to know which decisions must be retained as his or her sole responsibility.

Conclusion

Based on observations of multiple organizations, interviews with their leaders and with consultants, and from the literature, biopharmaceutical companies require leaders who are able to continually learn and adapt to the continuous change of permanent organizational whitewater likely to be present as technology organizations mature and develop [5,21]. This ability to continuously learn and adapt is the single most important requirement to lead biopharmaceutical companies to success. Without such a perspective, the leader and the organization will likely fail. To continuously learn, however, leaders must often suppress their own egos and relinquish control. Further, leaders need to embody the story and the vision of the organization. Part of that vision should include creating a learning organization where all employees are encouraged and expected to learn continuously ([23]; [24]; [25]; [5]). Such a learning organization should support and give confidence to employees so that they will take on leadership roles within their own jobs [22].

References

[1] Langer LJ. How scientist/founders lead successful biopharmaceutical organizations: a study of three companies [Ph.D. dissertation]. 2008.

[2] Langer LJ. Leadership strategies for biotechnology organizations: a literature review. In: Savage GT, Fottler M, editors. Biennial review of health care management: meso perspectives. Advances in health care management, vol. 8. Emerald Group Publishing Limited; 2009.

[3] Langer LJ. Moving beyond the start-up phase. Life Sci Leader 2011;3(3):60.

[4] Gritzo L, Fusfeld A, Carpenter D. Success factors in R&D leadership. Res Technol Manage 2017;60(4):43–51 https://doi.org/10.1080/08956308.2017.1325683.

[5] Vaill PB. Learning as a way of being. San Francisco, CA: Jossey-Boss; 1996.

[6] Prasay V, Mailankody S. Research and development spending to bring a single cancer drug to market and revenues after approval. J Am Med Assoc Intern Med 2017; Retrieved November 11, 2018 from: <https://jamanetwork.com/journals/jamainternalmedicine/fullarticle/2653012>.

[7] Stanford, Graduate School of Business. Biotech innovators and investors assess challenges, opportunities. Retrieved, June 6, 2007 from: <http://www.gsb.stanford.edu/NEWS/headlines/biotechnology.shtml>; n.d.

[8] Federal Reserve Bank of Dallas. A conversation with Nancy Chang, taking the pulse of biotech. p. 9. Retrieved June 6, 2007 from: <http://www.dallasfed.org/research/swe/2007/swe0702e.pdf>; 2007.

[9] Zhang J, Patel N. The dynamics of California's biotechnology industry. Retrieved May 29, 2007 from: <http://www.ppic.org/content/pubs/report/R_405JZR.pdf>; 2005.

[10] Greiner L. Evolution and revolution as organizations grow. Harvard Bus Rev 1998;55–66.

[11] Shukla A. Enduring edge: transforming how we think, create and change. Vitamita House; 2014.

[12] Joy L, Carter N, Wagner H, Narayanan S. The bottom line: corporate performance and women's representation on boards. Catalyst 2007.

[13] Perlberg H. Stocks perform better if women are on company boards. Bloomberg 2012.

[14] Bugeja M, Ghannam S, Matolcsy Z, Spiropoulos H. Does board gender-diversity matter in M&A activities? SSRN Electr J 2012; August.

[15] Carter DA, Simpkins BJ, Simpson WG. Corporate governance, board diversity and firm value. Financ Rev 2003;38(1):33–53.

[16] Marquis C, Lee M. Who is governing whom? Senior managers, governance and the structure of generosity in large firms. Harvard Business School; 2010.

[16a] Wilson N, Altanlar A. Director characteristics, gender balance and insolvencyrisk: An empirical study 2009. Retrieved from https://papers.ssrn.com/sol3/papers.cfm?abstract_id = 1932107.

[17] Catalyst Report. Why diversity matters. Retrieved June 14, 2016 from: <http://www.catalyst.org/knowledge/why-diversity-matters>; 2013.

[18] Catalyst. Catalyst consensus: women board directors. Retrieved June 14, 2016 from: <http://www.catalyst.org/knowledge/2014-catalyst-census-women-board-directors>; 2014.

[19] Arnaout RA. Amgen's CEO discusses company's secrets of success. The Tech Online Edition 1996;(6):116 Retrieved August 8, 2007 from: <https://www-tech.mit.edu/V116/N6/amgen.6n.html>.

[20] Grupp RW, Gaines-Ross L. Reputation management in the biotechnology industry. J Commer Biotechnol 2002;9(1):17–26.

[21] Heifetz RA. Leadership without easy answers. Cambridge, MA: Belknap Press of Harvard University Press; 1994.

[22] Wergin J, editor. Leadership in place: how academic professionals can find their leadership voice. Bolton, MA: Anker; 2007.

[23] Bennis WG, Nanus B. Leaders: Strategies for taking charge. 2nd ed New York: Harper Business; 1997.

[24] Gardner H. Leading minds: An anatomy of leadership. New York: Basic Books; 1995.

[25] Senge P. The fifth discipline. New York: Doubleday; 1990.

Further Reading

Amgen. Investors facts. Retrieved August 2, 2007 from: <http://www.amgen.com/investors/fact_sheets.html>; 2007.

Amgen. Awards and accolades. Retrieved November 12, 2018 from <https://www.amgen.com/about/awards-and-accolades/>; 2018.

Catalyst Report. Companies with more women board directors experience higher financial performance. Retrieved December 27, 2016 from: <https://sitatthetable.org/blogs/stats/117997059-companies-with-more-women-board-directors-experience-higher-financial-performance-catalyst>; 2011.

Section II

Overview of the Biotechnology Industry

Chapter 5

Unleashing the Promise of Biotechnology to Help Heal, Fuel, and Feed the World

The Honorable James C. Greenwood
President & CEO, Biotechnology Innovation Organization (BIO), Washington, DC, United States

Chapter Outline

Biotechnology is a significant part of our lives, often in ways we may not realize. Biotechnology has enabled the creation of breakthrough products and technologies to combat disease, protect the environment, feed the hungry, produce fuels, and make other useful products. We can see biotechnology at work each day in our homes, workplaces, and everywhere in between. Biotechnology enables and improves the production of the food we eat, the clothes we wear, the consumer products we use, and the medicines we take.

Humans have used some form of biotechnology since the dawn of civilization. The biotech products of today might seem like miracles to our ancestors, but they are developed on a foundation of hard-won scientific knowledge discovered by countless generations of researchers and visionaries. As a biotech entrepreneur or investor, you will build on this foundation and be part of the most transformative industry of the 21st century. Your work will help save lives and improve the quality of life for potentially billions of people around the world.

The modern biotechnology industry emerged in the 1970s, based largely on a new recombinant DNA technique published in 1973 by Stanley Cohen of Stanford University and Herbert Boyer of the University of California. Recombinant DNA and subsequent discoveries have enhanced and accelerated our ability to develop practical biotechnology products to help us live longer and healthier lives, have a more abundant and sustainable food supply, use cleaner and more efficient processes for industrial manufacturing [1] and reduce our greenhouse gas footprint. As of 2017, biotechnology is estimated to be more than a $400 billion global industry and projected to be $727 billion by 2025. In 2012 the US government released a *National Bioeconomy Blueprint* noting that bioscience industries are "a large and rapidly growing segment of the world economy that provides substantial public benefit." Nations around the world make large investments in the bioscience industry because they want the benefits of biotech innovation along with the good jobs and economic development that biotech brings.

Biotechnology Entrepreneurship. DOI: https://doi.org/10.1016/B978-0-12-815585-1.00005-X

The men and women of the biotechnology industry help heal, fuel, and feed the world. They also create immense economic value. This chapter will discuss a few of the many accomplishments of the biotechnology industry and some of the astounding breakthroughs on the horizon—new advances which you may play an important role in developing. It will also focus on the role that good public policy must play in supporting the biotechnology industry.

Health Biotechnology: Helping to Save and Extend Lives

Biotechnology product developments are transforming the practice of medicine and providing new and better ways to detect, treat, and prevent disease. These products provide targeted treatments to minimize health risks and side-effects for individual patients. Biotechnology tools and techniques open new research avenues for discovering how healthy bodies work and what goes wrong when problems arise.

The first biotech drug for human use, human insulin produced by genetically modified bacteria, was approved by the US Food and Drug Administration (FDA) in 1982. Today, the recombinant DNA technology that made production of human insulin and many other biologic medicines possible has been joined in the biotech tool kit by monoclonal antibodies, cellular therapy, gene therapy, RNA interference, stem cells, regenerative medicine, tissue engineering, new vaccine approaches, and other innovative technologies (see Fig. 5.1).

Biotechnology has revolutionized healthcare in many ways. Yet much more remains to be done in humanity's age-old battle against disease. Worldwide, more than 17 million people die each year from cardiovascular disease [2]. More than 9 million lives are lost to cancer [3]. More than a billion people, most of them in the developing world, are affected by deadly malaria, tuberculosis, and sleeping sickness [4]. Approximately 300 million people suffer from one of the more than 7000 known rare diseases [5].

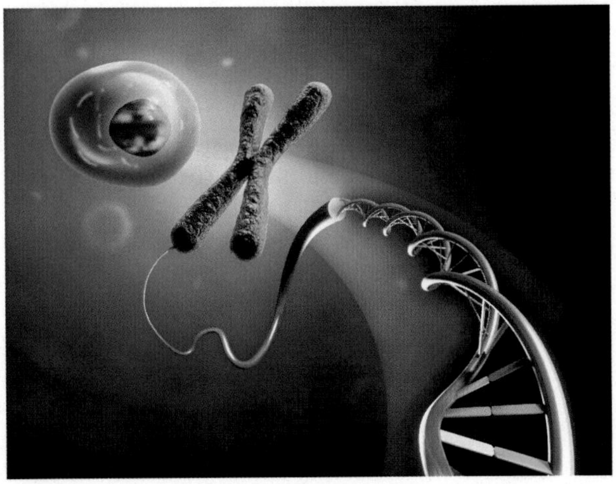

FIGURE 5.1 DNA is the genetic code for life.

The promise of biotech is to reduce suffering and extend lives by developing better ways to detect, treat, and prevent diseases at a genetic or molecular level. This will give us all a better chance to enjoy longer, healthier, and more productive lives. Let's look at some of the ways biotech has made a difference and where we might find the next lifesaving breakthrough.

Saving Lives with Vaccines

Vaccines and immunizations represent the greatest successes of biotechnology in sheer number of lives saved. Most people in the developed world take it for granted that their child will not die struggling for breath inside an iron lung due to paralysis from polio. We have little worry that our kids will be permanently scarred from the ravages of smallpox or die from complications of measles or from whooping cough. Diseases that inspired fear and ended untold millions of lives for most of human history are now nearly forgotten. Vaccines make this peace of mind possible.

By the beginning of the 20th century, vaccines existed for rabies, diphtheria, typhoid fever, and the plague. By the 1990s, smallpox and polio had been eradicated or nearly eradicated worldwide, preventing millions of deaths. Worldwide, 2.5 million child deaths are prevented each year by immunization. In this past decade alone, the biopharmaceutical industry has added to our arsenal new vaccines for shingles, pneumonia, human papilloma virus (which causes a common form of cervical cancer), and rotavirus (an infection fatal to many infants). Vaccine companies are now working to develop preventive vaccines against dangerous hospital infections such as group B streptococcus or *Staphylococcus aureus*; vaccines for neglected diseases such as dengue, malaria, and tuberculosis; and new pediatric vaccines. Immunology and vaccine development continue to be a promising and vital field of health biotechnology (Fig. 5.2).

Vaccines are among the most proven and studied public health interventions of the last century. The US Centers for Disease Control and Prevention reports that routine childhood vaccinations prevented 732,000 early deaths from 1994 to 2013. Vaccination continues to be the most effective wide-spread means to eliminate disease such as polio, small pox and other devastating diseases.

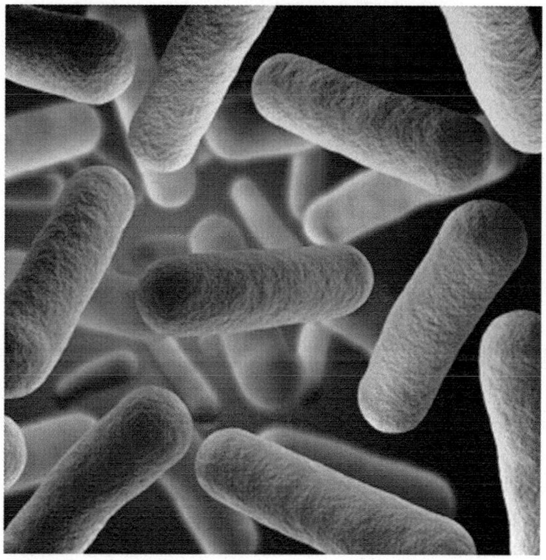

FIGURE 5.2 Vaccines are developed to combat infections from bacteria and other infectious organisms.

Surviving Cancer Like Never Before

Biotechnology is helping us make substantial progress in the fight against cancer. For more and more patients, a cancer diagnosis is no longer the death sentence it once was. Due to new, more effective treatments and other medical advances, survival rates have increased significantly for many types of cancer. For example, childhood leukemia is now cured in 80% of cases, testicular cancer in more than 90% of cases, and Hodgkin's lymphoma in more than 90% of cases. Cancer nevertheless remains the third leading cause of worldwide deaths each year, with global rates expected to double by 2020 and triple by 2030, resulting in 17 million cancer deaths that year.

Biotechnology is helping us better understand the molecular and genetic basis of cancer. We can now develop targeted treatments that use gene-based tests to match patients with optimal drugs and drug dosages.

Oncology is approaching an era when cancer treatment will be determined more by the genetic signature of the tumor than by its location in the body. For example, one therapeutic cancer vaccine in development aims to stimulate the immune system to attack cancer cells common to lung, breast, prostate, and colorectal cancer cells while leaving healthy cells unharmed. There are now more than 350 new biopharmaceutical cancer medicines in development [6]. Cancer treatment and prevention is another therapeutic area with high stakes and an urgent need for progress.

Improving Quality of Life

Even when biotechnology cannot yet offer a cure, biomedicines can greatly improve quality of life for patients with serious chronic illnesses. For example, innovative treatments are changing the outlook for multiple sclerosis (MS), an autoimmune disease that affects the brain and spinal cord. Due to nerve damage, MS patients can suffer severe symptoms in all parts of the body, including muscle loss, loss of bladder and bowel control, and vision loss. While a cure remains elusive, new biologic treatments have been shown to improve walking ability by 25% [7]. Similarly, a class of therapies called antiretrovirals has changed the prognosis for patients with HIV. Access to antiretroviral therapy has resulted in substantial declines in the number of people dying from AIDS-related reasons during the past decade. Mounting scientific evidence suggests that increased access to antiretroviral therapy is also contributing substantially to declines in the number of people acquiring HIV infection [8].

Other biologic medicines help some cancer patients avoid the debilitating side-effects of traditional chemotherapy, help certain cystic fibrosis patients breathe easier, and bring relief to many sufferers of rheumatoid arthritis and other immune disorders. Our ultimate goal is always to find cures and preventions for disease, but there is also great satisfaction in knowing that breakthroughs in biotechnology also help people with serious debilitating conditions move, breathe, and live a little easier.

Rare Diseases

If all of the people with rare diseases lived in one country, it would be the world's third most populous. Orphan drug development is especially challenging because of limited patient populations for required clinical trials. Rare diseases, by definition, impact fewer than 200,000 Americans—some impact hundreds or less. There are nearly 7000 such conditions. The vast majority of these conditions affect fewer than 6000 people each, but all of these rare diseases combined affect approximately 300 million people worldwide. Unfortunately, the healthcare needs of rare-disease patients are often unmet. The economics of developing a new drug for a small population are daunting and require strong public policy support, such as the incentives in the Orphan Drug Act, along with strong partnerships among biotech entrepreneurs, patient communities, healthcare providers, government, and others.

Today, fewer than 500 of the known rare diseases have FDA-approved therapies. But in 2018 the US FDA took important steps to bring more orphan drugs to market. Commissioner Scott Gottlieb cleared the backlog of hundreds of requests for orphan drug designations and now responds to such requests in 90 days or less. The FDA is also pioneering the use of innovative clinical trial designs and alternative data sources. The agency recently announced plans to develop clinical trial networks for rare diseases to better understand individual patient experiences, symptom progression, and clinical outcomes. This "natural history" model will help reviewers to boost orphan drug development.

After years of pressure by the patient advocacy community, the FDA is now systematically incorporating the patient perspective in the drug review process. Rather than occasionally consulting patients on drug efficiency and effectiveness, the FDA established Office of Patient Affairs to coordinate patient engagement across the agency. The goal is to collect statistically meaningful patient experience data that will be used to inform crucial regulatory decisions about new treatments.

Faster Detection, Better Accuracy, Greater Mobility

Biotech diagnostic tools have enhanced our ability to detect and diagnose conditions faster and with greater accuracy. There are more than 1200 biotech-based diagnostic tests in clinical use [9]. These range from faster and more accurate strep throat tests to tests that pinpoint-specific cancer cells to select treatment options. Genetic tests are available to detect approximately 2200 conditions, both common and rare, including tests for cancers, infectious diseases, and inherited genetic disorders [10]. Many require only a simple blood sample or mouth swab. Such tests can eliminate the need for costly and invasive exploratory surgeries. These tests analyze a patient's genetic material (DNA, RNA, chromosomes, and genes) as well as the molecular products of genes (biomarkers such as proteins, enzymes, or metabolites) that may indicate a disorder. Some newer molecular tests can also identify biomarkers indicating the presence of specific infectious agents, such as a virus, faster and more cost-effectively than can certain other existing alternatives (Fig. 5.3).

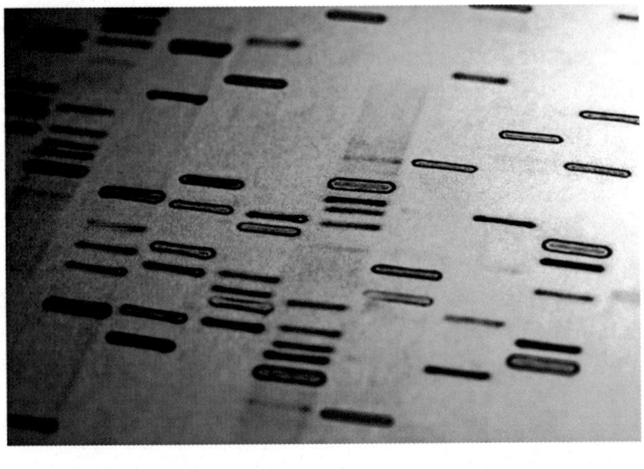

FIGURE 5.3 Genetic signatures and DNA ladders.

Many biotech diagnostic tools are portable, allowing physicians to conduct tests, interpret results, and determine treatment during an office visit rather than having to wait for results to be developed in a potentially distant lab. These tools have improved access to healthcare in developing countries, many of which lack a sufficient healthcare delivery infrastructure.

Personalized Medicine

It took researchers 13 years and more than $2.7 billion to sequence the first human genome. Some 15 years later, genetic sequencing breakthroughs have increased speed while decreasing costs, so now one individual genome can be sequenced in less than an hour for under $1000. New innovative technologies are incorporating algorithms and gate arrays that could soon lower the time to 20 minutes and the cost to $100.

Advances in biotechnology also can help healthcare providers tailor treatments to the individual patient, guided by genetic information and biomarkers. This is an example of *personalized medicine*: leveraging information from an individual's genome and other unique biological characteristics to guide healthcare decisions, rather than treating every individual such as the anonymous statistical average (Fig. 5.4). Genetic datasets have the potential to transform drug development. Biopharmaceutical companies face a 90% failure rate for novel drug candidates in the clinical pipeline, but those that utilize genetic data have a higher likelihood of achieving clinical success for their drug candidates. Thanks to the Human Genome Project, scientists can now mine the data and identify clinically relevant genetic targets—or biomarkers—to target with precision treatments. A 2016 analysis found that

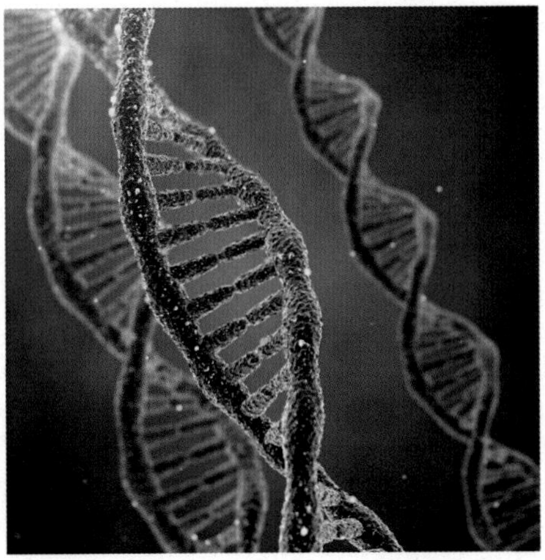

FIGURE 5.4 Personalized medicine utilizes the uniqueness of our genes.

the probability of clinical success increases from 8.4% with no biomarkers to 25.9% with biomarkers. Since the mapping of the first human genome, the private sector has seen a boom in direct to consumer (DTC) genetic testing with the growth of companies such as 23andMe and Ancestry.com.

The primary factors fueling the rise of DTC genetic testing are the public's inquisitiveness about early intervention in diseases, their lineage, and their health risks. The resulting health reports from these tests allow the consumer to glean a wide range of information, such as carrier status, ancestry, wellness, potential health risks for hereditary diseases, and interesting personal traits informed by your DNA. For instance, 23andMe can analyze whether you have genetic susceptibility to mosquito bites, a fear of heights, or tone-deaf musical pitch.

Genetic datasets have the potential to transform drug development. Biopharmaceutical companies face a 90% failure rate for novel drug candidates in the clinical pipeline, but those that utilize genetic data have a higher likelihood of achieving clinical success for their drug candidates. Thanks to the Human Genome Project, scientists can now mine the data and identify clinically relevant genetic targets—or biomarkers—to target with precision treatments. A 2016 analysis found that the probability of clinical success increases from 8.4% with no biomarkers to 25.9% with biomarkers. Of the 46 new molecular entities approved by the FDA in 2017, 16 new molecular entities and 3 gene therapies referenced specific biomarkers that were identified through diagnostic testing.

Consumers may opt in to allow the use of their genetic data to further scientific research. Notably, some 80% of 23andMe's users allow their genetic data to be aggregated for the good of humankind. These vast, new genetic data banks are a veritable bonanza for the medical research community. Drug developers are partnering with DTC genetic testing companies to gain new insights and find new genetic associations. Once the data is anonymized, scientists may analyze it to identify treatment targets and accelerate the discovery of new medicines. This was always the great hope of the Human Genome Project: to further the genetic understanding of ourselves so we can heal the sick and prevent disease.

Gene Editing

In 2018 three scientists won the Nobel Prize for the invention of the revolutionary CRISPR gene-editing tool, which may be the most consequential discovery in generations.

Genome-editing technologies hold tremendous promise to treat genetically defined diseases. Using genome editing, scientists and clinicians may not only treat the symptoms of a disease, but address its underlying root cause at the genetic level. Genome editing has the potential to someday mitigate, prevent, or cure genetically defined diseases. Depending on the disease and treatment in question, researchers expect that some genome-editing treatments might need to be repeated, whereas others may only need to be given once. In some cases, genome editing may be used to create healthy edited cells that divide, crowd out, and replace their unhealthy counterparts. It is hoped that these last cases lead to a permanent benefit.

In the agricultural space, gene editing can produce crops that withstand drought and disease or eliminate invasive species. It can produce foods that are more nutritious and create viral resistance in animals or increase their tolerance for heat in tropical climates. Bill Gates said, "Gene editing to make crops more abundant and resilient could be a lifesaver on a massive scale."

When it comes to human health, gene editing is still in its infancy. Research is under way to treat sickle-cell disease, cystic fibrosis, congenital blindness, and hemophilia. And the first gene-editing clinical trial started last year to treat a rare metabolic disorder known as Hunter syndrome. As scientists explore the myriad possibilities that come with being able to genetically repair cells, an emerging global ethical consensus has formed against germline editing, changing cells that can be passed down to the next generation.

Looking Ahead

Biotechnology companies continue to develop promising new tools. Gene therapy, tissue engineering, and other advances are further transforming how we think about and treat disease, injuries, and disabilities. Scientists can now engineer replacement human organs for transplant using stem cells cultured from a patient's own body. Relatively simple organs such as a bladder or trachea have been successfully used in surgery. Researchers are developing techniques to grow more complex organs, including hearts. The realm of the impossible gets smaller every day, thanks to dedicated biotech scientists and entrepreneurs.

Food and Agricultural Biotechnology: Helping to Feed the World

One of the challenges that biotech scientists and entrepreneurs are working to solve is how we address the needs of a growing world population. Today, there are more than 7 billion people living on our planet. However, by 2050, the global population is expected to reach 9 billion. That is many more mouths to feed. In fact, according to the United Nations Food and Agriculture Organization, we will have to double world food production to do it. With most of the world's arable land already in production, we'll need to make existing acreage much more productive. Biotechnology is helping us do so. The era of biotechnology-enhanced agriculture began in the 1990s with government approval for commercial deployment of biotech soybeans, corn, cotton, canola, and papaya. Because of their tremendous production advantages, biotech crops have become the most rapidly adopted technology in the history of agriculture, and in 2013, biotech crops were used by more than 17.3 million farmers on more than 420 million acres of farmland in 28 countries [11].

Biotech crops increase yields, thereby improving food security and enabling significant environmental, economic, and nutritional benefits. Animal biotechnology also contributes by increasing livestock production along with other benefits. A few examples of how agriculture biotechnology is helping to feed the world are found next.

Plant Biotechnology

Biotech tools enable plant breeders to select single genes that produce desired traits and move them from one plant to another. These tools can also move genetic traits between plants and other organisms to achieve desired higher yields and other benefits (Fig. 5.5).

- *Insect resistance (IR):* Biotech crops with IR traits reduce crop losses to insect pests. For instance, scientists have incorporated into corn, cotton, and other crops a gene from *Bacillus thuringinesis*, a common soil bacterium that produces a protein that effectively paralyzes the larvae of the corn borer and the cotton bollworm—the most destructive pests to corn and cotton crops. This gives the crops a built-in defense against their most threatening insect enemies without the need to use spray-on pesticides.
- *Herbicide tolerance:* Herbicide-tolerant (HT) crops have genetic traits that make them tolerant of certain herbicides. This allows farmers to spray herbicide to destroy the weeds without damaging the crops. This method saves labor and fuel for motorized equipment and also promotes no-till farming, which can cut soil erosion by up to 90%. The most common HT crops are cotton, corn, soybeans, and canola.
- *Resistance to environmental stresses:* Researchers are developing new products that have imported useful genes from other species to improve crop-plant tolerance for harsh conditions. Some of the products developed include plants with increased saline tolerance, drought tolerance, flood tolerance, and cold or heat tolerance. These traits will help farmers bring marginal lands into production and overcome some of the negative impacts of climate change.

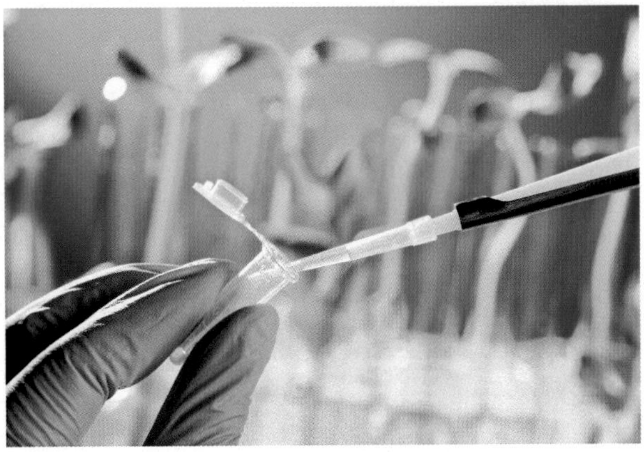

FIGURE 5.5 Genetic engineering for insect-resistant plants.

Other Traits

Other engineered traits can help deliver benefits to farmers and society. For example, increasing the nitrogen-use efficiency of crops reduces the need for expensive nitrogen fertilizers and delayed-ripening technology will give farmers more flexibility in marketing their produce, reduce spoilage, and provide consumers with "fresh-from-the-garden" produce.

Biotechnology also can enable plants to produce healthier and more nutritious foods. Over time, these developments could help improve the nutrition of billions of people in the developing world by fortifying their staple crops with the nutrients that are typically missing from their diets. One example is "golden rice" enhanced with β-carotene to help fight Vitamin A deficiency, a leading cause of blindness in the developing world. Other innovations that have been undertaken enhance the iron content of some foods, which could help prevent anemia that affects 2 billion people worldwide due to insufficient iron in their diet. For some other food crops, biotechnology is used to express positive oil traits, such as Omega-3 fatty acids associated with improved cardiovascular health. Omega-3-enhanced soybean has been approved [12] and other enhanced oil crops are in development. Scientists are also developing consumer-friendly improvements such as nonallergenic peanuts and improvements to the taste, texture, or the appearance of fruits and vegetables.

Stacked Traits

One of the most promising areas for the future of plant biotechnology is our expanding ability to "stack" traits, that is, to introduce more than one transgene into a crop to add multiple beneficial traits at once. The first commercial biotech crop with stacked traits was a cotton seed introduced in 1997 which had both IR and herbicide tolerance traits. By 2011, 26% of all biotech crops planted had stacked traits [11].

Benefits of Plant Biotechnology

Biotech crops help farmers increase yields, which is essential if we are to feed the growing world population. Today more than 90% of corn, 90% of cotton, and 93% of soybeans grown in the United States are biotech crops [13]. Farmers have increased corn yield by more than 33% and soybean yield by 22% in the United States since the introduction of biotech crops. Through 2010, biotech crops have helped produce an additional 300 million tons of canola, cotton, corn, and soybean (Fig. 5.6) [14].

Biotech crops also have significant environmental benefits. The adoption of HT crops has increased no-till agriculture by 69% [15], which reduces soil erosion and improves water quality. Through 2013, biotech crops have helped drive a 1.05 billion pound reduction in pesticide applications [14]. Reduced tilling and pesticide use also means less energy use and reduced greenhouse gas emissions. In 2011 biotech crops helped prevent the release of 23 billion kilograms of CO_2, the equivalent of taking almost 10.2 million cars off the road [14]. Biotech crops also increase farmer incomes. In 2011 biotech crops created a net economic benefit of $19.8 billion at the farm level. More than half of these farm income gains went to farmers in developing countries [14]. Of the 17.3 million farmers growing biotech crops, more than 90% are small, resource-poor farmers from developing countries. The additional income generated by the use of biotech crops makes a significant difference in their quality of life and ability to feed, care for, and educate their families.

In short, plant biotechnology helps feed the world, grow the agricultural economy, improve human health and nutrition [16], and make for a cleaner environment. Yet we are still in the early days of this technology, with many more potential benefits in store.

Animal Biotechnology

Rapidly rising global incomes and urbanization, along with population growth, is increasing the demand for meat and other animal products in many developing countries. Biotechnology contributes to meeting this rising demand by enabling healthier livestock populations and helping animal breeders better manage their herds for desired traits. Technologies such as embryo transfers, in vitro fertilization, cloning, and sex determination of embryos allow breeders to improve their herds. Biotech diagnostics, vaccines, and medicines help diagnose, treat, and prevent animal diseases in livestock. Other biotech products increase the digestibility of animal feed and improve animal nutrition, helping animals grow faster or, in the case of dairy cattle, produce more milk per unit of feed consumed.

Livestock can also be genetically engineered (GE) to use feed more efficiently and produce less manure. For example, the Enviropig, which was previously under development, is a GE pig uniquely able to digest the phosphorus in cereal grain. This limits the amount of phosphorus in the pig manure, reducing pollution. Other developments are improving disease resistance in animals, such as birds that don't transmit the H1N1 (avian flu)

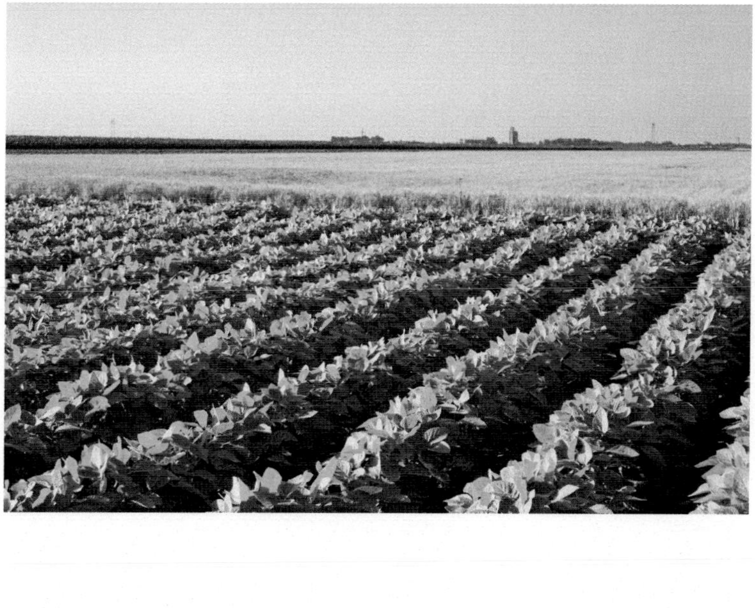

FIGURE 5.6 Biotechnology increases yields in soybeans.

virus or cattle resistant to bovine spongiform encephalopathy, BSE (mad cow disease) and common infections such as mastitis. In aquaculture, scientists have developed a GE salmon that can reach its market weight in half the time of conventionally raised salmon.

Animal Biotech: Beyond Food

Animal biotech, along with plant biotechnology, offers a nearly limitless range of new applications for the next wave of scientists and entrepreneurs to develop. Scientists have engineered animals for many nonfood applications. These include the following:

- Xenotransplantation, using biotech animals as blood, organ, or tissue donors for human patients.
- Production of therapeutic agents, such as human antibody production in cattle, or the production of novel proteins, vaccines, drugs, and tissues.
- Models of human disease, such as pigs that model heart disease or cystic fibrosis.
- In 2009 the FDA approved the first product from a GE animal. ATryn, an anticoagulant used for the prevention of blood clots in patients with a rare disease known as hereditary antithrombin deficiency, is made from GE goats [17].

Industrial and Environmental Biotechnology: A Better Way to Make Things

Industrial biotechnology is one of the most promising new approaches to help meet the global challenges of preventing pollution, conserving energy and natural resources, and reducing manufacturing costs. The application of biotechnology to industrial processes is transforming how we produce existing products and helping to generate new products that were not even imagined a few years ago. Industrial biotechnology uses natural biological processes, such as fermentation and the harnessing of enzymes, yeasts, and microbes as microscopic manufacturing plants, to produce useful products. Among the products being made with industrial biotechnology are biodegradable plastics, renewable chemicals, energy-saving low-temperature detergents, pollution-eating bacteria, multivitamins, and biofuels. With the growing adoption of industrial biotech, we are in the early stages of an emerging biobased economy that meets some of the most important needs of our global civilization.

Working with Nature

Industrial biotechnology is grounded in biocatalysis and fermentation technology. Industrial biotech involves working with nature to maximize and optimize existing biochemical pathways that can be used in manufacturing. Researchers first seek enzyme-producing microorganisms in the natural environment and then search at the molecular level for the genes that produce enzymes with specific biocatalytic capabilities. Once isolated, such enzymes can be characterized for their ability to function in specific industrial processes and, if necessary, can be modified for greater efficiency. Typically these processes are carried out using a controlled environment, a bioreactor, in which microorganisms or cell lines are used to convert raw materials into the desired products, such as chemicals, pharmaceuticals, biobased materials, bioplastics, and biofuels (Fig. 5.7).

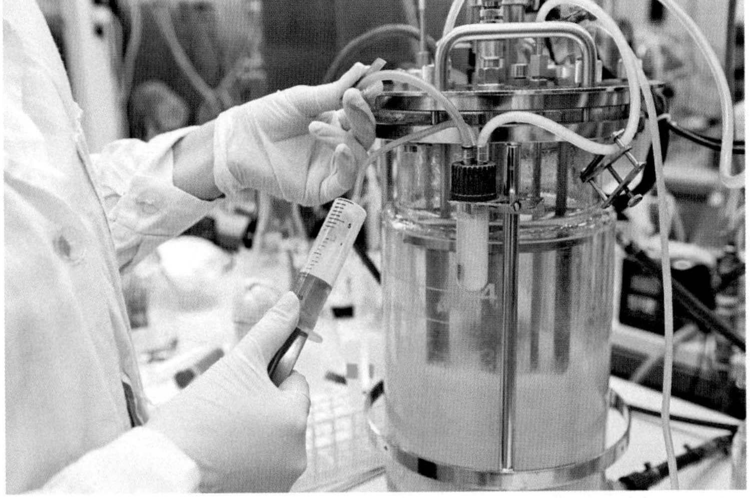

FIGURE 5.7 Lab-scale industrial biotechnology fermentation reactor.

Supporting Sustainability

Sustainability has become an important goal for society. For industry, sustainability means continuous innovation to make fundamental changes in resource consumption and product life-cycle management [18]. Companies are finding ways to reduce material inputs, save energy, minimize the generation of pollutants or waste in the manufacturing process, and either use renewable materials or produce recyclable or biodegradable products that minimize the end-of-life impact of products. Industrial biotechnology helps manufacturers accomplish these goals.

1. *Material inputs:* Many industrial products are petroleum-based. Petroleum is considered a nonrenewable resource that generates pollution, including greenhouse gases. Biotechnology enables manufacturers to reduce petroleum inputs by using biomass feedstocks. In most cases, this makes production cleaner and generates less waste.
2. *Saving energy:* Conventional manufacturing processes often require numerous energy-intensive steps, with many at high temperatures and high pressures. Industrial biotechnology can enable processing steps to be shortened or omitted altogether. This reduces energy requirements. For example, a biotech process for the bleaching of pulp for paper production has been demonstrated to cut related energy uses by 40%. Biocatalysts, particularly enzyme-based processes, also operate at lower temperatures than conventional chemical processes, further conserving energy for some manufacturing operations.
3. *Reducing pollution:* Replacing traditional chemicals with biobased alternatives helps cut pollution at the source. As an example, biotechnology has revolutionized and simplified the production of vitamin B-2 (riboflavin), by reducing a traditional multistep chemical synthesis and purification process to a one-step fermentation process that reduces waste by 95% and leads to a 30% reduction of CO_2 [19].
4. *Biodegradable products:* A significant amount of plastic and other waste is not properly disposed of and often makes its way into the environment. Petroleum-based plastics don't break down well and may last for centuries. Industrial biotechnology has produced biodegradable plastic materials to replace many nondegradable petroleum-based plastics. One such bioplastic is polylactic acid (PLA), a biopolymer that uses corn or sugar beets as a feedstock. PLA is recyclable, biodegradable, and can be composted. It is used in fabrics, plastic films, food and beverage containers, textiles, coated papers and boards, and many other packaging applications.

Advanced Biofuels

Our present standard of living is largely built on fossil fuels. But our children's future depends on our ability to shift over time to renewable energy sources to reduce our reliance on fossil fuels and reduce greenhouse gas emissions. Global energy demand is projected to grow 56% between 2010 and 2040 [20], making this transition all the more urgent. Biotechnology is helping us move toward biobased, low-carbon, or carbon-neutral fuels that are both renewable and better for our environment.

Conventional ethanol, typically produced from corn, accounts for most of the biofuel currently in use in the United States. Biotech innovation is helping to move us beyond the conventional biofuels to advanced biofuels such as cellulosic ethanol, biobutanol, isobutanol, and other drop-in fuels. These are being developed so they can be made from next-generation feedstocks such as algae; crop residues such as corn stalks, wheat straw, and rice straw; wood waste; switchgrass; and other dedicated energy crops—even household trash. Advanced bioethanol made from such cellulosic feedstocks has the potential to reduce greenhouse gas emissions by as much as 128%, compared to reference gasoline [21]. This is possible because managed energy crops, such as switchgrass (Fig. 5.8), are projected to become carbon sinks, since their root systems are generally undisturbed during harvest, which helps account for the estimated reductions of over 100%. The first several thousand commercial gallons

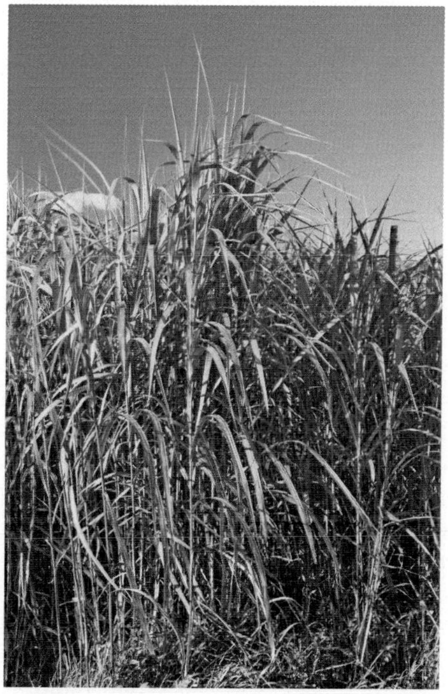

FIGURE 5.8 Switchgrass, a renewable bioenergy source.

of cellulosic biofuel in the United States were produced in 2012.

The key contribution of industrial biotechnology to the development of advanced biofuels is the identification of cellulases produced by microbes and fungi—and their production at industrial scales. Cellulases are enzymes that break down the cellulose found in plant cell walls into simple sugars that can serve as the raw materials for biofuels, as well as many of the biobased chemicals, plastics, and other materials discussed earlier.

Cellulose is the world's most common organic compound, estimated to make up half of all organic carbon on the planet. Biomass is therefore the most globally available and versatile renewable energy asset. There are enormous opportunities to tap this vast resource. Renewable fuels currently provide approximately 10% of US on-road transportation fuel needs. A 2005 analysis by the Natural Resources Defense Council found that ethanol from cellulose could supply half of the US transportation fuel needs by 2050.

The Biobased Economy

The big challenge for the industrial biotechnology sector is to develop a thriving biobased economy in which renewable agricultural feedstocks are converted to higher value products such as biofuels, renewable chemicals, and biobased materials with biotech-enabled processes. As discussed earlier, industrial enzymes, microorganisms, and microbial systems are used today to produce chemical intermediates or in the manufacture of consumer products. The challenge ahead is to accelerate the growth of this biobased economy to revitalize traditional manufacturing, create new manufacturing opportunities, and generate high-quality jobs.

Industrial biotech products have a significant market footprint today which is expected to grow to as much as $547 billion by 2025 [22]. There is already a more than $2.9 billion global market for industrial enzymes [23]. By some estimates the global sustainable chemical industry could reach $1 trillion within a decade. Manufacturers use industrial biotechnology in industries such as food processing, pharmaceuticals, plastics, fuels, specialty chemicals, textiles and paper, and advanced materials manufacture. In 2013, there are more than 75 biorefineries active or under construction across North America for commercial production of advanced biofuels and chemicals from renewable biomass. Industrial biotechnology is bringing new, high-paying, high-quality jobs to communities and will underpin future economic growth across the world.

Synthetic Biology: A New Approach to Engineering Biology

Synthetic biology is a new evolution of biotech innovation that enables biotechnologists to go beyond manipulation of one or two genes and apply engineering techniques to make changes in entire genetic pathways. Some of the earliest researchers in synthetic biology came from the engineering field rather than the more traditional life science disciplines. These scientists can now "write" DNA code in a technique analogous to writing computer code. Synthetic biology provides astounding opportunities to the industrial biotech sphere—most notably an ability to custom engineer microbes, such as bacteria or yeast, to produce specific chemical compounds that the microbe never previously made.

Innovation for any industry is enhanced by increased speed, efficiency, performance, and cost-effectiveness within product development. Synthetic biology enables this type of innovation by allowing more complex, multistep fermentation of organic chemicals and longer gene synthesis. Synthetic biology describes a set of tools that will aid the continued evolution of biotechnology, including applied protein design, the standardization of genomic parts, and synthesis of full genomes [24]. Synthetic biology may speed development of biotech solutions for clean energy and chemical production.

Transforming Industries and the World

With a boost from synthetic biology and other advances, industrial biotechnology can transform all of the industries mentioned in this section, and many more. The momentum for industrial biotech is driven by global needs. For both the developing and developed world, industrial biotechnology presents enormous economic opportunities. By converting locally produced biomass and biological resources into value-added manufactured products and energy, people from all parts of the world have the opportunity to participate in this new, global, biobased economy.

The Public Policy Environment for Biotech Innovation

The best scientists and the smartest entrepreneurs cannot succeed without the right public policy environment. Public policy affects the ability of entrepreneurs to raise capital, protect intellectual property, carry out research and development, receive timely regulatory review and approval, and earn a sufficient return on their investment of time and capital in the development of new products. America's flourishing biotechnology industry is aided by smart and effective public policy that supports innovation and scientific advances. For this trend to continue, those interested in the field need to be active, engaged, and informed about how legislative decisions affect the industry. You should be familiar with the policies that support biotechnology and stay informed about the decisions of Congress, state legislators, and other policymakers that could help—or hinder—the success and growth of the biotechnology industry.

A number of landmark laws and foundational public policies enabled the growth of a robust biotechnology industry in the United States. They include the following:

1. *National Institutes of Health (NIH):* The NIH funds much of the basic medical research in the United States, spending about $31 billion annually in recent years. More than 50,000 competitive grants from the NIH support more than 325,000 researchers at more than 3000 universities, medical schools, and research institutions, in addition to research the NIH conducts at its own facilities. The NIH has invested hundreds of billions of dollars in public funding over seven decades. This massive investment was a major factor in putting the United States at the forefront of biomedical innovation. NIH funding has helped scientists decipher the genetic code, sequence the human genome, and understand neurotransmitters and protein-folding, among many other fundamentals of biology.
2. *Bayh–Dole Act:* This law grants universities and nonprofit institutions exclusive rights to the intellectual property they produce through federally funded research. Since Bayh–Dole was adopted in 1980, more than 6000 US companies have been founded to commercialize university research. NIH-funded research and technology transfer under Bayh–Dole spurred the rise of research universities as the hubs of biotechnology industry clusters.
3. *FDA:* Another advantage for the US biotech industry is a favorable regulatory environment. New drugs and medical devices must receive FDA approval for safety and efficacy before entering the market. Globally, FDA approval is considered the "gold standard" of regulatory review—the most rigorous, predictable, and efficient system in the world. This has helped the United States to attract the vast majority of global biomedical research and development.
4. *Hatch–Waxman Act:* This law strikes a balance between the public benefits of introducing low-cost generic drugs to the market with the need to maintain the incentives for investment in new biopharmaceutical innovation. Because of the lengthy product development, testing, and review process, most drugs do not reach the market until a significant portion of their term-of-patent protection has already passed. Hatch–Waxman restores some of this effective patent life, while also creating a pathway for the eventual approval of generic drugs.
5. *Orphan Drug Act:* This law, passed in 1983, provides financial incentives to encourage companies to develop treatments for small patient populations. It provides developers with the exclusive right to market an orphan drug—a drug or biologic that treats a rare disease or condition—for that indication for 7 years from the date of FDA approval. According to the National Organization for Rare Disorders, more than 400 new drugs have been approved for treatment of orphan diseases since the signing of the Orphan Drug Act. In the 10 years preceding the approval of the Orphan Drug Act, only 10 new therapies had been developed.
6. *Patent protection:* Because the majority of biotech companies are small businesses with no products on the market, they must rely on outside private investment, often raised from venture capital firms, to fund their research and development work. Biotechnology drug development is a lengthy and expensive process. Strong patents provide the needed incentives to attract the private funding from investors necessary to fund biomedical research.
7. *Drug reimbursement:* In general, the United States does not limit or restrict prescription drug prices but allows the free market to work. With sound reimbursement policies in place, patients have greater and faster access to breakthrough therapies and medicines. Market-based drug pricing provides investors in new drug development with greater confidence that they will be able to earn a sufficient return on their investment. Conversely, government price controls reduce incentives for investment in new drug development. As the largest purchaser of prescription drugs through Medicare, Medicaid, and other publicly funded health programs, the United States government's pricing and reimbursement policies can have a huge effect on biomedical innovation.

These are only a few of many public policies that have helped the United States to lead the world in the development of new biotech medicines. The right public policies are just as important for innovation in other sectors of the biotech industry. For the United States to remain the agriculture production leader of the world, we need sensible, science-based regulations and a predictable review and approval process for agricultural biotech products that is based on scientific evidence and on the potential benefits to society and to the environment. Crops derived from modern biotechnology are among the most heavily regulated agricultural products.

Currently, biotech crops and animals undergo intense regulatory scrutiny throughout the development process, which can take 10–15 years. Agricultural biotechnology is stringently regulated, and depending on the product, the regulators are some combination of the FDA, the US Department of Agriculture, and the Environmental Protection Agency. Fair international trade policies and patent protection are also important to agricultural biotech, along with public funding for food and agricultural research.

Policies such as the Renewable Fuel Standard (which sets annual targets for the increased use of renewable fuels), tax credits, and other incentives have enabled the development of a biobased economy. These programs help companies attract the large investments needed to construct commercial-scale biorefineries by effectively guaranteeing a market for biorefinery products.

It is up to all of us in the biotech industry to educate the public about the value of biotechnology and to help policymakers understand the effects of their decisions on innovation. For instance, policymakers generally support developing new biologic treatments, but sometimes do not fully appreciate how expensive and high-risk biotech R&D really is—and thus how critical it is to have policies that maintain incentives for investors to back biotech innovation.

It is up to biotech innovators—those who understand the technology best—to share their experiences with friends, family, neighbors, and others. We should talk about our work and what we hope to accomplish for the world. It is up to us to educate people about the value of biotechnology and to present clear and accurate information about risks and benefits, so that public officials, and society as a whole, can make fully informed decisions. If we maintain and enhance public policies that support innovation, biotechnology will continue to fulfill its promise of offering powerful new solutions to some of the oldest human problems.

Promise for the Future

As the President and CEO of the Biotechnology Innovation Organization (BIO), I often have the opportunity to meet biotech entrepreneurs from across the United States and around the world. BIO represents more than 1000 innovative biotechnology companies and organizations. Many of our members are small, emerging companies involved in the research and development of innovative healthcare, agricultural, industrial, and environmental biotechnology products. I am constantly amazed by the ingenuity of biotech researchers and by the almost infinite possibilities for using the science of life to improve the lives of everyone on our planet. We are still in the early days of the biotech revolution, with an infinite amount to learn and boundless opportunities ahead. For you as an entrepreneur, the field of discovery is wide open, and much of the future is determined by the extent of our imagination. As we like to say at BIO, we feed, fuel, and heal the world.

References

[1] Ahmann D, Dorgan JR. Bioengineering for pollution prevention through development of biobased energy and materials state of the science report. Washington, DC: Environmental Protection Agency.

[2] World Health Organization. Top 10 causes of death, May 24, 2018. <https://www.who.int/news-room/fact-sheets/detail/the-top-10-causes-of-death> [accessed March 7, 2019].

[3] Globocan. International Agency for Research on Cancer, <https://onlinelibrary.wiley.com/doi/full/10.3322/caac.21492>; 2018 [accessed March 7, 2019].

[4] World Intellectual Property Organization. Neglected tropical diseases, July 11, 2019. <https://www.who.int/neglected_diseases/en/> [accessed March 7, 2019].

[5] Global Genes. Project estimates.

[6] PhRMA. Medicines in development for cancer, May 30, 2018. <https://www.phrma.org/report/medicines-in-development-for-cancer-2018-report> [accessed March 7, 2019].

[7] Goodman AD, et al. Sustained-release oral fampridine in multiple sclerosis: a randomized, double-blind, controlled trial. Lancet 2009;373(9665):732–8. <https://www.ncbi.nlm.nih.gov/pubmed/19249634> [accessed March 7, 2019].

[8] World Health Organization. Global HIV/AIDS response, progress report, 2011. <http://www.who.int/hiv/pub/progress_report2011/en/> [accessed March 7, 2019].

[9] Allingham-Hawkins D. Successful genetic tests are predicated on clinical utility. Genetic Engineering and Biotechnology News, August 1, 2008. <https://www.genengnews.com/magazine/96/successful-genetic-tests-are-predicated-on-clinical-utility/> [accessed July 16, 2019].

[10] Centers for Disease Control and Prevention. Evaluating genomic tests, December 20, 2016. <https://www.cdc.gov/genomics/gtesting/index.htm> [accessed March 7, 2019].

[11] ISAAA. Global status of commercialized biotech/GM crops: 2012, <http://isaaa.org/resources/publications/briefs/44/executive-summary/default.asp>; n.d. [accessed March 7, 2019].

[12] Monsanto. Omega-3-enhanced soybean oil, October 26, 2009. <https://monsanto.com/news-releases/worlds-first-sda-omega-3-soybean-oil-achieves-major-milestone-that-advances-the-development-of-foods-with-the-enhanced-nutritional-benefits/> [accessed March 7, 2019].

[13] USDA. Adoption of genetically engineered crops in the U.S. <https://www.ers.usda.gov/data-products/adoption-of-genetically-engineered-crops-in-the-us.aspx>; n.d. [accessed March 7, 2019].

[14] PG Economics. Press Release, <http://www.pgeconomics.co.uk/press + releases/6/Global + economic + benefits + of + GM + crops + reach + almost+ + + %26%2336%3B100 + billion/>; 2013 [accessed March 7, 2019].

[15] Conservation Technology Information Center. <http://www.ctic.purdue.edu/>; n.d. [accessed March 7, 2019].

[16] ISAAC. The ideal diet: sufficient and balanced, <https://docplayer.net/22411994-Rooting-out-hunger-in-malawi-with.html>; n.d. [accessed March 7, 2019].

[17] FDA grants first-ever U.S. approval of GE animal product, February 6, 2009. <https://www.bio.org/media/press-release/fda-grants-first-ever-us-approval-ge-animal-product> [accessed March 7, 2019].

[18] Ceschin, F., & Gaziulusoy, I. (2016). Evolution of design for sustainability: From product design to design for system innovations and transitions. *Design Studies, 47*, 118–163. <https://www.sciencedirect.com/science/article/pii/S0142694X16300631> [accessed March 7, 2019].

[19] OECD. Biotechnology for the environment in the future: science, technology and policy. In: OECD science, technology and industry policy papers, no. 3. Paris: OECD Publishing; 2013. <https://www.oecd-ilibrary.org/docserver/5k4840hqhp7j-en.pdf?expires = 1552013446&id = id&accname = guest&checksum = 1B64030-A6BD7A8A2CEB128468A46CACB> [accessed March 7, 2019].

[20] U.S. Energy Information Administration. International Energy Outlook 2018. July 24, 2018. Washington, DC. <http://www.eia.gov/forecasts/ieo/> [accessed March 7, 2019].

[21] U.S. Environmental Protection Agency. Renewable Fuel Standard Program (RFS2) Regulatory Impact Analysis, <https://www.federalregister.gov/documents/2018/07/10/2018-14448/renewable-fuel-standard-program-standards-for-2019-and-biomass-based-diesel-volume-for-2020>; July 2018 [accessed March 7, 2019].

[22] Department for Business Enterprise and Regulatory Reform. IB 2025: maximising UK opportunities from industrial biotechnology in a low carbon economy. London: Industrial Biotechnology Innovation and Growth Team. <http://beaconwales.org/uploads/resources/Maximising_UK_Opportunities_from_Industrial_Biotechnology_in_a_Low_Carbon_Economy.pdf> [accessed March 7, 2019].

[23] Erickson B, Nelson J, Winters P. Perspective on opportunities in industrial biotechnology in renewable chemicals. Biotechnol J 2012;7(2):176–85.

[24] Erickson B, Singh R, Winters P. Synthetic biology: regulating industry uses of new biotechnologies. Science 2011;333 (6047):1254–6.

Further Reading

Long G, Works J. Innovation in the Biopharmaceutical pipeline: a multidimensional view. Analysis Group with support from Pharmaceutical Research and Manufacturers of America, <https://www.analysisgroup.com/uploadedfiles/content/insights/publishing/2012_innovation_in_the_biopharmaceutical_pipeline.pdf>; 2013 [accessed March 7, 2019].

Medco. Mayo Clinic study reveals using a simple genetic test reduces hospitalization rates by nearly a third for patients on widely prescribed blood thinner. Press Release March 16, 2010. Available from: <https://www.prnewswire.com/news-releases/medco-mayo-clinic-study-reveals-using-a-simple-genetic-test-reduces-hospitalization-rates-by-nearly-a-third-for-patients-on-widely-prescribed-blood-thinner-87776257.html> [accessed March 7, 2019].

PhRMA. Medicines in development for rare diseases, March 1, 2017. <https://www.phrma.org/graphic/medicines-in-development-for-rare-diseases> [accessed March 7, 2019].

Chapter 6

Five Essential Elements and Regional Influences Required To Grow and Expand a Biotechnology Cluster or Hub

Craig Shimasaki, PhD, MBA

CEO, BioSource Consulting Group and Moleculera Labs, Oklahoma City, OK, United States

Chapter Outline

The first utilization of modern genetic engineering began in 1973 when Stanley Cohen and Herbert Boyer successfully excised a segment of frog DNA and transferred it into a bacterial plasmid to create a molecular factory for proteins. Just three years after those humble beginnings, Genentech was founded with $500 each from Robert Swanson, at the time a young venture capitalist, and Herbert Boyer, a University of California San Francisco professor. *The biotechnology industry had begun*. In the ensuing five years, only a handful of companies followed, such as Cetus (which began in 1971 but not based on genetic engineering until after 1976), Biogen and Hybritech in 1978, Amgen in 1980, and Genzyme and Chiron in 1981. Over the next four decades, the biotech industry grew to well over 10,000 public and private companies that collectively employ an estimated 1,000,000 individuals worldwide. Today, the biotechnology industry continues to expand as cities, states, and local governments vie for the creation of biotechnology clusters in their region. Although this industry is experiencing unprecedented growth, the particular expansion rate is not equal in all geographies but continues to be concentrated predominately in certain cluster locations, and in new regions where certain elements are present. Why is this the case? With the ensuing economic value of this high tech and clean industry, why is the biotech industry

Biotechnology Entrepreneurship. DOI: https://doi.org/10.1016/B978-0-12-815585-1.00006-1

biased toward growth and expansion in certain regions? In this chapter, I describe five essential elements and regional influences that are a requisite to fuel the growth, development and expansion of biotechnology clusters or hubs in a particular locale.

It's Not about the Climate, the Cost of Living, Culture, or the Scenery

One would think that the attractiveness of a location would be gorgeous weather, low cost of living, the culture, or the beautiful scenery. These qualities are great to have but they are tangential, and *not* the drivers of growth for a biotechnology hub. The Boston/Cambridge area and the San Francisco Bay Area are recognized as the top biotechnology clusters in the world. However, these regions both rank near the top in the United States for the cost of living, but this has not deterred the growth of these two biotech clusters. The frigid temperatures, long winters, and blizzards in Boston have not deterred the exponential establishment of biotechnology companies in this region. In fact, so many new companies are being established there, as well as big pharma locating into this region, that many outlying suburbs are creating biotechnology incubators to house the plethora of start-ups that cannot find space in the Boston or Cambridge areas. Despite the overcrowding, the ever-increasing traffic and the high cost-of-living, the San Francisco Bay Area continues to spawn multitudes of newly established biotechnology companies. Also, the growth and expansion of biotechnology hubs is not influenced by a particular culture or lifestyle. The Boston and San Francisco areas have vastly dissimilar cultures from each other (just ask anyone who has moved from San Francisco to Boston or vice versa), yet both regions continue to grow their respective biotechnology hubs at an unprecedented pace.

This may lead one to think that only locations with existing biotechnology hubs are capable of expansion. Indeed, many of the early biotechnology companies were started in the San Francisco and Boston regions, and today these are thriving biotechnology ecosystems, spawning new companies on a regular basis. It is estimated that approximately one-third of all US biotech employees work in the Boston and San Francisco Bay areas where the concentration of biotechnology companies eclipse that of all other regions. However, if you were to remove any two of the five essential elements we will discuss, from Boston or the San Francisco Bay Area, the expansion and growth of biotechnology in these regions would level off, and over time they would likely decline, as companies would find more suitable locations to start and grow. Yes, an existing biotech hub has momentum and this helps to accelerate growth, but that does not explain why locations previously less known as biotechnology hubs are moving up in the ranks as strong biotechnology clusters. Twenty years ago, Seattle, New York/New Jersey, Los Angeles/Orange County, Maryland/Virginia/DC Metro, Chicago, and many others were not thought of as biotech clusters, but now they typically rank in the top locations for biotechnology clusters in the United States.

What is it about these two distinctly diverse regions with their respective differences, that allows them to experience accelerated growth and expansion as the world's largest biotech hubs? In this chapter, we will examine five essential elements necessary for growing a biotechnology cluster, and we will discuss how a region or locale can create a tailored strategic plan for the establishment of a biotech hub in their area.

If we look at the history of the top two biotechnology hubs, it is insightful to understand what factors helped establish them in the first place, but more importantly, it gives us insight into these five essential elements that fueled the continued growth of these clusters over time. For instance, in the San Francisco Bay Area, one contributing factor that helped establish this location as a biotech hub was the colocation of the venture capital industry that previously funded the computer chip boom in the mid-1970s. Silicon Valley is proximal to San Francisco and is home to many entrepreneurial-minded leaders. Also, having several top-notch academic institutions conducting ground-breaking research all fueled the birth of numerous biotechnology companies there (Fig. 6.1). For the Boston and Cambridge regions, having top-ranked academic research institutions such as Harvard and MIT was key to Boston's transformation, as well as having proximity to a large concentration of well-established pharmaceutical companies (Fig. 6.2). The colocation of a mature pharmaceutical industry gave ready access to an abundant resource of industry leaders and drug development team members for fledgling biotechnology companies.

Biotechnology Clusters are Actively Developing Worldwide

Today, there are many other established and growing concentrations of biotech activity in diverse locations. A 2018 Jones Lang LaSalle Life Sciences Outlook Report [1] referenced and ranked the following as established clusters in the United States: Greater Boston Area, San Francisco Bay Area, San Diego Metro Area, Raleigh-Durham Metro Area, Philadelphia Metro Area, Suburban Maryland/Metro DC, Seattle Metro Area, New Jersey, Westchester County, Denver Metro Area, Chicago Metro Area, New York City, Minneapolis/St. Paul Metro Area, Houston, and Long Island.

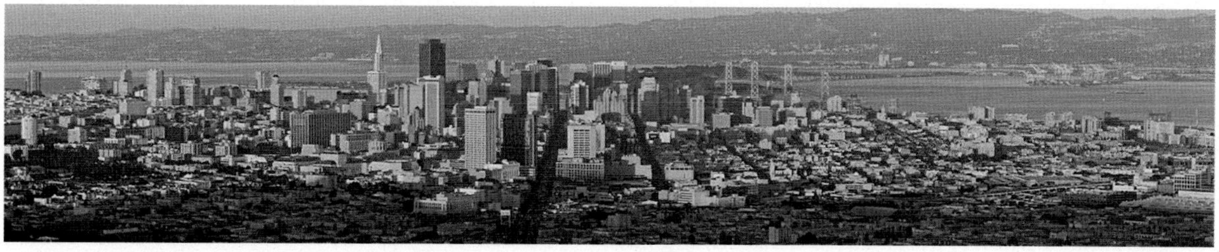

FIGURE 6.1 The San Francisco Bay Area, a major biotechnology cluster. *Wikipedia.*

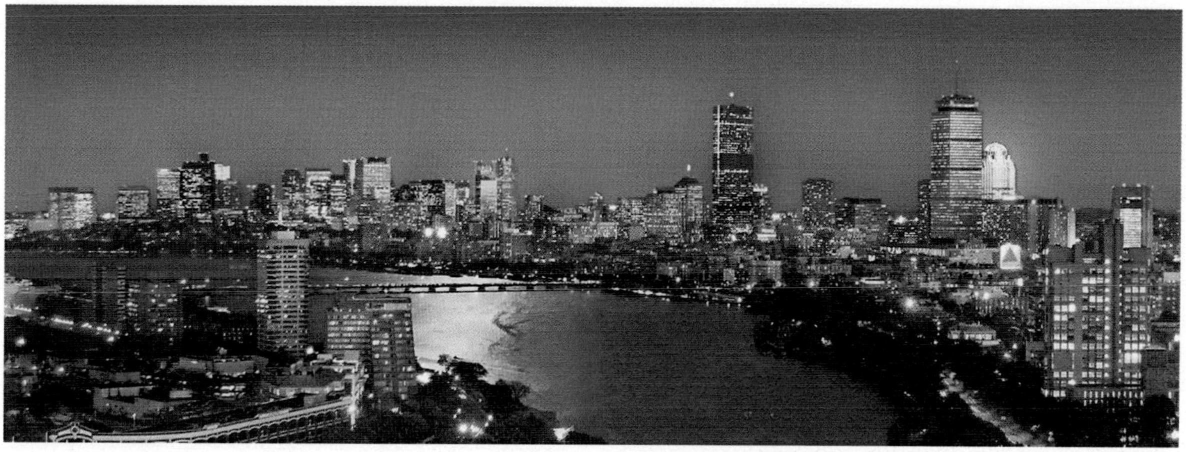

FIGURE 6.2 The Boston/Cambridge area, one of the top biotechnology clusters in the world. *Wikipedia.*

Biotechnology clusters are emerging around the globe. In 2018, Genetic Engineering and Biotechnology News listed the top 10 European biotech clusters [2] based upon public research funding, venture capital funding, patents, the number of biotech companies, and jobs. The top 10 European biotech clusters were led by the United Kingdom, then Germany, France, the Netherlands, Spain, Switzerland, Belgium, Sweden, Italy, and Denmark. The top 10 Asian biotech clusters [3] were based upon public R&D spending, patents, initial public offerings, number of biotech companies, and jobs. These were led by China, then Japan, South Korea, India, Australia, Taiwan, Singapore, Malaysia, Thailand, and Indonesia. Illustrative of this trend, epicenters, such as Medicon Valley, which straddles the border of Sweden and Denmark, are now home to over 350 biotechnology companies with over 40,000 employees, including biopharma companies, such as AstraZeneca, LEO Pharma, Baxter Gambro, and Lundbeck. Switzerland's BioValley connects academia and companies of three nations in the Upper Rhine Valley, namely France, Germany, and Switzerland, and is one of the leading European Life Sciences regions in the world with over 600 pharmaceutical and Medtech companies and 14 technology parks in this region. Australia has more than 400 biotechnology companies, predominately located in clusters in Sydney and Melbourne. There are more than 600 companies located in biotechnology clusters in Scotland, and in Oxford and London, biotechnology clusters are home to over 600 companies combined. Medcity, one of the United Kingdom's recent initiatives, is seeking to transform the London–Oxford–Cambridge life sciences sector into a world beating power cluster.

There is universal interest in establishing biotechnology clusters in most of the countries around the world, as evidenced by the major activities and initiatives over the past two decades. The providence of Ontario, Canada, has a Biotechnology Cluster Innovation Program where the government is focused on funding and developing a competitive biotechnology cluster. Europe INNOVA was launched in 2006 that ran through 2012 as an initiative of the European Commission's Directorate General Enterprise and Industry which aspires to become the laboratory for the development and testing of new tools and instruments in support of innovation with the view to help enterprises innovate faster and better. They have brought together public and private support and providers, such as innovation agencies, technology transfer offices, business incubators, financing intermediaries, cluster organizations, and others. The European Commission initiative

NETBIOCLUE was launched in 2006 to promote networking, cooperation and knowledge transfer between 14 partners from different bioclusters involved in the process of innovation in the field of biotechnology for health in Europe. The acronym stands for "NETworking activity for BIOtechnology CLUsters in Europe."

In 2006 the New York City Economic Development Corp. incorporated BioBAT (Fig. 6.3), a nonprofit organization that is leading the biotech development at the Brooklyn Army Terminal and converting it into a massive new bioresearch and manufacturing facility. BioBAT, a 524,000-square-feet center for commercial bioscience was the areas first biotech start-up incubator. The city invested $12 million in the project, and the state offered $48 million of funding. The Brooklyn Army Terminal is a 97-acre facility owned by the city and managed by the New York City Economic Development Corporation. In 2015 a new 26,000-square-feet space was officially opened to potential tenants. The Colorado Science and Technology Park at Fitzsimons is an example of what can be done to facilitate the organic growth of biotechnology in one's own state. A decommissioned army medical center was closed down a decade ago in Denver, and 18 million square feet is being converted to house 30,000 new employees with many of the companies being spin-off technology companies from the University of Colorado Health Science Center. The state's investment of $4 billion will become an economic generator for Colorado and stimulate the development of many new biotechnology companies. In order to reproduce this type of success, we need to understand the common denominators that continue to fuel the growth in these diverse but expanding biotechnology clusters.

What is a Biotechnology Cluster?

A biotechnology cluster is simply a very high concentration of organically grown biotechnology enterprises attached to a supportive ecosystem within a defined geographic region. Within this ecosystem, each of the biotechnology companies are not typically interconnected to one another; however, they are all interconnected to their local bioscience providers and are sustained by the presence of the five essential elements we will discuss. Often, a biotechnology cluster develops a subspecialty focus due to an inherent concentration of expertise and resources within that region. For instance, the greater Minneapolis, Minnesota region and surrounding areas are home to a high concentration of medical device companies, principally due to the historical presence of Medtronic (founded in 1949 with the development of the pacemaker), as well as 3M and Boston Scientific. High concentrations of therapeutic companies are located in the Boston area which was influenced by the large concentration of pharmaceutical companies clustered in New Jersey and the surrounding areas. A large number of agricultural biotechnology companies are clustered in Midwestern states of the United States, principally due to the high concentration of agricultural research conducted at local universities and academic institutions.

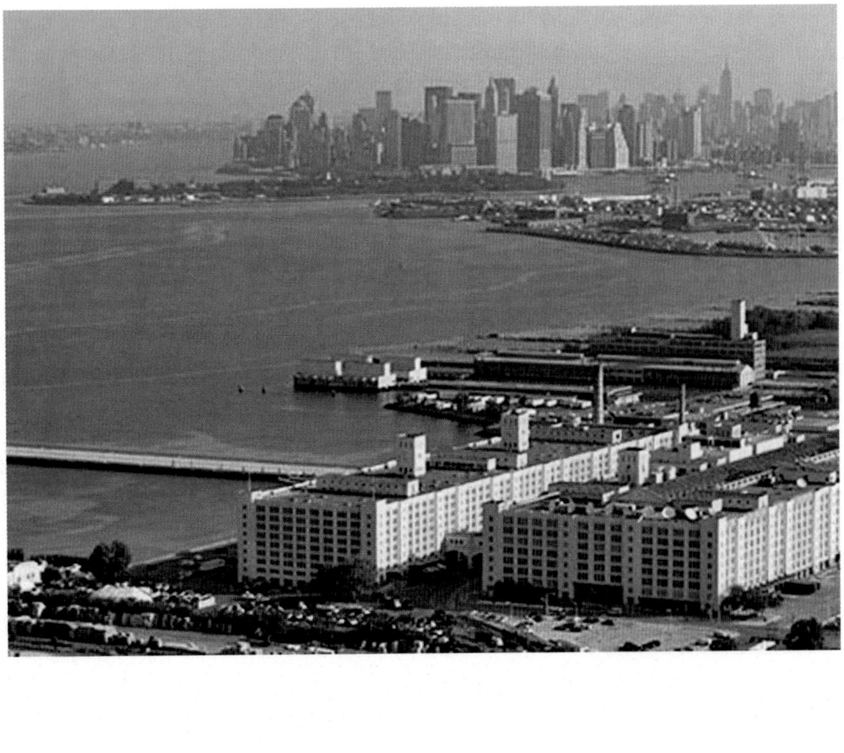

FIGURE 6.3 BioBAT at Brooklyn Army Terminal, a major biotechnology incubator in New York. *New York City Economic Development Corporation, NYCEDC.*

What are the Benefits of Having a Biotechnology Cluster?

In 2012 the US government released the *National Bioeconomy Blueprint* noting that bioscience industries are "a large and rapidly growing segment of the world economy that provides substantial public benefit" [4]. The economic benefit and quality-of-life impact of a mature biotechnology cluster in its municipality and local government are significant. The Biotechnology Innovation Organization (BIO) and TEConomy released a National Bioscience Industry Report in 2018 showing $2 trillion economic impact, accelerated venture capital investment, and the total impact of job growth in the United States of all biotechnology sectors [5]. Aside from the universal benefits of biotechnology products for health, agriculture, fuels, and energy, biotechnology clusters have much more to offer local regions and governments, with some of these benefits listed as follows:

1. ***The biotechnology industry creates clean and high-technology jobs:*** Regional municipalities and governments are searching for ways to attract and retain high-technology jobs which tend to be clean industries that generate fewer environmental issues. Based upon data from the US Bureau of Labor statistics, the bioscience industry in the United States has led in job creation during the 2001 to 2010 period when compared with other major knowledge-based industries critical for advancing high-quality jobs (Fig. 6.4A). This was in spite of a nationwide decline in most job categories. A primary reason for the resiliency of the bioscience industry is the diverse set of markets it serves. These markets span biomedical drugs, diagnostics and devices, agricultural products from animal health, to seeds and crop protection, and bio-based industrial products such as enzymes for industrial chemical processes and bioremediation, biofuels, and bioplastics. Over the expanded period of 2001 to 2016, jobs in the bioscience industry still grew at overall 18.6% but were outpaced during this period by the software and computer services industry (Fig. 6.4B). The biotechnology industry has fared much better than the overall economy through the recent US recession and recovery.

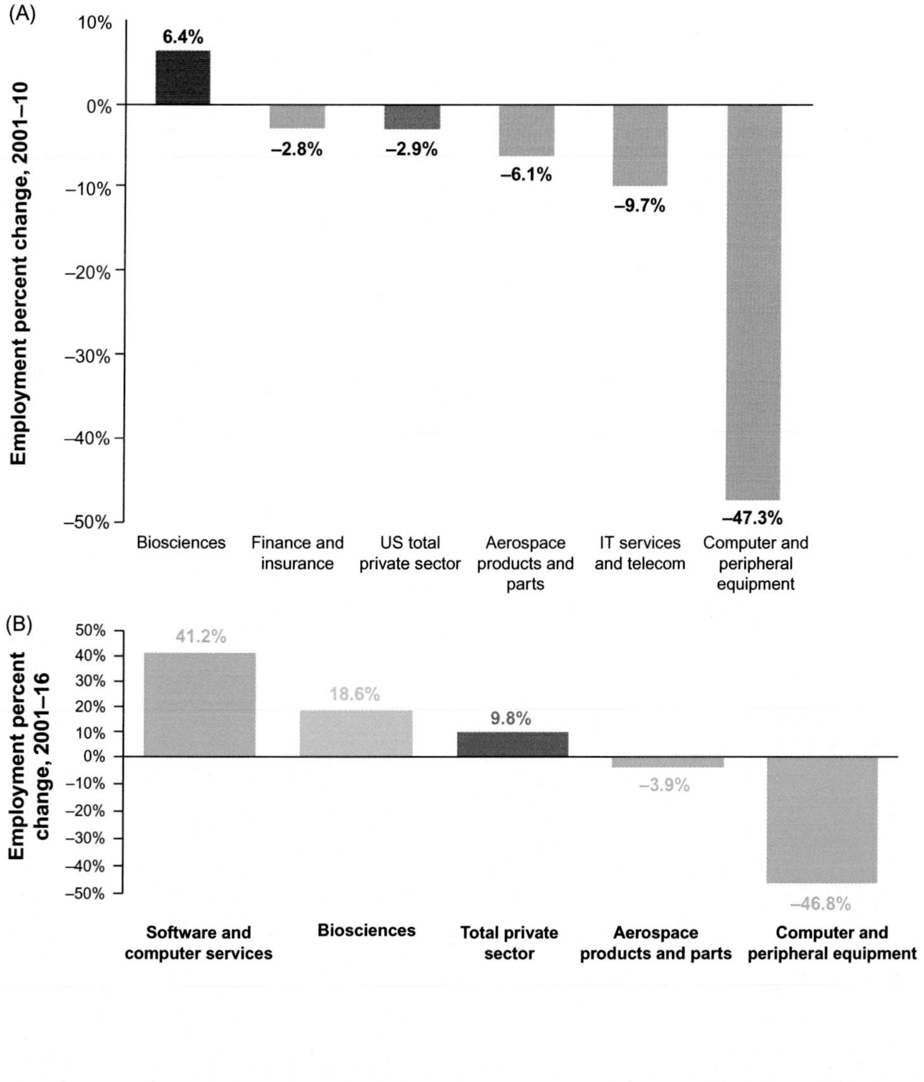

FIGURE 6.4 (A) Job growth in the bioscience compared to other knowledge-based industries, 2001–10. (B) Employment change—the US Bioscience Industry versus Other Technology Industries, 2001–16. *(A) Battelle analysis of Bureau of Labor Statistics, QCEW; enhanced file from IMPLAN; (B) TEConomy Partners analysis of U.S. Bureau of Labor Statistics, QCEW data; enhanced file from IMPLAN (2018 TEConomy/BIO "Investment, Innovation and Job Creation in a Growing U.S. Bioscience Industry" report).*

2. ***The biotechnology industry creates high paying jobs:*** The bioscience industry continues to be a source of high-wage jobs. Wages in the bioscience industry are consistently higher and growing faster on average than those for the overall economy. In 2016 the nation's bioscience workers earned nearly $99,000, on average (Fig. 6.5), which is more than $45,000 above the average for the nation's private sector. This wage premium earned by bioscience workers has grown from 64% in 2001 to 85% today. In the bioscience industry the average wage growth continued to outpace the private sector. Since 2001, inflation-adjusted (real) wages increased by 23% versus 9% for the economy as a whole [5].
3. ***New jobs and high paying jobs generate personal and sales taxes for local governments:*** Because biotechnology employees tend to have significantly higher salaries than the national averages, these employees on average purchase more goods and services, generating more tax revenue to the local economy. All local governments need tax revenue to operate and support their infrastructure services for their community. As these amenities and services improve and increase, this in turn can attract other industries to the region with more job relocations.
4. ***Biotechnology companies bring an innovative and skilled workforce:*** Biotechnology companies require diversely skilled employees who are experienced in various disciplines, including research and development, drug design, medical devices, mechanical and biomedical engineering, medical affairs, chemistry, molecular biology, regulatory affairs, clinical trials, and a host of other professional disciplines. Many times, industry professionals can contribute a portion of their time and resources to the local economy by participating in various local support and philanthropic activities in their community.
5. ***Biotechnology clusters attract collateral businesses and support services:*** Biotechnology companies require a host of collateral support groups in order to be successful. These support services also tend to employ positions that are higher paying than the national average and they tend to be in clean industries. Some of the support services and professionals include corporate and patent attorneys, prototype development companies, accountants, public relations firms, medical service providers, clinical trial coordinators, medical consultants, and research technologists.
6. ***Large talent pools bring cross-creativity and shortened development time:*** As the critical mass of biotechnology company employees and their service providers increase in a locale, the speed for development of company technology and products tends to accelerate. This is principally due to the availability and quality of cross-creativity experts with the necessary experience to support these companies' product development needs. This increase in product development momentum is attractive to other companies that want access to those same resources and talent pools. Concurrent with industry growth comes a greater expansion of support services and more professionals to support the industry—and the cycle continues.

Employment sector	Annual average wage
Drugs and pharmaceuticals	$113,815
Research, testing and medical labs	$106,942
Finance and insurance	$101,180
Total biosciences	**$98,961**
Information (IT, telecommunications, broadcasting, data processing)	$98,475
Bioscience-related distribution	$93,677
Professional and technical services	$90,950
Medical devices and equipment	$84,746
Agricultural feedstock and industrial biosciences	$80,961
Manufacturing	$64,860
Construction	$58,643
Real estate and rental and leasing	$54,959
Total private sector	**$53,354**
Transportation and warehousing	$50,443
Health care and social assistance	$47,955
Retail trade	$30,297

FIGURE 6.5 Average annual wages for the biosciences and other major industries, 2016. *TEConomy Partners analysis of U.S. Bureau of Labor Statistics, QCEW data; QCEW data; enhanced file from IMPLAN. (2018 TEConomy/BIO "Investment, Innovation and Job Creation in a Growing U.S. Bioscience Industry" report).*

The Five Essential Elements Necessary for Growing a Biotechnology Cluster or Hub

What are the key elements fueling the transformation of diverse locations such as Boston and San Francisco into two of the largest concentrations of biotechnology companies in the world? These same essential elements are the factors that drive the growth and expansions of biotechnology clusters irrespective of location. "Essential Elements" are the factors that when absent, or in limited quantity, inhibits a biotechnology cluster from developing and expanding in any location. The following five essential elements are necessary to establish, stimulate, and encourage continued growth of biotechnology companies within any geography in order to become a biotechnology hub. To the degree that any essential element is limited, to that same degree a region's biotechnology cluster growth will also be limited.

Five Essential Elements

1. ***Abundance of high quality, adequately funded academic research:*** This essential element is the basic academic research conducted at well-respected institutions, which are typically well funded and performed by high-caliber researchers, scientists, physicians, or engineers. These researchers are typically well published in top-tier peer-reviewed journals and are predictably scientific and technology leaders in their particular field. This includes the institution's technology transfer office, and how easy and efficient it is for licensees to work with them.
2. ***Ready resource of seasoned and experienced biotechnology entrepreneurs and mentors:*** This essential element is a supply of seasoned individuals who have the experience and expertise to shepherd fledgling companies during the difficult growth stages through to commercialization or corporate partnership. These individuals tend to be serial entrepreneurs who have founded previous companies or served in key roles at other biotechnology or life science organizations. Another experienced group consists of individuals with tenured experience in senior positions at large multinational pharmaceutical, medical device, agricultural, or venture capital organizations.
3. ***Ready access to at-risk, early, and development-stage capital willing to fund start-ups:*** This essential element consists of multiple funding sources, including angel investors, venture capital, or institutional capital located within, or proximal to, the local region. These are funding sources that actively invest in early- and development-stage life science enterprises. In addition, these sources can include local government-supported financing and granting programs directed to assist enterprises during the inception stages until significant value is realized.
4. ***Adequate supply of technically skilled workforce experienced in the biotechnology industry:*** This essential element is comprised of experienced scientists, technicians, and laboratory personnel who are well trained in the particular techniques and methods required to advance the technology from inception,

(Continued)

(Continued)

development, clinical testing, manufacturing, and commercialization within that biotechnology sector. Such a workforce is necessary in order to support product development for these companies without having to spend enormous amounts of time and resources for on-the-job training.

5. ***Availability of dedicated wet-laboratory and specialized facilities at affordable rates:*** This essential element is the supply of specialized facilities and laboratory space located in strategic areas that facilitate the incubation of nascent companies, so they can prove their biological concepts or build working prototypes. These facilities should be state-of-the-art and must be offered at affordable rates to allow these early-stage companies to make value-enhancing progress in order to attract more investor capital.

"Growing" biotechnology clusters

To understand the process of growing a biotechnology cluster, a helpful analogy is the corollary to a farmer who wants to reap a harvest of a particular agricultural crop on their land. Farmers know that they cannot "*make*" crops grow. However, farmers understand that they have the ability to greatly influence the likelihood of growth, the type of product produced, and the size of the harvest by ensuring that certain essential elements are present. For instance, if a farmer desires to harvest a crop of corn, he will plan corn seeds during the season that has adequate sunshine and water. The farmer must ensure that the soil is tilled, provided with adequate fertilizer, and then the farmer can expect a harvest of corn at the proper time. To carry this illustration further, if the farmer sows an abundance of fertile seed in nutrient-rich soil, provides an adequate supply of water and fertilizer, during a season of abundant sunshine, and removes destructive pests and weeds that inhibit growth, the seed will *naturally* flourish. Notably, if the farmer omits one or more of these essential elements, such as water or fertilizer, or if one essential element is in short supply, then it becomes very difficult, if not impossible, to reap the desired harvest even though other essential elements are in abundant supply (see Fig. 6.6). For this analogy, the "*farmer*" can be likened to seasoned and experienced biotech entrepreneur who watches over the budding seed and nurtures it to grow. As we will discuss later, the regional government or municipality that wants to establish or nurture a biotechnology hub, participates and influences the environment to be either conducive or detrimental for growth. Such an environment is produced by the joint efforts of both the public and private sectors.

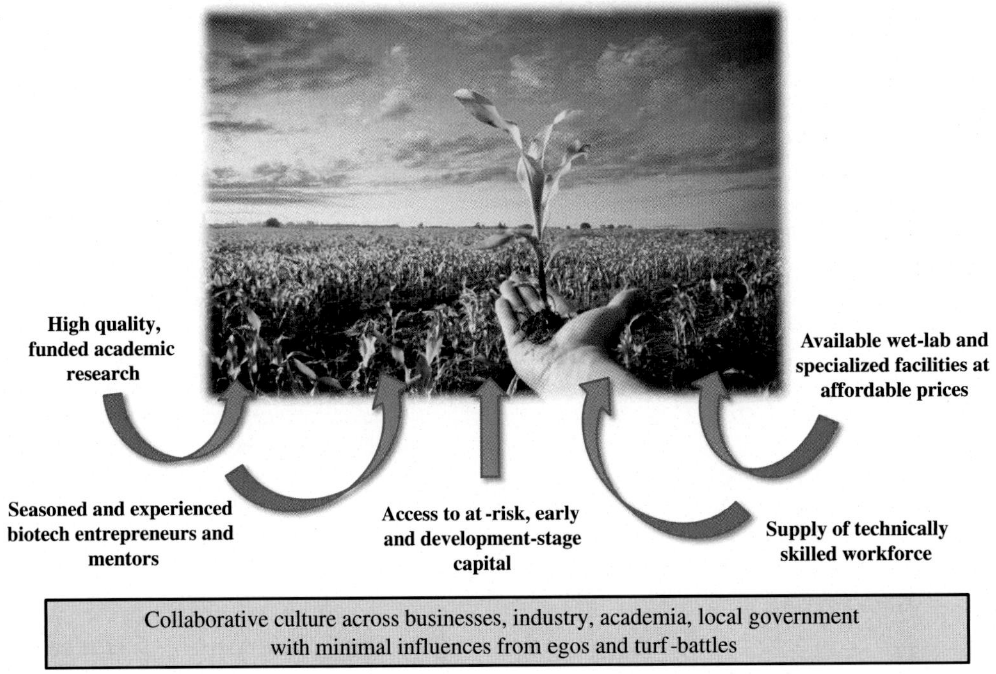

FIGURE 6.6 Five essential elements to growing biotechnology clusters.

Essential Element 1: Abundance of High Quality, Adequately Funded, Academic Research

This essential element of academic research must be plentiful, of high quality, and performed at local academic institutions by respected scientists, engineers, and physicians who are recognized as leaders in their field. Since the vast majority of all biotechnology products can trace their roots back to basic research originating at an academic institution, it is, therefore, necessary that within the planned region for a biotechnology hub, this element must be abundantly present. An abundance of high-quality academic research is the "***fertile seed***," and without seed, there will be no crop harvested. The number of companies that can grow within that region will be proportional to the amount of high-quality research conducted within that region. If the "***seed***" is insufficient in quantity or flawed in quality, a deficient or limited harvest will result. There is a direct correlation between the quality of a biotechnology company's products, and the quality of the underlying research from which it was licensed. Even though a company may still be formed from low-quality research, the underlying technology will be a detractor when trying to raise capital for product development. For the seed to be "fertile," both the research and the researcher(s) at these academic institutions must be respected in their field, be adequately funded, and have their results published in top-tier peer-reviewed scientific, medical, or industry journals. Without the abundance of high-quality seed, there will be very few biotechnology companies birthed within that region.

How is quality research assessed?

One measure of research quality is the researcher's ability to secure sufficient grant funding to support their work. This is because research grants are evaluated and awarded by peer review, then prioritized for funding by leaders in a related field, with the most innovative and competitive research typically funded. However, because of shrinking governmental budgets, *all* innovative research is not adequately funded. Still, in spite of grant funding limitations, these innovative and top-notch researchers should be successful in attracting funding, and often from multiple sources such as disease foundations, patient advocacy groups, and corporate donors. Another good measure of a region's likelihood of developing a biotechnology cluster is the amount of R&D spending within that region on a per capita basis. Fig. 6.7 shows the relative R&D spending around the world on a country basis, but the same measure can be applied to any specific geographic region.

Choosing the best product application based upon the research

Even when great research abounds, there still must be an efficient process to identify and transfer great technology opportunities from academic institutions to commercial

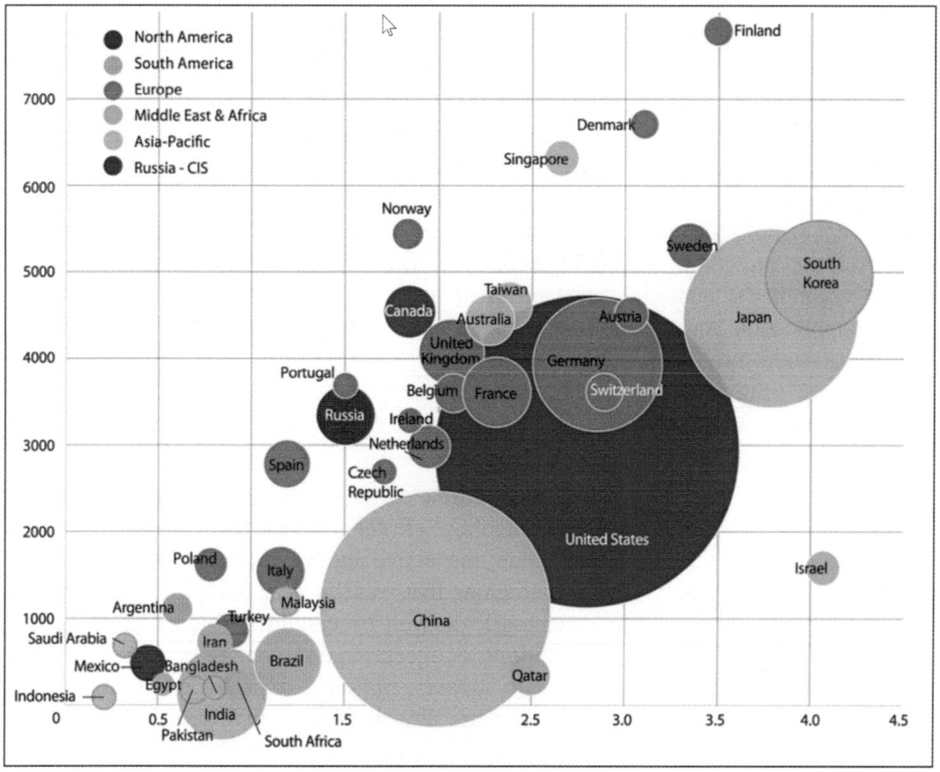

FIGURE 6.7 Summary of relative R&D spending by the indicated country. The size of the circles represents the relative amount of the country's annual R&D spending. *(Source: R&D Magazine 2017 Global R&D Funding Forecast).*

enterprises. Most of the universities and academic institutions have a technology transfer office that is charged with this objective. Within these offices, it is not uncommon for institutions to accumulate "shelves" of intellectual property and patents that are without a commercial home. On average, the number of patents that remain unlicensed at a typical university may be as high as 70%–85% of their intellectual property portfolio. In other words the majority of patented ideas do not receive a license for commercialization. I believe the reason that a large portion of these patents remain on university shelves is not because they are *not* innovative or because they are based upon poor quality science, but for three other reasons:

1. The product application that was chosen to demonstrate the underlying research or technology discovery is not of interest to potential licensees because it does not address a market need that would support commercial success.
2. The institution does not have the necessary support personnel or the incentives to adequately identify the most strategic and best opportunities or to actively solicit these to the most likely licensees.
3. The institution's academic researchers have limited interest, or minimal knowledge of the steps necessary for translational development of their basic research, or they do not know how, or want to spin-out a company on their own.

Overcoming these three challenges is not within the charter of academic institutions. However, because of shrinking educational budgets and the need to find additional sources of revenue, technology commercialization offices can play a major role in finding new sources of revenue. Academic institutions can help improve this dilemma by placing emphasis on the expansion of basic research to encompass applied or translational applications. Many academic researchers have found that by taking their existing basic research and extending experimentation toward the development of translational product concepts, they can build commercial value that attracts licensees to their technology. By incrementally advancing translational research to the next value enhancing milestone, academic institutions can realize higher values for their licenses or at least ensure that a greater percentage of their portfolio is outlicensed for future commercial applications.

For commercially minded researchers who desire to see products developed from their work, they need to understand that successful biotechnology products meet a vital need of a paying customer. When thinking about commercial applications, they should view their scientific technology as a *solution* seeking the *most acute problem* to solve. Therefore it is incumbent on the scientist or engineer to select the most critical problem having the largest market, with individuals who would gladly pay for their product or service to solve their problem. The selection of technology application is a conscious decision that is at the discretion of the researcher. This is true because most all technology concepts have diverse applications, whereas a researcher may select one particular application over another simply because they may be more familiar with it. However, from a commercial standpoint, their familiar application may be a poor market choice if it has many satisfactory products already serving that need. For example, let's say a researcher discovers a molecule that inhibits a metabolic enzyme vital for the growth of a streptococcal bacteria strain. The researcher's natural inclination may be to work on an application for the development of a new antibiotic to treat strep infections. However, unless that molecule works on drug-resistant strains of bacteria, there are already dozens of antibiotics that work effectively against strep—and inexpensively. This technology may be innovative and patentable but may never gain interest from a licensee or investor for future development. Alternatively, if that molecule could be found to inhibit other enzymes (let's hypothesize that it is a critical enzyme in the progression of Parkinson's disease), if the research was directed toward modifying that molecule and inhibiting *that* enzyme, there certainly would be licensee and investor interest in that application. Therefore, one method in which universities and academic institutions may increase their licensing opportunities is by training and informing researchers about how to evaluate commercial applications that align their technology with a real market need. This activity requires the help of individuals with both technical and business knowledge to assist in the disclosures and patent application when professors and scientists initiate filings. The earlier a technology transfer office works with researchers to teach or help guide them as they select specific applications of their discoveries, the higher the likelihood that these resulting patents and intellectual property will be licensed. For more information on bridging the technology licensing gap, see *Chapter 11, Technology Opportunities: Evaluating the Idea.*

Awareness of challenges with new discoveries

Because biotechnology products are based upon a current understanding of science at the time of discovery, occasionally our current understanding is inadequate or insufficient to optimally develop an effective biotechnology product. In other words the likelihood of success is not only the quality of the science but also how much is understood about the condition or disease at the time. For instance, when the AIDS virus (HIV) was first reported in humans in 1983, it was unclear how this virus replicated within the body and how it evaded the human immune system. Many strategies for therapeutics and vaccines failed simply because of our limited knowledge of the infectious cycle of the HIV virus, and an unclear understanding of the human immune system. However, as scientists later discovered how the virus replicated and evaded the immune system, effective therapeutics were successfully developed by many biotech and pharmaceutical companies. If a researcher desires to see their technology becoming a therapeutic application, there must be adequate knowledge available about the mechanism of the disease or condition, in order to support product development success. The better the understanding of the mechanism of a disease or condition, the more likely a therapeutic strategy will be successful when selecting a disease target.

Common goals

Leaders of municipalities who want to build and cultivate a biotechnology cluster must garner support for this goal from their respective universities and academic institutions. Regions that want to accelerate their cluster development will do well by convincing government agencies to facilitate or incentivize university technology transfer offices to support spin-out companies within their locale. Assistance can also include creative programs to improve or increase the academic and translational research quality. One noteworthy program that has run its course is Kentucky's Research Challenge Trust Fund also known as "Bucks for Brains," where they set out to recruit top talent to increase their research pool at local universities within their state. Bucks for Brains has enabled the University of Louisville to recruit and retain teams of research faculty from some of the best universities in the world.

Research at academic institutions verses commercialization at for-profit corporations

Although high-quality, adequately funded research is the fertile seed, a gap exists between the academic institutions that own them and the commercial enterprises that develop and commercialize them. The academic institutions' mission is that of gaining knowledge through basic research and teaching for the dissemination of knowledge, whereas a commercial organizations' purpose for conducting research is creating products and services to capture a financially profitable market. Between these organizations and institutions, each having different purposes, a gap must be bridged in order to increase the flow of research into commercially viable and needed products for society. To the extent that both academic and commercial organizations make concerted efforts to bridge that gap, it is to that same extent that greater numbers of biotechnology companies will be birthed within that locale.

Essential Element 2: A Ready Resource of Seasoned and Experienced Biotechnology Entrepreneurs and Mentors

Experienced management is one of the most significant factors in determining the success of start-up enterprises in *every* industry. For biotechnology companies, talented management is even more critical. Seasoned and experienced biotechnology entrepreneurs are likened to the "*farmer*" in our analogy. Experienced farmers know how to weather the storms and keep crops alive for harvest. Unfortunately, this essential element is in short supply almost everywhere, and this is one of the most critical rate-limiting essential elements in building biotechnology clusters. Biotechnology investors, particularly venture capital firms, invest in talented teams and experienced leaders who have expertise and experience within the biotechnology industry. These are individuals who can shepherd fledgling companies through the difficult growth stages in order to reach commercialization or partnering. Without an experienced biotechnology entrepreneur and talented team, there will be no company. One important characteristic of these individuals (who are entrepreneurs by desire or by necessity) is the ability to translate both science and business issues and to communicate effectively to both audiences. Some biotechnology entrepreneurs are former pharmaceutical and medical device executives with lengthy employment histories, or venture capital partners with past experience in leading start-up companies. Others are serial entrepreneurs that have started one or more biotechnology companies, or they may have served in senior roles at larger biotechnology companies. In the early days of the biotechnology industry, there were no serial entrepreneurs to lead these nascent companies. Management talent was recruited from the pharmaceutical industry, the finance industry, or they were scientists who learned by "on the job training." Interestingly, a good number of the early biotechnology leaders came from Baxter such as Ted Green, the first CEO of Hybritech, and late Henri Termeer, the former CEO of Genzyme [6].

In order to overcome the limited supply of these serial entrepreneurial leaders, many organizations within a region support an "Entrepreneur-in-Residence" program to recruit seasoned entrepreneurs who have started and exited previous biotechnology companies. The objective of such a program is that one seasoned entrepreneur leader can advise or manage multiple fledgling biotechnology companies until they gain enough intrinsic value to attract enough capital and can then hire a full-time CEO. Starting and growing a biotechnology company is not a straightforward process. There are many obstacles that line the path of would-be entrepreneurs, and it takes seasoned individuals to successfully navigate these obstacles and reach success. As the biotechnology industry continues to mature and companies birth leaders who can become future entrepreneurs, this industry will be better equipped for rapid growth and expansion.

Successful and Unsuccessful Companies will Birth Other Companies

Just as harvested crops become the seed for future crops, so do biotechnology companies give rise to seasoned entrepreneurs who then go out and start new biotechnology enterprises. Mature biotechnology companies will give rise to a fresh crop of biotechnology entrepreneurs who often start new companies in the same locale. An often-repeated scenario is where one biotechnology company grows over time, then many of the early employees leave to start new ventures within the same region. A single mature biotechnology company can become the training ground for a multitude of new entrepreneurs who often take experienced employees with them to accelerate the development of their new venture. This is principally how the San Diego biotechnology cluster was developed and expanded. In 1978 Ivor Royston, a professor at UC San Diego, and his research assistant Howard Birndorf, started Hybritech with $300,000 in seed funding. Hybritech was focused on developing monoclonal antibody diagnostic tests and gained enough momentum to go public in 1981. The company grew, and in 1985, Eli Lilly purchased Hybritech for an estimated $500 million. Unfortunately, the formal corporate structure of Eli Lilly with its policies and procedures was imposed on the informal energetic entrepreneurial culture of Hybritech and it created culture clashes. Within a year of the Eli Lilly acquisition, most of Hybritech's key talent left the company and many started new biotechnology enterprises in the San Diego area. More than 100 San Diego biotechnology companies can trace their roots back to Hybritech, such as Gensia, Gen-Probe, and IDEC. Fig. 6.8 lists a pedigree of some of these companies that trace their roots back to Hybritech. We see the same phenomena occur in other biotech clusters where the success and growth of one company breeds a large number of start-ups in the surrounding areas founded by former employees. Some serial founders also go on to be the financiers of new start-up biotechnology companies such as Ivor Royston, who became a Venture Capitalist and was an investor in many other companies in the San Diego area. This scenario is also true for Genentech in South San Francisco, where many of the biotechnology companies in the Bay Area were founded, or are run by former Genentech employees.

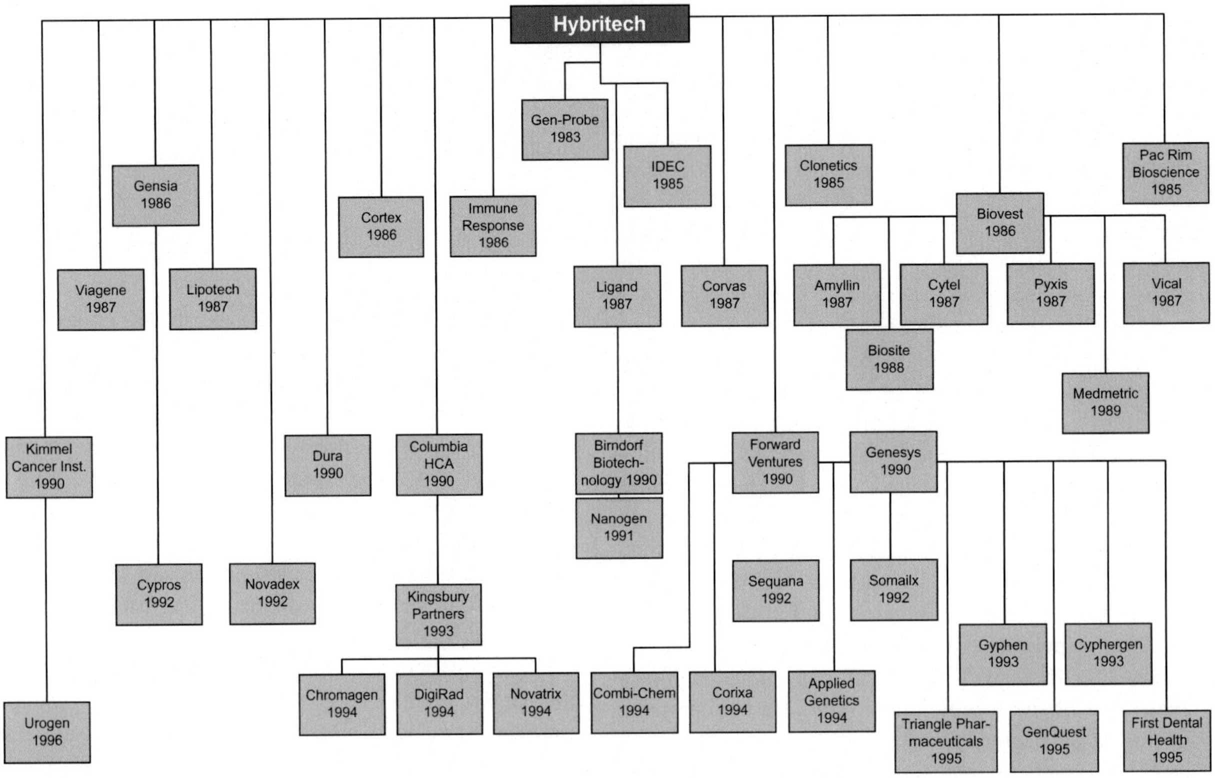

FIGURE 6.8 Companies founded by former Hybritech employees. (Begatting Chart Courtesy of UC San Diego Extension and UCSD CONNECT).

Essential Element 3: Access to Available Sources of at-risk, Early-Stage, and Development-Stage Capital Willing to Fund Start-ups

Without capital, even the best of ideas will not come to fruition. This essential element is one of the two major rate-limiting resources for the development of biotechnology clusters in any region. Capital can be likened to the "*rain*" in our analogy and is the fuel for the development of biotechnology products and services. Crops require an ample supply of water to grow, whereas the lack of rain, like capital limitations will hinder or delay product development progress and momentum, causing growth problems if funding is delayed too long. Notwithstanding, many companies simply run out of capital before they can complete product development, or they are unable to find investors soon enough before they are forced to downsize staffing. Occasionally, some funding issues have to do with poor planning on the leader's part by not understanding the length of time required to raise additional capital. However, seasoned entrepreneurs know that fundraising takes time. In other downturn situations the company may have missed an expected milestone and did not have enough capital to adjust or reposition their progress in time to find other interested investors. Apart from these situations, a major limitation for growth is the lack of early- and development-stage capital for companies within that region. It is a fact that capital is limited and there are not enough funds to support every start-up company that has a great idea. However, it is also true that many "fundable" enterprises never obtain enough funding simply because of the lack of access to capital in their geographical region.

In order for a biotechnology cluster to develop, it is not just capital in general that is needed, but a *continuum* of investment capital, which is capital directed to each of the different stages of growth for biotech companies.

Early/Seed Stage—Risk Capital Needed

Early-stage "risk" capital is generally considered grant funding, local government economic programs, angel investors and angel networks, and high-net worth individuals. A fledgling company needs access to risk capital to support their endeavors until significant valuation is realized. Various regions have implemented state or local funding programs to help fill this gap. Some programs are directed specifically toward life science or high-technology companies within their geographic region. Different financing mechanisms have been created by local governments, such as high-risk "loans," which are paid back (at a high premium) only if the company is successful, whereas if not, there is no further obligation. Other financing mechanisms include innovation grant awards that must be matched by private capital, thus incentivizing private investors to participate in the early-stage venture. Municipalities are also creating technology-commercialization centers to support their financing programs to add value with guidance, management, and board oversight for these young start-up companies. There are numerous ways that a regional government or municipality can support an early-stage biotechnology company's access to risk capital in their locale. The most important aspect is all of these sources must be readily accessible and directed toward early-stage financing of these innovative companies in order for a biotechnology cluster to be fostered. Many investors, particularly early angel investors, invest in companies in their local region, and some states and locales are supporting or creating independent angel networks, which are a group of angels that collectively meet together and evaluate a number of potential investment opportunities that are in or around their region. For more information about Angels and Angel Networks see *Chapter 19: Securing Angel Capital and Understanding How Angel Networks Operate*.

Needed Follow-On Capital during Development Stages

As discussed in *Chapter 17, Sources of Capital and Investor Motivations*, different investor groups have investing preferences for different stages of company development. Without a continuum of risk capital for companies within a locale, it is difficult to sustain a viable biotechnology hub. For instance, if a region has early-stage angel investors but little or no institutional investors or venture capital, companies may be started, but few will make it beyond the early stages of development. Without follow-on development-stage capital, what often happens is that the best organically funded companies relocate to other regions where access to capital is greater, or new funding is contingent on the company moving to that investor's locale.

Development-stage capital requires larger commitments of money than early-stage capital. Whereas early-stage/seed capital for a biotechnology company can be as little as $250,000–$750,000, during subsequent development stages, companies may require $3–$5 million in capital for a next round. Often this amount of money is too large for angel investors and may be too small, and too early, for large venture capital firms that manage $200–$500 million or more. However, there are a few development-stage friendly venture capital firms that do invest at these stages, but they are not as plentiful. In order to fill this development-stage funding gap, some local government agencies have allocated a portion of their funds toward development-stage companies, with private investor matching requirements. Depending on the fund size, these local government agencies have become "super angels" and can lead a funding round with a large group of individual angels matching the investment.

Regions that have the greatest access to innovation capital (early-stage) and development-stage (venture-type) capital are the regions that experience the greatest growth in their biotechnology cluster development. Fig. 6.9 shows regions in the United States with the most innovation capital and venture capital raised.

Essential Element 4: Adequate Supply of Technically Skilled Workforce Experienced in the Biotechnology Field

Start-up and development-stage biotechnology companies require *skilled and experienced teams of people* to develop their products. This essential element may be likened to "*fertilizer*" and comprises employees with specialized skill sets having the requisite expertise necessary to support the development of the company technology. Crops may grow sparsely without fertilizer, but in order to flourish they require ample fertilizer. A source of individuals with expertise in a specialized technology is required because these individuals are the ones who must overcome technical problems during the development of a product. Fledgling biotechnology companies require these types of skilled team members as they cannot afford to spend lots of time on lengthy on-the-job training. Each team member added to the start-up company must contribute in ways that are not limited by someone having to train them. Each new member becomes the growing critical mass of expertise that must help advance the technology into a developed product. Because biotechnology can become so specialized in any particular sector, it is very difficult for a single region to have an experienced workforce that spans expertise in all sectors of the biotechnology industry. This is one reason why many biotechnology clusters naturally develop a sector focus due to the workforce expertise located within that region. This workforce specialization phenomenon is evident in all industries, not just the biotechnology industry. For instance, auto manufacturing was originally clustered within the Detroit region of the United States, in part due to the high concentration of experienced autoworkers, whereas oil and gas clusters are strong in the Texas and Oklahoma regions. Having a supply of technically skilled workers is one reason that the existing biotechnology hubs of Boston and San Francisco continue to experience the rapid formation of new biotech companies. Such industry specialty focus

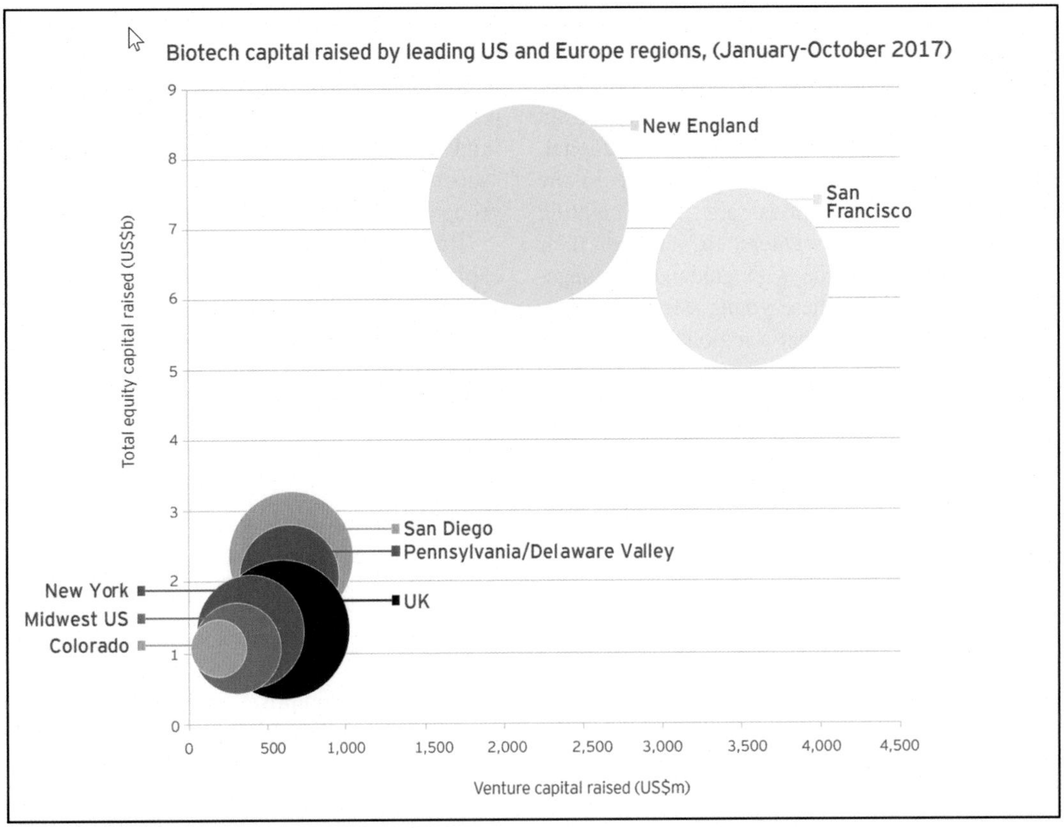

FIGURE 6.9 Capital raised by leading US regions, January to October 2017. Size of bubbles shows relative number of financings per region. Total capital excludes debt. *BMO Capital Markets, S&P Capital IQ, Dow Jones VentureSource, EY analysis in EY 2018 M&A Firepower Report: Life Sciences Deals and Data.*

is attractive for recruiting other individuals with the same skills because they know that if necessary, they can change jobs without ever changing zip codes.

Essential Element 5: Adequate and Dedicated Wet-Laboratory and Facilities at Affordable Rates

Biotechnology product development is highly specialized which requires specialized facilities and resources to service their product development needs. Adequate facilities are analogous to "*rich soil*" required for growing crops, and is essential to fledgling biotechnology companies, allowing them to efficiently conduct research and development, and prototype testing. Inadequate facilities hinder product development and makes a difficult product development timeline even more challenging. Many regional municipalities and academic institutions are addressing the facility needs of start-up companies in creative ways. Most frequently, this is accomplished through the creation of "incubators" which are often coupled with other resources. Incubators can assist young companies with the needed facilities and support to prove their scientific concepts or build working prototypes. The term *incubator* has been used to describe various types of facilities, but all incubators are not created equal. Some incubators provide subsidized rent along with support systems and personnel for a small fee. Other incubators are simply high-tech laboratory and office space at standard rates that are built and conveniently housed adjacent to an academic institution or university center. Ideally, an incubator program would be designed to support entrepreneurial companies by offering supportive resources and some assistance with nontechnical activities. In some cases, these programs can be bundled to provide access to seed funding. Incubator programs are usually region specific and have a mission to support local high-tech companies moving into their space for a period of time. Types of support can include nominal costs for access to common, but expensive equipment or usage of resources such as animal facilities. These types of support programs help start-up companies accelerate product testing to reach a value-enhancing milestone that increases the likelihood of more significant funding.

Many universities have built their own dedicated life science incubator facilities to support university spin-offs and give preference to serve their faculty or companies licensing their technology. In 1995 the University of Florida launched the Sid Martin Biotechnology Incubator with 40,000 square feet of labs, vivariums, greenhouses, fermentation facilities, and $1 million of shared scientific equipment and business-development services. In 2013 they were ranked the "World's Best University Biotechnology Incubator," based on an international study conducted by the Swedish-based research group, University Business Incubator. Other university-based incubator programs include the Harvard Innovation Lab, a 33,000 square-feet facility that includes all the Harvard schools, stimulating a cross-pollination of ideas, including biotechnology. For about a decade the University of Manchester in the United Kingdom has incubated start-up life science companies in its University of Manchester Innovation Center incubator building. At present, their state-of-the-art biotechnology R&D center includes over 86,000 square feet of bioscience incubator and related support facilities and includes turnkey laboratory suites with access to containment level 2 laboratories.

Irrespective of whether incubators are university or regional government-created and managed, biotech start-ups require specialized facilities and the supportive resources that these programs offer. For most regions, this essential element is one that can be easily remedied and should be a high priority, and not become a limiting factor. Creating incubators and support systems for these fledgling companies does require a large one-time capital commitment, with supplemental capital to offset the building and maintenance expenses until the incubator is fully occupied and profitable or at minimum breakeven.

Important Considerations

In our analogy, we likened the "***fertile seed***" to high quality, adequately funded, academic research. We likened the "***farmer***" to seasoned and experienced entrepreneurs. The more experienced the farmer is, the better they are at weathering the storms to protect the crops and nurture them to grow. Another important support group for the entrepreneur are experienced mentors. These individuals are essential to counsel and guide the entrepreneur along the way. *Chapter 9: "Mentorship: Why You Need a Team of Mentors to be Successful"* has more helpful information about this subject. In our analogy, we likened the "***rain***" to at-risk, early-stage, and development-stage capital. We likened the "***fertilizer***" to a supply of technically-skilled workforce experienced in the biotechnology field, and we likened the "***rich soil***" to dedicated wet-laboratory and facilities at affordable rates. In the same manner, these elements are essential for establishing, growing and expanding a bumper crop of successful biotech companies, which in turn, are needed to establish, grow and expand a biotechnology cluster or hub.

Another important principle to recognize is that an abundance of one essential element does not compensate for the lack of another. Often, there is a belief that a municipality or local government can simply provide more of an existing resource to overcome their cluster growth limitations. However, this is not the case for the establishment of biotechnology clusters. For example, specialized facilities and laboratories are essential to support biotechnology throughout the lengthy development process. However, providing an overabundance of state-of-the-art facilities, although they are needed, will not compensate for a lack of seasoned entrepreneurs with experience in starting and growing companies. All *five* of these essential elements must be present in sufficient quantities in order for a biotechnology cluster to take root and flourish.

Another important point to recognize is that there is a difference between "Convenience Elements," which are good, and "Essential Elements" which are *vital* to biotechnology cluster development. If a local government focuses a majority of its efforts on developing "nice-to-have" amenities but does not first focus on missing or limited essential elements, biotechnology cluster formation or expansion will not occur. For instance, focusing first on accessible airport transportation in and out of the local region without first dealing with the hindrances and limitations for universities to out-license technology to local companies will have limited impact on cluster development. Some companies may indeed enjoy those additional conveniences, but by themselves these conveniences do not result in an expansion of a biotechnology cluster if hindrances to essential elements remain in that locale.

Other Enhancers of Biotechnology Cluster Development

There are various enhancers of cluster development but remember that these are distinct from the essential elements. We will discuss two of them, which include

- having a risk-taking culture and
- having a collaborative spirit within the community.

"Enhancers" of biotechnology cluster development require something to enhance, so if the essential elements are not present, no enhancer will help with the development of a biotechnology cluster. Enhancers are certainly beneficial to the community and they help stimulate the attractiveness of that region; however, biotechnology clusters are unique in their requirements for establishing and flourishing. This, in fact, is what makes them more challenging to grow. Moreover, these two mentioned enhancers are not easily imported but rather are often characteristics inherent in the people living within a particular geographic location. As a region experiences biotech industry expansion, these enhancers may be self-generated or perpetuated concurrent with, or by, the growth of that cluster.

Risk-Taking Entrepreneurial Culture

Regions that have cultures of entrepreneurship and risk-taking are more successful than those without one. For any major work to be accomplished, there must be a champion and a team of people who believe in the vision. The development of a biotechnology cluster is no different. It requires that many groups buy into this vision. A key enhancer that is either present or absent in the local region is an innovative and entrepreneurial culture. This is an attribute that is characterized by the people located in that region. Risk-taking cultures are those that are not afraid to apply capital toward valuable, risk-based projects. In the state of Oklahoma, the city of Tulsa was once known as the "Oil Capital of the World," and there were many risk-takers living in the state. This risk-taking culture was prevalent throughout the majority of the state, and as a result, Oklahoma City built a large Health Sciences Center with a major Life Science Research Park, having approximately 1 million square feet of class A wet-labs and office space. When a population of people invest large sums of money to dig holes in the ground with hopes of striking oil, that risk-taking culture can certainly spill over into other industries within their region. As a result, Oklahoma City has frequently been named as one of the top places to start a business. Entrepreneurship is contagious.

Collegiality and Collaborative Spirit

In addition to a risk-taking culture, there must be an environment of collaboration within that region. Establishing and growing a new industry requires the support of organizations and teams of diverse individuals all cooperating together to achieve a common goal. Without a culture of collaboration, cross-discipline differences and conflicts can stall forward momentum and inhibit growth of a biotechnology cluster. If other industries within that region feel threatened by the focus or expansion of the biotechnology industry, there may be challenges to establishing a cluster. To avoid this, leaders should clearly and frequently communicate the collateral benefit to all stakeholders about the benefits of growing a biotechnology cluster within their region.

Maintenance Factors Versus Drivers

Municipalities may be able to tout their climate as one of the best in the world. They may also be able to point out that their region has one of the lowest cost-of-living indexes in the United States. These can be likened to "maintenance factors" for growing biotechnology clusters because they are supportive and helpful, but they are not drivers of cluster development. If these maintenance factors were effectors rather than supportive, Boston's cold winter weather and high cost-of-living would drive away every biotechnology company there. In fact, biotechnology companies still flock to regions where the winter weather is bitter and the cost-of-living is astronomical, as long as the five essential elements are in adequate supply in that region. Weather, cost-of-living, and transportation are truly supportive and helpful, but it is important to remember that they are not the drivers and effectors of biotechnology cluster development. That is not to say these maintenance factors do not need to be touted and even improved where humanly possible, but a region needs to be keenly focused on touting and enhancing each of the five essential elements that truly drive the development of biotechnology clusters in any given region.

Inhibitors of Biotechnology Cluster Growth

Just as there are facilitators of biotechnology cluster development, there can be inhibitors of development also. These inhibitors can be qualitative or quantitative factors, people, or policies. Inhibitors of biotechnology cluster development may include such things as high taxes on a small business for incorporation in a particular region and corporate laws that apply equally to large corporations and small businesses without consideration. Inhibitors may also be other industries competing for the same government dollars or for special attention. It is important that the leaders of cluster development identify these inhibitors and work to remove or mitigate them while focusing on the missing or limited essential elements within their region.

The Role of Government in Developing Biotechnology Clusters

Government must play a role in the development of biotechnology industry clusters. Traditionally, the ways they have participated has been in economic stimulation, financing, and incentives for companies and industries. Governments can stimulate private investments in biotechnology companies by providing investment tax credits for qualified investments in life science companies.

Government can also provide research tax credits for research-based companies in incubators, which help reduce the capital required for the research and development of their products. Other government initiatives can include matching of private investments or the matching of federal grants, such as Small Business Innovation Research (SBIR) and Small Business Technology Transfer, for start-up biotechnology companies. Municipal and civic leaders can assist by starting or supporting biotechnology focused industry trade associations. Federal governments can help by enacting supportive public policies that encourage biotechnology growth and expansion in all regions, such as the Bayh–Dole Act did in the United States and the SBIR grant program. Because the federal government funds a portion of public university's budget, they should also include or allocate incentives for university technology transfer offices that facilitate the creation and start-up of new companies using university-developed technology. Governments can also support or contribute to the development of incubators associated with universities or geographic regions.

Many state governments have undertaken initiatives to create biotechnology clusters. Florida is an example of a state seeking to diversify its industrial base by the wholesale development of a biotechnology hub within their state. They began a program of recruiting top-notch research institutions focused on life sciences and biotechnology. With a fund of $449 million, they recruited the Scripps Research Institute and the Sanford-Burnham Medical Research Institute to expand to their state. With matching local government money, they created a pool of $950 million for the development of a biotechnology hub. By 2006, Florida moved into the top 10 ranking of biotechnology business centers as determined by Ernst & Young's Global Biotechnology Report. Although Florida has had success, government by itself will not be successful in initiating and stimulating biotechnology hub development alone. The government must be a contributor and supporter of some of these essential elements but success requires that all stakeholders participate collectively.

Where do you to Start if you Desire to Build a Biotechnology Cluster?

For regional governments, municipalities, and chambers of commerce that desire to stimulate the growth of a biotechnology cluster in their region, there are discrete steps that can be taken to improve and increase the likelihood of that occurring. There is much detail to each of these steps, and I have outlined four key steps as a means to illustrate a starting point for a governmental or regional entity that has the vision and desire to build a biotechnology hub in their area. By following these steps, cities and municipalities can begin the process of establishing a long-term plan to grow a biotechnology cluster in their region.

Four Major Steps for Developing a Strategy to Grow a Biotechnology Cluster in your Region

1. ***Assess the five essential elements in your local region:*** The first step is to objectively assess the presence or absence, and the quality and strength of the five essential elements within your local region. In Fig. 6.10, I have outlined an example of a worksheet summary assessment to help initially rank your region in each of these five categories. This is only a summary of an assessment, whereas you will need a much greater detailed worksheet to accurately produce a summary assessment such as this. Within each category, you will have ranked your region on a 1–5 scale, where 1 is minimal or poor quality, and 5 is outstanding quality and strength. The ranking scale is a comparison to the best-established biotechnology clusters which may be near you or in other countries. Be aware that when comparing your situation to an established biotechnology hub in another country, there may be confounding factors that you cannot affect due to different norms. However, you have an opportunity to create an identity that is uniquely suited for your locale.
2. ***Develop a detailed gap analysis for your biotech hub:*** Next, a gap analysis should be conducted, and the key shortcomings should be listed for each essential element. Comprehensively list the major roadblocks and inhibitors of each element. Be aware that sometimes the roadblocks to an essential element may be clear, but there may be hidden inhibitors of those essential elements that are not obvious. The best way to uncover these hidden inhibitors is to interview many of the small biotech companies that are in your area and also those that have left your area, *and* especially those that are no longer in business. During these interviews, you will be surprised to learn many things you were not aware of which have impacted the growth and expansion of these fledgling companies. Be sure that you are identifying the real bottlenecks because you do not want to address a symptom, only to discover the real rate-limiting factor was not identified nor addressed. This is a very important point, as the action plan that will result from this exercise may be addressing something that does not really improve the essential element you desire.
3. ***Establish a written and prioritized action plan:*** Once the gaps and inhibitors are identified, verified, and well-understood, develop a prioritized plan with

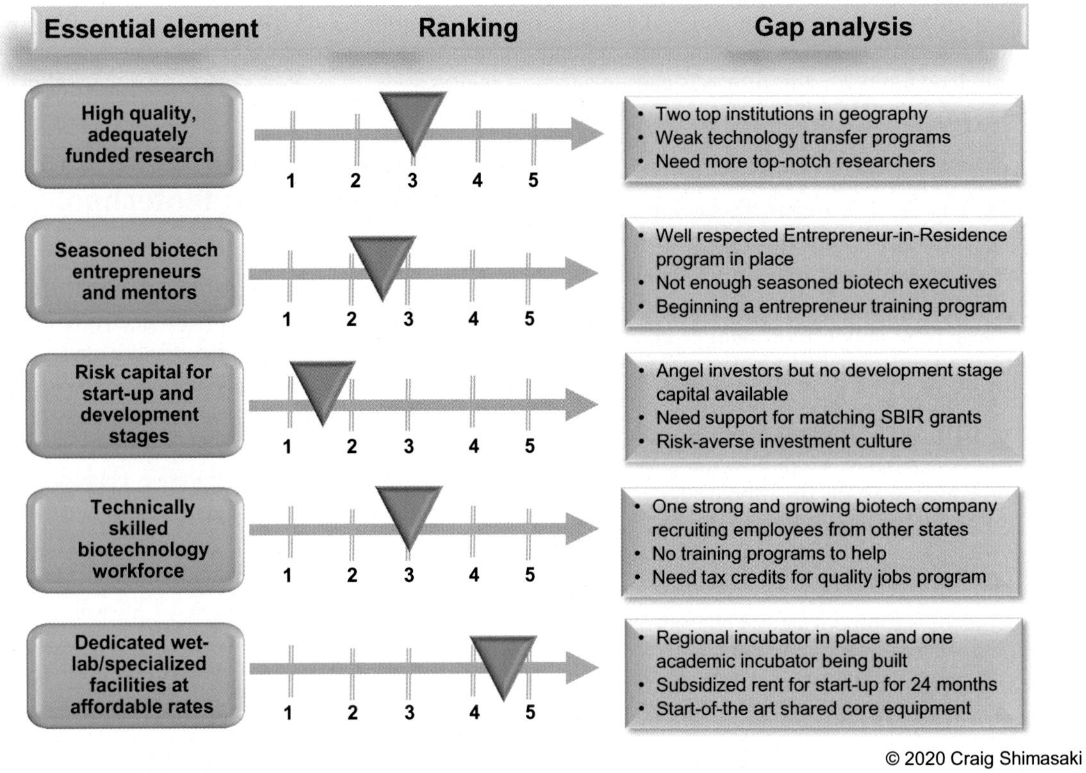

FIGURE 6.10 Example of a summary assessment of the five essential elements when building a biotech cluster.

creative solutions arrived by joint meetings among government officials, civic and community leaders, and the private sector in order to address these limitations. For any essential element that ranks a 3 or below, this should be a high priority and focus. In addition, many regions are implementing creative programs to address their cluster development limitations, and these best practices can be evaluated to help solidify the correct action plan that has some history of success or failure. Do not adopt and utilize a plan that was created by another region without first assessing your unique hindrances and limitations to biotechnology cluster development. Your region's limitations to these five essential elements can often be vastly different from another region's limitations, and your solutions should be directly tailored to your region's situation.

4. ***Agreement and ownership for stakeholder responsibilities:*** Once these strategic and specific solutions are identified for your region, create a timeline and jointly assign responsibilities to each stakeholder, with a time interval to report back with progress and improvements can be objectively measured. Remember that the stakeholders must include the local government leaders, civic leaders, industry heads, influencers in the community, and many of the biotech companies in your area. The various assignments and responsibilities must be agreed to by each stakeholder responsible for executing them. Recognize that your region's action plan will have different priorities and will likely focus on different limitations than another region. Be sure to set up reoccurring meetings with all key stakeholders to share progress and roadblocks to completion, such that these teams can assist each other in accomplishing their key goals.

Summary

The process of building a biotechnology cluster or hub within a geography can be tremendously rewarding and economically successful for the local region and for diversification of the local economy. Biotechnology jobs are high paying and employ a highly skilled workforce, and the biotech industry tends to be a clean industry. Companies that are organically started and established in a region tend to stay in their local region if these essential elements are present. As these companies grow, their employee base expands, and because they utilize local services, their impact on the local economy grows. In order for a biotechnology hub to successfully be established in a new location, the local government, academic institutions, industry, and civic leaders must share a vision for innovation and have a commitment for risk-taking in order for a sustainable biotechnology cluster to come to fruition. When each of these stakeholders are in the same proverbial "boat," rowing in the same direction, synergy will occur. Growing a biotechnology cluster in a new, or relatively new region should be viewed as a long-term growth plan and perceived in the same manner as a farmer views growing crops, except that it is a biotechnology cluster crop and must be measured in decades, rather than in seasons.

There are plenty of examples where regions have succeeded in growing and expanding their biotechnology cluster, such as in San Diego, Washington DC, Seattle, and Raleigh-Durham. Outside of the United States, there are good examples of biotechnology hubs emerging in Cambridge, United Kingdom; Berlin-Brandenburg, Munich; and more recently China. The recipe for growth in each of these regions is to ensure that all of these five essential elements are present in quality and breadth. Realize that there is no "one" essential element more important than the others, and in order to grow a thriving biotechnology hub, you need all five factors together. Others may point to additional elements and deem them "essential" but in some way, they may be iterations of these five. One thing is certain that without these five essential elements in abundant supply, regional growth of any biotechnology cluster will be limited, and likely declining. Recognize that biotechnology cluster development in new regions can take many years, possibly decades, so this is not necessarily a quick-fix program. However, by consistently focusing on targeted development of each of these elements, cluster development will eventually manifest and become self-perpetuating.

It is true that many early-stage biotechnology companies will fail, but business failure is normal in any industry and the employees of these companies tend to stay in the region. When these five essential elements are present, often some of these employees will start new companies that become successful. It is proven that regions which succeed in developing a sustainable biotechnology cluster reap dividends in their economy, in job creation, in diversification of an industrial base, and, more importantly, create products that improve the quality of life for millions. It takes much time and a sustained effort to see significant cluster development in a region that previously has been sparse in biotechnology. However, it can be done, and will be done by those with the fortitude, strategic leadership, and financial commitment to do so. Like any endeavor, success follows leadership that understands how to guide a team of people toward a big vision. Growing biotechnology clusters requires risk-taking and pioneering individuals. These individuals are the visionaries and drivers of future biotechnology expansion throughout the world. If your region has the motivation to undertake this type of visionary transformation to establish a biotechnology hub but does not know where to begin, you may contact me at cs@biosourceconsulting.com for some suggestions. Best wishes to you for your future biotech cluster success.

References

[1] 2018 Jones Lang LaSalle research report, life sciences outlook. <https://www.us.jll.com/content/dam/jll-com/documents/pdf/research/americas/us/US-Life-Sciences-Outlook-2018-JLL.pdf> (accessed February 8, 2019).

[2] GEN 2018 "Top 10 European biotech clusters". <https://www.genengnews.com/a-lists/top-10-european-biopharma-clusters-5/> (assessed February 8, 2019).

[3] GEN 2018 "Top 10 Asian biotech cluster", <https://www.genengnews.com/a-lists/top-10-asia-biopharma-clusters-2018/> (assessed February 8, 2019).

[4] Obama administration. National Bioeconomy Blueprint. p. 1., April 2012. <https://obamawhitehouse.archives.gov/sites/default/files/microsites/ostp/national_bioeconomy_blueprint_april_2012.pdf> (accessed February 8, 2019).

[5] Report: investment, innovation and job creation in a growing U.S. bioscience industry 2018 TEConomy/BIO. <https://www.bio.org/sites/default/files/TEConomy_BIO_2018_Report.pdf> (accessed February 8, 2019).

[6] Higgins M. Career imprints: creating leaders across an industry. Harvard Business School, Jossey-Bass, 2005.

Section III

The Human Capital Component

Chapter 7

Building, Managing, and Motivating Great Teams

Arthur A. Boni, PhD[1], Gergana Todorova, PhD[2] and Laurie R. Weingart, PhD[3]

[1]*John R. Thorne Distinguished Career Professor of Entrepreneurship, Emeritus, Tepper School of Business at Carnegie Mellon University, Pittsburgh, PA, United States,* [2]*Mihaylo College of Business and Economics, California State University, Fullerton, CA, United States,* [3]*Richard M. and Margaret S. Cyert Professor of Organizational Behavior and Theory, Tepper School of Business at Carnegie Mellon University, Pittsburgh, PA, United States*

Chapter Outline

This chapter focuses on the essentials of building and growing effective, diverse, collaborative, team-based organizations that are capable of creating both disruptive and sustained innovations in the biotechnology industry. Entrepreneurs and innovators, who found, build, and grow knowledge-based organizations that are technologically driven, must be market-focused. Although the technology is very important for the solution and may in fact define the company, it is the caliber and experience of the team that will determine whether or not the company is successful. Therefore it is critical for the entrepreneur to focus on developing collaborative teams with diverse skill sets and areas of expertise. We specifically focus on biotechnology organizations, but our approach is pertinent to most technology-driven businesses. The entrepreneurs pursuing opportunities in the biotechnology and biomedical fields are faced with special constraints that must be addressed by the leadership team and network partners. Biotechnology organizations are characterized by long industry life cycles and time to market. Moreover, they are highly capital and risk intensive, are regulated by a set of complex and changing government systems, and are constrained in their profitability due to reimbursement from third parties. These issues compound and confound the entrepreneurial challenges of any start-up. In any start-up organization, the founding team is challenged to reduce risk—technology, market, team, and business model. Due to this, we advocate building an interdisciplinary, collaborative team that can manage and balance the science with the business issues, while including the capacity to interact effectively with partners, investors, and a multitude of service providers to successfully commercialize and validate their business model.

Equally important are the following two issues that are related to any knowledge-based, human-intensive business. The first issue of importance is building and growing an entrepreneurial culture. The second and closely related issue is incorporating mechanisms to continually motivate the highly creative talent at the core of the enterprise. We present a framework for motivation that includes *ownership*, defined to include both *equity participation* for potential capital gain, and also *psychological ownership* of the direction and future of the organization itself. The culture created and nurtured by the founders and early employees and their investors evolves organically and guides the company through the changes

Biotechnology Entrepreneurship. DOI: https://doi.org/10.1016/B978-0-12-815585-1.00007-3

in team composition due to the diversity of challenges that occur across the company life cycle. The entrance and exodus of key personnel as the organization grows through its life cycle are the challenges the leadership team must address proactively.

In this chapter, we identify and discuss the principles and best practices for building entrepreneurial companies from two perspectives: (1) "experiential learning," and (2) "academic learning." Our perspective thus blends real-world lessons from building and growing early stage companies but filtered through and framed by a more scholarly approach based on case literature and research-based studies.

This balanced "theory and practice" of building a biotechnology company is framed to emphasize the entire company life cycle—start-up, development stage, clinical stage, market entry, growth, and exit. We want to begin with a description of the entrepreneurial process and note the importance of high-performance teams in building and growing the organization. We want to stress that an effective organization incorporates as a foundation, building and growing a culture that encourages and rewards collaborative interdisciplinary teams for their contributions to the success of the venture. The principles outlined are applicable to "fully integrated emerging and maturing companies" as well as to those organizations that employ "open-innovation" business models that are businesses that rely on partnering for outsourcing and developing new products and services, and for bringing them to market. We want to outline, from an academic and experiential perspective, those fundamental issues that must be addressed when building teams such as tasks to be performed, people/skills required, norms, and processes. We also include a "lessons learned" summary based on interviews and experiences with numerous early stage teams and their investors. This summary incorporates the principles that guide team formation, management, and motivation. In particular, how do you find, hire, and motivate teams that are effective or ineffective in the biopharmaceutical industry?

Fundamentals of Entrepreneurial Process Related to Teams

Building an entrepreneurial team for a biotechnology company incorporates a daunting set of challenges and tasks. We frame the *entrepreneurial process* on the following three components (as described by Timmons [1]):

1. Identifying the *opportunity* and developing a strategy capable of creating sustained and differentiated competitive advantage.
2. Acquiring the *resources* needed to develop the opportunity, thereby developing, creating, and capturing value in the marketplace, for example, financing and partnerships for market access (channels) and customer relations.
3. Building the *team* needed to exploit the opportunity. In science-based companies, teams must include people with expertise in science/technology, in business, and in other related "tasks," for example, product development, laboratory and clinical testing, and intellectual property (IP) development.

In addition, and most importantly, great *leadership* is essential to continually balance the opportunity with the resources and the team needed to exploit it. The entrepreneurial leadership team needs to evolve throughout the entrepreneurial process, continuously and seamlessly as the organization engages in the innovation process—inspiration, ideation, and implementation—and evolves through the company life cycle stages of start-up, development, clinical testing, and market introduction/growth. Another essential responsibility of the leadership team is to create the appropriate culture consistent with the vision and mantra and to maintain that culture through growth and "turbulence" expected during company development; for example, both internal and external factors must be managed.

Entrepreneurial leadership should not be viewed as a top-down vertical influence process but instead is seen to be a horizontal influence process shared among team members. Shared leadership is reflected by how much leadership influence and initiative are displayed by individual team members [2], and it is "an emergent and dynamic team phenomenon whereby leadership roles and influence are distributed among team members" [3]. In a recent study of start-ups, involving 166 creators and managers of new innovative businesses, Krieger showed that only 12% of start-ups are run with just one person making all of the strategic decisions, whereas in 72% of cases, these decisions are made by two or three partners [4]. Thus most of the leadership decisions and functions are often shared by entrepreneurial teams. Research demonstrates that shared leadership enhances team performance, and it is especially important for diverse entrepreneurial teams that incorporate "associative thinking" as an important component of the innovation culture. The distribution of leadership responsibilities and influence among multiple team members stimulates the sharing and elaboration of diverse information among those with different expertise and experiences (Fig. 7.1).

An important component of a strong leadership team is the presence, guidance, and mentoring provided by external parties such as advisors and the board of directors (BOD). It is essential that the founders and key management team members and their advisors create a vision that establishes the culture and strives to grow and maintain that culture. All organizations grow and adapt as continuing challenges are faced, handled, and new ones arise.

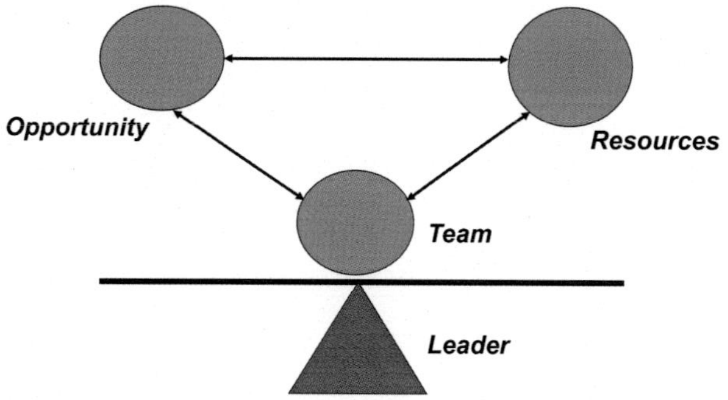

FIGURE 7.1 The entrepreneurial process model. *Adapted from Timmons JA, Stephen S. New venture creation, entrepreneurship for the 21st century. 7th ed. McGraw Hill Irwin; 2007.*

The competitive landscape, the financing environment, the regulatory environment, and the human motivations and ambitions are but a few of the variables that must be dealt with effectively and in a timely manner.

A key objective for the founders of the start-up organization is to create significant, differentiable, and sustainable value through the underlying technology. The entrepreneurial team is charged with the development of the business model to deliver the product or offering, and its inherent value to the marketplace, while returning shared value in the form of wealth and return on investment for the innovators, entrepreneurs, investors, and partners. We, as others, would argue that the team composition, incorporating the skills, wills, and fit, and leadership in new ventures are perhaps the most important determinants of the ultimate success of the venture. The entrepreneurial team must be developed with the ability to function as a successful leadership team in the entrepreneurial context of a high-risk competitive environment, dealing with complex incentive and financial structures.

Additional team-building challenges for entrepreneurs and innovators are emerging as a result of pressures in the pharmaceutical space such as diminishing product pipelines, regulatory failures, and the lack of capital availability. Therefore in today's economy, there is a recognition that the start-up team would be well served to utilize "open-innovation" approaches to leverage expertise, to gain the needed skills, and to commercialize complex technologies while preserving capital to ensure good returns on investment for all constituencies. An important corollary is that it is also important to ensure that rewards are apportioned to those who create value and who assume risk, that is, entrepreneurs and investors as well as partners and employees. We hypothesize that entrepreneurs and their organizational team members are more highly motivated by ownership that includes both psychological factors, such as the ability to influence the direction of "their firms," as well as financial factors via equity ownership.

Given the challenges to innovate, the industry is beginning to see a trend toward creation of more "virtual companies" (an "extreme" version of "open innovation") whereby a *small but highly experienced core team leverages the expertise and resources of an extended network of partners, collaborators, and resources.* Successful firms are increasingly reliant on open innovation, which involves interactions with outside agents such as investors, partners, customers, and experts to obtain ideas, technologies, expertise, and access to market channels. Accordingly, entrepreneurial firms may be nested or embedded within multiple external networks with different structures and flows of capital (human and financial) and services. Research on teams and innovation uses the term "boundary-spanning activities" to denote the interactions of team members with external agents including all activities of team members related to the flows of resources between the team and external agents. We illustrate some of these principles in a mini-case study later in the chapter.

A Kauffman Foundation study focused on collaboration surveyed firms in the first 4 years of their operations from 2004 to 2007 [5]. The authors reported that 25% of competitive advantage is attributed to collaboration with another firm, and 8% of competitive advantage was due to collaboration with a government laboratory or with universities, respectively. We would expect these numbers to be even higher in biotechnology (and in other industries with long, capital intensive commercialization pathways). While the Kauffman study [2] and other work discuss the trend toward the development and adoption of open-innovation business models, the literature does not discuss in any detail the motivation of entrepreneurial teams/firms to leverage and share expertise and capital returns within these networked models of innovation. The open-innovation framework [6,7] suggests that technology companies adopt a networked approach to high-performance innovation sustainably and efficiently—so that companies exchange ideas, information, and technologies and bring new products to market through alliances and other forms of interfirm collaborations. While ecosystems of shared values enhance innovation [8,9], these distributed or networked organizations are expected to add to the complexity of the team challenges involved (Fig. 7.2).

We have taken a team design perspective in our search for a better understanding of the interactions of entrepreneurial firms at both the firm level and extending to include interactions with external agents (i.e., boundary-spanning activities in networks). We have sought to better understand the motivational nature of teams and collaborations to highlight the internal and external predictors of success of entrepreneurial firms.

The Importance of Building and Maintaining an Entrepreneurial Culture

The onset of company formation starts with the vision of the founders and the articulation of the culture that they

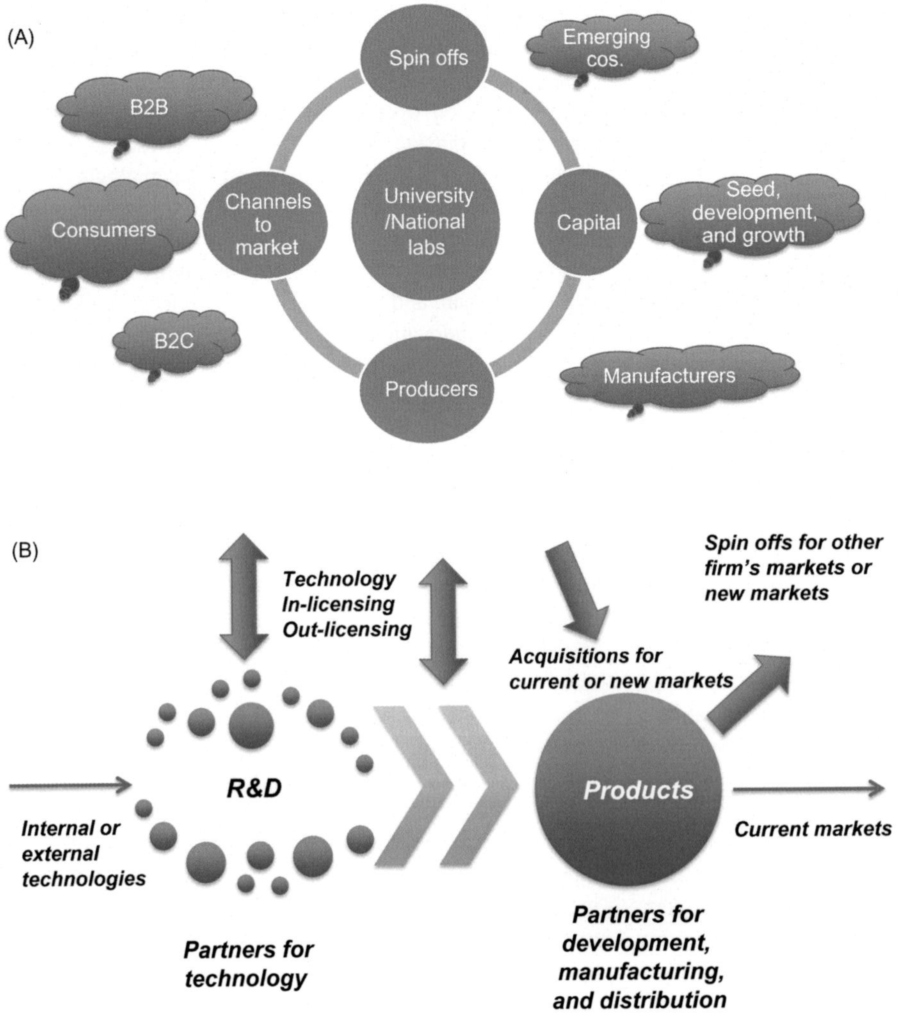

FIGURE 7.2 (A) The science-based innovation ecosystem and (B) an open-innovation network for sustained and disruptive innovation. *Adapted from Chesbrough H, Vanhaverbeke W, West J, editors. Open innovation: researching a new paradigm. Cambridge, MA: Harvard University Press; 2006.*

want to build into the "DNA" of the start-up organization. The goal is to build and then sustain that vision and culture as the company grows through its life cycle. While each company is different in regard to its culture and mission, the challenge faced by the founders can be reduced to the following ingredients articulated by Boni [10] in a review of the book written by the second chief executive officer (CEO) of Amgen, and Binder [11], who had the opportunity and challenge of following the legendary George Rathmann:

- Build a talented and balanced management team in a culture that incorporates an interdisciplinary, team-based, and collaborative approach with leadership throughout.
- Encourage and reward performance.
- Organize around autonomy and innovation.
- Tolerate risk and learn from failure.

All of us can learn a few lessons from Amgen that is arguably one of the most successful biotechnology companies in the relatively short history of the industry. We suggest that in building a management team, there are some best practices that have proven to be successful over the years. First and foremost is the challenge and principal objective to *build an entrepreneurial culture* that incorporates the necessary values and ingredients to capture and grow market share and utilize the principles of sustained or disruptive innovation including business model innovations. We focus on the "secret sauce of innovation" that is the *human capital and processes* needed to create and deliver innovations to the market and capture value for the organization sustainably.

The following additional cultural traits are required for successful organizations:

- A focus on the market is needed first, which comes from being close to the customer or user.
- Implementation of a reward system that values contribution and success and incorporates both psychological ownership of the outcome and equity ownership.

- Embrace an open-innovation model to take advantage of ideas and collaborations beyond the "borders" of the company itself.

The second challenge is to *imbue in this culture the following values* as identified in a recent Harvard Business Review article by Steve Prokesch, entitled "How GE Teaches Teams to Lead" [12] (Fig. 7.3).

- challenge and involvement,
- freedom,
- trust and openness,
- time for ideas,
- playfulness and humor,
- conflict (creative tension but not destructive),
- idea support,
- debate, and
- risk-taking.

These common principles form the basis for building an effective innovation team. Phil Jackson, the most winning professional basketball coach in history, said, "the strength of the team is each individual member—the strength of each member is the team."

McVicker [13] wrote "Starting Something: An Entrepreneur's Tale of Control, Confrontation & Corporate Culture" to illustrate his experience in building and growing an entrepreneurial culture. His company, Neoforma, was one of the first e-commerce companies in the healthcare space, so the lessons are applicable to biotechnology companies or to any other technology-driven but market-focused (or customer-centric) company. The book describes an insider's perspective that provides both the "dark and bright sides" of corporate culture. In a final chapter, titled *Afterthoughts*, McVicker includes 12 things (which we paraphrase next) to keep in mind when starting and growing something—most of which deal with corporate culture. McVicker advises aspiring entrepreneurs to focus on the team and the culture.

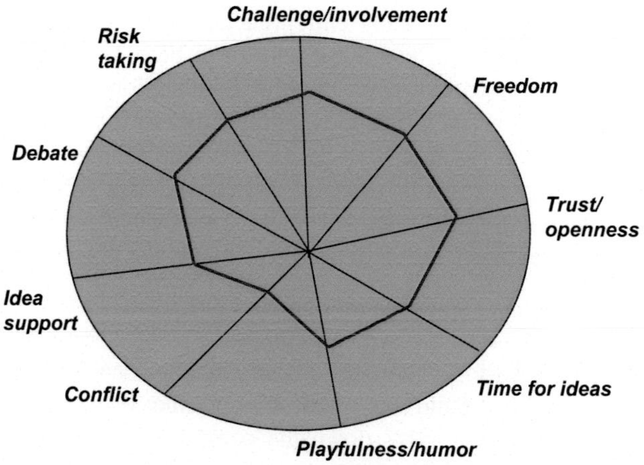

FIGURE 7.3 Attributes of an effective organizational culture. *Adapted from S. Prokesh,* How GE Teaches Teams to Lead Change, Harvard Business Review, *23 (3), 2009.*

1. Be who you are—otherwise your company's culture will suffer, as will you.
2. Hire for culture first, experience second—if someone feels wrong, they are.
3. Communicate empowerment—don't waste the potential of any employee.
4. Learn to release, without letting go—enable but monitor progress.
5. Balance is not always found in the middle—communicate decisions clearly, even if you need to change your position.
6. Do one thing well and then do it better—focus.
7. Regularly "wear your customer's clothes"—don't forget that's why you're in business.
8. The unsatisfied customer is the most important customer—that's where the opportunity lies.
9. Never let your competitors drive your business decisions—stay focused and listen to your customers.
10. Never let your investors drive your business decisions—keep the long-term view.
11. Listen to all advice, but trust what you know—ideas that require customers to change behavior often take 10 or more years to implement.
12. Enjoy yourself—it is fun to create something new and useful.

Summary of "Lessons Learned" (Further Experiential Perspective)

We provide, in this section, a "practitioner-originated" summary of issues regarding building and growing teams in biotech companies. In this regard, one of us (Boni) is the cofounder and national cochair of an Entrepreneurship Boot Camp started in 2005. It is hosted and logistically managed by the Biotechnology Innovation Organization at its annual meetings. One session deals with a moderated interview of a company CEO, chief technical or scientific officer (CTO/CSO), and one of their BOD members/investors. Different companies are incorporated into each boot camp, so the following represents a summary of the "hot topics" that are consistently discussed each year. Over the years the following topics and brief summary of recommendations gather most of the questions and discussion:

1. ***Virtual start-ups versus "bricks and mortar."*** Acquiring capital is very difficult if not impossible until a considerable amount of risk (technology, IP, clinical, and team) is reduced. However, progress must be made to interest investors and partners. Therefore founders

most often need to acquire nonequity resources (government, economic development, and selling of services) or funding from individual angels to raise limited seed capital. It is also beneficial to do so to increase market cap and reduce dilution. So, reducing the amount of capital needed is recommended by leveraging resources, for example, the use of academic facilities, outsourcing product development, and clinical work to others. It is recommended not to invest in facilities except for the bare minimum, instead invest in key people who may or may not join the company for full time, and have founders fill multiple functions on the management team. "Cash is king" so use it wisely. Eventually, you will need some facilities so consider locating in an incubator or leveraging common space with existing organizations in a research park. Invest in "hard assets" only when this is justifiable after evolving down the commercialization path.

2. ***The first hires and building a BOD.*** Start with a small core team that originally consists of the founders (two or three) and a few part-time consultants—noted earlier. Identify key advisors and directors who can provide you with good advice and credibility and pay them with equity (it's worth the dilution). Find an attorney that will work on a contingent basis (not always possible) and consult with them on creative and legal ways to handle compensation, stock, and corporate partnering issues. However, ensure that vesting is used for stock options. Alternately, issue restricted stock. Consider what happens to the stock if key people leave. If it is gone with the departing person, it will dilute those who remain since the person has to be replaced. Pay the core team less-than-competitive salaries until funds are raised—the early stage employees will make up for their reduced compensation with their stock grants. Hire for the essential tasks that need to get done but make sure the fit is good (see later). Use mentors to help you and to locate advisory board members and directors. Initially, you should have no more than three to five science/business advisory board members (nonfiduciary positions) and three board members (with at least one outside, credible, and experienced person). Advisors and directors surrounding and supporting (and mentoring) the core team will facilitate progress with commercialization and will lead to downstream success with fund raising and partnering.

   Hiring progression/priority will generally proceed in the following order of priority:
   - business, scientific/technical, market/business development leadership team;
   - clinical/medical, regulatory, and IP expertise (can be outsourced with inside leadership via a key employee at the appropriate time);
   - personnel to contribute to the scientific and business agenda associated with commercialization according to the organizational priorities (generally product development and customer/user development); and
   - financial management (once significant funds are raised, especially A-round financing).

   Keep in mind that as new team members join, they must buy into the culture that has been created by the founders. So, these first members are the key and will build and preserve the corporate culture. We highlight that "fit," shared values, and relevant experience and ability to execute are all important considerations.

   A subset of this discussion always revolves around the issue of "splitting the equity pie" and dilution. We could write an entire article on this topic; suffice it to say that the initial equity should be split among the founders and early hires (if any) based on what they have contributed to the company formation, what they will contribute going forward, and the level of risk each person takes. We encourage the founders to engage a good lawyer to help with this because it is always a contentious issue as to who contributed what and who will do so going forward. Most prominent among the contentious issues is the debate about the weighting of science versus business in equity participation. Make sure that the founders get rewarded for their founding contributions (value is attributed to both technology and business acumen), and make sure that those who take the risk and actually join the company are rewarded for that as well. Small equity pools are then created for advisors/directors and for stock options for employees to be hired prior to the next funding tranche—typically 15%–20% of the total for all parties. The pool will then be replenished prior to the next equity raise (investors will most often insist that the dilution will be taken by the insiders and not the investors). Many entrepreneurs worry excessively about dilution. For those who have been through this many times, however, there is a realization that creating value that builds the capitalization of the company is the key outcome to be pursued, and taking outside money is essential to value creation and risk reduction, that is, a "small piece of a large pie" is better than the alternative. Getting to the end game is the objective.

3. ***Balancing science and commercialization.*** In biotechnology and biomedical companies, there is always the need to continually advance the science (to prove principle, build the platform and the IP portfolio). However, progress down the commercialization pathway is necessary to generate the funding that will be needed to attract subsequent team members. Therefore priorities and a sense of urgency to advance the

technology and business have to be established early on at the founder and board level and managed carefully by the CEO and CTO/CSO of the company. Many organizations maintain close ties to a university where scientific advances can be handled (but be careful of IP and conflict-of-interest issues). Commercialization involves clinical demonstration in parallel with product development, which is difficult in a regulated environment. Once funding is raised make sure to allocate a small portion to advance the science and also consider some government augmentation (via the Small Business Innovation Research (SBIR) program) to achieve those objectives. While SBIR funding is nondilutive, sometimes the timing is not consistent with commercialization priorities.

4. ***Managing through transitions.*** Along the commercialization pathway, company leadership and the board will need to deal with evolution of the team as people join the team and leave the team—either voluntarily or involuntarily. Sometimes founders play "lesser roles" as new leadership is required to move forward thru the clinic and into the marketplace, or to raise venture capital and/or partnership funding. We have not found the perfect formula for dealing with these issues. One thing that can be counted on is that it will happen in virtually every company. In order to manage this process the right people must be on the board or on the advisory group to assist with the people issues—the addition or subtraction as well as the team remaining. Nothing can destroy team chemistry faster than a mismanaged transition. The best advice is to handle the situation quickly and professionally with good communication to all of the constituencies of the company appropriate to the specific situation. It is rare that a founder who becomes the CEO of a biotechnology start-up can survive through to the acquisition or Initial Public Offering (IPO).

We consider using more capital-efficient business models that can be achieved via various methods, for example, outsourcing, partnering, and use of agile methods borrowed from software development. Capital-efficient, agile development is essential for biotechnology and biomedical companies where it is important to reduce technical, market, and team risks prior to bringing in the extensive amounts of capital required. As noted, the formation of win–win partnerships, while maintaining the ability to share significantly in the value that has been created by the team, is recommended. For example, iterative product and market development can lead to lower capital expenditures and faster time to market (even though the regulatory authorities tend to slow down the cycle time—this is not as much of an issue for other technology companies where lean and agile methods are being employed). Also consider creating value and reducing risk via proof-of-principle demonstration in a clinical setting (even if offshore) prior to raising large amounts of capital. An extensive discussion on this topic is beyond the scope of the current article; however, suffice it to say that virtual companies can be created to leverage expertise by using open-innovation principles to partner for technology, market access, product development and clinical testing, manufacturing, and even management teams. Why build capacity that already exists? Sharing value might be a better option. The challenge is to build a core team that is equipped with the processes and networks to access and effectively manage these relationships. However, keep in mind that it will be necessary to have expertise on the extended team to manage the partnered or outsourced tasks. This will require the existence of talent that has experience with product development, clinical testing, etc. Keep in mind that the overall objective in building a team is to address one key component of risk reduction for the organization—*demonstration of the ability to execute*.

Key Questions to Ask When Building the Team—the Academic Perspective

Building a team is comprised of three phases summarized by Thompson [14], each of which must be revisited as the organization and the team transitions through development and commercialization stages, to market launch and growth.

Phase One—Task analysis. Specifically, what is the work that needs to be performed and what is its focus, how much authority and autonomy do the team have to manage its own work, what is the degree of interdependence among the team members, and are the team members' interests aligned or competitive?

Phase Two—People required. *What skill sets are needed* to perform the tasks to achieve at least the next milestone or two. Consider the blend of technical, task management; what interpersonal skills and diversity are optimal for the team?

Phase Three—Processes and procedures required. What are the explicit and implicit norms required for the performance, how are ineffective norms revised, and how much structure is required? We would suggest that a team contract be employed to provide a framework for the norms of behavior expected with the team (Fig. 7.4).

Underlying these tasks, people, and processes is the entrepreneurial culture that is desired. It indicates the organizational characteristics and norms noted previously and the "expected entrepreneurial style of the people engaged," for example, willingness to assume "some" risk, thriving on chaos, not controlling, positive,

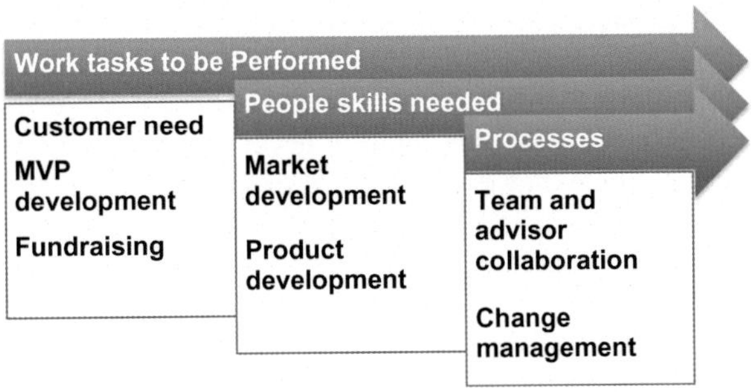

FIGURE 7.4 Three phases of building an effective team.

passionate, perseverant, and motivated to make an impact, or perhaps even to change the world.

Building a Biotechnology Organization

Most early stage biotechnology companies, as with most technology companies, start with two or three founders. The founders bring their passion, and vision for a new company, along with the needed expertise, skill sets, and networks to provide leadership for the two key and critical dimensions: (1) *technology advancement and* (2) *business/market development*. In effect, upon founding, the *task analysis* and *people required* phases occur simultaneously, and the founders form the kernel of a viable start-up. The focus on developing and advancing the technology and the market in parallel is the "essential task, or job to be done," and the founders are the key people who perform those tasks that are organization specific. This initial founding team (and their advisors added as needed) then evolves through Phases One and Two of the Thompson "model" in parallel where team members are acquired to evolve the technology and the market/industry dimensions while advancing the commercialization process and developing the business model. It is understood that they must also acquire the needed financial resources to move forward. In most biotechnology start-ups where both technology and business leaderships are essential, decisions are most often made informally and by consensus, with input and perspective from both dimensions, but overtime, these roles evolve into a more formal structure, with decisions by the CEO and CTO or CSO. In most technology-enabled organizations (including biotechnology) the task analysis indicates that leadership is required to

- provide vision, strategic direction, fund raising, team building, and overall leadership;
- lead scientific advancement, technology commercialization, and product development; and
- lead business development and partnering.

In addition, for biotechnology companies specifically, it will be necessary to add the capacity to deal with the following activities:

- regulatory compliance and clinical demonstration,
- IP development, and
- reimbursement.

Early on these tasks can be accomplished by the members of the founding team and/or by part-time talent and appropriate expertise from qualified consultants. These people expand from the kernel that comprises the core of the start-up and development-stage team—most often there are perhaps two C-level positions designated to handle *inside and outside functions*—these include simultaneous development of the product while working in parallel to more thoroughly understand and address customer/user need and the external environment/fund raising. Acquiring human assets in biotechnology/tech companies is as important as acquiring financial assets, but one is required to accomplish the other—while advancing the opportunity and proposed solution. In effect an additional key task is developing the organization—most often consuming a significant part of the CEO's time allocation, along with acquiring funding.

The team that comprises an early stage organization is not complete without developing its "periphery"—team members who serve in a more advisory function and contribute to the organization on an as-needed basis. It is critical for early stage organizations to develop a set of directors/advisors that bring specialized expertise, connections, and access to networks for funding, partnering, hiring, etc. Most important is the need to institute a formalized, but small, BOD of at least three people, including independent director(s) perhaps growing to five as equity investments occur. The BOD is responsible for fiduciary control, provides overview of strategic direction and operations, and also ensures that corrective actions based on internal and external changes and issues are addressed in a timely manner. Note that an advisory board is also important in that it performs different functions from a BOD. Although the BOD will have fiduciary responsibility, other boards can be formed, which are advisory only—most often providing specialized knowledge and guidance such as science/technology and clinical development. These bridges between the internal organization and the external environment also provide credibility and validation of the opportunity being pursued via the reputation of the people engaged with the organization. These directors and advisors are most often compensated via equity using industry norms as guidelines for a directors' and advisors' stock option pool.

Therefore the leadership team consists of both the core members (i.e., the people on the ground) who have committed and are willing to take risks to join the company, as well as the peripheral members, the BOD/advisory board. This extended team is expected to provide expertise, networks, perspective, and discipline as follows:

- Access to people, capital, partners, and markets/customers.
- Access to counsel and expertise for IP, regulatory, reimbursement, clinical trials, and corporate agreements.
- Advice, experienced perspective, and mentoring.
- Adherence to plan and fiduciary responsibility.

As noted earlier, the characteristics of this extended team include the knowledge, skills, and expertise, coupled with the requisite interpersonal skills (diversity, collaborative, and communicative), and a shared value system (a common purpose and vision, trust, and sense of humor). In addition, since in many technology-based organizations, one is dealing with large egos, it is advisable to be able to "check your egos at the door."

Finding and Hiring Good People

Finding and hiring good team members is the most important challenge faced by any company, let alone a start-up or early stage organization. Especially at the earliest stages of any organization, the CEO and other founders must be personally engaged in the hiring process since the "organizational DNA" or culture is imprinted starting with the hiring process. Selecting the right people "with the right DNA" is important to building the desired cultural norms—both spoken and unspoken. All start-ups should strive to hire only "A players," since excellence is essential to company success. Don't just hire to get the job done, make sure that the person "fits" and can also do the current task or job as well as grow with the organization. Hiring is expensive and time consuming, so do it wisely. A bad fit can be harmful for the organization, and replacing someone is also problematic as well as expensive. But if the replacement is necessary, do it quickly and professionally; otherwise, the "bad fit" will affect the organization itself.

Diversity is good since there are many skill sets required to build a successful company, and diverse perspectives and experience sets provide more enlightened and innovative solutions. In a biotechnology or biomedical company, diversity includes various scientific backgrounds, business development/industry knowledge, and expertise ranging from IP to regulatory to reimbursement. In addition, one must deal with perspectives gathered in small companies as well as in larger, more mature organizations, for example, pharmaceutical or large medical device companies. All of these key elements of the extended management team need to be integrated into the entrepreneurial and innovative culture being built. We advise embracing diversity, but not leaving the synergies to chance as the team is built up over the life cycle of the company. It is important to build mechanisms and processes to manage diversity not only internally but also across the boundaries of the firm as networked innovation and partnering emerge as a norm in the biotechnology/biopharmaceutical industry. This open-innovation business model is becoming increasingly important as industry convergence continues, blurring the boundaries between the pharmaceutical and the biotechnology organizations. The team, culture, and vision sharing are as important as skill sets so that there is trust, liking, and respect (unspoken norms) across the team and organization. Most successful organizations build this mentality into the hiring process and walk away from talented people if the cultural fit is not there.

It is important to understand and deal with factors that motivate entrepreneurs and to address them individually with team members as the team is built and expanded. We have previously discussed entrepreneurial characteristics that are pertinent to biotechnology and technology companies, including Boni's review of Binder's book [5].

What Makes Teams Work, or Not?

To discuss what works and what does not, from an academic perspective, we need to deal with three key factors: (1) the structure of the team, which includes roles and routines; (2) behavioral integration—managing the diversity; and (3) team norms—goals and shared values, team motivation, and processes for coordinating, communicating, managing conflict, making decisions, running meetings, and enforcing norms.

Larson and LaFasto [15] list the following necessary conditions for effective teamwork:

- a clear, shared, and elevating goal,
- a results-driven structure that includes the following:
  - clear roles and accountabilities,
  - an effective communication system,
  - monitoring of individual performance and providing feedback, and
  - fact-based judgments.
- competent team members (technical and interpersonal),
- unified commitment,
- collaborative climate,
- standards of excellence,
- external support and recognition, and
- principled leadership.

We refer the reader who is further interested in building effective teams to several good *Harvard Business Review* articles by Gulati and DeSantola [16], Haas and Mortensen [17], Billington [18], and Katzenbach and Smith [19]. While these articles are not targeted specifically at knowledge-based biotechnology companies, the authors address the issue of what makes the difference between teams that perform and those that don't. These are universal lessons. To be effective a team must go beyond just being a group or collective of individuals. The team is defined as "a small number of people with complementary skills (competence) who are committed to a common purpose, set of performance goals, and an approach for which they hold themselves mutually accountable." The Billington article points out that mutual accountability differentiates a team from a group. In a team, if the team fails (or the company), all fail together. If the team succeeds, all are rewarded in proportion to their contributions. Another way to keep motivation high, something that is important in any start-up organization, is for the leadership team (and its Board) to establish and maintain a sense of urgency. Kotter identifies the sense of urgency as the first and essential step in his eight-step process for leading change identified in extensive case studies [20]. From a practical perspective, we advise that the team consider spending a lot of time together outside of the workplace and inside (which is inevitable in a start-up environment).

Mini-case analyses of emerging open-innovation organizational structures in biotechnology

Previously, in this chapter, we emphasized the challenges faced by teams in "nontraditional" organizational firms. Historically, most biotechnology companies (and their pharmaceutical counterparts) have been built up and developed as "vertically integrated organizations"—most if not all functions of the organization accomplished internally with teams contained within the organization. However, it is important to recognize that a new paradigm has emerged with the recognition of open collaboration/innovation, and the introduction of virtual companies and networked organizations. We also note that the evolution of "the Pharma 3.0 model" is driven by the need to improve the efficiency of the biopharmaceutical innovation process through engagement of a broader set of ideas, technologies, resources, and capabilities. Collaboration across organizational and geographical boundaries is expected to provide a more capital-efficient, shorter development and approval cycle, with a higher success rate. However, no benefits are achieved without challenges. In this case the complexity of creating high-performance collaborative, cross-boundary teams adds new dimension to the challenge.

Next, we discuss several examples of promising models for bringing complex, high-risk, long development cycle biopharma products thru commercialization. We close with a short summary of selected issues dealing with building teams to lead and grow these new organizations. We also note that at the time of this writing, this new approach to innovation is still evolving, so whether or not these forms will be effective as a solution to the "biopharma innovators dilemma" is yet to be proven or demonstrated.

(Continued)

(Continued)

Inherent in these emerging organizational models is the ability to identify and source opportunities by assembling diverse and disparate resources that permit the identification and exploitation of promising disruptive technologies that address significant market need while validating the need, efficacy, and safety in close collaboration with corporate partners, for example, extant pharmaceutical organizations. As such, the market-first approach to commercialization proceeds in parallel with developing and validating key parts of the business model, including the partnerships, channels to market, and customer interaction components (channels and customer communications).

Team development in these new organizational forms also proceeds via a multistep process. However, now the leadership team can comprise the following:

- Industry leaders who are very experienced in commercialization and have thorough understanding of both the technology and the business aspects;
- Individuals who are well networked in the industry and financial communities (and perhaps academic community); and
- Those who really understand the market need and most probably include pharmaceutical partners.

These leadership teams can then build, acquire, and mentor multiple founding scientific teams who would then pursue specific commercialization opportunities with ideas, technologies, and capabilities acquired from the overall network (including clinical testing and manufacturing). The coupled management leadership team and scientific team (s) can then be linked to partner corporations (e.g., pharmaceutical companies) and early stage investors—both well known to the leadership management team.

We illustrate several promising emerging organizations using such an approach, but we highlight only two for brevity. The first organization highlighted, Enlight BioSciences [14], illustrates some essential features dealing with innovation in a networked environment. The second organization highlighted in this mini-case is summarized in some recent undertakings led by David U'Prichard and others—Druid BioVentures [15] and then BioMotiv LLC [16]. Taken together, they illustrate partnering across the entire value chain of biopharma and incorporate disparate sources of participants ranging from technology sourcing, to commercialization expertise, and to efficient channels to the market.

Enlight BioSciences, a Boston-based company, was founded by PureTech Ventures, a life science venture capital firm, and a team of industry leaders and academic luminaries in 2007 [21]. Enlight and PureTech provide the team leadership and early stage financing to identify new technologies to meet identified market need. They then develop the scientific leadership team to form a dedicated new company(s) to commercialize the opportunities in several areas of focus. Investment funding is provided by PureTech and a series of pharma partners that include Abbot, Johnson

(Continued)

(Continued)

& Johnson, Eli Lilly and Co., Merck, Novartis, and Pfizer. This investment and leadership group provided initial funding of $78M plus in-kind expertise to Endra Holdings, LLC, which then in turn invests in Endra, Inc. as the commercialization entity. Endra, Inc. is one of a series of companies that are expected to emerge to pursue specific commercialization opportunities in the suite of areas of interest identified by the Enlight BioSciences team and their partners.

For the start-up company, Endra, Inc., the venture creation model consists of a "seasoned management team" assigned from Enlight, coupled with a team of founding scientists who have been recruited from a laboratory (e.g., a university or government lab) as part of the founding team. Considering this specific case, we would highlight the challenges of team interactions, motivations at several, coupled levels, and "boundary-spanning activities" involving the management team from Enlight, PureTech Ventures, their partners and advisory boards, the science team from the start-up (i.e., the boundary-spanning activities), and teams from the supporting network of investors and corporate partners. Indeed, it is a very complex undertaking. All of the team dynamics are present here, but as noted, complicated by the various interests of the participating parties and their respective corporate cultures.

Other so-called virtual organizational models have been discussed and pursued in recent years. David U'Prichard, former Chair of Global R&D at SmithKline Beecham (now GlaxoSmithKline) and ICI/Zeneca, has pioneered two recent undertakings [22,23]. The need for these organizations is driven by several trends: (1) the lack of capital for pharmaceutical innovation in the "valley of death" (between early stage development and clinical validation), hence the need for capital efficiency; and (2) shrinking of the "pharma pipeline." There has been a shift from a fully integrated product company (FIPCO) model, in which the sponsor "owns" the entire drug development process from synthesis to marketing, toward a networked model of innovation, referred to as a FIPNet (or fully integrated pharmaceutical network). FIPNets engage all of the major stakeholders involved in the drug development process, blending the core competencies of each to leverage capabilities, enhance efficiency, and boost output.

The Harrington Project is a multihundred-million-dollar national initiative to accelerate breakthrough discoveries into medicines. A national consortium of academic medical centers (the Harrington Discovery Institute and an Innovation Center) translates promising discoveries into BioMotiv, which is a national bioaccelerator to promote commercialization and entrepreneurship in medicine. BioMotiv is a for profit entity that is an "evergreen" holding company that invests in and manages a portfolio of early projects, each structured as a virtual, single-asset development corporation. A full-time staff in Cleveland, Ohio is

(Continued)

(Continued)

complemented by a larger group of very senior pharmaceutical consultants in greater Philadelphia and in Oxford, the United Kingdom. BioMotiv "sources" the best opportunities from around the country, leveraging nonprofit assets, utilizes a team of experienced and connected advisors, and accelerates development to exit via partnership with pharmaceutical companies (at the late discovery stage thru Phase Ib). They anticipate significant and sustained financial returns from developing a portfolio of programs. Dr. David Pritchard is the CSO and Chairman of BioMotiv, Baiju Shah (former President and CEO of BioEnterprise in Cleveland) is the CEO, and they have assembled a very impressive team of consultants and advisors. The intent of the Harrington Project is to accelerate breakthrough discoveries into medicines and cross the valley of death with informed partnerships after reducing risk in the early development stages.

To summarize, in both mini-cases, we note boundary-spanning flows of knowledge, ideas, and financial resources across teams nested in networks. In these more complex organizational structures, it is important to understand the factors that enhance or inhibit these boundary-spanning flows with a focus on motivation. In particular, how does the role of employee ownership (psychological and financial) affect performance? It is our hypothesis that ownership structure and motivation in entrepreneurial firms affect the distribution of risk and reward across networks and value chains. Interest alignment that determines the competitive advantage [24] is particularly complex in highly novel, multiagent, and uncertain contexts such as these.

Understanding Factors That Motivate Teams

There are a variety of team-related motivational factors that lead to increased innovation throughput and capital efficiency in entrepreneurial firms. We have attempted to better define the role of team motivation through "employee ownership," both psychological and financial. We have focused first on how the team optimizes its performance. The approach outlined next incorporates a design that may be extended to deal with the more complex issue of how the performance is optimized in the supporting network.

Framework for an Entrepreneurial Team Motivation Model

In this subsection, we present a model that attempts to frame the issues involved in motivating team members and partners. Our basic assumption is that the young entrepreneurial firm can be modeled as an entrepreneurial

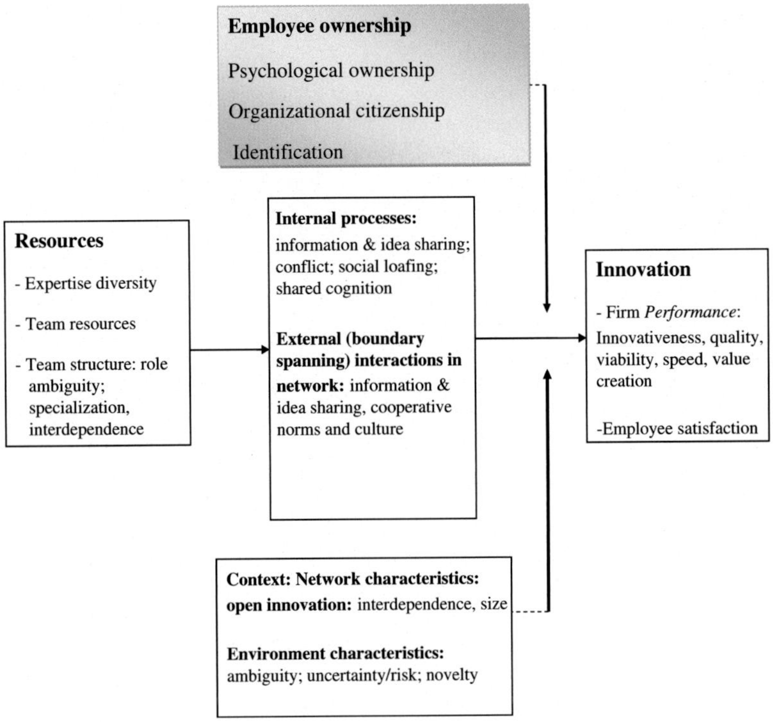

FIGURE 7.5 Framework for motivation of entrepreneurial teams incorporating employee ownership

team, because of its small size and the high interdependence of activities within the firm. Note that this approach could be extended to incorporate later stage companies and collaborative networks (Fig. 7.5).

We investigated whether employee ownership in terms of financial ownership was reflected in psychological ownership; that is, citizenship behaviors or voluntary contributions to the firm and identification with the firm/team. Based on the literature, and using the IPMO (input, process, moderators, and output) framework for the study of teamwork, we developed hypotheses about employee ownership (both financial and psychological) and its effects on team interactions and team performance.

We hypothesized that the choice of ownership structure plays a pivotal role in team motivation. Employee ownership was expected to promote value-creating dynamics of interactions of entrepreneurial firm/team members both with insiders and outside stakeholders.

We tested the following hypotheses about the role of motivation via employee ownership:

Hypothesis 1: Employee ownership (financial) leads to high *psychological ownership*, more citizenship behaviors, and higher identification with the firm.

Hypothesis 2: Employee ownership (both financial and psychological) enhances the *internal processes* of information and idea sharing, and divergent task conflict in the firm/team.

Hypothesis 3: Employee ownership (both financial and psychological) enhances *boundary-spanning (external) interactions (flows* of knowledge, ideas, and financial resources) between the firm/team nested in open innovation networks and the key external agents.

These hypotheses were tested using a quasiexperimental approach and two-group comparison. Group 1 was composed of start-up company teams initiated by the Carnegie Mellon University graduate students, and group 2 was composed of a parallel cohort of graduate students performing entrepreneurial projects sponsored by external companies [25,26]. The first group represented entrepreneurial firms with high employee ownership (financial), whereas the second group represented entrepreneurial firms with low employee ownership (financial). Our preliminary findings using statistical analysis are summarized briefly, which are as follows:

***Finding 1*:** In support of Hypothesis 1, we found that psychological ownership was significantly higher for the teams with high employee ownership (financial) than for the teams with low employee ownership (financial). Employee ownership (financial) also increased the voluntary contributions of team members (higher citizenship behaviors) and the identification with the team.

***Lesson learned 1*:** Employee ownership (financial) improves team motivation. It increases psychological ownership, voluntary contributions of team members (i.e., citizenship behaviors), and identification with the team.

***Finding 2*:** In support of Hypotheses 2 and 3, we found that higher level of employee ownership (both financial and psychological) led to enhanced team interactions. In teams with higher level of employee ownership, there were higher internal idea sharing, higher external idea sharing, and higher creative conflict.

***Lesson learned 2*:** Both financial and psychological employee ownerships improve innovation—enhancing team processes such as idea sharing (both internal and external) and creative conflict.

***Finding 3*:** In support of Hypothesis 4, we found that higher psychological ownership was related to higher satisfaction (both with the team and with the project). We also noted that team satisfaction is important because it predicts the willingness of the team members to stay with the team and thus enhances its longevity. Psychological ownership also had a positive effect on value added in terms of "usability" of innovation project outcome—whether the innovation outcome fills need, has utility, and has favorable timescale of return.

***Lesson learned 3*:** Psychological ownership represents an important motivating factor in teams because it improves team satisfaction and "usability" of innovations. Since employee ownership (financial) increases psychological ownership as per Finding 1, both financial and psychological employee ownerships represent essential motivating factors in entrepreneurial teams. In the future, we plan to examine how the open-innovation network characteristics influence the importance of ownership in enhancing innovation in extended networks.

Summary and Conclusion

In this chapter, we have discussed about building and growing collaborative, interdisciplinary teams that identify and commercialize promising biotechnology innovations and ultimately grow successful companies. From a practical perspective, we have emphasized one significant conclusion: the importance of the team in generating a successful outcome cannot be overemphasized. We also highlight the necessity of building and sustaining an entrepreneurial culture as a means to differentiate and sustain successful organizations. We further again stress that leadership must recognize and reward team (and partner) contributions to company value creation, and to incorporate mechanisms and processes to encourage employees to "own" and identify with their organization. The principles underlying building and growing high-performance teams apply in both traditional and emerging organizational structures. New organizational forms are evolving, and these require collaborative, networked partnerships that present human resource management challenges regarding (extended) team development, management, and performance.

Acknowledgments

The content of this article was previously published by Boni AA, Weingart LR. Building teams in entrepreneurial companies. J Commer Biotechnol 2012;18(2). doi:10.5912/jcb507 and is incorporated into this chapter as modified by the authors with the approval of the publisher of the *Journal of Commercial Biotechnology*.

The authors acknowledge that the framework for motivation of entrepreneurial teams incorporating employee ownership was supported by the Foundation for Enterprise Development (FED), La Jolla, CA. We appreciate the input and support of Mary Ann Beyster, CEO. Dr. Boni also acknowledges the leadership and team-building lessons learned early in his entrepreneurial career as part of the leadership team led by Dr. J. Robert Beyster, founder and chairman of FED and of Science Applications International Corporation (SAIC). During a decade of high growth at SAIC, spanning early stage to the largest US employee-owned technology-based company was a great learning experience on building and working with geographically dispersed high-performance teams.

References

1 Timmons JA, Stephen S. New venture creation, entrepreneurship for the 21st century. 7th ed. McGraw Hill Irwin; 2007.
2 Mathieu JE, Kukenberger MR, D'Innocenzo L, Reilly G. Modeling reciprocal team cohesion–performance relationships, as impacted by shared leadership and members' competence. J Appl Psychol 2015;100:713–34.
3 D'Innocenzo L, Mathieu JE, Kukenberger MR. A meta-analysis of different forms of shared leadership–team performance relations. J Manage 2016;42:1964–91.
4 Krieger E. The term 'entrepreneur' isn't usually associated with teams—how does an entrepreneurial team work? <www.ivyexec.com/executive-insights/2017/efficient-entrepreneurship-teams/>; 2017.
5 Robb A, Ballou J, DesRoches D, Potter F, Zhao Z, Reedy EJ. An overview of the Kauffman firm survey: results from the 2004 – 2007 data. Kauffman Foundation of Entrepreneurship webpage. <www.kauffman.org>; 2009.
6 Chesbrough H. Open innovation: the new imperative for creating and profiting from technology. Cambridge, MA: Harvard University Press; 2003.
7 Chesbrough H, Vanhaverbeke W, West J, editors. Open innovation: researching a new paradigm. Cambridge, MA: Harvard University Press; 2006.
8 Kramer MR, Pfizer MW. The ecosystems of shared value. Harv Bus Rev 2016;80–90.
9 Ihrig M, McMillan I. How to get ecosystem buy-in. Harv Bus Rev 2017;102–7.
10 Boni AA. Science lessons: what biotech taught me about management." A book review of Gordon Binder and Philip Bashe. J Commer Biotechnol 2009;15(1):86–91.
11 Binder G, Bashe P. Science lessons—what the business of biotech taught me about management. Harvard Business Press; 2008.
12 Prokesh S. How GE teaches teams to lead change. Harv Bus Rev 2009. Reprint R0901J.
13 McVicker WW. Starting something – an entrepreneur's tale of control, confrontation, and corporate culture. Los Altos, CA: Ravel Media, LLC; 2005.
14 Thompson L. Making the team. A guide for managers. 4th ed. Prentice Hall; 2011.
15 Larson CE, LaFasto FMJ. Teamwork: what must go right, what can go wrong. Newberry Park, CA: Sage; 1989.
16 Gulati R, DeSantola A. Start-ups that last. Harv Bus Rev 2016;54–62.
17 Haas M, Mortensen M. The secrets of great teamwork. Harv Bus Rev 2016;70–8.

18 Billington J. The three essentials of an effective team. Harv Bus Rev 1997. Reprint U9701A.
19 Katzenbach JR, Smith DK. The discipline of teams, Harv Bus Rev 2005. Reprint R0507P.
20 Kotter JP. Leading change. Boston, MA: Harvard Business Press; 1996.
21 Ernst & Young. In: Giovannetti GT, Gautam J, editors. Beyond borders, global biotechnology. Ernst & Young; 2010.
22 U'Prichard DC. Private communication from BIO Entrepreneurship Bootcamp organized by Boni and Steve Sammut; 2013. Held in Chicago, IL.
23 U'Prichard DC. New paradigms in drug R&D: a personal perspective. J Commer Biotechnol 2012;18(2):11–18.
24 Gottshalg O, Zollo M. Interest alignment and competitive advantage. Acad Manage Rev 2007;32:418–38.
25 Boni AA, Weingart LR, Evenson S. Innovation in an academic setting: designing and leading a business through market-focused, interdisciplinary teams. Acad Manage Learn Educ 2009;8:407–17.
26 Boni AA, Emerson ST. An integrated model of university technology commercialization and entrepreneurship education. In: Advances in the study of entrepreneurship, innovation and economic growth, Elsevier, vol. 16. 2005. p. 241–74.

Chapter 8

Building Human Relationship Networks

Tom D. Walker, MBA
CEO and President, Rev1 Ventures, Inc., Columbus, OH, United States

Chapter Outline

Biotechnology entrepreneurs face many challenges. It's a herculean task to research a new technology, successfully prove efficacy and safety through multiple levels of trials that may take decades, and then bring a new solution to market that improves, or perhaps, even saves people's lives. It's a race against time. Many biotech entrepreneurs may struggle with a problem situation that causes undue delays in development, difficulty in raising capital, or even failure of the company. They may not realize that there are experienced individuals who are ready, willing, and able to help. This chapter shares with biotechnology entrepreneurs how to build relationships with such individuals and organizations to overcome problems, or even avoid them completely, to advance and accelerate the creation and growth of a startup biotechnology company.

Within the personal relationships you already have, there likely are individuals who can casually offer connections and business advice; however, in this chapter, we are talking about an additional frame for relationships—*purposeful relationships*—defined as mutually beneficial connections that the entrepreneur develops expressly with a goal of making the business more successful. Some of these business relationships may eventually evolve into close personal relationships, but the primary reason for these relationships is to help a biotechnology company solve problems and achieve milestones that lead to growth.

Purposeful relationships can help make biotech entrepreneurs personally stronger as company founders and will help derisk the company. However, purposeful relationship building takes time, focus, and expertise. To be used to its best advantage, savvy entrepreneurs integrate relationship building into every biotechnology business plan from day one.

Biotechnology Entrepreneurship. DOI: https://doi.org/10.1016/B978-0-12-815585-1.00008-5

Purposeful Networking Expands Limited Resources

If You Don't Already Have a Networking Mindset, Develop One to Succeed

Every biotechnology entrepreneur needs to develop a *networking mindset*. Purposeful relationships with a diverse network of human beings and organizations (through formal and informal structures) are empowering. Throughout my career, I, and the companies I've invested in and led, have benefited from networked relationships that we built over time. Entrepreneurs with a winning mindset hold these following beliefs:

- I need outside help; without it my biotechnology company cannot succeed. I don't, can't, and won't ever know everything I need to know about company building. I don't even know what I don't know.
- There are many people who have traveled the path before me. Many are happy and eager to help.
- I connect with these people through intentional, deliberate relationships that provide benefits to all parties involved. It's my job to create a plan.
- My personal and company resources are limited. My startup will never have enough time, talent, or capital.
- In every area of my business, I need the most diversified and exceptional talent I can find.
- I am personally committed to a culture of inclusion and diversity because companies with diverse teams produce better results.
- I may or may not be the best person to be CEO. To advance my technology and startup through an exit strategy, my best contribution might be that of the chief technology officer (CTO). I will make that determination through a collaborative strategy of two-way trusted relationships with people who know me, know the company, and understand our intellectual property, our solutions, the people and markets we serve, and our exit strategy.

What Is Purposeful Networking?

In business, the term *network* describes the myriad of interconnected human relationships that exist between people and organizations. *Purposeful* networking is an intentional process of turning connections into cooperation and collaboration to accelerate discovery, advance research, and then help a biotechnology business grow, scale, and exit.

Human networks start when at least two people feel connected because they have something in common. They might meet casually, even accidentally—sharing a table at a coffee shop or because they are neighbors—or by each knowing the same person. They may be scientists or certified public accountants (CPA), patent holders or attorneys, or parents of an autistic child. With a strategy of purposeful networking, connections become more intentional: graduates of the same university connect through alumni organizations, a researcher reaches out to fellow researchers in a similar field, or a startup seeks candidates for clinical trials from international associations focusing on a certain disease. Purposeful networking also encompasses connections that come about with laser-like focus: an entrepreneur looking to acquire a specific technology; a CTO seeking an experienced investigator; a company founder raising capital to finance clinical trials, or a CEO exploring exit possibilities with a potential acquirer.

Why Is Purposeful Networking Important?

Human networks are a way for entrepreneurs and startup companies to accelerate and accomplish milestones that neither can accomplish alone. There is nothing one-sided, wrong, or misleading about building relationships to enhance your business. Purposeful networking leverages scarce company resources and helps entrepreneurs fill in the gaps in their own experience and capabilities. Seeking the coaching and advice of others helps entrepreneurs better manage the business as well as expand the company's reach into the marketplace so that it is easier to make productive contact with potential business partners, investors, and acquisitors.

The process of purposeful networking is especially critical in biotech because in the beginning stages of a biotech company, resources are always limited and achieving milestones is very, very difficult. Not only is funding limited in biotechnology startups, but the employee roster is very thin. Often, it is just the innovator/founder—the person who understands the science, knows his or her way around the research lab and academia, and who is often a relentless expert at experimentation, but likely doesn't know much about starting a business.

How Can Purposeful Relationship-Building Help a Biotech Startup Succeed?

The expertise and support that a biotechnology entrepreneur can gain from purposeful relationships falls into four categories:

1. ***Functional expertise in business operations and management***: Creating a company requires a range of cross-functional expertise, including finance, business development, product development marketing, sales, and human resources. As a biotechnology entrepreneur, the more specific your personal experience and

focus, the more you need outside advice and assistance. From incorporating the business, to licensing or protecting intellectual property, to managing hiring employees or contracting services, the day-to-day requirements of running a business grow larger and more pressing over time. Sit down with corporate business people to brainstorm challenges or ask for advice. They may not know what it is like to start a company from scratch, but they will know about operations. Talk with other entrepreneurs. They have been where you are and have done what you are trying to do. Ask them about their mistakes and about what they did right. Listen. Make notes. Ask them if you can talk to them again in the future.

2. ***Expert services***: Every business, no matter how small or new, needs the services of expert professionals, at a minimum to handle legal matters and for accounting and taxes. Budget for these services in the very first phases of your business plan. Enter into early professional services relationships with the intention of building trust and enduring partnerships. As the company grows and specific needs arise, your corporate attorney and CPA can be your pipeline to engaging professionals with more specific expertise. Outside experts in human resources, IT support, and business development can be useful and more affordable on a fee basis rather than as in-house salaried employees. Seek referrals from other biotechnology entrepreneurs, the technology transfer offices (TTOs) at local universities or research institutions, or from economic development organizations. Identify firms that specialize in working with startups. Attorneys, CPAs, and accounting firms sometimes offer reduced fee services to startup companies, recognizing that young companies that take hold and grow become long-term, profitable clients. Startup studios, accelerators, incubators, and economic development organizations may offer access to pro bono professional services. Ask.
3. ***Access to talent***: It is more challenging than ever for startups to recruit the diverse talent they need. Purposeful networking is virtually the only way that a biotechnology entrepreneur can build a culture of inclusion and diversity. Why is this important? Because companies with diverse founders, leaders, advisors, and teams typically outperform industry norms and achieve better financial results.[1] Racially and ethnically diverse companies are 35% more likely to outperform the national industry norm.[2] Gender-diverse companies are 15% more likely to exceed their peers.[3] If you, as a biotechnology entrepreneur, draw only on your own contacts and networks, you will likely hire people who look and think like you. It may seem more expedient to connect with people you already know, but that's the fastest way to miss out on the opportunities that an inclusive culture can bring to your startup. The more homogenous a company becomes, the more difficult it is to attract diversified candidates as the company grows. No founder should operate in a vacuum. If ever there was a place to ask for help, identifying and attracting talent is it. *Inclusive Entrepreneurship: Growing the Startup Economy through the Power of Inclusive Entrepreneurship*[4] is an excellent report on the impact of inclusion and diversity on young companies.
4. ***Access to capital***: While startups in other industries may be able to bootstrap for 24 months or more, the financial pressures on biotechnology startups are more immediate. Clinical studies and trials; licensing and protection for intellectual property, and dealing with FDA regulations are just a few of the very costly milestones that biotechnology startups must clear to be on track for the follow-on funding that is required to achieve milestones leading to a desirable exit or sustainability. Building contacts and relationships over time with the managers of public sector sources of capital, local bankers, angel investors, corporate venture funds, and venture capital firms that are participants in your region's entrepreneurial ecosystem is critical. Don't wait until the startup needs capital to establish and nurture these professional connections.

Using these four categories of required expertise, complete an honest self-assessment and then map out a plan to addresses your startup's particular needs. Prioritize timing based on the critical path milestones as defined by your business plan: What are your immediate needs? What help does the startup need in the future? And one more assessment: What help do you, as the entrepreneur and company founder, need personally to become the best founder and leader that you can?

A Roadmap to Creating Purposeful Relationships

In the interest of making this chapter as beneficial as possible, I want to directly address biotechnology innovators who find it challenging to connect, or who simply don't like talking with nonscientific folk. In a few words, get over it. Purposeful networking happens formally and informally for entrepreneurs willing and able to engage. Learn how to have conversations with people who are not scientists and may never have even been in a lab. Engage with people in finance, marketing, and sales. They likely will need high-level, nonscientific explanations of your research and technology, but they will know much more than you do about finance or marketing, personnel matters, culture building, and raising capital and structuring exit strategies. If you can't develop the ability to connect and collaborate with these folks, who often are very different in temperament, process, and mindset from scientists, then find another entrepreneur to start your company and take the role as chief technology officer.

With a networking mindset, you can recognize opportunities for purposeful relationship building every day. Most successful scientists and innovators have collaborated with other scientists. An entrepreneur founding a company can put those same techniques to work in building business relationships and networks that are sticky.

Prebuilt, Organized Support Networks: Build on Connections that Already Exist

With the emphasis on new company startups as a driver of economic growth, most regions have organizations that support new company formations. There are all sorts of ready-built entities and networking points: chambers of commerce, universities, incubators, and organizations responsible specifically for small business or broader economic development. Identify these organizations. Plot a roadmap of these to figure out how your company can benefit from the available programs and services. The more you become comfortable reaching into these groups, the faster you will build the unique foundation of human connections that your company needs.

Many regions these days have an economic development organization at least partially funded by the state. Those entities have teams that connect networks of other people—mentors, service providers, and even sources of capital. If you aren't naturally inclined to network, these intermediaries can make it easier for you with structured settings, receptions, and meeting formats. Some parts of the country even have robust entrepreneurial centers with websites that list the types of advisors that entrepreneurs can access once they become part of that center. For example, Rev1 Ventures' investor startup studio combines capital and strategic services to help startups scale. Our investor studio focuses on four areas that are critical to the business plan milestones that a startup must achieve to succeed. When connecting with entrepreneur centers, accelerators, or incubators in your region, ask about these four types of services which your biotechnology startup will need:

- ***Team***: Building the startup's human capacity through vetted service providers, mentors, or placing new talent;
- ***Connections***: Connecting to corporate partners that can provide market feedback, pilots, contracts, or capital;
- ***Infrastructure***: Shared or full-time office space at the center of the region's startup scene, and
- ***Capital***: A business plan that matches milestones to capital needs that positions the company for investment and then provides access to regional sources of capital.

Many entrepreneur centers serve diverse industries and broad markets as well as a range of entrepreneurs and innovators. Study the organization and decide which services are useful to you and your company and which you can skip.

Begin by setting up a brief 15-minute meeting with the head of the center—the president or the director. Offer a concise synopsis of who you are and the problem that your startup solves. Describe your business briefly and then express interest in how the center can help. The president or director of the place will likely steer you to someone else on the staff for the details or programs and the like, but it is always a good practice to make your initial contact with whoever is in charge.

Once you engage with a support organization, don't kill yourself by going to every meeting or event. Prioritize the time you spend at networking events versus building relationships one-on-one. It's often a matter of attending the next happy hour reception (easier) versus identifying and getting to know individuals who can help address gaps in your knowledge and expertise (requires more forethought and planning). Be targeted. Participate in the right things, not in everything. Pre–proof-of-concept startups don't need to focus on term sheets yet. Do build relationships with an eye to future needs *and* be smart about how you use your time.

Participating in regional support organizations isn't only about receiving, you are also giving back. By getting to know people in the community, you become part of other people's networks. It is a mutually beneficial process of building expertise and relationships that may lead to you becoming a mentor or an advisor with just the expertise that another person needs.

Investors Can Be Sources of Mentoring and Advice Before They Are Sources of Capital

Get to know angels and venture capitalists. Likely, no person understands more about the biotechnology entrepreneurial landscape than the angels and venture capitalists who invest there. Start when the company is at the concept stage, proving your business idea and developing your first business plan. Build relationships with individuals to help you gain access to the sources of equity capital that your business will need 18 to 36 months out. Entrepreneurs may be surprised at investors' willingness to share what they know with attentive and hardworking innovators. Investors, especially those who invest in medical devices or biotechnology, are always interested in scientific discovery. A bioscience entrepreneur may have perspectives and contacts with other scientists or institutions that can help make preinvestment relationships with angels and venture capitalists mutually beneficial.

Biotech entrepreneurs can use relationships with investors to seek advice about investor terms and an exit strategy. Exiting a biotechnology business is complicated and specialized. There are angel groups across the country that specialize in biotech deals. You will find many groups listed on the website of the Angel Capital Association.[5] This site and the site of the Angel Resource Institute[6] also provide extensive resources for entrepreneurs.

Sooner or later, every biotechnology business that survives will raise significant capital. If you have been wisely building connections to the individuals who are in this targeted and narrow industry, you will know how to talk with them. You will understand the vocabulary and common investment terms, and you will be better equipped to approach the capital-raising process with a CEO mentality when your company reaches that stage.

Engage Contacts and Associates at Universities and Research Institutions to Widen your Network

Innovators typically have deeply rooted associations in academic and research communities. These are natural networks for biotechnology entrepreneurs. University TTOs exist to help researchers transfer technologies to the commercial market. These departments strengthen their own networks by linking with alumni networks. Many research universities also have good business schools. More and more of these schools have entrepreneurship programs that extend across disciplines to bring the lesson of entrepreneurship directly into the course of study for science and engineering disciplines. Most entrepreneurship programs involve internships and company case studies. There are all sorts of opportunities for researchers to network with those entrepreneur programs, from engaging an intern, to mentoring student teams in business plan competitions.

Small Business Innovation Research and Small Business Technology Transfer Programs Are Vital Sources of Funding for Prototyping and Commercialization

The importance of the federal government's Small Business Innovation Research (SBIR) and Small Business Technology Transfer (STTR) programs to the landscape of biotechnology startups cannot be overstated. Competing for these awards (which range from $150,000 to millions of dollars) is arduous, but this funding can mean survival to biotechnology seed-stage companies. With at least 17 federal agencies offering this funding, the rules are varied and complex. The thing to remember about the federal government is that technologies cross agency needs. An innovative approach to treating a disease might be of interest to the National Institutes of Health as well as to the Department of Defense.

Winning approval is both science and art. There are multiple constituencies with which to build person-to-person relationships. Sometimes there is state funding for entrepreneurial assistance. Many regional incubators and economic development organizations have contacts and expertise. There are consultants who understand how to improve a company's odds of winning grant funding. An entrepreneur can also reach out to contacts within the agencies themselves. Federal procurement regulations allow you talk to people on the funding side. Their interests and needs are public information. Asking federal program managers to talk about what they are looking for gives the innovator an opportunity to talk about the company's technology and to build contacts and relationships for current and future opportunities.

Associations and Industry Groups Are a Source of Connections and Leadership Opportunities

Professional, industry, and trade associations are a great way to stay connected at a national or even international level with other people and companies in biotechnology and related fields. Associations provide website, event, and meeting access for entrepreneurs. Industry associations can be an avenue to find and forge strategic partnerships—from technical to marketing and distribution—and to seek out referrals for service providers. Serving on a committee or accepting a leadership role provides visibility and public relations (PR) opportunities for the entrepreneur and the company. If the group has a newsletter, volunteer to author an expert article. The trade-off between a more active or passive role is one of time management.

Members of the Media Can Be Your Friends

A startup company doesn't have the budget to pay for advertising or PR, but there are other ways to attract media attention. Local media are always looking for local stories about innovation. Figure out the local publications in your region and state—newspapers, business press, newsletters, and blogs from universities and economic development organizations. Offer your experience as an expert source. Reports are always looking for experts to quote. Sometimes newspapers run innovator awards. Look for those opportunities to get your name and your company name and story out early.

Community Leaders Are Always Seeking the Next Crop of Leaders-to-Be

In every community, there are people already doing the spadework of gathering together those in the region that want to be part of an entrepreneurial ecosystem. In that group, there will be individuals—often highly successful entrepreneurs themselves—who want to give back to fulfill a part of their own personal needs and goals, and who, in so doing, will also receive a benefit from the entrepreneurs they support and mentor. When you do connect with community leaders in meaningful productive ways, it can help in every other area of building relationships.

Networks Are Fluid and Change Over Time

The best human networks are dynamic. They change with different types of talent and different associations as the company gains traction and grows. There will be a small number of people that you will remain in steady contact with over time. You will be in less frequent contact with most others; however, you don't want to lose track of any the valuable contacts you've made.

Set up a system to capture the names and contact information of the people you meet. Obviously, you need an electronic address book to protect and keep backup. Invest time in creating a top-notch LinkedIn profile. The whole idea of networking is to build up your own personal directory of people who can help your business grow. Out of that, the entrepreneur with a fundable business will have the best chance of finding the right kind of resources and funding he or she needs.

Boards of Advisors and Directors Can Help Accelerate Company Success

Building an Advisory Board to Help Your Company in the Early Stages

A board of advisors is a group of at least three, but not more than five people, who you know and trust. Advisors participate at the invitation of the entrepreneur. They are there to provide insight, to offer suggestions, and to serve as a sounding board when you want to talk about a problem or opportunity through. Advisory boards, unlike boards of directors, do not carry legal or fiduciary responsibilities.

When it is time to start forming an advisory board, ask yourself: How do I supplement the skills and talents of my current team with volunteers who have expertise, interest, and are willing to prioritize advising my company for some period of time?

I've always found that entrepreneurs who seek advice *before* they begin asking people to serve as advisors build better boards. There are no hard and fast rules for setting up an advisory board, but here are some guidelines that contribute to a more successful experience for entrepreneur and advisors.

- Decide what kind of help you need from an advisory board. Seek talent, not bulk. If your strong suit is technology, then focus on experts in marketing, finance, or other disciplines where you have little or no experience. Expertise in regulatory considerations is always a plus. It may work well for a bioscience venture to begin with a clinical advisory board of one or two experts and then move into adding business expertise over time. One caution is that it is natural and more comfortable for scientists and researchers to interact with other scientists and researchers. The purpose of advisors is to supplement the knowledge you already have. Don't lose sight of this important principle.
- Have a timeline, but don't be in too much of a hurry to fill out your advisory board. Many successful advisory teams are created one member at a time. A slower approach gives the entrepreneur time to work with members as they come on board and to figure out where the gaps in expertise lie.
- When you talk to people about being advisors to your company, be clear about what you need and expect. Be straightforward about the importance you place on the board. Ask respectfully, *but ask*, if the individual will have the time and interest to participate at the level you anticipate. Ensure that there are no conflicts of interest.
- Choose people who will be able to work together, but resist building a team of people who are too like-minded. Seek a mix of strategic and tactical talent.
- It's logical to draw on your existing pool of mentors as well as professors or academic advisors. These individuals contribute in two possible ways. You may want to ask them to be advisors or you may ask them to suggest others who have the time, interest, and skills that match your needs.
- A bioscience company will benefit from having a recognized authority on the advisory team. A well-known name in the industry adds instant credibility and can open many doors.
- Friends and family members have their place in entrepreneurial ventures, but that place is not on the advisory board. The same is true for employees.

Following a few straightforward operating practices with your advisory board will produce more efficient and effective results as well as help you prepare for working with a formal board of directors if and when that comes about.

- When asking for help from an advisor, be clear about what you need. If you just want to brainstorm a problem or talk to think, frame the discussion that way. Your advisors are busy people. Help them help you by being specific as you can.
- Meet with the advisory board as a whole every quarter or so. These meetings can be face to face, via Skype, or on a conference call.
- Publish an agenda and stick to it. Update the group on company progress, but make the primary focus a time to discuss opportunities or issues to receive the benefit of the board's collective thought. It's your agenda.
- Summarize meeting discussions in advisory board notes. Include action items and owners. Promptly (within the same week) email the notes to board members. Create a follow-up process. Keep a retention file of these notes.
- Provide periodic email communications to keep the advisory board updated on company progress, key milestones, and challenges. Take the appropriate steps to ensure the confidentiality of these communications.
- Consider appropriate compensation for your advisory board. It's tough to pay board advisors when you lack the money to hire employees. There are degrees of compensation that evolve as your company and board evolves, including structured and common methods of providing options for board members that vest over time. Certainly, many advisors want to give back, but if you want to ensure priority and focus, compensation is one tool.
- The company always pays for any expenses the board incurs. That is part of the reason in the beginning to choose people who are local.
- Creating and working with a board of advisors is a great way to learn some things about how to work with a formal board.

The Right Board of Directors Can Help You and Your Company Succeed

Once the corporation has raised external capital, shareholder documents will require the company to have a board of directors. Everything the entrepreneur has learned from building and working with a board of advisors is applicable to working with a board of directors. It doesn't mean that the entrepreneur has learned everything there is to learn—for example, boards of directors have legal responsibilities—but experience with the board of advisors gives a biotechnology entrepreneur a great head start of working with a formal board.

Considerations for Selecting Your Formal Board of Directors

When you secure the first round of equity funding, your investors will require one or two board seats. If you are the founder/CEO, you will take a third. You have the opportunity to exert significant influence over the selection process for the remaining members of your board. When choosing directors, focus on those who have relevant experience. Typically, for a startup, boards of directors have three areas of contribution: (1) to coach, mentor, and, if necessary, fire and replace the CEO; (2) to never let the company run out of cash, and (3) to create and exit strategy that likely involves selling the company.

When it comes to recruiting board members, look for at least a couple of members who have experience on private boards. Being on the board of a public company just isn't the same. The boards of publicly traded companies typically, but not always, do not have to worry about the firm running out of cash. In a startup, that's the primary focus for the first two-to-three years. On the other hand, just because a startup is small doesn't mean that directors' challenges are necessarily less than those that face large company boards.

Extend the culture of inclusion and diversity that you are building in your company to the work you are doing to build your board of directors. Diverse teams drive successful companies. For every 10% increase in racial and ethnic diversity on a senior executive team in the United States, earnings before interest and taxes rise 0.8%. The reverse is also true. Companies that are at the bottom quartile in diversity are 25% less likely than average companies to achieve above-average financial returns.[7] Increasingly, research shows that businesses with women in leadership and on boards of directors perform better than companies that are less diverse.[8] Don't miss the opportunity to gain these benefits in the board room and through the additional connections that diverse board members bring.

Do not build the board with inside staff. Gain the benefit of outside perspectives and expertise. You can include the executive team in the open session of the board meeting. Create opportunities for them to present to the board and to participate in discussions. It's similar to being on the board, just without having a vote.

These guidelines can help make the board of directors experience a good one for your company and for you personally.

- Talk with other CEOs. Ask them how they built their boards. What criteria should you be thinking about?

Use the Internet to gain information and perspective. There is quite a bit of high-quality, easily searchable material on this topic.

- Before you seek additional board members, ensure that the financial and strategic expectations and objectives of the investors (via their representatives on your board), founder, CEO, and any other company officers are fully aligned and communicated.
- Pay particular attention to the exit strategy and also to investors' feelings about the experience and attributes of an operating CEO. In many biotechnology businesses investors recognized that a business-oriented CEO teamed with a founder/chief technology officer makes a more effective management team than one person wearing two or three hats. Understand this reality.
- Be proactive with board selection. Create and prioritize a list of candidates. Discuss these with your investors. Be prepared to talk about the skills you need and why you think these candidates could help the company achieve critical milestones.
- As you build advisory and board relationships, seek people who have relevant experience, especially experience that you don't have yourself. Build a diverse team in terms of professional skills, industry experience, gender, race, culture, etc. Companies with diverse teams and boards get better business results.

Now is the time that the mentoring and advisory relationships you have built so diligently really come into play. Use these human resources to help you figure out what type of expertise you need. What talent, experience, and contacts will complement you and the investor members? Do you need marketing, financial, engineering, or regulatory expertise?

Do you know people you want to ask to join the board, or do you want to use your relationships as a source of recommendations and referrals to people you don't yet know? You may choose to keep your advisory board intact, especially if their expertise is more on the scientific side, or you may choose one of these individuals as a member of your formal board.

- Investors may also require board observer seats. The corporate attorney may also be an observer.
- Whom your board members know can be as important as what they know. Would you benefit from having a board member who knows the industry, perhaps one who has contacts with the companies that could be players in your exit strategy?
- Be wary of egos—especially your own. The folks you will be considering for your board will be confident achievers in their fields. You want people who are able to work collaboratively and who will listen to different perspectives—people who can state their opinions and who also can modify their points-of-view when presented with alternative facts and opinions. Boards are most effective when the members are able to collaborate and work as a team to help the company achieve the key milestones of the business plan.
- Remain coachable. Collectively, your board knows more than you know. They have the power and authority to change your duties and responsibilities.

If your board is required to be a five-to-seven-member team, there will be two-to-four open seats depending on investors' terms. (Keep an odd number of seats on your board and not more than the number required by investment terms or to supply the expertise you need.)

The Role and Responsibilities of Boards of Directors Are Prescribed by Law

Boards of directors' legal responsibilities are very specific. You can and must learn the details of the fiduciary *duties of care and loyalty* from your corporate counsel. Be aware that boards of directors are bound to protect and grow the corporation, act in the corporation's best interest, and never engage in conflict of interest or use information obtained as a director for personal gain.

The board is in place to serve the company. The help that a company needs from the board varies from point to point on the entrepreneurial path. It's important to match the effort to the timing of milestones to be achieved. As the company evolves, the definition of the roles of the board, and for that matter the CEO, will also evolve. Boards are not authorized to sign contracts on behalf of the corporation, but they do elect the corporate officers (this includes you) who then have the responsibility for day-to-day operations of the company. Once you have a formal board, that board has the power to hire and fire the CEO. It is useful in the beginning to document the roles and responsibilities of the CEO and the board. Define which CEO decisions (including dollar limits) require board approval. Define term limits for board members and how the chairperson of the board will be chosen.

Set a Consistent Board Meeting Calendar and Format and Hold to It

Monthly board meetings are common for companies in seed stage to early growth stage. The CEO has the responsibility to set the tone and tempo of board meetings. Talk to your advisory board, other entrepreneurs, mentors, and board members to find out what, in their experience, has been effective. In-person meetings are the best. Convening online may save time and money, but board relationships aren't the place to cut corners. There is so much for the entrepreneur and the business to gain from getting board members together for a period of time to focus entirely on the company.

Invest the appropriate time and focus in preparing for board meetings. The CEO and the board chair should work together to develop meeting agendas. Discuss every topic with every board member ahead of time. Not only will you avoid surprises—which everyone will appreciate—you will also receive valuable feedback that may suggest ways to improve what you are doing (or the way you are doing it) before the meeting takes place.

Don't assume that board members will remember all the details from meeting to meeting. Provide updates. Send out board meeting materials at least two days ahead of the meeting. Include detailed financial information. Boards know how to read financial statements and can do that offline. Limit yourself to one financial chart in the board presentation. Use most of the meeting to talk about challenges and opportunities.

Standardize the format of your communications—board books, financial reports, capitalization table, and requests for grants of equity. As the company develops past the seed stage and adds employees or rewards contributors already on board, you will be requesting equity grants. Create a standard format that includes the capitalization table, whether it has changed or not. Set procedures and consistent report formats facilitate compensation discussions and cause the awarding of grants to proceed more smoothly and efficiently. Board minutes are important. They provide a continuous record of the company and can be used in legal proceedings. Get advice from your corporate counsel, investors, and board members who have served on other boards as to the level of detail.

Include your senior managers in board meetings. This gives the board and your management team an opportunity to get to know each other. The best board meetings are where the internal team can react with outside experts to get other views and advice. Management teams tend to become ingrown and don't always have the benefit of outsiders who have taken different approaches to solving similar problems. You can have a closed executive session to talk about personnel, compensation, or other confidential matters.

Directors' Compensation Usually Takes the Form of Options that Vest Over Time

The company will pay all directors' expenses. To have an engaged and enthusiastic board, the company needs to compensate them. Since cash is so limited, in seed and early stages, a common practice is to award directors with corporate options (typically 0.25% to 1% of outstanding shares), which vest in three-to-five years. Angels and venture capitalists who serve as a requirement of the investment do not receive additional compensation. Clearly define how the options vest. Ensure that the charter of the company defines the limits of the directors' liability. The company must also provide directors and officers liability insurance to protect the participants' assets.

Human Networks Lead to Mentoring

Thinking back over all the entrepreneurs I assisted in the last 20 years, most have one thing in common. They come in the door looking for money. It's the rare person who has said, "I need this kind of business mentoring." Instead, people say, "I'm looking for capital." Human relationships are third, fourth, or tenth on the list.

This is backward. Entrepreneurs need mentoring first; capital comes later. The first thing an entrepreneur needs is mentoring, not money. It is very difficult to start a company. Until they are knee-deep in alligators, most entrepreneurs don't realize how hard founding a business—especially a biotechnology business—actually is. A lot of it you have to learn for yourself, but there's also a lot that you can learn from entrepreneurs who have gone through this before and from experts in fields other than yours.

Overcome any reluctance to ask for help. Don't be afraid to sit down with someone and ask for advice. That's how to build off of what others have built for you. The second step is to map your networking plan, considering the critical milestones that must be achieved at your point on the entrepreneurial path. The more targeted you are on the type of mentoring you need, the greater success you will have in building a strong network to serve you over time. Say you are in the concept stage, still proving feasibility. Wouldn't it be cool to talk to the founder of a company who has been in your shoes? Someone who has done the exact same thing that you are trying to do—someone who has all kinds of life and business experience to help you grow and accelerate your company. That's the kind of thing targeted mentoring can do. However, mentors aren't foolproof. They know a lot, but not everything.

The most productive mentoring relationships are based on common objectives and expectations between mentor and entrepreneur. Mentors will expect entrepreneurs to listen to their advice and be coachable; however, an effective mentor will neither expect an entrepreneur to accept every suggestion nor act on every piece of advice. Mentors guide; they don't control. The best mentors provide information that entrepreneurs can use to make their own decisions about the direction of the company. It's the entrepreneur's day-to-day leadership that makes a company successful.

Just as entrepreneurs benefit from being respectful and engaged listeners themselves, they are best served by seeking out mentors who are good listeners, too.

Sometimes an entrepreneur needs to thoroughly talk through an issue to give a mentor a complete understanding of the challenges the entrepreneur is facing. It's better for the entrepreneur to air the situation thoroughly than to self-edit and omit a critical clue that may seem unimportant to the entrepreneur. When mentors ask questions, it's usually not to second guess. A mentor also needs to be a person who doesn't have an answer for everything. The best mentors are able and willing to say, I don't know. Let's work together to find someone who knows more than we do, someone who can help us out.

When challenges arise—as they certainly will—a mentor can help an entrepreneur prepare options and potential solutions to as a basis for discussion with the company's founding team, advisory board, and/or board of directors. An entrepreneur may find a certain freedom in working out the pros and cons of different scenarios with a trusted mentor.

Mentoring is the meaty part of the human resource network. Mentors provide advice and counsel based on their experience. Mentorships can be formal or informal, structured or casual. With mentors, you are adding to your personal expertise in the core disciplines that provide benefits immediately at the proof-of-concept stage and then carry through as the company progresses along the entrepreneurial path goals.

What Mentoring Does a Bioscience Entrepreneur Need?

Look for mentors who have been mentored themselves and who are motivated to "give back" as well as to share in the challenges and potential success of a startup company. Look for individuals who have experience in the areas where you need help. And don't be totally focused on winners. Entrepreneurs—especially first-time entrepreneurs—benefit from the wisdom of leaders who have failed. As for mentors who have been wildly successful, ask them why. Was it timing, functional expertise, serendipity, or leadership. Just what was their secret sauce? Another tip, if you are serious about gaining the benefits of an inclusive and diverse culture, seek out mentors who are different than you in education, gender, culture, race. For more additional information on the value of mentors, see *Chapter 9: Mentorship: Why You Need a Team of Mentors to be Successful.*

Biotechnology entrepreneurs are likely to benefit from mentoring in these areas:

- ***Company formation***: Entrepreneurs need someone to talk with about early-stage company formation in bioscience from a legal perspective. Should the company organize as a C-corporation or an LLC? What are the advantages and disadvantages of each? What kinds of capital can a bioscience entrepreneur raise and at what stage. Seek out individuals with an understanding of the continuum of capital—from federal grants to angel investment to venture capital (VC) funding. You aren't looking to raise capital at this point, just to understand how the decisions you make early on can affect investors' willingness to invest at a later stage. "I'm not trying to raise capital; I'm trying to learn" can open lots of doors.
- ***CEO perspective***: Most first-time bioscience entrepreneurs lack the CEO perspective, particularly if their formal training has always been in the sciences, and they haven't been to business school. Reach out to other people who have founded startups, especially those who have started more than one company. It's as important to talk to entrepreneurs who have failed as well as those who have achieved success.
- ***Technology experts***: This is the easy one. Scientists usually have their technology networks built out fairly well—sometimes to the extent that they extend far beyond a local region, even to being global. Most innovators are good at this. They understand these relationships—how to build them and how valuable they are. Build on that robust scientific network. How you built that network of technical cohorts can be your personal template for augmenting those incredibly talented people with others who have different expertise.
- ***Legal advice***: Good legal advice is never free and seldom cheap. This is one area where you need to budget early. Buy a few hours of time from an attorney who specializes in advanced technology startups. If the person has experience with biotechnology businesses all the way better, but this isn't a requirement. Sometimes attorneys have special rates for startup companies. Ask around for referrals. Economic development organizations can be a good source of information about people who work with early-stage businesses. Recognize that a biotechnology company will need different legal skills at different stages of development and that not all attorneys are created equal. I've always believed in building a diverse network of legal talent, especially for companies in the biotechnology industry. At a minimum, in addition to corporate counsel, you will need expertise in intellectual property (domestic and international) and in licensing. There is generally an attorney in every family. This is the attorney you should *not* use for legal advice. You can use family-member attorneys as business advisors and mentors, for referrals, or to point you in the right direction, but resist asking them for legal counsel.
- ***Talent acquisition and retention***: Limited time and lack of funds are a battle for startups—especially when it comes to acquiring talent. Most early-stage

companies don't have the budget to pay a recruiter, yet startups cannot rely entirely on online job boards to connect to the talent they need. Do not operate in a vacuum. Talk to everyone in your network—people you know from research institutions, your advisors, mentors, neighbors, your banker, attorney, anyone that you have a relationship with. Make sure they understand the skills you are seeking. Professional recruiters will tell you that many, many jobs are filled by candidates who are friends of friends who are hiring. Consider partnering with a university system to set up an internship that could turn into a full-time position. If you are looking for technologists (or will be) become a regular at software development or programming meetups. If you are looking for scientists, search for chief investigators and teams who are published in your area of discovery. List open positions on the free job boards in your area. Resist pigeonholing candidates based on appearance, alma maters, or prior jobs. Inclusive cultures are an excellent recruiting advantage, but to diversify, biotechnology entrepreneurs must reach beyond their usual networks. Compared to overall private industry, the high-tech sector employs a larger share of whites (68.5%) and men (64%).[9] Women make up 47% of the US workforce, yet represent only 26% of the people who work in STEM (science, technology, engineering, and math).[10] Deliberately expand access and networks to include organizations where women and minorities are. Build partnerships with grassroots organizations, such as i.c. stars, Bunker Labs, Venture for America, or Women for Economic and Leadership Development.

- ***Tactical financial*:** The single biggest problem that entrepreneurs face is running out of cash. Tactical financial mentoring can help you figure out how to make the money you have stretch as far as possible. For this, talk to entrepreneurs who have weathered the gap between proof-of-concept and Series A investment. Find out how they did it. From Skyping instead of traveling, to sharing office space, to stretching out the life of laptops and servers, talking to those who have done it will yield lots of useful ideas.
- ***Strategic financial*:** Every new business requires a capital strategy and plan. As a starting point, turn to the organizations in your region with services to support entrepreneurs. You will learn the vocabulary of capital markets and the sources and stages of capital that match the milestones in the entrepreneur's path. Work through your mentors, professors, and other contacts to meet angel investors—not to pitch your company, but to learn about the mindset of angels who invest in biotech.
- ***SBIR/STTR awards*:** There are companies in every state who have been successful with SBIR/STTRs. Seek them out. There are national consultants who are experts at developing SBIR/STTR proposals. Even if the company won't reach the grant-writing stage for months, we recommend seeking referrals and then talking to one or two of these specialists—even if you have to pay for their time. They can help you plan and structure your trials and reports to best match the information that agencies will require. The results of the trials will be the results, but agencies are very specific about the information they require and the formatting of that information. Compliance is usually straightforward—as long as the entrepreneur understands the requirements before trials start.
- ***Regulatory*:** Getting drugs and diagnostics to market requires an understanding of the legal and regulatory environment. University TTOs, research institutions, and individual innovators are all excellent sources of mentoring on how to manage the FDA process. It's important to speak to experts *before* you structure experiments and studies to ensure that the methods you employ and the way you structure the reporting of outcomes are synchronous with the requirements of the regulatory bodies you aim to convince.
- ***Business development and marketing*:** This is the Achilles heel for many innovators. Most have little experience in marketing and zero experience in sales. Yet these functions are the lifeblood of any successful company. Don't fall into the trap of thinking that the founder/innovator's job is only the science. While the company may literally be years away from business development and marketing, thinking about potential customers and markets, the problems they have that need solution, and about what the competition is doing or might do in the future—all these considerations help define the most appropriate commercialization path and help the innovator develop a mindset of application as well as research.
- ***Exit strategy*:** It may sound like strange advice to suggest that a bioscience entrepreneur who is thinking about starting a company also think about "ending" it, but that's what you must do. Because of the enormous investment required to bring medical innovations to the marketplace, successful bioscience startups are almost always acquired, so you want to anticipate that from the start. Biotechnology business models are well understood in the marketplace; however, there are also lots of subtleties. There may be angel investors in your region who specialize in bioscience. Ask them how they help their portfolio companies plan exit strategies. Ask them how you can learn the ropes.

Informal human networks can help you build the business in early stages, and you don't have to give up equity. At the proof-of-concept and seed stages, as the company progresses along the entrepreneurial path and you become engaged in the community, meet people, and interact with some of them as mentors, you might be ready for a more formal structure. Multiple heads are always better than one. The entrepreneur's goal: close and trusted working relationships that help the company achieve the milestones of the entrepreneur's path.

Personal Traits and Characteristics

All effective relationships are built on trust and mutual respect. In the entrepreneurial world, there is an extra something in the mix—the excitement that comes with invention, discovery, and building a whole business around the innovation of a new idea.

Do not be afraid to sit down with business people to brainstorm challenges or ask for advice. Start by talking with other entrepreneurs. They will be the easiest to reach; most will be empathetic. They've been where you are and have done what you are trying to do. They know how hard it is, and as a group are very willing to help the next entrepreneur.

It's easier to build relationships with individuals who are in close proximity. Start out by relationships that are within arms' reach. These will form the foundation of your network. Building a human network is a lot like building a house; if you have strong foundation, you can do a lot to that structure over the years. Networks are like that. Build them in layers.

Relationship building comes naturally to many entrepreneurs. For others, it is a learned skill. Either way, certain attitudes and behaviors foster relationships that can be as valuable to a company as assets on a balance sheet. Other traits can derail the best-intended connections between human beings, which are as follows:

- Operate with complete integrity. Follow the intent as well as the letter of the law. Match your words and deeds.
- Respect others, from the small to the large. Do what you say you will do. Be timely for meetings and with any other follow-up. Keep confidences.
- Remain coachable. Don't wait until you need to ask for help. Listen, especially when your first instinct is to disagree. Be willing to change your mind, say you were wrong, or stand your ground.
- Reciprocate. Give back to the relationship—in appreciation and expertise. There will always be entrepreneurs coming along behind you. Do for them what others did for you.
- Collaboration is the secret sauce of mutually beneficial relationships. Learn to work with others. Give credit where credit is due.

Conclusion

Purposeful and productive business relationships are assets that don't appear on the balance sheet. Formal and informal networks can help the entrepreneur grow the company. Even if the venture doesn't succeed, well-founded, purposeful business relationships endure.

The innovator's mantra of relationships is as follows:

1. I can't build a successful company without help.
2. Commercialization and science are two entirely different disciplines.
3. The attributes, skills, and experience that make me good at science may make me to be less effective in other disciplines.
4. There are many people with all kinds of experience and skill who are eagerly available to help entrepreneurs.
5. I can't count on the scientific method when it comes to building relationships with other human beings. I must learn new techniques.
6. It's my job to find mentors and advisors, meet them, and then demonstrate that I and my company are worthy of their attention and assistance.
7. I will be coachable and listen to what mentors and advisors have to say, recognizing that while I may be an expert in my field, great science is only the first step in great company formation.

Building and nurturing purposeful, diverse relationships is a critical success factor for becoming a successful entrepreneur. The benefits are enormous—from coaching and mentoring that money can't buy, to ensuring friendships that evolve and endure far beyond capital rounds, product launches, and profitable exits.

Anyone who has an interest in problem-solving, a thirst for learning, and a passion for his or her business can become a builder of meaningful relationships. I know because I've seen dozens and dozens of scientists and researchers do it successfully year after year.

Endnotes

1. Hunt V, Layton D, Prince S. Diversity matters. McKinsey & Company. <http://www.mckinsey.com/business-functions/organization/our-insights/why-diversity-matters>; 2015 [accessed 30.11.18].
2. Hunt V, Layton D, Prince S. Diversity matters. McKinsey & Company. <http://www.mckinsey.com/business-functions/organization/our-insights/why-diversity-matters>; 2015 [accessed 30.11.18].

3. Hunt V, Layton D, Prince S. Diversity matters. McKinsey & Company. <http://www.mckinsey.com/business-functions/organization/our-insights/why-diversity-matters>; 2015 [accessed 30.11.18].
4. Rev1 Ventures. Inclusive entrepreneurship: growing the startup economy through the power of inclusive entrepreneurship. <https://www.rev1ventures.com/entrepreneurs/inclusive-entrepreneurship/>; 2017 [accessed 30.11.18].
5. https://www.angelcapitalassociation.org.
6. https://www.angelresourceinstitute.org.
7. Hunt.
8. Burns J. The results are in: women are great for business, but still getting pushed out. Forbes September 22, 2017. <https://www.forbes.com/sites/janetwburns/2017/09/22/2016-proved-women-are-great-for-business-yet-still-being-pushed-out/#441c9b4b188b> [accessed 16.11.18].
9. U.S. Equal Employment Opportunity Commission. Diversity in high tech. U.S. Equal Employment Opportunity Commission. <https://www.eeoc.gov/eeoc/statistics/reports/hightech/> [accessed 30.11.18].
10. Pittman O. 7 Organizations working to promote women in STEM. College Raptor®. <https://www.collegeraptor.com/find-colleges/articles/college-majors-minors/7-organizations-working-to-promote-women-in-stem/>; 2018 [accessed 30.11.18].

Chapter 9

Mentorship: Why You Need a Team of Mentors to be Successful

Craig Shimasaki, PhD, MBA

CEO, BioSource Consulting Group and Moleculera Labs, Oklahoma City, OK, United States

Chapter Outline

One of the most critical, but least emphasized, factors for entrepreneurial leaders in becoming successful are multiple formal relationships with experienced individuals who have succeeded in doing what you want to accomplish. This chapter explains the value of mentors, the characteristics of good mentors, and how to engage them to help you in your success. Merriam-Webster defines "mentor" as a "trusted counselor or guide" or "tutor or coach." These are good definitions of mentors, but to an entrepreneurial leader, mentors are more than that. Mentors are individuals who inspire us to press forward even when circumstances appear difficult and the outlook seems grim. Mentors are individuals who unreservedly communicate the hard truths and tell us things we may not want to hear, but these are the things we know we need to be told. They identify our blind spots and share advice on how to keep these from negatively impacting our business or product development progress.

Throughout this chapter, I will refer to a "mentor" and "mentee." The term "mentee" is simply a generic reference to the person who is counseled, trained, and guided by a mentor. This *mentor–mentee* role is similar to a *coach–athlete* relationship or a *teacher–student* relationship in which we are readily familiar. However, there are differences in the mentor–mentee relationship that I will share with you as compared to these traditional examples. Without a doubt, you have heard inspirational stories of athletes who eulogize the impact their coaches had on their lives. One example is the legacy of Coach John Wooden who encouraged, challenged, and touched the lives of so many successful athletes and affected their lives in areas other than just sports.[1] Unfortunately, we also hear of negative experiences in these interactions, and consequently, this may inhibit our pursuit of mentorship relationships. We may shy away from mentoring influences altogether because we may incorrectly view this relationship as a taskmaster yoking us with a long list of impossible assignments in order to become a "Jedi Knight" under someone's demanding Yoda-type tutelage. A good mentor–mentee relationship is nothing comparable to this, but is the natural outcome of a learning and teaching trust relationship between an experienced individual and someone who is eager to learn.

The purpose of this chapter is to share with you the significance and value of purposely seeking and building good mentor relationships. These connections will be valuable to your overall success and will help you avoid potentially disastrous consequences. Choosing good mentors is vital to a successful career outcome, as you need individuals who have been there and done that, and know

1. Book: "Wooden: A Lifetime of Observations and Reflections On and Off the Court."

Biotechnology Entrepreneurship. DOI: https://doi.org/10.1016/B978-0-12-815585-1.00009-7

where the pitfalls are and the hidden "land mines" are buried. Remember the unknown—unknowns we discussed in *Chapter 1: What is Biotechnology Entrepreneurship?* Experienced mentors typically have encountered something very similar in their journey. I am a strong advocate of learning by reading books written by experts, but experience is an irreplaceable asset, and it is best shared in a two-way relationship.

Why do you Need Mentors?

Although you may have the technical and/or academic skills which make you very experienced in your field of study, mentors provide practical wisdom and can share consequences of decisions that can occur based upon their cumulative real-life experiences. Sometimes, just living longer and witnessing the cause and effect of decisions over time in an industry, yield advice that cannot be reproduced completely by textbook learning or cognitive reasoning. The quotation by Isaac Newton "*If I have seen a little further, it is by standing on the shoulders of Giants.*" is a good reference to the value of mentors. An earlier version of this phrase came from the 12th century theologian and author John of Salisbury in an 1159 Latin treatise called *Metalogicon.* One of the translations reads "*We are like dwarfs sitting on the shoulders of giants. We see more, and things that are more distant, than they did, not because our sight is superior or because we are taller than they, but because they raise us up, and by their great stature add to ours.*" The value of a good mentor is that they can enhance your capabilities such that you accomplish more than you could without their input.

How is it that Good Mentors Help You?

The basic process of mentorship occurs continuously throughout our lives and can be more broadly defined as any "influence" on our thinking about circumstances, events, and our beliefs. Whether or not we realize it, we are *informally* influenced by the books and magazines we read, the programs and events we watch, and the people with whom we have relationships and associate. But mentorship is a *purposeful* influence, in that we seek to be influenced by select individuals for their wisdom, experience, and knowledge in a two-way relationship through communication about issues we face. One who seeks out good mentors and purposefully gains from these relationships is a person who will advance in wisdom and one who models themselves after the proverb "*Where no counsel is, the people fall: but in the multitude of counselors there is safety.*" If you recognize that your thoughts and beliefs are constantly influenced by individuals, books, and events, you can purposefully enrich your life through those individuals and events that aid you in becoming successful.

One quote that I need to remind myself of more often is "*Learn from the mistakes of others, because you will never live long enough to make them all yourself.*" Often, I wonder if I have been the one that others can learn from my mistakes. Although I personally was not fortunate enough to know about engaging in formal mentoring relationships, I wish I would have understood this principle earlier as there were individuals in my life whom I learned from by observing, both good and bad events and outcomes. Learning by observation is also a wonderful teacher, but observation alone does not give you enough information about the issues, the decisions, and the motivation for these choices. You will be well served by making mentorship a way of life in your career, and these relationships will be invaluable to you for life lessons in other ways such as non-business relationships, marriage, finances, parenting, and many other aspects of life that are enriched by experience.

So, how can mentors help you? Good mentors can recognize your blind spots; things that you cannot see in your actions or character that is detrimental to your success. Good mentors provide encouragement when you encounter challenges and are short on motivation. Good mentors can connect you with other individuals in their network who can address specific problems in which you need specific answers. Good mentors share their experiences, so you can learn from their mistakes. Good mentors can be a sounding board for ideas and strategies before you move in different and strategic directions. Often, mentors can provide you with information that reveals an option you did not know existed. Good mentors can also hold you accountable for the things you said you would do. Mentors can give you an unbiased and external point of view which is something you may not always get from your employees, your board members, your investors, your service providers, or even your family.

What Would Keep you From Finding a Mentor?

For those who are new to the mentoring process, you may be reticent to show you are vulnerable or appear like you do not know what you are doing or know where you are going... but isn't this the truth? Resistance to appearing vulnerable can be a key reason why many individuals may avoid mentoring relationships. Mentorship may appear to be a dichotomy to entrepreneurs, simply because entrepreneurs have been trained to do everything themselves so they can survive until they can afford to hire help. In addition, entrepreneurs must possess a heavy dose of self-confidence in order to be perseverant, and they learn to be decent problem-solvers as they must figure out solutions to unanticipated challenges along the way. Seemingly contrary to this, in order to be a mentee, it requires that you internally acknowledge that you do not know all the answers, and you need help from others. This adjustment in thinking may appear to be a contradiction in the definition of an entrepreneur. In reality, this is not incongruent with true entrepreneurship, but it is an issue that must be resolved in order to gain the most value from a mentoring relationship. If you find that this is difficult, then it may be mostly an issue of pride. I admit that acknowledging to others you don't know something can seem humbling at first, especially for those who are experts in their fields of study and are used to having others come to you for information and help with their work. Realize that a successful entrepreneur is one who possesses subject matter expertise but does not let that interfere with their ability to learn from others about the things they do not know. A good way to learn to overcome this aversion in seeking help is to become comfortable asking questions from others, then finding value in the things you learn from them. The more you become comfortable with asking what may seem to be "dumb" questions, the more you will become comfortable with receiving information from literally anyone. One introductory point I repeatedly emphasize with my students in the Entrepreneurship Program at the University of Oklahoma is, the only "dumb" questions are the ones that everyone is thinking but no one is brave enough to ask. I teach students to purposefully interact with, and strike up conversations with someone in an industry they know nothing about. We encourage them to learn to ask questions about the issues these experts face and how things work in their industry. During this exchange, they learn about problems in other industries, methods for solving problems, and often these methods are portable to solve problems in a totally different industry. Those who know how to ask questions are people who can carry on a conversation with anyone, in any field, and on any subject, who will always be adding to their knowledge base and learning new ways to solve problems.

What to Look for in a Good Mentor?

Finding a good mentor is not as easy as it one may think. First of all, not everyone with experience would be a good mentor, just like not every great athlete will be a good coach. You should have many types of mentors, and one type of mentor should be someone with subject matter experience in your industry. Another type of mentor is someone with expertise in another industry who can give you some fresh ideas on solving problems that you did not think about. You should try to find someone in the biotechnology or life sciences industry who has decades of experience and has built or run biotech companies successfully. Because our industry is not historically old enough, we do not have masses of experienced mentors as is the case in other industries that have long histories such as the banking industry and the oil and gas industry. Other types of mentors are those who have built and run a successful company, someone who is responsible for the direction of an organization, responsible for meeting payroll, and having to solve business and personnel issues, as they will give you great insights. If they have built an organization and operated it successfully, sometimes individuals who are service providers to the biotechnology and life science industry may also be helpful mentors. However, recognize that it is also possible that some individuals who own service companies may have a strong interest in directing you toward their services. It does not mean that they cannot be objective; it is just important that you and your mentor discuss this topic before working together and taking their advice.

Ultimately, you want to identify individuals you trust, and those who you know truly have your best interest in mind. Someone who is knowledgeable and experienced in the area you are interested in, compassionate and caring about your success. You also want to work with someone in whom you feel comfortable and can talk with openly and candidly without fear of judgment or negative criticism. If you do not have that level of confidence in a relationship, you will be on your guard about sharing the real issues that you are dealing with in your organization. In this working relationship you need to have mutual respect, that the mentor has respect for you and what you are doing, and you have respect for what they have done and how they have accomplished their success. The mentors you choose should be individuals who are candid about telling you what you *need* to hear and not what you *want* to hear. Be sure to identify someone who is a good listener, as they have to understand what you are asking and doing before they can give advice. Avoid individuals who don't listen well and answer things before they understand what was being said. Below I have listed a number of characteristics I would recommend that you look for in a good mentor.

Characteristics to look for in a good mentor

- An individual that you trust, as this is a key characteristic of a mentorship relationship
- Someone you believe truly has your best interest in mind and does not see you as a potential customer for their business
- An individual who is knowledgeable and experienced in the segment of business or technology you are interested in learning from
- Someone who cares about your success
- Someone you feel comfortable around and with whom you can talk openly and candidly without fear of judgment or negative criticism

(Continued)

(Continued)

- Sharing a two-way relationship of mutual respect, that the mentor has respect for you and what you are doing, and you have respect for what they have done and how they have accomplished their success
- Someone who will be candid about telling you what you need to hear and not what you want to hear
- Someone who is a good listener. Avoid individuals who don't listen well and answer things before the understand what was being said

As you look at this list of recommended qualifications for good mentors, you likely will not know many individuals with *all* these characteristics. If you do, they are likely very busy and have others that they mentor already. Therefore you should find the key characteristics that you value in individuals and realize that you can learn something from everyone. Just be purposeful about choosing what it is that you want to learn from each individual.

Where to Find a Good Mentor?

Good mentors do not advertise and are busy individuals; therefore knowing how to find good mentors is important if you want to enrich your life through these relationships. Similar to when you buy a new car, it is astonishing how you notice that so many other people have purchased the same make and model, *after* you have purchased yours. When you look for potential mentors with these character qualities, you will be amazed that you may recognize several potential mentors in your current circle of interactions. Remember that mentors arise from relationships and common interests; therefore some of these individuals can be found from settings such as

- biotech or medical science networking events,
- various programs supported by universities and educational institutions,
- community or chamber of commerce events,
- nonprofit functions and societies,
- religious events or meetings,
- volunteer programs in the community, and
- entrepreneurship society meetings.

There are other ways to find mentors, but the key is to look for them within the social, public, business and industry events that you may already attend.

How to Scare off a Good Mentor?

The best way to be sure you will *not* have a mentor is to evaluate people, then pick the best one you want to be your mentor, then ask them the question "*will you be my mentor?*" This is a sure process that will scare good people off. Engaging someone to be a mentor is something that actually begins through a relationship and mutual connection to each other through events or associations, and is built over time until there is trust and comfort in the relationship. In some circumstances, calling someone your "mentor" or having them agree to be your "mentor" can be a title that may cause them concern about an unusual time commitment with someone they don't know very well. Unless you are in a formal mentorship program, or the person you want help from is not concerned about being called "your mentor," it may be best to refer to them as *trusted advisors* or someone who is helping you solve specific issues or problems that they have experience with. For busy executives, in their own mind there can be negative connotations about being a "mentor." In reality, you are simply having an ongoing and continuous dialog with an expert who is helping you solve issues over time.

You Need Different Mentors for Diverse Types of Assistance

I liken biotechnology companies to the melding of business and biology, which results in a business of uncertainty. Because you will never know all the answers, let alone know all the problems that you may encounter, you need help from those with experience There are individuals who have expertise in various aspects of what you will encounter and you will likely need many mentors that span different areas. These diverse types of mentors may include

- individuals with strategic and tactical knowledge in your industry,
- persons that can help with personal and motivational support,
- individuals strong in business leadership regardless of industry background,
- persons with sales and market or business development expertise,
- individuals with great interpersonal understanding in handling employee issues and culture building,
- persons with scientific knowledge in translating ideas and discoveries into commercial products,
- individuals with knowledge in raising capital and working with institutional investors, and
- persons with experience in reaching an exit and how to structure the deal.

It would be unrealistic to simultaneously have four to six mentors spanning different topics because you would not have time to do the work or follow up on the recommendations by all these mentors. You are best served by having a least one mentor who is experienced in the area that you are immediately dealing with in your organization or product development. For instance, if you are in the midst of raising your first round of capital, you would not want to be spending a lot of time in a mentoring relationship with someone who is an expert on building sales teams and business development. You should have mentors that fill a current or immediate need that you are dealing with at that time. Once you have accomplished that objective or satisfactorily overcome that particular issue, you can identify other mentors for other aspects of business, science, or corporate development for your company. It may seem impossible to think you can identify good mentorship guidance at the precise time that you need it for the various issues you face. However, you will find that when you are open to these relationships, and you are looking for them, you will be surprised to find that they are there.

The Mentoring Processes: How Does it Work?

The process of mentorship is a valuable exercise in itself. In many instances, the simple practice of verbalizing the details of key issues and dialoguing with others provides an opportunity for you to verbalize your own thoughts on the subject, which you may not have already done. Often this process brings clarity as you may not have verbalized the issues you are facing in a succinct manner and in a way that is understandable by others. I have seen on more than a few occasions that the entrepreneur has a "light bulb" moment after articulating the issue and fielding clarifying questions from the mentors. They somehow begin to understand what they need to do and often have formulated an answer which is solidified by further discussion with the mentors.

Before you embark on a mentorship relationship, you need to ask yourself the following questions:

- What do you want, or what are you looking for from this particular mentorship relationship?
- What do you want to learn from this person?
- What are the specific issues that you are struggling with and need help with?

The most common forum for mentoring is a formal face-to-face meeting. Prior to your mentor meeting you need to identify a specific issue or two that you want the mentor(s) to address and help you with. The mentoring session should revolve around solving or addressing the issue you have identified and verbalized. During this meeting, you should spend time answering clarifying questions that the mentor may ask so they can better understand the context of the issue and what things have been tried and what were the results. You should also give any background information such as restrictions that make some options not be available to you.

You should ask the mentor for their thoughts on the situation and if they have any suggestions on how to deal with this issue. One thing is sure, when you ask someone for their opinion about a topic that is in their area of expertise, you will get feedback. It is important that you *do not* dismiss any potential solutions being offered by your mentor. You should work through their thought process as if it is a "brainstorming" session, and see where it takes you during the interaction. Sometimes, just the discussion of options can help you clarify in your own mind what you need to do or what action you need to take. During your mentoring session, you should also ask if they have any contacts that they can put you in touch with, that could help with any of the tasks that are recommended by the mentor. Continue the dialog until it seems as if all the thoughts and options have been discussed or exhausted. Sometimes, these sessions are open-ended, and time is the constraint rather than exhausting things to discuss. Be mindful of the mentor's time and if there is a set time allotted for the meeting, do not go over that time limit. Mentors will be more willing to meet with you again if you honor and respect their time commitments.

Before your mentoring meeting is concluded, summarize the points or action items to the mentor to be sure that you have clearly understood the information and advice given to you. During the session, be sure to write down the advice as it is being given and repeat any information that may be unclear. In this way, your mentor also sees that you have listened to what they have said and made a commitment to follow up with these suggestions. Also, set yourself a date by which to have these action items completed. This is critical because without a due date, it is only an intention and not a measurable objective. By assigning dates to accomplish tasks, this will allow the mentor to follow up with you and hold you accountable for the things to want to get done. Basically, you want to share with them your plan of action of what you intend to do, and a date in which you commit to accomplish these tasks or action items.

Within a few days after your meeting, follow up with them by email, or whatever communication method is appropriate, about the results and the status of your progress toward resolution of the issue you were both discussing. Make sure that you understand it is your responsibility to keep your mentor updated and to have specific questions you want answers and help with. Be sure you value their time and be prepared, and they will want to continue to work with you. Remember that good mentors are very busy so respect their time. It is also good to think of ways to give back to your mentors. Thank them for specific things that they taught you that were of value to you. Although true mentorship is

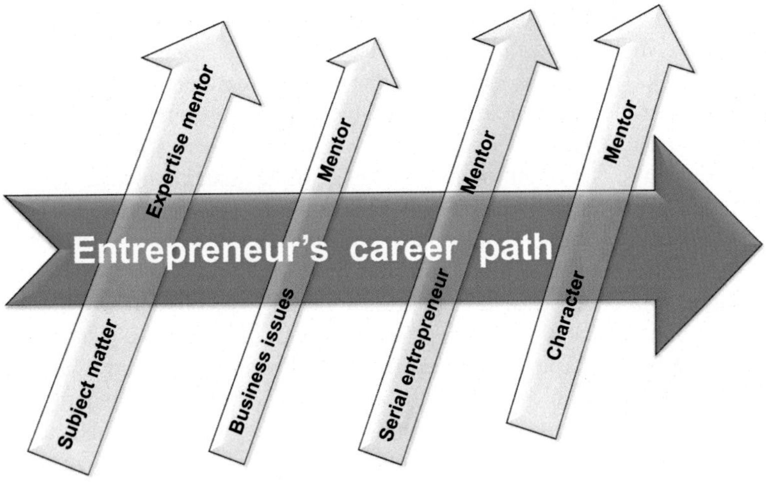

FIGURE 9.1 Illustration of how you should seek to have diverse mentors cross your career path over time.

technically free, you should expect to reciprocate, if not to them, to others that you can help in the future.

The image in Fig. 9.1 illustrates the concept that your career path should intersect with multiple mentors with expertise and experience in multiple areas. Over time you will intersect with many of them, who through their advice, guidance, and helpful prodding will enhance and expand your career path toward success. It is good to have multiple mentors to call upon because mentors are individuals with their own biases that influence their advice. When a mentee has several separate one-on-one mentors meetings, there arises the possibility that they may hear conflicting advice based upon the opinions of two different people, and the mentee will have to sort through the conflict. This is not always the case, but it is something to be aware of when seeking advice from several mentors individually. This is why a team mentoring program is an advantage when they are available.

Some Formal Mentorship Programs

Up to this point I have mostly been discussing one-on-one mentorship relationships, in which two individuals (mentor and mentee) establish a relationship and there is candid sharing of issues and solutions on an "as needed" basis. You should work to take advantage of as many of these individual mentorship opportunities as you can. For those who are fortunate enough to reside near an organization that has a formal mentorship program, you should take advantage of these when they are available. These programs typically have a formalized mentoring process, as well as a pool of qualified mentors who are able and willing to help. Recognize that not all mentorship programs are created equal and not all programs have subject matter expertise that can help a biotechnology entrepreneur with the technical details of their business. Most all these programs typically have excellent business and general entrepreneurship mentors who can help with these aspects of building a successful business. Most of these programs are nonprofit businesses and may not charge any fees, and mentors are volunteers. Because of this, you may not find extensive advertising about these programs, and there may be a selection process for mentees. Many universities have mentorship programs, so if you are affiliated with one, look to see if there is one that you can take advantage of in your area.

In Oklahoma, we are fortunate to have a couple of different types of mentorship programs. Each of these was started with the goal of supporting local entrepreneurs in their quest to be successful. One such program is called Oklahoma Entrepreneur Mentoring Program that is a licensed model from the Massachusetts Institute of Technology, Venture Mentoring Service (MIT VMS), a nonprofit organization affiliated with MIT and based in Cambridge, Massachusetts. This mentorship model began as a program serving the needs of MIT students and is now being used in over 80 different regions, institutions, states, and countries. It is a unique team-mentoring methodology with a strict code of ethics to assure objective, conflict-free, and confidential advice. They have developed a best practices model for recruiting, training, and retaining a community of highly qualified and committed volunteer mentors, with a formal operational processes and key focus on the entrepreneur. For more information on the MIT VMS model and its licensed locations, check their website at http://vms.mit.edu/home. One of the key elements of MIT VMS mentoring program is that mentoring session occurs in teams in which multiple mentors are present together in the same room during a session, and they address together the issue(s) that the entrepreneur has selected to be discussed. The opportunity to have a team of mentors discussing solutions to your issue often results in advice that is different from what any one mentor would have shared by themselves. I like what the team-mentoring approach brings to the mentee, in that the mentors, usually three or four, listen to each other and often the advice given to the entrepreneur results from an amalgam of the combined thoughts of all the mentors based upon hearing each others' personal opinion. The camaraderie that occurs in the team-mentoring process is energizing and informative for the mentors as they can interact, dialog, and learn from each other.

Another mentorship opportunity you may have available is through a technology commercialization center in your state, city or region, that provides assistance to local entrepreneurs and companies. Most cities, regions, locales have a vested interest in supporting the organic growth of economic development through local entrepreneurship. These entities are often nonprofit or government agencies whose mission is to foster entrepreneurial and economic development in your locale. In Oklahoma, we have two such agencies that work in tandem to provide competitive grant support for ideas and projects that could become high-tech products or services in the future (OCAST), and a commercialization center and venture funding source to assist with the development of these companies (i2E). Through these two government and nonprofit entities, scientists, engineers, physicians, and technical persons can win grants to help advance their projects into potential commercial products. Then, i2E can assist with mentorship programs, seed, and early-stage funding for feasibility and development capital for launching high-growth companies. Talk with those types of agencies in your locale, as you may be surprised to find that there are many opportunities you can take advantage of for mentoring help.

Other Ways to Get Mentorship Help

In addition to finding and recruiting individual mentors, there are other ways in which you can get insight and valuable advice from seasoned and experienced individuals. One way is to join a CEO peer advisory group such as Vistage, https://www.vistage.com. This is an international organization with CEO peer advisory groups located in many cities and countries around the world that meet monthly to exchange ideas, process issues, and listen to business experts. Vistage is an international organization in over 20 countries, with over 60 years of history and over 23,000 members. Although there may not be a "biotechnology" group per se in your area, these advisory groups typically comprise small-to-medium-sized company CEOs who are business owners and have dealt with various issues that you will find familiar in your organization. I have found that having CEO peers to listen to, and process issues with, is a valuable experience and provides insight into solutions that you may not have thought of previously. The Vistage issue processing method is helpful for entrepreneurs to practice as it allows them to frame a problem that they may not have been able to articulate previously. In a Vistage meeting session, when someone brings an issue to the table, the chairperson asks them to present the problem and state it as a "how do I?" question, After the "how do I?" question is stated, the person elaborates more on the specific issue by answering as many of the following:

- The issue/opportunity is . . .
- It is important because . . .
- My goal is . . .
- Relevant background information is . . .
- The options I have considered are . . .
- I am afraid that . . .
- The help I would like from the group is . . .

Once the issue is framed and the background information is presented, the members can only ask clarifying questions and cannot give any advice or suggestions. This prevents the "jump to conclusions" response until peer CEOs better understand the particular situation, the things that have been tried, and the reasons some actions have been avoided. I find that this process, when adhered to, provides great counsel and good ideas for options in which one or more will resonate as a viable solution to the issue or challenge faced.

What Mentors Cannot do for you?

One should never forget that a mentor is not a replacement for you making your own decisions. You should utilize mentors to help provide options for arriving at the best decision for your situation. Also realize that mentors provide information from their frame of reference, from their own individual experiences, and based upon their own core values. If you have not found this out already, you will soon find that the advice of some mentors will conflict with the advice of other mentors. This is a reminder that you are the ultimate decider of which direction you move in, and what actions you take. Mentors simply give you a perspective that you may not have considered, or they helped you become aware of risks that you may not have known. Obviously, mentors having many years of experience in the same situation and the same industry as you, can give you some worthy guidance, but remember that situations are not always identical, and the impact on others may not always be similar. You must weigh the options and make decisions based upon all the input from your mentors and choose the best path for your organization. Remember that mentoring is a two-way relationship, and it is important to provide some value to the mentor for giving of their time and sharing of their experiences with you.

For Those Considering Being a Mentor

If you are looking for a mentor, you may find these recommendations to mentors helpful to know. Some interesting results from 100 respondents to mentorship for tech startup in the San Francisco Bay area are listed in this website by First Company[2]:

They suggested that mentors should ask themselves:

- Can I clearly be helpful to this potential mentee? Have they reached out with clear reasons or intentions for why they'd like my help? Are there specific needs they have that I can address?
- Can this person be completely open and honest? Are they willing to provide deep context about their problems and vulnerabilities? Will they be able to share data, metrics, goals, slide decks, etc. that will help in the process?
- Is this person prepared? Do they tend to be proactive about setting up time and providing enough contexts or an agenda upfront? Do they direct conversations and ask specific questions? (Be wary of people who want more general help or to touch base without a topic in mind.)
- Does this person give me energy? Do I usually learn things from this person myself? Does talking to them allow me to reflect differently on my own business or path? Has talking to them in the past felt like a good use of time? Do they inspire me to think more deeply, even though they have less experience?

They suggested for mentees to ask themselves:

- Does this potential mentor remember key details about me? Have you had to continuously repeat yourself or remind them about who you are or the context of your job every time you see them? This doesn't bode well.
- Will it be hard to explain the concepts or context of my job? You should choose someone who is close enough to your industry and functional area so that very quick, even shorthand explanations, will do, and they can immediately dive in and understand your primary challenges and goals.
- Can this person give actionable advice? Have they told you something in the past that you've been able to apply right away? Are they a good teacher? Do they share tactics, or do they generalize? If they don't recommend specific actions to take, then pause. They might be too senior and removed from the day-to-day work. You might be better off with a skip-level above you than an executive.

Summary

Good mentors are vital to a biotech entrepreneur's success. Good mentors may or may not be in any mentoring relationships, but if you ask, they typically are willing to respond with help and advice. The mentor–mentee relationship is formed from existing common interests and a connection that has been built upon trust. For entrepreneurs, there are so many unknown–unknowns that you are best served by seeking out and learning from others in an informal or formalized program of mentorship. Remember that a key to receiving the most out of a mentoring relationship is to have a key issue that you have identified you want to solve and receive input, and always follow up with your mentor about your outcome or results. Also remember that mentors are doing something very important for you, therefore find ways in which you can do something for them, not in payment with cash, but by showing them appreciation for what they have done. Having a good eye for potential mentors, and formulating a strategy for integrating many of them into your life will help you as an entrepreneur leader to become a better person. We become like those we associate with, and we are influenced by the words and actions of those we look up to. Purposely have a plan for mentorship so you can become successful, and along the way, look for those whom you can mentor once you reach your destination.

2. <https://firstround.com/review/we-studied-100-mentor-mentee-matches-heres-what-makes-mentorship-work/> [accessed 01.10.19].

Section IV

The Innovative Technology Component

Chapter 10

Understanding Biotechnology Product Sectors

Craig Shimasaki, PhD, MBA
CEO, BioSource Consulting Group and Moleculera Labs, Oklahoma City, OK, United States

Chapter Outline

When we speak about the "biotechnology industry," we are referencing a broad and diverse group of therapeutics, biologics, diagnostics, medical devices, clinical laboratory tests, research tools, bioagricultural, industrial, and health-care information technology (IT) applications. The biotechnology industry encompasses many diverse sectors which are ever-expanding as new scientific and technical discoveries are made and new applications for these technologies are identified. The goal of biotechnology is to produce unique products, services, and processes that improve life, health, and well-being of individuals and society as a whole. On the surface, the biotechnology industry may appear to be complex because of the seemingly endless and diverse array of products that biotechnology is capable of producing. However, it is surprising how each sector utilizes many overlapping technologies and methods to create these diverse products.

The purpose of this chapter is to introduce you to the major sectors of the biotechnology industry and equip you with a better understanding of each of these segments. Each product sector has unique aspects, including specialized technical and regulatory hurdles. Understanding the many biotech sectors can also spark new ideas for novel product development within your own sector, and provide solutions to problems encountered during product development. Often, the convergence of these sectors produces products that are more effective than those that could be created by any single technology sector alone. For example, the category of combination device/therapeutics resulted from the introduction of vascular stents (metal scaffolds which are medical devices) which were later improved though the addition of anticoagulant drug coatings (therapeutics), resulting in more efficacious drug-eluting stents, which have now replaced the original stents used for coronary artery narrowing. New sectors within the biotechnology industry will no doubt continue to emerge. For instance, about three decades ago, there were no such things as "biochips" or "microarrays," whereas today, it is a commonly used tool in research laboratories, drug development and diagnostics. Possessing a working knowledge of each of these sectors is invaluable to biotech entrepreneurs, managers, and biotech executives. Regardless of the particular

Biotechnology Entrepreneurship. DOI: https://doi.org/10.1016/B978-0-12-815585-1.00010-3

sector you may be working in, having a basic understanding of all sectors will help relate the work of your organization to the broader biotechnology industry as a whole. This overview will provide a framework to aid you in later study of other product sectors. Should you find a particular biotechnology sector of interest, you are encouraged to seek out the many additional resources that can expand your detailed working knowledge of these sectors.

Biotechnology Product Sectors and Technology Sectors

Sectors in the biotechnology industry can be classified by *technology* or *product* category. For instance, genomics, proteomics, and metabolomics are indeed "sectors" of biotechnology, but these classifications are based upon the *technology* that they employ, rather than the resulting *product* that is produced from these technologies (Fig. 10.1). It is important to recognize that most *technologies* are capable of producing many different biotechnology products, which may belong to different *product sectors*. For instance, the use of *genomic technology* can result in a *diagnostic test* by measuring single-nucleotide polymorphism (SNP) or mRNA transcripts. Alternatively, genomic technology can also result in a *therapeutic* by utilizing siRNA to block or inhibit a disease process. *Genomic technology* can also result in a *research instrument* by utilizing specific sets of gene-based microarrays. Although genomic technology can result in a diagnostic, therapeutic, and research instrument product, each of these applications has vastly different development pathways, different costs, and different development time frames. Another example of a *technology sector* is "nanotechnology" that has significant promise and can be applied to a variety of product sectors from therapeutics to medical devices to diagnostics. Its applicability is so broad that nanotechnology can also be utilized in nonbiotechnology applications such as in the paint and electronics industry to name a few. Since our focus is on *biotechnology product commercialization*, in this chapter, we will discuss biotechnology *product sectors* rather than *technology sectors*. As we review these sectors, remember that any particular technology can span multiple product sectors, but the manner in which it is applied to a problem and solution, will determine the product category in which it resides. The categorization of sectors by *technology* has merit, especially for researchers, but in the context of this chapter, we will be focusing on *product* sectors and their commercialization aspects.

Biotechnology Product Sectors

In this chapter, I'd like to share with you 10 of the most common biotechnology product sectors. No doubt there may be more, and there are certainly other ways to subdivide these sectors. However, this categorization will provide a suitable framework for understanding the characteristics and features that comprise each of these sectors, including the differences in costs, development timeframe, and market applications for each of these categories. Within each product sector, we will discuss the function of products within this sector, pertinent characteristics of each product sector, product examples, and briefly describe how these products are regulated. The following are the biotechnology product sectors that we will use:

1. Therapeutics
2. Biologics and vaccines
3. In vitro diagnostics and personalized medicine

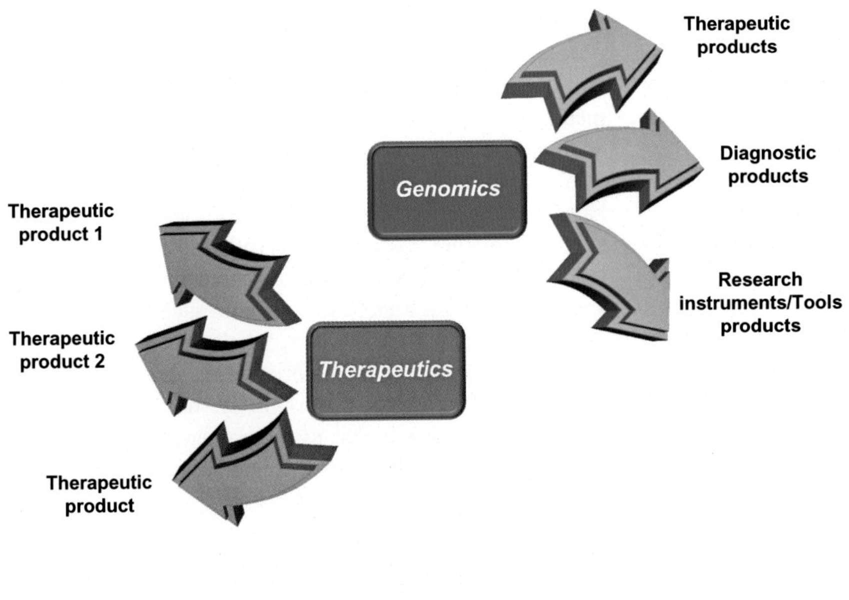

FIGURE 10.1 Technology sectors versus product sectors. Any one technology is capable of producing multiple products in different sectors, whereas one product sector focuses on multiple products within the same sector.

4. Medical devices
5. Combination device/therapeutics
6. Digital health IT products
7. Research reagents, instruments, and tools
8. Bioagriculture (BioAg)
9. Biofuels
10. Industrial and environmental

Product Development Sector Costs Vary Greatly

In general, biotechnology products and their development require enormous amounts of capital. Because of this, it is helpful to understand the general range of costs required to complete development and reach commercialization for each of these product sectors. There is no getting around the fact that *all* biotechnology product development is expensive and requires large amounts of capital to bring a product to commercialization. Many biotechnology companies have started with a great technology concept and novel product idea, but for lack of funds at a critical time period, these noble product applications have vanished. One of the many reasons for this shortfall can be attributed to poor financial planning and a lack of familiarity with the overall development costs and the need for continual fundraising. No one should undertake an endeavor, particularly a biotechnology enterprise, without first counting the financial costs, or at least *understanding* these costs before starting. An appropriate scriptural quote illustrates this: "*Suppose one of you wants to build a tower. Will he not first sit down and estimate the cost to see if he has enough money to complete it?*" Many biotechnology companies have shut their doors, not always due to the failure of the technology, but often it is because they could not raise the next round of capital needed to bring the product through a difficult development challenge and onto commercialization. At the outset of starting an enterprise, it is critical that the leader recognize and appreciate all the costs of product development, testing, and regulatory approval within their particular sector. Careful planning and timing for fundraising that is tied to meeting key milestones, along with proper fiscal management, can provide the greatest opportunity for a good product idea to reach commercialization. Few industries face the enormous expense, lengthy development time, and challenging regulatory hurdles inherent within the biotechnology product-development process. However, in contrast, few industries carry the medical impact that biotechnology has on the health and well-being of millions of lives. The reader will benefit by understanding the range of costs and the typical commercialization timeframes attributed to each of these product sectors.

Table 10.1 lists range estimates of the development costs for each of these product sectors. These ranges take into account the costs for research, development, clinical testing, regulatory, and approval costs prior to commercialization. Within some product sectors, the cost ranges are extremely broad simply because of the diverse types of products that can be produced within that particular category. For instance, within the in vitro diagnostics and personalized medicine category, there is a wide cost range of $25–$100 million. This is because follow-on diagnostics using existing platform technologies require less

TABLE 10.1 Product Sector Development Cost Estimates

Product Sector Categories	Development Cost Estimates[a]
Therapeutics	$250 million–$1.5 billion
Biologics and vaccines	$250 million–$1.5 billion
In vitro diagnostics and personalized medicine	$25–100 million
Medical devices	$25–100 million
Combination device/therapeutics	$75–250 million
Digital health IT applications	$250,000–$15 million
Research reagents, instruments, and tools	$10–75 million
Bioagriculture	$75–250 million
Biofuels	$50–150 million
Industrial and environmental	$15–75 million

IT, Information technology.
[a]*Ranges are estimates which are dependent on the actual product being developed, the underlying technology, the regulatory pathway, and the disease or indication targeted.*

development costs than a new diagnostic testing category using a relatively new technology platform. For instance, a hypothetical new diagnostic test for the detection of Lyme disease based upon several newly identified proteins utilizing existing point-of-care (POC) lateral-flow technology may be able to complete development and reach commercialization at the lower end of the cost range. Whereas a complex genetic test that uses RNA expression analysis to predict the likelihood of cancer recurrence and the prediction of breast cancer risk may require development costs at the upper end of the category. A general rule is that an improvement in an existing diagnostic test (one that is faster or more sensitive) than a test already on the market would most likely be at the lower end of the sector cost range, whereas totally new platforms and/or new diagnostic categories (tests not previously available) will typically be at the higher end of the cost range. For all products, the overall costs for development increases in proportion to the amount of laboratory, animal, and human clinical data that must be collected, and regulatory pathway in order to demonstrate safety and clinical efficacy of a product. In addition, each of these sector development costs are impacted by the technology utilized, the market, the regulatory pathway, and the disease or indication targeted.

For therapeutics, biologics, and vaccines, the "all-in" product development cost is now estimated to exceed \$2.5 billion [1], which takes into account the estimated number of research failures encountered when advancing one successful product to commercialization. In actuality, any one single therapeutic or biologic product-development program may have development costs that are lower than this, but no one can predict ahead of time which therapeutic will be successful in human clinical trials. Therefore, most large pharmaceutical companies make decisions on product development based upon certain cost estimates that include the typical failure rates incurred along the way. In the sector of BioAg, product development costs can vary based upon the type of product and the number and types of genetic traits incorporated into a product, including the amount of field testing required to prove safety.

Although I have listed general range estimates for development costs within each of these product sectors, it is essential to determine more precise cost estimates for your particular product when creating and establishing a product development plan and business plan. Precise product development cost estimates will help you assess the number and size of financing rounds required in order for your product to reach various development milestones and, ultimately, commercialization. Understanding the process required to arrive at accurate product development costs will help reduce the likelihood that you don't run short of capital, and it will also assure investors that you understand the capital requirements for bringing your product to the market. When calculating product development costs, be sure to build within your estimates an allowance for unexpected events and contingency plans. Rarely, if ever, do product development plans proceed exactly as anticipated. More often than not, unforeseen outcomes, delays, and development challenges arise which extend the originally estimated timeframe, which translates into additional costs. When estimating product development costs, consider adding a contingency factor of 15%–20% of the estimated costs to account for unexpected outcomes. Your goal is to arrive at the best and most reliable cost estimate of the entire development process from concept through to commercialization. You will not be raising all this capital at once. With this estimate in mind, you can plan out the stages in which you will want to raise incremental amounts that allow you to reach the next value-enhancing milestone, so you can raise subsequent rounds of capital at higher company valuations.

Product Development Timeframe Varies for Biotechnology Sectors

Just as the development costs vary, so do the product development timeframes. Each product sector requires varying amounts of time for R&D, prototype testing or animal testing, human clinical or field testing, and regulatory approval. It is equally important to determine an accurate timeframe required for your product to move from concept through each stage of product development and ultimately into the market.

Suffice it to say that all biotechnology product sectors (with the exception of digital health IT applications) require numerous years to move a product from concept through development, testing, regulatory approval, and into the marketplace. Table 10.2 lists a range of development timeframes for products within each of these sectors. Because of the expansion and mass adoption of digital and IT, many digital health IT applications have emerged which can potentially reach the market within 2–5 years of product concept, whereas therapeutics and biologics may require 12–15 years to reach commercialization. The product development timeframes listed encompass the time spent on research, development, prototype and clinical testing, regulatory, and approval processes.

Just as with sector costs, development timeframes vary between product sectors and within a sector depending on the particular product, the underlying technology, the market, the regulatory pathway, and the disease or indication for use. For the biotech entrepreneur or company leader, it is important to outline a timetable throughout each of the various development stages for your particular product. Mapping a development

TABLE 10.2 Product Sector Timeframe Estimates

Product Sector Categories	Timeframe Estimates[a]
Therapeutics	12–15 years
Biologics and vaccines	12–15 years
In vitro diagnostics and personalized medicine	3–7 years
Medical devices	3–5 years
Combination device/Therapeutics	5–10 years
Digital health IT applications	2–5 years
Research reagents, instruments, and tools	2–7 years
Bioagriculture	7–15 years
Biofuels	5–7 years
Industrial and environmental	2–5 years

IT, Information technology.
[a]Timeframes are estimates which are dependent on the actual product being developed, the underlying technology, the regulatory pathway and the disease or indication targeted.

timeframe for your particular product is essential because reaching certain product development milestones provide value-enhancing events for the company. In addition, as discussed in *Chapter 17: Sources of Capital and Investor Motivations*, there are certain company stages that investors prefer to invest in, and these are tied directly to product development milestones.

Examples of value-enhancing milestones for therapeutics and biologics:

1. Completion of basic and translational research
2. Completion of development and in vitro testing
3. Completion of lead identification/process optimization
4. Completion of preclinical testing in animals
5. Filing of an investigational new drug applications with the Food and Drug Administration (FDA)
6. Initiation or completion of each stage of clinical testing (Phase 1, 2, and 3)
7. Filing of a new drug application with the FDA
8. Scale-up and manufacturing
9. Regulatory review and product approval
10. Commercialization, marketing, and expansion

For medical devices and diagnostics, there are different value-enhancing milestones.

Examples of value-enhancing milestones for medical devices and diagnostics:

1. Completion of basic and translational research
2. Completion of the proof-of-concept phase
3. Completion of prototype development
4. Completion of clinical validation
5. Filing of a 510(k) or a premarket approvals (PMA) with the FDA
6. Completion of a regulatory review and approval or marketing clearance
7. Scale-up and manufacturing
8. Commercialization, marketing, and expansion

Each product sector has its own unique value-enhancing milestones. A company should recognize and outline each value-enhancing milestone that confers significant product development progress and increases interest and confidence in the company and its future. By outlining and achieving these milestones a company can progressively increase its value and continue to attract greater funding interest for the company throughout subsequent development stages of the product.

Creating Value

Regardless of the product sector, the goal of all start-up or early-stage biotechnology companies is to create value within the product being developed and within the company. Imperceptibly, throughout the entire product development process, value is created. Value is not created all at once, nor is it created proportional to the time or money invested. *Value is created incrementally every time a product development milestone is successfully reached.* Completing certain product development milestones confer more value than others and, with each successful milestone reached, risk is simultaneously reduced—value increases as risk is reduced (see Fig. 10.2). Steady progress through product development in a financially efficient manner creates a situation

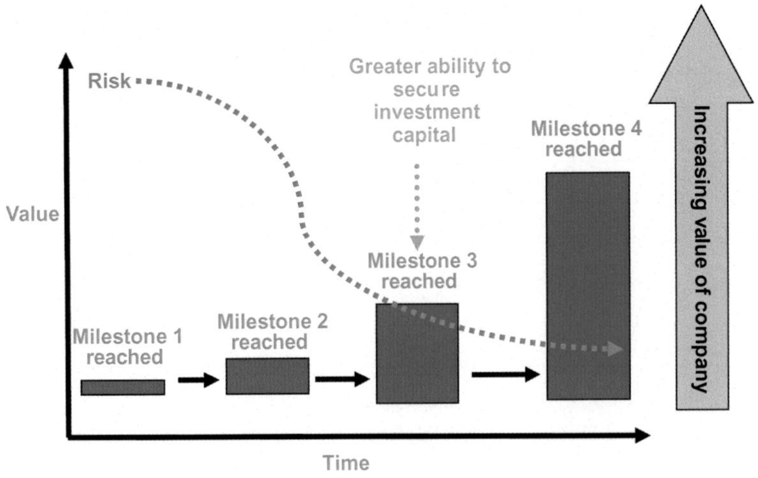

FIGURE 10.2 Value increases and risk reduces with each milestone reached.

where more investors will want to participate in your endeavor. Understanding the concept of value creation is important for entrepreneurs, because investors and future partners have expectations about product development progress, costs, and milestones. Everything the company does should be viewed in a way that it does not detract, but rather increases the value of the product and the company, and decreases the risk, thereby increasing the likelihood of raising additional capital. By properly estimating development costs and timeframes, and reaching value-enhancing milestones along the way, value is attributed to the company. As company value steadily increases, it makes the task of raising capital for subsequent financing rounds less difficult.

Overview of Product Sectors

Therapeutics

Therapeutics generally refer to any drug or medicine that is used to treat a disease or condition with the intent of curing or lessening its severity. The FDA does not list a definition of a "*therapeutic*" but does list a definition for a "*drug*" as "A substance recognized by an official pharmacopoeia or formulary; a substance intended for use in the diagnosis, cure, mitigation, treatment, or prevention of disease; a substance (other than food) intended to affect the structure or any function of the body; a substance intended for use as a component of a medicine but not a device or a component, part or accessory of a device." The word "*therapeutic*" as defined by *Merriam-Webster* states "relating to the treatment of disease or disorders by remedial agents or methods" or by others as "... pertaining to the treating or curing of a disease." The terms "*drug*" and "*therapeutic*" are often used synonymously in various contexts, and for this sector category, we will consider them the same. For the general public who first learns about the biotechnology industry, they most often associate this industry with therapeutic treatments for different diseases or conditions, such as AIDS, Alzheimer's, or cancer. Indeed, therapeutics comprise a very large portion of the development activity within the biotechnology industry, and this segment consumes the largest portion of the capital raised. However, therapeutic companies make up a limited portion of the total number of biotechnology companies within the industry, and they represent only a portion of the multitude of products produced by biotechnology.

***Overview* of the various sectors and a few examples of some subcategories:**

1. **Therapeutics**
   a. Small molecules
   b. Peptides and nucleic acids
2. **Biologics and vaccines**
   a. Oligonucleotides and antisense
   b. Proteins
   c. Monoclonal antibodies (Abs) (mAbs)
   d. Stem cells
   e. CAR T-cell therapy
3. **In vitro diagnostics (IVDs) and personalized medicine (PM)**
   a. In-vitro diagnostics (IVDs)
   b. Molecular diagnostic (MDx)
   c. Predictive and prognostic diagnostics
   d. Companion diagnostics
   e. Personalized medicine (PM)
   f. Clinical laboratory services—Clinical Laboratory Improvement Amendments (CLIA) laboratory
4. **Medical devices**
5. **Combination device/Therapeutic products**
6. **Research reagents, tools, and reagents**
   a. Sequencers
   b. Microarrays
7. **Digital health IT applications**
8. **BioAg**
   a. Biocrops
9. **Biofuels**
10. **Industrial and environmental**

Prior to the emergence of the biotechnology industry, therapeutics were developed and commercialized by the large pharmaceutical companies around the world such as Merck, Schering, Hoffmann-La Roche, and Burroughs Wellcome to name a few, whereas after numerous mergers and acquisitions, the names have changed along the way. Many of these companies originally started as chemical manufacturers, apothecaries, and pharmacies. Merck, in Germany, originated as a pharmacy located in Darmstadt in 1668 and was possibly the first company to move in the direction of pharmaceutical manufacturing. The main focus of the pharmaceutical industry has primarily been on the discovery and development of "small molecule" therapeutics which are chemical compounds that can be studied in isolated assays and synthetically produced by chemists (see *Chapter 24: Therapeutic Drug Development and Human Clinical Trials*). Many successful small molecule chemical entities were developed and produced by these pharmaceutical companies such as acetylsalicylic acid or aspirin. The pharmaceutical industry steadily grew as more small molecule drugs were successfully developed and commercialized such as analgesics (pain), antipyretics (fever reducers), barbiturates (acting on the central nervous system), and others.

These pharmaceutical companies experienced many successes and great demand for their products, which created the growth and expansion of these multinational mega companies. However, over time, the number of novel small molecule drug opportunities became less abundant as evidenced by the declining successes in finding and commercializing small molecule therapeutics. This issue, coupled with increasing drug-development costs, and changes in the patent exclusivity period laws, pharmaceutical companies sought methods and opportunities to create and develop more successful therapeutic products. Once biotechnology tools and recombinant DNA techniques emerged in the early 1970s, pharmaceutical companies saw the value of biologics. After many of these biotechnology products proved successful, pharmaceutical companies began acquiring biotechnology companies as a means of augmenting their biological expertise and acquiring access to biotechnology products. More and more pharmaceutical companies slowly began transitioning to the development of biologics and the acquisition of biotechnology companies. Further dissolving the distinction between pharmaceutical and biotechnology companies, we now have emerging a category of companies referred to as "biotherapeutics companies." Major biotechnology company acquisitions continue to occur such as in 2008 when Cambridge, Massachusetts, based Millennium Pharmaceuticals was acquired by Japanese Takeda Pharmaceutical for $8.8 billion. In 2009 Swiss-based Roche purchased the remaining shares of South San Francisco–based Genentech for $46.8 billion completing its full acquisition since it first acquired a 56% majority ownership in 1990. And in 2011, the French pharmaceutical giant Sanofi-Aventis acquired Boston-based Genzyme for $20.1 billion. More recently in 2018 Novartis acquired AveXis for $8.7 billion, New Jersey–headquartered Celgene acquired Juno Therapeutics for $9 billion, and Paris-based Sanofi-acquired Bioverativ for $11.6 billion.

It is important to recognize that in one sense, the term "therapeutics" includes "biologics" because biologics are also used for treating diseases and conditions. However, the reader should know that there are product development and regulatory distinctions between "therapeutics" and "biologics." We will discuss biologics in the next section but for now will elaborate on the differences and examine these two categories as clearly distinct entities. However, as time goes on, there appears to be less of a distinction between traditional therapeutics and biologics.

The vast majority of what is described as traditional therapeutics can be categorized as

- small organic molecules and
- peptides and nucleic acids.

Small molecules are chemical entities that are usually chemically synthesized, administered orally, and absorbed through the intestines into the bloodstream. The overall product development goal for a therapeutic is to produce a pill or capsule that contains the chemical entity which can be conveniently administered by mouth and quickly produce the desired effect within the body. As previously mentioned, small molecules, such as peptides and nucleic acids, can also be utilized as diagnostics and as reagents in clinical tests, whereas therapeutics utilize these types of molecules for the purpose of treating a disease or condition.

Mechanisms of Action for Therapeutics

Common mechanisms of action for many therapeutics are to block or interfere with a chemical reaction within the body, block a receptor, or to block or inhibit a process in an undesirable microorganism. These interferences and blockages can be targeted against critical enzymes that are involved in a disease process, or receptors on cells which trigger downstream events such as a transcription of RNA and translation of proteins. By interfering or blocking a specific biological or chemical process in the body or in a microorganism, therapeutics can "treat" a wide variety of diseases or conditions. To the degree that the therapeutic is specific enough and can target a single process or a single receptor, to that same degree therapeutics' "side effects" are minimized. However, within the body, many similar reactions occur simultaneously, and similar receptors can be found in various cells and organs throughout the body. As a result, almost all therapeutics have "side effects" which can range from minimal to very significant. The proper prescribing of a therapeutic is typically based upon an analysis of the risk/benefit to the patient by the physician. If the potential benefit of the therapeutic outweighs the risks of side effects or potential consequences, the clinician will prescribe the treatment. In certain therapeutics, side effects can be extremely severe or even life-threatening such as the case of chemotherapeutic drugs used in the treatment of certain types of cancers. However, in some cases, the physician may determine that the risk of no treatment may be worse than the risk of treatment side effects.

Therapeutics are created that can also target or interfere with biological processes that are not found in our own body, but rather in microorganisms that attack our body. For instance, antibiotics belong to a class of antiinfectives (which also include antivirals and antifungals), which are small molecules designed to inhibit a specific biologic process in the growth cycle in bacteria. Some of the processes that antibiotics target include inhibiting the synthesis of the bacteria's cell-walls or the synthesis of its protein, thus slowing down or stopping their reproduction. Antibiotics are developed with the intent of inhibiting or blocking bacteria-specific biological processes, and since bacteria possesses unique enzymes and proteins that differ from those in the human body, most of these drugs tend to be quite effective and usually elicit minimal side effects. However, because bacteria possess the ability to transfer genes to other bacteria and confer antibiotic resistance, this reduces the effectiveness of antibiotics over time and creates drug-resistant strains of bacteria. As a result, biotechnology can play an important role in identifying and creating antibiotics that may encounter minimal resistance from bacteria.

Therapeutic Categories

The number of therapeutic categories is large and growing as new biological mechanisms are discovered and new conditions emerge. The following list outlines 50 different therapeutic categories established by the US Pharmacopeia and listed on the FDA website [2]:

- Analgesics
- Anesthetics
- Antibacterials
- Anticonvulsants
- Antidementia agents
- Antidepressants
- Antidotes, deterrents, and toxicologic agents
- Antiemetics
- Antifungals
- Antigout agents
- Antiinflammatory agents
- Antimigraine agents
- Antimyasthenic agents
- Antimycobacterials
- Antineoplastics
- Antiparasitics
- Anti-Parkinson's agents
- Antipsychotics
- Antispasticity agents
- Antivirals
- Anxiolytics
- Bipolar agents
- Blood glucose regulators
- Blood products/modifiers/volume expanders
- Cardiovascular agents
- Central nervous system agents
- Dental and oral agents
- Dermatological agents
- Enzyme replacements/modifiers
- Gastrointestinal agents
- Genitourinary agents
- Hormonal agents, stimulant/replacement/modifying (adrenal)
- Hormonal agents, stimulant/replacement/modifying (pituitary)
- Hormonal agents, stimulant/replacement/modifying (prostaglandins)
- Hormonal agents, stimulant/replacement/modifying (sex hormones/modifiers)
- Hormonal agents, stimulant/replacement/modifying (thyroid)
- Hormonal agents, suppressant (adrenal)
- Hormonal agents, suppressant (parathyroid)
- Hormonal agents, suppressant (pituitary)
- Hormonal agents, suppressant (sex hormones/modifiers)
- Hormonal agents, suppressant (thyroid)
- Immunological agents
- Inflammatory bowel disease agents
- Metabolic bone disease agents
- Ophthalmic agents
- Otic agents
- Respiratory tract agents
- Sedatives/hypnotics
- Skeletal muscle relaxants
- Therapeutic nutrients/minerals/electrolytes

Other Characteristics of Therapeutics

Most therapeutic drugs have three or more names assigned to them. These names include the *brand name* or *trade name* which is given by the company, such as "Lipitor" by Pfizer. There is also a *generic name*

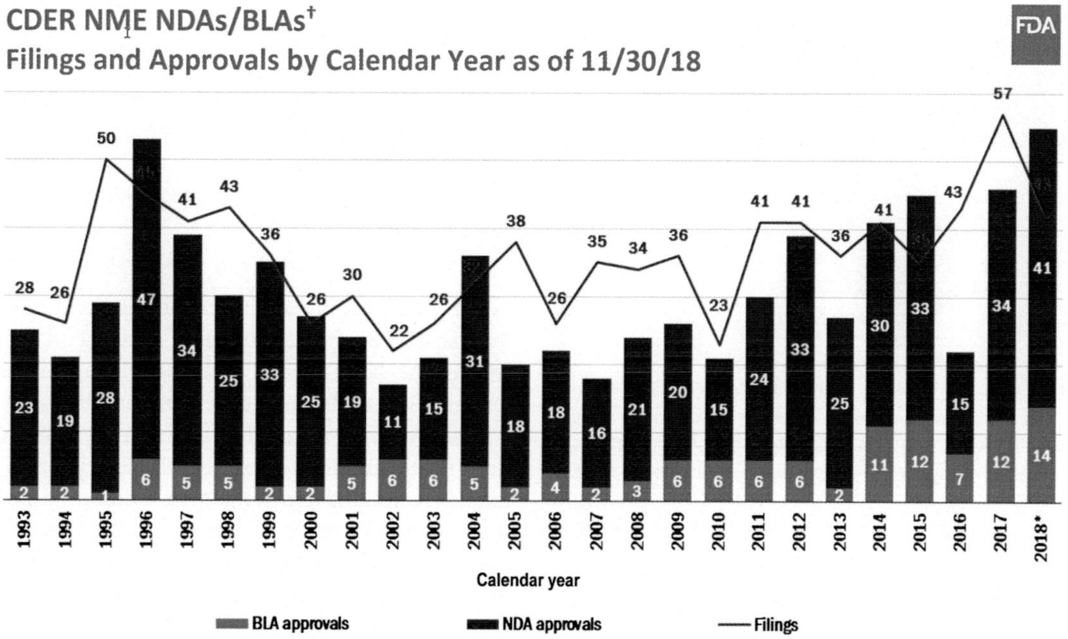

FIGURE 10.3 Annual new FDA-approved medicines since 1993. *CDER*, Center for Drug Evaluation and Research; *FDA*, Food and Drug Administration; *NDAs*, new drug applications.

†Multiple applications pertaining to a single new molecular/biologic entity are only counted once. Original BLAs that do not contain a new active ingredient are excluded.

*Information as of November 30, 2018. In rare instances, it may be necessary for FDA to change a drug's new molecular entity (NME) designation or the status of its application as a new biologics license application (BLA). Since applications are received and filed throughout a calendar year, the filed applications in a given calendar year do not necessarily correspond to an approval in the same calendar year. Certain applications are within their 60-day filing review period and may not be filed upon completion of the review. *FDA*.

"atorvastatin calcium," and a (usually long) *chemical name* "[R-(R*,R*)]-2-(4-fluorophenyl)-β,δ-dihydroxy-5-(1-methylethyl)–3-phenyl-4 [(phenylamino)carbonyl]–1*H*-pyrrole-1-heptanoic acid, calcium salt (2:1) trihydrate."

Regulation of Therapeutics

Therapeutics (and biologics) are some of the most stringently regulated sectors in any industry. Due in large part to the potential for unwanted side effects, the regulatory approval route for therapeutics, including the requirements for safety and efficacy in animal and clinical testing, is very strenuous and lengthy, often taking 10–15 years for a therapeutic product to reach the market. Whether the approval is in the United States under the FDA or in other countries through their own regulatory agencies, the therapeutic and biologic sectors have become the most costly segments in time and money to develop. Estimates for the cost of the development of a new therapeutic drug has escalated to be more than $2.5 billion [1].

Therapeutic Products in Development

There are a vast number of therapeutic drugs under development and in clinical studies. In a 2017 report [3]the Analysis Group identified 6300 drug products in clinical development for cancer to cardiovascular disease and diabetes to neurology to name just a few areas. They reported that about three-quarters of clinical phase products were *potentially first-in-class*—in other words, drugs that work by a unique pharmacological class distinct from any other marketed products. The pharmaceutical and biotechnology industries are continuously identifying new drug targets and new methods for treating some of the most chronic and debilitating conditions (see Fig. 10.3).

Biologics and Vaccines

Biologics can also be thought of as "therapeutics" in the sense that they are utilized to treat a disease or condition. The official FDA definition of "biological products" or "biologics" is any virus, therapeutic serum, toxin, antitoxin, or analogous product applicable to the prevention, treatment, or cure of diseases or injuries of man. The European Union regulations defines "biological medicinal products" as a protein or nucleic acid–based pharmaceutical substance used for therapeutic or in vivo diagnostic purposes, which is produced by means other than direct extraction from a native (nonengineered) biological source. Biologics differ from the above-mentioned therapeutic small molecule drugs in several characteristics. One of the most important characteristics of a biologic is that

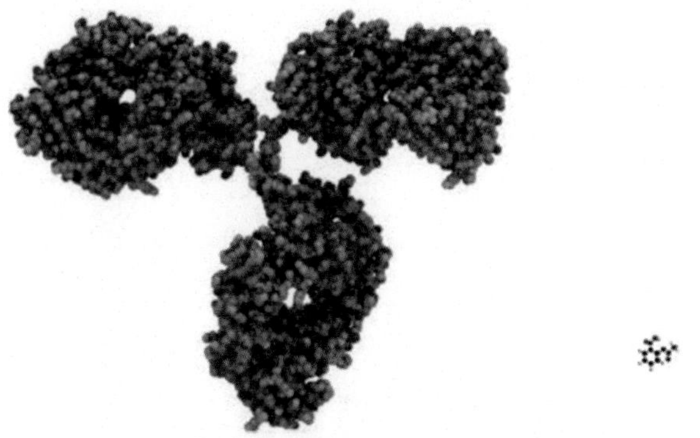

FIGURE 10.4 Biologic versus a small molecule drug. (Left) Biologic: molecular structure of a monoclonal antibody approximately 150,000 molecular weight. (Right) Small molecule drug: aspirin molecular structure approximately 180 molecular weight (approximate—not drawn to scale).

they are large complex molecules which require complex processes to manufacture and produce (see Fig. 10.4), whereas small molecule therapeutic drugs are often stable in most environments and can be chemically synthesized and administered orally. Biologics are usually fragile, and most often administered by injection into the bloodstream for treatment, as most biologics would be digested or broken down if administered orally. Rarely can a biologic be chemically synthesized because of their complexity and size (with the exception of oligonucleotides and antisense DNA) and they are often produced by a process that utilizes a protein expression system in a mammalian or insect cell line or in a bacteria. Biologics also rely on complex "posttranslational modifications" that are carried out by these living expression systems. Posttranslational modifications include different glycosylation patterns within these proteins which affect the activity (potency) of the protein, its three-dimensional structure (protein folding pattern), and rate of clearance from the body (elimination and half-life). Biologics are very complex and difficult to fully characterize, and for this reason, they are often characterized by their manufacturing processes. The manufacturing processes of biologics are complex, and slight changes in temperature during processing or other factors can impact the final product and affect how it works in patients. As a result, regulatory agencies require that changes in the manufacturing process or facility may require additional clinical studies to demonstrate safety, purity, and potency (see *Chapter 31: The Biomanufacturing of Biotechnology Products*).

Some examples of biologic categories include

- proteins, enzymes, and growth factors;
- monoclonal antibodies (mAbs);
- blood components such as blood factors, stem cells, or proteins;
- oligonucleotides and antisense DNA; and
- viral gene therapy.

It is important to remember that many of these same biologic entities can also be utilized in certain processes to identify disease conditions (diagnostics). For instance, mAbs, coupled or used with detection and signaling molecules, are commonly used to identify or capture molecular markers within the body or in a specimen. In this section, we differentiate the usage of these biologic products as treatments, whereas in the diagnostic section, we will elaborate on the usage of mAbs for diagnostics purposes.

Mechanisms of Action for Biologics

Most biologics are replacements or substitutes of actual human proteins that are either missing or at low levels within the body of the individual being treated. Genetic engineering tools have given us the ability to "cut" and "paste" various genes that code for human proteins, and transfer them into the genome of bacteria, insect, or mammalian cells and grow them in culture, so that they can express (produce) the desired human protein. Because most biologics are replicas of actual human proteins, their function is identical to the natural purpose of the original protein in the human body.

Examples of Biologic Products

Monoclonal Antibodies

Monoclonal antibodies are biologics that have shown increasing promise as candidates for treatments of diverse diseases because of their ability to bind specifically to almost any target molecule. Antibodies (Abs) are immune system proteins that recognize and bind to foreign substances, usually with very high affinity. mAbs refer to the fact that only a "single" antibody clone is being produced, as opposed to "polyclonal" where "multiple clones" or different Abs with different specificities are being produced. In 1975 Köhler and Milstein [4] discovered a method to produce mouse mAbs directed against any specific target. This provided the ability to engineer a mouse mAb directed against a desired target. For this monumental work and discovery, these scientists won the Nobel Prize in 1984. With the further advent of additional biotechnology tools, we can now genetically engineer and produce completely *humanized mAbs* that are directed against desired targets and thus eliminate the potential for rejection by the human immune system of an antibody from a mouse species. By 2013 a total of 33 mAbs were approved by the FDA as biologics for a variety of therapeutic targets. Biologic drug development of mAbs continued to accelerate such that by 2017, a total of 73 mAbs were approved by the FDA with about half being approve for cancer treatment. Because mAbs are specific enough to allow targeting of unhealthy cells without harm to healthy cells, they have been particularly important in fighting cancer, and more recently, have shown great promise for autoimmune diseases such as rheumatoid arthritis. Two successful mAb biologics include Herceptin produced by Genentech/Roche, which is a humanized mAb used in the treatment of certain types of breast cancer, and Remicade manufactured by Centocor/Janssen, which is a human mAb that binds and neutralizes TNF-alpha, an inflammatory cytokine overproduced in rheumatoid arthritis.

Vaccines as Biologics

Vaccines have been utilized as early as 1796 when Edward Jenner discovered that by injecting cowpox into an individual, he could create immunity to smallpox, the devastating viral disease that is now considered to be eradicated. Later, in 1885, Louis Pasteur successfully developed the first rabies vaccine. Since then vaccines have been developed against diphtheria, tetanus, anthrax, cholera, plague, typhoid, and tuberculosis (TB). The premise is that small amounts of attenuated infectious agents injected into the body can stimulate the natural immune system to develop immunity to these organisms and prevent future disease. Through biotechnology, vaccines are now being developed for HIV and even used as therapies for the treatment of cancer.

Therapeutic Vaccines

Therapeutic vaccines are different than those that are given for disease prevention such as measles, TB, and influenza vaccines. Therapeutic vaccines are used for treatment as they utilize a patient's own immune system to fight an existing disease rather than immunizing for protection against future disease. In 2010 the US FDA approved the first therapeutic vaccine, Provenge, manufactured by the Dendron Corporation, a novel method for treating prostate cancer. The treatment involves taking a patient's own white blood cells and using a drug that trains them to more actively attack cancer cells. The patient's white blood cells are collected and certain immune cells are isolated. The cells are then incubated with a protein often found on prostate tumors combined with an immune system booster. The treated cells are then infused back into the patient three times over the course of a month. Provenge is intended for men whose prostate cancer has spread throughout the body and it is personalized for each patient.

There are a number of therapeutic vaccines in development and many are directed against cancers such as glioblastoma, cervical cancer, skin cancer, lung cancer, breast cancer, cervical, and pancreatic cancers.

Stem Cell Therapy

Stem cells are unique from other cells within the body and have the potential to be utilized for many different applications. Stem cells are undifferentiated and have the potential to become any other specialized cell within the body and do so based upon various signals internal and external to the cell. Stem cells also act as a repair system for the body to replenish body tissues as cell turnover occurs. They have the capacity to divide for long periods of time, and they retain their ability to make all cell types within the body. All stem cells—regardless of their source—have three general properties: they are capable of dividing and renewing themselves for long periods; they are unspecialized; and they can give rise to specialized cell types.

There are a number of different types of stem cells:

1. *Embryonic stem cells* (ES) are isolated from tissues of a developing human fetus during the blastocyst phase of embryological development.
2. *Tissue-specific stem cells (adult stem cells or somatic stem cells)* are isolated from tissues of the adult body. Bone marrow is the most common source and is rich with stem cells that can be used to treat certain blood diseases and cancers.
3. *Mesenchymal stem cells (stromal stem cells)* come from the connective tissue that surrounds other tissues and organs. The first mesenchymal stem cells were discovered in the bone marrow and were shown to be capable of making bone, cartilage, and fat cells and now have been grown from other tissues, such as fat and cord blood. At this time is not certain whether these cells are actually stem cells or what types of cells they are capable of generating.
4. *Perinatal stem cells* that come from amniotic fluid and umbilical cord blood. These stem cells also have the ability to change into specialized cells.
5. *Induced-pluripotent stem cells (iPS)* are cells that have been engineered by converting tissue-specific cells, such as skin cells, into cells that behave like ES. iPS cells help us learn more about normal development and disease onset and progression, and are also useful for developing and testing new drugs and therapies.

Certain types of stem-cell usage remains an ethical debate primarily concerning the creation, treatment, and destruction of human embryos incident to research involving ES. An important point to know is that not all stem-cell research involves the creation, use, or destruction of human embryos as there are adult stem cells, amniotic stem cells, and induced-pluripotent stem cells which do not involve human embryos and are providing discoveries and answers for human health treatments. Stem-cell research is rapidly advancing and may soon result in treatments for Parkinson's disease, diabetes, cerebral palsy, heart disease, and many other chronic conditions (see Fig. 10.5).

Gene Therapy

Gene therapy is the insertion of genes into an individual's cells and tissues to treat or prevent disease instead of using drugs or surgery. In gene therapy, DNA is packaged into a "vector" that is used to transport the DNA inside cells within the body. Once inside, the DNA becomes expressed by the cell resulting in the production of a therapeutic protein, which in turn treats the patient's disease.

One gene therapy employs an adeno-associated virus (AAV) as a vector to deliver the gene neurturin, which has been found to restore cells damaged in Parkinson's patients and protect them from further degeneration. The first FDA-approved gene therapy experiment in the United States occurred in 1990 for the treatment of adenosine deaminase deficiency (ADA)—severe combined immunodeficiency (SCID); ADA is an inherited disorder that damages the immune system and causes SCID. Individuals with SCID lack immune protection from bacteria, viruses, and fungi. To date, over 2600 clinical trials have been conducted using a number of techniques for gene therapy (see Fig. 10.6).

Although gene therapy technology is still finding its way and has experienced some failures, it has also been used with success. In 2017 the FDA approved two gene therapies: Yescarta from Gilead, the first CAR T-cell therapy for non-Hodgkin lymphoma, and Kymriah from Novartis, a CAR T-cell therapy for acute lymphoblastic leukemia. There are other gene therapies that have previously been approved in Europe and China such as Glybera, Stremelis, and Gendicine. In 2018 the FDA approved another gene therapy product called Luxturna from Spark Therapeutics that used AAV to deliver a gene missing in patients suffering from an inherited eye disease. Currently, gene therapy is being tested for the treatment of diseases that have no other cures. Gene therapy holds promise for a number of diseases including inherited disorders, certain types of cancer, and certain viral infections. Gene therapy still has risks, and more clinical trials are underway to be sure that it will be safe and effective.

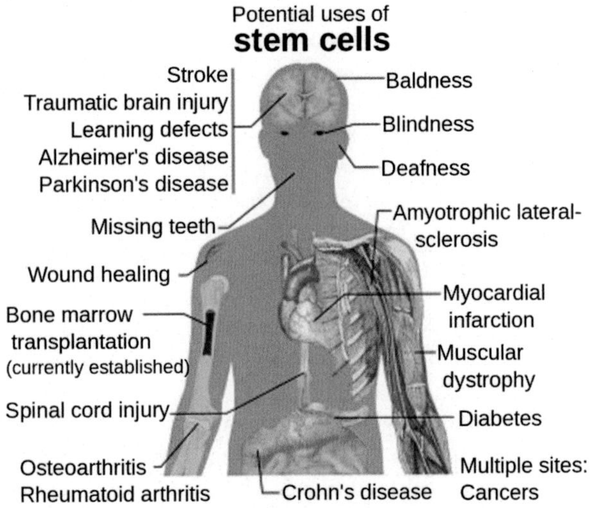

FIGURE 10.5 Potential uses of stem cells. *From: Wikipedia.*

Ribonucleic Acid Interference

RNA interference (RNAi) is a process in which RNAi molecules are used to inhibit gene expression. Specific

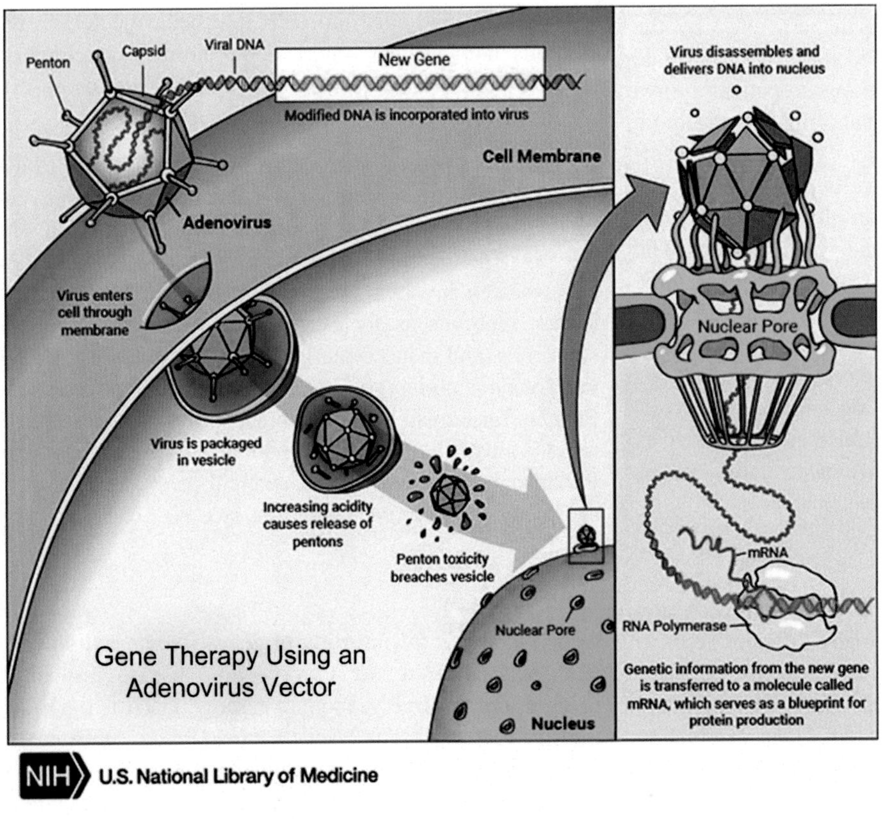

FIGURE 10.6 Example of viral-vector-based gene therapy. *From: US National Library of Medicine.*

RNAi sequences are introduced into the cell which binds to and destroys its mRNA target. RNAi molecules can either increase or decrease a gene's activity by preventing an mRNA from producing a protein or by blocking an expression inhibitor. Potentially, any disease-causing gene, cell type, or tissue can be targeted with RNAi. In 2006 Andrew Fire and Craig Mello won the Nobel Prize in Physiology or Medicine for discovering RNAi. Since its discovery, it has been used extensively in research, and finally, in 2018 the first RNAi therapeutic called Patisiran (Onpattro), developed by Alnylam Pharmaceuticals, was approved by the FDA. In patients with a rare genetic disorder called hereditary transthyretin amyloidosis, which is progressive and often fatal, this RNAi disrupts the production of a protein that causes nerve damage. There are scores of RNAi products in development, especially with indications for various forms of cancer, providing novel therapies for patients, especially those with genetic disorders.

Regulation of Biologics

In the United States, most biologics are regulated by the FDA through the Center for Biologics Evaluation and Research (CBER), whereas small molecule therapeutics are regulated by the Center for Drug Evaluation and Research (CDER). However, in 2003 the FDA transferred responsibility of certain biologics from CBER to CDER. The biologic products that are now regulated under CDER include mAbs for in vivo use, proteins intended for therapeutic use, including cytokines and enzymes, and immunomodulators such as proteins and peptides intended to treat disease. The types of biologics that remain regulated by CBER include cellular products such as whole cells and cell fragments, gene therapy products, human gene therapy; vaccines and vaccine-associated products; allergenic extracts used for the diagnosis and treatment of allergic diseases and allergen patch tests; blood and blood components such as albumin, immunoglobulins, and clotting factors to name a few. It is important to recognize that regulatory requirements and pathways continuously change, and it is incumbent upon the leader to understand current regulations and pathways for regulatory approval of their product in all countries where you intend to commercialize your product. Similar to traditional "therapeutics" described in the above section, the timeframe for biologic product development from idea to commercialization can require 12–15 years and cost upwards of $1.3 billion or more. Even though the costs are high and the time for development is lengthy, the value and potential payout for successful biologics are significant. Interestingly, of the top five therapeutic sales in 2017, all five were biologics and mAbs (Table 10.3).

Diagnostics

Diagnostics encompass a broad range of tests and testing methods. The most common term used to describe this product sector is IVDs. The word "*in vitro*" is a Latin term that means "*in glass*" and refers to the test tube experimentation of samples taken and tested outside of the body, as opposed to "*in vivo*" or "*in life*" or in the body. The entire diagnostic testing sector is often referred to as the "IVD industry." There are many subsectors of IVD products, and they can be categorized by the method that is utilized for testing (kits vs services), the purpose of the results (diagnostic vs predictive vs prognostic), whether they are paired with a specific treatment

TABLE 10.3 Top Five Therapeutic Annual Sales 2018[a]

Drug name	Type of product	Manufacturer	Indications	Est. worldwide sales ($billion)
Humira (adalimumab)	Monoclonal antibody	AbbVie	Rheumatoid arthritis, Crohn's disease	$18.43
Rituxan (MabThera; rituximab)	Monoclonal antibody	Roche, (Genentech), Biogen	Non-Hodgkin's lymphoma; chronic lymphocytic leukemia	$9.23
Revlimid (lenalidomide)	Monoclonal antibody	Celgene	Multiple myeloma	$8.19
Enbrel (etanercept)	Monoclonal antibody	Amgen, Pfizer	Rheumatoid arthritis	$7.89
Herceptin	Monoclonal antibody	Roche (Genentech)	HER-2 overexpressing breast cancer	$7.44

[a]*Sales revenue for 2017.*
Data from: Genetic Engineering and Biotechnology News, March 12, 2018.

(companion diagnostics), or by the targets that they identify (molecules vs genetics vs epigenetics). More industry focus is being directed toward identifying better, faster, and more novel diagnostic methods.

In this section, we will discuss:

- *In vitro* diagnostics (IVDs)
- Molecular diagnostics (MDx)
- Predictive and prognostic diagnostics
- Companion diagnostics
- Personalized medicine (PM)
- CLIA laboratory clinical testing

Most all diagnostic testing operates by determining whether a molecule, a set of molecules, or certain biochemical markers are present, absent, altered, or in higher or lower quantities than would be expected in a "normal" person. These markers are often referred to as "*analytes*" which are the substance being analyzed in an assay. Most often the analyte(s) being measured, whether in the body or in a specimen taken from the body, is in very low quantity. Various analytical methods and techniques have been developed to detect the smallest quantity of these analytes. Some of the methods and techniques used for IVD testing are detection platforms from the sector of research tools and reagents. There are a variety of detection and analytical methods. Some rely on complex and expensive equipment such as mass spectroscopy and flow-cytometers, whereas others rely on visual colorimetric reading called "lateral flow assays" providing a simple "yes" or "no" result (Fig. 10.7). All diagnostic tests intend to provide results that will give a clinician more information to know how to appropriately treat and/or monitor a patient's condition and or/make a proper diagnosis.

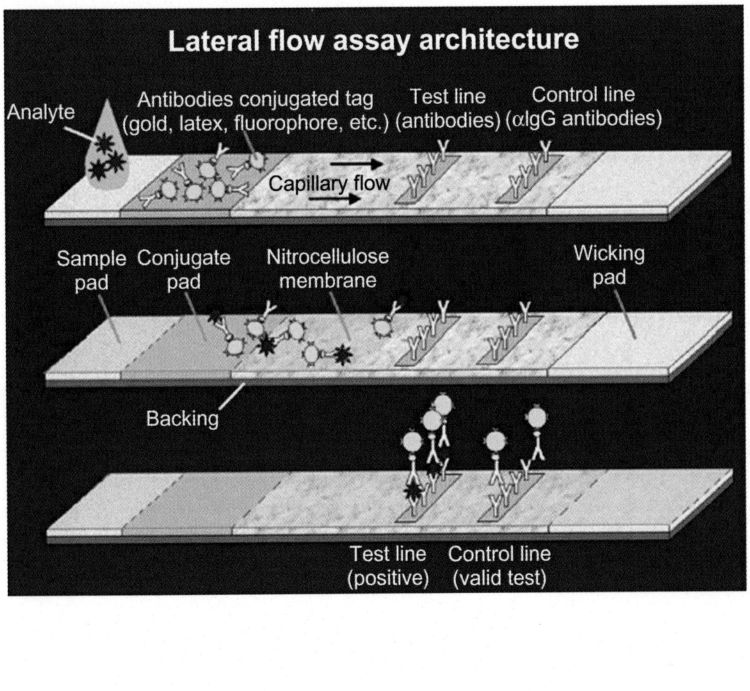

FIGURE 10.7 Lateral flow assay architecture for point-of-care testing. *From: Wikipedia.*

Performance measures for diagnostics

Although health-care costs of diagnostics comprise only about 2% of health-care costs, interestingly, diagnostics direct about 70% of the treatment costs [5]. Because of this, it is important to understand the reliability and limits of diagnostic testing results. There are several performance characteristics used to assess the value of a diagnostic test. These measures allow direct comparison of one diagnostic test to another. Although these performance measures can often be confusing and difficult to understand, knowing the reliability limits of a diagnostic test will help one assess the value of the results. Below is a brief description of the most commonly used diagnostic performance measures. The reader is encouraged to reference additional information about these and other diagnostic performance measures as it can also help you recognize opportunities for improvements in diagnostic testing methods.

1. ***Sensitivity***: This refers to the percentage of individuals who tested positive *and indeed have* the disease or condition. For instance, if a diagnostic test has a sensitivity of 87% it means that 87% of the time (in the population tested) a positive test was observed when the individuals truly had the disease or condition. These are called "true positives." However, it also means that 13% of the time (in the population tested) individuals who had the disease or condition *did not* show a positive test. These are called "false negatives."
2. ***Specificity***: This refers to the percentage of individuals who tested negative *and did not have* the disease or condition. For instance, if a diagnostic test has a specificity of 93%, it means that 93% of the time

(in the population tested) a negative test was observed when the individuals, indeed, did not have the disease or condition. These are called "true negatives." However, it also means that 7% of the time (in the population tested) individuals who did not have the disease or condition *did not* show a negative test. These are called "false positives."

Sensitivity and specificity are two important performance measures that help assess the reliability of a diagnostic test. Knowing these values helps the clinician make a more accurate clinical diagnosis, because they understand how reliable (or unreliable) the testing results are. Two other performance measures can be calculated from the same information, and these include

1. *Positive predictive value*: This refers to the chance (percent likelihood) that a positive test would be correct. In other words, it is the percent likelihood that an individual who receives a positive test truly *would have* the disease or condition.
2. *Negative predictive value*: This refers to the chance (percent likelihood) that a negative test would be correct. In other words, it is the percent likelihood that an individual who receives a negative test result *would not have* the disease or condition.

	Gold standard positive	Gold standard negative
New test positive	A	B
New test negative	C	D

Sensitivity = A/(A+C)
Specificity = D/(D+B)

Positive predictive value = A/(A+B)
Negative predictive value = D/(D+C)

FIGURE 10.8 Diagnostic 2 × 2.

	Culture confirmation positive	Culture conformation negative
New strep test positive	78	1
New strep test negative	22	99

Tested with *n*=100 positives and *n*=100 negatives

New point-of-care strep test sensitivity = 78/(78+22) = 78.0%
New point-of-care strep test specificity = 99/(99+1) = 99.0%

Positive predictive value = 78/(78+1) = 98.7%
Negative predictive value = 99/(99+22) = 81.8%

FIGURE 10.9 Hypothetical point-of-care strep test data.

Understanding the data

It is not uncommon to see the data used to calculate a diagnostic test's performance in a "two-by-two" (2 × 2) table with the total population of people (or specimens) used to determine these values. A 2 × 2 typically displays a comparison of the results between the diagnostic test of interest and a "gold standard" test. The gold standard is a test that is accepted to be the most accurate diagnostic measure currently available for that disease or condition irrespective of how difficult or how long it takes to perform. For instance, let's say you want to determine the performance measures of a new 15-minute Point-of-Care (POC) test to detect strep infections. Currently, for strep testing, the "gold standard" you would use for comparison is a laboratory culture confirmation test that would take 3–7 days to receive final results. The data from both of these tests would be presented in a 2 × 2 table with the sensitivity, specificity, and positive predictive and negative predictive values calculated based upon the formulas listed in Fig. 10.8.

In Fig. 10.9, you can see hypothetical data from our new POC strep test compared to the culture confirmation gold standard. We hypothetically used 100 positive samples and 100 negative samples. Of the 100 positive samples (patients with the disease or condition), 78 produced positive results and 22 produced negative results in the new test; therefore the sensitivity is 78.0%. Of the 100 negative samples (patients without the disease or condition), 99 produced negative results and 1 produced positive results; therefore the specificity is 99.0%. The positive and negative predictive values are calculated as shown in Fig. 10.9. A helpful reference for visually understanding diagnostic performance measures is "*Understanding sensitivity and specificity with the right side of the brain*" [6].

Reliable diagnostic tests should have sensitivities and specificities in the high 80‰ to the high 90‰ in order for them to have significant utility. However, depending on the purpose of the test, and the alternatives available, some tests with lower specificity but high sensitivity may be utilized for rapid screening of individuals. In this type of usage, screened patients that had positive results would benefit from more accurate, which are sometimes more costly and more invasive testing. For instance, the currently available PSA (prostate-specific antigen) blood test provides numeric scores of an individual's PSA level in the bloodstream. A cutoff score of 4.0 being positive has a reasonable sensitivity of 86%, whereas that cutoff is not highly specific for prostate cancer (specificity of 33%). What this means is that this test will generate a lot of "false positives" for individuals that really don't have prostate cancer. However, the relatively high sensitivity means that it will pick up most (86%) individuals who do indeed have prostate cancer. Although the specificity for current PSA testing is not great, it is an inexpensive monitoring diagnostic to identify potential prostate cancer patients who can later be screened with other tests and/or by biopsy. In applications like this, the subsequent tests are usually impractical, expensive, or unwarranted as a screening tool for the general population.

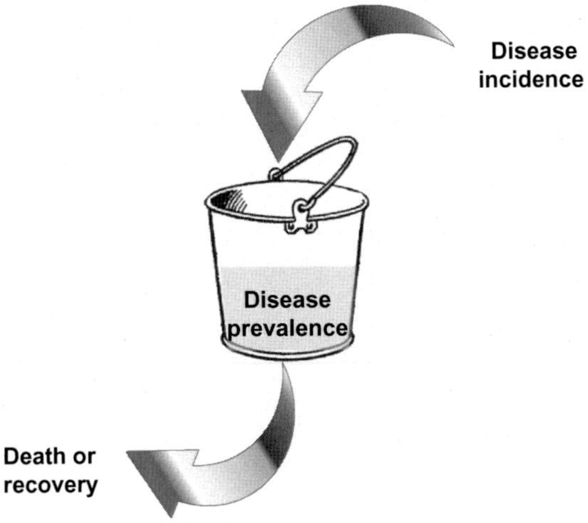

FIGURE 10.10 Disease incidence versus disease prevalence.

Incidence Rate and Prevalence Rate

Two values essential to properly evaluate the performance of a diagnostic test are the "incidence rate" and the "prevalence rate" of the disease or condition. Regulatory agencies will want to know these values because they affect the performance measures. If clinical testing was not performed in a manner that takes into account the disease prevalence rate, the calculated sensitivity and specificity may not be a reliable measure of the test's true performance in a real setting. For instance, if a disease or condition has a low prevalence rate, say 5%, meaning it is relatively infrequent among the population that will be tested, it is critical to also determine the performance measures using a similar frequency (5%) of positive samples. For example, suppose the sensitivity and specificity in a new test was calculated using 100 positive and 100 negative samples. If the new test only misdiagnosed one positive patient, this would not impact the sensitivity very much (99/100 = 99% sensitivity). Whereas if you clinically tested only five positive samples and misdiagnosed one positive sample, this would *significantly* impact the sensitivity results of the test (4/5 = 80% sensitivity).

"Incidence" is the number of instances of the disease or condition that occurs in a specified population *during a given period of time* (such as annually), whereas "prevalence" is the number of instances of a disease or condition in a specified population *at a designated time point.* These two terms may not seem very different, but they take into account the fact that individuals may recover or die from a disease or condition and are no longer counted in the disease prevalence (see Fig. 10.10).

Predictive and Prognostic Testing

For tests that are not "diagnostic" in nature, but rather predictive or prognostic, the sensitivity and specificity calculations and methods utilized will be slightly different. The performance measures for these types of tests are still evolving, because these test results are predictions of outcome or predictions of who will develop a disease or condition in the future. For the reader who wants to understand these predictive and prognostic tests better, a helpful reference to review is "*Systematic Review of Prognostic Tests.*" [7] In simple terms, for these types of tests the main premise of "sensitivity" and "specificity" is still the same:

- *Sensitivity:* Did the test correctly identify or detect those that have the disease or condition (or later contract the disease or condition).
- *Specificity:* Did the test correctly identify or detect those that do not have the disease or condition (or did not contract the disease or condition).

In Vitro Diagnostic Subsectors

The following are descriptions of the diagnostic *subsectors* and descriptions of these subcategories of diagnostic tests:

1. ***In vitro diagnostics:*** As mentioned previously, this category can, in a general sense, include all IVDs. Broadly speaking, the FDA describes IVD products as "those reagents, instruments, and systems intended for use in diagnosis of disease or other conditions, including a determination of the state of health, in order to cure, mitigate, treat, or prevent disease or its sequelae. Such products are intended for use in the collection, preparation, and examination of specimens taken from the human body." The size of the diagnostic market is

large and growing. According to a 2019 research and markets report, the global IVD market was estimated at approximately $69.6 billion in 2018 and is expected to grow by 4.75% compound annual growth rate, from 2019 to 2026. Factors likely to spur the growth include analytical laboratory automation, POC testing, MDx, immunoassays, hematology, flow cytometry, microbiology, and market expansion in emerging countries.

2. ***Molecular diagnostics:*** MDx comprises a category of diagnostics tests referring to the detection and analysis of nucleic acid molecules such as DNA or RNA that are used to provide clinical information. Although all IVDs measure or detect some type of "molecule," MDx is a specific category that detects and analyzes nucleic acids, DNA, and RNA as opposed to chemical, biochemical, and microbiological laboratory testing. MDx tests are available for detecting infectious diseases, cancer, genetic disease screening, human leukocyte antigen typing, coagulation, and PM.

3. ***Prognostic and predictive diagnostics:*** A *prognostic test* provides information about the patient's overall disease outcome, regardless of therapy. In other words, the results tell about the likely outcome of the disease in that individual. For instance, the Prolaris test developed by Myriad Genetics for the prognosis of prostate cancer in patients that are newly diagnosed, examines an "expression signature" consisting of 31 cell cycle genes and 15 normal genes. An expression score (Prolaris score) is provided which indicates the likelihood of prostate cancer progression based upon its genetic makeup. Whereas a *predictive test* provides information about the likelihood of an individual contracting a future disease or condition based upon their genetics. For example, BRCAnalysis, another test developed by Myriad Genetics, examines gene mutations in the BRCA1 and BRCA2 genes and estimates the risk of women with these mutations for developing breast cancer during their lifetime. The mutations in these genes are considered highly "penetrant," meaning a high proportion of individuals carrying a particular variant (allele or genotype) of this gene will also express the associated trait (phenotype). For example, if a particular gene or gene mutation has an 85% penetrance, it means that 85% of individuals with that mutation are estimated to develop the disease, while 15% should not. Because mutations in the BRCA1 and BRCA2 gene are considered to be highly penetrant, often, women testing positive for certain BRCA mutations adopt some proactive intervention such as more frequent screening with an MRI, or in some cases, prophylactic mastectomy.

4. ***Companion diagnostics:*** These are tests that are paired with a particular therapeutic. Companion diagnostics are developed and utilized specifically for determining whether one particular drug is appropriate, or could be the most effective, for treatment. Companion diagnostics are often developed in partnership with a therapeutic program, or more recently within a pharmaceutical company with the specific intent to provide a single test to determine if their particular treatment would be appropriate. More pharmaceutical companies are supporting programs for the development of a companion diagnostic as these tests can assist in assuring their therapeutic will be properly prescribed when the test is positive. For instance, Her-2 testing is a good example. If it is determined that a woman's breast cancer is over-expressing Her-2, this result indicates that Herceptin (a mAb targeted to that receptor) would be appropriate for treatment and have a high likelihood of effectiveness. The FDA maintains a list of the approved/cleared companion diagnostics on their website. The category of companion diagnostics is similar in some respects to the next subcategory of PM.

5. ***Personalized medicine:*** This refers to diagnostic tests that can tailor a treatment to the needs of each person individually. Many PM diagnostics are based upon an examination of an individual's genetics, and tailors their therapeutic dosage and frequency based upon their genetic results. The availability of rapid and cost-effective DNA sequencing, along with microarray DNA chips, have made it possible to identify a set of molecular markers or genomic signatures to produce a genetic fingerprint that correlates with effective treatment options. Some examples of PM diagnostics include a broad category of tests for determining SNPs such as those that occur in the P450 liver enzymes. The P450 liver enzymes affect a person's ability to process a number of different drugs. Certain individuals may carry particular SNP allele (genotype) within their P450 enzymes, and as a result, it affects their ability to metabolize certain drugs. These different SNPs are correlated with normal, increased, or decreased enzyme activity. Polymorphisms in the CYP2C9*2 and/or CYP2C9*3 liver enzyme genes have been associated with decreased warfarin metabolism. Warfarin is a medication used to treat blood clots such as in deep vein thrombosis or pulmonary embolus and to prevent new clots from forming in your body which reduces the risk of a stroke or heart attack. As a result, in August 2007, the FDA approved an update to warfarin labeling that highlighted the use of genetic testing to improve initial estimates of warfarin dosing. PM is a very broad category and includes all tests that identify specific treatments, or determine

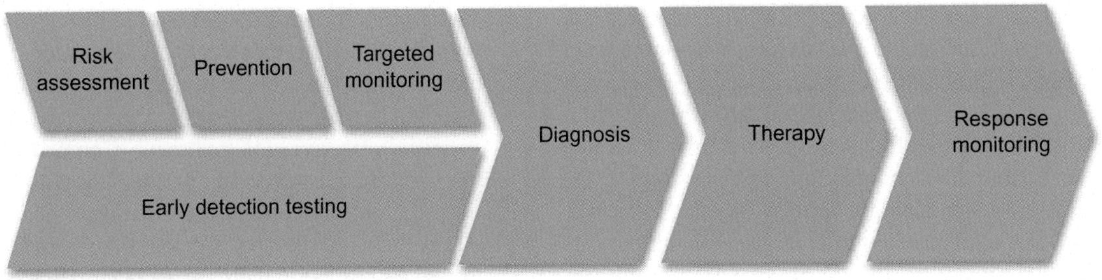

FIGURE 10.11 Personalized medicine goals. *Reproduced with permission from: Personalized Medicine Coalition.*

dosages of medicines, that are optimal for the individual taking them. Another term that refers to the practice of PM is the field of "pharmacogenomics" [8]. By performing PM testing prior to administering certain drugs, a physician can tailor the therapeutic dosage for safer prescribing and the most effective results for that particular patient. Whereas the traditional medical practice is to wait for individuals to present with a disease and then be diagnosed, a key goal of PM is to identify an individual's risk of future diseases and prevent it by employing risk-mitigating programs and/or early detection where treatment outcomes may be the greatest (see Fig. 10.11). More recently the term "precision medicine" is replacing "personalized medicine." There was concern that the word "personalized" could be misinterpreted to imply that treatments and preventions are being developed uniquely for each individual. Although these terms are used interchangeably, the evolution will be to use the term "precision medicine."

6. ***CLIA laboratory clinical testing:*** These are laboratory tests performed in a CLIA-certified laboratory as a service, rather than a diagnostic kit which is manufactured and sold. All laboratories perform diagnostic tests. In some laboratories the majority of the tests they perform have been developed, validated, clinically tested, achieved regulatory approval, and manufactured by another company which sells to them. Whereas some laboratories have developed highly specialized tests on their own, validated them, and they possess the unique skills internally to perform them as a testing service. These are known as laboratory-developed tests (LDTs), and they are services performed by a *single* laboratory in the United States, the one that developed it. Some advantages of LDTs are that the development time and regulatory path are usually shorter and less costly. However, the disadvantages are that the testing can only be performed by one laboratory. Examples of LDTs include Myriad Genetic's BRCA-1 and BRCA-2 test for identifying mutations in these genes that predispose for breast cancer, and Genomic Health's OncoType Dx, a prognostic test to identify a genetic signature for determining the outcome of breast cancer in women.

Regulation of Laboratory-Developed Tests and Clinical Laboratory Improvement Amendments Laboratory Services

In the United States, the regulation of laboratories performing diagnostic tests is the responsibility of the Center for Medicare and Medicaid Services (CMS) by authority of the CLIA of 1988. This regulation differs from IVD regulation under the responsibility of the FDA. The Food, Drug, and Cosmetic Act is a set of laws passed by Congress in 1938 that refers to the distribution of products through interstate commerce which is regulated by the FDA. Technically, laboratory services are not "distributed through interstate commerce," and there is an ongoing debate about which agency has regulatory authority in the United States for LDTs. The FDA has maintained that they have regulatory authority over LDTs but have exercised "enforcement discretion" and in doing so have deferred enforcement. Due in part to the of the growing number of direct-to-consumer genetic testing laboratories that have operated under the CLIA regulations, and the potential safety risk to the public, the FDA has been working on regulations for LDTs. CMS operates under the Department of Health and Human Services and has issued a report on laboratory-developed molecular tests for the readers who are interested [9]. In a 2007 Draft Guidance, the FDA describes "IVD multivariate index assay" (IVDMIA) as a segment of the LDTs that they regulate. IVDMIAs are LDTs that have unknown or undisclosed methods for which the assay results are determined when multiple analytes are examined. Some IVDMIA tests have been successful in navigating through the FDA process and receiving regulatory clearance. An example of an IVDMIA cleared by the FDA in 2008 is AlloMap developed by XDx in Brisbane, California. This test uses a multigene expression microarray to analyze the gene expression profile of RNA isolated from peripheral blood mononuclear cells. The results are an aid in the identification of heart transplant recipients who have a low probability of acute cellular rejection to predict heart transplant rejection. The majority of laboratories offering IVDMIAs are not FDA cleared, because at this time, clear regulations are not implemented, and these services are already compliant under the umbrella of a CLIA-certified laboratory. In 2010 the FDA announced its intent to reconsider its policy of enforcement discretion for LDTs and held a workshop to obtain input from stakeholders on such policy. FDA used this feedback to develop an initial draft approach for LDT oversight and published draft guidance in 2014. After subsequent input and public workshops, on January 13, 2017, the FDA issued a discussion paper on LDTs. On its website the FDA indicates that this is a synthesis of information and does not represent the formal position of FDA, nor is it enforceable. This area of regulation may be ongoing for a long period of time.

Regulation of all In Vitro Diagnostics

Laboratory test systems that are sold by a manufacturer or developed by a laboratory are known as IVD devices and fall under the oversight of the Office of In Vitro Diagnostic Device Evaluation and Safety (OIVD) within the Center for Devices and Radiological Health. OIVD performs its premarket review efforts through three subordinate divisions of immunology (including hematology and pathology), microbiology, and chemistry. Premarket review of IVDs for infectious agents that involve the blood supply and for retroviral testing is usually performed within the CBER.

There are two primary routes to the marketplace for new IVDs and medical devices. These include the following:

- ***Premarket notifications (PMN):*** These are commonly referred to as "510(k)" because it refers to that section of the law. A majority of new IVD assays enter the market through the 510(k) process.
- ***Premarket approval (PMA):*** This is a more lengthy and rigorous approval process compared to the 510(k) route. Products with greater safety risk to the public proceed through the PMA process.

The FDA terminology referring to commercialization and marketing approval is important to understand. Products that are authorized to be commercialized through the PMN route, or 510(k) route, are "cleared" for marketing. Products that reach commercialization via the PMA route are "approved" for marketing. This is an important distinction for the FDA and for labeling claims, as the FDA does not "approve" 510(k)s but rather determines them to be "substantially equivalent" to a product (a predicate device) that was placed on the market prior to May 28, 1976 (effective date of the Medical Device Amendments to the Food, Drug, and Cosmetics Act).

Regulation of IVDs through PMN and PMA allows the FDA to determine whether the device is equivalent to a device already on the market or on the market prior to 1976. Thus "new" devices (not in commercial distribution prior to May 28, 1976) that have not been classified can be properly identified. Specifically, medical device manufacturers are required to submit a PMN if they intend to introduce a device into commercial distribution for the first time or reintroduce a device that will be significantly changed or modified to the extent that its safety or effectiveness could be affected. Such change or modification could relate to the design, material, chemical composition, energy source, manufacturing process, or intended use. More information is provided in *Chapter 25: Integrating Diagnostic Products Into the Drug Development Workflow: Applications for Companion Diagnostics.*

Medical Devices

A medical device is any item used to diagnose a medical condition, prevent illness, promote healing, prevent conception, alleviate incapacity, replace anatomy or physiological process, and is not a medicine, cosmetic, or a food. The legal definition of medical device within the Food Drug & Cosmetic Act is "... an instrument, apparatus, implement, machine, contrivance, implant, in vitro reagent, or other similar or related article, including a component part, or accessory which is: recognized in the official National Formulary, or the United States Pharmacopoeia, or any supplement to them, intended for use in the diagnosis of disease or other conditions, or in the cure, mitigation, treatment, or prevention of disease, in man or other animals, or intended to affect the structure or any function of the body of man or other animals, and which does not achieve any of its primary intended purposes through chemical action within or on the body of man or other animals and which is not dependent upon being metabolized for the achievement of any of its primary intended purposes."

Examples of Medical Devices

There are a wide variety of medical devices, and many do not require biotechnology for their discovery and development. Products that are medical devices by classification include simple objects such as tongue depressors to complex machinery such as CAT scanners and X-ray imagers. Within the medical device industry, there is a need for biotechnology applications to improve and create needed medical devices. Examples of medical devices that biotechnology is helping to create include integrated insulin pumps and monitors that simultaneously measure and

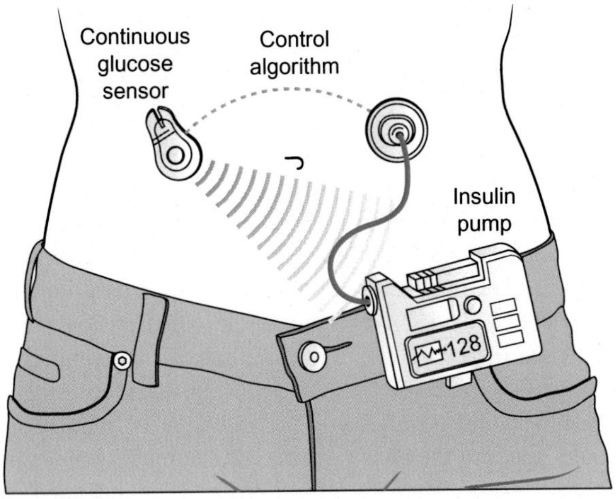

FIGURE 10.12 Integrated insulin pump with real-time glucose monitoring system. *Reproduced with permission from: Mayo Clinic.*

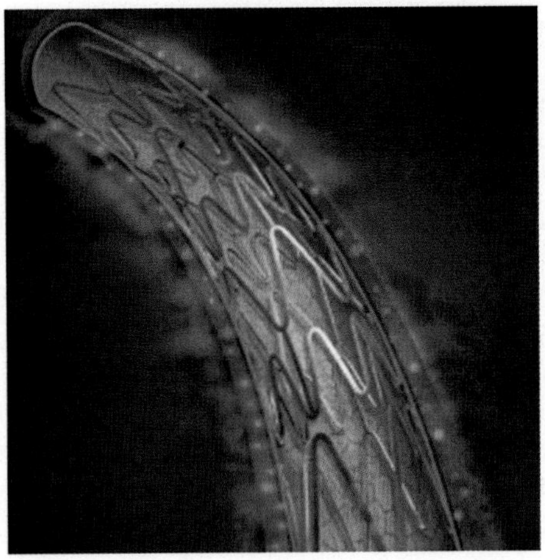

FIGURE 10.13 Combination device/Therapeutic: drug-eluting stent. *From: Boston Scientific.*

monitor real-time glucose levels in the body and signal an insulin pump to administer the proper amount of insulin for maintenance of proper levels in diabetics. These medical devices function for insulin-dependent diabetics as a type of "artificial pancreas" where the individual does not need to manually test their blood sugar and inject insulin according to the blood glucose results (Fig. 10.12).

Regulation of Medical Devices

The regulation of medical devices in the United States is through the FDA Center for Medical Device and Radiologic Health, the same center which regulates IVDs. The FDA classifies medical devices into classes I, II, and III, whereas regulatory control increases from Class I to Class III. The device classification regulation defines the regulatory requirements for a general device type. Most Class I devices are exempt from PMN 510(k); most Class II devices require PMN 510(k); and most Class III devices require premarket approval (PMA). In the United Kingdom, all medical devices that are placed on the market must comply with both European Union laws (the Medical Devices Directives and Regulations) and the UK laws (the Medical Devices Regulations). Each member state of the EU implements the directives into their own national law.

Combination Device/Therapeutic Products

Combination devices result from the combining of medical devices with therapeutics into one product. The purpose of these devices is to enhance their effectiveness by including a therapeutic within, or in association with, the medical device. One such example of a combination device is a drug-eluting stent. Vascular stents (stainless-steel scaffolds) were created to improve the flow of blood through the blood vessels in patients with ischemic problems and arterial clogging. These stents were implanted and served the purpose, but they were found less than adequate over the longer treatment studies due to the risk of thrombosis or clotting of the stent by normal platelet aggregation. Coating the stent with platinum or gold did not seem to eliminate the problem either. However, companies found that by coating the stent with a platelet inhibitor that was released slowly (eluting), they could concentrate this drug at the site and reduce the formation of scar tissue and platelet aggregation. Today the drug-eluting stent business is approximately $5 billion and operates in a product segment that did not exist about two decades ago (Fig. 10.13).

Regulation of Combination Devices

Because combination devices are considered both a therapeutic and a medical device, these are regulated by a section of the FDA that has access to both device and therapeutic reviewers. Combination devices require longer development times and greater amounts of capital to reach commercialization compared to typical medical devices. Combination products are assigned to a center at the FDA for review and regulation in accordance with the product's primary mode of action. When a product's primary mode of action is attributable to a type of biological product within CDER, the product will be assigned to CDER. Similarly, when a product's primary mode of action is attributable to a type of biological product assigned to CBER, the product will be assigned to CBER. For further information about combination products, see the "Combination Products" section of the FDA website.

Research Tools and Reagents

The sector of research tools and reagents encompass a broad range of equipment and specialty reagents used for product development in the biotechnology industry and for academic research. The development costs for these products are typically less expensive than therapeutics, diagnostics and medical devices, and the development time is much shorter. In general, research tools and reagents are not required to receive regulatory approval from the FDA or international regulatory agencies prior to commercialization if they are used solely for research and not clinical or therapeutic purposes. The number of products within this sector are growing rapidly as they are an essential source of materials, supplies, and equipment that biotechnology companies rely upon for the development and testing of their products. Examples of some products that comprise this sector are polymerase chain reaction instruments, DNA sequencers, gene chip analyzers, multiplex readers using various forms of fluorescent cell sorting and laser reading devices, mAb reagents, cytokines, cloning reagents and plasmids, and other specialty reagents used in biotechnology product development.

Sequencers

DNA sequencers play a vital role in the biotechnology industry. The ability to know the four-letter sequence of any gene or DNA segment is essential to conducting research and analyzing the genetics of individuals, organisms, plants, and animals. With the exponential improvements in sequencing DNA more rapidly and more cost effectively, there has been an explosion of genomic information which is giving us a greater understanding of disease. These astounding advances have made it possible to sequence the entire genome sequenced for about $1000 in less than a day. It is estimated that soon the cost for sequencing someone's genome can be done for about $100 and be completed within about one hour. Contrast this to the Human Genome Project which was launched in 1990 with multiple countries participating in sequencing the first human genome which took 15 years and cost about $3 billion.

The technology for sequencing has evolved since the initial work of Frederick Sanger in the mid-1970s, who developed techniques to sequence DNA using polyacrylamide gel electrophoresis and labeling to identify the four bases in sequence (see Fig. 10.14).

With the automation of DNA sequencing in the 1980s, new methods have produced equipment that have been very effective in more rapidly sequencing DNA. Much research and development has continued to be directed toward improving the chemistry, automation, and instrumentation

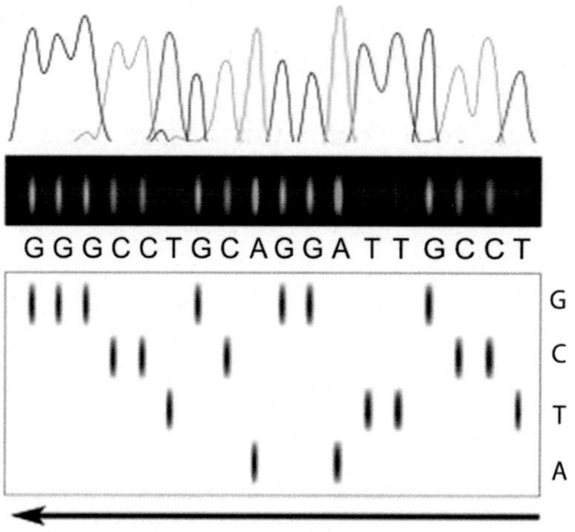

FIGURE 10.14 The Sanger method for sequencing DNA.

for DNA sequencing. The development costs and time associated with creating state-of-the-art instruments can approach the lower range of costs typically associated with therapeutics.

One such example includes the Pacific Biosciences sequencer which can sequence long regions of DNA from a single DNA strand. The basic premise is a single DNA molecule is sequenced by a single polymerase molecule anchored at the bottom of a tiny microwell with a volume measured in zeptoliters (the SI unit for 10^{-21} L). A strand of DNA is threaded to the polymerase while fluorescent-labeled nucleotides are incorporated, and individual color is detected when cleaved with the pyrophosphate group, and a Charge-Coupled Device (CCD) camera takes video as the DNA gets polymerized (see Fig. 10.15).

Microarrays

Many different methods have been developed for the study of gene interactions and gene recognition. These include microarray readers which allow the study of genes, so crucial to our understanding of the cell and its diseases (see Fig. 10.16). A microarray comprising a small support structure, such as a small silicon wafer, on which thousands to millions of DNA sequences from different genes are attached to the support in different locations. Samples of an organism's DNA can then be incubated on the microarray and analyzed using colored florescent tags for the sequences to which they bind. These instrument readers combine chemistry, computer science, biology, and robotics, allowing us to study interactions of genes and genetic material at one time.

Regulation of Research Tools and Reagents

Because products in this category are not directly utilized as therapeutics, diagnostics, or medical devices, and are

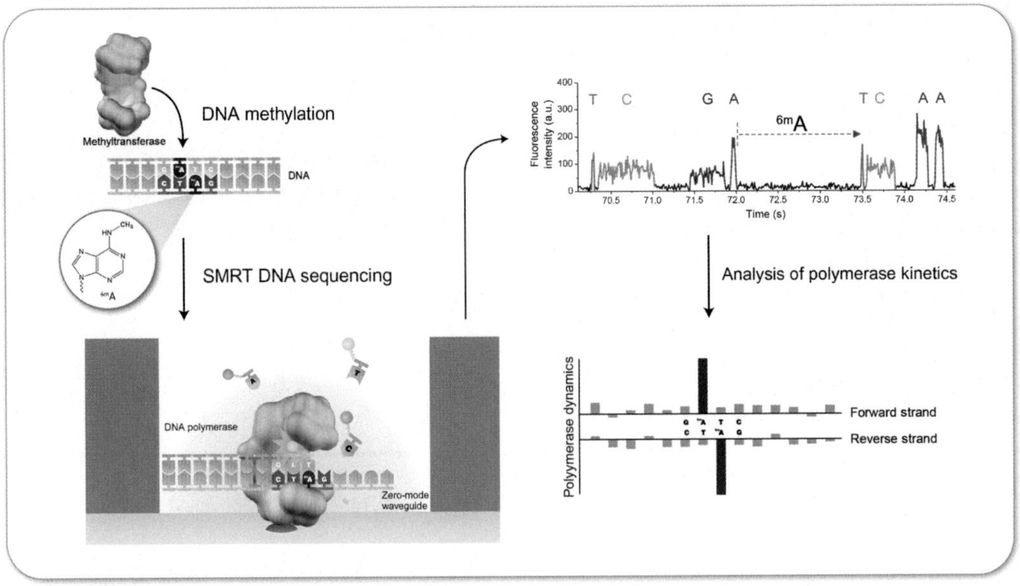

FIGURE 10.15 Pacific Biosciences sequencing method. *Reproduced with permission from: Pacific Biosciences.*

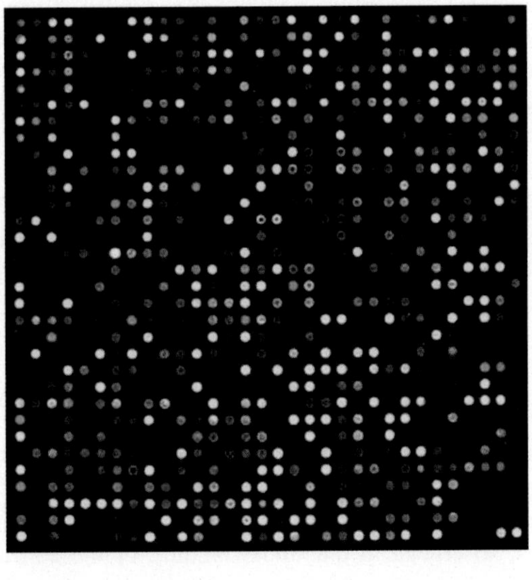

FIGURE 10.16 Microarrays. *Image reprinted courtesy of Promega Corporation.*

primarily used in research applications, in general, there is no official regulatory approval required prior to commercialization of these products. However, there are two categories of reagents to be aware of, that have regulatory requirements, and these are:

1. ***Analyte-specific reagents (ASRs):*** These are raw material components or reagents used to develop assays intended for use in a diagnostic application using human biological specimens. ASRs are considered medical devices that are regulated by FDA [10].
2. ***Research use only (RUO) and investigational use only (IUO):*** RUO refers to a product in the laboratory research phase of development and not represented as an IVD product. IUO refers to a product being shipped or delivered for testing prior to full commercial marketing (e.g., for use on specimens derived from humans to compare the usefulness of the product with other products or procedures) [11].

The FDA has developed these reagent categories, because some research reagents are utilized by companies in making their own diagnostic products, or these products are utilized as an essential reagent in a diagnostic laboratory process. The primary objective was to ensure that laboratories received high-quality building blocks for their in-house-developed tests. On September 14, 2007 the FDA Center for Device and Radiologic Health published a final guidance document governing the use of ASRs in certain IVD products and in-house laboratory assays [10]. On November 25, 2013 final guidance documents were published for RUO and IUO "Distribution of in vitro diagnostic products labeled for research use only or investigational use only" [11]. ASRs are only subject to regulation as medical devices when they are purchased by clinical laboratories for use in "Home Brews" or certain IVD tests. To control the use of ASRs, the FDA imposed a comprehensive set of restrictions. For example, ASRs may only be sold to (1) diagnostic device manufacturers; (2) clinical laboratories that are CLIA-qualified to perform high-complexity testing or clinical laboratories regulated under the Veteran's Health Administration Directive; or (3) organizations that use the reagents to make tests for forensic, academic, research, and other nonclinical (nonmedical) uses. In addition, ASRs may be sold only for use in home-brew tests that are ordered on a prescription basis. Additional information can be found on the FDA website.

The basic requirements of IUO are that all labeling for "a product being shipped or delivered for product testing prior to full commercial marketing (e.g., for use on specimens derived from humans to compare the usefulness of the product with other products or procedures which are in current use or recognized as useful)" must bear the statement, prominently placed: "For Investigational Use Only. The performance characteristics of this product have not been established." To be RUO, a product must be in the laboratory research phase of development and not represented as an effective IVD product. In addition, all labeling must bear the statement, prominently placed: "For Research Use Only. Not for use in diagnostic procedures." In addition, the FDA also advises manufacturers of products labeled as RUO or IUO that if they discover that one of their customers is a clinical laboratory using these IUO- or RUO-labeled products for a noninvestigational diagnostic use, "it should halt sales for such use or comply with FDA regulations for IVD products, including premarket review requirements." For more information, see the FDA website.

Digital Health and Health-care Delivery Information Technology

Digital health applications in biotechnology are diverse and expanding. With the ubiquitous nature of digital IT technology available at our fingertips and the adoption of digital IT technology in the medical and health-care setting, more opportunities are created utilizing some aspect of biotechnology. This growing sector is a convergence of IT technologies and life science problems. Mandatory compliance in the United States for making health-care records readily available to patients and the conversion of medical records to digital format have affected the way test results are delivered and the features imbedded within medical device products. Although every digital health and health-care delivery IT application does not necessarily utilize biotechnology processes per se, but they may involve biotechnology to develop, or it may lead to the utilization of biotechnology products. As 77 million aging "baby boomers" require health care and maintain more active lives, more pressure has been placed on keeping health-care costs from rising out of control. Integration of medical devices and digital health applications are one way of rapidly delivering and efficiently making health-care decisions quicker and providing more efficient health-care cost management.

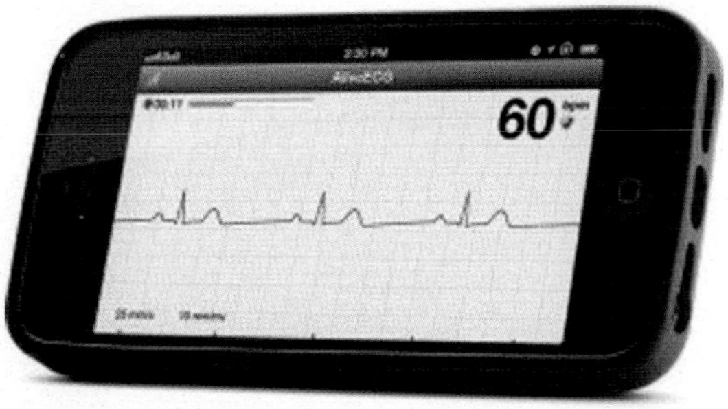

FIGURE 10.17 AliveCor heart monitor (digital ECG). *ECG*, Electrocardiogram. *Reproduced with permission from: AliveCore, LLC.*

Examples of Products

Many digital health products are methods that allow mobility and access to testing that previously could only be performed in a hospital or health-care setting. Today, with the advancement of "smart phones," wearable technology, and advanced materials, an arrhythmia patient can monitor, store, and transmit their electrocardiogram (ECG) directly to their doctor in real-time from anywhere in the world. A product developed by AliveCor utilizes conductive materials, wireless transmitters in a phone case, and sophisticated programming to create an FDA-cleared product called AliveCor Heart Monitor (see Fig. 10.17).

Regulation of Digital Health Products

The regulation of digital health products is determined by their usage and their claims. If a digital health product is used for, or has claims that include, diagnosis or treatment of a disease or condition, or any other claim that is listed above in the medical device section, these products will be regulated by the FDA under the same processes as therapeutics, medical devices, and diagnostics. However, if diagnosis or treatment claims are not made for these same products, FDA regulation is not required. The requirements for how these products are regulated are based upon their claims. As an example, the AliveCore ECG product was originally commercialized without a claim of usage for human health diagnosis or monitoring but rather for a veterinary-use product. During this time the company simultaneously conducted human clinical testing and completed the necessary regulatory requirements to ultimately receive a 510(k) marketing clearance from the FDA for its claims for human ECG monitoring.

Bioagriculture

BioAg refers to the use of biotechnology in agricultural products (Fig. 10.18). Some BioAg applications include creating crops with increased yields and insect resistance, developing biological pesticides, and microbial fertility enhancers to naturally produce healthier crops and

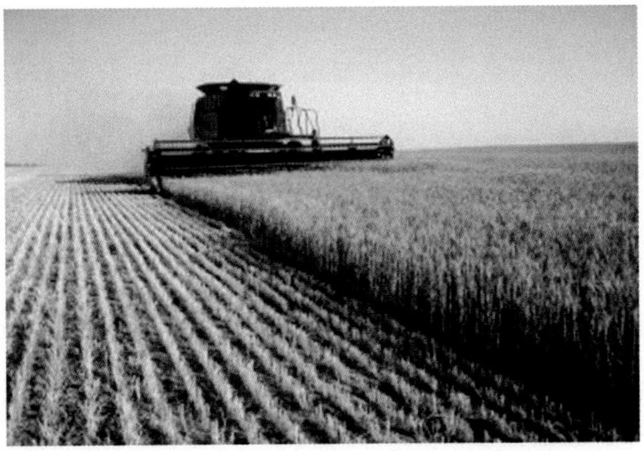

FIGURE 10.18 BioAg. Bioagriculture.

improved yields. The benefits associated with BioAg not only help the farmer, but also the environment and end-consumers. For centuries, farmers have made improvements to crops through selective breeding and hybridization by controlling pollination of plants. Agricultural biotechnology is an extension of plant breeding by using genetic engineering tools to transfer beneficial traits in a more precise, controlled manner.

Bioagricultural products can be divided into three major sectors: seeds, agrochemicals, and fertilizers. The seed sector is focused on crops such as corn, soybean, and cotton to improve these varieties through breeding applications, and now through adding or modifying biotech traits. The agrochemical products include combination of a biotech trait such as herbicide tolerance and crop protection along with novel herbicides based on new targets for herbicide screening. The fertilizer sector remains a commodity sector that awaits novel products that can reduce the amount of fertilizer required or increase the nitrogen uptake of crops. This opportunity awaits novel biotechnology products that lower fertilizer requirements which would result in reduced nitrogen pollution.

The benefits of agricultural biotechnology go beyond just the farmer to include consumers and also the environment. BioAg helps the farmers by providing more cost-effective crops with lowered maintenance costs. The consumers benefit from an affordable, abundant, and safe food supply. Some examples include foods with enhanced nutrition such as tomatoes enriched with the antioxidant lycopene, rice enriched with beta-carotene (the precursor to vitamin A), cooking oils with higher levels of vitamin E, lower levels of *trans*-fatty acids, and increased amounts of omega-3 fatty acids. BioAg helps the environment by the utilization of less pesticides and lowered tillage needs for crop production which decreases soil erosion.

There has been controversy in some areas of agricultural biotechnology for certain products, with the predominant issue being the concept of genetically altered food products. Like any other aspect of technology and science, including therapeutics, there are safety precautions and safety testing requirements that are performed prior to the introduction of any biotechnology product into the market. It is important for the reader and consumers to understand the issues when drawing conclusions about BioAg products. In some instances, certain BioAg products are equivalent to the way farmers and ranchers previously selected the best crops and breeds of animals, but without having to wait for stronger breeds and more hardy crops to spontaneously emerge. For more information on BioAg products, see *Chapter 27: Commercialization and Applications of Agricultural Biotechnology*, which provides more information on this growing and expanding sector.

Regulation of Bioagriculture Products

BioAg products potentially have three agencies in the United States that can require approval prior to commercialization depending upon the product's use and potential safety concerns. These regulatory agencies include the Environmental Protection Agency (EPA), the US Department of Agriculture (USDA), and the FDA.

Biofuels

Biofuels are important for a variety of reasons. The energy we use for transportation is dependent on a limited amount of fossil fuels such as oil and petroleum. Biofuels can offer an energy fuel resource that is both renewable and sustainable. Biofuels are fuels produced from living organisms such as plants or plant-derived materials and microalgae or from metabolic byproducts such as organic or food waste, often referred to as "biomass." Solar energy is first captured through photosynthesis by the plants and stored in the plants' cells. Biofuels are made by converting biomass into convenient energy containing substances in three different ways: thermal conversion, chemical conversion, and biochemical conversion. This biomass conversion can result as fuel in solid, liquid, or gas form. Another future advantage of biofuels is the reduced impact on the environment by the growth of plants used to produce biofuels. As these plants grow, they absorb carbon dioxide in a process called photosynthesis. This absorbed carbon dioxide from future biofuel sources may one day balance the carbon dioxide emitted when the biofuel is combusted, thus creating a smaller carbon footprint than oil. Biofuels have increased in popularity because of rising oil prices and the need for energy security.

Biofuels can be categorized into the following:

- ***Ethanol:*** Primarily used in cars, ethanol is a type of alcohol and is most commonly made from corn or sugarcane and is based on sugars.

- ***Biodiesel:*** A substitute for diesel fuel, which is used mostly in trucks in the United States but is also being used in an increasing number of diesel cars. Most commonly made from soybeans and is based on oils.
- ***Other biomass:*** Mostly used for the generation of electricity or heat. Examples: burning wood chips to boil water and create steam, which spins turbines and creates electricity; and collecting methane from manure piles to generate heat or electricity.

Bioethanol

Bioethanol is alcohol made by fermentation typically from carbohydrates produced in sugar or starch crops such as corn or sugarcane. Biomass, derived from cellulose and nonfood sources, such as trees and grasses, is also being developed as a feedstock for ethanol production. Although ethanol can be used as a fuel for vehicles in its pure form, it is usually used as a gasoline additive to increase octane and reduce vehicle emissions.

Biodiesel

Biodiesel is a renewable, clean-burning diesel replacement made from a diverse mix of recycled cooking oil, soybean oil, and animal fats. Biodiesel has been made by a chemical modification process called transesterification and has also been produced from microalgae and cyanobacteria (see Fig. 10.19). Although biodiesel can be used as a fuel for vehicles in its pure form, it is usually used as a diesel additive to reduce levels of particulates, carbon monoxide, and hydrocarbons from diesel-powered vehicles. The world's largest biodiesel producer is the European Union. By 2050 the International Energy Agency has a goal for biofuels to meet more than a quarter of the world demand for transportation fuels to reduce our dependence on petroleum and coal.

Regulation of Biofuels

Most regulation of biofuels is through the EPA in the United States, whereas in the EU the regulations that impact the EU biofuels market are the Biofuels Directive, the EU Climate and Energy Package, and the Fuel Quality Directive. On November 30, 2018 the US EPA finalized increasing volume requirements under the Renewable Fuel Standard program for 2019 for cellulosic biofuel, biomass-based diesel, advanced biofuel, and total renewable fuel, and biomass-based diesel for 2020 [12]. Because the needs, technology, and impact of biofuels continue to advance, these regulations will also be expected to change. As the availability and technology improve for production and utilization of biofuels so will the need to adopt less restrictive legislation for the development and commercialization of biofuels.

Industrial and Environmental Biotechnology

Industrial and environmental biotechnology products are applications of biotechnology used for industrial purposes such as manufacturing and production of biomaterials. The application of biotechnology to industrial processes is transforming how we manufacture products but is also providing us with new products by using cells or components of cells such as enzymes to generate industrially useful products. Industrial and environmental biotechnology is referred to the third wave of biotechnology, or as

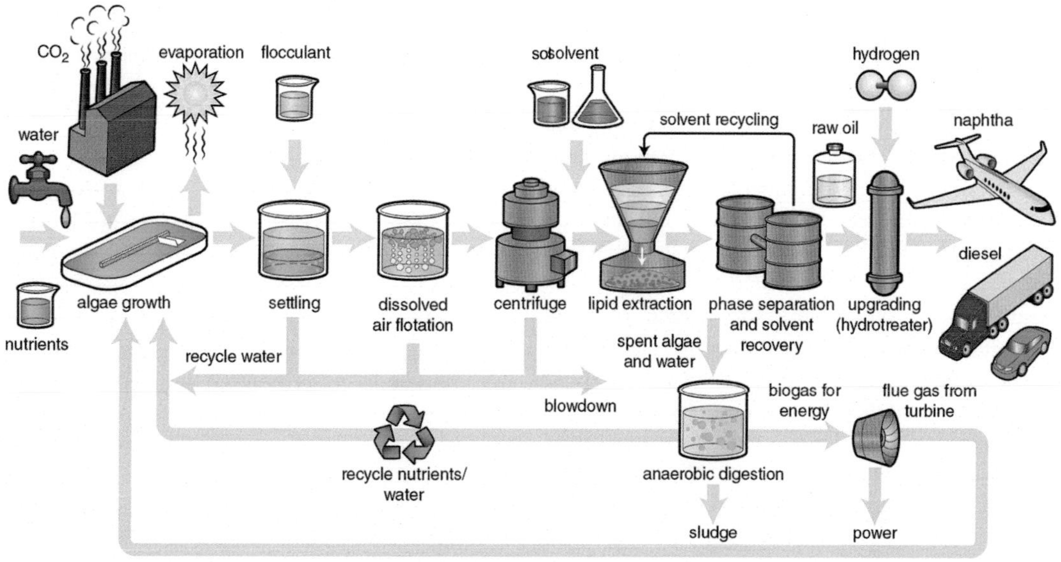

FIGURE 10.19 Production of biodiesel from algae. Illustration kindly provided by Barbara Aulicino with permission from American Scientist magazine

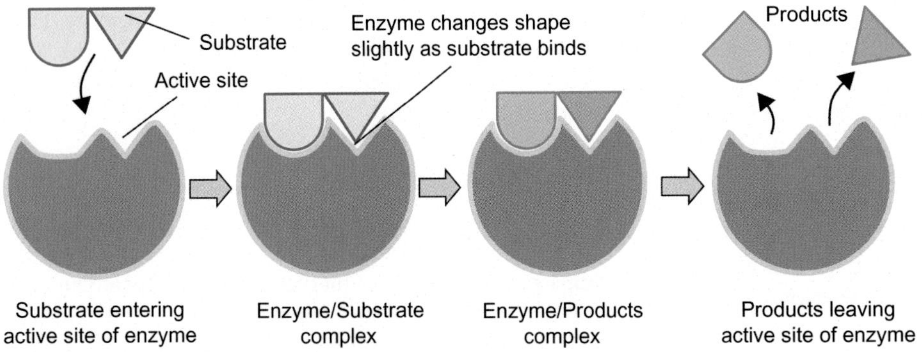

FIGURE 10.20 Enzyme reaction. *By Tim Vickers. From: Wikipedia.*

referred to in Europe as "white biotechnology," whereas agricultural, food, and plant are referred to as "green biotechnology," and the health and medical sector including diseases and pharmaceuticals and diagnostics is referred to as "red biotechnology."

For instance, industrial biotechnology has produced alternative industrial products that reduce pollution that has been a problem caused using phosphates in laundry and dishwashing detergents. Biotechnology companies have developed enzymes that remove stains from clothing that work better than phosphates, thus enabling the replacement of a polluting material with a nonpolluting bio-based additive while improving the performance of the end product. This innovation has dramatically reduced phosphate-related algal blooms in surface waters around the globe and simultaneously enabled consumers to get their clothes cleaner with lower wash water temperatures and concomitant energy savings. There are bio-derived polyester plastics such as biodegradable PHA, which had been demonstrated in a broad range of applications such as molded products such as cell phone cases.

Mechanisms Involved in Industrial Biotechnology Products

A large portion of industrial biotechnology products make use of enzymes that are involved in the metabolic processes of plants, animals, and humans. Enzymes are catalysts that speed chemical reactions which would take too long to accomplish normally. For example, proteases in our digestive tract are enzymes encoded by our DNA that rapidly break down proteins into their basic building blocks of amino acids from the food we eat. These building-block amino acids, in turn, are used by other enzymes to create our body's own specific proteins. Enzymes are now being used for hide degreasing in the leather industry and for metal cleaning in the electroplating industry. Biotechnology has utilized the genes that encode various important enzymes in plants, animals, and humans, and expressed these in large quantities to be used in industrial processes (see Fig. 10.20).

Examples of Uses of Industrial Enzymes

The capabilities of enzymes are utilized in washing and dishwashing machines. Proteases are incorporated into detergents to break down proteins responsible for soiling clothes, while lipases (lipid enzymes) are added to remove fatty acid stains even at low temperatures. Enzymes have become important ingredients that reduce the energy and time required to clean with laundry and automatic dishwashing detergents. Other enzymes such as lactases (enzymes that break down lactose) are utilized in the dairy industry to turn milk, ice cream, and cheese into "lactose-free" products for those individuals who are lactose intolerant. Certain dairy enzymes are used to substitute animal-derived microbial rennets (a complex of enzymes produced in any mammalian stomach) to enhance and produce the robust flavors and textures in cheese and accelerate the ripening of naturally aged cheeses. Biotechnology has also provided a ready source of various microbial enzymes that accelerate the breakdown of waste products in sanitation and waste treatment plants.

Bio-based Materials

Industrial biotechnology processes are being employed to create bioplastics. Common plastics are based upon fossil fuels and are derived from petroleum and produce more greenhouse gas. Bioplastics are plastics derived from renewable biomass sources, such as vegetable fats and oils, corn starch, pea starch, or microbiota. One goal of bioplastics is to provide biodegradable bioplastics that can breakdown in either anaerobic or aerobic environments, depending on how they are manufactured. Some of the applications of bioplastics include packaging materials, dining utensils, food packaging materials, and insulation.

Regulatory Approval of Industrial Biotechnology Products

There is variation on what regulatory agency, or if any agency, requires approval of industrial biotechnology products prior to commercialization. Some agencies within the United States that may regulate industrial biotechnology products include the FDA, the EPA, the USDA, and others. Regulation is dependent on the product and the use of the product. For instance, products that are used in manufacturing of nonfood items may not require approval, with the exception of the typical manufacturing process approvals and those that involve waste regulations from agencies such as the EPA. Whereas, industrial biotechnology products such as enzymes that are used in food production may have a particular FDA route or compliance requirement since the FDA also regulates food products. Industrial biotechnology products in general do not have the lengthy or costly regulatory approvals that are encountered in the therapeutic, biologic, diagnostic, and medical device sectors. It is important, however, to determine what the standard regulatory route for commercialization is of any particular industrial biotechnology product for the United States and non-United States countries prior to beginning development.

Summary

As you can see from the variety and number of products discussed, the biotechnology industry is diverse and encompasses a large number of sectors, each producing valuable products that contribute to improvements in human health, manufacturing, agriculture, and energy needs. The number of new product ideas is almost limitless as new biotechnology applications are being discovered continuously. Each of the various biotechnology sectors encompasses products having distinctive costs, development timeframes, and regulatory requirements. Yet each sector yields unique products that are enabled or produced by biotechnology methods and tools. Biotechnology entrepreneurs will be well served by having a working knowledge of all these sectors. By understanding biotechnology solutions to problems in one sector, similar problems in another sector can be solved by incorporating ideas and solutions from other sectors. Should any of these sectors pique your interest, I suggest that you delve further into the broad array of opportunities and benefits of products within these diverse sectors.

References

[1] DiMasi JA, Grabowski HG, Hansen RW. Innovation in the pharmaceutical industry: new estimates of R&D costs. J Health Econ 2016;47:20–33.

[2] USP Therapeutic Categories Model Guidelines, U.S. Food and Drug Administration Website. <https://www.fda.gov/RegulatoryInformation/LawsEnforcedbyFDA/SignificantAmendmentstotheFDCAct/FoodandDrugAdministrationAmendmentsActof2007/FDAAAImplementationChart/ucm232402.htm> [accessed February 10, 2019].

[3] Long G, Analysis Group. The biopharmaceutical pipeline: innovative therapies in clinical development, <http://phrma-docs.phrma.org/files/dmfile/Biopharmaceutical-Pipeline-Full-Report.pdf>; 2017 [accessed February 11, 2019].

[4] Köhler G, Millstein C. Continuous cultures of fused cells secreting antibody of predefined specificity. Nature 1975;256:495–7.

[5] Aspinall MG, Hamermesh RG. Realizing the promise of personalized medicine. Harv Bus Rev 2007;85(10):108–17 165.

[6] Loong T-W. Understanding sensitivity and specificity with the right side of the brain. Br Med J 2003;327(7417):716–19.

[7] Rector TS, Taylor BC, Wilt TJ. Systematic review of prognostic tests. J Gen Int Med 2012;27(Suppl. 1):94–101 Chapter 12.

[8] Kupiec T, Shimasaki CD. Pharmacogenomics. Remington: The Science and Practice of Pharmacy. 22nd ed. London: Pharmaceutical Press.

[9] Sun F, Bruening W, Uhl S, et al. Quality, Regulation and Clinical Utility of Laboratory-Developed Molecular Tests. Rockville, MD: Agency for Healthcare Research and Quality.

[10] Guidance for Industry and FDA Staff Commercially Distributed Analyte Specific Reagents (ASRs): Frequently Asked Questions. <http://www.fda.gov/downloads/MedicalDevices/DeviceRegulationandGuidance/GuidanceDocuments/ucm071269.pdf> [accessed February 15, 2019].

[11] Distribution of In Vitro Diagnostic Products Labeled for Research Use Only or Investigational Use Only. Guidance for Industry and FDA Staff, November 2013. <http://www.fda.gov/downloads/MedicalDevices/DeviceRegulationandGuidance/GuidanceDocuments/UCM376118.pdf> [accessed February 15, 2019].

[12] Environmental Protection Agency, 40 CFR Part 80, Renewable Fuel Standard Program: Standards for 2019 and Biomass<https://www.govinfo.gov/content/pkg/FR-2018-12-11/pdf/2018-26566.pdf> [accessed February 15, 2019].

Further Reading

Distribution of In Vitro Diagnostic Products Labeled for Research Use Only or Investigational Use Only. Guidance for Industry and FDA Staff, November 2013 <https://www.fda.gov/downloads/MedicalDevices/DeviceRegulationandGuidance/GuidanceDocuments/ucm376118.pdf> [accessed February 19, 2019].

Chapter 11

Technology Opportunities: Evaluating the Idea

Craig Shimasaki, PhD, MBA
CEO, BioSource Consulting Group and Moleculera Labs, Oklahoma City, OK, United States

Chapter Outline

Entrepreneurs in the biotechnology industry build companies based upon novel technologies that yield products they believe will be successful in providing value to a specific group of individuals. There are also venture capital firms that have a specific focus on identifying novel technologies in which they utilize to form start-up companies themselves. How do they choose which technology concepts and product ideas may be destined for success, and which ones to reject because they may not be future winners? The answer to this question is important for entrepreneurs, company leaders, and managers when determining which ideas have the best opportunity for success. These decisions have long-term impact because a group of individuals will then commit an enormous amount of time and resources to the development of this product concept. The information in this chapter will provide you with a framework to more effectively evaluate new product technology ideas and understand how to assess their likelihood for future commercial success. If you are an entrepreneur who is looking to license technology from an academic institution, or if you are a professor or postdoc wanting to know whether your discoveries are viable for starting a company and developing a desirable product, this chapter is for you. If you are working in an academic technology transfer office (TTO), this information will help you evaluate the potential opportunities you have in the pipeline and recognize which ones may, and may not be strong enough to go very far.

When one evaluates technology, an internal analysis must take place to determine whether or not the

Biotechnology Entrepreneurship. DOI: https://doi.org/10.1016/B978-0-12-815585-1.00011-5

technology product concept is more than just a good research project but has potential as a valuable product. Any technology evaluation process must include an examination of the soundness of the science, an appraisal of the supporting scientific and medical literature, and an evaluation of the scientific and technical team who will be participating in the early development of the product. If the underlying technology and product concept is not sound, no amount of marketing, capital, and team talent can overcome flawed science. The research and discoveries that support the product concept must be able to stand up to criticism, naysayers, and pessimists, all of whom predictably appear when individuals move forward with a new idea. In order to complete a technology assessment, it must also include more than just an examination of the technology and the research team. Once the underlying science is validated, before proceeding further, one must also evaluate whether or not this product concept will satisfy an unmet market need.

Sources of Biotechnology Product Ideas

The majority of innovative biotechnology products can be traced back to basic research that began at an academic or research institution over the course of several years, possibly decades. If you examine the original source of most successful biotechnology products, you will find that the vast majority of them originated from the basic research conducted by a scientist, professor, physician, or engineer at an academic or research institution. This is true because a fundamental goal of institutional research is the acquisition and discovery of new knowledge. Basic and academic research focuses on exploring new ideas, testing new concepts, and better understanding previously unknown processes in biology, science, and engineering. Unfortunately, for the commercially minded, academic research objectives rarely include product development or commercialization goals. As you will learn in the subsequent chapters about licensing and technology transfer processes at universities, increased efforts are being made to advance basic research ideas toward the early stages of product development while they are still at these institutions. Nevertheless, academic and research institutions do not typically possess the depth of expertise in biotechnology product development and often are not well equipped or experienced in assessing the potential for which technology concepts may become blockbuster products. Very few products have been fully developed within academic and research institutions. This is because their goals are not the same as in industry, and they possess limited experience in moving product concepts efficiently to product development and precommercialization prototypes. As a result, many good technology product concepts accumulate but lay dormant at these institutions.

Research to Commercialization Chasm

A great chasm exists between the large body of excellent research conducted within the laboratories of academic and research institutions, and the translation of these ideas into commercial products. One reason for this chasm is that basic research expertise and commercialization expertise are segmented, and the interface between these expertise holders is rarely linked. While the best scientific research is most often conducted at top-notch academic and research institutions, the finest product development work is most often performed in the commercial enterprises. These entities operate independently of each other and rarely overlap in any cross-functional way, and certainly not on a frequent basis. Due to this segmentation of expertise, knowledge and ability, academic institutions may have as much as 75%–80% of their entire patent portfolio sitting on their shelves with no commercial entity showing interest in these assets. During this time, these institutions pay patent prosecution fees on pending applications and maintenance fees, translation fees, and taxes on intellectual property (IP) that remains on shelves unrecognized and unlicensed.

Due to this chasm and the abundance of technology opportunities, academic and research institutions are the best places for entrepreneurs to uncover myriads of great ideas for future biotechnology products. For those interested in pursuing a path of biotechnology entrepreneurship, one great way to "discover" potential product ideas is to talk with the staff and management in TTOs at various academic and research institutions, including federal laboratories. There you can find some of the best life science, agricultural, and biofuel research being conducted. These institutions have numerous product opportunities for entrepreneurs who have the skill, seasoned experience, and drive to forge company opportunities based upon these technology and product concepts. When approaching a TTO, be sure to define the technology areas or market opportunities you are interested in and the fields where you believe you can recruit experienced help for your product development.

Technology Transfer Offices Manage Large Portfolios of Intellectual Property

Although every academic and research institution and federal laboratory will admit that a chasm exists, it is not necessarily because the TTOs are not actively soliciting potential suitors for their portfolio assets. Stanford University owns the IP that became "Google" and in the early days attempted to out-license this IP to many of the web companies over a period of time. The inventors, then graduate students, Sergey Brin, and Larry Page, were completing their PhD work and realized that none of the likely industry players were interested enough to license the IP. These inventors decided to commercialize the technology if no one else would. The TTO said that they were willing to grant a license, but they felt that the pair did not really know much about commercialization. These two nascent entrepreneurs learned some things along the way, and we all know the rest of the story.

Licensing offices at research and academic institutions are recognizing what methods work most effectively for out-licensing more of their technology assets. Stanford is one of the more prolific institutions in successfully licensing its technology and IP to commercial entities. It is interesting to note that Stanford's Office of Technology Licensing (OTL) employs mostly technical staff with backgrounds in industry and often individuals with MBA. The J.D.'s they have on staff appear to be managing contracts rather than negotiating licenses. It has been said of the Stanford's OTL office that while outside legal counsel is available, such oversight is not required if an agreement does not deviate from the university's standard practices of granting no warranty on an invention and total indemnification by the licensee. Ms. Katherine Ku has been the director of the OTL since 1992. She came from a small biotechnology company, and most of her associates have similar backgrounds. She has been quoted as saying, "We feel we are a marketing office, not a legal office." The technical background and training of her staff have been effective in negotiating licensing agreements because successful negotiations require an understanding of the technology. Several video lectures are available on the Stanford eCorner, which are helpful for other TTOs looking for help in building a successful TTO model.[1]

In an article by Fisher [1] about TTOs, Jeffrey Labovitz, who was the acting director of technology licensing at the University of California at San Francisco at that time, said, "A lot of technology-transfer offices are built around patent attorneys, and they lead with the agreement, as opposed to the deal, so it is very hard for them to negotiate. Deal-making is very much a creative endeavor, so the more you know about the variables, the more creative you can be."

So Why the Gap?

I believe that there are many reasons for the accumulation of IP at academic and research institutions in addition to those we have discussed. These include the following:

1. Seasoned entrepreneurs who possess the ability to build a company around a technology may shy away from licensing an academic institution's IP because of the perceived, or real, issues that hamper their ability to quickly and economically license a technology from the institution.
2. The most likely licensee organizations for these patent assets may not be interested in acquiring outside technology because they have already devoted internal research and development (R&D) resources toward internal projects that already address their market interest.
3. Industry executives may not be aware of the diversity of IP opportunities available in academic, research, and federal laboratories, or they may not be willing to pay a license or royalty on future products that their company would commercialize.
4. The IP assets are based upon excellent technology concepts but the product application chosen and tested by the scientist, engineer, or physician is not the ideal market opportunity due to existing competitive products in that market.
5. The TTO has the bulk of their resources focused on prosecuting patents filed with the Patent and Trademark Office and they have limited resources remaining to find and solicit licensees for the IP technology they have.
6. The TTO may not have the resources or budget appropriations to hire the type of staff with the skills and expertise, or their current staff may not have the liberty to effectively negotiate deal structures that would attract the type of licensee partners needed for their assets.
7. Many first-time entrepreneurs who may be interested in the IP assets do not have the skill set and experience to proceed with commercialization and may not demonstrate enough know-how for the institution to confidently license the technology to these individuals.

Due to these and other issues, the chasm remains. However, more TTOs are working to address these issues and facilitate the licensing of more of their IP assets to the best suitors. The issues still remain, so the commercial entities and entrepreneurial teams must avail themselves to these untapped opportunities because they possess the greatest ability to commercialize products from these IP assets. Together, the academic institutions and commercial entities and entrepreneurial teams must develop financial models that make licensing IP assets a viable alternative to conducting all of their own internal R&D. It is also helpful for entrepreneurs who are seeking to license technology from a particular institution to become acquainted with the individuals who are responsible for licensing technology. It is equally important for the potential licensee to outline their product development plans for the TTO as to how they intend to move a licensed

1. <https://ecorner.stanford.edu/> [accessed 12.02.19].

product concept toward commercialization. There are plenty of good product ideas waiting for good homes, and TTOs will be receptive to hearing from entrepreneurs who have credible commercialization experience and strategies.

Experimental Paths: Basic Research versus Translational Research

It is important to recognize that research conducted at academic research institutions by nature has a different goal than translational research performed at a biotechnology company. Academic research is performed for the purpose of gaining new knowledge, publishing discoveries, and securing grants to support further research. Whereas, the translational research conducted at companies is to develop a useful product. To casual observers, academic research experiments can appear, on the surface, identical to the translational research in commercial laboratories. However, the basic research and translational (or applied) research programs differ markedly in their decisions on the types of experiments to be conducted and the time spent on a particular experimental direction. For instance, in basic and academic research, a team may discover a new mechanism for cell signaling that triggers a unique inflammatory response. Future research choices by the academic research scientists may include identifying the receptor, determining the crystal structure and protein sequence, elucidating the triggering mechanism for stimulation, and uncovering the precise stepwise cascade involved in this inflammatory process. However, the ultimate experiments for industry researchers would be to screen chemical compounds that inhibit this inflammatory process for the development of drugs to treat rheumatoid arthritis or other inflammatory conditions. The industry researchers conduct similar types of experiments as academic researchers, but the underlying purpose is different—whereas they can use this knowledge to ultimately produce a product. Due to the difference in goals, the entrepreneurial team or evaluator of a technology must see beyond the actual experiments and look for the best commercial application of this research. For instance, if academic research has uncovered a new biological mechanism of action, ask youself the question, what potential applications would this mechanism-of-action have in other disease conditions, diagnostics, or new medical devices? In other words, what other applications can this discovery be applied toward?

Although all academic universities and research institutions have large IP portfolios that are idle, the *research* that underlies this IP is not necessarily idle. It is the *commercial development of the product* that is idle because the scientist or the professor will likely continue their focus on more basic research to uncover new discoveries and to better understand the science. This is where creative and experienced biotechnology entrepreneurs come in. There are vast technology opportunities housed within great academic institutions awaiting entrepreneurs who have the creative skill, technical expertise, and market understanding to develop desperately needed products. This academic research resource can be a treasure chest laden with valuable future biotechnology products (see Table 11.1).

Technology Is a Solution Seeking a Problem to Solve

Successful biotechnology entrepreneurs appreciate great scientific research, but what they keenly understand is that *technology is simply a solution seeking an important problem to solve*. If the problem that the technology can solve is extremely significant, there will be great interest from customers if this is a truly unmet need. If the problem this technology solves is minor and insignificant, there will be limited customer interest. Most people are amazed by the remarkable advances achieved in any field of technology. Moreover, it is true that sophisticated, leading-edge technology can enamor us with its novelty, complexity, and the amazing things that it can achieve. However, entrepreneurs must be cautious not to be overly charmed by the technology and forget that the most critical aspect of any product's value is the *problem* that it solves. It is helpful to keep this in perspective by realizing that the customer is not principally interested in the

TABLE 11.1 Basic research versus translational research.

	Basic research	Translational research
Driven by	Curiosity and questions	Developing useful products or services
Motivated by	Expanding and acquiring knowledge	Solving practical problems
Questions answered	How things work, why things work	What inventions can be made with this knowledge

technology or scientific method of *how* their problem is solved, just that your product delivered its promise and their problem *is* solved.

How to Determine if a Product Concept is Worth Pursuing as a Company

There are many technology projects that are worthy of consideration. These projects usually have a product concept in mind that may have some value. However, the entrepreneur must determine if this is simply an interesting research project or can this product idea establish the basis for a viable company. A research project will be considered successful if *the research idea is novel and the technology is interesting enough to be funded.* These criteria are not enough to consider a company successful. Although the company's product development must also be funded, the resulting product must also provide enough value to a target market of customers such that they would gladly purchase it and use it. Regrettably, some young biotechnology companies are founded with the belief that success will follow if *the research idea is novel and the technology is interesting enough to be funded.* The criterion used for determining a successful research project is not the same criterion required for building a successful company. Research projects are considered successful if they achieve their intended specific aims, whereas companies are only successful if they produce products that are successful in the market—these ultimate goals are different. The decision for the biotech entrepreneur is to carefully assess the product idea and determine whether it is simply a good research project or if it can become a great company. Properly assessing the technology is critical as once this is done the technology will move into product development, which will either result in "doing things right" or "doing the right things." In other words a company can be established upon *any* research project concept, but if the resulting product idea has limited market value, no amount of "right" method development or "right" project planning can solve the absence of a true market need for the product.

Three Initial Criteria for Assessing Technology Product Opportunities

The biotech entrepreneur must carefully evaluate (1) the underlying science, (2) the future product concept and the best market application, and (3) the people factor, which will be discussed at the end of this chapter. A scientific assessment of the technology is the first critical step, and it is the foundation upon which a future company will be built. If the science is not sound then no matter how great the market interest is for such a product, it cannot be delivered. However, scientific assessment by itself will not predict the likelihood of product success. One must also evaluate the market potential of a product in order to determine if it has a basis for a viable business. Initially, the following criteria should be evaluated when considering a product concept or a technology license from an academic institution. The evaluation of future product concepts must not end with only these two criteria but incorporate additional factors such as the company business model and the five criteria for assessing a company, which are discussed in *Chapter 12: Understanding Biotechnology Business Models and Managing Risk.* However, these criteria should serve as the basis for the initial assessment of the science and product concept.

Initial Assessment Criteria for Technology and Product Concepts

1. Evaluate the underlying science and the technology.
2. Evaluate the product's market potential for the best market application.
3. Evaluate the people factor (see Fig. 11.1).

Evaluate the Underlying Science and the Technology Team

What aspects of the science and technology make it worth creating a company to support the development of this

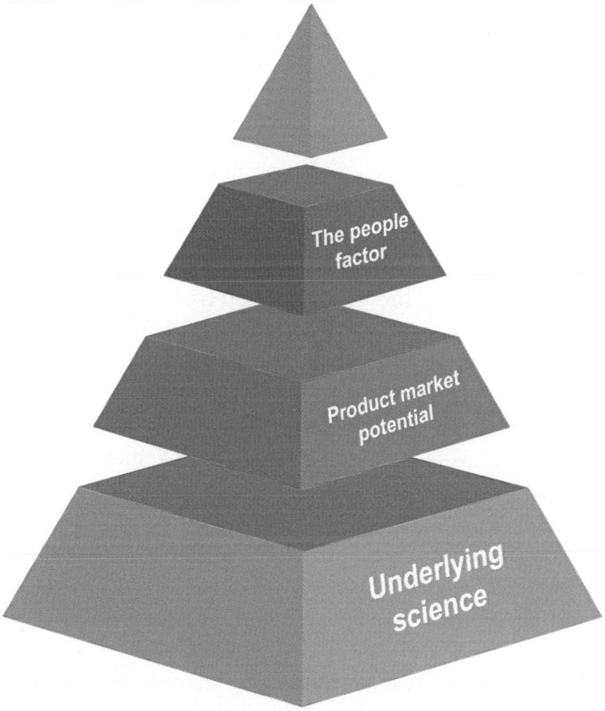

FIGURE 11.1: Three initial assessment criteria when evaluating technology product concepts for licensing.

product idea? I believe that there are several qualities that help determine a technology's viability as a product concept. These include

- the quality of the underlying research and the technical team involved;
- the breadth of scientific information understood about the disease or condition, or the biological certainty of the targeted application for the product;
- whether or not the product is capable of being developed within the knowledge and systems available today; and
- whether this is a single product idea or a platform technology with multiple future product applications.

The Quality of the Underlying Science Is Foundational

A thorough evaluation of the quality of the science and the underlying research is critical before making a decision to license or move forward with any product concept. Know that a major portion of a biotechnology company's early value is based on the science that underlies the product concept and the credentials of the inventors and researchers of the technology. Consequently, if the science is mediocre, the company will not have much value. If the science is top tier, then the company will be perceived to possess a great asset. As the company achieves and reaches product development milestones, additional value is apportioned to the company based upon the increased likelihood that the product will be commercialized.

One good method to assess the quality of the science is by reviewing published articles about the research in peer-reviewed journals. The originating scientist, engineer, or physician can provide you with some references to begin your search. You do not need to be an expert in this research, but you do need to be able to glean whether or not the conclusions are supported by the basic tenets of the underlying research. It is also important to conduct a literature search for other researchers working in this field, as you may also find out whether others are further ahead, or if they have disproved the research conclusions. Find out to what extent others cite this inventor's research papers and whether or not the conclusions are generally believed and supported by others. One noteworthy point is that any new research concept that is a sharp departure from previous understanding is often resisted by others until enough research is published, and many researchers are working in this field. When new or "radical" concepts are proposed in science, if they go against current understanding, they most often will meet resistance. This was true for Stanley Prusiner and his proposed existence of nongenetic infectious agents called "prions." He was greatly criticized for his theory and his experiments that were later proved to be true, and he received the Nobel Prize in 1997. When peptic ulcers were proposed to be caused by bacteria, there were challenges in the medical and scientific community until enough scientific evidence supported this theory leading to the ultimate identification of *Helicobacter pylori*, the causative bacterial agent. Although countercurrent research arises, most ideas and scientific concepts are built upon stepwise and incremental research advancements expanded from previous discoveries in science, biology, medicine, engineering, or physics.

When conducting a review of the scientific research, be sure to meet with the researchers and inventors themselves to assess the confidence they have in their research conclusions. Ask them about any conflicting research studies and whether the science has a controversial nature, and if so, what aspects. You can gain valuable insights by talking with them about their research. Another good way to assess the quality of the scientific research is to request to read any grant applications that resulted in awards to the researchers. Moreover, find out how many grants and granting agencies have funded their research. Having been awarded multiple federal grants is a good indicator that both the researcher and the research are respected by their peers. In addition to the scientific review and meeting with the researchers, for medical products, you should have discussions with academic and medical opinion leaders who would be prescribing, testing with, or utilizing the proposed product. If the proposed product is in the agricultural biotechnology industry, ask farmers, consumers, and regulatory agencies for their impressions of such a product idea. Key opinion leaders' impressions of a new product concept can impact the receptivity by others in the industry. Be sure to assess the receptivity of the key opinion leaders when making a technology assessment.

If *you* are the inventor and you are also considering being the future entrepreneur, it is too difficult to objectively assess your *own* technology, so the best advice is to get assistance in obtaining an unbiased opinion about the technical merits of your research leading to your envisioned product. Most researchers tend to *not* be as critical of their own research as others may be, so it is advisable to recruit the help of others for feedback. If the research is performed at an academic or research institution, it is possible that your TTO may have conducted some type of technology evaluation when they were preparing invention disclosures or patent applications. If the institution does not have this type of assessment available, find a business person, consultant, or even another entrepreneur in a similar biotech sector who would be willing to assess the merit and likelihood of the research resulting in a viable product. This can help you decide whether or not to pursue the product concept, modify the product concept, or obtain a license for the technology.

The Quality of the Researcher and the Technical Team

Great scientific research is associated with talented researchers who are of high caliber and respected in the scientific community. Typically, they will also have talented technicians, postdocs, and other researchers working in their laboratories. Practically speaking, the science and the scientists are not mutually exclusive. In other words, talented scientists tend to conduct impressive research. When you assess the science, you should also assess the quality of the research team who developed the underlying technology that supports the product concept you are considering. Often a good way to assess the team is to have face-to-face discussions, but when that is not possible, be sure to have plenty of telephone or video/Internet-based communications before making a decision to license a technology. Once you have concluded that the underlying science is solid, and the research team is of high caliber, you must be sure that this team is willing to spend time working on the commercial application you are interested in developing. If there is limited time for this team to devote to product development due to research and teaching responsibilities, grant commitments, or other administrative duties, it will be challenging to get the momentum you need to move the company forward. In the beginning, you critically need the expertise of the researchers who developed the technology so that they can help train or transfer the technology to others who can continue translational development of the product. The technology only remains viable as long as those who have developed it remain associated with its development in some capacity. It is imperative, for a period of time, to retain the inventors and researchers when negotiating a technology license. There are creative ways to work out arrangements with the discovering scientists even if they do not plan on being cofounders or employees of the company.

Be Sure the Underlying Biology of a Disease or Condition Is Sufficiently Understood

For instance, in the medical sector, there are several technology concepts being advanced for the treatment of Alzheimer's disease, which is a degenerative process albeit not completely understood. There is great market interest and need for products to treat this condition. However, to the degree that any product correctly targets the true underlying cause, to that same degree the product will have a high likelihood of being successful. When HIV was first discovered and its association with AIDS in the early 1980s, the infectious cycle of the virus and knowledge of immunology were not totally understood. As the mechanism of the HIV infectious cycle and its evasion of the immune system were elucidated, better and more effective treatments were developed. At the outset of any technology endeavor, you want to start with reasonable certainty that the future product is directed against the underlying pathway of the disease or condition.

Is Product Development Feasible Using Today's Knowledge and Systems?

Often a biotechnology product idea may appear initially intriguing, but as you delve deeper into the science and technology, you may uncover systems or methodology challenges that must also be overcome before the product can be developed. For instance, oral administration of peptide and protein-based drugs are typically degraded in the gut. If the market requires your product to be orally administered but there is no delivery method available for the drug to become systemic except by intravenous injection, the rest of the product development process is moot. In another example, if you are developing a drug that works effectively in the brain but you do not have a method that permits it to cross the blood–brain barrier, the product development process is academic. Ensure that there is not a major roadblock in product development, which cannot be solved or resolved by the knowledge and systems available today.

Is This a Single Product or a Core/Platform Technology with Multiple Products?

When assessing the technology, be sure to explore whether or not this is a single product or a technology platform that can produce multiple products. This may take some time to determine, but most product concepts in biotechnology have an underlying scientific basis that is applicable and transferrable to other applications. Spend some time to uncover the underlying scientific basis and work to identify additional product opportunities that have significant market value. Sometimes, it is subtle whether a technology can yield multiple applications. It is possible that the product development process may be the technology platform which can generate diverse products having related characteristics. For example, an innovative method for rapidly producing highly specific humanized monoclonal antibodies may be the core technology, and the original product application of the core technology may be, for example, a treatment for glioblastoma. There are multiple disease targets that would benefit from *highly specific humanized monoclonal antibody* treatments. In another example, the product application could be the development of a hepatitis vaccine, but the platform technology provides the ability to rapidly produce vaccines in mammalian cells in a fraction of the normal time. This core technology process could be adapted to rapidly manufacture influenza vaccines for the next season's strain since part of the problem for flu vaccine manufacturers is to quickly generate product once the World Health Organization and the Centers for Disease Control predict the next season's strain. For an example, in the molecular testing industry, let us say that a product application is a combination of gene signatures that predict the recurrence of breast cancer. However, the know-how generated during the development of this product could be leveraged to rapidly develop another gene signature for colon or prostate cancer recurrence. When you are searching for additional product applications, do not overlook the know-how generated during the development of the first product as an asset for accelerating other product opportunities. Often a single specific product application may have been the focus, but in reality, all biotechnology products operate with an underlying scientific basis that enables that product application to work. Your ability to attract investors increases with the likelihood that the technology can produce multiple products from the same research. Investor interest increases because they understand that follow-on products grow the future business, and a one-product company has limited long-term success. If the technology is absolutely limited to a single product, this does not mean that the technology is second rate, or that the company cannot raise capital for the product development. In fact, if the product is successful, there is a high likelihood that this single product may find other indications for use the longer it remains in the market. Spend time talking to individuals in the field such as scientists, physicians, clinicians, medical specialists, hospital staff, and laboratory directors, because these discussions can help you identify additional useful applications even for a single product.

Evaluate the Product's Market Potential in the Best Market Application

When evaluating technology, it is not uncommon to find that the research has a solid scientific basis, but sometimes, the initial product application is directed toward a subpar market, or to a market that is already filled with competitive products adequately serving the customer's needs. To produce a successful product the technology must be wisely applied to the best product opportunity that is directed toward an underserved market having a great need. Aspects of these criteria include the following:

1. Determine if the product application is directed toward an acute market need that is not currently being met or suitably addressed by other products or substitutes.
2. Determine whether the technology has the ability to deliver the market-needed product features.
3. Assess if there is an existing reimbursement pathway for the product.
4. Assess if the market is already saturated with multiple competitors having very little differentiation in value, even though all are meeting this need.

The Technology Must be Directed toward a Market with the Greatest Unmet Need

As will be discussed in more detail in *Chapter 13: Directing Your Technology toward a Market Problem: What You Need to Know Before Using the Business Model Canvas?*, understanding the market interest for a product is critical to the success of any biotechnology company. The choice of the first product application of any technology is key. Often biotechnology companies only get one chance to develop a product even though they may have a number of other good product application opportunities using the same technology. A single product failure for a well-capitalized pharmaceutical company will quickly get shelved, and another will take its place in the development without missing much of a beat. Whereas, development-stage biotechnology companies do not have cash reserves to support multiple product development programs through to commercialization. If a biotechnology company's first product fails anywhere along the development path, it is challenging to recover and have a second chance, irrespective of how great the other applications may be.

Ensuring that the first application of any technology is appropriately directed toward a market with the greatest unmet need is essential. For example, in the medical device and diagnostic sector, there is an unmet need for assay methods to determine the most effective chemotherapeutic agent prior to the treatment of a patient's cancer. These chemosensitivity assays could serve a great need by predicting the most effective chemotherapy for a specific tumor biopsied from a patient without having to resort to trial and error. If a researcher developed a chemosensitivity test that worked on a certain tumor tissue type, but selected a tumor tissue target based on the availability of tumors from collaborators, not based upon the market need (problem to be solved) the choice of this first product application will be directed toward a suboptimal market. For instance, in some cancers, there may only be one or two treatment choices that are effective, therefore, a chemosensitivity device specifically targeting for that type of cancer would not solve a significant market problem. Whereas, if this device tests for a tumor type that has 10 treatment options, each with varying degrees of success in different individuals, this would meet a significant market need. Be sure that the first product application of the technology is directed toward an unmet and significant need in the market.

Two additional criteria for evaluating the market potential of a product application include the following:

1. the acuteness of the market need for that product and
2. the competition or substitutes in the market now and in the near future.

These and other assessment criteria are essential to examine before starting a company or business based upon any product concept. Recognize that the greater the product market need, the increased likelihood that the company can also raise the capital to fund development. When choosing a product concept to build a company upon, be sure to optimize your chances of success and minimize your risk of failure.

Is There Market Demand That Is Not Met or Addressed with Substitutes?

Another key question to be answered before considering the licensing of any technology—is there significant market demand that is not addressed by competitors or substitutes for this product? World-class technology directed toward a product that is only "useful" will not guarantee that anyone will want to purchase the product once it is developed. For many biotech entrepreneurs, the analysis of market need and substitutes does not always rise to significance at this early stage, even though it should. This is a grave mistake because the level of market interest in the product impacts a multitude of other issues—especially your ability to raise capital for the company. For example, suppose you find a novel licensing opportunity with a product application for peptides that possess powerful antibiotic properties against a limited number of Gram-negative bacteria. The science may be novel and the results may be fantastic, yet there are dozens of antibiotics in the market (substitutes), which are very effective against Gram-negative bacteria and certainly economical to use. This project's lackluster market appeal makes it difficult if not impossible, to generate much interest from biotech investors, which hold the capital needed to develop any product through to commercialization. However, suppose the same technology produces a peptide with antibiotic properties against methicillin-resistant *Staphylococcus aureus* (MRSA). The market for such a product would be tremendous because of the lack of effective antibiotics that work against MRSA. Raising money for this product would be less difficult than the first. Recognize that no matter how stellar, novel, exciting, or ground-breaking the science is, if there is not a significant and acute market need for the resulting product, which is not addressed by substitutes, the endeavor will be futile.

How Big Is the Estimated Market for This Product?

Having a large market for a future product will help attract the type of investors needed to fund your product development. But there is also great interest in certain niche markets and especially those that can gain "orphan drug" status. If the product is for AgBiotech markets, the niche market strategy is not likely to be successful because of the low profit margins for most of these products. Regardless of where the technology is directed toward, whether it be AgBiotech, therapeutics, medical devices, molecular diagnostics, or industrial enzymes, be sure that you know the size of the total market for your future product and the size of the "target" market which is the highest likely group of customers who have the most acute need for that product. In the end, an acute need for a product is even more important than the size of the market. The need for a product must be acute and unmet in order for a future product to have great success. The greater the need for the product, the greater will be the receptivity. Conversely, if these customers are satisfied with the currently available products and substitutes, there will be minimal demand for your product.

When assessing the technology, determine if the proposed product features provide superior value to the target audience and that substitutes or alternatives are not already satisfying customer needs, or at least be sure the alternatives are inadequate or minimally effective in satisfying the needs of potential customers. This includes verifying that there is an existing unmet customer demand for your product because it is extremely difficult to sell a product for which you first have to create a demand. Successful products are launched to meet an existing unmet market need. If you must also create customer demand, it requires first educating the customer that they "need" the product when they do not know this. Creating market demand for a product is more difficult than producing a product that meets an existing unmet need.

Don't Be Too Far Ahead of the Market Need

Because of the lengthy biotechnology product development time frame, it is good to anticipate future product market needs. However, there is a potential problem in being *too* far ahead of any market need because products take time to be accepted if they are too far ahead of need. Technology adoption, customer interest, medical practices, and societal norms constantly change, and it is difficult to predict where demand will be far into the future.

Premature products move very slowly along adoption curves. Sometimes, these types of products may also create ethical concerns or face unknown consequences that would limit their market acceptance. For example, gene therapy has tremendous potential and should ultimately be effective for many debilitating conditions, but recognize how many decades it has taken to see the beginning of acceptance, whereas the first companies were too far ahead of medical adoption. Getting the timing right for a new product is just as important as choosing the right product application itself. Evaluate the market need for the future product before licensing any technology, and this will greatly improve your chances of success.

Is the Target Market Highly Competitive with Minimal Differentiation between Products?

You do not want to plan on entering a market that is currently saturated with products having minimal differentiating features because biotechnology products do not make good commodities. Biotech products are more complex, more expensive, and are breakthrough in nature. Companies with the most potential for success are targeting markets where there are very few, if any, existing competitors, or they are targeting markets where competitor's products do not fully meet the customer's needs.

Is There a Reimbursement Pathway for the Product That Is Readily Available and Accessible?

In the medical biotechnology industry, there are typically three customers who must see value in a product: the patient, the physician, and the payer. We discuss more about these three customers in *Chapter 32: Biotechnology Products and Their Customers: Developing a Successful Market Strategy*. In order for a medical biotechnology product to be successful, there needs to be a value proposition for the "payers" that cover some or all of the cost of these products ordered by the physician that are used on, or used by, the patient. Because most countries have some form of a third-party payer system, it is critical to know if each payer system has a mechanism to cover the costs of your future product and that they would be willing and inclined to do so. More information about reimbursement issues is covered in *Chapter 33: Biotechnology Product Coverage, Coding, and Reimbursement Strategies*. Even though there may be an unmet market need for your product, if there is not a reimbursement pathway that is available and accessible for your customers, this future product will likely have many challenges in the market.

The People Factor

Before you finally decide that you should proceed forward with a particular technology and product application, there is one intangible factor that also needs to be addressed and that is the "people factor," as it is the next critical predictor of success. What I mean by the people factor is the "chemistry" between you and the stakeholders in the entire process and value chain of the technology development and the building of the company. This is something that must be inwardly evaluated throughout the process when talking to the inventor, the research team, and others who are associated with the technology. This evaluation may include other individuals who have authority and responsibility for the development process throughout.

In reality, the majority of the real know-how for any technology is not contained within the IP, but inherent within the inventor and the technical staff. If you can communicate well with the inventor and the technical staff, and they are enthusiastic about the commercialization of their research, this is a favorable sign. If it is challenging to communicate with the inventor and their staff, or to get answers to various questions, it is not likely to get much better when the pressure of meeting product development goals is added. The ability to communicate, work well with, and to quickly resolve issues is important because there are a myriad of challenges a biotechnology entrepreneur will face during the product development, fundraising, and growth of the company. Therefore, the quality of this interaction and the cohesiveness of the team are vital. If there are constant disagreements resulting in the inability to quickly resolve issues, these are what I call "artificial problems." These are internally generated issues among the team members instead of external issues between the team and the environment. When artificial problems arise, they consume an inordinate amount of time and energy to resolve. Artificial problems detract from progress and reduce the ability to focus and resolve the true problems that the company will face during its product development. The ability to work effectively and efficiently as a team is like glue for a woodworking project. You may join all the right parts and pieces, but if they do not stick together, there will be no product. Knowing you can work well with all the stakeholders is an strategic advantage, and this will help accelerate rather than slow down the product development process.

It is rare, and highly unlikely, to find that all individuals within a group are happily cooperative and enthusiastic about every decision that is made. However, learn to recognize the situations and the individuals that create unresolvable disputes and insurmountable challenges. There are enough challenges you will face when developing a biotechnology product and building a company, you do not want to add more problems by creating teams that are not meant to work together.

If you determine that the people factor is positive, then before you are ready to move forward with licensing the technology, you need to have a discussion and agreement as to what level of involvement the inventors and research team will have. At a minimum, if the inventor and team are not part of the company, there needs to be an understanding that the inventors will consult for the company or possibly even conduct some product development activity within their own laboratory for a period of time, and for a fee.

What to Do Next?

Once you have made a decision to move forward with the technology concept and to obtain a license to the technology, you must then negotiate with the institution that owns the IP rights. Academic institutions that conduct basic research have a TTO or Technology Licensing Office staffed with individuals who are trained to license their technology and to work out a deal with the licensee. As mentioned previously, there can be significant differences in the philosophies of various TTOs. There are standard terms and conditions when licensing technology but there are also terms that are negotiable. You may be able to find out what to expect in the deal terms from a particular institution by talking to others who have licensed technology previously from that institution. Additional information about licensing terms and licensing conventions are reviewed in *Chapter 15: Licensing the Technology: Biotechnology Commercialization Strategies Using University and Federal Labs.*

Summary

The first step in starting a biotechnology endeavor is to be sure that the technology and product concept is foundationally sound and properly evaluated for the underlying science, literature support, and the inventor and technical team. This technology evaluation process is essential, and determines whether or not the future product will provide true value to the target audience and whether the concept has a high likelihood of success scientifically. A detailed analysis of the scientific merit of a technology is essential during a scientific review. If the basic research conducted at a particular academic institution is reputable and known for excellence, the majority of their IP available for licensing may likely be of high quality. That is why you should always work with high-quality and reputable institutions when seeking to license technology and future product concepts.

Of note, do not be misled into believing that high-quality research automatically guarantees a useful or marketable biotechnology product. In other words, entrepreneurs should understand that *excellent research is not a surrogate for medically useful or marketable products.* There are multitudes of laboratories filled with excellent research, much of which never results in a successful biotechnology product. This is because there is more to producing a successful biotechnology product than conducting great science. The most successful products absolutely are predicated upon quality science; however, conducting quality science alone does not assure a successful biotechnology product. Spend adequate time evaluating the science and consulting industry and clinical experts in the field.

Remember that the evaluation process must include an assessment of the future product's perceived value to the target audience. It is often the case that the technical staff and founders become enamored with their technology, but they must remember that *technology is simply a solution looking for a problem to solve.* If the problem that is selected is not selected based upon a true unmet need, then there will be limited opportunity and interest in the future product. The final and most telling assessment is the people factor: the ability to effectively communicate with each team member to address and resolve issues without creating "artificial problems" that are distracting and take away from the focus of the organization towards reaching its goal.

We have discussed three initial criteria that are important when evaluating a technology product concept or idea: (1) the underlying science and technology; (2) the product's market potential; and (3) the people factor. These three critera are critical when assessing any technology product idea and they serve as the basis for screening potential technology product ideas. When considering building a company around technology owned by academic or research institutions, be sure to evaluate the underlying science, technology, and market application. When building a company and raising capital, the investor and interested partners are also looking at the future product's value. If you build a company on sound science and the product addresses an acute unmet need, and the team can work together to quickly resolve problems, you will have minimized many of your early risks.

Reference

[1] Fisher LM. The innovation incubator: technology transfer at Stanford University. Strategy + Business. October 1, 1998 <http://www.strategy-business.com/article/13494> [accessed February 12, 2019].

Chapter 12

Understanding Biotechnology Business Models and Managing Risk

Craig Shimasaki, PhD, MBA

CEO, BioSource Consulting Group and Moleculera Labs, Oklahoma City, OK, United States

Chapter Outline

Biotechnology companies are started with the intent to commercialize products based upon novel technology concepts and ideas. In order to build a company that becomes profitable and generates sustainable revenue, it is critical to choose the right business model at the outset in order to give your company the best chance of success. Business models are important to both entrepreneurs and their investors, because business models are the method and manner in which a company makes, or intends to make money. Sophisticated investors are familiar with the required components for building competitive companies that generate sustainable revenue. If the company and its founders adopt a business model that is neither competitive nor sustainable for their type of product, there will be limited investment interest in the company.

Often, eager entrepreneurs believe that decisions about company business models and commercialization methods are made *after* the company has completed product development and has an approved product to sell. Entrepreneurs must resist the erroneous belief that business model decisions are deferred far into the product development future. Rather, entrepreneurs must identify and adopt a commercialization strategy at the outset of the business, because it will become a part of the value proposition of the company. Sometimes entrepreneurs may believe they "thought through" their business model choice, when in reality, they simply presumed a model that was familiar to them. If you do not understand the strengths, weaknesses, and strategic value of any business model, the model you choose for your company may result in limited success.

What Is a Business Model?

When describing business models, individuals often attempt to explain them in abstract concepts that are difficult to understand. In one sense, business models are abstract. However, in simpler terms I like to define a business model as, *the method by which a company makes and sells its products and services, which includes the interrelationship of all its component parts, and the manner in which the company creates value and makes money*. All companies operate with an underlying business model, whether recognized or not. Therefore, an

Biotechnology Entrepreneurship. DOI: https://doi.org/10.1016/B978-0-12-815585-1.00012-7

entrepreneur should purposefully select and adopt the optimal business model for their company, because a detrimental one may be entered into by default.

Building a company around an optimal business model can be likened to an engineer who draws a set of plans, then has a construction team erect the envisioned building according to a set of prescribed architectural drawings. Long before the first steel girder is laid, the designer conceives the structure and the architect draws out the plans based upon the desired functions and optimal usage of the structure. Based upon the proposed function of the envisioned structure, the architect draws an "internal frame" and determines the interconnectivity of each segment to all other segments of the whole structure. The internal frame predetermines the height, width, and breadth of the structure, and it also sets its limits (see Fig. 12.1). A team of builders then follows the plans and sets the frame in place, and the final exterior construction conforms to the limits of the structural frame. If the frame does not reach a necessary height or extends in a critical direction or have connectivity to another necessary component, no exterior work can compensate for these limitations. Your business model is analogous to this "internal frame" or structure, and it is the support upon which all the parts of the business (internal and external) are built and interconnected. As in this example, just as it is essential to predetermine the strategic and optimal frame prior to beginning construction, so it is vital to choose the right business model ***prior*** to building your business. This is because it is extremely difficult to change a business model once the organization is fully developed. Rarely can a company successfully change its business model once it is established, and certainly not without risking forward momentum and the company's future. Some companies have attempted to change their business model after commercialization with limited success; usually it is done because their current business model is not working. In reality, this is usually an attempt to salvage the most valuable parts of the business and jettison the parts that are not working. These efforts are usually a survival response rather than growth or expansion plans.

A development-stage biotechnology company has the opportunity to select and implement the ideal business model at the outset, and it should be one that fits their technology, products, and services and is optimized for their competitive advantage. To reiterate, a business model is simply the collective means and methods in which the company makes its products or provides its services, and the means by which the company makes money. It is the sum total of all the strategic business approaches and their interrelationship to other parts of the business and their relationship to the external world. A company selects a particular business model in order to give them a competitive advantage over other companies and their products.

In this chapter, we will review representative examples of business models used in, or adapted for, different sectors within the biotechnology industry. We will discuss representative business model and their benefits and limitations for certain products or services. The reader should realize that there are endless permutations of business models; however, at this time we will cover only a selected few. Fortunately, most business models follow a limited number of basic characteristics, and these will become familiar to you as we review this in the following sections. Before we delve into the various business model

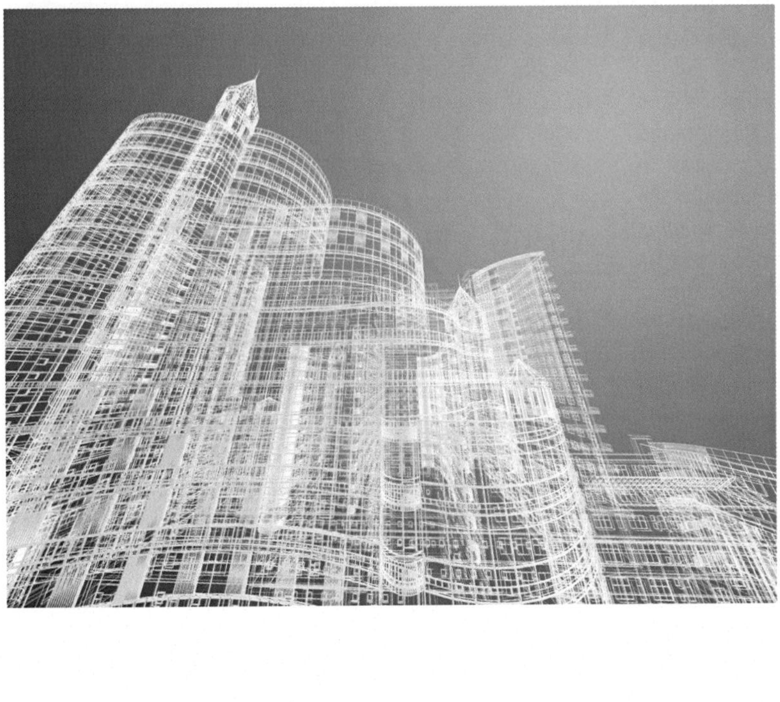

FIGURE 12.1 The internal frame determines the use and function of the future structure.

examples, we want to talk about a business model that almost all biotechnology companies (irrespective of sector) should operate under for a period of time during their early development.

The Virtual Company Business Model (A Temporary Start-Up Model)

A virtual company is an organization that outsources the majority of all its activities and owns or leases little, if any, physical space and possesses few full-time employees in order to keep overhead expenses at a minimum. There are extreme variations of virtual companies. Some can be quite frugal such as one that has no full-time employees, utilizes a home address or post office box to receive business mail, borrows equipment or barters for time on equipment, and leases facilities which may be the academic laboratories of the founding scientists. Operating as a virtual company means that the company does not *perform* all the necessary functions internally—yet the company still *accomplishes* all the necessary activities as if it was vertically integrated. I am a strong proponent of operating as a "virtual company" during the start-up phase, regardless if it is a biotherapeutic, diagnostic, medical device, Ag Biotech, or any other sector of biotechnology. The way this is accomplished is by carefully selecting outsourcing partners. For many early-stage companies the extent of outsourcing may be significant, and in some cases, most all development functions may be performed under contract by outside organizations. Because of the great expense associated with research and development (R&D), preclinical, and animal testing, most early-stage biotherapeutic companies operate as a virtual company until significant funding is acquired, which can support internal staffing, capital equipment, and in-house activities. Sometimes the type of R&D activities required by some early-stage biotechnology companies are so unique and specialized that their only option is to perform these functions in-house; however, the more common functions can still be outsourced to keep costs down.

During a start-up stage, capital is usually quite limited, and a company cannot hire many full-time employees, but substantial progress must still be made in order to gain interest from investors. Operating as a virtual company during the formative stage allows entrepreneurs to extend the time horizon of their operations, and it requires much less capital to maintain and sustain the company while their product is initially being developed. I know of companies that have successfully advanced their therapeutic product through animal studies and into early human clinical testing as a virtual company. These organizations may have only a few key employees, but they utilize many experienced consultants who are paid nominal fees and receive stock option incentives, while the company contracts out most of their activities. In order for R&D outsourcing to be successful, there must be a good working relationship with the contracted R&D group. For companies that are early-stage university spin-outs, the organization that performs the R&D may be the founder's/cofounder's own laboratory. This type of arrangement often works out well in the beginning because they have the specialized expertise and equipment to advance the translational research and advance the development of the product. In a virtual mode, additional R&D personnel may be contracted and operate under temporary agreements or work part-time. Typically, these individuals are compensated with a combination of incentives such as stock, stock options, or restricted stock for professional services, in addition to nominal salaries or fees. Be sure to discuss all employment and compensation commitments with your corporate attorney in order to draft the necessary documents that will protect intellectual property (IP) and avoid ownership issues in the future.

Virtual Companies Grow and Eventually Need Space

At some point in time, virtual companies grow and may need dedicated laboratory and office space in order to continue their pace of progress toward product development. When making a move to dedicated space, be sure to look into the availability of space within a technology incubator, since some incubator programs may subsidize a start-up company with reduced rates that escalate later when certain financial milestones are met. Many technology incubators may also have some support services and/or shared equipment available for a small fee. When deciding on space, be sure to anticipate your needs now and your growth needs into the near future but balance that by the current funding and the timeframe to reach your next product-development milestone. As you may already know, renting biotechnology space is not cheap. Depending on the geographic location of your company and the mix of laboratory to office space, rent may cost between $30 to as high as $90 per square foot per year. Often times incubators rent lab benches rather than rent space calculated by the square foot. If you can negotiate it, ask for month-to-month leases. If this is not possible, be sure to know the impact of any long-term lease and how these obligations may impact the overall burn rate of the company and the risk when raising another round of capital.

It is prudent for most start-up biotechnology companies to initially operate as virtual companies in order to efficiently utilize capital and create early value. By being a virtual company, it provides time to raise start-up, seed, or Series A financing, and it also provides time for the company to increase in value as product development progress is made. A virtual company can conserve cash which can then be properly deployed toward advancing the technology rather than supporting overhead that limits their existence. However, a virtual company business model is not a permanent or long-term business model choice for most companies. Virtual companies must still create internal value and ultimately possess some internal expertise that is not effectively reproduced by others. While most companies should start as a virtual company, this should be transitionary, and the company must have a commercialization business model selected and adopted that is long-term in nature.

Business Model Examples

In this section, we will review a few business model examples that are used in the biotechnology industry. Many of these examples can be applied to different sectors such as medical devices, agricultural and industrial biotechnology, digital health, and biofuels. These examples are presented to help understand the ways in which different models are applied to different biotechnology sectors. Later, we will discuss the different business model segments and how they are assembled to create new models. Some of the business models we will review include the following:

Therapeutic and Biologics Companies

- Fully integrated pharmaceutical or biotechnology company (FIPCO or FIBCO) business model
- Fully integrated pharmaceutical network (FIPNET) or biotechnology network business model
- Research intensive pharmaceutical company (RIPCO) business model
- Drug repositioning business model
- Enabling technology business model

Diagnostic and Research Tool Companies

- Platform instrument/menu content business model
- Clinical laboratory services business model
- Subscription business model

Therapeutics and Biologics Companies

Fully Integrated Pharmaceutical Company Business Model

The ***FIPCO*** model is a standard business model that was previously utilized by *all* pharmaceutical companies and is sometimes referred to as a "***vertically integrated***" or "***fully integrated***" model. In this model, the company performs (in-house) all the functions of the business—from initial R&D drug discovery, animal testing, human clinical testing, regulatory approval, manufacturing, and marketing of all their products. The advantage of the FIPCO business model is that the company can control *all* aspects of the development through to marketing and commercialization of the product. As a result, many of the early biotechnology companies wanted to follow this model. However, achieving this was attained by venerable pharmaceutical companies with 100 + years of history and resources, but it was challenging for early-stage biotechnology companies to become a FIPCO at the outset. Regardless, in the early days of the biotechnology industry, that is what most of all biotechnology companies aspired to become. It was soon discovered that it took an enormous amount of time, resources, capital (and good fortune) for a biotechnology company to become a FIPCO. Many failed along the way trying to achieve this goal. Some fortunate ones such as Genentech, Amgen, Genzyme, and IDEC became FIPCOs. However, over time, as companies were forced to focus on capital efficiencies due to the limitations in available capital and lowered sales revenue, even some major pharmaceutical companies realized that the FIPCO business model was not the most efficient one. Pharmaceutical companies recognized that without a continual source of innovative therapeutic ideas, drug development pipelines can quickly dry up, and the company is left with underutilized resources in regulatory, clinical trials, formulation, manufacturing, and marketing.

To be more competitive and efficient, these companies modified the FIPCO business model in ways that allowed them to continue generating the types of profits expected of these multinational companies. Some of these modifications include reducing downstream capabilities to base levels that can be efficiently utilized but can be outsourced beyond that capacity, and eliminating some functions entirely in favor of using contract research organizations (CRO). In addition, instead of attempting to internally discover *all* their drug candidates, pharmaceutical companies augmented their R&D capabilities by in-licensing development-stage products from other biotechnology companies, or by acquiring these companies outright. This alternate business model is called a ***Fully Integrated Pharmaceutical Network*** (***FIPNET***) or a ***Virtually Integrated Pharmaceutical Company Organization (VIPCO)***. FIPNET and VIPCO companies have realized improved productivity and increased efficiency, because they can outsource and/or contract for services at any point in their value chain and have access to complementary abilities outside the company. This model still allows a company to maintain control of the product development process and yet leverage the abilities of others at any point in the value chain. For biotechnology companies, FIPCO is referred to as FIBCO where the "B" refers to "biotechnology" or "biopharmaceutical" (see Fig. 12.2).

For start-up therapeutic and biologics companies, becoming a FIPCO is not the optimal business model choice; and at the outset it is *not* a realistic or believable one because doing this is even difficult for major pharmaceutical companies. Though it is possible that any start-up biotechnology company can become a FIPCO sometime in the future, it is hardly a business model that an early investor would take seriously. In fact, a start-up biotechnology company that is declaring a FIPCO business model would likely frighten sophisticated investors, and they would disappear quickly. However, becoming a FIPNET company can be a long-term business model realized for biotechnology companies focused on therapeutic and biologics. Over time, a few highly innovative research-intensive companies recognized that their strength was in their novel research functions and not their downstream activities. Hence, there arose another business model called a ***Research Intensive Pharmaceutical Company*** or ***RIPCO*** where they focused only on the R&D and licensed out all their product candidates to other organizations.

The Drug Repositioning Business Model

The ***drug repositioning*** business model (Fig. 12.3) is a therapeutic business model that focuses on repositioning abandoned drugs from other pharmaceutical or biotech companies (approved or not approved) and finds alternate intended use populations or finds a population in which the drug has fewer side-effects and greater efficacy. A biotech drug repositioning company uses specialized know-how to identify an alternate or narrower population that can benefit from a shelved drug and that is usually based upon understanding the drug's mechanism of action. These older or unused drugs are those that have already passed safety testing in humans. In order to speed up the development, some therapeutic biotech companies have adopted a drug repositioning business model to reduce the lengthy R&D timeframe and leverage the previously conducted drug safety profile. By adopting a drug repositioning business model, a number of biotech companies have shortened the drug development time and advanced rapidly into initial human safety testing. The support for the potential success of a drug repositioning business model came from the many drugs that failed for one particular indication but were later found to have success for use in another indication. One historically notable drug that failed as an antihypertensive drug and was later repositioned successfully was Viagra (sildenafil). Although human clinical studies did not demonstrate the desired antihypertensive effect, "side-effects" were noted by Pfizer scientists who then repositioned it as an erectile dysfunction drug. Other examples of successfully

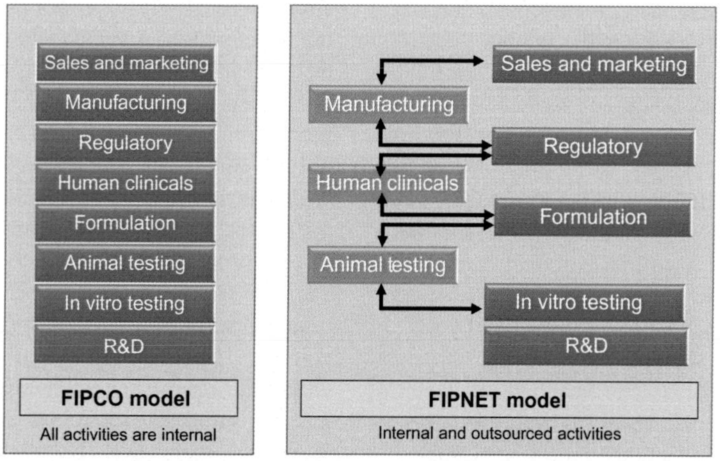

FIGURE 12.2 FIPCO and FIPNET business model structures. *FIPCO*, Fully integrated pharmaceutical company; *FIPNET*, fully integrated pharmaceutical network.

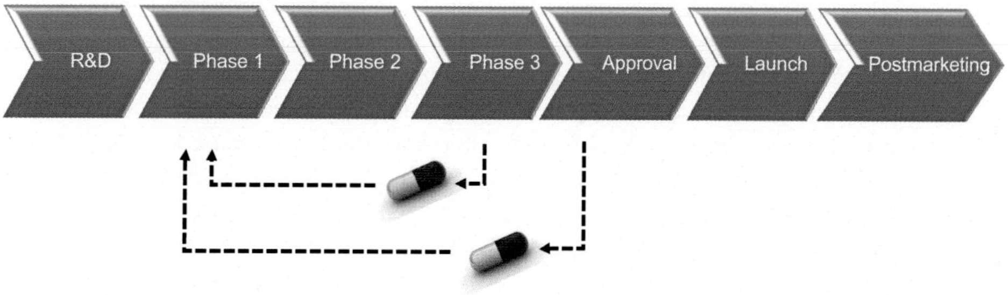

FIGURE 12.3 Drug repositioning model.

Drug	Original Indication	New Indication
Allopurinol	Cancer	Gout
Amantadine	Influenza	Parkinson´s disease
Amphotericin	Antifungal	Leishmaniasis
Arsenic	Syphilis	Leukemia
Aspirin	Inflammation, pain	Antiplatelet
Atomexetine	Depressive disorder	ADHD
Bimatoprost	Glaucoma	Promoting eyelash growth
Bromocriptine	Parkinson´s disease	Diabetes mellitus
Bupropion	Depression	Smoking cessation
Colchicine	Gout	Recurrent pericarditis
Colesevelam	Hyperlipidemia	Type 2 diabetes mellitus
Dapsone	Leprosy	Malaria
Disulfiram	Alcoholism	Melanoma
Doxepin	Depressive disorder	Antipruritic
Eflornithine	Depression	ADHD
Finasteride	Benign prostatic hyperplasia	Male pattern baldness
Gabapentin	Epilepsy	Neuropathic pain
Gemcitabine	Antiviral	Cancer
Lomitapide	Lipidemia	Familial hypercholesterolemia
Methotrexate	Cancer	Psoriasis, rheumatoid arthritis
Miltefosine	Cancer	Visceral leishmaniasis
Minoxidil	Hypertension	Hair loss
Naltrexone	Opioid addiction	Alcohol withdrawal
Naproxen	Inflammatian, pain	Alzheimer´s disease
Nortriptyline	Depression	Neuropathic pain
Premetrexed	Mesothelioma	Lung cancer
Propranolol	Hypertension	Migraine prophylaxis
Raloxifene	Contraceptive	Osteoporosis
Sildenafil	Angina	Erectile dysfunction; pulmonary hypertension
Thalidomide	Morning sickness	Leprosy; multiple myeloma
Tretinoin	Acne	Leukemia
Zidovudine	Cancer	HIV/AIDS
Zileuton	Asthma	Acne

FIGURE 12.4 Examples of repositioned drugs. Source: *Jaswanth K. Yella, Suryanarayana Yaddanapudi, Yunguan Wang and Anil G. Jegga "Changing Trends in Computational Drug Repositioning" Pharmaceuticals 2018, 11, 57.*

repositioned drugs include Eli Lilly's anticancer drug Gemzar (gemcitabine) that was originally developed as an antiviral agent, and Evista (raloxifene) that was originally developed as a birth control drug, then repositioned as a successful osteoporosis drug, and later, another indication as a prophylactic for the prevention of breast cancer. It is important to note that many drugs and biologics that were approved or launched in the United States were drugs repositioned for new indications, reformulations, or new combinations of existing drugs [1] (Fig. 12.4).

The advantage of a drug repositioning business model is that a company may be able to leapfrog over much of the safety and in vitro toxicity testing and have early support for safety in in vivo testing. This can save literally tens of millions of dollars and multiple years of development depending on the product's previous development stage and its new indication for use. However, as with any business model, there are weaknesses, and they must be evaluated in the context of the competition and based upon the proof that a model can be supported and become truly successful. One disadvantage of the drug repositioning model is that a company must convince enough investors that they can continue to reposition other company's previously failed drugs and biologics based upon some novel technology or idea that they possess. In addition, the drug repositioning business model does not *remove* all drug development risks; it just *reduces* some of them. In the early 2000s, there was a large number of biotech companies that started as drug-repositioning companies because of the heightened interest and the success of several repositioned drug examples. Today there are some companies that are doing well using this business model, but there are also a number of companies that are no longer in business or have switched to another model. This does not mean that the drug repositioning business model cannot be successful, it just emphasizes that the selection of your business model is an important component, but without a good technology application, IP protection, the right team, and adequate funding, no business model can guarantee success.

There are some biotechnology companies that do not operate as a drug repositioning company but they possess a repositioned drug candidate as their company product and are having great success. For instance, the repositioned drug idea is a fantastic concept, but starting as a company whose sole mission is to continuously identify successful candidates for repositioned drugs across a myriad of different indications may be quite challenging. However, there may be a sweet spot for an existing FIPCO therapeutic company that focuses on, for instance, rheumatoid arthritis anti-inflammatory compounds to reposition other company's failed drugs that also carry anti-inflammatory properties and develop them for different anti-inflammatory indications. In essence, they can leverage their internal anti-inflammatory drug screening capabilities and accelerate product development for their anti-inflammatory-focused indications.

For an example, Otologic Pharmaceuticals, a virtual therapeutic company, repositioned two different individual drugs as a combination drug and entered Phase 1 human clinical trials for the treatment of noise-induced hearing loss. One of the repositioned drugs was a novel free-radical scavenging compound that successfully completed human clinical Phases 1 and 2 but failed in Phase 3 as a stroke drug. They combined this drug and an FDA-approved product used for a totally different indication because the compound had a mechanism-of-action as a free-radical scavenger. When the combined product was tested in the new indication, the in vitro and animal testing showed synergistic results for the effective prevention of noise-induced hearing loss resulting from new noise insults. This company successfully completed Phase 1 and has advanced into Phase 2 human studies. The company reached this milestone using approximately 30%–40% of the typical expenses in about 50% of the typical drug development time. As a result, this combination product and other chemical derivatives of these compounds became the basis for a company with a technology having broad application for the treatment of hearing health. Although this company is not a "drug repositioning company," the genesis of its first product utilized one aspect of the "drug repositioning" business model, but they adopted an optimum business model for the future commercialization of their current product and future products for improvement of hearing health and for the growth of the company.

Enabling Technology Business Models

A company operating with an ***enabling technology*** business model is focused on a "**platform technology**" and can use it to enable or improve applications of other company's products. I have categorized this business model in the Therapeutics and Biologics Company section, but it can be applied to a number of other biotechnology sectors. Sometimes this business model is referred to as a "***horizontal model***" or a "***platform model***," because the company will focus on a single aspect or single segment of the value chain of a business. For example, drug delivery is a segment focus using the enabling technology business model delivering drugs into the body that otherwise would not have any application. One early biotech example of this type of business model was ALZA, a drug delivery company formerly based in Palo Alto, California, was founded in 1968 by entrepreneur *Al*ejandro *Za*ffaroni (hence the name ALZA), had a focus on drug delivery platforms and pioneered the transdermal delivery technology. The company successfully applied its skin-patch platform technology to existing drugs such as Nicoderm as an aid to help quit smoking, and Procardia XL for both angina and hypertension, Duragesic (fentanyl) for the management of cancer pain, and Glucotrol XL for the treatment of type 2 diabetes. In the mid-1990s the company added other segments of the vertical value chain and successfully transitioned to a FIPCO. ALZA eventually was acquired in 2001 by Johnson & Johnson for approximately $10 billion. By applying their technology for delivery of drugs across the skin barrier, they created an opportunity for their company to improve or expand access for many other products. Other applications of enabling technology business models include servicing companies that focus on certain types of drug screening, animal testing, and even CRO and contract manufacturing organizations (CMO), which all provide specialized services or technology as the value for their business.

Diagnostic and Research Tools Companies

Platform Instrument/Menu Content Business Model

A successful business model in the clinical diagnostic and molecular testing industry is the development of tests that run on proprietary platform instruments that are produced and manufactured by the same company. Diagnostic tools and instrument companies that use this ***Platform Instrument/Menu Content*** business model are Luminex, Becton Dickenson, Roche, Affymetrix, and Illumina to name a few. In this business model the company develops and markets content (different tests) that only operate on their instruments and cannot run on a competitor's testing platform. The success of their business model works when the company can develop or adapt the largest number of needed tests on their platform equipment and place them in the greatest number of clinical and research laboratories possible. In order for customers to have a desire to purchase these instruments, the company must develop a desirable menu of testing content that these customers want. The "Instrument and Test Menu" business model is an adaptation of the ***Razor Handle and Razor Blade*** business model because the principles are identical. The company creates and sells a tool, instrument, or platform and then perpetually sells to that same customer, specialized, high-margin consumables. Similar to the very early days in the shaving industry, Gillette and Schick understood they could essentially give away the razor handle and build a successful business. They understood that when a customer adopted their brand of razor handle, the customer was committed, and the company generated the majority of their profits on reoccurring purchases of high-margin disposable steel razor blades. Another similar business model is the ink-jet and toner printing industry. Companies such as Hewlett-Packard, Canon, and Epson compete for consumers to purchase their printers. Often they may even sell their printers at a loss because they know their profits come through the perpetual selling of branded high-profit margin ink and toner.

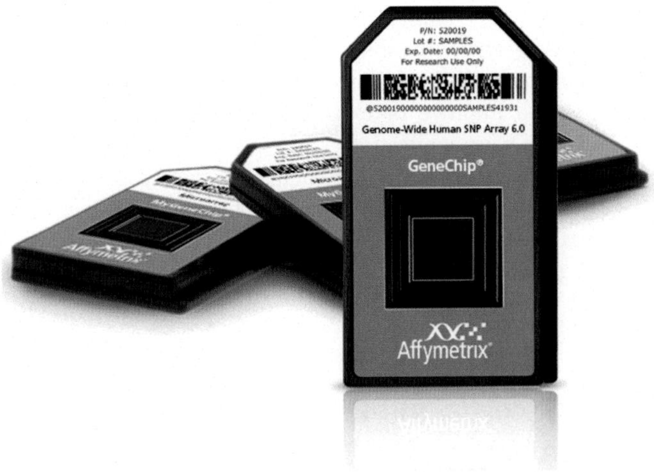

FIGURE 12.5 Affymetrix gene chip: example of instrument and menu content business model. Source: *(Courtesy of Affymetrix, Inc., Santa Clara, CA, USA).*

Another example of a biotechnology company using *Platform Instrument/Menu Content* business model is Affymetrix. The company designs, manufactures, and sells platform instruments based upon a microarray technology they have developed, which performs a variety of different types of genomic analyses. The chips are consumables that are purchased to run on Affymetrix's dedicated instrument platform and operate on their proprietary software (see Fig. 12.5).

The Platform Instrument/Menu Content business model can be applied to many other tools and instrument companies and also medical device and diagnostic companies. The advantages of this business model are that the company has a captive customer base with continual reoccurring revenue streams that would be proportional to the total number of instruments that are placed into the market. Often the company's consumable have a very high-profit margin and can offset even an initial loss on the instrument placement due to the long-term and perpetual purchasing of the company's consumables. One disadvantage of this business model is that competing technologies from other companies can sometimes quickly replace or even obsolete another company's platform technology, and therefore within a short period of time, the reoccurring revenue streams may disappear. It is therefore imperative for companies that adopt this business model to continually invest in R&D and improve, advance, and innovate so as to keep customers attached to their branded platforms and wedded to their expanding test menu.

Clinical Laboratory Service Business Model

In the diagnostics sector, a company will develop a detection technology for an analyte of interest (molecule, biomarker or chemical) then produce and manufacture a "kit" which is sold to commercial laboratories who perform these diagnostic tests. The ***Clinical Laboratory Service*** business model can be a viable alternative for these companies. In this model, molecular and diagnostic companies perform unique and proprietary tests as a *service*, operating through a single company-owned clinical laboratory, instead of manufacturing a "***kit manufacturing model***" which would be sold to others. There are several advantages to the Laboratory Service business model over the "kit manufacturing model" which include the following:

- shorter timeframe from inception of test technology to product commercialization,
- typically lower costs of product and service development,
- usually fewer employees required to begin commercialization, and
- an alternative regulatory path (Clinical Laboratory Improvement Amendments (CLIA)) rather than the FDA regulatory approval (note that the regulatory approval route is being evaluated and may change in the future).

There are also disadvantages to this business model over the traditional diagnostic kit manufacturing model, which include the following:

- The testing services can only be performed in *one* laboratory location, potentially limiting the volume of testing and potentially creating a bottleneck.
- Testing requires specialized employees who have the expertise to perform these testing services.
- Regulatory approval includes biannual laboratory inspections and proficiency testing which, if not compliant, can shut down or restrict all services for a period of time.

Diagnostic testing companies choose one business model over the other for strategic reasons and for competitive advantages. For instance, a very complex and highly technical test that is very difficult and labor intensive to perform may be challenging to reduce to a "kit" allowing others to perform these tests proficiently and accurately. Such a complex test may require specialized equipment that must be developed so users can adequately perform the test with consistent results. In this case, the Clinical Laboratory business model may be a better choice. Examples of companies using this business model include Myriad Genetics and Genomic Health. Myriad Genetics has research, development, marketing, and sales functions for its clinical laboratory molecular tests that are focused on predicting risk of hereditary-based cancers. They operate a single CLIA-certified clinical laboratory that is appropriately certified and accredited to perform these laboratory testing services. Because their tests cannot be licensed to other clinical laboratories, all testing is performed at the company's sole clinical laboratory in Salt Lake City, Utah—they also control and retain all the profits. Genomic Health, based in Redwood City, CA, also operates as a CLIA laboratory and performs its testing services using a similar business model. Both these companies have had tremendous success in using the Clinical Laboratory Services business model for their products. It is conceivable that both Myriad Genetics and Genomic Health could also create an instrument platform that could run their genetic tests as "kits" and sell their instruments to multiple laboratories under the Instrument/Content business model. However, their existing business model choice provides them with superior financial, market, and regulatory advantages and gives them the ability to rapidly introduce new testing services or make rapid modifications or improvements to their testing menu.

Subscription Business Model

Companies can have three options for the mode in which they deliver value to their customers: a product, a service, or a subscription. The ***subscription*** business model was utilized by many of the early genomic discovery companies in which they sold subscriptions to their valuable databases (Incyte Genomics, Millennium Pharmaceuticals, and Celera and Gene Logic). These organizations (some are no longer in business) sell/sold information, or access to information and data that is considered valuable to other companies. There are multiple options and iterations of the revenue portion of this business model which can include one or many of the following options:

- Charging an initiation fee or membership fee for initial access to data/information
- Charging ongoing subscription fees (annual or multiple years) for access to the data/information
- Adopting increased fees for increased number of "seats" or users that a company utilizes to access the data/information
- Implement future royalties on products developed from the data/information
- Charges for R&D for specialized data mining or data manipulation services
- Increased fees for access to additional or restricted data/information that is not available to those with a "regular" membership

The benefits of the subscription business model are that the company has predictability of ongoing revenue and low revenue risk for the period of time that the customer is committed. Also, the company usually receives their revenue upfront, and therefore the incremental cost of servicing another customer with the same information is nominal compared to the revenue received. In other words, the gross profit margins are extremely large for the company as they add additional customers. The risks of this business model are similar to those in the enabling technology business model in that competing technology companies can obviate or reduce the value of your service by providing more relevant or more valuable data. However, this risk is mitigated if the company holds unique, specialized, or proprietary data such as genomic information for certain types of tissues, diseases, conditions, microbes, or analyses of specialized information such as gene methylation patterns and copy-number variations to name a few. The risk comes when competitors have access to the same or similar data (possibly because it is in the public domain), or competitors provide significantly improved methods of data interpretation because of their developed algorithms or better software systems. One way to mitigate this type of risk for those who adopt this particular business model is to continue advancing product improvements to the point of even displacing their current products through perpetual improvements. In the biotech industry few companies were able to sustain this type of business model success over the long term, as several moved from providing access to data, to developing their own therapeutic products from their own data. One example is Incyte Genomics who changed their business model and moved to a business model of drug discovery and development based upon their own data and changed their name to Incyte Corporation.

How Do You Determine the Best Business Model for a Technology

Sometimes the product opportunity is straightforward and the business model is clear. However, remember there are multiple segments to a business that can result in hybrid models that are optimized for your specific business. Don't assume that your technology or industry sector will automatically dictate the best business model strategy. Always start by first examining the unmet needs in your target market and then think about the best way your technology can help meet these needs through your choice of business model. Examine the value provided by your current or future competitors and look for better ways that your value can be provided to your target market.

In order to identify the best business model strategy for a technology, the first step is to know the answers to the following questions:

- Who are the target customer groups that need and want your product?
- What are the needs your product will be satisfying for the target market? How will this be accomplished?
- Does your company have intermediaries in the value chain between itself and the end-user customers? Is there a way to leverage this relationship to improve the company's success?
- Are there any other external players in the value proposition to the customer that are required in order to sell your product?
- How does your company intend to reach these customers?
- What is the nature of the relationship between the company and its vendors and suppliers required to produce the product or generate the service?
- Are there relationships that can be leveraged and are synergistic?
- How will the distribution of the product be carried out and by whom?
- How does the company intend to make money?
- What is the process used to develop and produce the product?
- Are there alternative ways to reduce the time, costs, or risks during development of this product?
- Does a third party receive a benefit when the company sells its product or service to the target market? If so, can these relationships be leveraged to bring additional benefits to the company?

These questions simply represent a starting point to help you arrive at the best business model to leverage your technology and product opportunity into a market. There are a number of related questions that should be addressed when thinking about the optimum business model for your company. By knowing the answers to these questions, the optimal business model can be identified to maximize the benefits and efficiently deliver your product's value proposition to your target customers. Remember that some components of a business model are dynamic, and these can be optimized as the market evolves or new channels and methods become available or changes occur in the regulatory environment for your product. Who would have predicted 40 years ago the market value of the Internet on advertising, social media, and on sales strategies? Even though you can refine some of these business model components and adjust them to changes and improvements in the market, you still must first identify the most strategic model at the outset because this becomes the foundation of the business strategy, and all components are interconnected to this "frame."

The objectives for selecting a particular business model include the following:

- To maximize the profit potential of the company
- To minimize or reduce the commercialization timeframe and costs of product development
- To leverage your IP protection
- To provide a competitive advantage over other companies or products in the field
- To provide long-term sustainability in a changing market or regulatory environment

For more information on selecting the right business model for your company, see *Chapter 13: Directing Your Technology Toward a Market Problem: What You Need to Know Before Using the Business Model Canvas?*, in which I review a very useful tool called the Business Model Canvas [2] and discuss some of the things you need to know before applying this tool to your business.

Entrepreneurial Leaders Are Risk Managers

A key objective of the proper selection of an optimal business model is to maximize the opportunity for success of your company and to reduce the risks of failure. Throughout the process of establishing, building, leading, and managing a biotechnology company, the leaders and managers can be characterized as "*risk managers*." As a result of the many decisions that the leaders make, a course is chosen to reduce risk and improve success of the business. The business model selection is just one of those decisions. Every choice an individual makes, whether in business or in life, carries some measure of risk with consequences, and some measure of opportunity for success. For instance, when making a decision on purchasing an automobile, deciding on a particular make and model, whether new or used carries a risk as to reliability and repair frequency and costs, as well as safety and comfort. The level of risk for these choices is usually moderate and the consequences of these decisions are usually minimal—unless of course you are in a major accident and you chose a poorly designed or poorly maintained automobile. However, choosing a cardiac surgeon to operate and perform a coronary artery bypass surgery carriers a much higher degree of risk and potentially greater consequences than the previous example. Each decision a biotech entrepreneur makes requires a risk assessment, because there are differing consequences for a poor choice. The choice of a business model is critical, and the proper selection will greatly reduce the future risk to the business by selecting the best one. Spend the time necessary to select the proper business model for your company.

You Cannot Manage a Risk You Do Not Identify

Entrepreneurs and managers can greatly improve the odds of their success if they begin their business with a thorough understanding of the business and technology risks that they could face based upon the objectives they must accomplish. There are innumerable ways a company can fail but relatively few ways a company can succeed. One way to facilitate the success of your company is to identify and assess the risks, prioritize them as to the level of risk and impact, and address them by having mitigating plans for facilitating success. In order to do this, you must have a method of risk assessment. I have found that we can group the risks of biotechnology companies into five categories that are fundamental for success. These categories are

1. Management, leadership, and past success;
2. Technology robustness, applicability, and the scientific team;
3. Market demand and positioning;
4. Regulatory hurdles and barriers to entry; and
5. Future funding and financing suitability.

No doubt more than five categories of biotechnology company risks can be identified. However, if you examine the issues leading to failure of many biotechnology companies, you can trace their problems back to one or several failures within these five risk categories. Each of these risk categories is exceedingly important to success, and a company must be strong in each of the five areas in order to succeed. A company that possesses exceptional strength in four of these categories must recognize that this does not compensate for a weakness in the fifth one. A company must have strength in each of these five categories. The entrepreneur needs to integrate and manage all five risk categories in order to have the best opportunity for success. Integrative risk management is the ability to manage all risks simultaneously and understand how one risk impacts each of the other risks. Occasionally, activities or decisions in one area impact or cause challenges in another area as a consequence. Integrated risk management evaluates each decision in light of all the risks that must be managed.

Evaluating Your Company

Assessing your company's strengths and weaknesses is necessary before beginning to raise capital. Potential investors also evaluate a biotechnology business opportunity based upon similar criteria listed in the following evaluation tool. Therefore, I strongly advise utilizing this tool as it is likely to be similar to what investors may utilize when evaluating companies for investment interest. Such a tool is helpful when preparing for investor presentations and in writing your business plan and preparing your pitch deck. The Biotechnology Company Evaluation Tool is a worksheet I developed for assessing a company business and technology for the evaluation of investment advice, or potential for success and risks to be managed. When formally evaluating biotechnology companies, one can use a more detailed set of questions and analysis, but this list serves as the basis for an initial evaluation.

The purpose of the Biotechnology Company Evaluation Tool is to objectively rate your company as compared to others, and to identify your company's current strengths and weaknesses. Use this tool with the categorized questions to determine a ranking for your business. Score your company on a 1–5 scale, with 1 being the worst, and 5 being the best as compared to the best in the industry. After evaluating each question in each of the categories, average the scores in each section. A composite criteria score of 3.0 or below in any of these five risk categories reveals an unacceptable level of business risk that must be addressed. This tool can also measure the overall strengths of the company, as well as point to areas that need help. Another important purpose of this tool is that it provides a snapshot in time for your company's strengths and weaknesses.

Interpreting the Results

It is absolutely certain that a start-up or development-stage biotechnology company will not score well in all of these categories. When that happens, do not become discouraged—it does not mean that the company is destined to fail. Having a low score at one point in time can be transformed into a company strength years later if these risks have been addressed and overcome. It is essential to use this tool critically so you can identify your company's weaknesses, because it will direct your focus on what should to be done to improve and focus on over time. Remember, it is impossible to deal with an unidentified weakness. Once your company's areas of weakness are identified, draft a plan on how you will overcome these shortcomings with a timeline and responsible person(s) to manage them and their progress. Entrepreneurs don't do themselves any favors by overlooking problems or by using a biased ranking in this exercise. I would encourage you to be critically objective, because it is certain others evaluating your organization will. If the entrepreneur or leadership team has trouble being critically objective, enlist the help of others to give you feedback and comment on each of these categories. The opinion of outside experts can be very valuable when assessing your company's risk. This tool should also be dated and used at regular intervals, and the results periodically assessed throughout your organization's development to evaluate improvements and assess the effectiveness of changes made. If a company's key risks are properly managed, these scores will significantly improve over time. By demonstrating that you are successfully managing each of these risks, investors will be more favorable with your ability to lead your organization's development future.

Biotechnology Company Evaluation Tool

I. Management, Leadership, and Past Success

Score	Questions
	1. Does the CEO/entrepreneur/leader have previous successful experience in a *similar leadership capacity and demonstrated* that he/she is the right individual to *successfully* lead this organization?
	2. Is the Leadership Team passionate about their mission and work, and do they fully believe in its future success?
	3. Is the *Leadership Team* complete and in place with all members having directly applicable experience and success?
	4. If the management team is incomplete, are there *sound plans to bring on the remaining leaders*, and are the plans sufficient to overcome current weakness?
	5. Is there a *Core Leadership Team* in place, which is a group capable of managing the current and near term company needs and has previous experience and success?
	6. Are *all* the Leadership Team members *seasoned* and do they have *directly related expertise* applicable to this type of company and in this particular industry?
	7. Does the Leadership Team collectively have *complementary abilities* and expertise and do they share common core values and work extremely well together?
	8. Is the Leadership Team accustomed to a *start-up environment* and do they have past success accomplishments in a start-up situation?
	9. Does the Leadership Team have all the ability to *fully execute the current business plan and strategy*, and have they demonstrated performing these activities successfully in the past or through previous experience?
	10. Are all the Leadership Team members *aware of their weaknesses* individually and as a collective whole, and enthusiastic and willing to seek help to fill this gap?
———	***Total score*** ***Average score* (divide by 10) =**

II. Technology Robustness, Applicability, and Scientific Team

Score	Questions
	1. Is the technology and product application *truly innovative* relative to other new concepts and technologies in the industry?
	2. Are the *opinion leaders* in this field *positive, complementary, and excited* about this product and technology?
	3. Does the company have a team of *top-notch scientific and technical staff* who has *demonstrated scientific leadership* in this particular field?
	4. Has the scientific team members *published multiple* proof-of-concept studies or other supporting data and studies in *top-tier peer-reviewed journals?*
	5. Has this scientific team been *awarded multiple peer-reviewed government grants* which validate that their work is respected by their peers as this field?
	6. Is there a universally *clear scientific understanding of the biology of the disease or condition*, such that the target or product chosen has a high likelihood of success?
	7. Are the underlying technology, intellectual property, and product(s) protected by *issued patents*?
	8. Is there a *freedom-to-operate* opinion that has been performed, concluding that, the company does not have challenging intellectual property barriers?
	9. If the technology is licensed, is there a *perpetual exclusive license* having conventional royalty rates and reasonable milestone fees, and the freedom to sell the technology without approval from the licensee? (If the technology is wholly owned by the company outright, score 5.)
	10. Is this product based upon a core technology that has the potential to *produce multiple products* rather than just a one product idea?
———	***Total score*** ***Average score* (divide by 10) =**

III. Market Demand and Positioning

Score	Questions
	1. Has the company *selected the best target market* and demonstrated that there is significant *unmet demand* for their future product or service, without having to create this demand?
	2. Is the marketing strategy to the target market based upon *solid evidence* supporting that there is an *unmet market need* for this product where substitutes don't adequately satisfy the true need?
	3. Is the market *large enough* to support the types of *returns needed* for the company to become a *sustained success* once the product is commercialized?

☐ 4. Does the company understand the *real competitors and product substitutes* that could displace market demand for their product, and is there sufficient value proposition within their product to rapidly grow the customer base?

☐ 5. Are market forces *converging toward this product need* such that demand will increase rather than migrate away from where the product will be positioned in the future?

☐ 6. Is there an *existing and reliable distribution channel* in place to reach this market without having to create a new one for this product to be successful? (If the company is a traditional biotech therapeutic model that will be licensed to a pharmaceutical company, do not score this question)

☐ 7. Are the *Pro forma* projections based upon *tested assumptions* and are the market penetration plans for this product realistic and reasonable?

☐ 8. Does the company have the *necessary personnel and expertise* with the capabilities and know-how to lead and penetrate this market? (If the company is a traditional biotech therapeutic model that will be licensed to a pharmaceutical company, do not score this question)

☐ 9. Does the company have a *well-thought-out branding and positioning strategy* to successfully distinguish its product and services from others? (If the company is a traditional biotech therapeutic model that will be licensed to a pharmaceutical company, do not score this question)

☐ 10. Is the product offering *quickly scalable* and is there a worldwide need for the product offering?

______ ***Total score***
***Average score* (divide by 10) =** ☐

IV. Regulatory Hurdles and Barriers to Entry

Score	Questions
☐	1. Does the Leadership or Management Team have *previous experience with regulatory success* for approval of similar products or services?
☐	2. Does the Leadership or Management Team *know the process and the length of time* estimated to obtain regulatory approval?
☐	3. Does the Leadership or Management Team *know the risks for regulatory approval with this type of product,* having identified successful examples of others, without the possibility of classification into a totally new regulatory category?
☐	4. Has the Leadership or Management Team had recent and *direct communications with regulatory agencies or industry experts* who are intimately familiar with the current regulatory issues for their product?
☐	5. Are the regulations for marketing approval *clearly defined* without the possibility of dynamic and future changes anticipated for the product or the market the company is entering?
☐	6. Are there *impending regulation changes* for the company's product or market that are not yet completely defined? (If the answer to this question is "yes" rank this with lowered scores based upon increasing uncertainty).
☐	7. Does the company have a *well-developed and detailed plan* in place with the expertise in the regulatory strategy and process to assure that the regulatory steps are accomplishable by this team?
☐	8. Does the company possess *three or more significant barriers to entry* that have been identified such that these pose formidable challenges for competitors to successfully compete in this product market?
☐	9. Is the product offering free from *debatable ethical or unresolved societal issues* such that the product growth and market acceptance would not be hampered anywhere in the world?
☐	10. Is there *clear regulatory guidance* for the product offering in the major *countries throughout the world* such that the regulatory approval requirements are clearly understood?
______	***Total score*** ***Average score* (divide by 10) =** ☐

V. Future Funding and Financing Suitability

Score	Questions
☐	1. Is there very high potential for *continued funding* of the company based upon similar types of organizations and funding trends, or based upon expressed or stated interest of investors?
☐	2. Are the business, product, or target market *very good candidates for venture capital or institutional funding* based upon venture capital funding trends or directly expressed interest?
☐	3. Does the company currently have *Institutional Investors,* those with large cash investing reserves, or *Venture Capitalists* who are *positive* on the company and the product's future success potential?
☐	4. Is the exit strategy attractive enough to show a *potential greater than 10× return* on investment and is there a reasonable likelihood of achieving the exit goals based upon the current economic metrics in the industry?
☐	5. Is there sufficient *cash on hand* to carry the company at least 18 months at its projected burn rate, or well past the next significant value-enhancing milestone?
☐	6. Has the company identified fundable *value-enhancing development milestones* that can be reached which will significantly improve the valuation of the company and the likelihood of securing follow-on funding?

☐ 7. Are the *outlined use-of-proceeds* for the development of the organization reasonable and effective throughout the product development cycle?

☐ 8. Are the current *investors supportive of the company, product, and Leadership Team* such that they would add to their investment or recommend this investment to others?

☐ 9. Does the company reside in a geographic location that historically has access to Venture Capital or Institutional Funds and/or located in a geography that is considered a *biotechnology cluster or hub*?

☐ 10. Does the Leadership Team have *experience in successfully raising the total amount of capital* projected to reach the exit or to reach profitability?

____ ***Total score***
***Average score* (divide by 10) =** ☐

Summary

These biotechnology business model examples show how a business model can help a company become competitive with their technology or product. Recognize that there are numerous business models in the therapeutic, biologic, diagnostic, medical device, clinical laboratory, and research reagent industry, and many are adapted and modified for a company's competitive advantage. The process of selecting the optimal business model must involve the collective assessment of all the various business segments essential for your business, while taking into account all their associated risks. Choosing the best business model provides your company with the greatest opportunity for success, and it is the first step in managing the business risk and should be selected and implemented during the company's inception stage. It is important to know the business models of your competitors in the industry and to identify what aspects of their model make them successful. There are multiple components within any single business model. Some components may be strengths, and some may be weaknesses, so understand what they are before making a choice. Study alternate business models in adjacent sectors and in totally different industries and consider if portions of these may be adaptable and improve competitiveness or reduce business risks for your company. As with the razor-handle/razor-blade model, portions of old business models may be applicable and transferable to new products or technology depending on your needs or objectives. Identify the reasons why one model works in one particular business and why the same business model might be a failure in another business. Think about the overall strategies that give a company a sustainable competitive advantage over the competition and lead the company to sustained profitability.

As an entrepreneur or company leader, you are also the risk manager of the business. In order to manage the risk, you must first understand what they are, and then actively manage them. Leaders can reduce risks by making sound decisions and identifying ways to mitigate these risks. Remember that in the early stages of any business, many decisions have long-term impact such as determining your product development pathway, protecting your IP, determining the method and timing of financing, deciding upon which individuals to hire, and choosing your marketing strategy. To help assess your company's risks, utilize the Biotechnology Company Evaluation Tool to rank the five risk categories. Be sure to objectively assess your strengths and weaknesses and then develop a plan for how to bring those areas to a level of excellence. This tool will be helpful when preparing to raise capital, and it will also establish a reference point during your company's development that will help you gauge future progress and your overall improvement. The information gained from critically answering the questions in each of these categories will be helpful when creating your business plan as discussed in *Chapter 22: Your Business Plan and Presentation: Articulating Your Journey to Commercialization.*

No entrepreneur can be expected to completely eliminate risk, but it is extremely hazardous if the leader does not even know what the risks are to the company. The entrepreneurial team's objective is to understand the risks associated with accomplishing the core objectives of the company and to identify ways to mitigate these risks. It is important to recognize that success does not come solely by making the right choices when presented with decisions. Much of the success is influenced by one's creativity in finding ways to effectively and resourcefully circumvent challenges rather than simply by choosing the path holding the lowest risk.

References

[1] Yella JK, Yaddanapudi S, Wang Y, Jegga AG. Changing trends in computational drug repositioning. Pharmaceuticals 2018;11:57.

[2] Osterwalder A, Pigneur Y, Smith A. Business model generation. Hoboken, NJ: John Wiley & Sons, Inc; 2010.

Chapter 13

Directing Your Technology Toward a Market Problem: What You Need to Know Before Using the Business Model Canvas?

Craig Shimasaki, PhD, MBA

CEO, BioSource Consulting Group and Moleculera Labs, Oklahoma City, OK, United States

Chapter Outline

In this chapter, I'll describe a helpful tool for optimizing your comapny's business model that is frequently used in many business schools, entrepreneurship training program, and even in the National Science Foundation's i-Corps program. If you are not already familiar with it, this tool is called the *Business Model Canvas* and has made the building, evaluating, and optimizing of business models easier and much more efficient. However, I will also share one pitfall that frequently occurs with biotechnology products if the Business Model Canvas is applied ***prior*** to identifying the most strategic product application and target market for your technology. We will discuss how most novel biotechnology products have an underlying technology platform and how it should be utilized to identify the best product application ***before*** applying the Business Model Canvas. Once the underlying technology platform is recognized, I will share how to recognize the optimal market application(s) for your technology. We will then review the key points for optimizing your business model using the Business Model Canvas.

An Innovative Technology is Agnostic to the Product Application

Most medical and biotechnology research discoveries are not beholden to a single specific market application. For instance, a genomic discovery could technically be applied to diagnostics, therapeutics, or research tool or research reagent product applications. For example, a scientific discovery that was identified as a rapid cell culture method for producing influenza vaccines could technically be applied to *Zika virus*, *Ebola virus*, or in military applications to biological warfare viruses (Fig. 13.1), whereas a cell cycle checkpoint inhibitor that was identified while studying breast cancer could technically be applied to ovarian cancer, lung cancer, or glioblastoma (Fig. 13.2). No doubt these applications would have additional technical hurdles, but the point is that although the discovery may have been identified in a certain targeted application, with additional work these discoveries can be applied to a broader array of market applications. Why is

Biotechnology Entrepreneurship. DOI: https://doi.org/10.1016/B978-0-12-815585-1.00013-9

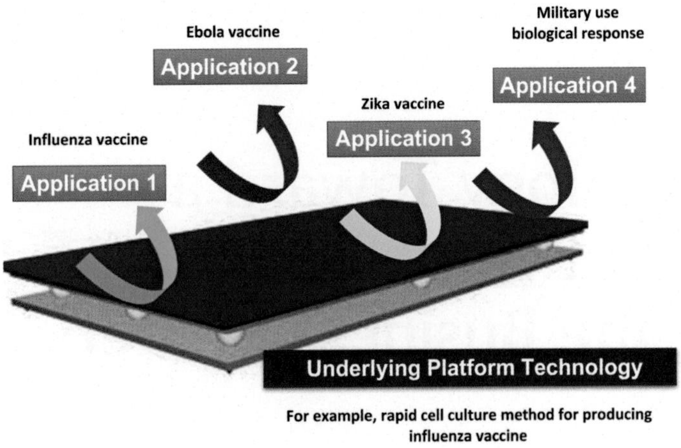

FIGURE 13.1 Most scientific discoveries have an underlying platform technology that gives rise to multiple applications. Used with permission C. Shimasaki

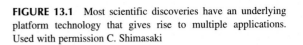

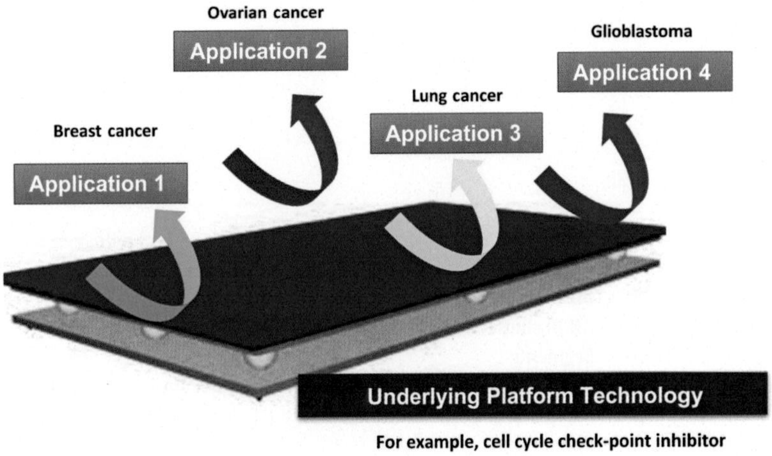

FIGURE 13.2 By identifying your underlying platform technology, you can direct it toward strategic market applications. Used with permission C. Shimasaki

this important to understand as a biotechnology entrepreneur? It is because the market for each of these applications has vastly different values, needs, and competitors. When choosing to start a company, entrepreneurs must first seek to align their technology with an acute market need if they intend to build and grow a successful company because investors understand this principle and so do the strategic partners. If you direct a novel technology to a lackluster product market application, you will have difficulty gaining interest from prospective partners and venture capital investors; and without capital, you cannot develop your product.

Seek to Identify Your Underlying Platform Technology

The basis of a biotechnology product originates from a novel research discovery that may be a unique mechanism-of-action for a chronic disease, a new composite material that can be inserted into the body for a specific use, a new marker that can monitor disease progression, or a variety of other discoveries. The technology that lies beneath the product application making this product work can be referred to as its ***underlying technology platform***. In practice, entrepreneurs utilize this underlying technology platform and direct it toward a particular market application, such as a diagnostic, medical device, therapeutic, then more specifically to a particular application within these sectors. The selection of an application is often a subconscious decision. All too often, the entrepreneur may not recognize that they are working with an *underlying technology platform*, but rather presuming it to be a ***single product opportunity***. The choice of market application for your technology is one of the most critical early stage decisions that an entrepreneur makes, and often they may not even know that they are making a decision. One reason for this occurring is a belief that the underlying technology and the product application are one and the same. This can occur because the validation of the technology may have been extensively performed on that specific target application.

Let me share with you an example similar to what occurs in many early stage biotechnology company start-ups. A company called Selexys Pharmaceuticals in Oklahoma City was built upon a key discovery of the role of P-selectin in inflammation, in which the founding scientists developed a blocking anti-P-selectin antibody. In the beginning the company identified and targeted logical applications of asthma and arthritis, which seemed obvious because of the tremendous market size. However, over time, the company struggled to gain investor interest and momentum even after a subsequent pivot to ischemia and thrombosis. In spite of such a breakthrough technology discovery and large markets for arthritis, asthma, ischemia, and thrombosis, the company labored for many years to gain traction and investor interest. With the recruitment of a successful serial entrepreneur to be CEO, Scott Rollins, cofounder of Alexion purposefully migrated away from asthma/arthritis and ischemia/thrombosis, which are crowded markets with many good products and therefore *not* an acute unmet medical need. They turned this technology toward vaso-occlusive pain crisis in sickle cell disease, an application that had *no* good treatments and was a severe unmet medical need in which patients sought medical care in hospital emergency rooms. This lesser known and smaller market had no adequate products to address the underlying problem that was also associated with inflammation and the role of P-selectin impacted this process. In response, the company was able to raise $35 MM in grants and investor funding to complete Phase 1 and Phase 2 with an ultimate buyout by Novartis in 2016 for $665 million dollars in upfront, acquisition, and milestone payments. As a result, the entrepreneurial team has been able to move forward to targeting other follow-on targets such as Crohn's disease using the same underlying platform technology (Fig. 13.3).

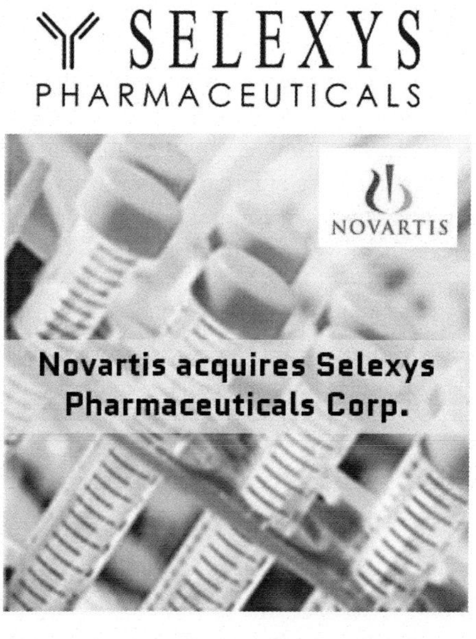

FIGURE 13.3 Selexys Pharmaceuticals acquired by Novartis for $665 million.

A strong admonition to all biotechnology entrepreneurs is to spend time identifying their underlying technology platform, to explore all possible market applications based upon the presence of an unmet medical need and the absence of good products for these conditions. Knowing this, you can then select the most strategic application based upon a critical unmet market need. Sometimes, recognizing your underlying technology platform is not easy, as it may be subtle. Just remember, your underlying technology is agnostic to its application and the target market experiencing that problem. In the biotechnology industry the vast majority of product ideas originate from basic research and discoveries in academic institutions. Therefore, it is incumbent upon the entrepreneur to first select the best application and the right target market before refining their business model. This would be analogous to a situation in business where someone believes that by improving a process, the problem will be solved, when in reality, they should be focused on making the right choice on what problem to work on. It is like mapping the fastest and most economical driving route to Columbus, Ohio, when you need to be in San Francisco, California. You want to first decide the right things to do before you improve the way in which you do them. Why is this point *so important*? It often makes the difference between a nonstarter business versus one in which there is high receptivity by investors, partners, and future acquirers.

A strategic early stage mistake is to have identified a great technology platform but the choice of market application be based upon the entrepreneur's familiarity with one particular problem—or shall we say—a lack of familiarity with more acute problems. This pitfall is described in *Chapter 41: Common Biotechnology Entrepreneur Mistakes and How to Avoid Them* (see "*Common Mistake 2: Misalignment of Technology Toward a Lukewarm Market: A Technology solution in search of a problem to solve*" section). At the outset, entrepreneurs must first seek to align their technology with an acute market need in order to be successful.

Basic research discoveries made in academic institutions and research institutes are usually tied to an application for a specific disease, a proposed treatment, cure, a diagnostic, or tool for improving or supporting health. As these discoveries are made, the academic institution will file patent applications tied to a market application that the inventor identified and worked on as a description of its use. Large gaps exist in translating these discoveries made in academic institutions into needed products in the medical and biotechnology industries. It is not unusual to find that approximately 70%−80% of issued patents sit on university and academic institution shelves unlicensed. A great majority of these patents go unlicensed, not because the underlying technology is inferior or have no value, but more often the target application chosen was not directed toward a market with a compelling unmet medical need.

Advice to Entrepreneurs

A strong admonition to all biotechnology entrepreneurs is to spend time identifying their underlying technology platform, to explore all possible market applications based upon the unmet medical need and the absence of good products for these conditions, and to select the most strategic application based upon a critical market need.

The Drawback in Using the Business Model Canvas *Before* Selecting the Optimal Application for Your Technology

The Business Model Canvas is an excellent tool for assisting entrepreneurs in optimizing their business model and improving its execution. If you are not familiar with the Business Model Canvas, I share an overview of this tool below. As with the use of any tool, the most important step is knowing when and what to use the tool on. No matter how innovative a tool is, if it is not used for the appropriate problem, and at the appropriate time, it is of little value. The Business Model Canvas has been implemented in many biotechnology entrepreneurship training programs and has exposed many scientists, physicians and engineers to important aspects of marketing, segmentation, value proposition and other key business model elements. However, when taking scientists and engineers through these programs they start with a presumption of a market application for their underlying technology which is then run through the Business Model Canvas, and the business is optimized for that application. For biotechnology entrepreneurs there is a problem that occurs if this tool is applied ***prior*** to defining the optimal target market application. The problem is ***not*** with the Business Model Canvas, but with the application of the technology which may not have been selected based upon greatest market need and the most acute market pain. Therefore, no amount of optimization of a business model will overcome a misdirected market application of the technology. Identifying the optimal application of the technology must occur ***before*** using the Business Model Canvas in order for this tool to be most effective. For consumer products, IT, and products that fill a clear unmet need, the Business Model Canvas has helped untold numbers of entrepreneurs in avoiding unforeseen problems by refining their model prior to execution. The challenge for biotechnology and life science technology is that the application of this model ***assumes*** that the entrepreneur has selected the best commercial application for a technology to a particular disease, disorder, or condition. When a tool such as the Business Model Canvas is used for its suited purpose, it becomes a strategic advantage; whereas a tool utilized for an application where it is not suited, it will not be beneficial (Fig. 13.4). The Business Model Canvas is a tool for creatively improving and maximizing your business model when your technology is directed toward a strategic application, but you must ensure that it is applied toward the optimal application ***first***.

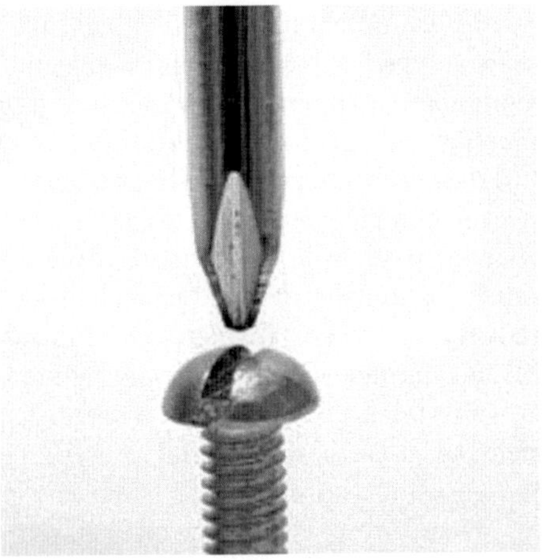

FIGURE 13.4 No matter how great a tool, you must use a tool for the purpose it was intended.

What you Should Evaluate *Before* Using the Business Model Canvas?

If you are starting a company based upon a novel technology, and have a specific product or target application in mind, think of technology as a platform that is agnostic to the application. If you have a development-stage company but you are facing trouble gaining traction and interest from investors and strategic partners, this exercise may be important to ensure that you are not missing a better market application of your technology. The following steps are outlined to help you identify and connect the underlying platform technology with any and all plausible market applications. Follow these steps to help you identify the most strategic market application of your technology.

Feasibility Analysis on Applications of Your Underlying Platform Technology

1. ***First assess and identify the underlying core platform technology.*** Reduce the technology you are utilizing in your product to its simplest concepts. Sometimes, this is difficult to do at first. If you take your product

application out of the picture, what are the unique and valuable features that this technology is *capable* of delivering, doing, or providing. For example, if your product is positioned as an antiviral that can inhibit viral replication in Nipah virus, and it is based upon a protein–protein interference mechanism, can this same technology be directed toward a related virus having a greater and more acute need such as respiratory syncytial virus (RSV) in infants? Can this technology have an application in blocking protein—-protein binding in a cancer pathway? Although the application of your technology may seem endless, there will be certain limitations in your choices, such as if an application would require much more basic research in order to really be viable. You want to be sure that you identify applications that are reasonable for the technology without having to go back to basic research and start over. This exercise should be performed with the scientists involved in the technology and the businesspersons working with your company. If you dig deep into the capabilities of the technology rather than the specific product application, you will begin to see the underlying platform technology.

2. ***Use this information to talk to individuals with expertise in different areas of science and medicine.*** Once you have clearly identified the *underlying platform technology* and have reduced it to its simplest concepts, ask colleagues and experts what they think could be good applications of this underlying technology. The best applications are those that have few, if any substitutes or there are no adequate products for that purpose. Start by talking with those who have expertise in other areas of science and medicine, and only discuss the underlying technology platform and listen intently. Another way to identify different potential applications of your technology is to branch out and listen to problems in other related fields of medicine, health, and science. Once you clearly understand your technology platform and have reduced it to its simplest concepts, imagine other applications as you hear talks, listen to seminars and communicate with others; you may find that this will trigger ideas for other applications of your technology.
3. ***List all potential applications for this technology.*** Over a period of time, you will create a growing list of potential applications for your technology platform. Write all these down, prioritize your list based upon the amount of work and likelihood that these pivots can be accomplished, and then quantify them in decreasing order. The next step is to eliminate those that may not align with what the technology can truly deliver with reasonable efforts.
4. ***Begin a market analysis of the remaining applications.*** Ask or hire a young research analyst who works in the life science industry to help you by researching and finding top-level information such as:
   a. Number of individuals impacted by this disease, disorder, condition, or problem.
   b. What is the current medical practice for these disorders?
   c. List the number of competitors or substitute products
   d. How acute is the need for products for this application?
   e. Categorize the barrier to entry as low, medium, or high, and then define it.
   f. Evaluate the difficulty in bringing a safe and effective product to the market for these conditions: moderate, difficult, and next to impossible.
   g. When you talk to potential investors or partners, do they get excited about these potential applications for such a product?
5. ***Ask an insurance reimbursement expert.*** Based upon the above answers, inquire if there was a safe and effective product to diagnose, mitigate, support, treat, or cure, would insurance companies be willing to reimburse? Are there Current Procedural Terminology (CPT) or reimbursement codes for these products? What does the insurance reimbursement environment look like for products in this category? How competitive are the products in this category, and is there a unique need for your product that other products and substitutes cannot fulfill. How acute is the need?
6. ***Rank your market applications into the top three.*** List the top three applications of your underlying technology based upon the factors in the above analysis. Through continued assessment, determine the best option to leverage your platform technology and save the others for additional follow-on applications and future product development.

By conducting this analysis first, you can be sure that there will be market interest and customers who need the product you will be developing. If you have followed this process, you will have evaluated the market interest ***prior to*** choosing the target application for your technology platform. There are other additional strategic market and business factors that you will want to include to support your competitive advantage such as describing your points of differentiation, setting up barriers to entry, evaluating market adoption hurdles, and timing to the market for your product. However, by strategically identifying the best market application first, you can be sure that you have the optimal opportunity to go with a product that has a clear market need, rather than one that is only presumed. In working with many entrepreneurial-minded professors over the years who have made great research discoveries, I have found that the choice of application for their technology as a market strategy is not foremost on their minds. Often, the most convenient and readily accessible application is reasonable in their minds to use for validating their research discovery. Whereas, building a successful commercial biotechnology product business requires a different assessment that is not often considered during the process of advancing the technology in an academic setting. Once you have carefully and thoroughly identified your top market application, you can then begin to apply the Business Model Canvas to optimize your business model.

With the Optional Market Application of Your Technology, Apply the Business Model Canvas to Optimize Your Business Model

As described in *Chapter 12, Understanding Biotechnology Business Models and Managing Risk*, all companies rely on a business model that allows them to be competitive and one that fits with their product or service offering. In simpler terms *a business model is the method by which a company makes and sells its products and services, which includes the interrelationship of all its component parts, and the manner in which the company creates value and makes money*. Because business models and their terminology can be idiosyncratic and can mean different things to different people, it is challenging to explain abstract concepts to others when there is little common language. Choosing the right business model for your company is critically important, and a framework is needed to identify and share a common language.

The Business Model Canvas is an innovative tool used to build, understand, and visualize the components that make up a business model. The Business Model Canvas was developed by Alexander Osterwalder as his PhD thesis and is a template that allows you to view a business as a whole and then to evaluate it in discreet but interconnecting parts. In the model, there are multiple key building blocks or segments that are divided into the customer facing building blocks and the infrastructure building blocks. For those who are interested in learning more detail than we will cover in this chapter, see the book *Business Model Generation* [1]. One of the key benefits of the Business Model Canvas is that it has made it easier to collaborate with others in the building of business models such that it is creative and iterative. Many business schools, entrepreneurship programs, and accelerator programs have adopted the Business Model Canvas to help entrepreneurs think through and build out their value chain for their product development idea. This has been tremendously helpful and successful as it forces the entrepreneur and team to acquire customer feedback, understand their target market, and the value proposition to their target audience. In addition, it illustrates to the entrepreneur the need to understand the value chain of distributors, providers, and the complex interaction in these relationships that create value.

All Business Models Have Transferable Component Parts or Segments

There are an endless number of permutations to each business model. The reason the number of business models grow is that they are comprised of transposable segments, each of which can be assembled in a variety of combinations to produce variations of any single model. Most business model segments can be "lifted" from one to create a hybrid business model for another application. The Business Model Canvas is a method to visualize and think about the parts of a business allowing you to optimize and improve the way your business creates, captures, and delivers value to its customers. In order to use the Business Model Canvas, you need to understand the nine business model segments. These are as follows:

1. ***Customer segments***—These include all the groups of people and organizations for which you are creating value, which include users and paying customers. For more information on the segmentation of customers, see *Chapter 32: Biotechnology Products and Their Customers: Developing a Successful Market Strategy*.
2. ***Value proposition to each segment***—These are the values, features, and benefits provided to each customer segment. It is the value your product provides to your target customer segments and how you solve the problem or the "pain" that they have.
3. ***Channels to reach customers***—These are all the "touch-points" that are necessary to reach customers and deliver value to them. They include the ways and methods in which you reach your customers and connect with them.
4. ***Customer relationships to establish***—This is a description of the type of relationship you need to establish with your customers. It is the way that your customers interact with you over time and during the life of the product you provide.
5. ***Revenue streams generated***—This one is pretty clear, and it includes all the ways in which you generate revenue from your products and/or services. This includes a description of how, and through which pricing mechanism your business is capturing value.
6. ***Key resources required to create value***—This is a description of the infrastructure required to create,

deliver, and capture value, and the key resources that are indispensable to your business model. This includes key assets that you need in place to deliver your value.

7. ***Key activities required to create value***—This is a description of the things you need to perform well. It encompasses the critical things the company needs to do to deliver on its value proposition to its customers.
8. ***Key partners***—This is a description of who you need to help you leverage your business model. These include key partnerships that help you bring the value you deliver to your customers.
9. ***Cost structure of the business model***—The cost structure of the entire business model for delivering value to each customer segment. How are the costs aligned with delivering the value to your customers, and can they scale?

Fig. 13.5 illustrates the Business Model Canvas and the relationship these nine segments have to each other. For first-time entrepreneurs and those who are not familiar with business models and business strategies, it would be worthwhile to take the time to familiarize yourself with and thoroughly understand each of these segments. Once you have a working understanding of all the segments, it is easier to optimize your strategy for each of these segments as you build your business model. A great benefit of using the Business Model Canvas is that it requires the entrepreneur and leadership team to identify and agree upon their target customers, their value proposition to each, and the manner in which they will deliver value. Don't forget that, in the biotechnology industry, your product typically has three customers (physician prescriber, the patients or users, and the payer or insurance company), each of them require a different value proposition. Although there are some biotechnology sectors that do not have all three customers, such as BioAg, research reagents and tools, typically there are at least two different customers for your product or service, and each of them have different value propositions that need to be satisfied.

Interacting with your Team to Optimize your Business Model

These nine segments become the building blocks of your business model, and it allows you to innovate, ideate, and optimize each of these segments. It is simply a method to improve how your company will create, deliver, and capture value for the product and service it sells. There are many ways to start using this model, but most of them involve bringing together a group of individuals who have a vested interest in your business, typically your team and supporters. What you need to start this process:

- A large whiteboard or image of the Business Model Canvas on a large background.
- A stack of sticky notes of different colors.
- A creative and collaborative environment.
- A group of individuals who are intimately involved in building your company.
- Each person should have previously reviewed and understands the nine business model segments. For a

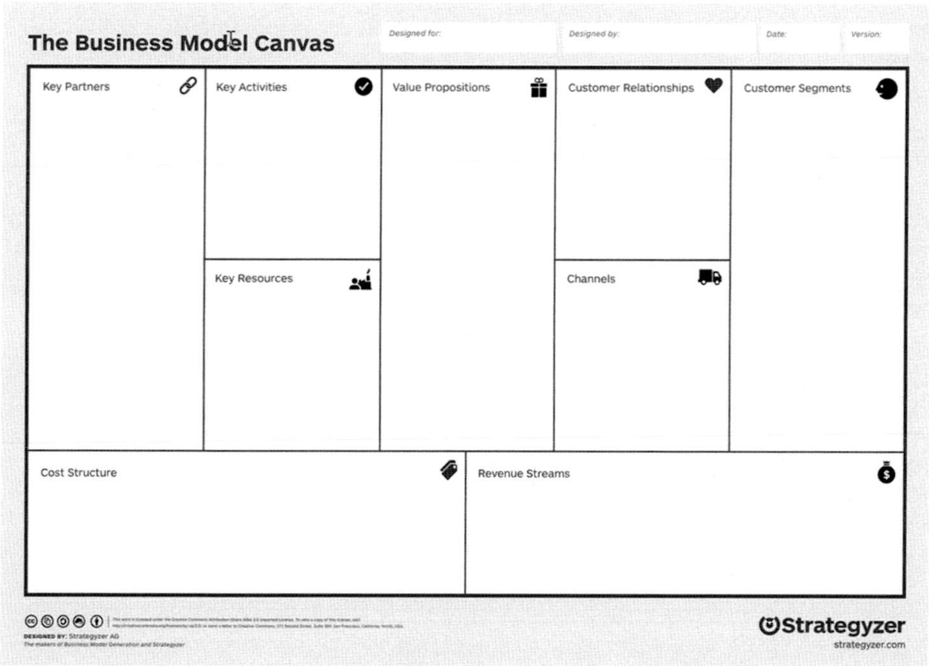

FIGURE 13.5 The Business Model Canvas nine segments. *Reproduced with permission from Strategyzer.com.*

short video explanation, see "Business Model Canvas Explained" [2].
- Someone to lead the team in this brainstorming and ideation session.

For this exercise, you will start with an open discussion about the first segment (customer segments). You will talk about this segment and generate ideas and suggestions of who these individuals are and why they should be placed within this segment. Throughout this process, you will use the sticky notes to post the information from participants into each segment while you brainstorm all the possible and likely inclusions into these boxes. This process is intended to create discussion, challenge your thinking, and create homework to verify your assumptions. For an example of the Business Model Canvas for an influenza vaccine application, see Figure 13.6. To stimulate ideas and discussion, you should ask yourself questions such as "who, what, and why." Some of the questions for different segments may include the following:

- Who are our customers and what are their demographic and behavior characteristics?
- Are they key customers who will influence other customers?
- What are the acute needs we are meeting or problems we are solving with our product?
- Why would these customers purchase our product?
- Describe the pain we are alleviating in our target market?
- How are we alleviating this pain in the market?
- What is our value proposition to each of these identified customer segments?
- How can we increase our value proposition such that they would pay more for our product?
- What strategic relationships do we need in order to deliver this value to our customers?
- How will these strategic relationships be built?
- How will we reach our maximal revenue projections?
- What are our most effective market channels we need and why would they be effective?
- What are the costs of our resources and can we find lower cost resources that are more effective for our market channels?

Once you have exhausted all the ideas for a particular segment, you move to the next segment. Often, you will find the need to go back to change or include additional information in a segment or move sticky notes into different segments as your overall business model begins to

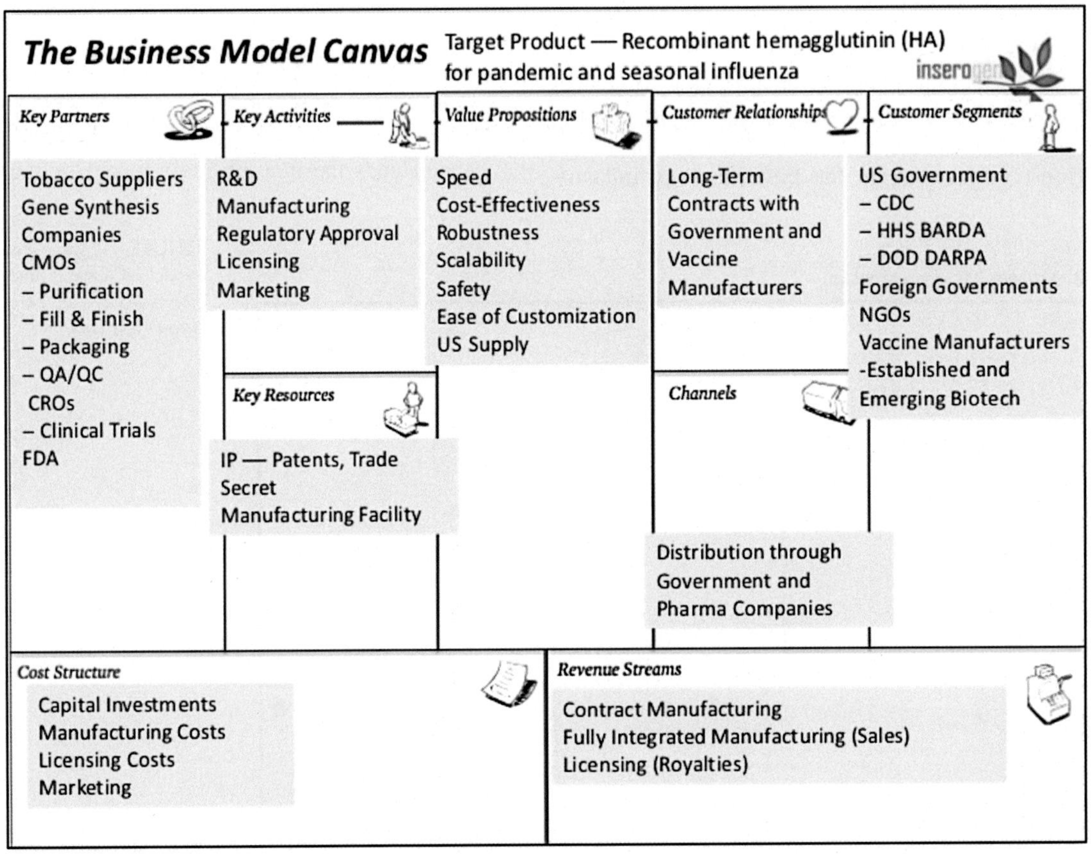

FIGURE 13.6 Example of a Business Model Canvas exercise. *https://www.slideshare.net/sblank/canvas-examples.*

build. It is important to realize that this exercise will *not* be completed in one session but rather it will be an open-ended process that continues to evolve as you learn more about your customer segments, gain more information about your product's value, and find opportunities that you did not recognize initially. At some point, you will feel confident that you and your team have identified the optimal business model and at that point you formalize and freeze the plan. Realize that over time, your market may evolve, competition may arise, your market need may change, and you should use this process to improve your business model again.

As you work through this process, there is a weakness in this approach, which is that all the building blocks must at the end be assembled into an integrated whole. In order to finalize an integrated model, it requires that all the building blocks or segments be joined into a cohesive system where the component parts do not conflict, and the integrated whole is the most efficient and effective method for competitively delivering the product and company value. Sometimes, this final integration requires the individual segments to be adjusted or modified to fit within an integrated strategy. This business model planning exercise is a process that is valuable and essential for any start-up or development-stage biotechnology company. Having a sound and well-thought-out rationale for a company business model will help improve the likelihood of investor interest and your ability to raise the needed capital during the formative stages of the product development.

Summary

We have reviewed a valuable tool, the Business Model Canvas, for optimizing your business model that is directed toward a particular market application in the biotechnology industry. The most important point to come away with is that this tool should be applied to your business ***after*** you have identified the optimal market application for your technology. By first uncovering your underlying technology platform, then using the six steps listed, you can be confident that the market application of your technology is one that has the best chance of success in the market. Then, by applying the Business Model Canvas to your best market application, you can optimize each of these segments to deliver the greatest value to your customers and thus generate greater interest from funding and strategic partners who recognize a true need for your product.

References

[1] Osterwalder A, Pigneur Y. Business model generation: a handbook for visionaries, game changers, and challengers. 1st ed. Hoboken, NJ: John Wiley & Sons; 2010.

[2] YouTube. YouTube video: Business Model Canvas explained. <https://www.youtube.com/watch?v = QoAOzMTLP5s> [accessed March 9, 2019].

Section V

The Emerging Biotechnology Enterprise

Chapter 14

Company Formation, Ownership Structure, and Securities Issues

Craig C. Bradley, JD
Much Shelist, P.C., Chicago, IL, United States

Chapter Outline

The choice of the form of entity that is going to be used to operate the business is an important one for a biotech entrepreneur. A number of factors as described later should be carefully considered in making this decision. If the formation of the business is not properly documented, then the ownership of the entity and the intellectual property and tax issues can create great and sometimes insurmountable problems. Care should be taken to use a seasoned counsel who is experienced in working with technology start-up companies. You should get recommendations from successful executives in your area, and you may also get leads from accounting firms, bankers, and your nearest biotech or other technology association. It is best to interview at least two or three lawyers in order to increase your chances of finding a good "fit." Almost all attorneys will agree to a 1 hour meeting with no obligation.

Law firms charge by the hour, which can range from $200 on the low side to up to $1000 for senior partners at large law firms. Of course, some start-up company's needs are relatively simple and straightforward, while some can be complicated and time consuming. A good start-up lawyer should be able to give you a fairly narrow range of estimated costs. Many firms offer discounts and deferral arrangements for promising start-up companies.

Part 1—Entity Formation

Entities are formed to conduct business principally in order to limit the personal liability of the owners. It is the nature of businesses to incur liabilities. If formed and operated appropriately, creditors cannot attack the personal assets of the owners, instead the assets of the entity. These basic requirements include the formal organization of the entity in one of the states of the United States (this chapter is limited to US law), observing certain formalities (e.g., maintaining certain company records), avoiding being too thinly capitalized and the commingling of assets between the company and the owners, and certain other elements. As these conditions, to avoid "piercing the corporate veil" are easily met, the discussion of them is briefed here. One thing is for certain that is it almost is

Biotechnology Entrepreneurship. DOI: https://doi.org/10.1016/B978-0-12-815585-1.00014-0

never advisable to conduct business without the benefit of forming an entity to shield the personal assets of the owners—sometimes referred to as "bet your house" liability.

There are a limited number of types of entities to choose from the following:

1. corporations (both C and S, and so-called benefit corporations);
2. partnerships (both general and limited); and
3. limited liability companies (LLCs).

Corporations

Corporations are franchises granted by a state. A corporation is formed by filing a document with the state, generally as either a "certificate of incorporation" or "articles of incorporation." The owners are issued stock and are referred to as stockholders or shareholders. The stockholders elect a board of directors who are charged with the general management of the corporation. The board of directors in turn elects the officers—usually a president, one or more vice presidents, a treasurer, and a secretary. The officers are charged with the day-to-day operation of the corporation.

The common practice in the industry of start-ups is to form entities, whether corporations or LLCs in the state of Delaware. One reason is that the Delaware statutes are well written, and the case law interpreting these laws is well developed. It is not expensive to organize in Delaware even if the entity's operations are in another state. Another key reason is that corporate lawyers across the country are familiar with Delaware corporate law. The lawyers who represent investors prefer dealing with a company that is governed by Delaware law. Many states have quirky provisions that are traps for the unwary. The formation of a start-up technology business in a state other than Delaware is usually an indication that the entity is not well advised.

One of the most critical issues to consider in the formation of an entity is the fact that a corporation is subject to two levels of taxes: (1) the corporation itself is taxed at the entity level for income earned and for any gain on the sale of its assets and (2) the stockholders are taxed on dividends (amounts received other than in liquidation) and on distributions (amounts received from the corporation as a result of the sale or liquidation of its assets). The dreaded "double tax!"

The double tax on corporations can be contrasted with the single-level taxation of "pass-through" entities, which are the S corporation and the LLC, as well as partnerships. Note also that an LLC or S corporation can always change to a C corporation with no adverse tax consequences. However, switching from a C corporation to an S corporation or an LLC is a deemed liquidation and a taxable event.

S Corporations

"S corporations" are the same as regular corporations, sometimes referred to as "C corporations" in all operational respects, except that an election is made under subchapter S of the Internal Revenue Code of 1986, as amended (the "IRC"), to be taxed as a partnership. Being taxed as a partnership means that the entity is disregarded for tax purposes, and all the tax attributes (e.g., profits and losses) of the entity are passed through to the owners, the stockholders. When income is earned, the S corporation owes no tax—the stockholders are liable for the income tax. When an S corporation sells its assets to a buyer, the S corporation owes no tax on the gain—the stockholders are liable for the tax.

The S election was enacted for small businesses. Accordingly, there are limitations on S corporations, such as (1) a maximum of 100 stockholders, (2) only individuals can be stockholders (other than certain trusts and charities, and also S corporations can wholly own other S corporations), (3) stockholders cannot be nonresident aliens, and (4) only one class of stock is permitted, for example, no preferred stock is permitted (although there can be voting and nonvoting stock).

Because of these limitations, S corporations rarely are used for technology start-ups. For example, universities, which often receive some equity in exchange for the licensing of technology, cannot be stockholders in S corporations. Most angel investors insist on a preferred equity position, but preferred stock cannot be issued by an S corporation. If a pass-through entity is desired, LLCs are invariably preferred over S corporations. Keep in mind that if the S corporation runs afoul of one of the S corporation limitations, then it is disqualified and immediately becomes, without any further condition or action, a C corporation, which can cause disastrous consequences.

Benefit Corporations

Benefit corporations, as well as so-called L3Cs, are organizations which embed in their charter provisions that the company must legally account for nonfinancial considerations, for example, the public good and the environment. There are third-party organizations which issue certifications stating that a company meets certain qualifications. Very few start-up technology companies want to travel down the road of being a benefit corporation.

Partnerships

Partnerships can be general or limited. General partnerships have no limitation on personal liability. Entities can be the general partners, so most often, the partners in a general partnership are corporations or LLCs. Limited partnerships require the filing of a certificate with a state. The owners of a limited partnership comprised a limited partner or partners and must include at least one general partner. Limited partners have limited personal liability, as long as they don't meaningfully participate in the management of the partnership. How much they can "manage" varies from state to state.

Partnerships are almost never used by start-ups—LLCs are invariably preferred over partnerships. Nowadays, the only partnerships you see in the technology start-up world are long-standing venture capital (VC) firms that are limited partnerships and that have not changed over yet to an LLC structure.

Limited Liability Companies

LLCs are a hybrid of the corporation and the partnership. Most critically, LLCs are pass-through entities, taxed as partnerships (although in rare cases an LLC will elect to be taxed as a C corporation). LLCs are formed in a state by the filing of a "certificate of formation," and in some states "articles of organization." The owners are referred to as "members." The LLC can be managed by its members or the LLC can opt to be managed by a "manager" or "managers" or even by a "board of managers," analogous to a board of directors in a corporation. Ownership usually is not certificated, that is, there are usually no paper certificates representing ownership, like a stock certificate in a corporation, although issuing certificates is permitted. Like a partnership, ownership is a percentage, with all the percentages, not surprisingly, adding up to 100%. Often, for ease of reference, the term "units" is employed. Like shares of stock, use of the nomenclature of units makes the calculations on a cap table much easier.

LLCs are governed by their "Limited Liability Company Agreements," also referred to as "operating agreements" in some states. These agreements are analogous to bylaws and stockholder agreements for corporations. These agreements, for pass-through entities such as LLCs and S corporations, should always contain a provision requiring that cash be distributed to the owners in amounts sufficient to pay their respective income tax obligations. As with stockholder agreements in corporations, they can contain the following:

- *Rights of first refusal*—If an owner desires to sell equity to a third party, it must first be offered to the company and/or the other owners.
- *Cosale rights*—If rights of first refusal are not exercised, then the other owners can elect to sell a pro rata portion of their equity.
- *Drag-along rights*—If a majority (or another specified percentage) of the owners want to sell the company, then all the other owners must sell their equity too.
- *Market standoff*—If the company does an initial public offering, then, generally, the owners can't make any transfers for 180 days.
- *Voting agreement*—The owners can agree to vote their equity to elect a certain manager or managers.
- *Supermajority voting*—The owners can agree that certain important actions require the prior written consent of a supermajority percentage (e.g., two-thirds or 75%, or even unanimous consent), such as sale of new equity, sale of the company, sale or licensing of the company's technology, borrowing money, new hires, and salaries.

LLCs have none of the limitations of an S corporation. There are no limitations on the nature of its owners, on its equity structure, or with regard to how the LLC is governed. Not only LLCs can have a preferred equity structure, profits and losses can also be allocated on a basis other than ownership percentage. For example, say a senior scientist started the business and invested $25,000 of his own funds but now desires to return to the lab and let others run the company. The LLC could be structured to return the first $25,000 with interest at the prime rate to the scientist, then the scientist could receive 50% of the first $1 million and then 10% after that. The scientist could retain some or all management authority until the receipt of a certain amount of funds or until the LLC raised a certain amount of investment. Cash investors can be allocated a greater amount of the losses than noncash investors (keep in mind that losses can be taken only to the extent of "basis," that is, cash invested plus certain recourse loans).

Making the Choice of Either a C Corporation or a Limited Liability Company

C corporations are subject to a double tax but LLCs are not. S corporations have some strict limitations but LLCs do not. An LLC or an S corporation can be changed to a C corporation with no adverse tax consequences, but not vice versa. So why ever choose to be anything other than an LLC?

If your business model requires to obtain funding from a VC firm within the next 2 years, then it is likely that you should forego an LLC and start out as a C corporation. VC firms only invest in C corporations and will not invest in pass-through entities, including LLCs. The investors in most VC firms include entities with 501(c)(3) status, such as pension funds and endowments. These are nonprofit organizations, and in order to retain their tax-free status they are not permitted to earn "unrelated business taxable income" (UBTI). Funds that pass through an LLC to the VC firm and then to the 501(c)(3) organization constitute UBTI. Funds that are distributed by a C corporation, sometimes referred to as a "blocking C corporation," do not constitute UBTI. Many investors in LLCs like the fact that they get the benefit of deducting losses, as most early-stage technology companies incur losses for several years. However, some investors don't like dealing with the K-1 tax reporting forms that are issued by LLCs. Corporations are not required to issue any tax reporting forms to stockholders unless dividends are paid, which is rare for an early-stage technology company.

Another disadvantage of an LLC is that they cannot issue "incentive stock options" (ISOs), which are options to purchase equity. ISOs have certain tax advantages that are explained later. The inability to grant ISOs is greatly ameliorated by the ability of LLCs to issue "profits interests," explained later.

Members of LLCs who are also employees are deemed to be self-employed and must pay all of their social security taxes. This is, in contrast, such corporations, in which the corporation pays half of these taxes. Rank-and-file employees in the lower salary ranges are often shocked to learn this, and they certainly don't appreciate it. And it is possible to avoid by having the employee hold the LLC interest in an S corporation, but this is more than cumbersome. Often an LLC will pay the employee some sort of bonus to lessen the burden (although a complete "gross-up" is expensive!).

Finally, it is worth highlighting the advantage of the single-level taxation of LLCs in two contexts. One is with respect to a life sciences or other technology company that is going to earn its income principally through the licensing of its technology. In this case, there will be revenue streams, which are far greater than minimal operating expenses, resulting in the generation of significant cash income. Adopting an LLC rather than a C corporation would be much more advantageous in order for income to be distributed currently to the owners at only one level of income tax. Second, buyers of early-stage companies generally want to buy assets, not equity. The purchaser of the equity of an entity takes the entity subject to all of its liabilities. Buyers are afraid that there may be "wayward founders" who come out of the woodwork and claim to have an unrecorded ownership interest in the company. There could be other undisclosed liabilities that rear their ugly heads as well. The buyer of assets can specify the assets purchased and the specific liabilities assumed and thus insulate itself from claims on equity and most other liabilities associated with the selling entity (buyers sometimes cannot escape successor liability for certain items, e.g., pension and environmental liabilities).

Because a gain on the sale of the assets of a C corporation would be subject to double taxation, an LLC is a better choice for a company that may be sold early in its history and desire to be in a better position to sell assets. Of course, sales of C corporations happen all the time, and buyers can protect themselves by insisting that the stockholders personally indemnify them from undisclosed liabilities and increased escrow funds. However, as buyers are aware, such indemnifications outside of the escrow are only as good as the wherewithal of the sellers.

Why Choose a Limited Liability Company?

- Only one level of taxation—best if
  - will receive a stream of licensing revenue or
  - may sell assets.
- Investors can deduct losses.
- Profits interests are a great way to grant equity to nonfounders.
- Can change to a C corporation if needed without tax consequences.
- Flexible with respect to the allocation of profits and losses and governance.

Why Choose a C Corporation?

- If likely to get VC funding in the next 2 years.
- If employees won't accept paying their own half of social security taxes.
- If afraid employees just won't understand owning equity in an LLC.
- If you don't want to spend the (not much) greater expense of being an LLC.

An Interesting Life Sciences Limited Liability Company Asset-Centric Paradigm

Albert Sokal, a partner of mine at Edwards Wildman, has pioneered the implementation of utilizing an asset-centric parent LLC holding company with C corporation subsidiaries. This structure is most advantageous in situations where the company owns a platform technology that can be employed in a number of separate fields and thus separate businesses. Stakeholders, including founders, employee participants, and investors, own interests in the parent LLC. A C corporation subsidiary holds the company's operating assets and is the employer. Other C corporation subsidiaries hold licenses to the technology (and may have their own separate technology). This is cutting-edge law and requires a thorough analysis of tax, governance, ownership structure, investor requirements, and other factors.

Part 2—Ownership Structure

The initial issuance of equity to those who start the business, the so-called founders' transaction, should not be taken lightly. One risk not to be overlooked is a finding by taxing authorities that the equity was issued not in consideration for payment of fair value but for services to the company, resulting in the receipt of stock taxed as ordinary income compensation. The problem is that the value of the equity may skyrocket from almost nothing to 1 million or several million dollars (e.g., based on the premoney value given in a financing round). If the formation papers recite only a de minimis dollar amount paid for the founders' equity, the difference between that amount and the far greater fair market value a few months later may be deemed to be compensation.

To mitigate against this, usually the tangible technology owned by the founders, such as the business plan, patentable inventions (although in a university setting these may be owned by the university), trade secrets, and software, can be contributed to the company in exchange for equity. This is accomplished so as to qualify as a tax-free incorporation under Section 351 of the IRC (IRC Section 701 in the case of an LLC). Tax counsel should be consulted in this regard. In any event, care should be taken to document the transfer of all pertinent technology from the founders to the company.

Restricted Stock (Corporation) or Restricted Units (Limited Liability Company)

What if one of the cofounders, whom everyone assumed was going to spend a lot of time working on company matters, takes a job in another state and announces his intention to have nothing further to do with the company? Is it fair for him to retain some or all of his equity? In the case of more than one founder, it is often advisable to impose restrictions on the equity so that if the owner's service to the company ceases for any reason, then the equity is forfeited or repurchased for a nominal amount. This is referred to as "reverse vesting." An example is a cofounder who received 100,000 units in an LLC, which reverse vests over a 4-year period.

A standard vesting schedule is 25% on the first anniversary (a so-called 1-year cliff) and equal monthly increments over the following 3 years. If service terminates prior to 1 year, then all equity is forfeited or repurchased. If service terminates after 18 months, then 18 months of equity is retained, and the balance is forfeited or repurchased. These numbers are not set in stone. For example, founders often get to retain a certain percentage of their equity no matter what, say 25%, and only the rest is subject to vesting. Often, a portion or all of the vesting is accelerated upon a sale of the company, a so-called single trigger, or less favorably to the stockholder upon termination by the acquiror without cause within 1 year after the acquisition, a so-called double trigger.

These vesting provisions usually are reflected in a Restricted Stock Agreement in the case of a corporation and a Restricted Unit Agreement in an LLC. With restricted equity, the owner is the beneficial and record holder and is entitled to voting and dividend/distribution rights. Importantly, the capital gains holding period commences upon the issuance of the equity.

An election pursuant to Section 83(b) of the IRC should almost always be made by the holder of restricted equity. Without an 83(b) election, ordinary income tax is assessed at each time that restrictions lapse in the amount of the difference of the fair market value at the time of the lapse less the amount paid for the equity. Thus an owner could find himself owing a lot in taxes due to a rapid rise in the fair market value of the company (e.g., a successful financing round) with no way to pay the tax (generally equity in a private company is illiquid until the company is sold). When an 83(b) election is made, tax is paid up front on the difference between the fair market value and the amount paid for the equity, usually a very minimal amount, and then no tax is due upon the lapsing of any restrictions. Tax is due when the equity is sold, and if that's more than a year later, then it is subject to the lower tax rate on capital gains, not ordinary income. Very critically, *an 83(b) election must be made within 30 days after the issuance of the equity*. There are no exceptions or alternatives for relief.

Profits Interests in a Limited Liability Company

So-called profits interests are a profound tax-efficient manner of getting equity in an LLC to nonfounders. A profits interest is an ownership interest in the LLC entitling the holder to the specified percentage of the value of the company *after* the preexisting value of the company is distributed to the prior owners. There is no tax on the grant of a profits interest (!). Like restricted equity, it is a live interest in the LLC and needs to be held for only over 1 year in order to receive capital gains treatment on the sale.

An example is helpful in the explanation of profits interests. Say that the founders contributed $100,000 in cash upon the start of the LLC. The company is now determined to have a fair market value of $1 million. The founders want to bring on a senior executive and grant him a 10% ownership interest. If a 10% interest were to be granted outright, then the executive would be subject to tax on $100,000 of ordinary income, representing the fair market value of the equity. With a profits interest, the executive is entitled to a 10% interest after the founders' capital accounts have been "booked up" to the company's value at the time of the grant of the profits interest. If the company is later sold for $10 million, the executive would be entitled to 10% of $9 million.

Because of the advantages of the profits interest in an LLC, it rarely makes sense to grant options to purchase an LLC interest. This is because the exercise price for the option must be equal to at least the fair market value (according to IRC Section 409A), and the equity must be held for at least 1 year after the option is exercised in order to qualify for capital gains. Many tax advisors recommend a "protective" 83(b) filing for profits interests. Technically, an 83(b) filing is not required for a profits interest, but if for whatever reason, the interest is determined not to qualify as a profits interest, then the 83(b) filing may save the day. For example, IRS Revenue Procedure 93-27 provides for a safe harbor for profits interests which, among certain other conditions, are held for at least 2 years. Profits interests held for less time do not meet this test and are susceptible to losing their status.

Incentive Stock Options and Nonqualified Stock Options

A stock option is a contract for the purchase of a certain number of shares, at a certain price, during a certain period of time, and subject to other terms and conditions. Like restricted equity, options are almost always subject to a vesting schedule. Options that qualify for treatment as "ISOs" under IRC Section 422 (ISOs) enjoy certain tax advantages.

An ISO can only be granted by a corporation (not an LLC and not a stockholder) to an employee (who can be full or part time). They cannot be granted to nonemployees such as consultants or nonemployee directors. ISOs must be granted at an exercise price of at least the fair market value of the underlying stock (110% for owners of 10% or more). The maximum exercise period is 10 years (5 years for owners of 10% or more). The maximum value is $100,000 per year and $1 million in the aggregate (determined at the time of the grant).

There is no tax on the grant of a stock option, whether it is an ISO or a nonqualified stock option. The advantage of ISOs is that there is no tax on the exercise of an option. And if the stock that is purchased is held for a minimum of 1 year and for at least 2 years after the grant of the ISO, then a sale of the stock is entitled to capital gains. One caveat is that although the exercise of an ISO is not subject to a regular tax it is subject to the alternative minimum tax provisions of the IRC.

As alluded to above section, IRC Section 409A mandates that options must have an exercise price equal to at least the fair market value of the underlying stock. If this fair market value requirement is not met, then very punitive taxes are imposed. For companies that are less than 10 years old (and are not expecting a liquidity event within 90 days or an IPO in the next 180 days), the fair market value can be determined by a written internal valuation analysis. This analysis need not to be prepared by a person or entity independent from the company, but the preparer must have at least 5 years of relevant experience in business valuation, financial accounting, investment banking, private equity, secured lending, or another comparable experience.

Phantom Stock

I refer to the so-called phantom stocks as "fake equity." It's nothing more than a contract requiring the company to pay the executive money upon the occurrence of an event, usually the sale of the company. In this regard, it's more like a typical salesman commission plan. Most importantly, capital gains treatment is never available. In addition, the holder of phantom stock does not really hold any equity and is not owed any fiduciary duties by the board of directors or any of the company's equity holders.

Employment and Consultant Issues

The transfer of all intellectual property rights from the founders to the company by a written Technology Assignment Agreement should not be overlooked. Moreover, the founders, as well as all employees and consultants, should sign an agreement, often referred to as a "Proprietary Rights Agreement," which assigns all inventions to the company and confirms that the individual will maintain the confidentiality of the company's information.

Generally, it is in the company's interest to require employees (and often consultants) to agree and not to compete with the company after termination. The maximum posttermination noncompete period varies from state to state. The provisions of noncompetes must be carefully drafted to be enforceable, and experienced legal counsel should be consulted. It is worth noting that such noncompetes in the state of California are per se invalid.

Most start-ups can get by without formal employment agreements, although it is advisable to use written offer letters setting forth the basic terms of employment and reciting that employment is "at will," among some other basic matters.

What's the Downside if You Wait?

You might think: "There's too much to do, and I don't want to spend time or money on lawyers." And: "I'm not sure who's going to work out, so I don't want to resolve things now." Finally: "I'll fix it all later."

To this I say, "There's a very real risk you will suffer substantial harm, and you might even lose everything." One risk is the "wayward founder." By not having solid agreements regarding equity, someone may claim more than what they're entitled to. This may cause an investor to make the other founders liable for this claim or to walk away. Worse, a sizable threat to the cap table may result in the company just not being financeable.

Another problem is delaying the grant of equity until a term sheet has been presented—and then the equity has to be granted at the new, higher value. Talk about upsetting your fellow team members! In a successful start-up, millions of dollars can be at stake.

And here's my favorite most easy mistake to avoid: the company not owning its intellectual property! All founders, contractors, and employees must sign confidentiality and assignment of inventions agreements. Try getting a former disgruntled employee to sign such an agreement after the fact. Do you think they might try to hold you up?

The issues mentioned earlier are just a few of the problems if you let the legal things wait. And fixing problems is so much more expensive than just getting them right in the first place. It reminds me of my childhood friend who is a dentist in Florida. He tells me that he makes far more money on patients who ignore their routine cleanings and occasional fillings and then have to come in for crowns, implants and gum surgery. You really don't want to be like that patient.

Part 3—Fundraising

Selling Equity Versus Convertible Debt or Convertible Equity

Most life sciences companies are formed in university labs and often receive a healthy amount of grants and other nondilutive funding. At some point the decision is made to spin out a company with an exclusive license from the institution (see *Chapter 15: Licensing the Technology: Biotechnology Commercialization Strategies Using University and Federal Labs*). Whether or not the company was conceived in an institutional setting, in order to commercialize the technology typically outside "seed" or "angel" financing is necessary or desirable.

The first issue to confront is the "premoney" valuation of the company. In other words, what percentage of the company's ownership should the investors get for their money? For example, if the premoney valuation is $2 million, and the investors pay $500,000, then the investors would receive 20% of the equity (500,000/2500,000). Sophisticated investors will insist on a "preferred" instrument, meaning preferred stock in a corporation, or preferred units in an LLC. Preferred means that the investors have a preference with respect to getting their money back first—before the founders, as well as employees and consultants. In the abovementioned example, if things didn't go well and the technology was sold for $700,000, the investors would get their $500,000 back before any other distributions.

More often than not, the premoney valuation of the company is not easy to resolve between the founders, who believe the company deserves a very high valuation, and the investors, who may be optimistic but are aware of the downside risk. Convertible notes to the rescue!

The convertible note is technically debt, but typically the note is automatically converted into equity on the same terms and conditions as the next "qualified financing." A "qualified financing" is the next round of equity financing of at least a certain dollar amount, which can range from as low as $500,000 to as high as $3 million. Qualifications can also include that it be a preferred instrument and/or that the lead investor(s) must be institutional investors. The maturity date is typically between 1 and 2 years.

If a qualified financing has not occurred by the maturity date, then alternatives may include (1) the ability of the investors to foreclose on the assets of the company, (2) the note is convertible into equity at a predetermined "backup" premoney valuation, or (3) the note is convertible into equity at an agreed premoney valuation or, if not agreed, then by an independent appraisal.

Most convertible notes include a "valuation cap," so that the premoney value of the conversion is capped at a certain dollar amount, notwithstanding that the qualified financing premoney valuation is higher. As a result, the existing equity holders (usually the founders) absorb this dilution.

In exchange for the risk taken by the note holders, they are given a discount on the price paid by those leading the qualified financing—a 20% discount is market, although it can be as low as 5% if a qualified financing is expected soon, or as high as 30%–40% if the deal is perceived as riskier. Sometimes it's a sliding scale by the number of months it takes to complete a qualified financing.

The stated interest rate for convertible notes in years past was usually 8%. In recent times, with interest rates so low, the common rate has drifted down to 5%. A new concept, called "convertible equity" has been advanced in which no interest is payable and there is no maturity date. "Convertible equity" is like convertible debt, except that it has no maturity date and no interest rate. Another advantage to the company is that the investment is moved from the liability side of the balance sheet to the equity column, thus making the balance sheet appear in much better health to customers, suppliers, and employees. For the investor, it's live equity, so the capital gains clock starts running. However, in my experience, convertible equity is just too new, and most investors resist it.

Convertible Note Checklist

- Amount offered, and the minimum amount, if any.
- Maturity date—usually 1–2 years.
- Interest rate—usually 5%–8%.
- Definition of the "qualified financing" which triggers conversion of the notes often $1 million priced round, can be more or less.
- Percentage discount note holders receive in the qualified financing—often 20%.
- Notes can be secured by the assets of the company.

What happens if a qualified financing has not occurred by the maturity date? It can (1) have a "backup" premoney valuation, (2) provide for the premoney valuation to be determined by an appraisal, and (3) be silent, thus giving the note holders the right to foreclose.

What happens if the company is sold prior to conversion or the maturity date? Often, note holders are paid 2 or 3 × principal.

Securities Laws

Whether it's a priced equity round or a convertible note round, the issuing company must be cognizant of federal and state securities laws. Some make the mistake of thinking that convertible notes are not securities because they are not equity instruments, or that interests of LLC are not securities since they are not "stock." This almost always is not the case, and the securities laws apply.

Section 5 of the Securities Act of 1933, as amended (the Securities Act), requires all securities transactions to be registered with Securities and Exchange Commission (SEC). Section 4(2) provides an exemption for the offering of securities in a transaction, which is "not a public offering." But you can scour the Securities Act and won't find a definition of a "public offering."

The US Supreme Court settled this question in the landmark case of *SEC v. Ralston Purina Co.*, 346 US 119 (1953). In short the holding was that in order for an offering to be private, and not public, and thus exempt from registration requirements: (1) same kind of information that otherwise generally would be available in a registration statement must be provided to investors and (2) the investors themselves must be sophisticated, that is, able to understand such information.

What's an entrepreneur to do, be a scholar of US Supreme Court cases? Here, it's the SEC to the rescue in the form of Regulation D (Reg. D). Reg. D is not exclusive, meaning the case law of *Ralston Purina* and its progeny can be relied upon. However, if case law is relied upon then the issuing company has the burden of proof that the offering is indeed private. If a company complies with Reg. D, then the presumption in a court of law is that the offering is private.

Without getting into a detailed discussion of Reg. D, the fact of the matter is that Rule 506 of Reg. D is almost always used for private offerings. One great advantage of Rule 506 is that it preempts state securities laws and has no dollar limit on the amount of funds raised. Requirements of Rule 506 include an unlimited number of accredited investors and not more than 35 unaccredited investors, no general solicitation or advertising, and certain resale limitations and the filing of Form D within 15 days of first sale of securities (form D must also be filed in each state in which securities are sold).

Very importantly, there are rigid disclosure requirements to investors if there is even one investor who is not "accredited." Generally, it is best to offer securities only to accredited investors. Nonaccredited investors often are referred to as "widows and orphans" and have no business participating in an investment in a start-up company, by definition it is a very risky endeavor. The following are the categories of "accredited investor":

- Individuals with a $1 million net worth (exclusive of primary residence) or $200,000 in income (or $300,000 with his or her spouse) in past 2 years and expected in the current year.
- Entities in which all investors are accredited investors.
- Directors and executive officers of the issuer.
- Corporations or trusts with assets in excess of $5 million (not formed for the purpose of making the investment).
- Institutional investors such as banks, savings and loans, broker–dealers, insurance companies, and investment companies.

If there are no nonaccredited investors, then no specific written disclosure is required, but the antifraud rules still apply! Because the antifraud rules always apply, it is advisable (read obligatory) to provide to investors a written disclosure document—usually referred to as a "private placement memorandum," which includes the terms of the offering, risk factors, capitalization, use of proceeds, a description of the business, and the bios of management—in other words all information material to an investment decision.

Advertising and general solicitation with regard to the sale of securities is now (since September 23, 2013) permitted under Rule 506(c) of Reg. D. This is as a result of the Jumpstart Our Business Startups (JOBS) Act and a game-changing departure. Unfortunately for entrepreneurs, the SEC specified in the rule that the securities can be sold to only accredited investors and that their status as accredited investors must be stringently verified—income by W-2s, 1099s, etc. and net worth by bank statements, appraisals, etc. (although an attorney, accountant, or broker–dealer can furnish a certification).

Finally, the JOBS Act permits the sale of securities through certain qualified Internet portals. To be clear a company cannot set up its own portal to sell its securities—it must sell through an approved intermediary (SEC-registered broker–dealers and certain other registered entities). These portals are permitted to advertise and publically solicit the sale of securities. Companies are limited to raising no more than $1 million per year. Unlike Rule 506(c), *investors need not be accredited.* Individuals with less than $100,000 in income can invest up to $2000 or 5% of their income or net worth. Individuals with more than $100,000 can invest up to 10% of their income or net worth. In addition unlike Rule 506(c), no strict income or net worth verification requirements are included in the proposed Regulations (although they may be included in the final Regs).

The previous description is not an exhaustive presentation of the US or state securities laws, and prior to offering securities a company should obtain the advice of an experienced securities attorney.

Finding Legal Counsel; Legal Costs

Care should be taken to use seasoned counsel who is experienced in working with technology start-up companies. You should get recommendations from successful executives in your area, and you may also get leads from accounting firms, bankers, and your nearest biotech or other technology association. Almost all attorneys will agree to a 1 hour meeting with no obligations.

Law firms charge by the hour, which can range from $200 on the low side to up to $1000 for senior partners at large law firms. Of course, some start-up company's needs are relatively simple and straightforward, while some can be complicated and time consuming. A good start-up lawyer should be able to give you a fairly narrow range of estimated costs. Many firms offer discounts and deferral arrangements for promising start-up companies.

Summary

The choice of an entity for a start-up should not be made without a thorough understanding of all the implications, including tax, founder, management, and employee considerations. Invariably, the choice is between a C corporation and an LLC. An LLC most likely is the default selection, unless investment by a VC firm is on the near horizon. There are no tax consequences when converting from an LLC to a C corporation, but converting from an LLC to a C corporation is a taxable event.

The "founders' transaction" should be carefully considered. It almost always makes sense to institute a vesting program for founders and employees. Finally, great care should be taken to comply with federal and state securities laws. All of these matters requires sound legal advice and should be discussed with a seasoned attorney having extensive experience with start-up issues for companies in the biotechnology industry.

Chapter 15

Licensing the Technology: Biotechnology Commercialization Strategies Using University and Federal Labs

Steven M. Ferguson, CLP[1] and Uma S. Kaundinya, PhD, CLP[2]

[1]Special Advisor, Office of Technology Transfer, National Institutes of Health, Rockville, MD, United States, [2]Vice-President, Corporate Development, Goldfinch Bio, Cambridge, MA, United States

Chapter Outline

The Federal Government's Investment in Basic Biomedical Research

For many years the United States has led the world in government funding of nonmilitary research and development (R&D), notably support for basic and clinical research that directly relates to health and human development. While new biotechnology entrepreneurs often rely upon the "Three Fs" of founders, friends, and family for advice, assistance, and financing during the early years of their company, they often overlook a "Fourth F" that can be of major assistance during many phases of their growth—that being federal, especially federal labs and federally funded research in universities and academic medical centers (AMCs), also referred to as academic medical organizations (AMOs) across the United States. A longtime focal point for such federal investment by the US government in biomedical research has been the National Institutes of Health (NIH) through its intramural laboratories and the funding provided to most academic and university- or hospital-based research programs. Funding provided by the NIH alone reached $37.3 billion in the fiscal year 2018; approximately 10% of this funding was spent on internal NIH R&D projects

Biotechnology Entrepreneurship. DOI: https://doi.org/10.1016/B978-0-12-815585-1.00015-2

(intramural research) carried out by the approximately 6000 scientists employed by the NIH. The balance was distributed in the form of grants, contracts, and fellowships for the research endeavors of more than 300,000 nongovernment scientists (extramural research) at 2500 colleges, universities, and research organizations throughout the world [1]. Each year, this biomedical research leads to a large variety of novel basic and clinical research discoveries, all of which generally require commercial partners to develop them into products for consumer, scientist, physician, or patient use. Thus federal laboratories and universities need and actively seek corporate partners or licensees to commercialize their federally funded research into products to help fulfill their fundamental missions in public health.

AMCs, with their dual components of research and clinical care, are in a unique position of being at the very beginning and very end of the science-to-business and product-to-patient chain. For example, the University of Massachusetts Medical School (UMMS) in Worcester receives $250 million in federal funding for its nearly 1100 investigators and Partners Health Care at Massachusetts General Hospital (MGH) and Brigham and Women's Hospital receives about $1.4 billion in federal funding for its approximately 1300 investigators. These AMCs use the very therapies and diagnostics that its researchers invent, for clinical care.

Translation of Academic Research to Products for the Public Good

Most biotechnology products have some history of their R&D that can be traced back to a basic research institution, most often funded by federal grants. Licensing and technology transfer programs at nonprofit basic research organizations provide a means for getting new inventions to the market for public use and benefit. From a research institution's perspective, this is quite desirable since the public and commercial use of inventions typically come with new recognition of the value of basic research programs at the university or organization that originated it. These inventions also serve as helpful means to attract new R&D resources and partnerships to these laboratories. Through licensing or other technology-transfer mechanisms, these institutions also receive a "return on investment" whether that is measured in terms of financial, educational or societal parameters, or some combination thereof. A recent study by the Brookings Institute [2] offers useful insights about the academic innovation enterprise.

Universities and AMCs are known as centers of education, patient care, and basic research. This basic research, fueled largely by the curious mind and funding from the government, has transformed our understanding of important fundamental phenomena. This research activity results in publications that dictate the careers of those in academia and defines the institution's academic culture and spirit. Important discoveries are made at each of these institutions, but they are largely confined to the research realm. Starting from the early 1960s, the need to maximize the benefits from such intense and groundbreaking research was felt thanks to Jerome Wiesner, the scientific advisor to President John F. Kennedy. He recognized that most of the innovations which impacted everyday people were left primarily to the large companies of the day—Lucent Bell Labs, Kodak, Johnson & Johnson, to name a few—which held the most patents, and their products were known all over the world.

Bayh–Dole and the Birth of Technology Transfer (1980)

Picking up from the momentum of the policies of Presidents John F. Kennedy and Richard Nixon in 1980, Senators Birch Bayh and Bob Dole enacted legislation that gave universities, nonprofits, and small businesses the *right* to own inventions made by their employees for federal government-funded research. The Bayh–Dole Act of 1980 (P.L. 96-517) reversed the presumption of title and permitted a university, small business, or nonprofit institution to elect and pursue ownership of an invention in preference to the government. The underlying spirit of this important piece of legislation was to maximally utilize the outstanding research at these universities and other nonprofits for the good of the public who funded the research through their tax dollars.

The ownership right that universities have to these inventions comes with obligations. Primarily, it is the obligation to actively market and attempt to commercialize the invention, preferably through US-based business enterprises including start-ups to benefit the public. Thus was born the field of "technology transfer" and the mushrooming of technology-transfer offices (TTOs). Prior to Bayh–Dole, 28,000 patents were owned by the US government, less than 5% of which were commercialized. It has been reported that since the enactment of Bayh–Dole, 5000 new companies have been created, resulting in billions of dollars of direct economic impact within the United States and close to 600 products put in the market during these 40 years—all based upon university research.

Because a substantial portion of the inventions that arise from basic research programs are supported by research that is federally funded, there are also substantial legal obligations incurred by universities and AMOs to promote commercial development of such new inventions. Similarly, in the 1980s, federal intramural laboratories were also given a statutory mandate under the Stevenson-Wydler Technology Innovation Act (P.L. 96-480), the Federal Technology Transfer Act (P.L. 99-502), and Executive Order 12591 to ensure that new technologies developed in federal laboratories were similarly transferred to the private sector and commercialized.

Commercialization of inventions from nonprofit basic research institutions typically follows a multistep process as academic and federal laboratories typically do not provide technology commercialization themselves. The inventions made by these researchers are converted into products and processes by for-profit companies. In the case of AMCs the clinical products often return to these AMCs for clinical collaborations including clinical trials. Thus these AMCs contribute twice at the very beginning, at the birth of the invention and at the end toward approval by regulatory authorities. For example, U Mass Medical School and several other academic medical centers conduct compassionate use clinical trials for the discoveries arising from their own biomedical research. The TTOs act as key liaisons to link these important connections between the academic/government, clinical, and the commercial world. In some cases, these inventions, protected through intellectual property (IP), are "transferred" to the company for product development via license agreements that give the company the rights to make the products or use these processes. In other cases, as a prelude to the license agreement or concomitant with it, a collaboration agreement or a sponsored research agreement (SRA) is negotiated by the TTO that allows a period wherein the research institution and company researchers jointly work on the invention prior to its complete transfer to the company. In exchange, financial consideration or other benefits are received by the research institution through what is often an agreement with a small company, which may bring in a large corporate partner during a later stage of development. This process has been likened to a relay race where there may be several baton transfers.

Since the 1980s, federal labs and universities have developed a strategic focus for their technology-transfer activities and they are particularly interested in working with bioentrepreneurs. This is because revenue enhancement from licensing is no longer the sole institutional goal. Instead, institutions find themselves also looking to increase company formation and new jobs based upon academic inventiveness, support faculty recruitment and retention, enhance research funding, create an entrepreneurial culture, attract venture investment to their regions, and the like. The economic development aspects of research are being recognized as a "fourth mission" for such institutions—going along with education, research, and public service. Bioentrepreneurs play a key role in this "fourth mission" by establishing companies driven by new research discoveries.

Accessing Academic Technologies and Collaborations

Generally, bioentrepreneurs can directly access research and inventions for product development from three main sources as shown in Table 15.1. For research funded by grants and contracts from NIH or other federal agencies (extramural research), the individual university or small business would control commercial rights, with only standard reporting and utilization obligations to the federal funding agency. Biomedical research conducted by the federal laboratory (intramural research program) is licensed directly through the TTO at the federal lab.

According to a 2016 annual survey from the Association of University Technology Managers (AUTM) [3], this incentivized approach, which dates from the Bayh–Dole Act, has contributed to the annual formation of more than two new products, and nearly three new companies each day through university technology transfer. Table 15.2 provides trends from the 2016 annual survey and underscores the volume of licensing activity that goes on in the United States from reporting universities and AMCs.

Each of these institutions has a robust research program "pipeline" that provides novel, fundamental research

TABLE 15.1 Federally funded technologies can be licensed from several sources.

- Federal lab research (from lab technology transfer office)
- University grantee research (from specific university technology transfer offices)
- SBIR and STTR small business programs (from small business awardees)

SBIR, Small Business Innovation Research; *STTR*, Small Business Technology Transfer Research.

TABLE 15.2 Volume of license activity at universities and academic medical organizations.

2017 AUTM survey figures	
Exclusive license agreements	2037
License option agreements	1566
Nonexclusive license agreements	4195
Active license agreements	45,657
New products launched	755
Licensing income	$3.14B

AUTM, Association of University Technology Managers.

discoveries available for commercial applications. NIH, for instance, as both a large-scale provider and consumer, represents a sort of "supermarket" of research products or tools for its commercial partners and suppliers. In addition, overall product sales of all types by NIH licensees now exceed $6 billion annually. As mentioned previously, most technology transfer activities at NIH and other federal laboratories date from the Federal Technology Transfer Act of 1986 which authorized formal research partnerships with industry and provided incentives to these programs to license technology by allowing the federal laboratory to, for the first time, keep its license royalties and share them between the individual inventors and their laboratories or institutes.

Research collaborations or research assistance with research institutions can take several forms as these researchers and clinicians can work with industry under different collaborative modalities. For example, research institutions may need to access technologies developed by industry—an imaging tool, a sequencing platform, or a drug discovered and in development by a company. The TTO then works with companies and clinical partners to memorialize the understanding between the scientists and/or clinicians to allow the collaborations to happen. Of course, as with all arrangements, each party desires to obtain terms that they feel are the most equitable for the party they represent. The key components of a collaboration agreement that are often the subject of most negotiations are terms related to inventions, rights to inventions, confidentiality versus publication, managing conflicts of interest, and, finally, indemnification. Indemnification (having one party to bear the monetary costs, either directly or by reimbursement, for losses incurred by a second party) is very important to research institutions when working with new biotech technologies that will be used in patient care.

Academic–Industry Collaborative Research Agreements

There are several types of research or collaboration-related agreements that biotech companies will commonly encounter in working with universities and federal laboratories:

Confidential Disclosure/Nondisclosure Agreements

Prior to engaging in any collaboration, each party may need to disclose to the other party some proprietary information that if passed on to third parties might be detrimental to the interest of the disclosing party. Such a discussion is a necessary first step to determine the interest in, and the breadth and scope of any potential collaboration. The parties will negotiate a confidential disclosure agreement (CDA)/nondisclosure agreement that ensures the information disclosed is held confidential, is only used for establishing the collaboration, stipulates a term of how long the information needs to be held confidential, and describes the consequences of nonadherence to the terms of the agreement.

Material Transfer Agreement, Sponsored Research Agreement, and Cooperative Research and Development Agreement

Companies, both small and large, have invested a lot of R&D dollars toward developing drugs or other biotech products. Research institutions have several programs that are geared toward understanding the fundamental biology underlying a wide variety of commercial products. When these two entities want to collaborate, they have very different things at stake. For the company, they are hoping to learn more about their product concept, get mechanistic insights they can exploit to position their product better in the marketplace, and have discoveries come out of this collaboration related to their product, which may extend the patent life of their eventual product. In the case of collaborations with AMCs, companies would like access to patient samples in addition to the valuable clinical insights they hope would guide them through the process of clinical validation of their product whether it be a drug, medical device, or diagnostic. For the academic and clinical investigator, they would like to test various drugs from various companies to build a scientific story or medical knowledge that they can publish. Even more importantly, with the dwindling of federal funds for academic research, their activities can be supported through cash from the company.

Material Transfer Agreements (MTAs) and Sponsored Research Agreements (SRAs) dictate the terms of transfer of material and money respectively, from company to the academic institution. Similarly, at federal labs, research projects for basic research or clinical studies are called cooperative research and development agreements (CRADAs). Due to their clinical hospitals and centers as well as other networks and facilities, the NIH and at least some universities can take some of their medical discoveries (or those of their partners) into clinical trials through clinical trial agreements (CTAs).

Key Elements of Collaborative Agreements

Provided in the following are key elements that are at the heart of the negotiation of these agreements:

1. ***Inventions***—The definition of "invention" is crucial. Academic centers will typically require that any inventions can be both conceived *and* reduced to

practice during the term of the collaborative research using the company material and/or money. Companies want it to be conceived "or" reduced to practice. The problem for the TTOs with agreeing to "or" is simply that academic researchers collaborate with lots of companies, often at the same time on similar broad programs but with different individualized projects. If institutions agree to the "or" language, it creates several issues: (1) it is nearly impossible for the TTOs to police when the conception of the invention happened and when it was reduced to practice and (2) the institution may end up with conflicting arrangements with companies. Federal laboratories (by statute) use the language "conceived or *actually* reduced to practiced" in their agreements. Practically speaking, TTOs may only hear of inventions when the researchers decide to disclose them as investigators at research institutions are not under as tight control as their counterparts in industry.

2. ***Ownership of inventions***—Companies may want academic researchers to assign their inventions to the companies. This is a hard one for academic TTOs to accept since in the instance of an MTA, there will likely be funding from the federal government, and under the terms of the grant, such assignments are prohibited without specific permission from the funding agency. Even under the terms of an SRA where the company is providing money in addition to providing the material, given the large amount of federal dollars that most academic institutions receive with the lab resources and several personnel being funded by the government, universities are unable to agree to the assignment of inventions to companies as it would again be in violation of the terms of the grant from the federal agency. Instead, typically the company will be granted the desired license options by the research institution to new discoveries during the collaborative or sponsored research program.
3. ***Rights to inventions***—Freedom to operate (FTO) rights are very important to a company. They have invested a lot of money into their drug discovery or device-development programs. Biotech companies do not want the academic research collaborator to make important inventions that are somehow related to their drug or device in development and then not have the needed rights to the inventions that they helped with their material and money to discover. There is often no right or wrong answer to this question and it can be subject to negotiation depending on what each party feels is equitable for the specific collaboration and can vary from a royalty-bearing to a nonexclusive royalty-free license or option to a license.
4. ***Confidentiality and publication***—An important aspect of the academic mission and spirit is to publish and disseminate the results of research widely to the public. This is typically at odds with the company's best interest which may need to keep things under cover until they are very sure and ready to disclose especially to their competitors. A typical compromise is for the publication/public disclosure to be provided to the company ahead of time and for the company to remove its confidential information while still providing for a meaningful publication in the journal of choice by the investigators. For example, if the journal required publication of the structure of the compound to make it meaningful, then if that were not already in the public domain through publication (journal or patent) of the company, then that constraint should be discussed at the time of the negotiation of the contract.

Technology Transfer Office Set-Up and Licensing from Universities and Federal Laboratories

Technology Transfer Office Operations

Fig. 15.1 provides an overview of the core operational elements and activities of TTOs at research institutions. There are several key areas of importance to the industry. In addition, several TTOs house an internal venture group or work with some outside venture funds for commercialization of their technologies in the form of a new company/start-up. The internal funds often serve several functions including educating the investigator/inventor as they work with outside venture capital (VC), bringing together several outside ventures, given their connections and expertise and work with the licensing staff within the TTO to help get the start-up off the ground.

Inventions and Intellectual Property Strategy

Inventions made by the research center's investigators are the currency that drives the licensing operations of a TTO. As summarized later in Fig. 15.2, the TTO personnel has the huge responsibility of reaching out to their research community to educate them about the process, evaluate and access patentability of inventions, devise simple to complex IP strategies for the inventions, and finally to work with attorneys to protect these inventions.

Disclosure of Inventions

When research findings are disclosed to the TTO, it typically goes through a triage process that involves accessing/scoring its scientific strength, its patentability in light of prior art, including the investigators' own prior public disclosures, its market potential, and commercial path. The TTO will also look for the investigators' availability

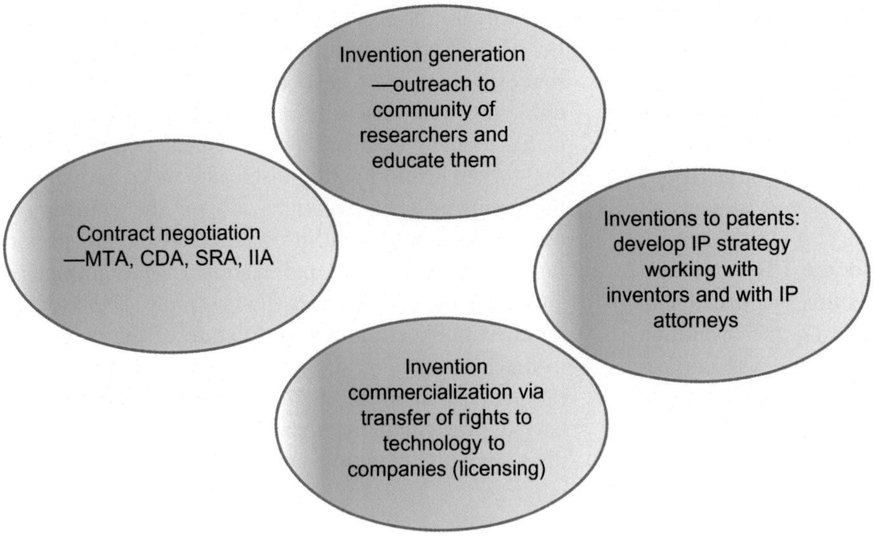

FIGURE 15.1 Core elements of a tech transfer office.

of resources including funding as well as their commitment to work with the TTO to move the invention through the next steps of validation that would add to its commercial value.

Some key challenges that TTOs face are (1) lack of control of the overall disclosure process since disclosure of inventions is purely voluntary—furthermore, investigators differ widely in what they would consider to be valuable inventions; (2) investigators do not sign documents assigning their inventions to their employer at the time of employment, rather they are obligated to do so under the institution's IP policies; and (3) investigators vary widely in their aptitude to work with the TTO to commercialize their inventions and get it into the marketplace. At UMMS, innovative initiatives are underway to address these challenges. The goal is to increase collaboration with investigators, throughput in processing disclosures, and the workflow overall.

Marketing of Inventions and Business Strategies

For companies looking to work with a TTO, there are both push (when the TTO reaches out to companies to license/partner the technologies) and pull (when companies contact the TTOs) marketing. Companies contact TTOs typically following a public presentation—a publication that's either in a journal or a patent. For companies seeking a license from a TTO the following outlines a good approach: (1) identify the university's technology that is of interest; (2) provide a path for diligent development of technology, if licensed, along with an estimated timeline; and (3) indicate if the technology will add to, replace an existing product, or be a new line of products for the company. Having this basic information available will accelerate the time to a term sheet and eventually a completed license.

Licensing Technologies—Working with the Technology Transfer Offices

From Universities and Academic Medical Centers

Once the academic and company feel there is a path forward to bring the technology into the company, then it proceeds to a license. Oftentimes, the company is not sure and needs to bring the technology in under an evaluation license to ensure that the technology works before they can commit to a license. This is accomplished via an option agreement that would (1) obligate the academic to hold the rights to the technology for a certain period of time within which it will execute a license to the company and (2) grant the company rights to test/evaluate the technology. These agreements are accompanied by nominal fee arrangements, oftentimes to cover patent costs previously incurred and/or that would be incurred during the option period. Once the parties are engaged in negotiations, it is typical to start with a term sheet. It is good to get all the deal breakers addressed in the term sheet and get a verbal understanding of the key terms before committing to paper. For universities and AMCs, a typical concern is companies not committing to diligent development of technologies they license. This would be an issue that is best addressed early on in the negotiation. A combination of an exchange of a written draft agreement and periodic verbal communication will ensure that things are proceeding on track.

Time periods to complete these transactions can vary widely. Option agreements typically take a few days to a month. Agreements for nonexclusive license to technologies take on average about 2–6 months to finalize.

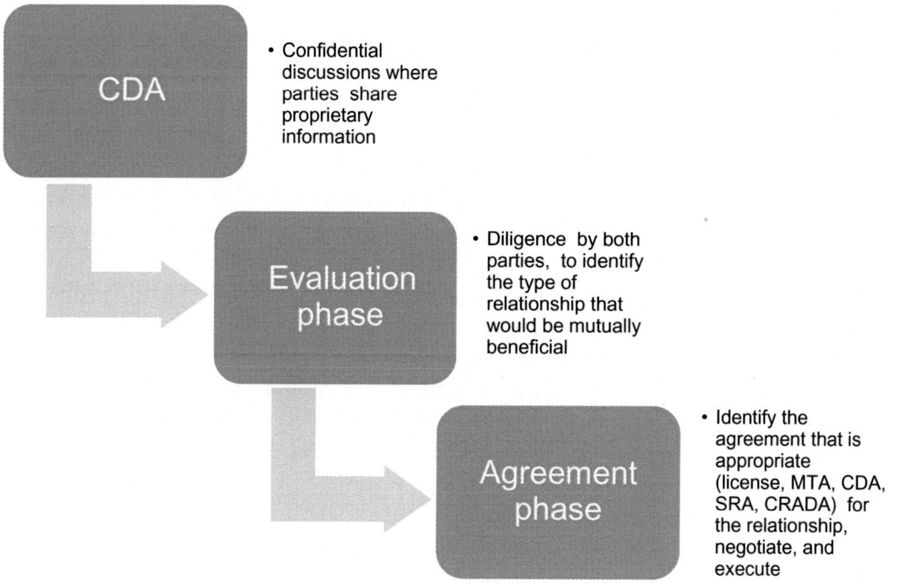

FIGURE 15.2 Fundamental steps leading to agreements with research institutions.

For exclusive license agreements the period varies quite widely. If there are two committed parties that want to get a deal done, it can be as quick as 3–4 months. An average deal would probably take 6–9 months to complete. In all instances of licenses, TTOs always prefer to start from their template. Given that companies' license agreements are designed for company-to-company transactions, it is very cumbersome and time-consuming for the academic licensing professional to adapt the company template to fit the academic's needs. If the institution has previously licensed the technology either nonexclusively or exclusively in another field, there would be a constraint to using terms they have agreed to with the other parties on the same technology. Moreover, if that company and the academic have a prior license agreement, the quickest way to a deal would be to start with that as a template for at least the nontechnology-specific terms.

From the National Institutes of Health

As is the case with universities, the NIH is not able to commercialize its discoveries even with its considerable size and resources—it relies instead upon partners. Commercializing technologies, such as vaccines or drugs and then marketing them successfully in a worldwide market, thus cannot be the responsibility or mission of research institutions or government agencies. Companies with access to the needed expertise and money are needed to undertake continued development of these inventions from the NIH or other research institutions into final products. Typically, a royalty-bearing exclusive license agreement with the right to sublicense is given to a company from NIH (if NIH-owned) or the university (if university-owned) to use patents, materials, or other assets to bring a therapeutic or vaccine product concept to the market. Exclusivity is almost always the norm for the US Food and Drug Administration (FDA)-regulated products due to the risk involved in time, money, and regulatory pathways to companies and their investors. Financial terms of the license agreement are negotiable but do reflect the nascent, high-risk nature of the discovery. Because the technologies coming from NIH or NIH-funded research are most typically preclinical inventions, most licensees are early-stage companies or start-ups rather than larger firms that typically want more proven ideas for new products. In addition to the license agreement, there will often be research collaborations between the licensee and the NIH or university to assist with additional work needed on the product technology. When the licensee can sufficiently "de-risk" the technology through its various efforts, these companies then sublicense, partner, or get acquired by larger biotech or pharmaceutical firms for the final, most expensive stages of development with the large company expected to sell the product once it reaches the market.

Since the 1980s, federally funded health research institutions, such as the NIH and AMCs, have developed an active but increasingly strategic focus on improving public health through technology-transfer activities. As such, they are particularly interested in working with start-ups and other early-stage companies in the health-care area which are looking to develop and deliver innovative products. Rather than just seeking a financial return through revenue generation, these institutions are looking to utilize licensing of nascent inventions to increase new company formation, support faculty recruitment and retention, enhance research funding, and create in general a more entrepreneurial culture within the organization, attracting venture investment and development to their specific region (universities) or to the health sector in general (NIH).

Start-Ups and Other Licensing Vehicles for Technology Transfer

The licensing practices for most nonprofit research institutions including federal institutions and universities have changed significantly over recent years with respect to biomedical inventions [4]. With its ever-increasing consolidation, large pharmaceutical firms are typically no longer looking to directly license early-stage technologies for commercialization, whereas the number of licenses signed with start-ups as well as small-to-medium-sized biotechnology companies is on the rise. Indeed, typically around 70% of the total license executed by universities and AMCs are to start-ups and small biotech firms. Unlike 15–20 years ago, when all or most of the high-revenue medical products based on licenses from university or federal laboratory research came from direct agreements with large pharmaceutical firms, most of the latest success stories tend to be from those originally partnered with biotech or other smaller companies at the time of the original license agreement. Some examples from the NIH licensing program are Kepivance (a human growth factor used to treat oral sores arising from chemotherapy licensed to Amgen), Velcade (a small molecule proteasome inhibitor used to treat multiple myeloma from Millennium), Synagis (a recombinant monoclonal antibody for preventing serious lung disease caused by respiratory syncytial virus in premature infants from MedImmune), Prezista (an HIV protease inhibitor used to treat drug-resistant AIDS patients from Tibotec), and Taxus Express (a paclitaxel drug-eluting coronary stent used to prevent restenosis from Angiotech). Although these firms or their successors are all substantive, well-known companies now, at the time the underlying technology was licensed to them, they were not large corporations. The UMMS is unique in its structure in that it includes not only the medical school and the powerful biomedical research powerhouse but also Mass Biologics, the world's only Good Manufacturing Practices (GMP) biologics manufacturing facility operated by a nonprofit, and Commonwealth of Medicine, a unique health-care consulting operation. Further, UMMS has 40 + cores and a voucher program that allows start-ups to use these facilities at a steep discount. Companies with 1–10 employees get a 75% discount and companies with 10–50 employees get a 50% discount.

Many products developed at UMMS are already creating impact. Rabishield (Rabies vaccine, approved for sale in India) and Zinplava (*Clostridium difficile* infections, Ph 2) are monoclonal antibodies developed at Massbiologics and licensed to Serum Institute of India and Merck, respectively. Spinraza that treats spinal muscular atrophy was discovered at UMMS. It was partnered with Biogen that launched the product in 2017. Other recent products impacting patients include gene therapy technology to treat Canavan's disease—one patient was successfully treated. Technology was basis of the UMMS start-up Aspa Therapeutics (2018). Also, Onpattro—the first siRNA therapeutic launched by Alnylam in 2018—includes vital technology from UMMS.

Many models of licensing are used with a goal to get technology in the hands of commercial entities so there can be an impact on patients. In certain instances, licensing offices prefer licenses to a start-up company because unlike big companies, start-ups are motivated to rigorously work on their founding technology to raise funds from VC and are unlikely to "shelve" technology. Most of the time, this option is viewed more favorably to licensing the technology to a very large company where several similar technologies would typically be developed concomitantly. The risk is that the university or federal research institution's technology may get scuttled due to business factors or viewed as being of a high-risk nature. The biggest challenge of licensing the technology to a start-up company, however, is "cash uncertainty," that is, whether the start-up company will be able to secure future capital to develop the technology in a timely fashion. It is, therefore, important that bioentrepreneurs do the right thing in the right way at the right time to keep a strong relationship with the federal lab or university/AMC and its venture fund group as described in later sections of this chapter. One vehicle for bioentrepreneurs to engage with universities/AMCs is to work with them as an entrepreneur-in-residence that allows them to do prediligence on the technology working closing with the academic innovators and bringing in a business perspective that kick-starts the eventual start-up.

Basic Licensing Principles of University and Federal Laboratories

Compared to biomedical licensing from corporations, the federal laboratories and universities bring a different focus and perspective to the table when negotiating its technology transfer agreements. Because these agreements are used to further overall institutional missions, representatives from such nonprofit institutions consider the public consequences of such licenses as their first priority, not the financial terms that may be involved.

For example, federally funded nonprofit institutions, compared with their peers in the industry, have the mandate to make new technology as broadly available as possible. This means that there is a strong preference to limit the scope of a license to only what is needed to develop specific products. Exclusive licenses are quite typical for biomedical products, such as vaccines, therapeutics, and others, where the underlying technologies require substantial private risk and investment (and a prior public notice and comment period in the *Federal Register* in the case of federal laboratories). In their agreements, federal laboratories and universities would also typically expect to retain the right to permit further research use of the technology whether to be conducted either in the intramural program, universities, or companies. Because the commercial rights granted represent institutional (and often public) assets, these agreements have enforceable performance benchmarks to ensure that the public will eventually receive the benefit (through commercialized products) of the research it funded. Regulations governing the license negotiation of federally owned technologies and their mandated requirements are described in more detail at 37 Code of Federal Regulations (CFR), Part 404, while those for federally funded technologies can be found at 37 CFR Part 401.

Fig. 15.2 illustrates the fundamental steps that lead up to a license or other types of agreements with research institutions. In a license agreement the academic entity essentially grants rights to a company to make, use, and sell products that were it not for the license would infringe on the patent rights that the academic center owns and/or controls. In some instances the academic center also grants the company rights to use technological information/know-how or materials that go together with the information in the patent application and that is valuable to the company as it hopes to commercialize the technology into products. Licensing is at the heart of operations of a university TTO and is the core of its set-up, post-Bayh–Dole. However, both academic centers and federal labs function as nonprofits and do not and cannot have a product commercialization arm and so cannot themselves convert inventions into commercial products and processes. They must partner with industry to do that. Hence these out-licensing activities are the key to fulfilling the core of Bayh–Dole and other federal mandates of commercializing inventions that arise from federal funding.

Characteristics of Typical Biotech License Agreements

Generally, it is considered good business practice in licensing from a research institution that the organization would standardize license terms to the extent possible. Standardizing nonfinancial license terms levels, the playing field for licensees (an important concept for public institutions), and creates a common understanding of the balance of risks acceptable to a research institution (which may differ markedly from the for-profit sector).

Royalty rate negotiations with these institutions are influenced by factors (Table 15.3) commonly encountered in other negotiations of early-stage biomedical technologies. Unique to federal laboratory and university negotiations are factors relating to the public health interest in the technology being licensed and the products to be developed from it (so-called white knight clauses). Examples of this may include supply back of materials for clinical use, indigent patient access programs in the United States, commercial benefit sharing for natural product source countries, or incentives for developing world access to the licensed products.

The royalty payments (Table 15.4) consist of license payments received for execution royalties, minimum annual royalties (MARs) (received regardless of the amount of product sales), earned royalties (a percentage of product sales), benchmark royalties, and payments for patent costs. To date the NIH has not sought equity payments in licenses or directly participated in company start-ups due to conflict of interest concerns. Instead, in lieu of equity, the NIH can consider equity-like benchmark royalties that track successful commercial events at the company. However, many universities do take equity payments in their license agreements to assist a

TABLE 15.3 Factors influencing royalty rate negotiations with research institutions.

- Stage of development
- Type of product
- Market readiness and value of product
- Uniqueness of biological materials
- Scope of patent coverage
- Research institution "Content"
- Public health significance

TABLE 15.4 Typical types of fees and royalties in licenses agreements with research institutions.

- Execution fees
- Minimum annual royalty (regardless of the amount of net sales)
- Earned royalties (fixed percentage of net sales)
- Benchmark royalties
- Patent costs
- Sublicense fees (percentage of income)
- Equity (varies by institution)

new start-up company even though there is considerable risk in accepting equity in lieu of cash payments since such equity is illiquid and has no present value at the time license is executed.

Licensing institutions will often opt to take an equity or equity-like position when available from their licensees for several reasons. For example, equity would provide for additional revenue in addition to the licensing royalties, especially if the licensed product failed in development but the company itself later became successful. Equity also can be seen as a risk premium for the research institution that provides additional inducement to grant the license to a new start-up company verses a more-established firm. Importantly, and perhaps most important for bioentrepreneurs, equity allows a licensee who is cash poor but equity rich to substitute an ownership position for a cash payment (in full or in part) for an up-front licensing fee and/or a reduced royalty rate. Finally, research institutions accept this risk to support its mission to assist in commercialization of early-stage technologies, which may not be turned into marketable products otherwise and to encourage small business development. However, universities and AMCs recognize that holding ownership rights in a start-up company creates a potential conflict of interest and adopts various internal policies that mitigate and/or manage such conflicts.

Unlike their corporate counterparts, inventors at nonprofit research institutions do receive a share of the royalties generated from the licensing of their inventions. However, each institution might have a slightly different revenue-sharing policy with respect to the percent of licensing revenues that are shared with inventors. Next, we discuss what might be some of the typical license agreements that a bioentrepreneur would come across in dealing with a nonprofit research institution.

Types of License Agreements

Universities and federal research institutions negotiate a variety of different types of license agreements for use and development of biomedical technologies. Besides offering exclusive and nonexclusive commercialization agreements for patented technologies, commercialization agreements are negotiated for unpatented biological materials. Being increasingly more selective as to what type of technologies they seek to patent, both types of institutions are unlikely to patent research materials or research methodologies that can be easily transferred for commercial use by biological material license agreements or publication. For patent rights or materials that are not to be sold as commercial products but are useful in internal R&D programs, both federal research institutions and universities would typically negotiate nonexclusive internal use license agreements. In addition, companies may obtain evaluation agreements to new technologies as well as specialized agreements relating to interference or other patent dispute settlements. Finally, for bioentrepreneurs interested in a technology that was jointly invented by two or more institutions, an interinstitutional patent/licensing management agreement would be negotiated so that the bioentrepreneur would be able to obtain an exclusive license by only dealing with one party.

TABLE 15.5 Major types of licenses agreements involving research institutions.

- Commercial evaluation/Option license agreement
- Internal commercial use license agreement
- Research products commercialization license agreement
- Vaccine, diagnostic, therapeutic, or medical device product commercialization license agreement. Increasingly, there are evolving models of agreements for access to data and health apps developed by universities and academic medical centers.
- Interinstitutional agreements (for joint inventions)

Typically, federal research institutions and many universities have the types of license agreements shown in Table 15.5 and described in the following [5]:

1. ***Commercial evaluation/option license agreements*** are short-term nonexclusive license agreements to allow a licensee to conduct feasibility testing but not the sale of products developed from a technology. These typically run no longer than a few months, have a modest cost associated with them, and include relevant materials that are supplied by inventor(s). Screening use is not permitted but the agreement has proven to be ideal for feasibility testing of new technologies that have a wide variety of possible useful (but unproven) applications. "Screening use" implies use of the licensed material in the discovery or development of a different final end product. For example, a reporter cell that expresses an oncogene can be tested to screen drug candidates that could potentially be effective in certain cancer therapeutics. Some universities may also use this type of agreement in the form of a short-term exclusive option agreement for a nascent technology with the hope that a long-term diagnostic, vaccine, or therapeutic product commercialization license agreement will later be completed.
2. ***Internal commercial-use license agreements*** are another nonexclusive license arrangement that allows a licensee to use (but not sell) technology in its internal programs. Here materials (either patented or unpatented) are provided, and screening uses are permitted. The financial structure of this agreement can be either

a "paid-up" term license or annual royalty payments each, however, without any "reach-through" royalty obligations to other products being used or discovered by the licensee. A "paid-up term" license would be a license in which the company makes a one-time lump sum payment to obtain the rights to use the licensed technology for the duration of the license. On the other hand, "reach through" royalty provisions in a license agreement create royalties to the licensor on the future sales of downstream products that are discovered or developed using the licensed technology, even though the final end product may not contain the licensed technology. In other words, reach-through royalties are royalties that are due to a licensor even though manufacture, use, or the sale of the final product does not infringe any patents claiming the licensed technology. Internal commercial-use agreements themselves historically have been very popular with medium-to-larger biomedical firms who are eager to acquire reagents to speed their internal development programs. Popular technologies licensed in this manner include animal models and receptors.

3. ***Research products commercialization license agreements*** are another nonexclusive license agreement but allow a licensee to sell products to the research products market. Here materials (either patented or unpatented) are also generally provided with smaller firms predominating as licensees. For federal laboratories, US manufacturing is required even for nonexclusive product sales in the United States unless a waiver is granted. Waivers are granted based on a lack of manufacturing capacity in the United States or economic hardship for the licensee. The financial structure of these licenses generally involves low up-front royalties but relatively high earned-royalty payments since the materials provided are frequently close or very close to the finished product that is to be sold. Popular research products licensed in this manner include a wide variety of monoclonal or polyclonal antibodies or other research materials used in basic research.
4. ***Vaccine, diagnostic, therapeutic, or medical device product commercialization license agreements*** are agreements that can be exclusive if such is necessary for product development due to the capital and risk involved for the licensee. Important for bioentrepreneurs is the fact that by law, small, capable biomedical firms receive preference from federal laboratories and federally funded universities as exclusive licensees. At NIH and other federal laboratories, all prospective grants of exclusive licenses (identifying the licensee and technology by name) are published in the *Federal Register* for public comment or objections for a minimum period of 15 days. A detailed development plan with product benchmarks or milestones is expected for licenses in this area. Collaborative research with federal laboratories regarding further preclinical or clinical development of the technology is encouraged but not required to obtain a license and is negotiated separately by the individual laboratory program. These agreements also have a requirement for US manufacturing for US product sales unless a waiver is granted. The federal laboratory can typically grant waivers only when US manufacturing sites are unavailable or manufacturing in the United States is economically infeasible. The financial structure of these licenses can involve substantial up-front royalties, but much more moderate-earned royalties (since the technology is typically not close to a finished product) and appropriate benchmark payments. Other provisions to be negotiated include a share amount of sublicensing proceeds, any of the public health "white knight" provisions described earlier, as well as licensee performance monitoring and audit requirements.
5. ***Interinstitutional agreements (IIAs) or joint invention agreements (JIAs).*** Many commercializable technologies will often have inventors from more than one university or federal laboratory due to the collaborative nature of science. The institutes will often execute an IIA or JIA so one entity takes the lead in working with the external partner. This mitigates risk for investors, since, especially for US patent rights, all owners have the ability to license separately. In addition to mitigating risk, IIAs or JIAs help bioentrepreneurs since they would have to negotiate with only one research institution to secure an exclusive license to the technology.
6. ***License agreements with non-US firms*** are an increasingly common occurrence from NIH and universities due to the global nature of healthcare markets and the growing biotechnology sector in a number of areas of the world. While for US federally funded inventions there is a preference for US firms, this would typically be applied only in instances of exclusive license agreements—meaning that nonexclusive agreements such as those for research materials and tools would be available to all firms. In addition, some medical technologies only have patient populations and markets outside the United States, so license agreements for these types of inventions are often most appropriate for non-US firms. This is because the US manufacturing requirement required (unless a waiver is granted) in federally funded technologies applies to only products to be sold in the United States. Products to be sold outside the United States can be thus manufactured anywhere. Special circumstances can allow for a waiver of the US

manufacturing requirement, such as documented lack of manufacturing capacity for the product within the United States or the risk of an economic hardship for a licensee of replicating an existing FDA-approved manufacturing facility outside the United States within the United States solely to make the new product in question.

Universities and AMCs have had to adapt to increasingly global nature of the biotech world. Many international companies and investors, particularly from China, are interested in working with US universities and AMCs.

Components of a Biotechnology License Agreement

1. ***Breadth of rights***—This depends on the technology that is being licensed and the size and need of the company. If the patent rights/technology is specific to a certain company's drug, for example, something that arose from a SRA (described earlier in this chapter), then it would be typical to give the company exclusive license rights to all fields available within the patent rights. For platform technologies that have broad uses in very different medical applications—for example, micro-fluidic IP—field specific but still exclusive licenses would be appropriate.
   a. For diagnostic technologies, the trend is to grant nonexclusive rights to the technology, but with an eye toward incentivizing the companies to invest into developing the technology. For research-tool technologies, it is typical to grant nonexclusive access to use the technologies in their internal research, for example, in their drug discovery, programs.
   b. There is another dimension to consider in addition in the case of start-ups—for the fledgling company to attract investment, a broader field of use is appropriate. But if it is a small company, a recent start-up from another university perhaps and a second university's technology is offering a solution to a specific problem, then only narrow rights to the company from the second university would be appropriate.
2. ***Signing fees and patent costs***—Having invested in the technology through IP protection, the academic institution would typically reimburse themselves for the patent costs incurred to date. A license is their exit, and the minimum terms of this exit is to recoup patent costs, and further, a modest signing fee is appropriate at the time of signing of a license.
3. ***Sublicense fees***—The statistics are that most technologies are not developed by the first licensee of the technology but by the company's further licensee (the "sublicensee"). Typically, this sublicense happens when the original company licensee has developed and validated the technology further. Depending on the situation, a fixed percentage or a sliding scale of percentage sublicense income back to the original licensor is considered equitable.
4. ***MARs/Milestone fees***—A certain percentage of royalty on net sales of the product comes back to the licensor (academic institution). To ensure diligent development, having a set annual payment is customary. Sometimes this is termed "annual maintenance fee" that is credited against royalty upon product launch. The diligent development of the product, covered next, is a key element to the contract. Payments to the academic institution upon reaching key milestones in the path to the product are customary.
5. ***Diligent development of the licensed technology***—For technologies that are funded in whole or in part with federal funding, this is an absolute requirement. Companies are required to give the TTOs their product development plan along with the expected timelines. The consequence of not meeting these diligence goals is termination. A key item to remember is that research institutions have the flexibility to work with licensees and can accommodate changing needs. The key is to have a mechanism of communication and cooperation between both parties. If the company is really "shelving" the technology, the university or federal lab needs to be able to get it back to seek and find another licensing partner to commercialize these technologies.
6. ***Reserved rights***—As per Bayh–Dole for government-funded technologies, academic centers are required to reserve rights for their continued use of the technology for further academic research. Typically, the academic center reserves rights not only for its own use but also for the research use of other academic centers. For hospitals, this would include clinical research use as well, since patient care is part of the institutional mission. The reason for this clause is for licensees not to block anyone from continuing research on the technology that could benefit the public given that it was funded by the tax dollars from the public in the first place. For government labs, the reserved right is for any governmental purpose and is required by statue.
7. ***Enforcement***—Patent rights are enforced by the owner or in cooperation from the owner. An "infringer" of the technology is hurting the market share of our licensee. As the patent owner, universities and federal labs are affected since the patent licensees are affected. Typically, exclusive licensees seek to get first rights to go after infringers but the actions by licensees might drag the TTOs into lawsuits and potential invalidation of the patent claims. Academic

centers do not have the appetite (or the money) for lawsuits. A common approach is, therefore, to have the first right to pursue infringers when informed by our companies to encourage them to take a license from our licensees. Failing this, it is typical to have licensees pursue infringers.

8. ***Indemnification and insurance***—AMCs have to protect themselves from lawsuits that may arise from patients who may be injured by the products that companies make, market, and sell. When sponsored research is performed and broad access is given to all results that arise from the collaborations, judicious use of the results in the drug-development process is the company's responsibility and the terms of the agreement in this section are designed to protect the TTOs. Thus, in their agreements, companies are required to provide evidence that they have the necessary backing via insurance protection. This is a requirement from institutional insurance carriers and therefore this term is typically nonnegotiable from the TTO's side.
9. ***Conflicts of interest***—This is a very significant and real issue particularly for teaching hospitals, AMCs, and federal laboratories that are doing both clinical and basic research. Conflicts are managed by ensuring that at the time of the licensing of inventions to a company related to a certain drug, the medical center does not have any sponsored research collaboration on the same drug with the same investigator whose invention(s)/technology was licensed. Moreover, the investigator cannot consult for the company whose drugs are in clinical trials under his or her guidance. Additional conflict of interest rules apply to federal scientists. The conflict of interest policies of research institutions are typically available on their public websites.

Financial terms for nonexclusive license grants including license grants to research-tool technologies can vary widely. These licenses would not have all the elaborate terms described earlier but rather would have a fixed annual fee-type structure or even have a one-time "fully paid-up" financial structure. Table 15.6 gives some ranges of financial terms for exclusive licenses. Note that while these terms are typical ranges, when an AMC has a clinical candidate that is being licensed, as in the case of gene therapy with Adeno-associated virus (AAV) vectors being the clinical candidates, the up-fronts can be in the millions.

Advantages for a Biotech Start-Up to Work with the National Institutes of Health and Universities

Why Start-Ups Should Work with National Institutes of Health and Universities

National Institutes of Health's New Low-Cost Start-Up License Agreements

To better facilitate this "fourth mission" of economic development in conjunction with increased development of new therapeutic products, the NIH has developed a new short-term Start-Up Exclusive Evaluation License Agreement (Start-up EELA) and a Start-Up Exclusive Commercial License Agreement (Start-up ECLA) to facilitate licensing of intramural NIH and FDA inventions to early-stage companies. Similar "express" or "start-up" agreements are available at many universities as well. The NIH start-up licenses are generally provided to assist those companies that are less than 5 years old, have less than $5 million in capital raised, and have fewer than 50 employees, which can obtain an exclusive license from the NIH for a biomedical invention of interest arising from the NIH. NIH start-up licenses are offered to those companies developing drugs, vaccines, therapeutics, and certain devices from NIH patented or patent-pending technologies that NIH determines will require significant investment to develop, such as those undergoing clinical

TABLE 15.6 Common ranges of financial terms for exclusive license agreements.

Term	Diagnostic	Therapeutic
License signing fee[a]	$25–$50k	$50–$200k
Sublicense fees[b]	10%–40%	10%–40%
Annual fees or annual minimum royalties	$10–$50k	$10–$100k
Earned royalties[c] (percentage of net sales)	2–15	2–6
Total milestone payments	$1–$3m	$1–$7m

[a]*Start-up or express agreements may have substantial milestone, liquidity, or equity payments in lieu of early fees.*
[b]*Higher percentage in payments maybe appropriate if the company intends to monetize the technology through further licensing rather than through product development.*
[c]*Stacking of royalties to allow company to further in-license other technologies for the development of product is typical. With stacking/offsets the lower end of the range may be applicable.*

trials to achieve FDA approval or Class III diagnostics. The new company must license at least one NIH-owned US patent and commit to developing a product or service for the US market. The licensee may also obtain in the license related NIH-owned patents filed in other countries if the company agrees to commercialize products in those countries as well.

Financial terms for the start-up licenses are designed with the fiscal realities of small firms in mind and feature either a 1-year exclusive evaluation license with a flat $2000 execution fee (this license can be later transitioned to become an exclusive commercialization license) or an immediate exclusive commercialization license. The Start-Up Exclusive Commercial License includes the following:

- A delayed tiered up-front execution royalty, which would be due to the NIH upon a liquidity event such as an initial public offering (IPO), a merger, a sublicense, an assignment, acquisition by another firm, or a first commercial sale.
- A delayed MAR or a MAR that is waived if there is a CRADA with the NIH (or FDA) concerning the development of the licensed technology and providing value comparable to the MAR. In addition, the MAR will be waived for up to 5 years during the term of a Small Business Innovation Research (SBIR) or Small Business Technology Transfer Research (STTR) grant for the development of the licensed technology.
- An initial lower reimbursement rate of patent expenses that increases over time to full reimbursement of expenses tied to the earliest of a liquidity event, an IPO, the grant of a sublicense, a first commercial sale, or upon the third anniversary of the effective date of the agreement.
- Consideration by the NIH of all requests from a start-up company to file new or continuing patent applications if the company is actively and timely reimbursing patent-prosecution expenses.
- A set earned royalty rate of 1.5% on the sale of licensed products.
- A set sublicensing royalty rate of 15% of the other consideration received from the grant of a sublicense.
- An antistacking royalty payment license provision can be negotiated by a company if it encounters a stacking royalty problem. A stacking royalty problem could potentially occur when a licensee's third-party royalty obligations add up to such a high total royalty percentage such that the project becomes unattractive for investment, sublicensing, or self-development due to low profit margins. Royalty stacking can especially be a problem in the development of biologics due to the breadth of a possible third-party IP that may be needed compared with traditional small molecule drugs.
- Mutually agreed-upon specific benchmarks and performance milestones that do not require a royalty payment but rather ensure that the start-up licensee is taking concrete steps toward a practical application of the licensed product or process.
- NIH start-up commercial licenses represent a significant front-end savings in negotiation time and money for new companies. An exclusive license, for a new technology (even early-stage), might have expectations prior to negotiations (for a large-market indication) of an immediate execution fee of up to $250,000 or more, a MAR due in the first year and beyond of up to $25,000 or more, immediate payment of all past patent expenses and ongoing payments of future patent expenses, benchmark royalties in the range of up to $1 million or more, significant sublicensing consideration, and earned royalties in the range up to 5% or more depending on the technology.

Because many, if not most of the technologies developed at the NIH, are early-stage biomedical technologies, the time and development risks to develop a commercial product are high. Depending on the technology and the stage of formation of the potential licensee, the company may prefer to enter into the Start-up EELA to evaluate their interest before committing to a longer-term Start-up ECLA. Bioentrepreneurs can identify technologies of interest by searching licensing opportunities on the NIH Office of Technology Transfer (OTT) website [5], by email notification via Real Simple Syndication (RSS) feed and by getting in touch with the listed licensing contact. Usage of the start-up agreements varies by institute TTOs at NIH, including a new "Start-Up 2.0" Agreement version at the National Cancer Institute (NCI). Details for the start-up licenses and other information on the licensing process are published on the OTT "Start-up Webpage" and the NCI "Start-up 2.0 Webpage" [6].

Unique Features of Biotech Start-Up Licenses

While start-ups can be seen to have the potential to produce significant opportunities for the inventors, investors, the research institution, and regional economies, such projects involve more work and are riskier than a traditional license to an existing, capitalized company. Although research conducted at federal laboratories and universities is not specifically designed to lead to a new company formation, such activities are a way for such institutions to support the economic development aspects of their licensing- and technology-transfer programs as previously described. Successful start-up companies and bioentrepreneurs are highly prized because of the direct benefits to the community, region, state, and country in terms of new employment and tax revenue. Because of this, some research institutions have in-house business development professional dedicated to working with inventors as they consider start-up opportunities for their technology. However, many institutions handle this as part of the activities of the regular TTO staff. Several institutions have in-house incubators and bridge funds due to the "valley of death" in funding for academic technologies.

A typical practice for a research institution that is licensing to a start-up company is to first confirm that there is no other prior claim of rights from a commercial sponsor and to then execute a confidentiality agreement, a letter of intent or other indication of interest, which should be followed quickly thereafter with an option agreement to a future exclusive license. If the bioentrepreneur has substantial resources already in place it may be possible to grant the license directly in place of an option when it is merited. Whatever the nature of the agreement, it is generally expected that the negotiation be with an officer of the new venture (or their attorney) and not a university faculty member who may hope to be involved in the company. Agreements should also contain clear timelines to enforce the diligent development of the technology toward commercialization. Particularly critical are deadlines for raising predetermined levels of initial funding to establish and operate the venture. To avoid conflict of interest problems at the research institution, the new company should operate separately from the inventor's lab, with a local incubator or business park space being ideal. Most research institutions have policies around faculty inventors not holding fiduciary responsibility at the companies they help start. Generally, a federal laboratory inventor is not able to have an active role in the company without leaving federal employment. The share of equity held by a university in these circumstances can vary by the type of technology.

The actual share amount held by the research institution, or the equivalent value to be paid to it, is often not that critical as the overall goal for the university or federal laboratory to develop a robust local, regional, or national corporate research community that closely complements and interacts with ongoing research at the institution. It is also a way to support university or former federal faculty members who are themselves entrepreneurial and willing to commit their time and often their own money to bringing their inventions to the marketplace.

Advantages to Working with Universities and Federal Laboratories

Within these basic licensing structures, however, there are several advantages that bioentrepreneurs can utilize in their product development efforts since federal laboratories and universities offer favorable treatment to small businesses to create an attractive playing field for them to get into new areas of product development. For example, start-ups can utilize the expertise of the patent law firm hired by the institution to manage the patent prosecution of the licensed technology. This is particularly useful for small firms that may not yet have internal patent counsel or the resources to retain a top IP law firm.

Another useful example is that license agreements with federal laboratories and universities (in contrast with corporate license agreements) do not require bioentrepreneurs to cross-license existing rights they may own, give up any product marketing rights, nor forsake any downstream developmental rights. Also, research-tool licenses negotiated through the NIH and many universities carry no grant-backs or reach-through rights. For instance, when a research-tool technology is licensed to a company by the NIH, the licensee is not required to grant back any usage rights to the improvements that it may develop after the license agreement. Also, the licensee is not required to share with the NIH any future profits that may be made because of improvements to the original discovery. In other words, IP derived from new discoveries made with NIH-licensed tools will remain clear and unencumbered.

Another advantage for a bioentrepreneur to license a technology from a nonprofit institution is the flexibility in the financial terms. While the NIH and many research institutions have "Start-up" or "Express" template agreements with favorable terms already in place, these can typically be negotiated separately. For example, reimbursement of back patent expenses, which the licensee typically pays upon the signing of the license agreement, could be deferred for a certain period. Similarly, the license deal could be structured to be heavily back-end loaded and/or equity-based to allow the bioentrepreneur to apply its cash toward R&D. Unlike many research institutions that take equity in lieu of cash, federal institutions and some universities do not consider equity-based license deals but do take roughly equivalent equity-like benchmark payments. The resulting lack of equity dilution may become an important feature as the bioentrepreneur looks to raise capital through additional rounds of financing.

A bioentrepreneur could also take advantage of the capabilities and technical expertise residing in the licensor's laboratories by collaboration and/or sponsorship of the research needed to expedite the development of the technology. While sponsoring research at the inventor's laboratory may in some circumstances raise conflict of interest issues, many institutions are willing to put together a conflict management plan with the engaged parties in order to help the start-up to exploit all the resources offered by the licensor. Many research institutions would, however, execute an agreement separate from a license agreement to formalize, such an arrangement.

At a basic level, the success of a new biotechnology venture depends on six key ingredients: (1) technical expertise, (2) IP assets, (3) business expertise, (4) physical space, (5) human capital, and (6) money [7]. Institutional scientists or faculty entrepreneurs themselves can provide the needed technical expertise (especially if students or postdocs can be hired by the new venture) and the research institutions of course can license key patent rights to the company. But business expertise, space, and money are often more difficult to come by. Research institutions often try to help new firms bridge this gap by providing more than just IP licensing and technical expertise. This is because commercial partners, especially small, innovative ones, are essential to the role of federally funded research institutions in delivering novel health-care products to the market. There is now an attractive array of available options or opportunities for new biotech firms beyond just traditional licenses or start-up license agreements, and several of these options will be examined in more detail.

Research Collaboration Programs for Start-Ups

For some entrepreneurs, there is a misperception that NIH scientists (unlike their university counterparts) are not allowed to interact with private-sector firms due to the implementation of strict government ethics and conflict of interest rules. While it is true that NIH investigators, in general, cannot engage in outside consulting with biotechnology and pharmaceutical companies in their personal capacity, the fact is that technology transfer–related activities are actually among the "official duties," in which NIH scientists are encouraged to participate. These activities may include the reporting of new inventions from the laboratory and assisting technology-transfer staff with patenting, marketing, and licensing interactions with companies. NIH scientists can also officially collaborate with industry scientists through the use of various mechanisms, including more complex CRADAs and CTAs as well as simpler CDAs and MTAs.

In a CRADA research project, which could run for several years, NIH and company scientists can engage in mutually beneficial joint research, where each party provides unique resources, skills, and funding, and where either partner may not otherwise be able to solely provide all the resources needed for the successful completion of the project. In such an arrangement, the details of the research activity to be carried out and the scope of the license options granted to discoveries emanating from the joint research are clearly spelled out in advance. A CTA would typically involve the clinical testing of a private-sector company's small molecule compound or biologic drug. The company gains access to the clinical trial infrastructure and clinical expertise available at NIH; however, unlike what occurs with a CRADA, the company partner does not have any licensing rights to IP that is generated during the clinical research project. The NIH usually enters into these agreements only in cases where such trials would be difficult or impossible to run in other places. The NIH is particularly interested in clinical trials involving rare or orphan diseases that affect 200,000 or fewer patients per year in the United States. An MTA is a popular mechanism for exchanging proprietary research reagents and is used by scientists worldwide. NIH investigators actively use this mechanism to share reagents with scientists in other nonprofit organizations. Proprietary and/or unpublished information can be exchanged between NIH researchers and company personnel in advance of making a decision to enter into a formal CRADA or CTA via the use of a CDA.

Of the collaborative mechanisms described earlier, a CRADA is perhaps the most comprehensive and far-reaching agreement for federal laboratories. Such agreements can provide additional funds for an NIH lab while providing the collaborating company with preferential access to the NIH scientist's future discoveries and access to scientific and medical expertise during the research or clinical collaboration. A CRADA is not, however, intended to be a means for the NIH to provide funding for a new company; in fact, the NIH cannot supply any funding to its CRADA partners. The easiest way for an entrepreneur to access this expertise is to simply approach the agency officially either by contacting a scientist directly or by contacting the institute TTO and/or technology development coordinator [8].

If an early-stage company needs access to NIH materials for commercial purposes outside a formal collaboration, this usually would be done utilizing an Internal Commercial Use License Agreement rather than MTA. As noted before, these are nonexclusive license agreements to allow a licensee to use (but not sell) technology in its internal programs. Here, materials (either patented or unpatented) are provided, and drug screening uses are permitted. The financial structure of this agreement can be either a single payment, a paid-up term license, or annual royalty payments, though the second structure is more popular with start-up companies.

Funding Opportunities for Start-Ups—Small Business Innovation Research Programs

In addition to contracting opportunities, the NIH and other federal labs can provide private sector entities with nondilutive funding through the SBIR and STTR programs [9]. The NIH SBIR program is perhaps the most lucrative and stable funding source for new companies and unlike a small business loan, SBIR grant funds do not need to be repaid.

Other noteworthy advantages of SBIR programs for small companies include retention by the company of any IP rights from the research funding, receipt of early-stage funding that doesn't impact stock or shares in any way (e.g., no dilution of capital), national recognition for the firm, verification and visibility for the underlying technology, and the generation of a leveraging tool that can attract other funding from venture capital or angel investors.

The SBIR program itself was established in 1982 by the Small Business Innovation Development Act to increase the participation of small, high technology firms in federal R&D activities. Under this program, departments and agencies with R&D budgets of $100 million or more are required to set aside 3.2% (for FY 2017) of their R&D budgets to sponsor research at small companies. The STTR program was established by the Small Business Technology Transfer Act of 1992 and requires federal agencies with extramural R&D budgets over $1 billion to administer STTR programs using an annual set-aside of 0.45% (for FY 2017). In FY 2017 NIH's combined SBIR and STTR grants totaled over $971 million.

The STTR and SBIR programs are similar in that both seek to increase small business participation and private-sector commercialization of technology developed through federal R&D. The SBIR program funds early-stage R&D at small businesses. The unique feature of the STTR program is the requirement for the small business applicant to formally collaborate with a research institution in Phases I and II (see description later).

Thus the SBIR and STTR programs differ in two major ways. First, under the SBIR program, the principal investigator must have his or her primary employment with the small business concern at the time of the award and for the duration of the project period. However, under the STTR program, primary employment is not stipulated. Second, the STTR program requires research partners at universities and other nonprofit research institutions to have a formal collaborative relationship with the small business concern. At least 40% of the STTR research project is to be conducted by the small business concern and at least 30% of the effort is to be conducted by the single "partnering" research institution.

As a major mechanism at the NIH for achieving the goals of enhancing public health through the commercialization of new technology, the SBIR and STTR grants present an excellent funding source for start-up and other small biotechnology companies. The NIH SBIR and STTR programs themselves are structured in three primary phases:

Phase I—The objective of Phase I is to establish the technical merit and feasibility of the proposed R&D efforts and to determine the quality of performance of the small business prior to providing further federal funding in Phase II. Phase I awards are normally $150,000, provided over a period of 6 months for SBIR and $150,000 over a period of 1 year for STTR. However, with proper justification, applicants may propose longer periods of time and greater amounts of funds necessary to establish the technical merit and feasibility of the proposed project.

Phase II—The objective of Phase II is to continue the R&D efforts initiated in Phase I. Only Phase I awardees are eligible for a Phase II award. Phase II awards are normally $1 million over 2 years for SBIR and $1 million over 2 years for STTR. However, with proper justification, applicants may propose longer periods of time and greater amounts of funds necessary for the completion of the project.

SBIR-Technology Transfer (SBIR-TT)—Under this program (SBIR-TT) undertaken at the NCI at the NIH and other NIH institutes, SBIR Phases I and II awards are given in conjunction with exclusive licenses to selected underlying background discoveries made by an intramural research laboratory at the institute.

SBIR Phase IIB Bridge—The NCI SBIR program has created the Phase IIB Bridge Award for previously funded NCI SBIR Phase II awardees to continue the next stage of R&D for projects in the areas of cancer therapeutics, imaging technologies, interventional devices, diagnostics, and prognostics. The objective of the NCI Phase IIB Bridge Award is to help address the funding gap that a company may encounter between the end of the Phase II award and the commercialization stage. For any single year of the project period, budgets up to $2 million total costs may be requested. However, the combined budget requested for the entire project period must not exceed $4 million total costs. To incentivize partnerships between awardees and third-party investors and/or strategic partners, a competitive preference and funding priority will be given to applicants that demonstrate the ability to secure substantial independent third-party investor funds (i.e., third-party funds that equal or exceed the requested NCI funds). This funding opportunity is open to current and recently expired SBIR Phase II projects.

Fast track—Fast-track incorporates a submission and review process in which both Phases I and II grant applications are submitted and reviewed together as one application. Because both phases undergo review at the same time, the NIH Fast-Track mechanism can reduce or eliminate the funding gap between phases.

Direct to Phase II—This recently reestablished program provides authorized NIH that may issue a Phase II awards to a small business concern that did not receive a Phase I award for that research/R&D. This type of award is appropriate for technologies where the phase flexibility studies have already been completed.

Phase III—The objective of Phase III, where appropriate, is for the small business concern to pursue with non-SBIR/STTR funds the commercialization objectives resulting from the Phase I/II R&D activities.

In addition to receiving funding through the SBIR and STTR programs, small companies may also be eligible for technical and management assistance programs designed to increase their chances for successful commercialization of the funded technology. These would include the following:

Niche Assessment Program—*For SBIR/STTR Phase I Awardees*—The Niche Assessment Program is designed to help small businesses "jump start" their commercialization efforts by providing market insight and data that can be used to help such companies strategically position their technology in the marketplace. The results of this program can help small businesses develop their commercialization plans for their Phase II application and be exposed to potential commercial partners.

I-Corps at NIH—The I-Corps program provides funding, mentoring, and networking opportunities to help SBIR Phase I awardees commercialize promising biomedical technology. During this 8-week, hands-on program, companies learn how to focus their business plans and get the tools to bring their treatment to market. Program benefits include funding up to $55,000 to cover direct program costs; training from biotech sector experts; expanding professional networks; creating a comprehensive business model; and gaining entrepreneurial skills.

Commercialization Accelerator Program (CAP)—NIH CAP is a 9-month program open to SBIR/STTR Phase II awardees that is well regarded for its combination of deep domain expertise and access to industry connections, which have resulted in measurable gains and accomplishments by participating companies. Offered since 2004 to address the commercialization objectives of companies across the spectrum of experience and stage, 1000 + companies have participated in the CAP. The program enables participants to establish market and customer relevance, build commercial relationships, and focus on revenue opportunities available to them.

SBIR/STTR key points—Those who hope to receive an SBIR or STTR grant from the NIH must convince the NIH that the proposed research is unique, creates value for the public at large through advancements in knowledge and treatment of disease, and is relevant to the overall goals of the NIH. It is important to contact the program officials ahead of time within the component of the NIH from where funding is sought to determine whether the proposed research plan fits these criteria. For start-ups, generally SBIR applications are most successful when they include an entrepreneur-founder with experience in the field, a highly innovative technical solution to significant clinical needs, an end product with significant commercial potential, a technology in need of more feasibility data that the proposed research project would generate, and finally a project that, if successful, would have reduced risk and become more attractive for downstream investment. At the NIH, grant applications are currently reviewed three times a year (April 5, August 5, and December 5) and contract proposals the first week in November. Note that both programs are subject to periodic reauthorizations and changes by the US Congress.

New and Innovative Programs as We Move Toward "V2.0" of Technology Transfer

Basic and Clinical Research Assistance from the National Institutes of Health

Basic and clinical research assistance from the NIH institutes may also be available to companies through specialized services such as drug candidate compound screening and preclinical and clinical drug development and testing services, which are offered by several programs. These initiatives are particularly targeted toward developing and enhancing new clinical candidates in the disease or health area of focus at various NIH institutes. The largest and perhaps best-known programs of these types at the NIH are those that currently run in the NCI [10]. The NCI has played an active role in the development of drugs for cancer treatment for over 50 years. This is reflected in the fact that approximately one half of the chemotherapeutic drugs currently used by oncologists for cancer treatments were in some form discovered and/or developed at NCI. The Developmental Therapeutics Program promotes all aspects of drug discovery and development before testing in humans (preclinical development) and is a part of the Division of Cancer Treatment and Diagnosis (DCTD). NCI also funds an extensive clinical (human) trials network to ensure that promising agents are tested in humans. NCI's Cancer Therapy Evaluation Program, also a part of the DCTD, administers clinical drug development. Compounds can enter at any stage of the development process with either very little or extensive prior testing. Drugs developed through these programs include well-known products such as cisplatin, paclitaxel, and fludarabine.

In the beginning of 2012, the NIH established a new center called the National Center for Advancing Translational Sciences (NCATS) that is designed to assist companies with the many costly, time-consuming bottlenecks that exist in translational product development [11]. Working in partnership with both the public and private organizations, NCATS seeks to develop innovative ways to reduce, remove, or bypass such bottlenecks to speed the delivery of new drugs, diagnostics, and medical devices to patients. The center is not a drug development company but focuses more on using science to create powerful new tools and technologies that can be adopted widely by translational researchers in all sectors.

NCATS was formed primarily by uniting and realigning a variety of existing NIH programs that play key roles in translational science along with adding key initiatives. Programs of note for bioentrepreneurs at NCATS include the following:

1. ***Bridging Interventional Development Gaps (BrIDGs)*** enables research collaborations to advance candidate therapeutics for both common and rare diseases into clinical testing. Investigators do not receive grant funds through this program. Instead, selected researchers partner with NCATS experts to generate preclinical data and clinical-grade material through government contracts for use in Investigational New Drug applications to a regulatory authority, such as the FDA. In general, BrIDGs provides synthesis, formulation, pharmacokinetic, and toxicology expertise and resources to its collaborators.
2. ***Clinical and Translational Science Awards (CTSA)*** support a national network of medical research institutions—called hubs—that work together to improve the translational research process to get more treatments to more patients more quickly. The hubs collaborate locally and regionally to catalyze innovation in training, research tools, and processes. CTSA program support enables research teams including scientists, patient advocacy organizations, and community members to tackle system-wide scientific and operational problems in clinical and translational research that no one team can overcome.
3. ***Chemical Genomics Center (National Chemical Genomics Center (NCGC))*** is one of the centers in the Molecular Libraries Probe Production Centers Network. Through this program, biomedical researchers gain access to the large-scale small molecule screening capacity, along with medicinal chemistry and informatics necessary to identify chemical probes to study the functions of genes, cells, and biochemical pathways. These chemical probes may also be used in developing of new drugs.
4. ***Therapeutics for Rare and Neglected Diseases (TRND)*** offers collaborative opportunities to access rare and neglected disease drug-development capabilities, expertise, and clinical/regulatory resources. Its goal is to move promising therapeutics into human clinical trials. Selected applicants can partner with TRND staff on a joint project plan and implement a drug-development program. Applicant investigators provide the drug project starting points and ongoing biological/disease expertise throughout the project. A collaboration agreement is established between TRND and successful applicants.

NCATS-supported programs and projects have also produced numerous tools to help basic and clinical researchers advance translational science. These resources include clinical research tools and resources to aid in such activities as patient recruitment, clinical study management, and public–private partnership development as well as preclinical research tools and resources to help researchers explore the functions of cells at the genome level, including more than 60 chemical probes.

There is additional assistance available from other NIH institutes to firms in a variety of disease areas including infectious diseases, drug abuse, and others—many more than can be highlighted here. All in all, such efforts can provide a wide variety of technical assistance (often at modest or no cost) for preclinical and even clinical development of novel therapies or other biomedical products by start-up firms.

Selling Products to Universities and Federal Labs

One of the most commonly overlooked opportunities by biomedical-focused companies is the ability to sell products and services to the NIH and similar research centers. Indeed, for start-up companies looking to develop new products used in conducting basic or clinical research, the NIH may be their first customer. With an intramural staff of about 18,000 employees, laboratories in several regions of the country (with the Bethesda campus in Maryland home to the majority), and an annual intramural budget of more than $3 billion, the NIH is perhaps the largest individual institutional consumer of bioscience research reagents and instruments in the world. A variety of mechanisms for selling products and services to the NIH are possible, including stocking in government storerooms. Selling to the NIH can be seen as a daunting task for new companies because of the US government's complex acquisition process. However, there are a few simple steps that companies can take, such as establishing a Blanket Purchase Agreement (BPA) with the NIH and getting their goods and services into the NIH stockroom. Once these hurdles are cleared, it is much easier for NIH scientists to buy from such companies, and if the quality of goods and services provided by a biotech company is superior, an NIH scientist can justify buying solely from that very source.

Companies that provide products and services to NIH laboratories can not only generate cash flow and revenues to fuel R&D but also begin to demonstrate their commercial acumen to would-be partners and investors. Being a large research organization, the NIH has numerous R&D contracting opportunities. For specific information on such opportunities, visit the NIH Office of Acquisition Management and Policy website [12].

The annual NIH Research Festival is also an excellent starting point for companies hoping to sell products to the NIH [13]. This event is held every fall at the Bethesda, Maryland campus and every spring on the Frederick, Maryland campus. Part scientific, part social, part informational, and part inspirational, this 3-day event draws a variety of small-to-medium-sized bioscience companies. These events attract almost 6000 NIH scientists, many of whom come to these gatherings to learn about and potentially purchase the latest research tools and services.

Translational Research Center—A Newer Model of Technology Transfer

AMCs such as the MGH are also evolving into this new model of technology commercialization that places a greater emphasis on the translational aspects of research. In the traditional technology transfer model, as you recall, the academic entity has used its intellectual capital to make breakthrough, cutting-edge discoveries, protecting them with patent picket-fences, and "transfers" it out to the company for them to develop these stellar scientific discoveries into products. These institutions recognize that to have the best patient outcomes for these new inventions, there is also a need to participate further in the translation of the early discovery to actual products.

The pictorial in Fig. 15.3 illustrates this model of a collaboration with a company that was used at the MGH and it is evident from this depiction that the huge advantages can be had from the utilization of the complementary strengths of the two parties in such a translation research effort. As illustrated, the research center brings to the table the technology, the IP, the know-how, and deep understanding of the inner workings of the technology, and in the case of MGH, significant biological and clinical insights. The company would provide the funding, the product development expertise, the regulatory expertise, and finally and importantly the marketing and product-positioning expertise. One such center was established at MGH with funding from a large company in the fall of 2010. The product is a next-generation diagnostic for cancer care—one that may fundamentally change therapeutic decisions for cancer patients. For this program, the TTO was instrumental right from the start in nurturing/protecting and maintaining the IP from its early days, working with the investigators to attract companies to the table, doing the deal with the company, and of course helping see this technology being translated into a product.

Impact of Technology Transfer

Licensing has Spurred Biotechnology Industry Growth

As mentioned before, the economic development potential of biomedical research is being recognized as a "fourth mission" for research institutions—going along with education, research, and public or community service. Thus it is in this "fourth mission" that bioentrepreneurs and research institutions find themselves again sharing the

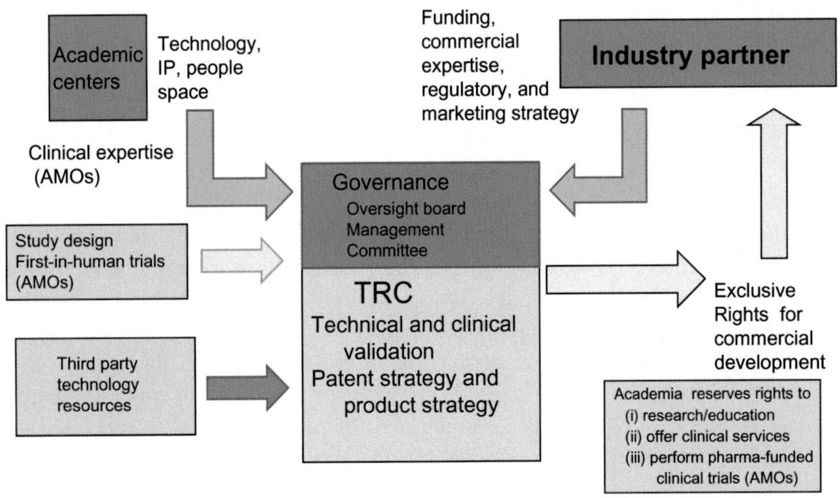

FIGURE 15.3 A business model for tech transfer: TRC. *TRC*, Translational Research Centers.

common goal of having new companies established based upon innovative research discoveries.

The economic importance of licensing and technology transfer has become better recognized during the recent recessionary period and some of the figures can be quite striking. For example, the overall product sales of all types by licensees of NIH intramural research is now reported by the NIH OTT as being over $6 billion annually, the equivalent of mid-tier Fortune 500 companies. Economic development also was the focus of the October 28, 2011 US Presidential Memorandum entitled "Accelerating Technology Transfer and Commercialization of Federal Research in Support of High-Growth Businesses" [13]. This directive from the White House recognized the economic aspects of innovation and technology transfer for federal research in the way it fuels economic growth as well as creating new industries, companies, jobs, products and services, and improving the global competitiveness of US industries. The directive requires federal laboratories, such as the NIH, to support high-growth entrepreneurship by increasing the rate of technology transfer and the economic and societal impact from federal R&D investments over a 5-year period. During this period, federal laboratories, such as the NIH, will be (1) establishing goals and measuring progress toward commercialization, (2) streamlining the technology transfer and commercialization processes, especially for licensing, collaborations, and grants to small companies, and (3) facilitating the commercialization of new technology and the formation of new start-up firms through local and regional economic development partnerships.

Looking at the university and AMC figures reported by the AUTM, we find similarly strong figures for the economic impact of technology transfer. In 2016, AUTM reported that license income generated almost $3 billion and an additional $4 billion came in through industry-sponsored research. In 2016, more than 1000 start-ups were formed of which approximately 750 were doing business in the same state as the university/nonprofit from which the technology arose. By the end of 2016, 800 new products were introduced into the marketplace. In addition to the employment created by these start-ups, the tech-transfer industry itself has created significant employment both directly and indirectly through the related businesses it has helped to spawn.

In addition, many universities and the NIH have set up or have access to educational programs that train scientists and engineers to have a greater appreciation as to the importance of commercialization. These include entrepreneurship centers and small business assistance programs at many universities [14], and such things as the "Advanced Studies in Technology Transfer" program given at the Foundation for Advanced Education in the Sciences Graduate School at the NIH [15].

Maximal Leveraging of Technologies from Universities and Federal Labs

With their leading-edge research programs and focus in the health-care market, the federal laboratory and university-based research programs have an exemplary record in providing opportunities for bioentrepreneurs to develop both high-growth companies and high-growth medical products. Indeed, a preliminary study from 2007 has shown that more than 100 drug and vaccine products approved by the US FDA were based at least in part on technologies directly licensed from university and federal laboratories with federal labs (NIH) providing nearly 20% of the total [16]. Further, another study from 2009 has shown that university-licensed products commercialized by industry created at least 279,000 jobs across the United States during a 12-year period and that there was an increasing share of the United States GDP each year attributable to university-licensed products [17]. In addition, a study published in the *New England Journal of Medicine* [18] in 2011 based upon the earlier 2007 preliminary study showed the intramural research laboratories at the NIH as by far the largest single nonprofit source of new drugs and vaccines approved by the FDA. This is an indication that the impact of licensing by universities and (by extension) federal laboratories will be increasingly effective and important in the future. Even with this success, there is movement toward a new, more collaborative horizon, especially with a "bench-to-beside" style collaboration as show in Fig. 15.4.

With the rising costs of traditional drug discovery and mounting pressures on health-care costs, companies are starting to adopt the model of a joint venture with academia. For example, Pfizer has embarked on a novel academic–industry partnership paradigm with the establishment of its Center for Therapeutic Innovation (CTI) program. By the end of 2011, CTI has established partnerships with 20 leading AMCs across the United States and supports collaborative projects from four dedicated labs in Boston, New York City, San Francisco, and San Diego. Another example is the establishment of Innovations Centers by Johnson & Johnson in Boston, San Francisco, Shanghai, and London. Scientists from academia are embracing this model as well given the pressures of funding their research as well as their drive to see their work not only published in leading journals but also seeing the products of their research turn into a product that can benefit the public at large.

Although this commercial success has been a model in showing the value of technology transfer from federal laboratories, universities, and similar nonprofit research institutions, it is not the entire story. The final tally must include not only the full societal value and economic impact both of new companies but more importantly as

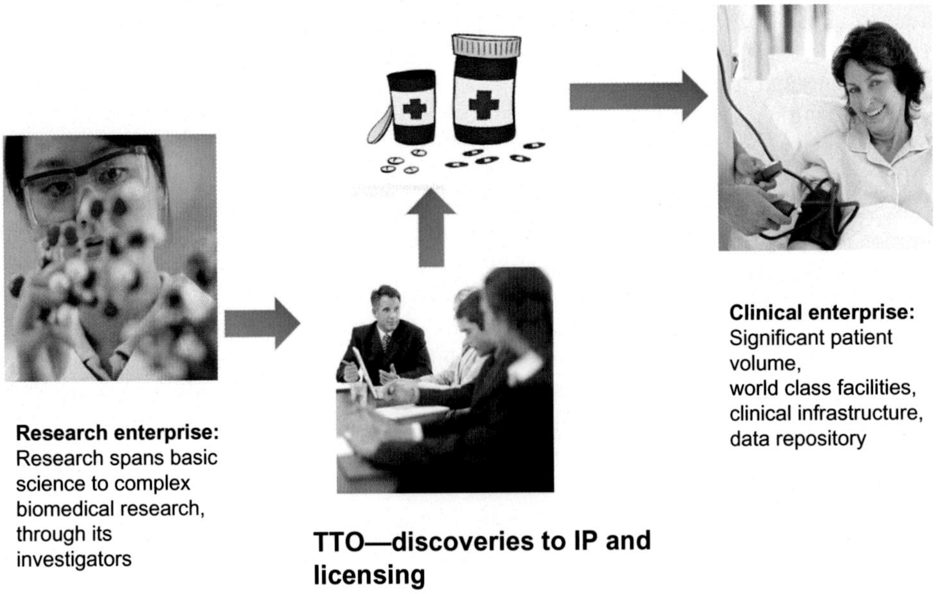
Research enterprise:
Research spans basic science to complex biomedical research, through its investigators
TTO—discoveries to IP and licensing
Clinical enterprise:
Significant patient volume,
world class facilities,
clinical infrastructure,
data repository

FIGURE 15.4 NIH and academic medical centers: Bench—bedside collaborations. *NIH*, National Institutes of Health.

well as the life-saving or enhancing therapeutics, vaccines, diagnostics, and other biomedical products on the market that have origins in this federally funded research. This is believed to be the truest measure of the value and importance of licensing and technology transfer from research institutions.

Case studies in biotech commercialization using university and federal labs

Case study 1: licensing of human papillomavirus vaccine technology

The human papillomavirus (HPV) vaccine is a vaccine that prevents infection against certain species of HPV associated with the development of cervical cancer, genital warts, and some less-common cancers. Although most women infected with genital HPV will not have complications from the virus, worldwide there are an estimated 470,000 new cases of cervical cancer that result in 233,000 deaths per year. About 80% of deaths from cervical cancer occur in poor countries.

The research that led to the development of the vaccine began in the 1980s by groups primarily at the University of Rochester, Georgetown University, the German Cancer Center (DKFZ), Queensland University in Australia, and the NIH. This work, and the work of others, eventually became the basis of Gardasil (sold by Merck) and Cervarix (sold by GSK)—blockbuster products in terms of public health and market impacts.

MedImmune, Inc., then a very small development-stage vaccine company based in Gaithersburg, Maryland, licensed the HPV vaccine technology available from all US institutions as well as the DKFZ in the early 1990s. GSK later received a license to all the rights held by MedImmune; Merck received a license from the NIH as

(Continued)

(Continued)

well as to the Queensland rights. All of the license agreements were exclusive; those granted by NIH (who had been conducting separate clinical trials) were nonexclusive. The discoveries made at the research institutions were all very close in subject matter in what was then a relatively small research field and thus overlapping in terms of patent applications. Multiple patent interferences and patent oppositions resulted in patent offices around the world.

While patent interferences and oppositions can be expensive and difficult to resolve, the underlying technology proved to be extraordinarily successful in its clinical applications by both Merck and GSK—results that were confirmed in separate trials by the NIH. Given the strong clinical efficacy for these vaccines based upon the underlying technology discovered at the research institutions, a comprehensive settlement agreement was reached (regardless of the procedural outcomes at the patent offices around the world) whereby both Merck and GSK received coexclusive rights to the patent rights of all the research institutions, permitting the launch of similar (but slightly different) versions by both companies of these very important cervical cancer vaccines.

Discussion questions

After reading this chapter along with others in this book:

1. consider the role of MedImmune in the development of this vaccine. How risky was the strategy to acquire either control or access to nearly all the available license rights at a preclinical stage?
2. how did the strategy of the NIH work out, conducting some independent clinical trials and licensing both major developing parties originally on a nonexclusive basis?

(Continued)

(Continued)

Case study II—sponsored clinical research agreement

The company in this case study was providing drugs as well as money (to the tune of millions of dollars over a few years) to the hospital. The drugs were in development at the company and were poised to enter the clinic (company's prized "Clinical Candidates"). The collaboration with the TTO was going to be in two phases—a preclinical research collaboration and a clinical collaboration in that order. The terms described later apply for the preclinical research collaboration.

Inventions were defined as those that were made during the term of the collaboration with funding from the company. Because inventorship follows US patent law, it was decided that ownership would follow inventorship making for three categories of inventions—company solely owned, hospital solely owned, and jointly owned. The parties would work together to protect inventions via patent applications. The company would pay for patent protection for all inventions in these three categories and in exchange would receive the rights later described. If the company did not see the value in any hospital solely owned inventions, then they would not pay for the protection of these inventions nor receive rights to these inventions.

The company retained full rights to use their own inventions. For jointly owned inventions, they had nonexclusive rights to access the inventions for internal research and all commercial purposes by virtue of their joint ownership. For hospital solely owned inventions, they received free rights for their internal research purposes. As compensation for paying for the patent costs to support the inventions, they also received an option to license the inventions at a later time. As the collaborative research informs them about the commercial prospects of this clinical candidate coupled with their separate ongoing internal efforts in this program, they would make a decision during a defined option period about exclusive or nonexclusive licensing. The option period had a time window of 2.5 years from the time of the initial filing of the patent application to protect the invention. This coincides with an important decision point in the life of a patent application, the decision to file for patent protection in specific individual countries—a very cost-intensive decision. Notably, through the option to license, the academic center is providing a route to obtain rights to the inventions developed in the collaboration or the FTO rights that is a must-have for the company as described earlier.

The terms of the license would be standard between academia and industry for such technologies (see Table 15.6). Such a license would involve the hospital's rights in both jointly owned inventions as well as in its solely owned inventions.

Publication versus confidentiality

Being clinical candidates, the company was very averse to any publications until the collaborative research was completed. This would mean publications could not happen for 2, maybe even 3 years from the start of the work. While this may be the actual timing of the publication, as an academic

(Continued)

(Continued)

institution the hospital could not agree to an apparent delay of the publication for a very long time. As per the guidelines under which academic research institutions operate, they cannot "withhold" publications for longer than 2–3 months. This issue was resolved by tasking the steering committee that was set-up with members from both institutions with finding a reasonable solution at the time when publication of the work is imminent. It was likely that the work will be published only when it is complete which may be 2 years from the start of the research anyway, so there will be no issue to resolve. But if there was a disagreement and a long 2–3-year delay to provide for patent protection, then the committee will come up with a reasonable compromise.

Discussion questions

1. What were the sensitive issues during the negotiation of the research collaboration agreement between the two parties and how did they resolve their differences?
2. Do you think either of the parties had to unnecessarily compromise on any basic principles in order to reach agreement? Discuss these points in more detail.

References

[1] National Institutes of Health. NIH overview, 2018. <http://www.nih.gov/about/budget.htm/> [accessed December 19, 2018].

[2] Brookings Institute. University start-ups: critical for improving technology transfer, 2013. <http://www.brookings.edu/research/papers/2013/11/university-start-ups-technology-transfer-valdivia> [accessed December 19, 2018].

[3] Association of University Technology Managers (AUTM). AUTM U.S. annual licensing survey highlights, 2017. <https://autm.net/surveys-and-tools/surveys/licensing-survey/2017-licensing-activity-survey> [accessed January 1, 2019].

[4] Ben-Menachem G, Ferguson S, Balakrishnan K. Doing business with NIH. Nat Biotechnol 2006;24(1):17–20.

[5] Ferguson S. Products, partners and public health: transfer of biomedical technologies from the U.S. government. J Biolaw Bus 2002;5(2):35–9.

[6] National Institutes of Health. Office of Technology Transfer. Startups, 2019. <http://www.ott.nih.gov/nih-start-exclusive-license-agreements> [accessed December 19, 2018].

[7] MacWright R. The University of Virginia Patent Foundation: a midsized technology transfer foundation focused on faculty service, operated using a deal-based business model. In: AUTM technology transfer practice manual. 3rd ed. 2(2.3a), pp. 1–21, 2019.

[8] National Institutes of Health. Office of Technology Transfer. Public health service technology development coordinators, 2019. <http://www.ott.nih.gov/technology-development-coordinators> [accessed December 19, 2018].

[9] National Institutes of Health. Office of Extramural Research. Small Business Innovation Research (SBIR) and Small Business Technology Transfer (STTR) Programs. <http://grants.nih.gov/grants/funding/sbir.htm> [accessed 12.19.18].

[10] National Institutes of Health. National Cancer Institute. Developmental Therapeutics Program and Cancer Therapy

Evaluation Program, 2018. <http://dtp.nci.nih.gov/> and <http://ctep.cancer.gov/> [accessed December 19, 2018].

[11] National Institutes of Health. National Center for Advancing Translational Science, 2018. <http://ncats.nih.gov/> [accessed December 19, 2018].

[12] National Institutes of Health. Office of Acquisition Management and Policy, 2018. <http://oamp.od.nih.gov/> [accessed December 19, 2018].

[13] National Institutes of Health. NIH Research Festival, 2018. <http://researchfestival.nih.gov/> [accessed December 19, 2018].

[14] Johns Hopkins University, Carey Business School. Discovery To Market (D2M) Program, 2019. <https://carey.jhu.edu/current-students/carey-life/experiential-learning/experiential-courses/discovery-to-market/> [accessed 01.01.19].

[15] Foundation for Advanced Education in the Sciences (FAES). FAES Graduate School at NIH Certificate Program, 2018. <http://www.faes.org/grad/advanced_studies/technology_transfer> [accessed December 19, 2018].

[16] Jensen J, Wyller K, London E, Chatterjee S, Murray F, Rohrbaugh M, et al. The contribution of public sector research to the discovery of new drugs. In: Personal communication of poster at 2007 AUTM annual meeting, 2007.

[17] Roessner D, Bond J, Okubo S, Planting M. The economic impact of licensed commercialized inventions originating in university research, 1996–2007. In: Final report to the Biotechnology Industry Organization, 2019. <http://www.bio.org/articles/economic-impact-licensed-commercialized-inventions-originating-university-research-1996-200> [accessed January 1, 2019].

[18] Stevens A, Jensen J, Wyller K, Kilgore P, Chatterjee S, Rohrbaugh M. The role of public-sector research in the discovery of drugs and vaccines. N Engl J Med 2011;364:535–41.

Further Reading

National Institutes of HealthNational Institutes of Health. Office of Technology Transfer. Licensing opportunities, 2018. <http://www.ott.nih.gov/opportunities> [accessed December 19, 2018].

The White HouseThe White House. Office of the Press Secretary. Presidential memorandum—accelerating technology transfer and commercialization of federal research in support of high-growth businesses, 2011. <http://www.whitehouse.gov/the-press-office/2011/10/28/presidential-memorandum-accelerating-technology-transfer-and-commerciali> [accessed December 19, 2018].

Chapter 16

Intellectual Property Protection Strategies for Biotechnology Innovations

Gerry J. Elman, MS, JD[1] and Jay Z. Zhang, MS, JD[2,3]

[1]*Elman Technology Law, P.C., Media, PA, United States,* [2]*Shuwen Biotech Co. Ltd., Deqing, P.R. China,* [3]*China Jiliang University Law School, Hangzhou, P.R. China*

Chapter Outline

Biotechnology companies typically begin with ideas for products or services that have a technological and beneficial advantage over other products in the market. As these improvements, or new product concepts and ideas, are implemented into practical commercial use, they will attract attention. The better they are, the more likely others will desire to copy them. Strategies for achieving exclusivity or at least a head start in this regard include the use of legal tools in the category of intellectual property (IP). These strategies are the focus of this chapter, wherein we provide an overview of the tools available to protect one of your company's most important assets.

Much of the early value that investors attribute to a development-stage biotechnology company is the "ownership" of these technological concepts and new product ideas as embodied in the company's IP. Also important will be your ability to communicate and collaborate with patent counsel who will be advising you about IP strategy and providing support throughout this process.

Biotechnology Entrepreneurship. DOI: https://doi.org/10.1016/B978-0-12-815585-1.00016-4

The Intellectual Property Toolbox[1]

To gain a competitive advantage, your company will endeavor to provide something unique. If the technology you'll be implementing is an in-house discovery that can't be reverse-engineered by analyzing the product, the first order of business may be to keep the details secret. In that event, you'll take advantage of legal principles that protect *trade secrets*.[2] And if it's likely that, sooner or later, the technology will become publicly accessible, you'll consider other methods to fend off imitators, such as *patents* and other methods from a legal toolkit relating to *IP* as well as regulatory regimes pertinent to the subject matter, for example, drugs or agricultural products.

Generally, the more traditional term *industrial property* [1] (as distinguished from "IP") refers to *patents*, *design patents* or *industrial designs*, *utility model patents* or *petty patents*, and *plant patents*, as well as *trademarks*, *service marks*, and layout designs of integrated circuits, commercial names and designations, geographical indications, and protection against *unfair competition*. *IP* is a more recently coined term that subsumes the various forms of the industrial property mentioned earlier, plus *copyright*. *Copyright*, also known in certain other jurisdictions as *authors' rights*, traditionally relates to artistic creations, such as poems, novels, music, paintings, and cinematographic works, as well as photographs, the text of scientific papers, and more recently, computer software [2].

Each country, as a legal jurisdiction, has its own set of principles and practices applicable to IP. Although they have a lot in common, the details of IP law vary from jurisdiction-to-jurisdiction, and even from time-to-time. In February 2013, for example, the Federal Court of Australia ruled that isolated polynucleotides embodying naturally occurring genetic sequences are potentially patentable subject matter, whereas in June of that year, the US Supreme Court took the opposite tack. Then, in October 2015, the High Court of Australia overturned the earlier decision of the Federal Court [3]. More about this is mentioned later.

Patents

Let's take a closer look at some of these legal tools, starting with patents. The word *patent* means "open and apparent." In the present context, it is shorthand for *letters patent* and refers to a public document granting rights to the owner, or *holder* of the patent, to exclude others for a limited time from practicing the invention as recited in any of a series of numbered *patent claims*. Below we provide some examples of biotechnology patent claims:

Amgen's patent claims for erythropoietin:

- A purified and isolated DNA sequence consisting essentially of a DNA sequence encoding human erythropoietin.[3]
- A nonnaturally occurring erythropoietin glycoprotein product having the in vivo biological activity of causing bone marrow cells to increase the production of reticulocytes and red blood cells and having glycosylation which differs from that of human urinary erythropoietin.

Cetus/Roche's Foundation patent claim for polymerase chain reaction (PCR):

- A process for amplifying at least one specific nucleic acid sequence contained in a nucleic acid or a mixture of nucleic acids wherein each nucleic acid consists of two separate complementary strands of equal or unequal length which process comprises the following:
  - Treating the strands with two oligonucleotide primers for each different specific sequence being amplified under conditions such that for each different sequence being amplified, an extension product of each primer is synthesized which is complementary to each nucleic acid strand, wherein said primers are selected so as to be sufficiently complementary to different strands of each specific sequence to hybridize therewith such that the extension product synthesized from one primer, when it is separated from its complement, can serve as a template for synthesis of the extension product of the other primer.
  - Separating the primer extension products from the templates on which they were synthesized to produce single-stranded molecules.
  - Treating the single-stranded molecules generated from step 2 with the primers of step 1 under conditions that a primer extension product is synthesized

1. This chapter is presented for educational purposes and not as actionable legal advice. Any opinions expressed herein are those of the individual authors and not of any business, institution, or client. Due to the rapid change in this field of law and practice, the authors, editor, and publisher cannot warrant that a particular item of information is necessarily current. We recommend the reader seek up-to-date advice from counsel practicing in the relevant jurisdiction. We welcome any updates or discrepancies that readers wish to call to our attention. Direct such correspondence to elman@elman.com. We acknowledge with thanks the research assistance of Michael Donnini and M.P. Moon.

2. Throughout this chapter, we'll present in italics certain "terms of art." They're the building blocks that identify concepts you'll want to keep in mind.

3. This claim was granted before the US Supreme Court's decision in Association for Molecular Pathology v. Myriad Genetics, Inc., June 13, 2013. Almost certainly, it wouldn't be enforceable since then. See text after Ref. [4,16–18] and note 4.

using each of the single strands produced in step 2 as a template.

Thomas Cech's patent for ribozymes:

- An enzymatic RNA molecule not naturally occurring in nature having an endonuclease activity independent of any protein, said endonuclease activity being specific for a nucleotide sequence defining a cleavage site comprising single-stranded RNA in a separate RNA molecule and causing cleavage at said cleavage site by a transesterification reaction.

"Harvard Mouse" patent claim:

- A transgenic nonhuman mammal whose germ cells and somatic cells contain a recombinant-activated oncogene sequence introduced into the said mammal, or an ancestor of the said mammal, at an embryonic stage.

University of Wisconsin Alumni Research Foundation's stem cell patent claims:

- A purified preparation of primate embryonic stem cells which (1) is capable of proliferation in an in vitro culture for over 1 year; (2) maintains a karyotype in which all the chromosome characteristics of the primate species are present and not noticeably altered through prolonged culture; (3) maintains the potential to differentiate into derivatives of endoderm, mesoderm, and ectoderm tissues throughout the culture; and (4) will not differentiate when cultured on a fibroblast feeder layer.
- A preparation of pluripotent human embryonic stem cells comprising cells that (1) proliferate in vitro for over 1 year; (2) maintain a karyotype in which the chromosomes are euploid through prolonged culture; (3) maintain the potential to differentiate to derivatives of endoderm, mesoderm, and ectoderm tissues; (4) are inhibited from differentiation when cultured on a fibroblast feeder layer; and (5) are negative for the SSEA-1 cell surface marker and positive for the SSEA-4 cell surface marker.
- A method of isolating a pluripotent human embryonic stem cell line, comprising the steps of:
  - isolating a human blastocyst;
  - isolating cells from the inner cell mass of the above blastocyte;
  - plating the inner cell mass cells on embryonic fibroblasts, wherein inner cell mass–derived cell masses are formed;
  - dissociating the mass into dissociated cells;
  - replating the dissociated cells on embryonic feeder cells;
  - selecting colonies with compact morphologies and cells with high nucleus to cytoplasm ratios and prominent nucleoli; and
  - culturing the cells of the selected colonies to thereby obtain an isolated pluripotent human embryonic stem cell line.

Cornell University's "gene gun" patent claim:

- A method for introducing particles into cells comprising accelerating particles having a diameter sufficiently small to penetrate and be retained in a preselected cell without killing the cell, and propelling said particles at said cells whereby said particles penetrate the surface of said cells and become incorporated into the interior of said cells.

Merck's Fosamax patent claims:

- A method of treatment of urolithiasis and inhibiting bone reabsorption which consists of administering to a patient in need, thereof an effective amount of 4-amino-1-hydroxybutane-1,1-biphosphonic acid.
- A pharmaceutical composition comprising a pharmaceutically effective amount of alendronate, in a pharmaceutically acceptable carrier and a sufficient amount of a buffer to maintain a pH of the composition in the range of 2–8 and complexing agent to prevent the precipitation of alendronate in aqueous solution.

What Is a Patent?

The patent grant is sometimes viewed as a quid pro quo exchange for the patent holder's making public the subject matter taught in the *patent specification*, which otherwise might have been kept secret indefinitely. In other words, if the inventor fully discloses to the public how to make and how to use the invention, the government grants to the patent owner a right to exclude others from making, using, selling, or importing the invention as defined by any of the *claims* recited in the patent. In the United States, patents are granted by the US Patent and Trademark Office (PTO), an agency of the Department of Commerce, in accordance with laws passed by the Congress and signed by the President. In turn, the power of the Congress to enact laws governing patents and copyrights stems from the US Constitution.[4]

To seek a US patent, an applicant prepares and files with the PTO a *patent application* intended to comply with various legal requirements, for example, that it includes a *disclosure* that's detailed enough to *enable* a person skilled in the technical field to make and use the invention. To provide a *written description* of the inventive subject matter, the applicant desirably has become cognizant of the characteristics that distinguish the present invention from subject matter that's already publicly known or otherwise in the legal category referred to as

4. US Constitution, Art. 1, sec. 8, cl. 8: "Congress shall have the power . . .. To promote the progress of science and useful arts, by securing for limited times to authors and inventors the exclusive right to their respective writings and discoveries."

prior art.[5] Typically, this includes a *patentability search*, which seeks to uncover various forms of the pertinent prior art, not only patents. Yet, even if the subject of a proposed patent claim is clearly *novel*, as compared with all the prior art in the world, that isn't enough to establish that the claim fulfills the requisites of patentability. *Patent eligibility* and *nonobviousness* are also required.

Patent Eligibility

A threshold question identified by the US Supreme Court is whether the subject matter is *patent-eligible*, that is, something which can be protected within the patent statute. For many years a fundamental principle of patent law has been that an inventor who's merely characterized a novel composition of matter isn't entitled to a patent, regardless of whether the inventor isolated it from a natural source or synthesized it from scratch. Rather, for a newly generated composition to be patentable, the inventor would need to identify a "practical utility" for it as well. During the past decade, the Court has continued to revisit this issue, raising the hurdle against patentability and seemingly creating chaos in what had previously been considered well-settled principles of law.

At this writing, three Supreme Court decisions impacting patent eligibility of biotechnology inventions are *Mayo Collaborative Services v. Prometheus Laboratories* (2012), *Ass'n for Molecular Pathology v. Myriad Genetics* (2013), and *Alice Corp. v. CLS Bank International* (2014). *Mayo* summarized the judge-made carve-outs from what might otherwise seem to be patentable. Products of nature, natural phenomena, and abstract ideas are not patent-eligible subject matters. However, applications of these subjects may be patented, provided that the claims include recitations of elements that are not routine, conventional, or well known.

Myriad extended the principles set forth in *Mayo* to include the isolation (or chemical state) of otherwise unaltered gene sequences as patent-ineligible subject matter. For more about this, see starting at note 10.

Alice provided a rubric for assessing patent ineligibility of claimed subject matter—articulating a two-part test. First is the subject matter of the claim directed to a patent-ineligible concept (i.e., law of nature, natural phenomenon, or abstract idea)? Second is there something other than well-understood, routine, or conventional claim elements that transform the nature of the claim to something significantly more than the ineligible concept itself? If this "something more" is present, then the claimed subject matter would be patent-eligible.

A 2018 decision of the Court of Appeals for the Federal Circuit is also pertinent—*Vanda Pharm. Inc. v. W.-Ward Pharm. Int'l Ltd*. The *Vanda* case suggests that the addition of an "action step" in a recited diagnostic method claim could impart patent eligibility to a claim.

"Characterization of an invention as using a law of nature or using a natural relationship (as opposed to detecting the presence of the law or relationship)" or "inventions which are claimed as improvements on existing technology" are more likely to be deemed patent-eligible. Consult the PTO's current guidelines on patent eligibility for additional information on what may or may not be effective claim strategies for such subject matter [4].

Nonobviousness or Inventive Height

In addition to patent eligibility and novelty, a valid patent claim is required to define an invention that would not have been *obvious* to a person having ordinary skill in the pertinent art. For the US patents governed by pre-America Invents Act (pre-AIA) law, this hypothetical inquiry is to be performed as of the date that the patent applicant made the invention. For the US patents governed by post-AIA law, an obviousness question is posed as of the *effective filing date* of the patent application. In general, if a hypothetical worker having such skill, who is deemed to have assembled examples of all pertinent prior art, would arrive at the claimed invention without hindsight reconstruction but just using reason and common sense in combining different aspects of them, then the invention as claimed would fail to meet the "nonobviousness" requirement of patentability under the US law.

In some other jurisdictions a similar analysis is performed under the rubric of "inventive height" or "inventive step."

The Patenting Process

Since 1995 there have been two kinds of US patent applications you could file for a useful invention: (1) a provisional patent application (PPA) and (2) the traditional, formal patent application (sometimes called a nonprovisional patent application or NPA) (Fig. 16.1).

The current government fee for a PPA filing is $280 plus a surcharge if it is lengthy. A 50% discount applies to filings by "small entities," which include businesses with fewer than 500 employees. A discount of 75% applies to "micro-entities," which include universities and newly minted private inventors whose income in the previous year was less than the stated cap.

A PPA does not ever get published, so it doesn't have to meet the stringent format requirements of an NPA. The drawings can be informal and it's okay to omit formal

5. Recall that the Constitution refers to the "useful arts" for what today we'd call "technology."

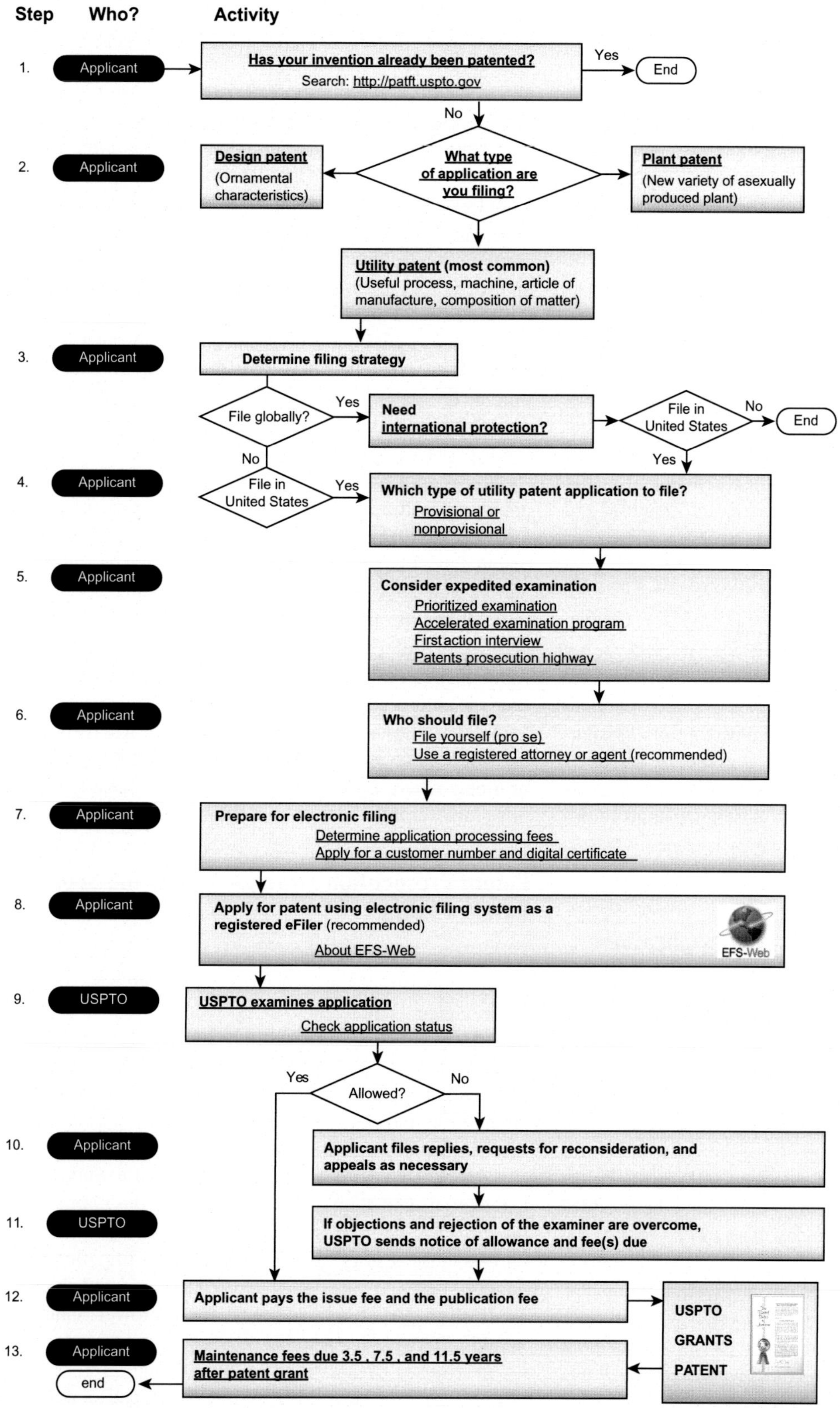

FIGURE 16.1 A flowchart for a US patent application. *From The US Patent and Trademark Office. <https://www.uspto.gov/patents-getting-started/patent-basics/types-patent-applications/utility-patent/process-obtaining>.*

claims. But beware, the law requires a valid PPA to include an enabling disclosure and written description of the invention.

To get a US patent on an invention disclosed in a PPA within a year from the filing of the PPA, you would typically generate and file an NPA which claims "benefit" of the PPA. If this 1-year deadline is missed, a later filed NPA would not be entitled to claim the benefit of the PPA's filing date, so another year or so of prior art would become available to constrain the patentability of the NPA's claims. Each PPA automatically becomes abandoned a year after its filing date and in some circumstances, it may be desirable to formally abandon a PPA before then.

As research and development (R&D) on a project progresses during the year after filing a PPA, it's likely that your technologists will make improvements to the invention(s) described in the PPA. It is often convenient to file additional PPAs that include the new information and then to claim the benefit of all of them in an NPA filed within a year of the first PPA.

Design Patents (Industrial Designs)

A different kind of patent is available to protect the "look" of useful objects. This may be a surface ornamentation or some or all of the overall configuration. Designs are examined to confirm that they are novel and not obvious from the prior art, and thereupon a design patent is granted with a term of 14 years. Design patents don't have "claims," rather the drawings define what is protected.

Pregrant Publication of US Patent Applications

Most foreign countries have been publishing patent applications 18 months from their respective priority filing dates, but until 2000, the law in the United States was that a patent would be published only when it was actually granted. However, a significant fraction of US patent applications filed from then on are automatically published approximately 18 months from their respective filing or priority dates. Since March 2001, new Patent Application Publications, or "PA Pubs," have been added to the PTO website each Thursday. The PTO website is at https://www.uspto.gov/.

If you elect to have your patent application published, once your PA Pub appears on the PTO site, you will have certain "provisional rights" in the subject matter of your pending patent claims. That is, if a company in the United States makes, uses, sells, or imports something that infringes a published claim of your PA Pub, it would be opportune to direct your patent counsel, if appropriate, to send a formal notice to them. Then, if that claim eventually is included in your granted patent, you would be entitled to money damages not only for their infringement from the date of the patent grant but including as well their infringement from the date of your notice up to the patent grant date. If the claims are amended to read differently from the way they have appeared in a PA Pub, it is sometimes advantageous to request the publication of the application as amended to enhance the provisional rights described earlier.

However, automatic pregrant publication of US patent applications is subject to a certain exception. That exception is for patent applications which the applicant does *not* wish to have published, wherein the applicant states at the time of filing that he *does not intend* to file a corresponding application in any foreign countries. For such applications the applicant can get the benefit of secrecy until the patent is granted, the same as under previous US patent law. Because the PTO currently makes the docket entries and ongoing papers filed in pending applications once they are published available on the Web, some applicants prefer to forego the option to obtain provisional rights through a PA Pub and instead opt for the traditional secrecy until a US patent is granted.

In the alternative, there are scenarios where it would be desirable to request early publication of an application or others where it would be desirable to request republication, for example, where the claims have been amended.

Patent Prosecution Strategy Affects the Scope of Patent Claims

During the past few years the federal courts by various judicial decisions have increased the implicit "penalty" against patent applicants for presenting subject matter in patent applications that is not eventually included in granted claims. A "dedication to the public" is said to arise when an applicant includes disclosure in a patent application and does not eventually obtain claims reciting the subject matter. Similarly, an "estoppel" arises when an applicant presents a claim to the patent examiner, gets a rejection, and then acquiesces, letting the claim wither on the vine without arguing against the rejection. Such "prosecution history" is typically used in litigation by an adverse party to assert that any claims granted from the application (or a related one) are narrower than they would otherwise seem to be.

In a series of decisions on how to interpret, or "*construe*,"[6] patent claims, US courts developed a policy of

6. The process of analyzing the meaning of a patent claim, determining its legal metes and bounds, is called *claim construction*. Note that this term does not refer to "constructing" a claim from scratch, but rather to *construing* its meaning after it has been written.

allowing claims to "stretch" to cover certain variants that would otherwise have been outside the scope of the patent claim. This policy came to be known as the *doctrine of equivalents*. Understand that a patent claim can be considered to recite a collection of "elements." For years, when patent claims were interpreted in court, each such element might be deemed to include not only things within its literal wording but also some things that were outside a literal interpretation but which were still "equivalent."

Increasingly, the courts have taken heed of public outcry arising from perceptions that certain patents were overly broad. In a landmark case a few years ago, the US Supreme Court redefined the scope of such equivalents as "mere inconsequential differences," and in another case, it held that there is a presumption that no equivalents would be allowed for any claim element that was amended during the prosecution of the patent. Later, the Court of Appeals for the Federal Circuit surprisingly held that this adverse presumption applies even where the applicant merely cancels an independent claim and rewrites a preexisting dependent claim in independent form. Thus the doctrine of equivalents is now more of an exception than a general rule.

The upshot of these cases is to increase the importance of "getting it right" as early as possible during patent prosecution. The more variations of your invention that are disclosed in the patent application, the broader the literal scope of the claims you file at the outset can be. Endeavor to set forth all the variations of the invention that you contemplate, not only what your company might provide but also what your competitor might do if they are precluded by your patent from copying your invention.

Patent Reform Legislation

Over the past decade, the Congress has taken a hand in "reforming" some of the principles of US patent law. Aspects of patent *reform* were enshrined in the AIA of 2011, the various provisions of which took effect in stages culminating in March 2013 [5]. The most publicized of the "reforms" was to change the uniquely American practice of "first to invent"—awarding a patent sought simultaneously by two or more different inventors (or *inventive entities* composed of two or more inventors acting jointly) to the members of the entity who could prove that they were first to form a mental conception of the claimed subject matter and then act diligently to reduce it to practice, regardless of whether they beat the others in a race to file a patent application. The administrative minitrial at the PTO to make this determination was known as an *interference proceeding*, and the dice was loaded in favor of evidence originating in the United States. In contrast, foreign patent laws favored those who first filed their patent application in the pertinent patent office, typically taking into account a *right-of-priority* that was accorded to filings in the inventor's home patent office by the Paris Convention on Industrial Property.

The AIA eliminated interference proceedings for the US patent applications filed after May 15, 2013, which disclose new inventions. Those new applications will be examined for novelty over, and nonobviousness from, a subtly redefined universe of "prior art." Nevertheless, applications filed after that date that claim subject matter fully disclosed in previously filed applications (i.e., with an effective filing date before May 16, 2013) will be examined under pre-AIA patent law. So during the next 20 years, some US patents will have had their patentability determined against one body of prior art, whereas others will have had patentability determined by another. For patent applications filed during this transition period, an applicant should consider carefully whether to "check the box" on the application form that would direct the patent examination toward one track or the other.

The AIA also created a new procedure for challenging the validity of granted patents, called *Inter Partes Reviews* (IPRs) [6]. These reviews are conducted at the Patent Trial and Appeal Board of the PTO rather than through the courts. The goal of IPRs was to provide a process to eliminate weak or improperly granted patents in a quicker and more cost-effective manner than court litigation. An IPR allows a petitioner to challenge the validity of a patent by presenting evidence to support unpatentability.

IPRs have been criticized as unfairly disadvantaging the patent owner. And since multiple IPR challenges can be entered against a given patent, inventors and patent owners with limited funds can be financially overwhelmed to defend against them. A patent owner who challenged the constitutionality of the IPR procedure took the case all the way to the Supreme Court. But, on narrow grounds, the Court held that IPRs do not violate Article III or the Seventh Amendment of the Constitution. There remains a possibility that a future challenge to IPRs on grounds of either due process or retroactive application of the IPR to pre-AIA patents might lead to a different result. In 2018 some salutary changes to IPR procedure were made [7].

Foreign Patent Filing

You may also be interested in making a decision regarding strategies for filing foreign counterpart patent applications either under the Patent Cooperation Treaty (PCT) or otherwise. These foreign patents would be intended to provide similar rights in various foreign countries you may select. Because there is no such thing as a worldwide patent, it is necessary to obtain a patent for every country in which protection is desired. However, certain regions, namely, Europe, the former USSR (Eurasia), and certain groups of countries in Africa, also have their own patent offices.

The date that a patent application is filed is important, for example, because anything appearing in publication after that date is not "prior art" that can be used to show that the claimed invention is not new. As mentioned earlier, the Paris Convention for the Protection of Industrial Property, which has been in force since 1883, created the concept of a "priority date" that could be applied to a patent application based on a previously filed application. (The Paris Convention also pertains to design patent applications and trademark applications.)

If a first patent application is filed in any of the countries that are members of the Paris Convention, then a copy of that first application that is filed in another member country (translated into the local language) can claim as a "priority date," the filing date of the first application, provided that the copy meets the requirements of the convention. The main requirement is that the copy be filed within *12 months* of the date of the first application. (However, for *design* patents and trademarks, foreign counterparts must be filed within 6 months.)

Although the AIA has modified the *grace period* somewhat from what it used to be, the United States permits inventors up to 1 year from the date of their own public disclosure before their own actions make it too late to file a US patent application. After that time, we say that the patent application is "time barred." However, beware that most foreign countries *do not* provide such a "grace period" (though the 11-member Comprehensive and Progressive Agreement for Trans-Pacific Partnership of 2018 does). The best strategy to preserve your rights internationally is to file a US patent application *before* making a nonconfidential disclosure of the invention or offering to sell the product to anyone. Then, within the prescribed period, file counterpart applications for the countries where you desire patent protection, claiming the priority date of the US application.

At present, 177 countries (from Afghanistan to Zimbabwe) have signed one or more versions of the Paris Convention and thus have joined an International Union on Industrial Property. Taiwan also grants similar priority rights to applicants from the United States due to a bilateral agreement.

The Patent Cooperation Treaty

At present, 152 members of the Paris Convention also belong to the *PCT*, first signed in 1970. Members in the PCT include the United States, Canada, virtually all European countries, Mexico, Australia, Brazil, China, Israel, Japan, Korea, India, South Africa, and many others. (Countries that are still *nonmembers* include Taiwan and various countries in the Middle East, South Asia, Africa, and Central and South America, as well as numerous island nations.)

The PCT provides a procedure whereby a single patent application in English can be filed to start the patenting process for any of the countries that are "designated" in the "PCT application" by marking a checkbox on the form and paying the requisite fee. Under the Paris Convention, a PCT application filed within 12 months of a corresponding US patent application (the first of either a PPA or an NPA) could get the benefit of its priority date.

The following strategy is typical for an applicant in the United States that wishes to defer (for up to a total of 30 months) the high cost of widely filing foreign patent applications. This can provide enough time to evaluate the market and to obtain financing. The strategy is to file a US patent application first (often as a PPA) and then to file a PCT application 12 months later. Typical costs of filing a PCT application range from about $3500 to about $8000, depending on the number of pages in the application and whether revisions to the previously filed text and drawings are desired.

Under PCT procedure, everything starts with the "priority date," which in this example would be the date the original US application was filed, for example, a US PPA. Within about 16 months from that date, an International Searching Authority examiner is supposed to issue the results of a patent search for the claimed invention (ISR) plus a preliminary "written opinion" on patentability pursuant to international standards. The PCT application is published with the ISR about 18 months after its priority date (Fig. 16.2).

At 18 or 2 months from the ISR, an applicant may optionally amend the claims. At 19 months the applicant may optionally request a supplementary international search to cover claims not searched by the ISA or to seek to turn up prior art in a language not used by the ISA. An applicant may optionally file a formal "demand" for an International Preliminary Examination pursuant to Chapter II of the PCT within 3 months after the ISR, or 22 months from the priority date, whichever is later. During the exam under Chapter II by an International Preliminary Examining Authority (typically an examiner at a selected national patent office), the applicant gets one or more chances to respond with an argument in favor of patentability and optionally submitting amendments to the claims.

For most countries, 30 months from the priority date is a crucial time. That is when the PCT procedure ends and the application is submitted for entry into a "national phase" patent prosecution. This typically means that the application is translated into the local language and filed

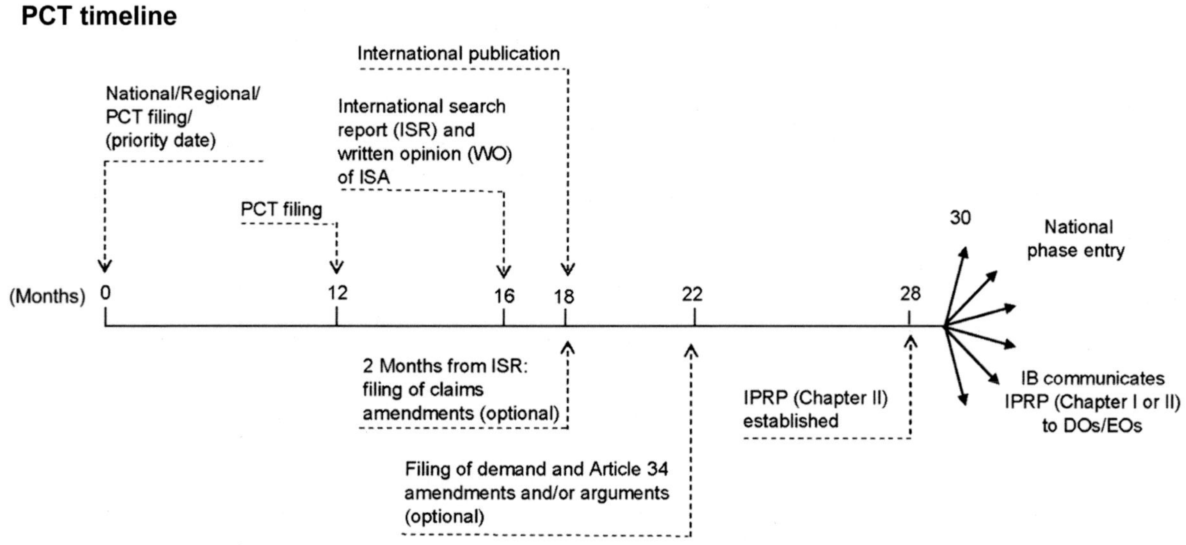

FIGURE 16.2 PCT timeline. *PCT*, Patent Cooperation Treaty.

with the local patent office by local patent practitioners pursuant to instructions from your patent counsel.

However, there are some small deviations from this rule-of-thumb. Some non-English-speaking countries, such as Israel, nevertheless accept English-language filings, avoiding translation costs. Other patent offices, including the European Patent Office, the Eurasian Patent Office, India, and Australia, accept such filings up to 31 months from the priority date. At this point, costs for patent filings typically range from about $1500 for an English-language application in Canada or Australia to about $6000 or more for a European, Chinese, or Japanese application. Thus to seek wide geographic coverage in, say, two dozen countries requires an investment of well over $100,000. Note, too, that most foreign countries impose annual fees ("annuities" or "maintenance fees") to maintain a patent application or patent in force, and many also require that a patent be "worked" or licensed locally. Typically, a patent expires 20 years from its local or PCT filing date, provided that maintenance fees are paid for the duration.

Freedom-to-Operate Studies of Third-Party Patents

At some point, your investors or board of directors may ask whether a proposed product comes within the claims of a particular patent of a competitor or other identified party. In that event, consider engaging patent counsel to determine the scope of the claims by obtaining and reviewing a copy of the prosecution history of the patent and the cited prior art. If the proposed product is not clearly outside the scope of the issued claims, the patent attorney would next seek to determine if any of the claims might be invalid (e.g., because of additional prior art not brought to the patent examiner's attention or perhaps due to a change in the law regarding patent-eligible subject matter since the application was examined). If counsel is able to provide an opinion that the proposed product does not infringe any valid claims of the patent, then it would benefit your company because generally a court would decline to award additional damages for "willful infringement," even if the court were to disagree with your counsel and find that the patent is infringed.

In 2007 the Federal Circuit stated in *In re Seagate* that enhanced damages for willful infringement of a patent requires clear and convincing evidence (1) that the infringer acted despite an objectively high likelihood that its actions constituted infringement of a valid patent and (2) that the infringer had knowledge (or should have known) of this risk.

Also, as part of the AIA, the Congress created a variety of new pathways for a business to challenge its rivals' pending applications and granted patents. It will be advantageous for your company to monitor patent applications as they are published to the Web (PA Pubs) for optimum advantage in selecting among the available options.

Patent Expiration

It used to be relatively simple to say when a US patent would expire: look at the date it was granted and add 17 years. (Except that the term could be truncated by a *terminal disclaimer* filed in the case to match the expiration to the term of a related patent.) But a law that took effect in 1995 has made the calculation more complicated, and another one that took effect in 2000 has created further changes.

Now, a newly issued patent generally expires 20 years after the date of filing of the earliest nonprovisional US patent application on which it relies, unless it is subject to a terminal disclaimer as mentioned earlier or unless it is entitled to *patent term adjustment* (PTA), for example, because the PTO took too long in some phases of patent prosecution while the applicant acted with relative diligence, or because the grant of the patent was delayed by an appeal or an interference proceeding in the PTO. Another way the patent term may have been extended would be because marketing was delayed by the Food and Drug Administration (FDA) clearance procedures—*patent term extension* (PTE) authorized under the Hatch-Waxman Act. For a drug first approved for marketing in the United States the term of a patent covering the drug may be extended by up to 5 years provided that certain conditions are met. After the PTE the patent term remaining at the date of FDA approval must not exceed 14 years. An application for PTE must be filed within a certain time limit after the FDA approval. Other countries including the EU countries, Japan, and others also have similar laws to allow PTE for delays by regulatory approval. The PTA and PTE calculations also presume that maintenance fees are paid within, respectively, 4, 8, and 12 years after the date the patent is granted. *Note:* it is often possible to reinstate a US patent if a maintenance fee deadline is inadvertently missed.

Contracts Relating to Intellectual Property

Who Owns the Invention?

When drafting, negotiating, or signing contracts involving your IP, beware that even a single word could make the difference between owning and not owning rights to a valuable technology. For example, in 2011 the US Supreme Court decided that Cetus Corporation, rather than Stanford University, had acquired the right to patent an invention by a Stanford faculty member that applies the PCR technique to test for HIV, the AIDS virus. When he began work for the university, the inventor had signed a form whereby he *agree[d] to assign* to Stanford his "right, title and interest in" inventions resulting from his employment at the University. On this basis, Stanford had filed and obtained three US patents relating to the invention.

The university technology transfer office had a rude awakening when it sought patent royalties for the HIV test from Roche (the successor to Cetus). Roche asserted in court the counterintuitive argument that a Cetus document governed ownership of the invention, even though the inventor had signed it *after* he had signed the Stanford University document.

The agreement with Cetus that the inventor had signed when he started the project had included language reciting not only that the inventor "will assign" but also that he *does hereby assign* to Cetus his "right, title, and interest in each of the ideas, inventions, and improvements" made as a consequence of his access to Cetus. Surprising to many, the courts held that even though the inventor had originally agreed with Stanford to make a future assignment of ownership of inventions, the Cetus document, worded in the present tense, was effective, *immediately upon signing*, to transfer to Cetus the inventor's ownership of any pertinent inventions he would *thereafter* make. So, although the inventor had later signed documents purporting to transfer to Stanford his ownership rights in the inventions, it was too late—he had already divested himself of those rights by the operation of the Cetus document.

The takeaway is to ask your IP lawyer to review even "boilerplate" forms to ensure they embody the latest version of the language that the courts have held to be effective [8].

Trade Secrets

As patents in the United States become more elusive for some biotechnology innovations, another tool for legal protection rises in ascendancy: *trade secrets.* To the greatest extent possible, biotechnology entrepreneurs should seek to protect their unique technological and marketing expertise. But because there isn't a government agency that registers trade secrets or a mandated form for recording them, the tools of *trade secrets* can be overlooked unless you keep it in mind. These tools are in the form of legal principles that apply in state courts, and now federal courts [9], and in virtually all foreign countries.

In general, a *trade secret* is information (including a formula, pattern, compilation, program, device, method, technique, or process) that (1) derives independent economic value from not being generally known to, and not being readily ascertainable by proper means by, other persons who can obtain economic value from its disclosure or use and (2) is the subject of efforts that are reasonable under the circumstances to maintain its secrecy.

The often-overlooked catch is that the company won't be entitled to enforce its trade secrets in court unless it can prove that it has used reasonable efforts to maintain secrecy. These efforts should include having pertinent confidentiality provisions in contracts with employees, contractors, suppliers, and sometimes customers. And it's essential to create a culture of respect within the company for the confidentiality of pertinent information.

Joint Research Projects

Most biotechnology start-ups collaborate with researchers from other companies or universities at some time during the development of their inventions. Federal law includes a curious judge-made doctrine called "secret prior art" that can disqualify from protection certain inventions that involve different people contributing to the invention over a timeframe, especially if they happen to work for different employers. In September 2005 the PTO issued its regulations implementing the CREATE Act, a law passed in December 2004 that permits such inventions to avoid the pitfall, but only if a qualifying joint research agreement was in place beforehand and the agreement is properly cited in the patent application.

Although the AIA now allows a business to be named as an *applicant* for a US patent, the law still requires including in the patent application as an inventor everyone who contributes materially to the subject matter of even one claim of the patent. And, as mentioned earlier, it may be appropriate to inform the PTO if your company has a joint research agreement in the field of the invention.

Copyrights

Good news: The *Stanford v. Roche* case (with its counter-intuitive result discussed earlier) doesn't apply to ownership of copyrights. Rather, your company automatically owns the copyright in the works of authorship (including text, graphics, and computer code) generated by its employees in the course of their assignments, even if they haven't signed an agreement about the subject. Bad news: the same isn't true for copyrightable subject matter generated by *independent contractors*, whether individuals or at another company. If a transfer of ownership of copyrighted subject matter is desired, it must be in writing, and optionally may be recorded at the US Copyright Office (an arm of the Library of Congress). Alternatively, a license, or *grant of permission* to use a copyrighted work, may be appropriate.

As soon as a work of authorship is fixed in a tangible medium of expression (e.g., written on paper or saved on a computer disk), it is protected by the US Copyright Act. The protection is automatic and does not require that you take any further action. However, it's desirable to take two steps (which are optional for new works) to gain additional protection. These two steps are (1) place a copyright notice on your work and (2) register the copyright with the US Copyright Office.

A copyright notice should look like this:

Copyright © [Year of first publication] [Name of copyright owner]. All rights reserved.

If the work is not published (i.e., offered for distribution to the general public), then leave out the year of first publication. Although a copyright notice is not absolutely required for any work first published on or after March 1, 1989, it's still desirable to put copyright notices on all copyrightable works generated in the United States.

The second step is to register your company's copyrights. You aren't required to register a copyright, but the law provides additional benefits to those who do so promptly. Moreover, you cannot sue an infringer in court unless and until you have received a certificate of copyright registration for your work. If you file an application for copyright registration before someone infringes your work, or within 3 months of the date your work is first published (if your work is published), then you receive two additional benefits that you would not otherwise have.

The first additional benefit is that the federal court may award you money toward your *attorney's fees*. The second additional benefit is that you may request the court to award "statutory" damages instead of any actual damages that your company proves to have suffered. *Statutory damages* are preferred when you cannot prove that you actually lost money or when you have lost a relatively small amount. The judge may then award statutory damages somewhere between $750 and $30,000 per work. If you prove the infringer *willfully infringed* the copyright, then the judge may award up to $150,000 of statutory damages per work.

As mentioned earlier, if the work of authorship is created by an independent contractor, your company does not automatically own the copyright. Make sure that agreements with independent contractors fully protect your business if you wish to own the copyright outright. Unfortunately, this fine point is frequently overlooked with independent contractors developing computer software, sometimes leading to misunderstandings and expensive litigation.

Trademarks

Attorneys use the term "trademark" to refer to any design, word, or combination of words and designs used in connection with the products or services of a business. Technically, the term "service mark" is used for designations of services, but a service mark is just one type of trademark. One kind of trademark that we've mentioned earlier is a *brand name*, especially as contrasted with the generic name that's also adopted for the active ingredient or new chemical entity (NCE) (see next for further discussion).

As soon as you start using your trademark, your company may customarily employ the symbol "TM" to designate a trademark for goods and the symbol "SM" to designate a service mark for services.

If you desire to protect your trademarks, engage your IP counsel to do a search to find out if the proposed marks are available. It's typical to search not only the database of federal trademark registrations and applications but also state trademark registrations and selected foreign jurisdictions. Many of these databases are organized for searching alphabetically for "direct hits" and also phonetic sound-alikes as well as for suffixes and prefixes. Your attorney will use the search results to initially evaluate whether your proposed trademarks are "confusingly similar" to the trademarks of your prospective competitors.

It's desirable to supplement those search results with other databases and Internet search engines to look for similar marks used by companies that haven't yet *registered* their marks. Under US law, these companies may have developed *common law* rights by using their trademarks.

Bases for Filing a Trademark Application: Intent-to-Use or Actual Use

The US trademark law was amended in 1989 to allow you to file an application based on your *bona fide* (good faith) intent to start using your trademark in the future. You may file an *intent-to-use* application even before you place your trademark on goods. By comparison, you may only file an *actual use* application after your company has used the trademark in interstate commerce, such as by shipping your goods to a customer in another state or by advertising your services to those in another state.

Trademark Prosecution

Within about 6 months after your application for trademark registration is filed, an attorney in the PTO searches registered marks and pending federal applications for any that may be confusingly similar to your trademark. The PTO attorney also examines the application for compliance with various technical and legal standards. Many times, the PTO attorney raises questions or objections to one or more aspects of the application, and your attorney may file a response. When and if the PTO attorney finds no further barriers to grant your application, the PTO will publish your mark in the *Official Gazette of the PTO*. Then, for a month or so, others who may have adopted a similar mark will have the opportunity to challenge your right to register your mark. If your mark is challenged, then the PTO conducts an administrative trial to determine the matter. If there is no challenge, your application would proceed to the next stage.

If your company has filed an "actual use" application, then the PTO registers your trademark and issues a certificate of registration. If the application is an "intent-to-use" application, then the PTO will not register your trademark until your attorney files your sworn statement documenting that the mark has actually gone into bona fide use in interstate commerce.

The ® Symbol

Once the PTO issues the certificate of trademark registration, your company may then use the symbol ® in connection with the mark, or alternatively the term *Reg. U.S. Pat. and T.M. Off.* (which is more cumbersome). Until you receive a certificate of trademark registration, use the TM and SM symbols.

This completes the registration process. Once the PTO issues a registration, you generally won't need to bother with this registration for another 5 years. Between the fifth and sixth anniversaries of the registration date, you would need to file an affidavit that your company is still using the trademark in connection with the same goods and services. If the "affidavit of use" is not filed during that time, the registration is canceled (although you could afterward seek to reregister your trademark).

US Trademark Affidavit of Use and Incontestability

Further, if your trademark had not been found invalid or was not in litigation at the time that you filed the affidavit of use or at the end of any 5-year period, your attorney could file an "affidavit of incontestability," either by itself or as part of the same transaction as the affidavit of use. An affidavit of incontestability provides additional rights in case your company needs to sue a trademark infringer. The infringer would have a higher standard to overcome to battle you in court as the validity of your trademark would be "incontestable."

Trademarks for Pharma/BioTech Products

There are a few additional requirements in order to clear and adopt a particular product name for the pharmaceutical industry. Drug products must satisfy not only prohibitions against deceptiveness and likelihood of confusion examined by the PTO, but they must also satisfy requirements administered by the US FDA [10]. Each of these agencies conducts a distinct and independent review, and only when all parties are satisfied, is the proposed mark fully cleared for use. The reason for the extra scrutiny is safety. Pharmaceutical mistakes have the potential to cause serious damage, illness, or death when drug names look alike or sound alike, or there is a carelessness, lack of knowledge of drug names, poor handwriting, or human error between physicians, pharmacists, and patients.

The PTO recognizes the need for safety regarding pharmaceuticals and applies the doctrine of greater care[7] in the prosecution of trademark applications for ethical pharmaceuticals because confusion here may have life-and-death consequences.

As the naming process runs its course, each new pharmaceutical product would acquire three names: a chemical name (the CAS registry number for the compound, e.g., 85721-33-1); a generic, nonproprietary name (e.g., ciprofloxacin); and a trademark or brand name (e.g., CIPRO).

The applicant must first propose to the United States Adopted Name (USAN) Council a *generic (or nonproprietary) name* for the product, providing chemical information and medical indications [11]. The USAN Council reviews the proposed generic name for characteristics, such as appropriateness for the drug, adherence to nomenclature rules, suitability for routine use both in the United States and internationally, not being misleading or confusing or implying efficacy or application to particular anatomical parts, and being distinctive from other drug names.

When the USAN Council assigns a generic name to the product, that name is sent for final approval to the World Health Organization International Nonproprietary Name (INN) Committee [12]. The INN suggests that word elements from biochemical nomenclature (such as *feron* from interferon or *leukin* from interleukin) be used as stems for generic terms within a scheme of drug nomenclature adopted by the INN. In contrast, drug trademarks should avoid incorporating such INN stems.

The selection of trademarks for pharmaceutical products in the United States is complicated by the requirement that two different federal agencies—the PTO and the FDA—review and approve such marks. The PTO examination has been described earlier. The review process at the FDA starts when an applicant files a *request for proprietary name review*, coordinated by the Division of Medication Error Prevention and Analysis (DMEPA). The DMEPA would look at similar trademarks for products currently on the market and those in the development pipeline. They often perform studies with simulated prescriptions to guard against the misreading of handwritten prescriptions and consider similar terms among common medical terminology.

As the pharmaceutical approval cycle can be a lengthy process, consider registering a trademark first for R&D services as well as for the drug product itself.

US Trademark Renewal

A US trademark registration is valid for 10 years provided that the registrant documents continuing use of the trademark by the end of the sixth year. To renew the registration a renewal application with an affidavit of continued use must be filed between 1 year before the anniversary to 6 months after the anniversary.

Foreign Trademark Registration

It's desirable to register your trademarks in other countries in which you plan to do business. There is a European Trademark Office in Alicante, Spain. In 2003 the United States became a party to the Madrid Protocol, a trademark treaty that corresponds somewhat to the PCT. There are certain advantages and disadvantages of the procedures available under the Madrid System. Moreover, if a trademark application is filed in a foreign country within 6 months from the day it is filed in the United States, it is generally able to get a right-of-priority under the Paris Convention based on the filing date of the US application. Thus it is desirable to make such choices within this timeframe.

Recording Trademarks, Copyrights, and Trade Names With US Customs

To help protect against the importation of products that infringe your IP rights, your business may record your rights with the Bureau of Customs and Border Protection (CBP) in the United States Department of Homeland Security. This option is available for trademarks registered on the principal register at the US PTO, copyrights registered with the US Copyright Office, and trade names (i.e., the names of businesses) that have been in use for at least 6 months.

An application to record your trademark, copyright, or trade name can be submitted on paper or electronically. As mentioned previously, trademarks and copyrights must be federally registered before they are eligible for recordation, and the CBP automatically accepts such registrations as valid.

Pharmaceutical Patents and Market Exclusivity

Every new drug can cost hundreds of millions of dollars to develop and the risk of failure is very high. Thus there must be adequate patent exclusivity for a new drug to incentivize investment in drug development. Indeed, that

7. See TMEP §1207.01(d)(xii) re Pharmaceuticals or Medicinal Products.

patents stimulate innovation and reward risk-taking is best exemplified in the pharmaceutical area. In 1984 the Congress enacted the Drug Price Competition and Patent Term Restoration Act of 1984 (a.k.a. the *Hatch-Waxman Act*) that provides the most important components of the regulatory frame for pharmaceutical exclusivity in the United States.

Notably, the Hatch-Waxman Act provides significant incentives for generic drug makers to challenge drug patents long before their expiration dates. With minimal cost associated with generic drug approval contrasted with the significant investment required for de novo drug development, it is no wonder that patent challenges by generic drug companies became the drug developers' nightmare and are the main focus of their patent strategies.

As mentioned earlier, a *generic drug* is a copycat of a *brand-name drug*. It has the same active pharmaceutical ingredient (API) as the corresponding brand-name drug and is supposed to be bioequivalent to it. A generic drug is approved by the US FDA based on a so-called Abbreviated New Drug Application (ANDA), which relies on the preclinical and clinical data of the copied brand-name drug generated by the original developer.

In fact the FDA requires the prescription drug labeling of the generic drug to be largely identical to that of the brand-name drug. For this reason, unlike many other technical areas, patents for an innovative drug having relatively narrow claims may provide adequate protection against generic drug competition. Innovative drug developers should not overlook incremental inventions and should endeavor to obtain patents covering as many as possible novel inventions reflected (or to be reflected) in the prescription drug labeling of a new drug.

Examples of such patentable inventions include the API and variants thereof (including advantageous racemates or enantiomers, polymorphs, salt forms, solvates, and prodrugs, as well as metabolites of the API produced in the patient's body), pharmaceutical compositions containing the API, methods of use (based on use of the API or pharmaceutical composition in specific disease indications, patient populations, lines of therapy, combination therapies, biomarker-based or personalized treatment, dosing regimens, administration route, advantageous pharmacokinetic profiles to be achieved, etc.), formulations (immediate or extended release formulations, special delivery forms such as transdermal or buccal delivery forms and nasal spray), dosage units, coformulations for combination therapies, advantageous purity or impurity characterization of the API or pharmaceutical compositions, methods of making the API or formulations or dosage units, advantageous packaging, etc.

Even if the recent *Myriad* decision was to be read to cast doubt on the patent eligibility of purified natural products (e.g., natural proteins, isolated genes, and small molecules discovered in natural sources), pharmaceutical compositions comprising them should still be patent-eligible. New drug developers should create and seize every opportunity to seek patent protection on all drug-related inventions at every stage of the drug-development process. In this way a comprehensive patent portfolio may be established to provide multiple layers of patent protection around the new drug.

Strategically, for a new drug with an NCE, it is preferable to postpone the publication of the chemical structure or identity of the NCE, typically until after completion of a Phase II trial, lest the publication be construed as prior art that interferes with patenting later incremental inventions.[8] Delaying publication of the chemical structure may also reduce the possibility that third parties experiment with the same compound and publish or seek to patent their results. Such publications by third parties would also create prior art adverse to the developer's future patent filings. In addition, third-party patents may interfere with the innovator's patent strategies and even impinge upon the innovator's freedom to commercialize the drug.

To maximize patent terms, drug developers should make full use of the PTA and PTE provisions of the US patent law. Specifically, the US patent statute requires the PTO to adjust the term of a patent to compensate for certain delays during patent prosecution caused by the PTO. In addition, the Hatch-Waxman Act provides for an extension of a selected patent covering a newly approved drug to compensate for the regulatory delay in the FDA. For a drug with an annual sale of $365 million, each extra day at the back end of the patent term means the protection of $1 million sales. It is no wonder that *The Wall Street Journal* proclaimed "The most profitable activity an NDA holder can engage in is delaying approval of a generic" [13].

Importantly, the FDA publishes the *Orange Book* listing specific patents the new drug developer certifies to cover the approved new drug [14]. A generic must overcome all patents listed in the Orange Book for a particular new drug before its ANDA for a generic drug can be approved by the FDA. So it is important to list as many drug-related patents in the Orange Book to create more barriers to generic competition. Not all kinds of patents related to a new drug can be listed in the Orange Book. Patents covering the drug compound, formulations of the drug, or methods of treating diseases by administering the

8. If you pursue an international patent strategy, keep in mind that you won't be able to avoid having your own disclosure published 18 months from its priority date.

drug may be listed. But patents claiming manufacturing processes, metabolites, intermediates, or packaging are not listable.

Market Protection via Regulatory Exclusivity

New drugs may also be protected by *regulatory exclusivity*, that is, exclusive marketing rights granted by the FDA under certain conditions. Regulatory exclusivity is independent of patents and can run concurrently with patents. There are several important types of regulatory exclusivity: orphan drug exclusivity, pediatric exclusivity (PE), and data exclusivity. *Orphan drug* exclusivity is granted by the FDA under the Orphan Drug Act of 1983 for products to treat rare diseases and conditions affecting fewer than 200,000 patients in the United States. It prohibits approval of another application "for such drug for such disease or condition" for 7 years after the initial product approval, except for a "clinically superior" product that uses the "same active moiety." *PE* is granted by the FDA to extend by 6 months the expiration dates of other forms of exclusivity (e.g., patent, orphan exclusivity, or data exclusivity) if the new drug developer conducts pediatric trials of the drug.

Data exclusivity granted by the FDA is another important aspect of the new drug protection framework. Also sometimes referred to as *marketing exclusivity*, this form of protection prohibits, during a defined period of time after new drug approval, any reliance by a third party on the data generated for the new drug for purposes of obtaining approval of a generic. Data exclusivity is independent of, and supplements, patent protection. An NCE approved for the first time for commercial marketing in the United States is entitled to a 5-year data exclusivity.

When the FDA approval of a new drug is not the first permitted commercial marketing or use of the product in the United States, a 3-year marketing exclusivity is granted. The FDA grants a 3-year marketing exclusivity for a combination drug if one of the coformulated APIs was previously approved for marketing or use in the United States. Similarly, an enantiomer drug is entitled to only 3 years of marketing exclusivity from the FDA if the racemate was previously approved for marketing in the United States. An exception to this is that an amendment to the Food Drug and Cosmetic Act in 2007 provides a 5-year marketing exclusivity for a new drug wherein the API is an enantiomer of a previously approved racemate drug, provided that the enantiomer drug has undergone independent clinical trials and is approved for a completely different indication from that of the racemate drug.[9]

With a 5-year data exclusivity, a prospective competitor seeking approval of a generic may not file an ANDA during the 5 years after the FDA's approval for marketing of the brand-name drug. But if a patent covering the brand-name drug is listed in the Orange Book, a generic manufacturer may file an ANDA 4 years after the FDA's approval of the brand-name drug, certifying that the patents in the Orange Book are either invalid or not infringed or that approval to market the generic is not sought until after the patent expiration. Once a certification of patent invalidity or patent noninfringement is made, the brand-name developer is empowered to start a patent infringement suit in a US district court against the ANDA filer. If such a patent litigation is initiated, the FDA by law must stay the approval of the ANDA for 30 months. The stay may be extended by a court to provide a total of 7.5 years from initial NDA approval to the time of ANDA approval.

With 3-year data exclusivity, a prospective competitor may file an ANDA with the FDA, but the ANDA may not be approved until 3 years after the marketing approval of the brand-name drug. The filing of an ANDA may also trigger patent infringement litigation under the Hatch-Waxman Act as described earlier.

Generic drug makers have a strong incentive to challenge the relevant patents in the Orange Book, as the first filer of an ANDA who successfully challenges the patents will be entitled to a 180-day exclusivity to market the generic. So a developer of new drugs needs to implement comprehensive strategies to build a strong patent estate, erecting as many entry barriers as possible to protect market exclusivity (Fig. 16.3).

Regulatory Approvals for Biologics and Biosimilars

Note that *biologics* are approved under a different regulatory regime. Biologics are biological products including, for example, recombinant proteins, antibodies, vaccines, gene and cell therapies, and blood and blood components. Commercial marketing of biologics requires the approval by the FDA of a *biologic license application.* In addition to patent protection, the orphan drug exclusivity and PE discussed earlier are applicable to biologics. The Biologics Price Competition and Innovation Act enacted in 2010 for the first time provides an abbreviated regulatory pathway for *biosimilars* and a regulatory framework similar to that for new drugs under the Hatch-Waxman Act.

The FDA has issued three guidance documents to help sponsors comply with the BPCIA. First, on December 28, 2016, the FDA issued Guidance for Industry on Clinical

9. Public Law 110-85, codified as 21 U.S.C. § 355(u)(1) (Supp. II 2008)

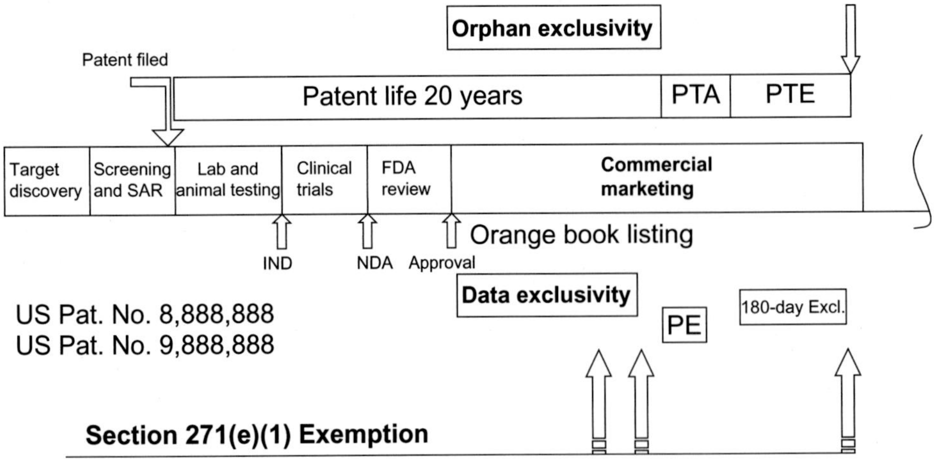

FIGURE 16.3 Market protection via regulatory exclusivity.

Pharmacology Data to Support a Demonstration of Biosimilarity to a Reference Product, which assists sponsors with the design and use of clinical pharmacology studies to support that a proposed product is biosimilar to a known reference product. Nonproprietary naming conventions for products are discussed in the January 12, 2017 FDA document *Nonproprietary Naming of Biological Products*. On January 17, 2017 the FDA issued a guidance document *Considerations in Demonstrating Interchangeability with a Reference Product* regarding what is required to demonstrate that a proposed biosimilar is interchangeable with its reference product (see Ref. [15]).

Diagnostics and Personalized Medicine

The advent of personalized medicine is making the diagnostic industry ever more attractive to investors. By definition, personalized medicine requires that preventive or treatment measures be tailored to a particular patient. This customized approach necessarily depends on molecular diagnostic tests to determine a patient's genetic or molecular markers which are *correlated* to clinically useful disease characters. The significant investment and substantial risk involved in the discovery, development, and implementation of diagnostic tests mandate strong patent protection. Ironically, some recent court decisions in the United States have significantly weakened patent protection in the field and will tend to impede future efforts to patent some aspects of such tests.

Generally speaking, diagnostic tests have two fundamental components: (1) one or more biomarkers to be detected or measured and (2) the correlation between the biomarker(s) and disease characters. Patents on the composition of matter of a biomarker molecule would essentially exclude others from making or using the same biomarker and thus would offer the strongest protection for a diagnostic test.

In addition, patent claims to the use of a correlation for diagnosis (not limited to any specific detection technique) could also provide strong protection for a diagnostic test. Many times, a biomarker can be detected by many different alternative techniques or equipment. Thus patent claims reciting a specific detection technique or equipment often can be circumvented (*designed around*) and thus might not provide the desired exclusivity for the overall diagnostic test. See the discussion below the US Supreme Court decision in March 2012 of *Mayo Collaborative Services v. Prometheus Laboratories*.

In this post–Human Genome Project era, almost the entirety of the human genome, and most of its encoded proteins, as well as the general methods of analyzing such molecular markers, are public knowledge (prior art). Thus most molecular markers, for example, genes or proteins, wouldn't be patentable as novel molecular entities.

Exacerbating the situation, the US Supreme Court's 2013 case *Association for Molecular Pathology v. Myriad Genetics, Inc.* excludes from patent-eligible subject matter even newly discovered and isolated genes. Specifically, in *Myriad*, the Court was asked to review claims to various "isolated and purified nucleic acids" and address the question whether such molecules are eligible for patenting under the US patent law.[10] In the 1990s, Myriad Genetics and its collaborators (including the NIH, the University of

10. Section 101 of the US Patent Law, 35 U.S.C. § 101, provides, in part: "Whoever invents or discovers any new and useful process, machine, manufacture, or composition of matter, or any new and useful improvement thereof, may obtain a patent therefore, subject to the conditions and requirements of [title 35 of the U.S. Code]." Court decisions interpreting this provision include man-made organisms within patent-eligible subject matter but expressly exclude laws of nature, abstract ideas, and mathematical concepts.

Utah, and others) successfully located in the human genome the *BRCA1* and *BRCA2* genes and identified particular mutations that are associated with the predisposition to breast and ovarian cancer. They determined the nucleotide sequences of the genes, filed patent applications, and were later granted patents for isolated nucleic acids including those gene sequences. For years, these patents provided exclusive rights for Myriad to perform mutation testing in *BRCA1* and *BRCA2* genes (i.e., its BRCAnalysis test).

However, in 2009, a group of plaintiffs including several medical associations and clinical geneticists filed suit seeking a declaration that Myriad's patents are invalid under 35 U.S.C. §101 [16]. The plaintiffs asserted that the isolated genes have the same sequence information as the corresponding genes or mRNA in cells and are products of nature that are ineligible for patenting. The Supreme Court, in a unanimous decision, held that while cDNA different from naturally occurring DNA is eligible for patenting, isolated genes are not eligible for patent protection because they are not "new 'with markedly different characteristics from any found in nature.' " The decision concludes that "Separating that gene from its surrounding genetic material is not an act of invention".[11] Thus under *Myriad*, isolated, naturally occurring DNA is no longer patent-eligible in the United States, and most previously granted claims to isolated genes are invalid.

Even though the *Myriad* decision applies expressly just to isolated genes, characterizing them as unique due to their information content, it also renders uncertain at this point the patent eligibility of other naturally occurring biomolecules, such as isolated or purified peptides, proteins, mRNA, miRNAs, siRNA, metabolites, antibodies, organic molecules, and others [17]. Under that rationale, mere isolation and purification of natural substances would not make such substances patent-eligible in the United States.

As the law of the land in the United States, *Myriad* has generated a significant impact on the diagnostic industry [18]. The *Myriad* decision essentially precludes the patenting of molecular biomarkers as most biomarkers for diagnostic tests are molecules naturally occurring and detectable in human tissue or bodily fluid samples. Inventors and their patent attorneys would need to be really creative to gain meaningful patents on naturally occurring biomarkers. For example, if a novel protein as a biomarker has to be detected immunologically with an antibody, then a protein–antibody complex could be patent-eligible if it does not exist in nature. Similarly, one may patent an artificial complex of an mRNA or miRNA with a primer or probe if the complex necessarily forms in a diagnostic test. In tests that require multiple biomarkers, such as prognostic gene signatures, a composition comprising two or more biomarkers, may be claimed, although such patent claims may be circumvented by the separate measurement of the biomarkers before combining the results in the same computer analysis algorithm. Of course, one may also patent diagnostic kits containing a combination of multiple components required for performing a diagnostic test. While these patent claims are not as strong as a composition of matter claim for a single biomarker, they can provide extra layers of picket fences around the exclusive territory of a diagnostic test.

As discussed previously, beside biomarkers, the other fundamental component of a diagnostic test is the correlation between the biomarker(s) and disease characters. When strong patent protection for biomarkers is unavailable, it would have been important to obtain broad patent protection for the application of the correlation in diagnosis. Before the Supreme Court decided the *Mayo v. Prometheus* case in 2012,[12] it was commonplace to obtain a patent claim to a diagnosis method based on a newly discovered correlation in the following format:

> *A method of diagnosing disease X, comprising determining the presence or absence [or amount] of a biomarker Y in patient, and correlating the presence [or the amount above a level W] of the biomarker Y with disease X in the patient.*

Note that this patent claim would be infringed regardless of what technique is used in analyzing the biomarker Y in a patient sample. However, the *Mayo* decision made claims such as this essentially ineligible for patenting.

According to the Supreme Court, the correlation between the biomarker and the disease is an unpatentable law of nature, and "simply appending conventional steps, specified at a high level of generality, to laws of nature, natural phenomena, and abstract ideas cannot make those laws, phenomena, and ideas patentable." After *Mayo*, the method claim in the earlier example would most likely have to be modified to recite additional details with specificity in order to become patent-eligible. Any additional specifics would necessarily narrow the scope of the claim and thereby detract from the protection that otherwise would have been afforded by the patent.

The PTO and courts are still struggling to articulate a clear standard to determine the patent eligibility of method claims that appear to embrace a "law of nature." As the case law and guidance from the PTO evolves, you'll want to seek ongoing advice from a trusted patent attorney who keeps abreast of such developments.

In the era of companion diagnostics, diagnostic method claims may be alternatively drafted in the form of

11. Association for Molecular Pathology v. Myriad Genetics, Inc., 569 U. S. 576 (2013) (citing Diamond v. Chakrabarty, 447 U. S. 303, 310(1980)).
12. Mayo Collaborative Services v. Prometheus Laboratories, Inc., 566 U. S. 66; March 20, 2012.

the method of treating diseases. The following is a hypothetical example:

A method of treating breast cancer, comprising detecting Her2 expression in a breast tumor tissue sample from a patient using an antibody immunologically reactive with Her2 protein, and administering trastuzumab to the patient if Her2 expression is detected to be positive.

Such a method-of-treatment claim may be eligible for listing in the FDA's Orange Book and thus provide an effective entry barrier against generic drug competition. Note that the abovementioned method claim includes two steps that, in reality, often are practiced by two different entities. The first step would typically be done by a diagnostic lab and the second by a doctor or patient. However, for a patent claim to be infringed, US courts generally require that all steps in the claim be performed by a single entity or at least by related entities acting in concert. Under that rubric, it would appear that none of the pertinent actors is infringing the patent claim.

This dilemma was posed in a series of court decisions involving the case of *Akamai Technologies, Inc. v. Limelight Networks, Inc.* The ultimate decision (*Akamai V*) held that in order for direct patent infringement to be established when different actors perform steps of the claim, a single entity is responsible for the performance of the steps and that entity "directs or controls' others' performance," or when "the actors form a joint enterprise." Further, directing or controlling others' performance includes circumstances in which an alleged infringer (1) "conditions participation in an activity or receipt of a benefit upon performance of a step or steps of a patented method" and (2) "establishes the manner or timing of that performance." The takeaway is that it's desirable to craft claims with steps that are all going to be performed by an individual or single entity but that sometimes "direction or control" or a "joint enterprise" can be proven under the circumstances.[13]

This issue arose in a medical context in *Eli Lilly v. Teva Parenterals Medicines Inc.* [19]. In that case the Federal Circuit agreed that both physician prescribing information and patient information can be used as evidence to show direct and induced infringement.

Other than biomarkers and general methods of using correlations, there may be many other patentable aspects in a new diagnostic test. Examples may include detection techniques, hardware equipment (e.g., chips, machines, and magnetic beads), reagents, labeled probes and primers, synthetic primers and probes with nonnaturally occurring nucleotide sequences, and diagnostic kits. Depending on the circumstances, patents on these aspects can also provide valuable protection for a diagnostic test. One dramatic example is the original patents on the PCR technique issued to Cetus Corp., which were sold in 1991 to Hoffmann-La Roche for $300 million (for all uses except DNA forensics).

It is also important to bear in mind that although isolated genes and other biomolecules have been ruled to be unpatentable in the United States and Australia, carefully crafted claims to pertinent inventions and discoveries may still be patent-eligible in some other countries, such as the EU countries, Canada, China, Japan, and South Korea. When in doubt, check with local patent counsel on a current basis.

As a generality, patent claims to methods of using correlations, although unpatentable in the United States, are routinely granted by the European Patent Office and in other countries [20]. In China, although methods of diagnosing diseases as a category are unpatentable subject matter, such method inventions may be patentable when presented in so-called Swiss use claims. For example, if a previously known mutation in a gene is discovered to be correlated with an increased risk of cancer, then a claim may be drafted, for example, as follows:

Use of a primer or probe hybridizing to gene X for the manufacture of diagnostic reagents useful for detecting mutation Y in gene X and for diagnosing an increased risk of cancer in a human subject.

As an entrepreneur seeking to fashion a worldwide IP strategy to develop and market a novel biotechnology product or service, you may come to envy the relative certainty of the croquet match in Wonderland fantasized by Lewis Carroll, even though Alice had to use a flamingo as a mallet seeking to strike a live hedgehog as the ball [21].

In summary, recent changes in the US patent law have significantly weakened patent protection in the diagnostic field. Nonetheless, with creative strategies and attention to detail, entrepreneurs and businesses may still be able to obtain patents on their diagnostic tests and erect significant barriers to entry by their competitors. If foreign markets are part of the business strategies, then comprehensive foreign patent claims should be actively pursued.

Corporate Intellectual Property Management

For entrepreneurs starting a biotechnology business, IP is often the most important asset that attracts investors and

13. Akamai Technologies, Inc. v. LimelightNetworks, Inc. (Akamai V), 797 F.3d 1020 (Fed. Cir. 2015) (en banc)(per curiam).

justifies the endeavor. Entrepreneurs should ensure that the core IP asset is adequately protected. Ideally, entrepreneurs should seek help from experts in patent law even before the formation of the business, and of course as the business grows. It is often valuable to have an experienced patent attorney as a close adviser, for example, as an interested cofounder, on the board, or as a regular consultant of the biotech start-up. Comprehensive patent strategies should be designed and implemented from the very beginning of the start-up business. A law firm or an outside attorney should be hired to advise on patent issues and prepare and prosecute patent applications. As the start-up grows, there will be an increased amount of IP-related legal work, and at some point it might be time to hire an in-house counsel. There are two main factors to consider to justify hiring an in-house IP counsel: cost saving and value creation. For example, when outside IP legal fees (excluding government fees) per year become high enough, say about US $200,000–300,000, it might make economic sense to hire an in-house IP counsel. However, the more important factor to bear in mind is the value added by having a patent attorney stationed in the office, proactively managing IP assets and providing practical IP advice.

Indeed, an in-house IP attorney or IP department may perform a wide variety of functions within a biotechnology company. These include working with management to establish IP policies and strategies, setting up and managing necessary IP-related infrastructures and procedures, providing necessary IP-related training to the relevant company personnel, conducting patent preparation and prosecution, providing IP-related counseling to inventors and business people, resolving IP disputes and enforcing IP rights against infringers, reviewing and negotiating IP-related agreements, and, in some cases, participating in business development and licensing negotiations.

To begin with, a biotechnology company should establish IP-related policies and strategies that are tailored to the business strategy and needs. For example, IP-related policies and strategies may include policies on rewarding inventors for their inventions, ownership of inventions and patents, confidentiality obligations, invention reporting obligations, policies on scientific publication and public announcement of R&D results, patent clearance and noninfringement policies, legal fee policies, general patent filing strategies, and IP dispute resolution strategies. The IP department needs to set up the necessary infrastructures and procedures to implement the policies and strategies. For example, employment agreements should be prepared and signed by all employees clearly defining the ownership of inventions by employees, employees' confidentiality obligation, and, if appropriate, a noncompete covenant. Procedures should be in place to prevent the publication of valuable inventions before a patent application is filed to protect them. In addition, a company should also have a customary procedure for inventors to disclose their inventions to the IP department to be considered for patenting. The IP department may also want to conduct regular training sessions for employees to promote awareness of their IP-related obligations and ensure timely disclosure of inventions.

In many companies, in-house patent attorneys do little hands-on patent drafting and prosecution before the US PTO but farm out most of such work to outside law firms. In this approach the in-house patent attorney acts as a liaison between the inventors within the company and the outside law firm and supervises the outside attorneys' work. However, companies increasingly move patent preparation and prosecution work in-house. This is especially true in medium-to-large biotech and pharmaceutical companies whose IP departments can match small-to-medium patent law firms in size and functions. Biotech and pharmaceutical companies typically rely on patents much more than businesses in any other industries, and a large in-house patent preparation and prosecution group is often justifiably economical and adds substantial value: in-house patent attorneys are integrated closely with the R&D departments within the company and are narrowly focused on the company's technologies and business and thus have a better understanding of the technologies and business goals in the company. In addition, they are not so constrained by billable hours and profit margins that outside attorneys have to be concerned about. Of course, outside counsel have their own advantages in that they deal with a wider variety of clients and gain more diverse experience which may prove beneficial in problem-solving and creative patent strategies.

A biotech company should encourage in-house counsel to integrate closely with its different functional groups, such as the R&D, business development, manufacturing, and marketing teams, and to have regular meetings and exchanges with these groups. In the process, in-house counsel will be able to keep up with the company business, contribute their patent expertise and perspective, and capture inventions to strengthen the company's IP portfolio. To illustrate, ideally in-house counsel should participate in R&D projects by regularly attending R&D meetings even at the project's planning stage and follow through the entire process of the project. This way, the patent counsel will be able to gain a good understanding of the project, the technologies, and the marketing and business strategies. In turn, the counsel can advise the R&D group during the entire process, helping to further the business goals. For example, at the planning stage, the in-house counsel can help the R&D group make informed decisions for pursuing the project, for example, by raising issues, such as potential patent infringement risks associated with the technology to be used or with the expected product to be developed, competitive intelligence on patent landscape, or the patentability of the expected product. These factors may either strengthen or undermine the justification for the project. During the project, by close interaction with the R&D group, the counsel will be able to timely spot potential IP risks and capture patentable inventions that scientists might otherwise miss. Creative patent counsel should even be able to suggest certain experiments to do to generate new patents or support existing patent strategies. While some scientists might view such advice as "the tail wagging the dog," patents are so crucial to most biotech and pharmaceutical companies that sometimes the dog had better be wagged by the little tail.

Many in-house patent attorneys also spend a significant amount of time providing legal advice to the company on diverse issues such as freedom-to-operate patent clearance to avoid patent infringement, patent due diligence in business transactions, and IP-related contract negotiations. In many biotech companies, it is the patent attorneys who are put in charge of licensing and business development functions besides IP responsibilities. Indeed, as IP is the underlying basis in most licensing and business alliances in biotech, business-savvy patent attorneys are a natural fit for such functions—in-house patent attorneys understand the technologies, the sophisticated IP strategies, as well as the business goals, and thus can have a better grasp of the IP-related subtleties and pitfalls in such business negotiations. Moreover, negotiation skills fostered in law school and honed by experience in the field can also be put to good use in this function.

Patent Strategies and Product Life Cycle Management

Patents are crucial to biotechnology companies in recouping the significant investment often required to get a product developed and marketed. Patents are also critical in maintaining a competitive edge in the face of competition. Thus it is important for entrepreneurs and biotech companies to build a strong patent portfolio around their products and manage product life cycle to maximize the exclusivity on the products. These require sophisticated patent strategies and expertise. Close collaboration between R&D personnel and patent attorneys is also needed. Biotech businesses should avoid becoming complacent when a first patent covering a product is granted but rather would do well to strive to build a portfolio of multiple patents and patent families covering the product. Ideally, the company will pursue multiple patents with stacked patent terms in an effort to extend the life of patent protection. Timing for filing patent applications is also important. For products that take a long time to develop, consider delaying the filing of some patents so as to maximize the overlap between the patent term and the commercialization stage of the product life. But beware that delayed patent filing incurs the risk of losing the first-to-file priority status and thus the right to obtain such a patent vis-à-vis another worker in your field. Timing in filings is also important in minimizing prior art, as well as avoiding creating prior art against the company's other patents covering the same product.

Roche's PCR patent portfolio is a good example of successful IP strategies. After Hoffmann-La Roche acquired the fundamental PCR patents from Cetus Corporation, it proceeded to acquire and file additional patents and built a comprehensive patent portfolio. In particular, this patent portfolio includes a large number of patents with different expiration dates covering different aspects of the PCR process and its various applications, including the basic PCR method, the PCR process using thermostable polymerases, purified *Taq* polymerase enzyme, recombinant *Taq* polymerase and fragments, PCR machine and method for performing automated PCR amplification, thermostable reverse transcriptase, real-time PCR, *Taq*Man probes, *Taq*Man-based real-time PCR method, and others. These patents formed thick picket fences around the PCR technology since the late 1980s, with patent expiration dates between 2005 and 2017 or later. This patent portfolio has largely withstood patent challenges and generated hundreds of millions of dollars for Roche.

Merck's patent coverage on Fosamax illustrates a sound pharmaceutical patent strategy in a difficult situation. Fosamax was Merck's blockbuster drug for treating osteoporosis. Its active ingredient alendronate sodium was already publicly known by the time the Italian company Instituto Gentili, Merck's licensor, discovered its use in treating osteoporosis in 1982, and thus there was no patent available on the chemical compound itself or even a pharmaceutical composition thereof. Instituto Gentili filed for a "method-of-use" patent in 1984 and was granted a US patent in 1986. After Merck licensed the program, it created multiple patents with stacked patent terms, extending exclusivity until 2008. In addition to the original method-of-use patent it licensed, Merck filed a number of patents on processes for the preparation of alendronate. It also obtained patent protection on the crystalline trihydrate form of alendronate monosodium, the final form of the active ingredient in the Fosamax drug.

A patent was also granted claiming the formulation of the oral tablet drug and the method of preparing the tablet. Moreover, a patent was also filed and granted on a weekly dosing regimen based on the discovery that a weekly dosing of a high-dose alendronate sodium was well tolerated in patients and alleviated a great deal of the side effects associated with the original daily dosing. While some of these patents eventually were invalidated or revoked in litigation or oppositions, the portfolio as a whole was sufficient to protect Fosamax for an extended period of time even though the chemical entity of the drug was not protected by a claim to the compound itself. Of note, even before Merck lost exclusivity for Fosamax, it developed Fosamax Plus D [a combination of alendronate sodium and vitamin D (cholecalciferol)], a second-generation product. Fosamax Plus D is covered by patents listed in the Orange Book.

Many biotechnology developments that showed promise to blossom into lifesaving products nevertheless were aborted at the research stage, never to be fully developed, largely due to lack of the patent protection that would have justified the enormous investment required. The foregoing example of Fosamax illustrates that sufficient patent protection may sometimes be established in difficult situations, provided that patent strategies are created and followed through the drug-development process. Entrepreneurs and biotech managers should work closely with experienced patent counsel and stay vigilant in capturing and creating patentable inventions through the entire process of product development and even thereafter for second-generation products. Collective effort and creative strategizing among the IP, R&D, and even the marketing teams increase the likelihood of such a payoff.

References

[1] The granddaddy international treaty on this subject was first adopted in 1883, in Paris, France. Read the "Paris Convention for the Protection of Industrial Property". <https://www.wipo.int/treaties/en/text.jsp?file_id = 288514> [accessed January 3, 2019].

[2] Similarly, the major international treaty on copyrights was adopted in 1886 in Berne, Switzerland. Berne Convention for the Protection of Literary and Artistic Works. <https://www.wipo.int/treaties/en/text.jsp?file_id = 283698> [accessed January 3, 2019].

[3] *D'Arcy v Myriad Genetics Inc* [2015] HCA 35 (7 October 2015). <http://www8.austlii.edu.au/cgi-bin/viewdoc/au/cases/cth/HCA/2015/35.html> [accessed January 3, 2019].

[4] USPTO web page on subject matter eligibility. <https://www.uspto.gov/patent/laws-and-regulations/examination-policy/subject-matter-eligibility> [accessed February 7, 2019]. *Mayo Collaborative Services v. Prometheus Laboratories*, 566 U.S. 66 (2012); *Ass'n for Molecular Pathology v. Myriad Genetics*, 569 U.S. 576 (2013); *Alice Corp. v. CLS Bank International*, 573 U.S. 208 (2014); *Vanda Pharm. Inc. v. West-Ward Pharm. Int'l Ltd.*, 887 F.3d 1117 (Fed. Cir. 2018); *Athena Diagnostics, Inc. v. Mayo Collaborative Services, LLC* (Fed. Cir. 2019). <http://www.cafc.uscourts.gov/sites/default/files/opinions-orders/17-2508.Opinion.2-6-2019.pdf> [accessed February 6, 2019]. See Holman CM. Vanda v. West-Ward Pharmaceuticals: good news for the patent eligibility of diagnostics and personalized medicine, with some important caveats. Biotech Law Rep 2018;37:117–25. <https://www.liebertpub.com/doi/abs/10.1089/blr.2018.29069.cmh> [accessed January 3, 2019].

[5] America Invents Act of September 16, 2011. <https://www.uspto.gov/aia_implementation/index.jsp> [accessed January 3, 2019] One of the more significant changes to U.S. patent law wrought by this Act was to subtly redefine "prior art." Compare the currently amended version of § 102 of the patent law with its predecessor. Also, on December 5, 2013, yet another "patent reform" bill was introduced in Congress, as H.R. 3309, dubbed the "Innovation Act." passed the House.

[6] 35 U.S.C. §§ 311–319. <https://www.uspto.gov/patents-application-process/appealing-patent-decisions/trials/inter-partes-review> [accessed January 3, 2019].

[7] *Oil States Energy Services, LLC v Greene's Energy Group, LLC*, 584 U.S. ___ (2018). See Stoll R. A review at five years: inter partes review; 2017. <http://www.ipwatchdog.com/2017/09/12/five-years-inter-partes-review/id = 87424/> [accessed January 3, 2019]; Carmichael J, Close B. Despite *oil states*, inter partes review may still be held unconstitutional; 2018. <https://www.ipwatchdog.com/2018/04/25/despite-oil-states-inter-partes-review-may-still-be-held-unconstitutional/id = 96406/> [accessed January 3, 2019]; Mahanta S. To shift or not to shift: burden shifting framework and the PTAB; 2018. <https://www.ipwatchdog.com/2018/12/03/burden-shifting-framework-ptab/id = 103496/> [accessed January 3, 2019]. Iancu A. Remarks by Director Iancu at the American Intellectual Property Law Association Annual Meeting; October 25, 2018. <https://www.uspto.gov/about-us/news-updates/remarks-director-iancu-american-intellectual-property-law-association-annual> [accessed January 3, 2019].

[8] See Supreme Court Affirms CAFC in Stanford v. Roche on Bayh-Dole; June 6, 2011. <http://www.ipwatchdog.com/2011/06/06/supreme-court-affirms-cafc-in-stanford-v-roche-on-bayh-dole/id = 17594/> [accessed January 3, 2019].

[9] Defend Trade Secrets Act of 2016. Pub.L. 114–153, 130 Stat. 376, enacted May 11, 2016, codified at 18 U.S.C. § 1836, et seq. Note that the DTSA includes an exception to permit whistleblowers to disclose trade secrets to government agencies without the company's permission. Confidentiality provisions won't be enforced in federal court unless they notify employees of the *whistleblower exception*. For more info on trade secrets, see <https://elman.com/gerry-elman-and-josh-waterstons-dpac-presentation-on-trade-secrets-december-18-2018/> [accessed January 3, 2019].

[10] Flax S. An introduction to pharma trademarks. Maryland State Bar Ass'n IP Section Newsletter 2009;1.

[11] The timeline for development of a non-proprietary drug name. Drug Name Development Timeline <https://www.ama-assn.org/about/united-states-adopted-names/drug-name-development-timeline> [accessed July 26, 2019].

[12] *Guidance on INN*, World Health Organization. Available from: <http://www.who.int/medicines/services/inn/innquidance/en/>. The WHO created the INN based on concerns during the international conference of drug regulatory authorities in 1991, thereafter adopting resolution WHA46.19 on nonproprietary names for pharmaceutical substances. For guidelines, see <https://www.ama-assn.org/about/united-states-adopted-names/united-states-adopted-names-faq>.

[13] Wall Street Journal, July 12, 2000.

[14] The Orange Book is available at the FDA. <https://www.accessdata.fda.gov/scripts/cder/ob/default.cfm> [accessed January 3, 2019]. See also <http://wikidelphia.org/wiki/Orange_Book_Companion> [accessed January 3, 2019].

[15] Information on biosimilar rules and regulations is available at the FDA. <https://www.fda.gov/drugs/developmentapprovalprocess/howdrugsaredevelopedandapproved/approvalapplications/

therapeuticbiologicapplications/biosimilars/default.htm> [accessed January 3, 2019]. Papageorgiou A. New guidances from FDA for biosimilars and interchangeables. Biotech Law Rep 2017;36:17–21. <https://www.liebertpub.com/doi/full/10.1089/blr.2017.29002.ap> [accessed January 3, 2019].

[16] Powell SR, Elman GJ. ACLU Lawyers Face Off Against the U.S. Patent Office and Myriad Genetics. Biotech Law Rep 2010;29. <http://online.liebertpub.com/doi/abs/10.1089/blr.2010.9987> [accessed January 3, 2019].

[17] Elman G. What subject matter is patentable? Reading Myriad Genetics while waiting for Bilski. Why is this molecule different from all other molecules? Biotech Law Rep 2010;29:167. <https://elman.com/what-subject-matter-is-patentable/> [accessed January 3, 2019].

[18] Experts Debate MDx Industry Impact of AMP v. Myriad Three Years After Court's Decision; Nov 15, 2016. GenomeWeb <https://www.genomeweb.com/business-news/experts-debate-mdx-industry-impact-amp-v-myriad-three-years-after-courts-decision> [accessed January 3, 2019]. In the interest of full disclosure, co-author Jay Z. Zhang was the Senior Vice President of Intellectual Property at Myriad Genetics leading the *Myriad* litigation in the district court and the Federal Circuit Court of Appeals before it was appealed to the U.S. Supreme Court.

[19] *Eli Lilly v. Teva Parenterals Medicines Inc.*, 845 F.3d 1357 (Fed. Cir. 2017). See Steffe E, et al. *Divided Infringement After Eli Lilly v. Teva.* Law360; Apr. 18, 2017. https://www.law360.com/articles/914062/divided-infringement-after-eli-lilly-v-teva [accessed January 3, 2019].

[20] See, for example, European Patent Office Decisions *EPO* G1/04; EPO T310/99. Cold Spring Harb Perspect Med. 2015;5(5). <http://perspectivesinmedicine.cshlp.org/content/5/5/a020891> [accessed January 3, 2019].

[21] Carroll L. Alice's Adventures in Wonderland and Through the Looking-Glass (Signet Classics, The New America Library 1960). p. 79.

Some Resources and General Information

World Intellectual Property Organization (WIPO). <https://www.wipo.int/>.

American Intellectual Property Law Association (AIPLA). <https://www.aipla.org>.

US Patent and Trademark Office, Manual of Patent Examining Procedure (MPEP). 9th edn. Rev. 08 (Jan 2018) <https://mpep.uspto.gov>.

Understanding Industrial Property. World Intellectual Property Organization (2016)—WIPO publication no. 895(E). ISBN 978-92-805-1257. <http://www.wipo.int/edocs/pubdocs/en/wipo_pub_895_2016.pdf>.

Rai A. Intellectual property and biotechnology. Edward Elgar Publishing. (2011)

Castle D. The role of intellectual property rights in biotechnology innovation. Edward Elgar Publishing. (2011)

Rimmer M. Intellectual property and biotechnology. Edward Elgar Publishing. (2011)

Hine D, Kapeleris J. Innovation and entrepreneurship in biotechnology, an international perspective. Edward Elgar Publishing. (2008)

Litan RE, Luppino AJ, editors. Law and entrepreneurship. Edward Elgar Publishing. (2013)

Göransson B, Pålsson CM. Biotechnology and innovation systems. Edward Elgar Publishing. (2012)

Cooper I. Biotechnology and the law. Revision ed. Clark Boardman Callaghan. (2000–2019)

Wellons HB, et al., editors. Biotechnology and the law. American Bar Association Section of Science and Technology; 2007.

Elman GJ, founding editor. Biotechnology law report, 1982 to present. Mary Ann Liebert, Inc. <https://home.liebertpub.com/publications/biotechnology-law-report/6>.

Pappas MG. The biotech entrepreneur's glossary. Shrewsbury, MA: M. G. Pappas & Co.; 1998.

Mark Halligan R, Weyand R. Trade secret asset management 2018: a guide to information asset management including RICO and Blockchain. Weyand Associates, Inc.; 2018.

Patent searching

U.S. Patent & Trademark Office. <https://www.uspto.gov/>.

WIPO PatentScope. <https://patentscope.wipo.int/search/en/advancedSearch.jsf>.

Esp@cenet Search. <https://worldwide.espacenet.com/advancedSearch>.

Google Patents. <https://patents.google.com>.

Free Patents Online. <http://freepatentsonline.com>.

Section VI

The Financial Capital Component

Chapter 17

Sources of Capital and Investor Motivations

Craig Shimasaki, PhD, MBA
CEO, BioSource Consulting Group and Moleculera Labs, Oklahoma City, OK, United States

Chapter Outline

Capital is the lifeblood of every biotechnology company. Without capital, product development ceases irrespective of its potential value and market need. Because biotechnology companies require an enormous amount of capital in order to advance their product toward commercialization, it behooves the company leader to develop a well-thought-out fundraising plan tied to a detailed strategy for the use of this capital. Knowing which capital source is optimally interested in your stage of development is essential. For instance, during the inception stage when your product idea is a basic research concept, and the company does not have a full management team, it is unlikely that a venture capital (VC) firm would be interested in listening to a pitch about your enterprise. Your time would be wasted trying to secure a meeting with a disinterested VC firm as they need to deploy a larger amount of capital in each company than you can justify at an early stage. In this chapter, we will review the different sources of capital available, the stages that they are most likely to invest, and list some of the factors that influence their decisions. For more information on how investors are influenced in their decisions, see *Chapter 18: How Investors* Really *Make Decisions: What Entrepreneurs Need to Know When Raising Money.*

Understanding Investor Criteria and Limitations

Before we discuss the various of capital sources and their preferred company investment stages, it is important to know that each group has investing preferences and investing limitations. These criteria include preferences for a particular biotechnology sector (see *Chapter 10: Understanding Biotechnology Product Sectors*), minimum and maximum investing limits, and a specific investing

Biotechnology Entrepreneurship. DOI: https://doi.org/10.1016/B978-0-12-815585-1.00017-6

time horizon. It is an advantage to understand the interests, motivations, and limitations of each of these sources of capital prior to raising money. For instance, it would be futile to try to raise $5 to $10 million from angel investors, as this amount is typically beyond their capacity and interest for investing. Possibly, some angels may appear interested in your technology and your market opportunity, but if you don't realize that angel investors are unlikely to be able to collectively invest $5 to $10 million dollars, you will be wasting your time trying to interest them in your opportunity. Late-stage investors, such as VC firms, can also have preferences for specific biotechnology sectors in which their partners or principles have subject matter expertise. It would be better to pitch your medical device opportunity to a VC group whose portfolio already contains other ***non***-competitive medical device companies, rather than to try to pitch to a VC firm mostly comprised of GreenTech companies. If a VC has a medical device company in their portfolio, you can be sure they will have at least one VC partner with a preference and expertise in evaluating medical device deals; and they would be a likely source to consider investing in another medical device company. Therefore, be sure to align with the right investor group for your company, understand the investor group you are targeting, and know the biotech sector stage of development that is of interest to them.

Recognize that each funding source has an investing time horizon in which they need to have their capital deployed and also returned. Some investment firms have a 5–7-year time horizon in which they expect to see a return, whereas others have shorter time horizons for an investment. If your business does not anticipate having an exit opportunity (exits are discussed later) until 8 years, it would be futile to spend any time trying to pitch your company to an investor group that wants an exit in 3–5 years. When you understand the interests and limitations of different capital sources, it helps you to focus your efforts on sources with the highest likelihood of interest in investing in your company. It is important to know that each group's investment criteria may not be written down, but it is certainly understood by their partners. Always be sure to ask about a group's investing criteria and limitations when considering an investor group; this will help reduce the time you spend on fundraising and increase the likelihood of investment success.

Understanding Investors' Expectations for Return on Investment

Investors in biotechnology companies expect to receive a return that is significantly greater than a mutual fund, certificate of deposit, or other lower return investment opportunities. Most investor groups have well-defined expectations for returns on their investment, and these expectations are commensurate with the level of risk they are taking. A return on investment (ROI) is often stated as a multiple of the amount originally invested such as a 5×, 10×, or 20× return. Investment returns are also expressed as an "*internal rate of return*" (IRR). An IRR is the percent increase in the original investment calculated on an annual basis. IRRs are related to a specific investment time frame without referring to that time frame. For instance, an opportunity can be expressed as having an IRR of 30%, but you don't know whether the exit is in 3 or 7 years. In general, biotech investor's interest perks up with IRRs in the range of 30%–40%. When asked, most investors typically describe their expectations as a multiple of their investments, and also within the number of years they expect to exit.

As we discuss in greater detail later, angel investors are early stage investors. Because angels typically invest before VCs do, they may have higher ROI expectations for their money than VCs. This is because early stage investors bear a greater risk than a late-stage investor does. Therefore, it is not unusual for angels to have an expectation of 10× to 20× return on their investment for the greater risk they take on an investment, whereas at least a 10× return initially gets the attention of a VC. Both angels and VCs require high-return multiples because biotechnology investing is high risk, and many of the companies in their portfolios may not return any money at all. In order to compensate for the failures, investors have extremely high expectations for returns on *every* deal they make. As an entrepreneur, make sure that your product and business model support the level of investor return necessary for the particular group you desire to interest (see Table 17.1).

Understand What Comes With Invested Money: Motivations and Interests

All the sources of capital invested into a company spends the same. In other words, a dollar from one investor spends the same as a dollar from another investor, and both last the same amount of time in a company's bank account. However, there can be vastly different ties, values, and benefits that come with each investor who puts that dollar into your company. For instance, if you are at an early stage and need to raise $750,000 to reach your next value-enhancing milestone, this amount of capital is an amount that multiple angels can cumulatively fulfill. However, each angel investor, as well as each angel group has differing philosophies about investing, and how a business should be managed. In addition, each investing source can have differing perceptions about how a business should be run, what is expected from a management team, and how much they expect to be involved. Along

TABLE 17.1 The internal rate of return (IRR) relationship to the number of years an investment is held before an exit, and the return multiple.

	Exit year for investment and its corresponding IRR									
Return multiple on invested capital	1	2	3	4	5	6	7	8	9	10
1.0×	0%	0%	0%	0%	0%	0%	0%	0%	0%	0%
2.0×	100%	41%	26%	19%	15%	12%	10%	9%	8%	7%
3.0×	200%	73%	44%	32%	25%	20%	17%	15%	13%	12%
4.0×	300%	100%	59%	41%	32%	26%	22%	19%	17%	15%
5.0×	400%	124%	71%	50%	38%	31%	26%	22%	20%	17%
6.0×	500%	145%	82%	57%	43%	35%	29%	25%	22%	20%
7.0×	600%	165%	91%	63%	48%	38%	32%	28%	24%	21%
8.0×	700%	183%	100%	68%	52%	41%	35%	30%	26%	23%
9.0×	800%	200%	108%	73%	55%	44%	37%	32%	28%	25%
10.0×	900%	216%	115%	78%	58%	47%	39%	33%	29%	26%

Data from: Industry Ventures LLC.

with these varied expectations, there are different intangible benefits that accompany each investor. In other words, each capital source brings a different value to your company. For instance, some angels may be former entrepreneurs who have worked in a similar sector developing a similar product. Investors like these, if you can find them, are familiar with the issues your start-up company will face, and they can advise the management team about the ways they overcame similar issues. Whereas other investors who are not familiar with the biotechnology industry, may come with unrealistic expectations on how to develop, test, and market your future product even though they not have invested in a life science deal before. The entrepreneurial leader should evaluate each investor's expectations and their perceptions of business conduct, as well as their business acumen to understand their benefit or detriment to the company. Doing this prior to accepting capital can prevent or mitigate problematic issues and operational challenges that the entrepreneurial leader may face when interfacing with these investors over time. In a sense, you are screening your investors for fit with the goals of your business and the core values of your company. All too often this "investor fit" is not evaluated, which can lead to conflicts when decisions about methods for reaching company goals are made.

When the company's management and investors are aligned, there is synergy in motivation and acceleration in the company growth and development. Harmonious alignment brings added value and enhances your ability to reach goals that may otherwise be difficult to achieve without these types of investors. Conversely, an incongruent investor will sooner or later precipitate conflicts with the company, taking a toll on its management, which hinders your focus on product development and advancement. When investor misalignment occurs, more energy is devoted to resolving internal conflicts than is expended on making product-development progress. As a result, wasted energy and resources detract from the future success of the organization. I have observed in real life where investor conflicts became so severe that there was an unexpected departure of the management and entrepreneurial leaders. Always examine the interests, motivations, and core values of potential investors to ensure that they are aligned with those of the company and its founders before closing a financing round: I call these *"funding alignment principles,"* (Figure 17.1). The entrepreneur should recognize that it is natural to have differing opinions about methods for reaching company goals, but there should still be alignment in the interests, motivations, and core values of both parties. Having value-adding investors provides an opportunity for the management to gain wisdom from like-minded individuals who have more experience and resources than they do.

Finding the ideal funding partner is not easy but the likelihood increases in finding the right fit by the following funding alignment principles. These include the following:

1. Select the right capital source for your company at its particular stage.
2. Make sure that the target capital source has interest in the product sector and development stage of your company.
3. Make sure there is alignment with your company's financial needs and the criteria and limitations of the funding source.
4. Make sure that your opportunity can provide the necessary return that your target funding source is seeking.
5. Make sure there is alignment with the motivations and core values of the potential funding source investors and the company.

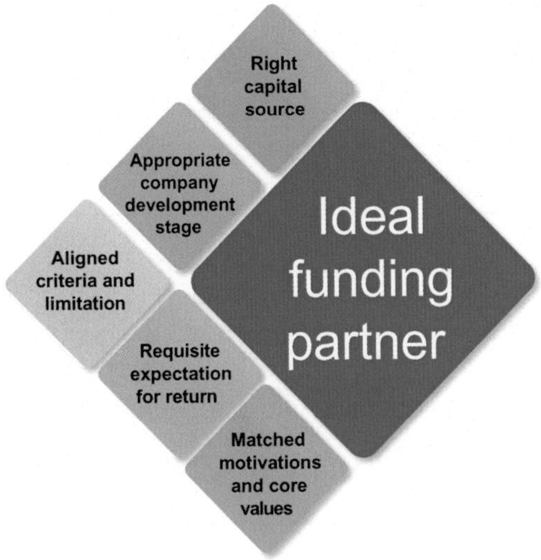

FIGURE 17.1 Funding alignment principles

What Are the Capital Sources Available to Biotechnology Companies?

A variety of capital sources are available to finance product development and grow biotechnology companies, and these sources have a preference for the stage at which they invest in a company (see Table 17.2 and Fig. 17.2). In this section, we discuss the most common sources of capital available to this industry. There are additional sources of capital other than those described later, such as bank loans, but those sources are not known for investing or financing biotechnology companies. The following list contains the sources most common to this industry:

1. Personal Capital
2. Friends and Family
3. Grants: Local and Federal–SBIR/STTR
4. State Financing/Funding Programs
5. Angel Investors/Family Fund Offices
6. Nonprofit Foundations
7. Venture Capital
8. Corporate Sponsors or Partnerships
9. Private Equity/Institutional Debt/Mezzanine Financing

Personal Capital

It is not unusual for the founders of a new company to initially operate for a period of time utilizing their own personal funds. Often, founders will invest some of their own money to operate their company as it shows that they are serious and committed to the enterprise. Subsequent investors have a more favorable impression about the company founders knowing that they have some "skin-in-the-game." Investors realize that founders are not likely to walk away or shirk their responsibilities if they have their own hard-earned capital riding on the success of their company. Depending on the stage of the company and the sector, the amount of personal money an entrepreneur invests can vary. Sometimes the amount invested can be symbolic, like the $500 invested by both Rob Swanson and Herb Boyer when they founded Genentech. For others, their investment can accumulate to tens of thousands of dollars as you build the organization prior to other investors participating. A good personal rule to follow is that a capital investment of 5% of your net assets would be favorably viewed by other investors, whereas 20% or more of your personal assets invested in your start-up may seem naïve and can be viewed as a poor business decision. Even though it may sound noble to

TABLE 17.2 Biotech funding stages, valuation ranges, and estimated ranges for amounts raised.

Stages	Product characterization	Valuation ranges (MM)[a]	Amounts raised (MM)[a]	Funding sources
Start-up (preseed)	Concept	$2–$10	$25,000–$1	Entrepreneur/friends and family/SBIR/STTR/local grants
Seed	Proof-of-concept	$3–$15	$0.5–$5 or more	Entrepreneur/friends and family/angels/some VC/SBIR/STTR/local grants/institutions
Early and development stage Series A/B preferred	Development	$10–$50	$3–$25 or more	Angels/VCs/private equity/institutions/SBIR/STTR/local grants/institutions
Later stage Series C/D preferred	Development/clinical testing	$25–$100	$15–100	VCs/private equity institutions/local grants/institutions
Mezzanine	Market launch	$50–$500	$25–$150	VCs/investment banks/private equity/institutions

SBIR, Small Business Innovative Research; *STTR*, Strategic Technology Transfer Research; *VC*, venture capital.
[a]*Valuation ranges and amounts raised* vary greatly *with respect to the specific biotech product sector, the type of product in development, the management team, and the competitive nature of the market the company is targeting.*

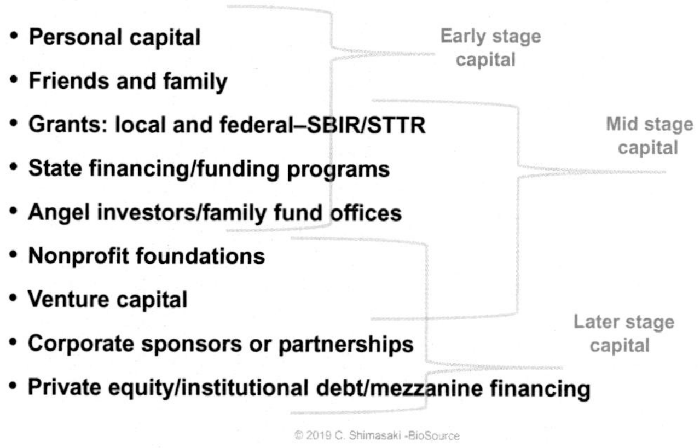

FIGURE 17.2 Traditional sources of capital for a biotechnology company.

have a large portion of your assets invested in your company, it is not a financially wise thing to do. Be sure the amount committed is something you can afford to lose. Unsuspecting founders think that their investment is simply a loan to the company until new investors join, and they can then be paid back. New investors, however, rarely agree to let their capital be used to pay back previous investors or company debt. New investors want their fresh capital to go toward building value into the business rather than paying off past debt obligations.

Another reason that founders will invest their own money into their companies is to purchase their stock outright. Paying a nominal amount of money for founder's stock (different types of stock are discussed in *Chapter 14: Company Formation, Ownership Structure, and Securities Issues*) is not unusual, and there can be a tax advantage to paying for your stock when the company has minimal financial value. Frequently, start-up entrepreneurs do not possess significant amounts of capital to contribute to their new company venture. And it is not unusual for founders to work for minimal, and sometimes no salary for a period of time while the company matures. Underpaid or nonpaid effort is referred to as "*sweat equity*," and this is, in essence, a tangible contribution to the company. As the enterprise grows and additional investment capital is secured, the founders may still earn lower than average wages, but they still should be compensated by holding significant amounts of equity (stock) in their company.

Friends and Family

Early stage capital for your venture can also come from friends, family members, and close associates. These individuals may not always be sophisticated investors, and their major motivation for investing is because they know you, and they believe in what you are doing. The amount of money raised from friends and family varies, but it is usually small compared to the amount of money you need to make a significant product-development process. Often this capital is used along with personal capital to initiate company formation and make some progress toward product development while seeking investments from other sources of capital. Sometimes an entrepreneur may be fortunate to have very knowledgeable family members with industry and investing experience. However, more often than not, these "*experienced*" family members are less experienced in the biotechnology industry than one may think. Unfortunately, sometimes friends and family can have even greater expectations than traditional investors who are aware of the risks associated with this industry. Although friends and family can be a ready and familiar source of capital, do not forget that Thanksgiving and Christmas are annual holidays when your friends and family may be sitting across the dinner table expecting to hear good news about their investment. If friends and family invest, it is always a good idea to be sure that it is money they can afford to lose. The amount one can expect to reasonably raise from friends and family varies from thousands of dollars to tens of thousands of dollars. In rare cases, you may find that the combination of your personal money and capital from friends and family could total hundreds of thousands of dollars. Just be cautious if you are considering asking friends and family to invest, because a good relationship with them is more valuable than the money they provide.

Grants: Local and Federal Agencies

It is wise to seek and apply for various types of grant funding to help offset your research and development (R&D) costs. Grant funding is competitive, but it is an excellent source of funding that can be directed toward making significant R&D progress. I know of an early stage biotechnology company that was successfully awarded enough state and federal grants to advance their therapeutic product through animal studies and into a major portion of early human clinical trials. One medical device company has been so successful in winning federal grants that they funded almost all their R&D costs for the new products they developed and commercialized. Grant funding is also known as "*non-dilutive*" capital. Grants are "non-dilutive" because you are not giving away equity (stock) in exchange for this capital. As will be discussed later in this chapter, each time you raise dilutive capital you must give away equity in return. When you do this, you simultaneously reduce the percentage of ownership for all the existing shareholders. Even though previous shareholders, including founders, may still hold the same number of shares that were originally issued, the percent ownership tied to those shares becomes "diluted" when additional shares are issued to others.

Local and federal governments are aware of the economic benefit in supporting the development and growth of technology businesses, and as such there may be special incentives in your area that support biotechnology companies. Be sure to allocate time and effort towards finding and applying to these non-dilutive sources which are supportive of your business. Even though grants are "free" money, the time from application to receiving grant awards can be quite lengthy, on the order of 6-9 months. In spite of this time lag, careful planning for grant opportunities can make a difference in the success and future of your company and product development.

Academic and Small Business Innovative Research/Strategic Technology Transfer Research Grants

There are different types of grants that biotechnology companies can access. Academic professors and scientists in the United States are familiar with the National Institutes of Health (NIH) grant program that funds basic research and keeps their laboratories active with graduate students and postdocs. Traditional academic research grants are a great way for scientists who are contemplating a spin-off company, to advance their product idea as far as possible on grant funding. My most recent company, Moleculera Labs, licensed a panel of five clinical assays that had completed basic research but not ready to be commercially offered through our clinical laboratory. The R&D was advanced far enough through numerous research grants that the principal investigator was awarded over the many years of research testing.

For-profit companies are not often recipients of academic research grants; however, there are 11 federal agencies in the United States, which have other grant programs to fund science-based, high-risk commercial product development. This granting program is called the Small Business Innovative Research (SBIR) program, which is operated similarly to the basic research programs that award basic research grants. These same federal agencies have a parallel grant program called the Small Business Technology Transfer (STTR) program, which awards grants to partnerships between the academic institutions and for-profit companies that codevelop high-technology commercial products. The SBIR and STTR programs grant money to for-profit companies that are developing products and services considered to be "high risk" but have high potential economic payoffs. Each year, US federal agencies with extramural R&D budgets that exceed $100 million are required to allocate 3.2% (FY 2017) of their R&D budget to these programs. SBIR Phase I grants can provide up to $150,000 or more for 6 months to 1 year, whereas SBIR Phase II grants can provide up to $1,000,000 or more for 2–3 years. More detailed information about SBIR/STTR grants can be found in *Chapter 15: Licensing the Technology: Biotechnology Commercialization Strategies Using University and Federal Labs*. As an added incentive, it is not uncommon to find local government programs that will provide a one-to-one match for companies that receive SBIR and STTR fundings. Even if you are not a proficient grant writer, there are free SBIR workshops to assist in improving your grant writing skills. There are also webinar-based support groups such as The National Council of Entrepreneurial Tech Transfer (NCET2) [1] that offer help to first-time grant applicants of SBIR. Alternatively, you can hire proficient grant writers to assist you in these efforts, but realize that good grant writing is not a substitute for having a top-notch R&D strategy with a novel and significant product.

Another significant value of winning peer-reviewed government grants (aside from the nondilutive benefit) is that these awards indirectly provide validation from peer reviewers and scientists, especially if the company has won more than one award. Funding sources such as VCs look favorably on companies that have been successful in winning Phase II SBIR and STTR grants. More information on these government programs can be found on the SBIR website [2].

Local Grant Programs

Cities, states, and regional governments have become increasingly interested in creating biotechnology clusters in their locale. The biotechnology industry is attractive because it creates high-technology and high-paying jobs, is a clean industry, and brings in knowledge-based and highly skilled laborers. As described in *Chapter 6: Five Essential Elements and Regional Influences Required to Grow and Expand a Biotechnology Cluster or Hub*, one of the significant missing elements is access to capital for these companies. As a result, local governments have created various programs, including grant programs to fund start-ups and early development–stage technology companies as a means to jump-start their local bioscience industry. Hundreds of millions, even billions, of dollars in funding initiatives have been set aside by various governments in support of local biotechnology growth initiatives. Entrepreneurs should familiarize themselves with their own local grant-support programs. These programs are usually tailored to support technology companies located in a specific region. The number of applicants to these programs is usually fewer than for federal programs and, as a result, they usually have higher award rates because of the smaller pool of applicants. If you are not aware of regional government-funding programs in your area, start out by asking your local Chamber of Commerce and your State Department of Commerce to find out what is available for your type of company and stage of development. Moreover, some municipalities have designated underdeveloped areas where the government offers financial assistance to companies that will locate in these less commercialized areas.

As an example of local government-supported grants, the state of Oklahoma passed an Economic Development Act in 1987 creating the Oklahoma Center for the Advancement of Science and Technology (OCAST) to spur economic growth and diversity. OCAST adopted an NIH-type peer-reviewed grant system using subject matter experts external to Oklahoma. Over the past 30 years, since 1988, OCAST has invested $285 million in 2700 projects that have returned $6.5 billion to the state for science and technology research that translated into companies creating technology products developed in the state of Oklahoma. At a previous company, we received over $900,000 from OCAST's competitive grant program, and at a subsequent company, we won another $850,000 to fund our company's product development. Because entrepreneurs need as much financial help as they can get, spend time learning about your local government-assistance programs. You may be pleasantly surprised at the funds that are available directly from your own state or local government.

State Financing Programs

In your state, there may be government-backed and government-funded programs that support biotechnology and high-technology companies in a particular geographic region. The difference between government *financing* programs and government *granting* programs is that financing programs may take equity in the company or have a security interest in the company in exchange for funding, whereas government grants are non-dilutive, and the company does not give anything in exchange. These financing programs often operate similarly to other institutional sources that take stock in exchange for capital, or issue debts that must be paid back. Often these government financing programs are mission or industry driven, and there may be some favorable terms given in order to stimulate the growth of the biotechnology industry in your state or local region. Sometimes there may be no difference in terms compared to other sources of capital, just that it is available to companies in a locale limited in capital resources for biotechnology companies at developmental stages. Check for local technology commercialization programs that may have government-backed financing for your company. In 1997 the state of Oklahoma created a Technology Commercialization Center after the oil bust, as a means to help stimulate the organic development of new technology companies and to diversify the state's economy. The center is managed by I2E, an acronym for Innovation-to-Enterprise, where trained staff and funding sources are made available to shepherd and guide promising but fledgling high growth technology companies to be successful. To date, they have provided government-backed and government-financed fundings, making 266 investments totaling more than $50 million, served 700 client companies and entrepreneurs, and have managed six early stage investment funds. Through this state-sponsored program, they have leveraged an additional $591 million from private investors for Oklahoma companies. I2E has become a recognized model organization for technology development across the country. Just remember that sometimes you may find government-backed or government-funding sources of capital that you were not aware of right in your own neighborhood.

Angel Investors/Family Fund Offices

This investor group is more purposeful in their investing than most friends and family. Private individuals who invest early in a company and meet certain investing criteria are called "*angel investors*." The term ascribed to these individuals is not necessarily related to their generosity or their spirituality, but rather these investors are considered to be "angelic" or "heaven sent," in a sense, rescuing a company at critical times by providing life-support financing. Angel investors generally invest at early stages of product and company development which is typically before VC funds invest. Because of the early investment risk, their expectation for return ranges from $10\times$ to $20\times$, and some have higher expectations of $30\times$ or more. Most angel investors do not coinvest with VC funds or institutional investors. The typical angel investor invests from $25,000 to $250,000 in any one deal, and in rare cases, some can invest multiple millions depending upon their interest in the technology, and their capital resources. Sometimes angel investors will collectively pull together their investment with other angels and form a limited liability corporation for a larger pooled investment in a company.

The term *angel investor* is used synonymously with, or interpreted to mean, "*accredited investor.*" The US Securities and Exchange Commission (SEC) defines an accredited investor [3] as an individual (or individual and spouse) with a net worth of over $1 million, or an individual with an annual income of $200,000 or more for the past 2 years, or $300,000 with a spouse for the past two years, and a reasonable expectation of the same income for the current year. In the United States, there are over 400,000 active angels investing in various companies.

They may invest in companies individually or in formalized groups called "*angel networks*." Well-established angel networks have formal meetings and participation requirements in order to be a member. Membership dues are usually required, and there are formalized structures with defined funding review systems that assist with due diligence and mechanisms for following their investments. Some examples of angel network groups that invest in life sciences include the St. Louis Arch Angels that was founded in 2005, has about 85 active members and invested over $100 million in over 90 companies. The Tech Coast Angels in California is one of the largest angel networks with over 300 members who collectively invested over $180 million in over 300 companies. The Tech Coast Angels invests in a broader sector of high technology, including IT and life science. The biotech entrepreneur should know that the competition for investment from these groups is high. For example, in 2017 the Tech Cost Angels received over 500 applications and funded 42 companies with $14.2 million. Two very active angel groups with a specific focus on biotechnology and the life sciences are the Life Science Angels (LSA) located in Sunnyvale, CA and the Mass Medical Angels (M2A) located in Boston, MA. Since 2005, LSA has invested nearly $50 million in over 40 companies and the M2A, according to CrunchBase, has invested in 14 companies. More information about angel investors and angel networks can be found in *Chapter 19: Securing Angel Capital and Understanding How Angel Networks Operate*.

Angel investors are motivated to invest in companies because they are either familiar with the market need for a product, or have a desire to support a local company, or because they believe in the entrepreneur and their ability to make it successful. Sometimes angels may require more time to learn about the business and science if they have limited exposure to biotechnology. However, as this industry expands and matures, there are increasing numbers of experienced angels who were former entrepreneurs that became successful through exits from their own biotech companies. In general, angels typically prefer to invest in local companies, and they may limit their investments to their local geographic region. The reason for this is a combination of the desire to see local companies succeed , coupled with the lack of interest in traveling long distances to monitor their investment. Increasingly, however, more angels and angel networks are branching out to "syndicate" or coinvest with other angels to diversify their portfolio, and this requires that angels consider nonlocal deals.

For the most part, for a higher likelihood of interest, seek angels in your own geographic region who may know you or have heard about your company. Finding these investors can be challenging because they do not advertise their activities, and investing is not their full-time job. A good way to find angel investors is by networking with people who know them and by asking them for introductions. Other ways include checking with your local university or research institution's technology transfer office for names and contacts, as they may know many of the local angels. Also check with the local Chamber of Commerce, your regional economic development agency, or a technology commercialization center or equivalent—these may be good sources of angel contacts that invest in biotechnology. Do not forget that most angels are connected to other angels. Once an angel has invested, ask them for help and introductions to others. A motivated and excited angel investor telling your company story is very effective. There are many angels out there—just be persistent in locating them.

Family offices can also be another source of funding at this stage for biotechnology companies. They are businesses run by, and for a single family, or in some cases, multiple families. These are high net-worth families with an office that invests the family's money, manages the family's assets, and disburses payments to family members as required. Family offices typically have a focused mission to invest in organizations that have a tie to their interests as a means of generating returns for their family funds, so it is helpful to find out this information prior to approaching them. These family offices do not typically advertise, therefore finding them can require work. However, one good resource for finding specific types of investors is the Redefining Early Stage Investments (RESI) database and conferences that provide a wealth of information on various types of investors, including VC and family offices. Their conferences are the one-on-one type 30-minute meetings that are scheduled ahead of time, similar to the format that the Biotechnology Innovation Organization (BIO) and other organization use. Whereas RESI collects large amounts of data on a variety of investor groups and makes selective information available through the conferences, but you can access more information for a fee. If you are looking for more practical helps on targeting investors, check out "*The Life Science Executive's Fundraising Manifesto: Best Practices for Identifying Capital in the Biotech and Medtech Arenas*" by RESI CEO Dennis Ford [4].

Nonprofit Foundations With a Focus in Your Sector

In the recent decade, nonprofit foundations focused on certain disease conditions have become an increasingly more common funder of biotechnology product development. These foundations are focused on improving the health and advancing solutions for individuals afflicted with a specific condition or disease. In the past, they have had a major focus on funding small research grants to very early stage academic and basic research. However, these projects are usually many years, possibly a decade, away from a treatment or diagnostic solution for the constituents they are working to help. Foundations have begun to make much larger investments in individual companies that are already advancing a product, treatment or diagnostic toward commercial development. This, in turn, supports their mission by advancing a future commercial product by helping the company reach the market with a product sooner. Entrepreneurs should search to see if their focus is aligned with a nonprofit foundation that may be interested in funding your company's product development. Some examples of disease foundations that have funded product development include the Bill and Melinda Gates' Foundation, the Cystic Fibrosis Foundation, the Juvenile Diabetes Research Foundation, and the Michael J. Fox Foundation for Parkinson's Research to name just a few.

Venture Capital

VC is comprised of funds managed by professionals who invest in high-risk ventures with the expectation of producing higher than average rates of returns. Most VC firms raise money for their fund from institutional investors, such as foundations and endowments, pension funds, insurance companies, and high net-worth families and individuals. The investors who invest in VC funds are referred to as "*limited partners*." Venture capitalists who manage the fund are referred to as "*general partners*." The general partners have a fiduciary responsibility to their limited partners and are supported through a management fee from the fund, but they make their money on what is called a "carry," typically 20% of the profits after the principal is returned to their limited partners. For more information on VC investors, see *Chapter 20: Understanding and Securing Venture Capital: An Entrepreneur's Perspective*.

The size of any venture fund varies greatly, from $20 million to over $5 billion per fund with over 1000 VC funds in existence. There are VC funds directed to most types of industries such as life science, therapeutics, diagnostics, medical services, IT, software, and some large funds invest in all of the above. In 2017, $9.7 billion was invested in biotechnology companies in the United States. VC continues to provide a large portion of the funding for the biotechnology industry, especially during the later development stages of product development where large amounts of capital are consumed during clinical trial testing. Fig. 17.3 shows that over the years, an increase in the size of funding rounds from VCs (in millions of dollars) for companies in the life science sector.

In order to understand the motivations of VC, one must understand the constraints and limitations of VC

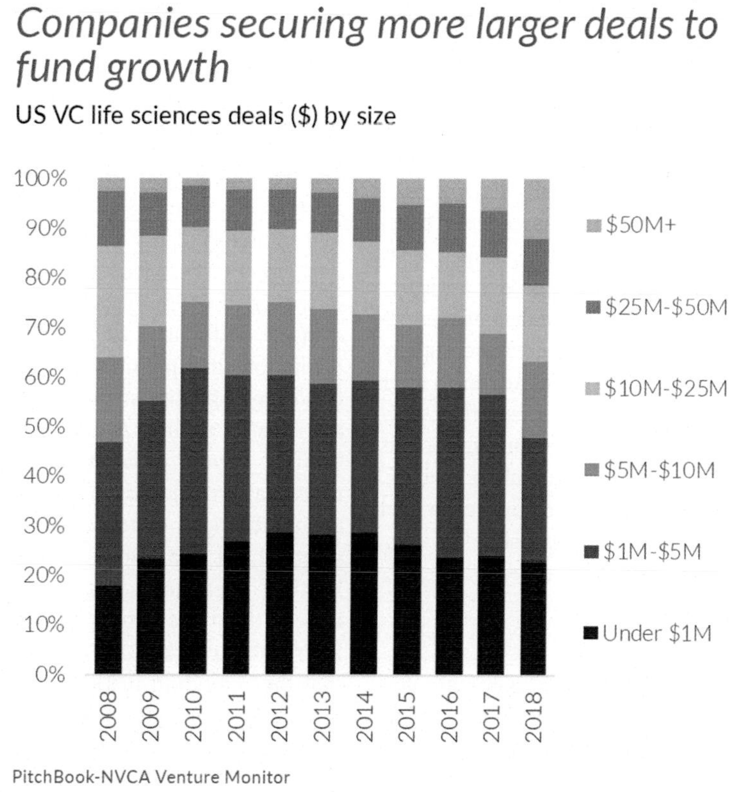

FIGURE 17.3 US VC life science deals by ($) size.

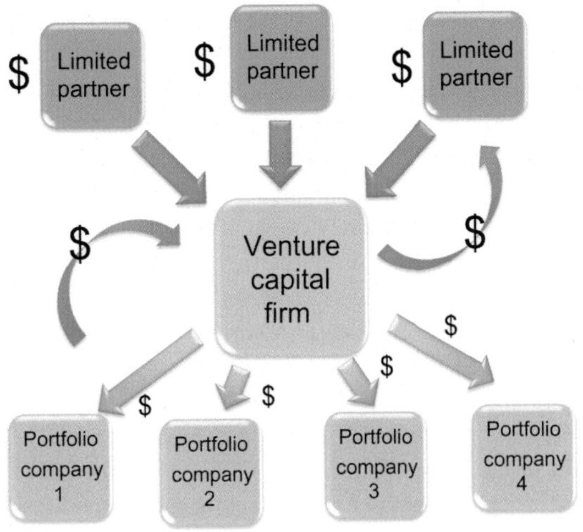

FIGURE 17.4 The venture capital funding cycle

funds. As shown in Fig. 17.4, the VC firm receives money from its limited partners for a defined period of time. The limited partners have an expectation for return within that time frame. The VC firm must then identify a portfolio of companies in which to invest with the expectation that these companies each return a significant profit before the fund life cycle is over. All companies are not successful nor do they all bring extraordinary returns to their investors, so the VCs must build into their plan an assumption of the number of failures, while still meeting their investors' expectations for returns. There is pressure on the VC firm to have their portfolio companies perform and meet expectations. Fund managers that are not successful at this may not be able to raise a follow-on fund.

The general partners of a VC firm usually devote 100% of their time investing and managing their portfolio of companies, compared to angels who typically have a "day job" and invest on the side when they have time. Even though general partners work full-time at finding investments and managing their portfolios, their time is typically limited and in great demand due to the number of companies they manage and the number of issues each company faces. General partners must also answer and report to their limited partners, raise capital for their fund, find new investments, and manage their existing companies. For this reason, it is vital when trying to gain the attention of a VC that you make your pitch and value proposition clear and concise so they can quickly assess their interest.

Corporate Sponsors or Partnerships

In addition to traditional financing, another source of capital for biotechnology companies is corporate partnerships. The biotechnology company possesses something of value to the corporate partner that they cannot provide on their own. It may be that the biotechnology company's product could help increase sales of the corporate partner's existing products, or it gives them a complementary product they need in their existing market, or the new product leverages their current sales and distribution channel, or it is a way for them to remove a competitive product from their existing market. Biotechnology company partners may be pharmaceutical companies, vaccine manufacturers, medical device companies, large national laboratories, or chemical companies depending on what the biotechnology company has in development and in their pipeline. The formation of a corporate partnership most often occurs during the later stages of product development. However, it does not hurt to solicit interest from these organizations early on as they may have a special interest in your earlier stage of development. Often, a corporate partner may have a longer term goal which may be to acquire your biotechnology company sometime in the future.

A common exchange between these partners is that the biotechnology company receives cash, milestone fees, reimbursement for development costs, and future royalties on their product (Fig. 17.5). The corporate partner usually receives an exclusive license to the biotechnology company's future product and a right to market and sell that product in all countries (or selected countries). In the case of therapeutics, biologics, and vaccines, the corporate partner may also take over responsibility for the remaining stages of human clinical testing and regulatory approval since they have the capital, resources, and the expertise.

Private Equity/Institutional Debt/Mezzanine Financing

Private equity, institutional debt, and mezzanine financing are typically funding vehicles that are utilized for late-stage biotechnology companies that already have a commercialized product or service, or at the very least, near-market introduction. These funding sources are rarely available to start-up and early stage biotechnology companies. The institutions that provide this type of financing are interested in lower risk investments and are looking to deploy large amounts of capital. Although VC is technically a form of "*private equity*", this term is usually referred to organizations that provide private companies with large amounts of capital during commercialization or near commercialization stages. Debt financing is a debt instrument that is also utilized at later stages because the lending institution must believe that the company is a very low risk and there is collateral that can be used to secure the debt. The collateral that these lending institutions require must be worth significantly more than the loan amount should the institution have to "call" the debt because of nonpayment or default. Early stage and development-stage biotechnology

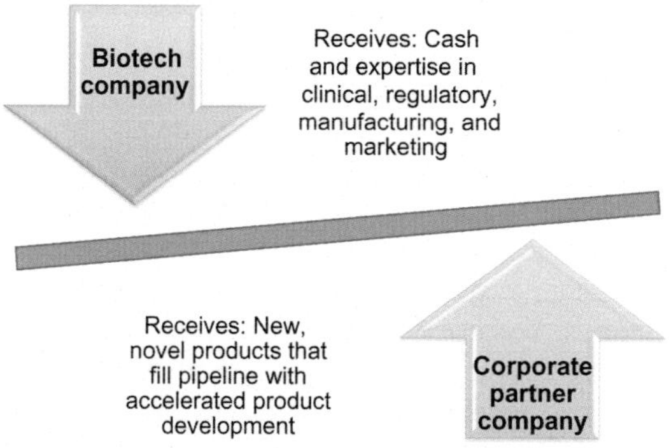

FIGURE 17.5 The value exchange between corporate partners

companies possess very little in the way of "tangible" assets to use as collateral. Because of this, debt financing is really only available to those companies that have commercial products and services on the market, and collateral becomes accounts receivable, inventory, equipment, facilities, or land. For companies that qualify, there are organizations that provide debt financing for the biotechnology industry, which include Silicon Valley Bank, Comerica, and GE Capital to name a few.

Another way to free up cash for working capital is to finance existing equipment if it is already paid off and owned by the company. Cash can be be provided through a loan for security interest in the paid-off equipment, which would free up more cash for operations. Occasionally, other creative debt-financing methods may be possible. Sometimes an early stage company may obtain a line of credit from a local instuitional lender if a local high-net worth investor is willing to guarantee the loan. Obviously, the investor would need to believe that there is some assurance that the company can make the payments on the note, and that there will be more value for the investor who backs the note. As a general rule, it is not advisable to use debt financing as a means of funding product development for an early stage biotechnology company. This is due to the high risk, the long development times, and the large amount of capital needed to sustain the company through to commercialization.

Mezzanine financing is a typical combination of debt and equity (or warrants) reserved for companies with a track record of revenue to provide them with capital for expansion, acquisitions, or an initial public offering (IPO). The interest rate is usually high (12%–30%), and the company that receives mezzanine capital is leveraging its return while contributing less of its own capital. These types of financing vehicles and instruments are often utilized in some combination for companies at later stages that need access to large amounts of capital but have significant upside to make these terms reasonable to undertake.

Determining the Value of Development-Stage Biotechnology Companies

In order to complete a financing transaction and raise capital, all companies must address the question "*how much is your company worth?*". The answer to this question determines the percentage of the company given to new investors in exchange for capital. Valuation also determines the percentage of the company retained by the founders, employees, and existing shareholders. Because of this issue, reaching agreement with potential investors on company valuation is often a debated and contentious process for the entrepreneurial management team. For every company, there is a valuation range where any amount within that range can be justified by each party. Most founders and entrepreneurial management teams want to value their company as high as possible. However, *overvaluing* your company beyond a reasonable range can be counterproductive and detrimental to attracting institutional and VC in the future. There are standard and universally accepted methods for determining the value of a company that has product revenue history. Unfortunately, development-stage biotechnology companies do not have product revenue and must raise significant amounts of capital prior to reaching commercialization.

A brief overview of the various valuation methods for biotechnology companies is provided. This will give you a starting point should you desire additional and more detailed information on company valuation methods. When assessing the valuation of *later development-stage companies*, the following methods are utilized, each of which can provide differing valuations, but the best valuation is an estimate determined by referencing all four methods.

1. ***Valuation by comparables***: Identify similar organizations in similar sectors at similar development stages that have been recently valued at a financing round within the last 12 months. Although valuations of private companies are not publicly disclosed, there are available resources (for fees) you can access to obtain this information. Moreover, if you know or have worked with VC firms or institutional capital firms, an individual working there may be able to help you obtain this type of information. Ideally, one would want to have three or more comparables for reference, with those transactions being closed within the past 12 months. Frequently, exact comparables are not available but there may be related comparables in a related segment that could be used as a surrogate reference. When that occurs, one would use this valuation as a reference, then make any appropriate adjustments (see number 4).
2. ***Valuation by public and private exits***: This method is similar to the previous one except that the calculation is performed on mature companies that have had an

exit. For instance, one would use the value of mature companies in a similar sector (therapeutic, diagnostic, medical device, clinical laboratory, bioagriculture, and biofuel) determined at the time the company either completed an IPO or an acquisition by a publicly traded company. This "exit" value is then divided by the return multiples required by a typical institutional investor. For instance, if an institutional investor today requires an 8 to 10× return on their investment in order to invest, then based upon an IPO or acquisition value of $250 million for the mature company in the same sector, divide by 8–10, for an estimated ceiling valuation range of $25–$31 million. Knowing this would be a maximum range, you would then make adjustments and reductions for your stage and risk level to arrive at an estimated range.

3. ***Valuation by risk-adjusted discounted cash flow (DCF) (rDCF)*:** This is determined by first estimating the company's future revenues minus the costs associated with generating those revenues, then discounting these by an appropriate interest rate. So, starting with a *DCF* or *net present value* of those future earnings, the value of those future earnings is then discounted again by the risk of successfully completing the remaining phases of product development and the FDA approval. This final value is called an *rDCF*. Although this method sounds complicated, there are good mathematical programs available for calculating these values. The uncertainty comes predominately from the estimation of the risks associated with successfully completing the remaining product-development phases and regulatory success. Although this method is relatively straightforward to calculate, it is not recognized as a reliable and trusted valuation method for pre-revenue biotechnology companies.
4. ***Valuation adjustments*:** There are several value-adding or value-detracting factors that warrant adjustments to an estimated valuation. Examples of valuation adjustment factors include the experience and caliber of the management team, the acuteness of the medical need for their product (e.g., HIV, Alzheimer, and cystic fibrosis), the likelihood of follow-on product applications, the strength of existing financial and development partners, and the current financing window, to name a few. There are certainly other considerations to valuation such as if a biotech company urgently needs capital but doesn't have readily available resources, their valuation is often reduced. Conversely, for an organization that is adequately funded with adequate resources to reach their next value-enhancing milestone, the valuation may be enhanced.

Before performing a valuation exercise, biotechnology companies should be segmented into two separate groups: *early development*– and *later development–stage companies*. Early development–stage companies are pre-seed, seed, start-up, early stage and mid-stage organizations, or those having products that are in preclinical development prior to commercialization. The latter development-stage includes later stage, mezzanine, and publicly-traded companies, or those that have products in human clinical trials or beginning commercialization for nontherapeutics and diagnostics. For early development–stage companies, one can use all the previous methods *except* the rDCF method. Early development–stage companies have many more financial and scientific uncertainties that weaken the ability to confidently utilize the rDCF method. These companies lack certainty of successfully reaching the next stage of development and uncertainty in securing adequate funding to continue progress toward the clinical testing and regulatory phases. Moreover, the cost, risk, and time associated with the R&D phase of any one particular biotechnology product is uncertain. Once a company receives the FDA approval to begin human clinical testing (for a therapeutic or medical device), there is a better understanding of the development path risks associated with these products reaching commercialization. More importantly, recognize that VCs do not use rDCF for the valuation of early development–stage companies, and the VCs are the most common investors at later stages of development. A company's value can also decrease over time even though the valuation was fairly assessed at one point. Decreases in value can occur for a variety of reasons that are under the company's control and for reasons that are out of the control of the company. Since a biotech company's value is closely tied to its product-development progress, if the company consumes much more capital than originally anticipated and does not reach any new value-enhancing milestone, this will negatively impact valuation.

Accurately determining the valuation of a development-stage biotechnology company is important for attracting investors, issuing stock at "fair-market" value, and ensuring that future financing partners are not soured by an unrealistically high-valued company. The key to arriving at a fair valuation is by using the appropriate method for your company's stage of development. Having a realistic valuation for your company will increase the likelihood of financing your enterprise. In reality, after utilizing all these valuation methods, never forget that *valuation is ultimately determined by the investor who writes the check*.

Financing Stages for a Biotechnology Company

All companies transition through discrete capital financing stages that are tied or related to the product-development stage of the company. As discussed in the previous section, each investor group has preferred stages at which they invest, and they have limitations as to the amount of capital they can invest, and a specified time frame. In this section, we describe the most common financing stages of a company and tie them to the investor groups that most often invest at these stages. Financing stage terminology may vary but these are some of the terms most commonly used. For those that are more familiar with product-development stages rather than financing stages, a product-development stage is implied by the financing stage, and I briefly mention the product-development stage associated with these terms. I also discuss the most common order in which they occur and review the typical exit strategies for a company.

Start-Up or Preseed Capital

"*Start-up capital*" is also known as formation capital or preseed capital, which is usually the smallest amount of money raised at any one time. Typically, the funds raised are used to establish corporate operating and employment agreements, file and prosecute intellectual property, and incrementally advance the technology. Most often these are the funds that allow the full development of a business plan and marketing strategy. Sometimes these funds will be used to pay early salaries for a few individuals and pay for a website and logo. Usually the company is already incorporated into an appropriate business entity or soon to be incorporated prior to the receipt of the funds. The product that the company is developing will be at a very early stage of inception. Sometimes the R&D may still be performed at an academic institution, and it is possible that the entrepreneurs may not yet have a license to the technology. The amount of capital raised during this stage can be as little as $25,000 or as much as $1 million. The sources of capital usually come from the entrepreneurs, friends and family, and occasionally personal loans secured against personal assets of the entrepreneurs. If a large enough round of capital is raised at this stage, there may not be any distinction between the start-up capital and the next stage of seed capital.

Seed Capital

"*Seed capital*" is sometimes called proof-of-concept capital, which is the next larger round of capital after the start-up capital. The money raised in this round can range between $500,000 and $5 million or more depending on your biotech sector. This money is typically used to advance the technology or product to a stage that would increase the value of the company and reach a value-enhancing milestone. Other uses of capital go toward expanding the target market research, hiring consultants, subcontracting to contract research organizations, and often to hire part-time or temporary employees. At this stage the entrepreneurs may take a nominal salary. Capital sources at this stage include the entrepreneurs, friends and family, government grants, existing or new angel investors, and local funding programs.

Convertible Notes

It is worthwhile to discuss at this stage what is given in exchange for cash. During these very early development stages (start-up, preseed, and seed rounds), when the valuation of the company is unclear, it is difficult to ascribe, or agree to, how much the company is worth to an investor, and to the company. However, the company still needs the capital. An investor can invest in the company through the use of "*convertible notes*." A convertible note is essentially a "loan" to the company with the intent to convert that "loan" into equity at a subsequent round of financing, usually when institutional capital or VC capital is raised, and the value of the company is more reasonably determined. Convertible note holders are usually given an annual accumulated interest rate, accrued but not paid, which can range from 8% to 12% depending on the market and need of the company, and they are given a discount into the next round (typically in the range of 20%) depending on the industry and the stage of the company. By issuing convertible notes, the noteholder has a preferred position, and they have the option of converting at a discount when the next round of capital is secured. The holders of convertible notes have a priority position in the event of any downturn in the company, as noteholders are usually ahead of shareholders when it comes to a liquidation of the company assets in the event of bankruptcy. Although the most common method of accepting funds at this stage is through convertible notes, direct equity investments are also made at this time. A direct equity investment means that in exchange for cash, the company gives up a percentage of ownership to the new investorsin the form of stock.

Early Stage Capital: Series A/B Preferred Rounds

Early stage capital rounds are considered to be "*Series A preferred*" and "*Series B preferred*" rounds. This is the next significant funding round for the organization. This money may come from angels or a group of angels and local government–funding or financing programs. Early stage capital will occasionally come from institutional investors such as VC groups that focus on early stage investing. These rounds can range from a million dollars to multiple millions of dollars; if the product is a therapeutic, a diagnostic, or a medical device, it can range up to tens of millions of dollars. Money invested at this stage is exchanged for equity in the company and comes with certain "*preferences*" that are above all other investments previously made into the company. In other words a Series B investment takes precedent and has preferences over Series A investors, and Series A preferred investors have preferences over holders of common stock such as founders, management, and key employees. These "preferences" are spelled out in a "term sheet" that contains the terms of the investment. Sequential preferred financing rounds are labeled alphabetically and each subsequent round receives preferences over all previous rounds of capital raised. For more information on term sheets, see *Chapter 21: Financial Ramifications of Funding a Biotechnology Venture: What You Need to Know About Valuation and Term Sheets.*

Private Placements

At this point, we should discuss "*private placements*" because raising money for a biotech company is, in essence, selling underlying securities (stock or equity) in your company. As such, these activities are regulated in the United States by the SEC. When a company raises capital, particularly when they exchange stock for capital, these offerings are called "private offerings" or "private placements." Most individuals have heard of public offerings such as an IPO, whereas a private offering or a private placement is made to only a select group of individuals. When a private placement of stock is made, specific offering documents are required, and a securities or good corporate start-up attorney will know what documents are required and how to handle the regulatory filings after the capital is raised. There are specific exemptions in the Securities Laws, and the most commonly used exemption is called "Regulation D," which is a safe-harbor exemption. Under these laws, a company may be exempt from many securities requirements, but there are still obligations and legal requirements for disclosure. Your securities attorney should advise the company on how to comply with these disclosures. When raising money from individual or angel investors, it is wise to accept money only from accredited investors because this assures that your investors understand the risks associated with their investment. Moreover, by raising money only from the accredited investors, if the company is unsuccessful, the amount the investor loses would not significantly impact their livelihood. Some of the requirements under the SEC exemptions are to provide, a "private placement memorandum" (PPM), when soliciting investments from individuals. Basically, the PPM contains your complete business plan along with your financials, your sales projections, a potential ROI, and a lengthy list of potential risks associated with this endeavor. Your securities attorney should review these documents and ensure that the investment risks are adequately described, whereas it is the company's responsibility to write the business plan. For more information on private placements, see *Chapter 14: Company Formation, Ownership Structure and Securities Issues.*

Mid-Stage or Development-Stage Capital: Series C/D Preferred Rounds

Series C and D preferred rounds are follow-on rounds and usually involve some or all of the investors in the previous preferred rounds plus new investors. The money that comes in at this stage, is mostly institutional capital such as VC and corporate partners. There are more VCs that invest in mid-stage development companies than in early stage development companies. The number and size of these rounds vary, and the letter designations C and D are only examples. There are no hard and fast rules on round designations, so if a company's product has progressed far enough in development, sometimes a Series B preferred round can be considered a "mid-stage round." This could occur if the product is either a molecular test, diagnostic, or simple medical device, where the capital needs for product development are smaller, and the time for development is shorter compared to human therapeutics. The amount of money usually invested in these rounds typically is in the tens of millions of dollars.

Filling the Funding Gaps With Bridge Loans

There are often gaps between funding events for a company. A development-stage company can be very close to running out of money in-between any of the abovementioned capital rounds; whereas the company can still be making significant product-development progress and generating interest from investors. One financing instrument used to close this funding gap is a "*bridge loan*". Bridge loans sometimes fill the funding chasm between angel funding and the closing of VC and larger equity investments. Bridge loans are notes that bear a risk-appropriate interest rate, whereas convertible notes are bridge loans that have a right to convert their principle and interest into the next financing round at the same terms that the next investors determine. A company may consider a bridge loan because either they do not have long before they run out of money, or they know they will be raising a larger round later, and the valuation is difficult to assess or agree upon by the company and investors. These bridge loans will often come with an extra incentive to the investor in the form of stock warrants based upon a percentage of the amount loaned. A warrant is like a stock option that gives the holder the right to purchase shares in the company over an extended period of time at a set price. Depending upon the strength of the company's product development and progress, the bridge loan holder may want it to be structured with an option for converting just like a convertible note with a discount into the next round. When a company has interested investors who cannot put up the full amount of capital needed to make all the progress a company desires, bridge loans and convertible notes provide a way to support the company and still advance product development to later secure funding from larger investors.

Later Stage and Expansion Capital: Series E/F Preferred Rounds

Therapeutics and biologics require large capital investments and more funding rounds compared to diagnostics, medical devices, molecular tests, and some agbiotech products. However, there are greater numbers of VC firms that invest in these later stage rounds because fund managers can deploy more capital (tens of millions of dollars vs a few million dollars) and product-development risk is lower than at early stage development. Usually these later-stage rounds are for therapeutics and biologics, and by this funding stage, the company is usually in human clinical trials and potentially for more than one indication for use. Some very complex genetic expression tests and combination medical devices may also require later-stage capital to reach commercialization. If more capital is required, series designations continue alphabetically such as G and H, and each subsequent round has preferences over all previous rounds. One reason that VC investors in previous rounds will participate in subsequent rounds is to maintain their position and ownership percentages. They usually also syndicate investment participation so that responsibility for funding these subsequent and larger rounds is not borne by any one VC.

Mezzanine Capital

For companies that need it, "*mezzanine capital*" is usually the last round of capital before an IPO, an acquisition of the company, or an exit for the investors. VC funds are plentiful at this stage when product-development risks have been greatly reduced. Investors at this stage enjoy a shorter time from investment to exit than for those who invested at early or development stages. Not surprisingly, the returns on investments at this stage are lower than when investing at earlier stages of company development. For this reason, VC funds may balance their portfolio with some early, later, and mezzanine capital investments.

Initial Public Offering or Acquisition

An IPO or an acquisition of a company is an event where all the investors and shareholders can reap a financial reward for their work and perseverance. However, for drug-development and biologics companies, the requirement for capital is so high that often an IPO really becomes another later stage financing round for the company rather than solely an exit for investors, although it does accomplish both. Given the tremendous amount of capital required for drug development—up to $1 billion or more—and the length of time to reach the market—up to 15 years—it is not feasible for any single investor group to fund a company from start-up to commercialization without a public financing event or a corporate partnership or acquisition. Large amounts of money can be raised in an IPO with availability for follow-on public financing rounds. This is what makes an IPO an attractive event for the company and its investors.

What Is an "Exit" Strategy?

All investors invest with a purpose in mind—there will be a time when they can recoup their investment ***and*** a sizable profit. Until there is an exit event, all shareholder value is locked within the company, and the investors have no viable means to convert their shares back into cash. Although entrepreneurs may plan on staying with their company for the long haul, the investors are not in it for the same reasons. Yes, your investors will believe in the mission and the goals of the company; however, they are investors, and they want to know the company's exit strategy and the potential financial return. Investors have expectations that in the not-too-distant future they will part ways with the company and receive significant monetary benefit for financing that endeavor. Therefore, before an investor commits to investing, they want to know the company's exit strategy and when the company anticipates that to occur. During an exit the investors and shareholders exchange their shares for cash or, sometimes they may hold on to them anticipating that their shares may increase in value in the future.

Investors, by definition, invest for returns. The expectation of their level of return varies with the type of investor and the stage at which they invest in, which can range from 5 × to 40 × the original investment in a time period of 3–7 years. If your potential returns are not attractive enough to a particular investor, they will not invest. So when writing a business plan and before raising any money, the company leader should have a well-researched plan explaining how future investors will receive a return on their capital. For the entrepreneur, this exercise may seem premature and nearly impossible to calculate, but to an investor, it is not an unreasonable expectation. Exit planning is essential in order to attract investors because it is the means by which shareholders exchange their holdings for cash and are rewarded for their participation in the company.

What Are the Exits for a Biotechnology Company?

The most likely exit options for a biotech company are an acquisition by a larger corporation that is either private or public, or through a public offering (IPO), or a merger with another company (including reverse merger). For a number of years, there were many successful biotechnology company IPOs. When the IPO market is favorable it is possible for biotech companies to get their investors a 10× or greater return typically sought by VC investors. One historic example is that of Genentech's IPO on October 14, 1980. The stock went for sale on the NASDAQ exchange at $35 a share, and within hours the share price reached $89 before closing at the end of the day at $71.25. Genentech raised $35 million that day. In its second public offering of shares on July 20, 1999, 20 million shares were sold at $97 per share raising nearly $2 billion and the closing price that day was $127 per share.

Although an IPO can seem glamorous, being a publicly traded company also comes with certain financial governance requirements and expenses of compliance with Sarbanes–Oxley estimated to cost between $0.5 and $2 million. There are also costs of going public, it is estimated that about 15%–30% of gross proceeds are consumed when a company goes public. Compliance costs annually are projected to range between $2 and $4 million for most publicly traded companies [5]. In addition, there are daily fluctuations in market value, which can add pressure to make short-term decisions by the management that may be counterproductive to long-term product-development and market expansion progress. Publicly traded biotechnology companies also become subject to the same scrutiny that highly profitable Fortune 500 companies face daily. The attractiveness for a biotech IPO depends on many factors such as the general market conditions for IPOs, investor interest in the high-technology sector, the success of other biotechnology companies in a similar sector, and the overall economy.

What is the Typical Sequence of Funding Events?

There is no universal funding formula for all biotechnology companies to follow. However, a typical sequence may follow something similar to this:

1. ***Start-up capital*** may be provided by founders, friends, and family.
2. ***Seed capital*** may be provided by founders, friends, and family and local government entities, and grants directed toward funding the early R&D.
3. ***Series A Preferred capital*** may be provided by angel investors and/or local government entities, interested foundations, and possibly early stage VC and grants directed toward funding the early R&D.

(*Continued*)

(Continued)

4. ***Series B Preferred capital*** may be provided by angel investors, interested foundations, and syndicated VC.
5. ***Series C Preferred capital and later stage capital*** may be provided by syndicated VC and corporate partnerships.
6. ***Mezzanine capital*** may be provided by VC and large financing institutions or investment bankers.
7. ***Acquisition or strategic partnership*** with a large corporation brings capital from the parent company or *IPO* capital that comes from the public and institutional investors purchasing shares on the open public market.

There are additional ways for a privately held company to become publicly traded, such as a reverse merger with another publicly traded entity or a "shell" company. A reverse merger is less expensive than an IPO, which is relatively easy for a company to accomplish when there is a suitable shell company to reverse merge into. This transaction provides liquidity for shareholders, as their shares would be exchanged for publicly traded shares of the joined company. More recently, it has been challenging to have an IPO and maintain a stock price well above the initial pricing, and due to this, there have been more biotechnology companies opting for being acquired by larger corporations. Some investors believe that mergers and acquisitions (M&A) provide a better avenue for exit and better valuation, but it also depends on the amount of corporate interest in your company and its products. Spend time researching the M&A or IPO market for comparable companies in your sector. Become familiar with the valuations received for these companies, and learn to calculate a potential return for investors by knowing the comparable company values at each type of exit.

How Much Money Is Raised at Each Funding Stage?

The average amount of capital raised during each funding stage can vary greatly within each biotech industry sector. The amount of money that is raised during any stage is influenced by the following:

1. ***The type of product being developed.*** Therapeutics, biologics, and vaccines generally require greater amounts of capital during each round than do most medical diagnostics, medical devices, point-of-care tests, clinical laboratory tests, and many bioagriculture products. Therefore companies developing the former products will be raising larger amounts of capital in each round compared to the latter group.

2. ***The financial market's interest in a disease segment at the time of raising capital.*** Investor interest in certain disease segments changes over time. In the past, anti-sepsis therapeutics were being funded relatively quickly. Due to multiple clinical trial failures, today there is cautious interest for these types of companies. More recently, cancer immunotherapy, gene therapy, and RNAi companies have received high interest and have raised great amounts of money. The success and failure of similar predecessor products influence the value placed on the company and affect the eagerness of investors to fund these companies.
3. ***The strength of the IPO and acquisition market at the time of raising capital.*** When financial markets as a whole increase or decline, it impacts the amount of money that can be raised for any development-stage company. During 1999 and 2000, valuations for all biotechnology companies significantly increased because the IPO market was strong with exits available for the investors who provided excellent returns, and many companies raised significant amounts of capital. Later, the stock market downturn reduced valuations of early stage companies because the exits were not returning the profits investors expected, and the funding rounds were much smaller and more difficult to close. The strength of the financial market impacts the number of companies that can go public. Between 2008 and 2012, there were only 42 biotech companies that went public over that 5-year period, whereas in 2018, there were 60 biotech IPOs. Recognize that the general condition of the economy and financial markets impact the amount of capital you can raise and at what valuation because the investors are also looking at the financial markets for exits.

How Much of the Company Is Given Up in Each Round?

Each time your company raises capital from the investors it simultaneously gives away a portion of the ownership of the corporation. Because biotechnology companies require significant amounts of capital to reach commercialization, over time there will be significant ownership dilution to founders, early shareholders, and the management of the company who built it. Although dilution may be undesirable, without investor financing, there is little consolation in owning the majority of a company with no value.

In a survey that was completed by VentureOne with 75 respondents, Table 17.3 shows the mean, median, minimum, and maximum percentages of the company sold on a fully-diluted basis in each round (fully-diluted basis means all stock outstanding plus any options and warrants issued or granted, such that all were converted into shares). Most of these companies gave up approximately 25%−35% of the company each time they raised new money. Giving up 35% of the company three times does not mean there is nothing left after three rounds. Ownership gets recalculated each time for everyone, so investors in the previous round also get diluted if they don't participate in the next round.

TABLE 17.3 Percentages of company sold on a fully diluted basis.

	1st round	2nd round	3rd and later
Mean	41%	35%	27%
Median	40%	33%	26%
Minimum	8%	6%	4%
Maximum	82%	73%	70%
Total respondents	**97**	**65**	**79**

Data from: VentureOne deal terms report. 4th ed. (rounded).

For a theoretical example, if in the first round, 50% of the company is given away, 50% remains with the existing shareholders. If the founders originally owned 70%, then after the first round, they would own 70% of 50%, or 35% of the company after the first round. If the company raises capital in a second round and gives up 40%, then 60% is owned by all the prior shareholders, including those that participated in the first round. After each financing round a percentage of the company is given to the new shareholders, and all subsequent shareholders are diluted. Unlike a family-owned small business where the original founders can expect to retain the majority ownership of the organization, building a biotechnology company is a team project. The founder needs to realize that by the time the company is ready for an exit, they will typically own a minor percentage of the organization. Depending on the biotechnology sector and number of financing rounds, founder ownership at the time of an exit can range from 5% to 15% (see Fig. 17.6). This re-emphasizes the importance of accomplishing as much as possible with as little early money as possible, and reach significant milestones to increase valuation, which reduces the equity given up in each financing round. Founders should not be too discouraged because 5% of hundreds of millions is much better than 100% of nothing.

Summary

Capital for biotechnology product development comes from a variety of sources, and each source has their own

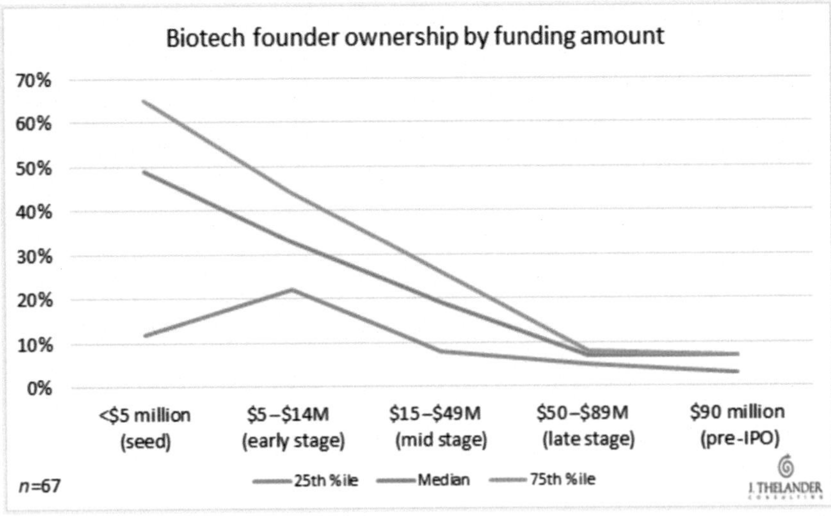

FIGURE 17.6 The average percent ownership of biotech company founders by funding stage. *From J. Thelander Consulting's private company option pool and ownership survey, which includes responses from 380 private venture backed companies in the United States.* https://pitchbook.com/news/articles/3-charts-that-show-the-effect-of-venture-fund-raising-on-founder-ownership

preference for the stage at which they invest. Each of these investor groups has different investment risk tolerances along with differing motivations and limitations for investing. Moreover, each group tends to focus on a particular segment or sector where they are familiar and comfortable with the investment risk. It is essential for the management team to understand these motivations and limitations prior to a fundraising campaign. By doing so, you can decrease the time spent on raising capital and increase your likelihood of finding the right partner for your product at your particular stage of development. At some point in development, most biotechnology companies will need VC or corporate partnership funding in order to reach commercialization. Start early and do some homework to identify the VCs that favor your company's technology space and target market. Be sure to target VCs and corporate partners who bring more than just money; seek a true partner who will provide experienced help along the way.

The biotech entrepreneur and management team are responsible for ensuring that the company continues to make steady product-development progress. Since the likelihood of raising the next round of capital is dependent upon scientific and developmental milestones made, make sure to hit most, if not all of them—on time. If your organization is consistently making progress toward its development goals, and these milestones are significant, it will be easier to continually attract the needed capital for the company at all stages. Once capital is raised, be extremely efficient in managing capital irrespective of how much is raised or how much you have left. The efficient use of capital is one hallmark of successful biotechnology companies.

A tremendous amount of time and effort will be put forth to secure funding at the right time from the right financing partner. As a result, it may be tempting to relax when fundraising is completed. Securing funding just means the hard work can begin in earnest. The company leader must always maintain the organization's *intensity* toward reaching the next value-increasing milestone if they hope to have a successful biotechnology company. Never forget that a funding event is a means to an end, and not an end in itself. The company goals are product development, market development, and business development milestones that increase the value and reduce the risk of the company. Keep your focus on your real goals and make progress so that you won't lack for future funding.

Cash is a precious and a limited commodity to a start-up company. It is like gas to a vehicle; even though you may have a high-performance automobile with the most powerful engine, when it runs out of gas, you go nowhere. When you accept money from others, there is a shared level of involvement and an increased level of responsibility to others. After a funding round is completed, you will have new investors or new partners, and your responsibilities broaden to more individuals than just those within the company. The hard fact is that there is not enough investment capital to fund all the good ideas conceived by every biotechnology company. Securing biotech funding requires perseverance and the ability to learn from each investor meeting to improve your chances of funding the company at subsequent junctures. The greatest idea imagined, the most amazing drug ever conceived, or the greatest life-saving medical device dreamed is of no consequence if you cannot finance its development to commercialization. Someone once said, "*a vision without execution is a hallucination.*" To have a vision without funds to execute it is an exercise in frustration and futility. Perseverance, flexibility, creativity, and working with exceptional people are key ingredients to successful fundraising.

References

[1] National Council of Technology Transfer (NCET2). Research Commercialization and SBIR Center. <https://ncet2.org/> [accessed January 26, 2019].

[2] Small Business Innovative Research. <http://www.sbir.gov/> [accessed January 26, 2019].

[3] U.S. Security and Exchange Commission, Accredited Investors. January 31, 2019. <https://www.investor.gov/additional-resources/news-alerts/alerts-bulletins/investor-bulletin-accredited-investors> [assessed January 26, 2019].

[4] Ford D. The life science executive's fundraising manifesto: best practices for identifying capital in the Biotech and Medtech Arenas. Boston, MA: Life Science Nation; 2014.

[5] PriceWaterhouseCoopers. Considering an IPO: the cost of going public may surprise you? November 2017. <https://www.pwc.com/us/en/deals/publications/assets/cost-of-an-ipo.pdf> [accessed January 26, 2019].

Chapter 18

How Investors *Really* Make Decisions: What Entrepreneurs Need to Know When Raising Money

Konstantin S. Kostov, PhD

Cantina Angels, Chicago, IL, United States; Life Science Angels, Sunnyvale, CA, United States

Chapter Outline

Introduction

Decisions are the result of a complex psychological process. Although certain decisions may seem rational at the time, they do not all lead to favorable outcomes. Amusing examples are provided by Bessemer Venture Partners, a venerable venture fund with more than 50 years of investing experience that has resulted in more than 120 initial public offerings (IPOs). In their antiportfolio web page, they describe the reasons they turned down investments opportunities, sometimes more than once, in numerous, ultimately very successful companies. David Cowan, one of Bessemer's partners, had a college friend who rented her garage to Sergey Brin and Larry Page during the first year of their company, Google. In 1999 she tried to introduce Cowan to "these two really smart Stanford students writing a search engine." Students? Search engine? Cowan asked her, "How can I get out of this house without going anywhere near your garage?"

In this chapter I want to share with you some historical background about how biases and behavior can impact investors and their decisions. I also want to share with you some common cogitative biases, and then illustrate how these can influence investors. In concluding, I would like to give you some advice on how you can avoid, counteract, and possibly leverage these biases so that you can have an opportunity to be fairly evaluated when presenting to investors.

The modern age of reason began with the Enlightenment in the 18th century. One of its major figures David Hume famously declared in *A Treatise of Human Nature* "Reason is, and ought only to be, the slave to the passions, and can never pretend to any other office than to serve and obey them." More recently, starting with the publication of von Neumann and Morgenstern's *Theory of Games and Economic Behavior* in 1944, economic science entered a period that focused on the idea that human beings acted and made decisions as fully rational agents which could be expressed using mathematical models. This culminated with the works of Eugene Fama and other economists at the University of Chicago on efficient markets theory, namely that stock market prices were the result of all available public information. These approaches were expressed by elegant mathematical formulas due to the belief that human behavior could be reduced to a sequence of consistent and predictable actions.

Biotechnology Entrepreneurship. DOI: https://doi.org/10.1016/B978-0-12-815585-1.00018-8

The common assumption was that individuals had complete information about all relevant facts, including all actions available to them, the strategies that others could adopt, and the probabilities of certain consequences resulting from their choices. Based upon this assumption, it was believed that stock market prices would be driven only by unanticipated events that could not be predicted.

The assumption of "unbounded rationality," the belief that all things are connected by right decisions, might hold true in modeled game theory and only in the simplest repetitive interactions. It also appears to be true at the macroeconomic level—where asset price movements in the public markets are indeed largely unpredictable. Because of this, *consistently* making money in excess of the markets as a whole by using unstable patterns that are subtle to infer, are very difficult. However, when it came to common human actions and decisions, in the 1970s some psychologists and economists began pointing out many cases that deviated from what one would expect rational people to do. So many deviations were discovered that in 1984 a pioneer in the field, the economist Richard Thaler (now a recipient of the Nobel Prize in Economics), began publishing a series of articles called "Anomalies" in the *Journal of Economic Perspectives*. Since 1991 these articles have appeared only occasionally, not because of the lack of anomalies but because choosing which anomaly to publish was taking up too much of Thaler's time.

The author of this chapter went through a similar personal evolution. I started my career as a theoretical and computational chemist studying the motions of protein molecules using sophisticated mathematics and large-scale computer simulations that required the highest computational precision. Eventually, the path of my life led me to become an investor in early stage science-based companies. The one translatable skill I acquired in my scientific career that I thought would be useful for investing was my quantitative and rational thinking and the ability to dive into a given topic and perform a deep analysis. I subsequently joined angel groups comprised of highly sophisticated and accomplished people, and developed relationships with venture capitalists—professional investors of the highest intellectual caliber and business success. I thought that the environment I became a part of would consist of the analytical and rational business people implied in Eugene Fama's and von Neumann's models—people who make decisions based on facts and logic. I was so wrong.

As I observed the manner in which my fellow investors and I made decisions, it became apparent that while we made every effort to be analytical and data driven, and there was no shortage of analysis, many of our decisions were inconsistent, random, and based on preconceived notions and biases. Early stage investing involves making judgments about a multitude of uncertainties and complex issues. Given the time constraints involved in making an investment decision, it is impossible to reach conclusions in a fully rational fashion. Moreover, the inherent randomness in future events means that the probabilities of their occurrence are difficult to estimate, a problem further compounded by the fact that many of these probabilities also evolve with time.

The remainder of this chapter will review in more detail the foundations of behavioral economics and decision-making psychology and hopefully provide some practical guidance to entrepreneurs who are raising capital.

Primer on Behavioral Economics

Behavioral economics is rooted in cognitive psychology. Major developments in this field occurred simultaneously with the development of rational agent economic models but initially were not well known to economists. A systematic framework was first created by the work of the Israeli psychologists Amos Tversky and Daniel Kahneman, working as a team. Their research brought together different concepts from psychology and statistics and constructed the framework of cognitive biases in decision-making that serves as the foundation of behavioral economics. This chapter can only provide a brief overview of these concepts, for further information I strongly recommend reading Daniel Kahneman's elegant and only slightly technical book *Thinking Fast and Slow* [1]. Amos Tversky died prematurely and therefore was ineligible to receive the Nobel Prize in Economics together with Kahneman in 2011. Another book worth reading is *Misbehaving* by Richard Thaler [2].

Research has established that humans have two cognitive systems that operate side by side and interact with each other in intricate ways that are called in shorthand "System 1" and "System 2". Knowing how these systems work is essential to understanding how people, and investors in particular, make decisions. System 1 controls automatic and almost effortless decisions—it takes priority in emergencies where fast actions are essential and is the default system that responds to the sensory inputs that we receive from the surrounding world. System 2, on the other hand, is involved in activities that require effort, concentration, and self-control. Each of these two systems have a natural pace—System 1 is quick, impulsive, and fast at reaching conclusions. System 2 is slow, deliberative, and reasoned. The two systems are in constant interaction with each other—if System 1 determines that a task is both vital and complex, it engages System 2 for further processing.

It is important to note that these two systems are a conceptual oversimplification aimed at—what else—our System 1. There are no currently known regions in the brain that physically correspond to either system. Most likely, our reaction to any given situation is a mixture of the two systems operating simultaneously. Yet, this oversimplification is essential in revealing how human beings make decisions.

Central to this understanding is the realization that each individual has a more or less fixed pool of mental energy or capacity. Moreover, this energy pool is shared between cognitive, emotional, and physical efforts. For example, walking at a slow tempo allows simultaneous thinking about other things. However, as the pace is increased it becomes more difficult to pay attention to anything except the act of the physical activity itself. This also holds true when performing sequential tasks. For instance, if one had to force themselves to perform a task requiring a tremendous amount of concentration or effort, and they had to do this repetitively they would perform poorly on subsequent challenges, a phenomenon called ego depletion. The size of this mental energy pool varies between individuals, thus individuals with high intelligence quotients (IQs) have larger mental energy pools or they expend less energy in solving a problem that requires significant mental effort. Systems 1 and 2 exist simply to regulate the use and allocation of this mental energy pool. If System 2 were engaged all the time this pool would be quickly depleted, leaving an individual unable to make other decisions when required. Fundamentally, people differ in how they make decisions depending on when and why they choose to engage their System 2.

The key to understanding how System 1 makes quick judgments is the process of **substitution**. Whenever someone is faced with a demanding task or challenging question, there are two broad choices—either activate System 2 immediately or else substitute the question at hand with one that is much easier to solve. Certain questions such as solving a moderately complicated mathematical problem almost always require the engagement of System 2. But other questions are very amenable to substitution—either because the question is deceptively simple or because we can easily recall a piece of information that we think provides the right answer. The process of substitution involves the use of *heuristics*—simple mental rules-of-thumb or procedures that provide adequate, though often imperfect, answers to difficult questions. The use of these mental shortcuts frequently happens automatically and even subconsciously with little effort. When used consciously this approach is in fact a great strategy to solve difficult problems; to quote the mathematician George Polya: "If you can't solve a problem, then there is an easier problem you can solve, find it." Most of the time, the automatic use of heuristics provides adequate answers to routine and inconsequential problems; however, this approach frequently fails when dealing with critical issues and leads to the formation of *cognitive biases*.

There is a subtle but important distinction between heuristics and cognitive biases. Since it is outside of the scope of this chapter to review the psychological literature on this topic, I will oversimplify the subtleties involved. Cognitive biases arise when imperfect heuristics become habitually used in processing certain information and result in a *systematic* error in decision-making. Perhaps the most important finding of behavioral economics research is that most of the errors people make in their thinking and decisions are not random, but systematic and predictable.

It is also important to note that not all cognitive biases involved in making decisions are the result of using heuristics—many biases are derived from deeply held beliefs or aspects of one's personality. Cognitive biases are strictly speaking biases that result from faulty reasoning. Arguably, every bias has a cognitive component; however, many cultural biases such as sexism or racism are due to the unconditional acceptance of certain beliefs and not meant to short-circuit mental reasoning; by their nature, System 2 is never invoked.

Common Cognitive Biases

Wikipedia lists over 100 cognitive biases, whereas John Manoogian [3] published a cognitive bias codex using 189 biases by positioning them in a circle with two major axes. We already discussed that in order to act fast, there is a need to filter a lot of information quickly and the circular arrangement highlights two other reasons for having biases: to fill in the gaps of filtered information by creating stories and to decide what information to remember. The experienced angel investor John Huston [4] identified 17 cognitive biases that impact an investor's first investment decision, with another 29 cognitive biases that influence follow-on financing decisions, for a total of 46. In the remainder of this section, I will review some of the most common ones.

The availability heuristic is the process of making assessments based on the ease with which analogous situations quickly come to mind (System 1) rather than engaging in a detailed and rigorous analysis of the data and the situation at hand (System 2). With investors, this is most frequently expressed when recalling unsuccessful, or conversely successful, investments that they have made in the past, serving as a quick template to assess the current opportunity. In extreme cases, this may involve random, but recent news events that can cast positive or negative light on the company being considered. Sometimes, well-informed investors might recall statistics about industry trends and neglect evaluating whether changes in the market are occurring that would soon invalidate the status quo.

Representativeness bias involves making judgments about the frequency or likelihood of occurrence of an event based on the degree of similarity to a typical case or a certain stereotype—"representativeness." This bias ignores the likelihood that an event may occur based only on prior information as well as the degree of accuracy of the new information. The likelihood is substituted by a similarity. If the statistical prior probability is very different or the new information is unreliable or inaccurate, this bias can lead to seriously flawed conclusions.

Anchoring involves arriving at an estimation using an initial baseline number derived from insufficient data or irrelevant past events that are then not adequately adjusted. Frequently, the baseline is suggested or mentioned by somebody else to his or her advantage, such as the asking price or a company valuation in a business transaction. The baseline need not be a number but instead may be a negotiating position or a concept that one considers the default or the most likely one. The objective is to get the other side to accept your "ask" or point of view as the baseline. It turns out that two mechanisms are responsible for anchoring effects—System 2 uses a deliberative process of adjustment, whereas System 1 works via an automatic priming effect. Anchoring is so ubiquitous in investment pitches and negotiations that every entrepreneur should use it in a measured way, and at the same time be on the alert to avoid being anchored themselves.

Confirmation bias results from the active search for evidence or information that conforms to one's preformed notions about a certain topic while at the same time actively ignoring or not seeking evidence that would challenge these notions. That is, there is bias to seek confirming evidence and not disconfirming one. This is perhaps the most commonly occurring bias in venture investing especially in combination with the availability heuristic. Investors initially evaluate deals they see based on their System 1 by doing a quick screen to recall patterns of success or failure in their memory. Since a given investor can only invest in a limited number of companies in the screening stage, he or she is a skeptic—the bias is toward finding evidence confirming that the investment opportunity being considered is weak and finding reasons to reject it.

However, once a company passes this initial screen and generates investor excitement as a deserving investment candidate, a positive mode of thinking takes over. Whether it is the partner in a venture capital (VC) fund or the deal champion in an angel group, the investor(s) conducts further diligence that is structured so as to confirm the superiority of the investment opportunity. Interviews are conducted, information is collected, and research performed, but the difficult questions are either not probed or else the negatives are diminished by favorable considerations. In VC funds, this phenomenon is at least partially attenuated since the partner sponsoring the deal has to persuade the other partners in the fund to support the investment (this is one reason why most VC investment decisions are made unanimously). The problem of course is that the other partners bring their own biases and prejudices so the decision-making process still remains somewhat random and suboptimal. In angel groups where every investor makes their own decision, the deal champion(s) are typically committed to investing in a given company, and very infrequently have I observed the champions withdrawing a deal after going into diligence. More commonly, the company is rejected because very few additional angel group members are persuaded to invest.

In order to counterbalance confirmation bias, some angel groups such as the Ohio Tech Angel Fund assign a "devil's advocate" position to one of the members of the diligence team [4]. Sometimes, they will conduct a "pre-mortem" analysis by enumerating the ways in which the target company may fail by trying to evaluate the likelihood of those scenarios occurring [4].

"I like how you think"—research by Murnieks et al. [5] has shown that venture capitalists (VCs) more favorably evaluate opportunities presented by entrepreneurs who "think" in ways similar to their own way of thinking. This effect is distinct and in addition to other personality assessment and interaction biases that may exist such as age, gender, race, common educational background, or referral source. The investment decision-making may most broadly be defined as evaluating founder-quality "the jockey" and economic-quality "the horse" characteristics. The authors find that the presence of this "thinking alike" similarity impacts the founder-quality component by increasing its influence in the overall investment decision. While the economic-quality component is not changed directly, it is diminished by effectively receiving a smaller weight in the final decision.

Overcoming Investor Overconfidence and Ego

Since this is a book about biotechnology entrepreneurship, some comments are in order about whether cognitive biases are present or even applicable at all in what is a highly technical and data-driven part of the start-up economy. Most participants in this field are scientists, medical doctors, engineers, and otherwise very rational individuals with several advanced degrees. Still, perhaps the most important conclusion of behavioral economics research is that no one is immune to cognitive biases, even the smartest and most technical, accomplished, and rationally thinking people.

The phrase *We Are All Competent Idiots* comes from the title of an article by David Dunning [6], now retired psychology professor at Cornell University. In the late 1990s he and his student, Justin Kruger, conducted a study describing a phenomenon now known as the Dunning–Kruger effect. They documented how incompetent people do not recognize, and actually cannot recognize, just how incompetent they are. Instead of being confused, perplexed, or cautious in their conclusions, they display inappropriate confidence sustained by a false sense of something that seems to them like knowledge.

This is by itself not surprising. About the same time as this study appeared, in a regular segment on the Tonight Show the comedian Jay Leno interviewed people in the Los Angeles area asking nonsensical and fabricated questions to which many gave confident responses. What is surprising is that the same phenomenon is observed among the most highly educated and competent individuals. In fact, many studies have found that those who assess themselves as having moderate competence were the most doubtful about the accuracy of their answers and the limits of their competence. We tend to think education is the opposite of ignorance, however, education and ignorance are alike in one important respect—education can produce confidence that is illusory.

Dunning mentions several reasons that may explain these observations. First, many of our deepest intuitions are formed when we are babies and small children and they remain with us for the rest of our lives; education fails to overturn them. What education often appears to do is to instill in us confidence in the errors we have internalized. Second, we frequently use knowledge we have acquired in one context in a very different setting where it is inappropriate, that is, we use *substitution* in combination with the *availability* bias. The last major category of misbeliefs according to Dunning stems from values and philosophies we hold as individuals such as hierarchist versus egalitarian or individualist versus communitarian. For example, when people who were initially uninformed about nanotechnology were asked to comment on its risks and benefits, their opinions did not correlate with their values. When another group was given a brief but carefully balanced description of the promises and perils of nanotech, their opinions split and aligned with their worldviews. Hierarchists viewed nanotechnology favorably as they respect authority, while collectivists worried about the industry's effect on the environment and public health.

The Ego as a Cognitive Bias and Its Role in Making Investment Decisions

Some of the beliefs outlined in the preceding section go to the core of not only who we are as individuals, but also *being* individuals where the ego plays a central role. One important group of cognitive biases, usually classified as social biases, involves our egos. Even if we act out of selfishness most of the time, most of us believe that we are good and caring persons, and any evidence that contradicts these notions is resisted and discarded. Perhaps somewhat less strongly, most of us believe that we are capable and competent in what we do. While that may be the case in our immediate professional activity, too often this sense of confidence expands to encompass adjacent fields and areas that are far out of our core expertise. Believing that one is smart can frequently deepen the effects of many of the biases described earlier. People who believe that they have arrived at the right solution commonly become insulated and disregard contradictory evidence, as such evidence would undermine their belief in their intelligence. Nobody likes to admit they are wrong, but this is especially pronounced when being "right" becomes part of one's persona. I have observed that a common trait among venture capitalists in particular is their internal belief that they are special, very talented, and intelligent. When raising money for their funds, VCs have to externally project an extremely high degree of confidence in their investment thesis and ability in front of potential and their existing investors called limited partners (LPs), as well as internally to the other partners in the fund. The "smartness" as an essential part of their ego starts to dominate their personalities. Errors and poor decisions are rarely acknowledged as that would challenge these core beliefs. Bad outcomes are instead attributed to external factors outside of the VCs control or to the inherently high failure rate in the industry (not everything works).

We can see the difficulty that many entrepreneurs face. By and large the investment community consists of people who are highly qualified and educated, yet too much education frequently leads to illusory knowledge and overconfidence which is really difficult to overcome as doing so would challenge deeply held notions about their self as being competent and rational. Sometimes, there is alignment between the business concept of the company seeking funding and the knowledge—actual or illusory—of the investor. Many times there is not. In these situations, it is best not to become argumentative or challenge sacrosanct notions of the self as these cannot be changed. Psychological research has showed that what works better is to accompany such a difference in perspectives with statements that will make the investor proud of their competence, values, or character.

The Role of Cognitive Biases, Emotions, and Intuition in the Investment Decision Process

There are numerous articles and surveys that describe the criteria different types of investors use in order to make decisions [7,8]. The majority of them are descriptive and do not attempt to explain why a particular set of criteria was used and the relative weights chosen for each of these criteria, nor why a particular company or entrepreneur was judged to meet, or not, those criteria. Broadly speaking, these criteria fall into two categories: business viability (industry, market size, adoption likelihood, stage and risks of product development, sales strategy, business model) and perceptions about the quality of founders and/or management. Studies that focus on cognitive biases primarily address the founder-quality category. In fact, biases may, and likely are, present in the more quantitative analyses of business plan aspects such as projections of future market adoption rates of a product or the market size growth. Biases in the economic-quality dimension of the decision-making have been scarcely studied.

Venture Capitalists

Being a venture capitalist must be one of the most demanding occupations that exist. It requires a high degree of intellectual capability as well as intensive multitasking and juggling of different responsibilities. Venture capitalists are entrepreneurs just like the individuals in the companies they invest in as they are almost continuously raising money for their funds by pitching to potential LPs. They also have to spend significant amounts of time not only for managing their firms but also to participate in the management of their portfolio companies as board members, and sometimes operationally on a day to day basis. Of course, VCs have to devote most of their time to the core aspect of their business—developing a high volume/high quality deal flow and choosing a handful of companies to invest in.

This means that VCs are inundated by business plans and pitch decks. Over the years they develop a large network of trusted sources that continuously refer to them new investment opportunities. In addition, they receive many unsolicited business plans and pitch decks "over the transom" or learn about opportunities from secondary sources such as the news media and attending conferences. Engaging their System 2 for each and every business plan they receive is plainly not possible (though the larger funds have teams of associates that are involved in this screening process). Thus VCs rely heavily on their System 1 to perform a quick triage of the incoming deal flow and pick deals that are either outright exciting or merit further work by System 2. In the process of doing this, investors use a number of heuristics to separate incoming deals into those that are rejected and those that merit further consideration. Understanding this process, the heuristics used most frequently, and in particular the aspects of this process that the entrepreneur can control, is the key to increasing the likelihood of a favorable funding decision.

Gompers et al. [7] conducted a survey of 680 VC firms and nearly 900 investors about the criteria they use to source deals and select the ones to invest in. Of the incoming companies, one member of the fund investment team met with the company management 28% of the time. They then reviewed 36% of those deals (10% of the total) with other partners at the firm. About half of those companies entered due diligence and a third of the companies in diligence were offered a term sheet. The average firm screened 200 companies in a given year and ended up investing in four of them. By far, the most important factor for investment selection was the team. When evaluating a team, VCs focused most on skill, domain expertise, passion, entrepreneurial experience, and teamwork. The second most important factor was product/technology, and among other important factors were industry, market, and business model (obviously fit with the fund strategy is an important criterion as well).

Most VC funds articulate their "investment thesis" on their websites. Some investors also post their decision-making process in blogs on the Internet that provide insights into the decision trees they use to make investment decisions. For example, Rob Go [9] uses founders and product–market-fit as the most important criteria. In his blog post, he states that the first step of evaluation is to determine whether the company has an "awesome founder" (in a later version of the post the founder is termed "exceptional"). The investor would then consider if the market is "attractive." A "top 0.01%" founder can overcome an "unattractive" market. Never mind why such a genius would choose to start a venture in an "unattractive market," at least we know that an "awesome" or "exceptional" founder is in the 0.1% or perhaps the 1%, however that is determined. Eventually, the need for "strong" data to show "product–market-fit" is considered.

Korver [10] presents an elaborate quantitative decision-making model whose creation is motivated by the work of Tversky and Kahneman as he acknowledges the difficulty in making unbiased venture decisions. In an attempt to mitigate cognitive biases Korver proposes an *a priori* risk assessment process of the stages of a company's development that requires quantification of the major risk factors at each stage. This decision framework is intended to complement "the art of decision-making" by allowing for subjective judgment, intuition, and pattern matching based on experience. There certainly is power in simplification and identifying the key factors that matter for the success of early stage ventures. However, in the end, these factors are not that different from those used by Go, and they contain another set of qualitative descriptors—"capable" CEO, "viable" business model, "healthy" team dynamics, "predictable" sales cycle—whose evaluation is subject to the cognitive biases that the method is designed to avoid. Further, the weight assigned to each risk factor is itself subjective and prone to biases.

The problem with all of these studies and decision trees is that they while they do outline an overall decision-making framework that appears very rational and makes sense they are superficial and only scratch the surface. The determinations of whether the founder is "exceptional," the market is "attractive," and the fit between product and market is "great" remain subjective and potentially influenced by all the cognitive biases discussed in this chapter. Certainly, everybody would want to invest in a great team that is building a product with tremendous product–market-fit in an enormous and fast growing market. These schemata are starting points, not the end of a decision-making process that involves a lot of subjectivity and cognitive biases. No matter what the prior industry experience and professional success of the management team, gauging its true strength involves a psychological evaluation.

Angel Investors and Angel Groups

Interactions with angel investors involve a different dynamic that is more varied and unpredictable than communicating with VCs. Many angels invest individually which means that there are fewer checks-and-balances to minimize cognitive distortions aside from perhaps their spouses or any help they obtain on their own. These independent angels typically invest during the earliest stages such as friends-and-family or seed stage rounds. A key element of their investment strategy is to rely on the competency and trustworthiness of the founder(s). In many cases, these angels feel almost as business partners or cofounders in the enterprise and expect to work closely with the entrepreneur. Some invest infrequently and do not have robust deal flow or a reference point of comparison about deal terms, valuations, and the relative merits of different investments. They might consult legal or finance professionals, but rarely interact with other angels for an exchange of opinions.

For those angel investors who invest with angel groups, in most cases each investor makes their own decision with regard to a given investment and they are completely free to heed or ignore the input of other investors in their network. There are two general types of angel investors—professionals that are still working full time (attorneys, physicians, traders, senior business executives) and those that are semi- or fully retired but would like to remain active. The first category is just as busy as VCs and thus relies primarily on their System 1 in making quick decisions with limited time to engage System 2 in performing in-depth analysis and diligence. The second group is seemingly the opposite—they have the time to engage System 2. However, they lack the inclination since this involves mental stress and effort, and retirement after all is about relaxation and enjoyment of one's free time. Therefore more often than not investors in angel groups are influenced by someone else in the group who happens to be a domain expert as their opinion provides an easy shortcut eliminating the need to do their own diligence work. In my experience the most frequent reason for the rejection of companies that have passed screening and are invited to pitch to an angel group is when an expert stands up and gives an authoritative negative opinion—whether it is true or completely misses the mark—that almost everybody in the room accepts unconditionally. On the other hand, I have found that enthusiasm is not nearly as contagious, probably due to the phenomenon of loss aversion. Most people including many investors are biased toward acting to avoid a loss rather than obtaining a financially equivalent gain.

Carpentier and Suret [8] analyze the decision process and rejection reasons of a Canadian angel group by monitoring its screening and diligence process over a period of several years. They evaluated objectively each team's experience based on three categories—industry, management, and start-up experience, and three levels (none, moderate, extensive) and then cross-referenced these rankings to the companies that were funded. Industry and management experience were most important—no companies were funded if the team was lacking experience in those categories. Multiple companies received investment despite their teams having no or moderate start-up experience. Surprisingly, the angel group explicitly noted the team's inexperience as the main rejection reason in only a few cases. The authors conclude that the lack of industry experience was reflected in the poor quality of the business plans presented, and thus the rejection was based on the weakness of those proposals and insufficient capacity to formulate a credible market strategy. If true, this means that lack of experience by itself is not disqualifying: even entrepreneurs with no or little industry experience can get funded provided they spend the extra time and effort to develop a deep knowledge of the industry that is then reflected in their pitches.

The other key factor in the angel group assessment of the team is agency risk—all other reasons associated with the quality of the team excluding experience. Agency risk may be viewed as arising from information asymmetry, e.g. the founders or managers have information that the investors lack. This leads to the possibility that entrepreneurs will pursue their own interests at the expense of those of the investors. Examples include potential dishonesty, insufficient motivation, acting only in their self-interest, evasive answers/behavior, poor communication/responsiveness, perception of whether the founders or management work well together as a team, and similar psychological factors. Agency issues are best evaluated through face-to-face contact and tend to be most important for ventures in the very early stages. Carpentier and Suret find that companies are most frequently rejected for market, product, and financial reasons and relatively infrequently for experience or agency reasons.

Many investors rely on a combination of expertise-based intuition and formal analysis when making decisions in situations of extreme uncertainty. What is commonly called "gut feel" in investment decisions is a complex process of dynamic emotion–cognition in which analysis and intuition are blended such that intuition trumps analysis. The dominance of intuition over formal analysis was demonstrated by Huang and Pierce [11] who asked investors to rate four versions of a business plan combining strong versus weak plan-based business viability and positive versus negative founder perceptions. They found that experienced angel investors have a higher likelihood to invest in situations where they had a positive assessment of the entrepreneur and a weak assessment of the business than vice versa. Although this might seem as a trivial finding that simply echoes the "bet on the jockey not the horse" theme, there is richness in the interplay between these two major aspects of investment decisions. The "gut feel" is a holistic judgment that includes both factors and where both emotion and cognition play a role. Investors rely heavily on their prior experience and previous investments while simultaneously focusing on their intuitions about the character of the entrepreneur. As an angel investor colleague likes to say "Before I invest I have to look into the whites of the founder's eyes."

Comparing Investors

Both the angel investors and VCs place a lot of importance on the quality of the team, an area where emotions, subjectivity, and biases play a large role. Nonetheless, there are significant differences in how they arrive at their judgments. These differences stem from the fact that angels invest their own money and have no one to report to (well, aside from their spouses) whereas VCs are investment professionals who manage the money of others and thus are responsible for their investment performance to third parties. Consequently, the decisions of VCs are based primarily on what they believe to be rational analysis. To the degree gut feelings or emotions play a role they are downplayed, if admitted at all, as that would negatively impact the image they have cultivated with their LPs. VCs also have more resources to perform diligence and better access to key opinion leaders (KOLs) to inform them in their decisions and enable a data-driven decision approach.

Another important difference is that while VCs place a lot of importance on the team, they frequently invest in entrepreneurs or management they have already worked with; the quality of the team is known, to them. They also typically invest in later stages where the founders have either stepped aside or have surrounded themselves with a team who has the requisite industry and professional expertise. Although VCs will fund first-time entrepreneurs, compared to angels they have much more influence and control over the path and strategy of the company due to the large amount of capital they invest and their presence on company boards. I have heard anecdotally that some VCs require inexperienced founding CEOs to sign an undated resignation letter at the time of investment that is kept on file. Given their influence, what matters most to VCs in first-time founders is that they are coachable, responsive and proactive communicators, and willing to defer to the VCs key decisions when divergence of views occurs.

Some Personal Reflections

I avoid investing in sectors such as consumer products where I have strong biases and personal preferences that I find hard to overcome. I also avoid areas not well aligned with my ethical or moral beliefs, as the dissonance would dominate my investment decisions. Investing in biomedical and other advanced science technologies, subject to a proper cost–benefits analysis, is aligned with my values and allows me to make a positive contribution to society. I prefer to consider technologies where I have a basic scientific and business knowledge and proficiency but am not a subject matter or domain expert. Apart from learning new things, I feel that my System 2 is more engaged and alert in such situations and as I don't have the calcified biases of a veteran of the field I do not take things for granted and am better able to discern faulty assumptions and paradigm shifts. As an added bonus I have the liberty to ask basic and dumb questions without embarrassment, and sometimes they are the better ones to ask.

I personally believe that character is destiny, and therefore I focus on aspects of the character and personality of the founder(s) more than on their experience. I would classify these aspects into three groups: (1) innate intelligence, general competency, and a balanced character; (2) honesty, integrity, and trustworthiness; and (3) commitment, perseverance, and tenacity. My biggest disappointments and failures to date in early stage investing have all involved misperceptions of the founder(s)—a pair who could not work together, a CEO who misrepresented the true capabilities of the software, another CEO who was an affable domain expert but incapable of financial planning, and others whose actions were driven more by their ego and reluctance to recognize their mistakes.

I do not fool myself into believing that I can read someone else's soul or true capability in a few meetings. In one of my favorite chapters in *Thinking Fast and Slow*, Kahneman describes his experience as a psychologist in the Israeli army assessing the leadership abilities of candidate officers based on observing their performance in an artificial training exercise. Initially confident in the strength of his predictions, he soon realized that when comparing them with the true performance of the soldiers over a period of time in realistic conditions, his predictions were only marginally better than random guesses. I am therefore cautious in developing too strong opinions and heavily relying on only one of the above three factors. Rather, I would like to feel reasonably comfortable about all three. I ask pointed questions and frequently like to engage the founders in a debate on their assumptions—this gives me a window into their thinking and depth of knowledge. Shallow and evasive answers disappoint, as well as carefully rehearsed rebuttals that do not address the question. I do not underestimate the need for industry specific experience; however, I believe that a truly exceptional founder—the kind I am looking for—will be able to recruit people who have it. The founder who sold their home in order to bootstrap their business impresses me. Founders who have put everything on the line and persist for half a dozen years without any momentum strike me as foolish and naïve. I try to avoid founders who are overly ambitious in a narrow way and those who are focused entirely on their own achievement, as that type of ambition can be blinding and lead to fraud ... as described in the following section.

Case Study on Biases: The Story of Theranos

The story of Theranos has been well publicized in the press and in the book "Bad Blood" by Carreyrou [12], so I will present only a very brief summary for the purposes of this chapter. Elizabeth Holmes, a charismatic young woman who dropped out of Stanford University at age 19, raised over $700 M in an attempt to achieve her vision of enabling inexpensive and ubiquitous blood tests that could be performed in retail locations utilizing only a pin prick of blood. In the process, she recruited a board of luminaries (Secretaries of State Henry Kissinger, William Perry, and George Shultz; the former Senators Sam Nunn and Bill Frist; Larry Ellison CEO and cofounder of Oracle; Robert Shapiro, ex-CEO of Monsanto, G.D. Searle, and Pharmacia; Richard Kovacevich former Wells Fargo CEO; Gen. James Mattis; and many more). She persuaded numerous ultrawealthy investors to invest, including members of the Walton family, Betsy DeVos, Rupert Murdoch, New England Patriots owner Bob Craft, Tim Draper of Draper Fisher Jurvetson (he likely invested since his daughter and Elizabeth Holmes were high school friends), the Mexican billionaire Carlos Slim, to name a few. The key assumptions for her vision to be feasible were (1) that blood from a finger-prick and venous blood would provide identical results, not just for one or two but for the hundreds of analytes and biomarkers used clinically, and using all four major types of diagnostic tests and (2) manipulating the tiny sample would not impact the accuracy of the test results.

Arguably, the esteemed investors and board members of Theranos initially made a rational decision—investing in a high risk, high-reward opportunity that could transform the diagnostic testing industry by enabling blood testing at such low prices that it would become a consumer-driven commodity allowing anyone to test their blood anywhere and at any time without needing a doctor's prescription. While these investors were fully aware that technology development carried risk, they likely calculated that the rewards would outweigh those risks.

This would be plausible had these investors eventually asked for and analyzed the data that supported Holmes' bold idea. Even granting that the initial seed and Series A investment rounds were by nature speculative and aimed to demonstrate early proof of concept, $700 M was invested over the 10 years that followed. In interviews and public presentations, Holmes was vague in explaining how her scientific innovation worked, using generic terms like "we are able to handle these tiny samples thanks to miniaturization and automation." There was only a single non-peer-reviewed article supporting the technology, published in 2008 in Hematology Reports (since withdrawn) that contained a cohort of six patients. According to Carreyrou, Holmes explained her penchant for secrecy by the paramount necessity to prevent Quest Diagnostics and LabCorp from stealing her technology. It is not publicly known what level of detail was presented to potential investors and Theranos' Board about the technology and data collected by the company. It could be possible that she provided data and explanations that were falsified and difficult to expose. During investor and partner presentations, Holmes made numerous false statements about business traction and provided plenty of financial projections that had no basis in reality. When her CFO Henry Moseley objected, he was fired on the spot. Whatever the scientific data that she provided, it is known that at least one board member—Avie Tevanian, the former Chief Software Officer of Apple who joined in 2006, quickly developed strong concerns and after his third board meeting privately met with the board chair Don Lucas and provided him with a memo of over 100 pages elaborating those concerns. No action was taken and Tevanian soon resigned. Clear signals existed on all levels. Holmes was eventually exposed by Tyler Shultz, the grandson of

Board Director George Shultz, whom she hired in 2012. When Tyler confronted his grandfather with his findings that the low accuracy and high imprecision of Theranos' test results would endanger patient health and safety, George Shultz sided with Holmes.

It is particularly astounding that big companies such as Walgreens and Safeway would engage in partnerships with Theranos that involved hundreds of millions of dollars possibly without conducting a thorough technical verification of how well the technology worked. Notably, hardly any VC firms specializing in the life sciences invested in Theranos. Perhaps, one day a comprehensive book will be written on all the cognitive biases that enabled Holmes to gain the investment support she did. Here, I can only suggest a few that potentially were involved, as well as some lessons learned.

First, there is the broad cultural context in America that glorifies the visionary young entrepreneur who is a force for good and disrupts the world while becoming a multibillionaire. For example, Bill Gates, Mark Zuckerberg, Ken Griffin, Sergey Brin, Larry Page, all left their college or graduate program to start companies that transformed society and became rich at a young age. Elizabeth Holmes fit that mold—Stanford college dropout with a far reaching idea who created a persona down to wearing the same type of clothes as Steve Jobs, leading to a bias that she belonged to this selected group of young visionaries.

This appeal was enhanced by her use of social bias. Perhaps, key was the support of one of her Stanford University chemical engineering professors—Channing Robertson, who himself had established a public image as an expert witness against Big Tobacco and medical device companies. His claims that Holmes was once-in-a-generation genius comparable to Newton or Einstein, as well as him leaving two endowed chairs at Stanford to join Theranos' board of directors and become a consultant to the company, were instrumental in attracting luminary directors from the Hoover Institute at Stanford. This, in turn, made it easier to attract other directors, as well as investors whose concerns were no doubt diminished or even eliminated by the presence of a world-class cast of supporters.

Holmes was further able to enhance the "social proof" aspect by using another psychological bias—the fear of missing out. Walgreens may have been persuaded to enter into a partnership with Theranos without conducting the detailed technical analysis that would have revealed the limitations of its technology knowing that CVS might be interested.

Both the investors and directors suffered from the "desirability bias"—the strong desire that a scientific breakthrough would create big health-care benefits for patients and improve the life of humanity. This likely led them to suspend deeper diligence that would otherwise be conducted for more mundane technologies of limited societal impact.

From Theory to Practice

Deciphering the cognitive biases and the operation of System 1/System 2 in individuals you have never met may seem like an insurmountable task. Each person has his or her own idiosyncrasies and specific biases that are difficult to discern in brief meetings and conversations. Nonetheless, some general approaches listed below can be very productive. The task of the entrepreneur seeking capital is to exploit the weaknesses of the investors' System 1 by taking advantage of positive cognitive biases and steering System 1 away from what could be negative biases, and further attempt to influence the transition between their Systems 1 and 2 thinking (or at least be aware of when it happens). This requires carefully observing people and having a lot of flexibility in your approach and presentation. Fortunately, many cognitive biases are widespread and easy to identify. Much of this advice may seem redundant to that given by other investors. However, I believe that knowing and understanding the deep psychological reasons of how investors act and decide is empowering and enables a greater flexibility in dealing with specific situations, thus it is likely to produce a better outcome.

Get noticed by System 2— In both the angel groups and VC funds, 70%–90% of investment solicitations don't pass the prescreening or initial screen stages and never get seriously considered. As mentioned earlier, at this stage of evaluation, System 1 is most active and in rejection mode. Further, many VCs believe that their deal flow is so good that they shouldn't worry if they miss good opportunities and instead focus on the performance of the ones they have already selected. While a large number of capital solicitations are either too weak or are not a good fit to the investment strategy or interests of the group or firm, many potentially strong opportunities do not advance to the diligence stages. The best strategy to ensure receiving at least a fair consideration is to find an appropriate referral source rather than applying for consideration "over the transom." VCs have a trusted network of deal flow sources whose opinion or endorsement they respect—this includes the current and former CEOs, senior management from the companies they have invested in, coinvestors in their portfolio companies, scientific founders who are in academia, and even attorneys and accountants. Given that there are typically only a small number of VC funds or angel groups that represent a fundraising fit with your organization, if you do not know any partners of the VC fund directly or through common contacts, it pays dividends to conduct a broader search and find a source they trust that will be able to make an introduction. The same applies to angel groups where most commonly the introduction will be made by one of the group members or one of the sponsors of the group. Once engagement occurs, the next step is to cultivate a champion of your company—in an angel group that would usually be one or more of the group's members, whereas in a VC fund, it could either be one of the partners or an associate in larger funds. While associates do not make the final investment decisions, they do have a lot of influence in the diligence process and can help one to ensure that your company receives a fair and thorough consideration.

Keep things as simple as possible especially in initial communications—As I have mentioned earlier, the key goal of an entrepreneur who is raising capital is to navigate the heuristics used by System 1 of the investor to make judgments and engage their System 2. Kahneman calls System 2 "the lazy controller"—presenting too much detail to an investor in the beginning might inhibit System 2 engagement altogether.

Storytelling—We all have gaps in our recollections and understanding that we have a need to fill with meaning and we have to decide what to remember out of the overwhelming stream of information we encounter daily. Whether it is in a slide deck or a face-to-face meeting, weaving a story that can be remembered is essential. Stories of stereotypical patients who will be helped by a treatment have become somewhat trite. But there is a story in everything—it could be a personal story, the story of the scientific discovery, the story of a mechanism of action, or the story of an evolving market. Elizabeth Holmes created a convincing story—from being the genius college dropout, down to her motivation due to her fear of needles and her uncle's blood draws trauma. The problem was that her story was lacking substance, but if the substance is there, a good story would help.

Framing—Framing is also under the full control of the entrepreneur—it involves providing a context that is aimed at triggering heuristics that have a favorable impact on the investor's perception of the business opportunity while avoiding the activation of heuristics that will lead to a negative decision. As an example, I recently heard a pitch starting with "My husband and I recently moved our company from the northern tip of Queensland, Australia, to Denver and are excited to start our business here." I immediately thought: husband and wife team on a temporary visa who are trying to make a living in the United States on my dime. A much better use of framing, which I later found out was true would be "After we won a green card through the visa lottery and my husband received a job offer in the marketing department of Coors I decided that moving to the USA would allow me to scale the proven success of my telemedicine business in Australia in a much larger market."

Social proof—Having so-called KOLs supporting your company and on your clinical or scientific advisory board helps significantly. It is even better if these KOLs are founders of the company and involved in its operations. Mentioning names of reputable funds looking into your company helps too, so does mentioning large and well-known companies that have engaged as your partners.

List the objections upfront—This a technique commonly used in sales and marketing. Raising money is nothing more than selling the vision and the potential of your company, and more narrowly, selling equity to investors. Any investor group you are selling to will have easy objections that you should know and anticipate. If you don't bring them up and they don't bring them up, then they will not buy your product, that is make an investment. If they bring them up before you do, it appears as if you were hiding something and are wasting their time by forcing them to ask about these issues. The best approach is to address all of the *easy* objections upfront by weaving them into the presentation and providing persuasive counterpoints. This should be done concisely and subtly as the target is System 1. Lengthy justifications and rebuttals are not necessary and are counterproductive.

Scarcity—You are selling equity (a limited commodity) and access to an outstanding investment opportunity. A sense of urgency can be created by sizing up the investment round so that the limited room left is commensurate with the expected investment amount from a given investor, introducing a time deadline, or mentioning the strong interest from others that will oversubscribe the round. Overplaying this hand could backfire—having such-and-such investors almost ready to sign a term sheet is the most frequent lie in fundraising, and if several months have passed without the funding materializing, the credibility of the entrepreneur is significantly diminished.

Conclusion

Scientists are trained to perform research on narrowly defined topics that is driven by, in most cases, quantitative analysis of the evidence collected in order to prove or disprove hypotheses or reach conclusions. Commercializing research requires leaving academia and persuading investors that making an investment in an early stage company is worth the risk. While presenting robust scientific evidence remains an important part of the capital raising process for biomedical science-based companies, investment decisions are frequently and substantially influenced by cognitive biases of the investors and are not fully rational. Discovering the biases that each investor might harbor during limited interactions such as pitches and investment meetings might seem like an impossible task. Fortunately, following a few simple steps can go a long way toward this goal. First, the general awareness of the psychological aspects of decision-making and existence of biases makes one more alert and receptive of cues during meetings with investors. Second, there are a handful of biases shared by most people. Understanding what they are and focusing on overcoming them can be very valuable during fundraising. Third, while the existence of biases might frequently be a detrimental factor that must to be overcome, do not forget that the reverse is also true—the entrepreneur can actively exploit such biases to their benefit. However, these tips are only provided to assist entrepreneurs in presenting information about their company or themselves in a positive light and to improve their chances of successfully eliminating negative biases. They are not provided for finding ways to falsify information about your company in order to manipulate individuals into investing in your company. One of the most important tenets about investor relationships is the trust between the investor and the entrepreneur. If an entrepreneur falsifies or embellishes information given to investors, not only does this jeopardize their trust relationship but in many cases it can eventually result in serious legal implications, as happened with Theranos.

In conclusion, nothing can help more to understand the biases of others than to observe one's own. Kahneman, Tversky, and Thaler created a new scientific field by observing the biases in themselves and the very educated people around them and realizing that they are common to all people.

Acknowledgments

I would like to thank all the angel investors and venture capitalists from whom I learned the art of early stage investing. The list would be too long to include everyone, but I would like to extend special thanks to John Huston for sharing his thoughts and materials on cognitive biases and his entertaining summary of the story of Theranos, and to Bill Houston for the many discussions of investment opportunities that focused me on my own cognitive biases.

References

[1] Kahneman D. Thinking fast and slow. New York: Farrar, Strauss and Giroux; 2011. 499 p.

[2] Thaler R. Misbehaving: the making of behavioral economics. W. W. Norton & Norton; 2016. 415 p.

[3] <https://commons.wikimedia.org/wiki/File:Cognitive_bias_codex_en.svg>, June 6, 2018, [accessed 10.04.19].

[4] Huston J. Personal communication.

[5] Murnieks CY, Haynie M, Wiltbank RE, Harting T. 'I like how you think': similarity as an interaction bias in the investor-entrepreneur dyad. J Manage Stud 2011;48(7):1533–61.

[6] Dunning D. We are all confident idiots. Pacific Standard Magazine, October 24, 2014.

[7] Gompers P, Gornall W, Kaplan SN, Strebulaev IA. How do venture capitalists make decisions? In: National Bureau of Economic Research working paper no. 22857; 2016.

[8] Carpentier C, Suret J. Angel group member's decision process and rejection criteria: a longitudinal analysis. J Bus Venturing 2015;30:808–21.

[9] Goblog R, Available from: <https://robgo.org/2013/10/29/a-seed-vcs-decision-tree/>, October 29, 2013, [accessed 25.02.19]; Next View Ventures. Blog. Available from: <https://nextviewventures.com/blog/flowchart-vc-decision-making/>, April 28, 2015, [accessed 25.02.19].

[10] Korver C. Kauffman Fellows Report, Volume 3, Spring/Summer 2012. Available from: <https://www.kauffmanfellows.org/journal_posts/applying-decision-analysis-to-venture-investing> [accessed 25.02.19].

[11] Huang L, Pierce JL. Managing the unknowable: the effectiveness of early-stage investor gut-feel in entrepreneurial investment decisions. Admin Sci Q 2015;60(4):634–70.

[12] Carreyrou J. Bad blood: secrets and lies in a Silicon Valley startup. New York: Alfred A. Knopf; 2019. 339 p.

Chapter 19

Securing Angel Capital and Understanding How Angel Networks Operate

Robert J. Calcaterra, DSc

Founder, St. Louis Arch Angels; Co-founder and Managing Director, Exeteur Group, LLC; StartUp Partners International, LLC, St. Louis, MO, United States

Chapter Outline

What is an Angel Investor?

An angel investor is an individual who is willing to put some of their financial assets at risk by investing in early stage private equity companies. The term "angel investor" is often interpreted to mean an "accredited investor." The Securities and Exchange Commission defines an accredited investor as an individual with a net worth, or joint net worth, with a spouse of over $1 million excluding their home, or an individual with an annual income for the past 2 years of $200,000 or more, or $300,000 with a spouse, and a reasonable expectation of the same for the current year. Because angel investors tend to invest at very early stages of a company, this group will most likely be one of the first or earliest investors in a start-up biotechnology company business. However, experienced angel investors tend to "keep their powder dry" and reserve some money to invest numerous times during the life of an enterprise.

Angel investors may work alone or within organized angel networks which I will describe in more detail later. There are many well-established sophisticated angel networks throughout the United States and some have specific industry focuses. In the United States, there are over 600,000 active angels investing in various companies. Most of the time, an entrepreneur can find an angel network somewhere close to their geographic location. In general, most angel investors usually prefer to invest in companies within their local region to help local companies and for the convenience of monitoring their investment company.

Typical Background of Angel Investors

The make-up of angel investors varies depending upon where you are located. In hotbeds of entrepreneurship such as Silicon Valley, Boston, or Boulder where I lived for a number of years, the backgrounds of angels are

Biotechnology Entrepreneurship. DOI: https://doi.org/10.1016/B978-0-12-815585-1.00019-X

people who have already succeeded as serial entrepreneurs themselves and are supporting others who are trying to do the same. Unfortunately, many of these people invest independently of angel networks. They might invest as an independent syndicate, but it tends to be with others who invested in their deals. I don't know if it is their self-assuredness that motivates them to be independent or if it is not wanting to be responsible for making recommendations to a group of people they don't know very well. This is unfortunate because being exclusive and reclusive can reduce the number of sources of money available to the start-up community. This leads to less thorough due diligence in deals they invest in.

How Much Does a Typical Angel Investor Invest?

In a later section, I will talk about teaching angel investors "to keep their powder dry." What we are talking about here is that companies you invest in will inevitably return for a second, third, and potentially fourth round of investment. You need to keep back at least two-thirds or three-fourths of the total money you ultimately want to invest in a given deal when you make your first investment. Of course that dollar amount is dependent on a particular angel investor's assets and how many companies they think they will invest in over the years.

All of that said from my experience and discussions with other angel network managers, the most common angel investment is normally around $25,000 with follow-on rounds comparable. I have seen very few investments less than that and very few at $50,000 per round and higher, especially after the first year or two of the network. The amount of money invested in specific companies by one angel group varies depending on the investment round and stage of the company. Seed rounds typically are $150,000–$300,000. With companies that have progressed through milestones and may have reached a Series A or B round investment, the total amount raised from a single angel group can be in the $700,000 to $1 million level.

Angel Investor Motivations

Experienced and savvy angel investors, or members of angel funds or networks, tend to want to invest in highly scalable companies (i.e., companies that can reach very high value with a relatively low level of initial investment). This is the case with agriculture and life sciences biotechnology companies, in particular device, diagnostics, and IT-based opportunities. By that I do not mean that these companies will *not* need large amounts of invested capital but that they can reach high multiple values compared to the size of an investment, whereas nonscalable companies will not be able to reach those kinds of multiple valuations. Agriculture and life science angel investors tend to be driven by motivations that include value proposition, relative scientific risk of succeeding, and emotion. The emotional aspect of investing in agricultural and life science-related deals deserves further thought. Bioagricultural investors tend to be driven by altruistic motivations related to animal health and treatment, nutrition, food safety, and feeding the world through increased yields and sustainable practices. In the life sciences, many angel investors are driven by the potential to prevent, better diagnose, treat, or cure specific illnesses. Frequently, this includes having a family member suffering from a particular disease or condition where the start-up company has a product that will treat or diagnose this condition. Angel investors tend to invest in companies within their geographic region as they are interested in supporting economic growth within their city or locale. Investing in local companies also allows them to be able to follow more closely their investments and the progress the company makes.

Angel investors typically are very early investors in companies, before most venture capital (VC) firms consider investing, commonly in seed and Series A rounds. Although there are some very early stage VC firms that do invest in start-ups, the majority of the VCs invest in later stages of the company development. Seed stage investing firms are rare. Angels are usually willing to take more risks and as a result they have very high-return expectations. In the 1970s and 1980s, angels had a reputation for making ill-advised investments and not making money on the deals they invested in. The reason was that they were not concerned enough about the management team, the value proposition, marketing barriers, regulatory issues, financial needs, etc. And of course they then overvalued the company. Today, angel investors are much more sophisticated and their investing practices are much more refined.

What Does it Take for an Angel Investor to be Interested in Investing?

Angel investors are not unique in their requirements for investing in a biotech company compared with institutional investors, such as VC. That is, we all look for unique science and/or technology that has a great value proposition, a strong experienced management team across all disciplines, a reasonable marketing and reimbursement strategy, a clear and defined regulatory path, strong intellectual property position, a well-defined timeline and financing, and an exit strategy. Companies will succeed in raising money if they present a compelling case around all of the abovementioned items. Companies commonly fail to raise money by not demonstrating that the management team is knowledgeable enough during the question and answer sessions of a presentation and during due diligence. In addition, fundraising is negatively impacted by not demonstrating that the company has a significant-enough technical and proprietary position and value proposition. In addition, investors will be on the lookout for naïve marketing strategies versus competitive products, a lack of understanding who their customer is, and a reasonable path to payee status.

As a cofounder of numerous start-up companies, angel investors are of major importance to me for the following reasons:

1. They tend to be less risk-averse than institutional investors and more willing to invest at the earliest and most risky proof-of-concept stage of companies (although this is changing the more sophisticated angel groups become).
2. They tend to be more patient than institutional investors with respect to exit, especially in biotech-related companies where there is an emotional-related driving force.
3. They tend to be less punitive with their terms for investing in early rounds compared to institutional investors.
4. They tend to be more willing to be flexible in terms of investment in subsequent investment rounds.

There is a significant danger for entrepreneurial companies caused by abovementioned items (1) and (3). Entrepreneurs need to be extremely cautious in the early seed stages of investment in their company. They must avoid overvaluing their company because subsequent Series A and Series B round VC investment terms can lead to severe negative impacts on early investors and founders for companies where this has happened. This can lead to negative feelings between founders and their most supportive stockholders.

A good solution to the overvaluation problem is to use convertible notes for early investment in companies in order to avoid the need for valuing the company at this early stage. A convertible note is simply a debt (note) that is owed to the investor but has a conversion feature that will convert the debt into equity, usually at a larger investment round. This investment vehicle will typically offer the investor a premium at conversion of 15%–20% (i.e., acquiring equity during conversion for 85%–80% of the stock price) and interest on the investment of 8%–10% per annum and a forced conversion when a qualified Series A round investment occurs. With the St. Louis Arch Angels where I have been a member for 14 years, I have participated in note conversions where venture funds accepted and upheld these previously agreed terms when they came in for the subsequent round.

Entrepreneurs need to know that with every form of early investment, there are issues that can usually occur. For convertible notes, they work well if conversion occurs quickly. However, problems occur when conversion does not occur soon but drags on with multiple rounds of small seed investments. Many times that will lead to an unrealistic capitalization table. I always recommend in convertible notes that conversion should be forced at modest conversion prices if a qualified investment does not occur within the first year or two of seed investment. Most Series A and Series B round investors also recognize accumulated interest in convertible notes as "double dipping" and normally will negotiate the elimination of the interest at conversion or a reduction of the rate in exchange for accepting the premium price. I have had both occur in investments I have made using convertible notes.

In recent years, another form of note called a SAFE (Simple Agreement for Future Equity) instrument has become popular in certain regions of the country that involves no interest and no conversion deadline to the note. I have seen SAFE agreements with and without conversion premiums. In fact, I have a company that I have cofounded that has two such investment instruments. A SAFE is an agreement between an investor and a company that provides rights to the investor for future equity in the company similar to a warrant, except without determining a specific price per share at the time of the initial investment. The SAFE investor receives the future shares when a priced round of investment or liquidation event occurs.

Individuals, Networks, and Funds

Angel investors come in all forms and invest through many different approaches and organizations. Each form has its own advantages and disadvantages.

Individual investors who don't participate in formal funds or networks tend to be somewhat reclusive and as a result very hard to find. Introductions to them come from very close trusted friends or through lawyers or financial advisors they have hired to manage their investments. They are reclusive because they do not want to have large numbers of people bother them with "deals" to invest in. I am aware of and have received investment into companies I have cofounded from individuals or families who have created formal funds to just invest their personal assets in early stage companies. Their motivation is purely seeking returns on investment higher than they can get in the public markets or for personal reasons associated with family susceptibility to certain diseases (i.e., cancer and heart disease). This occurs with very wealthy individuals with a net worth at a nine-figure level. Finding individual angel investors can be challenging because they usually do not do this full time and they certainly do not advertise. The best way to find individual angels is by networking with people who know them and by asking them for introductions. Check with your local university or research institution technology transfer office for names and contacts, as they may know some of the local angels. Moreover, check with the local Chamber of Commerce, regional economic development agency, or a technology commercialization center or equivalent, as these may be good sources of angel contacts who invest in biotechnology. Most angels are good sources for names of other angels. Once an angel has invested, ask them for help and introductions to others, because having a motivated and excited investor first tell the story is more effective than the entrepreneur doing it cold. There are many angels out there—be persistent in locating them.

Some angel groups create and invest in *angel funds*. Angel funds are set up by people who don't have the time or inkling to get involved in the due diligence and day-to-day oversight of the companies they invest in. This requires either the hiring of professional staff to run the fund or more likely a volunteer member who does due diligence on deals and does the negotiation of investment terms with the companies. Decisions in these types of funds are commonly made by an appointed investment committee. The advantage of this approach is that angel members get their investment spread over a large portfolio of opportunities in diverse industries much like investing in a mutual fund. The disadvantages are that you are relinquishing decision-making to a committee that may or may not be good at deciding what to invest in. In addition, everyone participating gets a normalized return for the whole portfolio which may have some very good returns and some very bad returns.

The most common form of angel investing today occurs through *angel networks* where each member of the angel group invests only in the deals they are interested in. The Angel Capital Association (ACA) has well over 260 member groups representing over 140,000 angel investors. This is an indication of at least a minimum number of groups of people doing these types of investment nationwide. Membership in angel networks can be as low as 5–10 people and up to as many as 100–200 people in some groups in Los Angeles and Boston. In addition, some angel networks have established "side car funds" to allow members to also invest in a fund that matches investments from members; this allows members to diversify their portfolio.

Angel networks in locations that are less known for being entrepreneurial have very diverse memberships: for example, some are composed of doctors, lawyers, accountants, and people who own their own companies that are either family or self-made. Other members come from large companies and tend to be retired from a mid-management level. We found out in our early recruiting for the St. Louis Arch Angels that the general councils of major international technology-based corporations would not allow top-level management (CEO, CSO, CIO, board of director members, etc.) to participate in angel networks because of the fear of conflicts of interest. They even strongly discouraged participation from spouses and offspring of those executives. The industry background of members also tends to be very diverse. One absolute requirement, however, is that there have to be a few members in the early stages of a network who have experience in investing and managing early stage IT- and biotech-related companies. These people become the bell cows for early investments. Without their leadership, angel networks will fail in the very first couple of years of formation because of a lack of investment or bad investment decisions.

Locating Angel Networks

Finding individual angels can be difficult because they usually have full-time jobs and do not advertise. However, locating angel networks is becoming easier as their groups are organized and more networks are emerging constantly. There are two good sources for finding angel networks in your region, these include the ACA [1] and the Angel Resource Institute [2]. These organizations have databases containing the various angel network groups and are listed by geographic location. Another way to find interested angel networks is through Gust [3], an Internet platform that facilitates the connecting of entrepreneurs and start-up companies based upon profiles that a company creates and then sends to those groups that have an interest in investing in your sector. One important point for entrepreneurs is to learn about your audience and screen the angels and angel groups that you target. You will be wasting your time if you are working to get a meeting with a group that only invests in IT and you are in biotechnology, or the group only invests in local companies and you are out of their region. By researching an angel group, you are considering approaching you can also learn if it is a group that tends to kick the tires and then not invest or also is difficult to work with because of punitive deals or constant oversight issues with management. You should do due diligence on them just as they do with you.

How to Get an Audience with an Angel Group

Getting an audience with an angel fund or network is normally quite easy. They have been formed for the sole purpose to find opportunities for the group to invest in. Some groups have a much-formalized application and matriculation process and some are very informal. Whatever the process, it will be something very readily available on their website or in the local media. In both cases, it is best to identify the leadership and key influencers within the organization. I have found that administrators for these organizations are very willing to identify those people for you because that is their job. Making a full PowerPoint presentation to those key people is critical to finding a champion that will help you through their process. Without someone championing your cause within the group, it is very difficult to succeed in raising money.

The advantages for entrepreneurs in engaging angel networks are numerous:

1. One point of contact with a large number of potential investors at a fairly high level of investment.
2. The ability to find knowledgeable members of your science or industry who can influence unknowledgeable members to invest in your opportunity.
3. Once invested, one point of contact that streamlines communications to your investment group.
4. Access to a very large network of people and services in your community who have been screened that might be of value to your company going forward.

Things to Know When Presenting to Angel Investors

When you, as a biotechnology entrepreneur, are presenting your case to an angel network for the first time, all you are doing is trying to whet their appetite to hear more. You will only have at best 20 minutes to present. Most likely 10. You need to remember that 90% of the listeners may not understand the science you are presenting. Therefore you need a very concise and understandable lay summary of what your science is and what it does compared to current methods. Spend most of your presentation justifying the huge value proposition over any others' approach and selling your management team's qualifications and ability to execute. Before the management team slide, which should be last, spend very little time letting your audience know that this is a huge market and that you have a proprietary position. If you have accomplished your goal of striking interest, you will then have much more time in due diligence to present your plan in-depth, elaborating on all of these sections and getting into your roadmap (required tasks to complete, costs, and timing) and financial proformas. Angels will turn down an investment if they spot certain risks because they know that companies fail because of these key reasons:

1. Poor management team
2. No market
3. Lack of capital
4. Bad science

Of course if you talk to those failed entrepreneurs, many times they feel that lack of capital and bad science was the reason they failed rather than a poor management team or the lack of a market. It's human nature *not* to blame yourself.

When I think about the hundreds of examples of companies I have observed that successfully raise money, and then assess why some succeed and others do not, it tends to be in all of the factors I have mentioned above. However, it is my impression that most companies that do not even make it through the first investment screening fail because they can't explain the value proposition of their idea well enough. Those that make it into due diligence but fail are normally because the management team does not convince the angel group that they have the ability to execute the plan. Their answers to questions don't seem to demonstrate the knowledge and experience expected. Essentially, it is a trust issue. Trust of the management team is the one thing, with everything being equal, that correlates with investment occurring. We all know the old adage "invest in companies with a top management team and average science, over a company with mediocre management and world class science." In other words, its management, management, management; good management is the biggest indicator of successful companies above all other factors. Finally, in a very few cases where companies make it through the due diligence stage and fail to close on an investment, it is usually because the management team has extreme views as to the value of their company or an inordinate fear of dilution.

Understanding Angel Networks and How They are Formed

Understanding how an angel network is formed may help you appreciate some of the issues, motivations, and factors that angels are dealing with to find good investments. Also, you may be a successful entrepreneur or businessperson and may consider starting your own angel network in your region. There are numerous methods for starting and developing a successful and thriving angel network. I am presenting for your consideration a case study of an approach I was intimately involved in creating—the St. Louis Arch Angels in conjunction with Bob Coy who in 2004 was an executive with the Regional Commerce and Growth Association in St. Louis. Bob is currently the President of Cincy Tech, a public–private seed fund in Cincinnati, Ohio.

The St. Louis Arch Angels, where I am currently president, has succeeded beyond my fondest expectation with investments approaching $100 million over 14 years, from its founding in 2005–19. We have invested in approximately 90 companies in a region where prior attempts to develop robust angel funding failed and where angel investing in 2004 was very low. Keep in mind that this investment has occurred during a 3-year period when there was a recession.

Angel networks tend to be different in the types of deals they favor. The Arch Angel network, for example, is partial to IT deals that require a partnering relationship to gain traction, such as retail chains, sports teams, manufacturing, or research partners, with less interest in attracting direct consumer plays without a combined benefit to the partner and consumer both. With respect to agricultural and life science deals, we tend to become enamored with very big opportunities that have huge value proposition advantages over the current gold standard which is not a final solution. The process we used to build the St. Louis Arch Angel network is as follows.

Building Consensus and Structure

A task force of approximately 10 people spent all of 2004 researching angel network structures used by others throughout the country. We agreed on a model similar to the Tech Coast Angels in Orange County, California. We rejected a fund or side car fund approach. However, a very unique venture group using a very innovative structure called Cultivation Capital was formed by some of the members of the Arch Angels. It has also been quite successful.

Key features are not insignificant: a $1000 initiation fee, $1500 annual membership fee, and a required minimum $50,000 investment yearly.

Selecting and Enlisting Key Leadership

We very deliberately hand-picked the first 10 people we sought as members because of their previous leadership and because of their successful investment history.

An Efficient Process

Our process is very structured and clear to entrepreneurs, and that process is managed by an administrator and a deal due diligence part-time employee:

1. Apply online.
2. Initial screening and culling of applications by angel network management.
3. Presentation to the selection committee of membership (invitation to all members to attend). Average of around five to eight members attend with one to two companies matriculating to the membership meeting.
4. Company presenters mentored by selected volunteer members before presenting to the full membership meeting.
5. Membership meeting 10 times per year always on the same date (i.e., last Wednesday of the month). No meetings in July or December.
6. Immediate member feedback and statistics using technology regarding interest.
7. Due diligence membership team set up with a designated leader.
8. Regular progress updates from invested companies at membership meetings.

The number of applicants to our website average 5–10 each month, which would be equivalent to approximately 700–1400 deals over a 14-year period. We average 2 presentations at our monthly membership meetings so that would represent about 300 deals we listened to in 14 years, and we are now approaching 90 investments. This process continued to occur during a period of about 3 years of recession. Investments have ranged from $150,000 to $6 million per deal. Our current membership is around 70 members.

Entrepreneurs should realize that angel investing is highly dependent on building personal relationships. The smart entrepreneur should attempt to meet key members of the network to present their deal before they apply. If that member is impressed by the opportunity and management team, he or she will become champions in the selection committee and membership meetings. Accepting early coaching from angel members is key to succeeding in raising money in angel groups. Early contact between entrepreneurs and angel members can also help manage entrepreneur expectations.

The Arch Angel Network goes out of its way to participate in workshops in the community to educate entrepreneurs about our process.

Educating Angel Investors

Educating first-time angel investors is very much an apprenticeship approach. However, there are numerous workshops around the country that are available. In general, the best programs are managed by the ACA and cover basic topics and in some cases, in-depth workshops on specialized subjects, such as due diligence and term sheets.

First-time angels commonly make the following mistakes:

1. Becoming too enamored by the science and technology.
2. Becoming too focused on the benefit to society of the science and technology (e.g., a cancer cure).

3. Not concentrating enough on the qualifications of the management team.
4. Not factoring in risk and timeline in relationship to rewards associated with the investments they make.
5. Not "keeping their powder dry," that is, investing too much of their available assets in the first seed round of the investment and not having reserves for follow-on rounds.

For that very reason the Arch Angels use the initiation fee from new members to encourage them to attend angel-investing workshops. If they do so, we pay their registration and expenses from those fees. Unfortunately, not many people use this available asset. Another educational opportunity is during due diligence where we match experienced members with less experienced members on the due diligence teams.

Member Retention and Building Esprit-De-Corps

Angel networks historically have a huge amount of turnover; approximately 20% of the membership each year. This of course can lead to a lot of uncertainty with the networks. This has not occurred as severely with the St. Louis Arch Angels. The members we had leave the group left very early and they were self-selected by realizing they were not comfortable with the risk profile and exit timelines for companies they were seeing. Or, they have left because exits have not met their expectations and these members are "tapped out." Our membership has gone from 35 in 2005 to near 70 today with many existing members being replaced by new members. We have never had to invoke the minimum investment rule. We have members who have not met the minimum $50,000 investment in a given year but they have been people who have invested substantially more money in previous or later years. I attribute our current investment success to an esprit-de-corps (feelings of loyalty) within the group and our ability to build subtle trust among members. As is normal, the quality of deals has improved with time and we have seen more deals throughout the Midwest. I believe it is also driven by our screening, training, and selection of members. We allow prospective members to attend due diligence meetings with companies as well as membership meetings numerous times before asking them to commit. Obviously, our initiation and annual fees force members to make a serious reassessment every year.

Defining Success for Angel Networks

Defining success for angel networks is very difficult because it is a constant rolling fund with no defined beginning and end. Clearly it has to be related to the return its members receive from investments they make. That could be defined by the networks total internal rate of return over a defined period of time. I think a better measurement would be related to the number or percentage of companies invested in, which returned positive money to its investors, the number of failed companies or percentage, and a substantive number of examples of companies that can be highlighted which have returned significant multiples to member investors. During its 14-year life, the St. Louis Arch Angels had 8 exits and 10–12 failed companies out of 90 investments. That is a pretty good record but we certainly can't claim success quite yet. It is my belief that we are going to have a few very large exits within the next 2 years.

I personally have invested in 23 Arch Angel deals and have had 4 failures and 2 significant exits of 2.4-fold in 1.5 years which is a 40% return on investment (ROI) and the second at 4.2 times in approximately 7 years. I have 2–3 companies that may have substantial exits within the next 12–18 months. One is in negotiations for a possible 7× return over 7 years at this time, with another in the process of filing for an IPO. I have another four to five that look like break even in a longer timeframe with more risk of failure, and the rest which are less promising. Of course the ace in the hole card for everyone in the investment business is that the companies that fail early have less money invested in them than the ones that look like they are good because they have had multiple investment rounds. My portfolio looks pretty good, right? We shall see. The big question is, am I representative of the other 69 members of the network or not? In other words, the success of angel networks is very hard to define. It will be different for each member.

I must say that the biggest issue in the angel network community is the lack of exits in timeframes that their membership expects. That is the primary reason for some networks failing and for membership attrition.

Angel Expectations

In my opinion the old VC model is dead. That is, portfolios populated solely with perceived high-risk, high-return (greater than 20-fold) deals with expectations of 1-out-of-10 company success rates that drive the success of the fund, while dropping nonhomeruns quickly from their portfolio. Many institutional investors and analysts that I have talked to recently say they have modified their strategy to invest in companies with a higher probability of success and potentially more modest (such as 10-fold or more) expectation of return. This of course necessitates an optimization strategy regarding the whole portfolio and not just the big winners. This strategy closely mirrors the strategy that has been used by angels.

Reporting and Follow-up

One of the most frustrating experiences for angel investors is the lack of communications from companies they have invested in. This can lead to the lack of follow-on investment from angels. For me, by definition, top entrepreneurs provide all of their investors, not just board members and institutional investors, quarterly updates on their companies' progress or lack thereof. This is not optional. It is required.

Risk, Reward, and Myths

If you are interested in securing angel capital, you should go through an exercise I did recently and Google "private equity investing risk vs. reward" or "VC investing risk vs. reward," or many other variations thereof. You will literally find hundreds of sites and articles. Let me summarize this for you. The general sense of what you will read is that angel investors are investing a similar total amount of money every year as are VCs. The difference is that angels are investing in 10 times the number of companies as VCs and getting twice the return. Obviously this means that angel investors are investing earlier in deals at a time when the risk is much higher where VCs are being more cautious and investing at a later stage and not earning as much. Interesting! The corollary to this of course is that it is a sad indication of the lack of Series A and B round money in the market and the difficulty companies are having raising money after their seed rounds. Those of us in the game of raising money for our start-ups don't need to be told this through articles on the Web or in newspapers. We are experiencing it.

Of course, another belief is that biotechnology investors typically do not make as good a return as people investing in other industries, in particular the IT industry. This of course is due to the risk of science and regulatory issues and the high cost of science. Not so. It turns out that investment in biotech deals on a number of fronts and is not as bad as we all have been led to believe, and returns are better than in other industries. Good deals are getting funded and are succeeding and are giving great returns at exit.

I have been intimately involved in the creation, raising funds, staffing, managing, and leading as a board member for 10 companies over the last 10 years and advising over 100 companies for 30 years. It is an exhilarating experience and the most fun I have had in my whole life. I love the chase. Of course if you succeed it's all the more satisfying, as well as financially rewarding. Needless to say, you don't get a financial reward from every company you invest in; however, it is still fun even if you fail. You learn from the experience and you can try again.

Therefore if you personally have "the fire in your belly," nurture it and feed it and whatever you do—enjoy it.

References

[1] <http://www.angelcapitalassociation.org/> [last accessed February 18, 2019].

[2] <http://www.angelresourceinstitute.org> [last accessed February 18, 2019].

[3] <http://gust.com/> [last accessed February 18, 2019].

Chapter 20

Understanding and Securing Venture Capital: An Entrepreneur's Perspective

Craig Shimasaki, PhD, MBA
CEO, BioSource Consulting Group and Moleculera Labs, Oklahoma City, OK, United States

Chapter Outline

Venture capital (VC) continues to play a vital role in the building of biotechnology businesses as well as the development and commercialization of innovative products. If you are an entrepreneur or work in a biotech start-up in the biotechnology industry, it is likely that you will at some point require the finances and support of VC. In this chapter, we examine, from both the entrepreneur and the VC firm's perspectives, what is involved in finding and working with a great VC partner. The information presented in this chapter has been taken from my own experience and the advice of successful venture partners. The goal is to help entrepreneurial teams become more effective in raising capital from the partners that are right for your organization and at the right time in your company development. As we have discussed in the previous chapters, no matter how groundbreaking and world class your technology and product opportunity are, without a steady and uninterrupted source of capital, your innovative product will not be developed. Conversely, capital alone will not create these products; rather, it is the combination of skilled and experienced management, enabling technology, targeting a market with an acute unmet need, and having a great partnership with an experienced VC firm. In this chapter, we will review some background information about VC, their objectives, how they make money, how to help you find the right partners, how to approach them, and a few of the best ways to ensure a higher likelihood of closing a deal.

What Is Venture Capital?

VC is money that is managed by fund professionals used for the purpose of investing in high-risk ventures with the

Biotechnology Entrepreneurship. DOI: https://doi.org/10.1016/B978-0-12-815585-1.00020-6

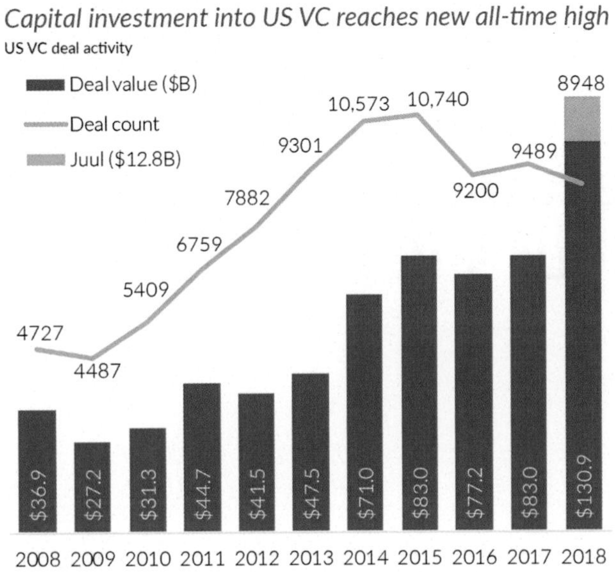

FIGURE 20.1 Venture capital investments in the United States from 2008 to 2018. *Q4 2018 PitchBook NVCA Venture Monitor—Overview.*

expectation of producing high rates of returns. Professionals that manage VC funds are called *general partners* (GPs), and the money in these funds typically comes from institutions or high-net-worth individuals and even from other funds. Individuals or institutions that invest money into a VC fund are called *limited partners* (LPs). These resulting funds are usually set up under limited liability companies for the protection of the LPs and for certain tax treatments. The National Venture Capital Association indicates that there are approximately 800 VC firms in the United States, defined as those funds that invest at least $5 million in companies. The size of a fund can vary widely, anywhere from $20 million to over $5 billion. There are VC funds that are directed toward almost every type of industry such as software, biotechnology, medical devices, media and entertainment, wireless communications, Internet, and networking, and some large funds invest in all of the above. According to Pitchbook [1], 2018 ended up being a banner year for the VC industry with $130.9 billion invested across 8948 US venture deals, the first time that annual capital investment eclipsed the $100 billion watermark set at the height of the dotcom boom in 2000 (see Fig. 20.1).

For the VC firms that invest in biotechnology, their GPs will have a specialized focus on one or more sectors such as therapeutics, diagnostics, medical devices, bioagriculture, or biofuels. In addition to the sector focus, each firm will have a preference for investing at a particular stage of development such as start-up, early or late development stage, human clinical trials, or expansion stages. And finally, in addition, all VC firms have distinct investment philosophies that are implemented by GPs who have different backgrounds and expertise such as cardiology, biomedical engineering, clinical laboratory, and immunology to name just a few examples. An important point to remember is that there is *great* diversity among VC firm's investing interest and philosophy, not to mention their geographic focus, their fund size, and the timing and availability of investment capital. Therefore, it is critical for biotechnology entrepreneurs who are seeking a VC investment to find out who their most likely venture partners would be before approaching any firm. Recognize that a good percentage of VC funds typically focus on later stages of company development when more capital can be deployed into each deal. However, there are also VC funds that focus on early stage deals, but it is important to do your homework prior to approaching a VC so that you are not wasting your time on a futile endeavor if your company is not at a stage of interest to them.

Most VCs are extremely active in their portfolio companies, and they integrate themselves in their company's strategic decisions, and even in certain operational activities as needed. These proactive VCs see themselves as part of the company rather than as simply investors. Other VCs operate somewhat passively, although I do not think the terms "venture capital" and "passive" can truthfully be used in the same sentence. However, compared to VC firms that "actively" integrate themselves into most of the company operational activities, there are others that participate predominantly through the company's board meetings and as needed based upon the issues facing the company. The entrepreneurial leader should determine what type of help and participation they want from a VC partner, and then seek those that provide that type of support.

How Do Venture Capital Partners Make Money?

An important question that entrepreneurs need to know the answer to is, how do venture capitalists make money? Understanding this helps the entrepreneurial leader with some background that drives many financial decisions made by VC. There are primarily two ways in which VC firms make their money; these are as follows:

1. **Management fees**—depending on the size of the fund, about 2%–2.5% of total money under management is allocated each year to cover operating expenses, salaries, overhead, legal, and costs associated with evaluating and managing the portfolio.
2. **Carried interest**—also known as "*carry*." Generally, about 20% of the profits from the fund are shared with the VC. In other words, there is a 20/80 split of any profits *after* the principal is returned to the LPs from

their fund. This is typically the most significant way that the VCs make money. It also means that they must produce significant returns on their fund in order to cover management fees and make a sizeable return to pay back the principle and receive a carried interest of the profits. This is the incentive to the GPs to significantly increase the value of the fund, and use their expertise to create and increase value.

Capital Is a Commodity, Whereas Experienced Investing Partners Are Not

Inexperienced entrepreneurs tend to view VC firms as strictly a capital resource that they need to accomplish their product-development goals. In reality, a good VC investment will come with much more than just cash. The ideal VC investment brings with it valuable expertise, which helps in navigating product-development and growth challenges, key contacts, senior management recruits, and—money. If given a choice between a $5 million investment from a group of individual investors, or $5 million from a top VC firm in your industry, going with the VC firm can be an advantage even if it means giving up a bit more equity. A key reason the value of investor's help and expertise, and the resources they bring which can improve the likelihood of success for your company. In addition, VCs have working relationships with other VCs, so if your company runs into development or market challenges that require larger financing rounds later, VCs can bring others to the table to help. Whereas individual investors and angel networks do not typically have the funding capacity to support the next level of expansion capital required for the growth of an organization. However, recognize that angel investors will typically invest at earlier stages than VCs do, and often do not require a board seat upon investing.

Search for the Right Venture Capital Partnership

The way I like to describe this relationship is a "*partnership*." Just as a company desires to partner with the best collaborators, they should also seek the best VCs as their partners. Finding the right VC partnership is critical to the ultimate success of a biotech enterprise. Here is some advice for those looking for the right VC partner:

- First, identify all the venture firms that have funded successful deals in your product sector or market space.
- Examine their track record, and research the backgrounds of their partners and associates.
- Narrow this list down to your top 5 to 10 VCs. Within each of these firms, find out which partners have complementary backgrounds, knowledge, and expertise that will help improve the decisions your company is expected to face.
- Talk with other entrepreneurs and CEOs who are running companies held within their portfolio. Ask them questions about their working relationship with the VC partner to see if that partner has brought value through their participation.
- Ask these entrepreneurs if the VC partner has the patience to listen to problems and if they offer helpful solutions and sound advice.
- Ask the entrepreneurs if the VC partner has used their contacts to help with any development challenges for the company.

The Start-Up Stage and Venture Capital Investments

In general, it is true that most large VC firms do not focus on start-up companies unless they form them themselves. However, this can vary depending on the economy and capital markets. Some VC funds do allocate a portion of their fund to early-stage development. But for the most part, if your company is a start-up, do not focus *all* your efforts on attracting VC at this stage as it could be a time-consuming, low-payoff, and disappointing endeavor. Before approaching a VC, you need to show product-development progress, and you need to have reduced the scientific development risks. If you are a start-up company, a good use of your time at this stage is to keep certain VCs informed of your development progress and apprise them as you move through product-development stages and achieve key milestones. Let these VCs know that you are *not* seeking funding at this time but want to know if they would be interested in being updated on the growth and development of your organization for potential future discussions. Work on preparing future prospective opportunities and establish some history and credibility with these organizations.

Another reason that most VCs do not typically invest at the start-up stage is that they have specific time horizons for their fund, and the typical fund life cycle is 10 years. Therefore if you are a start-up company and the VC is in the last half of their fund cycle, the length of time for your company to exit may be beyond their ability to invest. Ideally, seek a VC fund that is in the first third of its fund cycle (first 3 years of their fund) because they will have the longest investment horizon and typically will be seeking good investment opportunities. A VC fund in the middle of its investment cycle is starting to be choosier as to the stage of the company and the length of time to a potential exit. A VC fund in the final third of its life cycle is focused predominantly on follow-on investments in existing portfolio companies and liquidations.

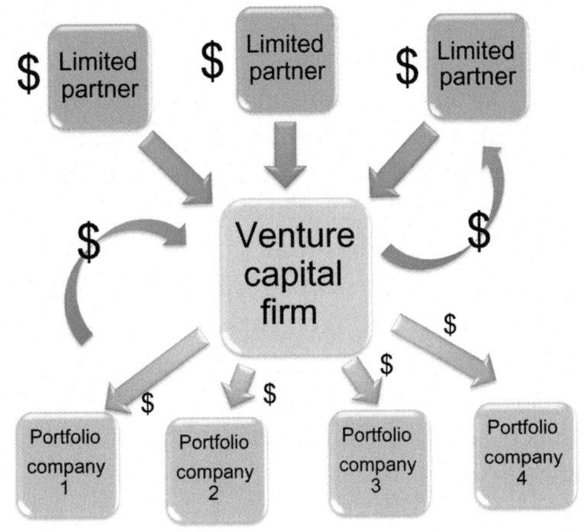

FIGURE 20.2 Understanding the Venture Capital Cycle.

Moreover, be sure that your capital requirements are in sync with the VC's fund requirements because the amount of money that a VC needs to deploy is enormous. A $1 million dollar investment from a $200 million fund is not a wise, or likely decision for the VC. That is because a $1 million investment in any one company requires the same amount of time to manage as a $20 million investment. For a graphical illustration of money flow into and out of a VC firm, see Fig. 20.2. The VC fund receives investments from LPs to deploy into their portfolio companies, and the VC fund managers, or GPs, are accountable to the LPs and they must return their investment with reasonable profits (see Fig. 20.2).

In short, seek a VC partner that plays two roles—a strategic advisor *and* an investor. A good VC must possess the experience and insight to add value to grow your enterprise better than the management could without them. Unfortunately, sometimes, a company does not have a choice in VC partners if only one avenue for financing presents itself. This is a good reason to start a VC search early and target only those VC firms that fit with the organizational goals of your company. Ideally, search for a venture fund with GPs that share similar goals, ideals, and values because these individuals become partners who will be providing help, expertise, and guidance to your team.

Venture Capital Partners Are Time Constrained

It is helpful to understand the time constraints of GPs at successful VC firms. These individuals are extremely active and usually pressed for time. They typically sit on multiple boards for their portfolio companies, each of which has needs and problems of their own that require the VC's help. VCs also have LPs to report to and communicate the progress of their portfolio and their fund's returns. VCs also have families. They have limited time and attention, so be sure to cut to the chase and give them the most important information about your company and product, and any other information that is of interest to them. However, do not forget the personal nature of this relationship, and ultimately, if you expect to have a chance of them funding your deal, the VC partner needs to like, rather than loathe, working with you.

Dana Mead, the former partner at Kleiner Perkins, Caufield & Byers, tells listeners during a talk he gave at Stanford [2] that VC partners at his firm spend their time predominantly in the following areas:

1. ***Reviewing investments***—Mead says, individually they look at between 200 and 300 ventures each year, whereas each partner invests in only one or two deals per year. The point is that all VC firms invest in a very small percentage of opportunities that they review, approximately 1%–2% of all venture opportunities.
2. ***Participating on boards***—most VC partners who have an established portfolio will sit on multiple boards and therefore will have less time to focus on looking at new ventures.
3. ***Networking***—they spend time meeting many people and with other VCs that they syndicate with, or may syndicate with in the future. They have 10–15 select VCs that they work with out of the whole cohort of VCs. The reason is, these are the people they trust, the people they like, the people they want to work with, and it is a collaborative environment.
4. ***Working with their portfolio companies***—they assist in recruiting good people for their companies. They apply their network to whatever challenge is faced by the company and they help raise capital during the next round.

Confirming the point about the enormous number of opportunities reviewed, Tom Dickerson, a private equity partner, shared that they see on average 1000 business plans each year, then do further research on about two dozen. Of those 20–30 plans, they invite 10 for presentations and invest in 2–3 deals annually (see Fig. 20.3).

Venture Partners Are Incentivized to Build Successful Companies

VC managing partners are the individuals who manage the funds, and the success of their fund is dependent on their ability to identify opportunities that have the best success potential. They also must assist in mitigating risks and helping the company management navigate through

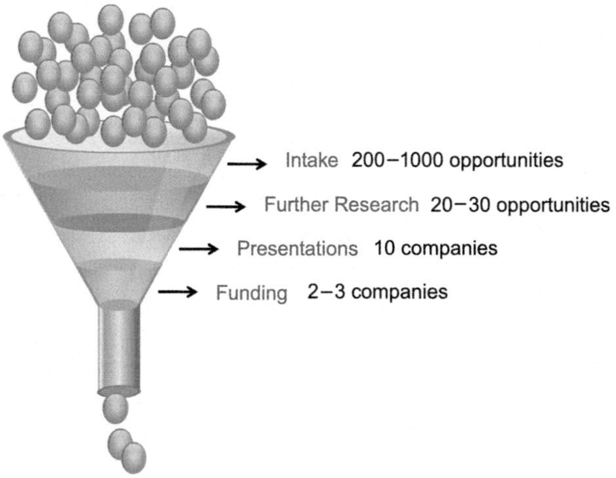

FIGURE 20.3 An Example of a Venture Capital Investment Funnel.

product- and corporate-development obstacles. Each VC fund typically has a 10-year cycle, which is the time expected for a return by the LP's investment. The better they are at helping to build companies with successful exits, the more profit they will receive from their carried interest, and their reputation improves for raising subsequent funds and aids in attracting the best companies who will want to work with them.

What Are Venture Capital Partners Looking for?

VCs like to invest in big ideas that make a difference. Beth Seidenberg, founding partner at Westlake Village BioPartners and former partner at Kleiner Perkins, Caufield & Byers, in a short interview describes what she looks for in biotechnology investments [3]: *"I'm looking for big ideas to disrupt the delivery of health care. KPCB is looking for people who are focused on what's possible and people who dream big and drive change. The millennial generation is frustrated and disenchanted with the current delivery of health care. We're looking for entrepreneurs who will apply the best tools, smart business models and inventive design to connect the silos of health care in creative ways and drive the transformation of the US healthcare system."*

Dana Mead describes what they do when they see a venture opportunity, breaking all the different risks into the following three major areas:

1. ***The technical and clinical risk and Intellectual Property (IP)***—they try to figure out what the technical risks are and put some boundaries around that risk to see if there is a way with a reasonable amount of capital to mitigate those risks.
2. ***The market risk***—at KPCB, he says they are willing to take certain technical risks, but they do not like market risks. They do not want to solve a really difficult clinical or technical problem only to find out later that the market is only moderately interested. If they go through the time, the risk, and the hard work, they want the product to be a commercial success.
3. ***The management risk***—for a young company with few management personnel, they also look at who is associated with the venture. Who are the people that have given them money? Who are people giving them advice? Will they be able to attract great talent as they move forward as a team?

These are the three most important things they look at in a new venture:

1. **Technical and/or clinical risk and IP.**
2. **Market risk (unmet critical needs).**
3. **Management.**

How Can an Entrepreneur Improve Their Chances of Securing Venture Capital?

Dana Mead says that the number one thing that sours their interest is entrepreneurs who are imbalanced. VCs understand that early-stage companies have lots of risks, so do not be afraid to talk about what these risks are. He says to be passionate and optimistic about what you are doing, but don't be afraid to talk about the risks; but at the same time, having some balance is good. You want to show passion that is contagious and have a big vision for the company. Moreover, he tells listeners, entrepreneurs should really leverage their available connections and connect with experienced individuals in their locale because they want to help. In summary, his admonitions to entrepreneurs are as follows:

- **Be balanced,**
- **Show passion for your idea and vision,**
- **Leverage networks and seek free counsel,**
- **Do not focus on the exit,**
- **Be persistent,**
- **Focus on attracting top talent and advisors, and**
- **Have fun.**

Beth Seidenberg exclaims that the biggest mistake entrepreneurs make is overpromising and underdelivering. She admonishes entrepreneurs to find the right balance between dreaming the dream and being realistic about what they can deliver within a specific time frame. "*Then do what you do best: Set up a plan and do more than anyone believed was possible.*" She continues, "*The best entrepreneurs always meet or beat their plans—and have fun doing it. Although entrepreneurs have to be optimists and believe in their mission, they also need to highlight the risks and communicate bad news faster than good*" [3].

When and How to Approach a Venture Capital Firm

Know Their Preferences for a Company Investment Stage

It is important to know the preferred investing stage of the VC firm that you are interested in working with. You should approach a VC firm when your development stage matches their preferred investing stage. If you are too early or too late for their fund, you will spend a lot of unproductive time that will likely result in little success. Most VC firms are latter-stage investors, some are in early stage, and some actually participate in start-ups or even form companies around a technology themselves. However, these seed-stage VCs are rare. Most VCs that participate in early-stage investing typically participate in Series A preferred investment rounds. A Series A Preferred round is usually the first "*institutional capital*" round. Prior to this round, your company will have secured a start-up and/or a seed round of capital that typically comes from the founders themselves, friends, family, and angel investors (as discussed in *Chapter 17: Sources of Capital and Investor Motivations*). Typically, the company will have been established, a corporate structure formed, a talented team of scientists, advisors, consultants, and possibly partners will be working together in some capacity, but usually the company will be somewhat "virtual." There will be key proof-of-concept work or preprototypes produced and a suitable target market defined with an acute unmet need. The product will have met some early development milestones that reduce the future risk of the technology. For those interested in specific product-development stages and examples of milestones, you can find more information in *Chapter 6: The Product Development Pathway: Charting the Right Course*, in the book *The Business of Bioscience: What Goes Into Making a Biotechnology Product* [4].

Have a Proper Introduction and Understand the Venture Capital's Financing Stage

From experience, and from talking and listening to VC partners, your introduction to a venture firm matters. The manner of introduction to a VC is a good predictor of whether or not the firm will initially have interest, or even read your information. Very early on in my entrepreneurial career, I erroneously presumed that the larger the number of venture firms that I contacted, the better my chances of attracting a firm that would invest. To me, it was simply the "*law of large numbers*" so the more I contacted, the higher the likelihood of success. Based upon this presumption, I purchased an expensive email contact list of all VC firms operating in the life science industry in the United States and overseas. I carefully crafted a (lengthy) email explaining what I was looking for and what our start-up company had plans to do, I attached what I thought was a stellar (lengthy) executive summary and sent this to over 200 VC firms I thought would be interested in my start-up. I eagerly and anxiously awaited their responses. Over a period of one week to as long as four months later, I began to receive responses. Of the 200 solicitations emailed, I eventually heard from about 60 individuals, and the vast majority of them gave me a very polite, and often apologetic, "*no*." I eventually received seven "*maybe*" responses, but after more correspondence and an occasional phone conversation or two, I received one weak interest for a presentation. I boarded an airplane and flew to their office to give the presentation, but this effort resulted in no investment. The partner I was talking with had only moderate interest that was not shared by any of his partners due to our early start-up stage. At the end of this 10-month process, I had no VC partner and no money. After this disappointing but eye-opening experience, I focused on high-net-worth angel investors located in my geographic region and raised two rounds of capital, \$1.25 and \$2.4 million each. The point of this example is to emphasize the importance of approaching VCs at the right stage of your development and to target the ones that would most likely invest based upon their investment criteria and philosophy . Be sure to secure an introduction from an individual who has contact with partners in the firm you are interested in. If I had understood this ahead of time, it could have saved me about 10 months of futile effort.

Bruce Booth, a partner at Atlas Venture, discusses in an article on *LifeSciVC* [5], the subject of getting an introduction to a VC, and he reiterates that cold calls, or more commonly "cold emails," are ineffective in getting attention from their firm. Moreover, hiring a regional or boutique investment advisory firm to raise your initial round of funding is also not typically a productive way to reach a top-tier venture firm. He recommends that you be creative in finding ways to get an introduction to the venture firm partner you want, such as reaching out to the companies already within the particular VC's portfolio. These portfolio companies can be easily contacted via social media. He also says that he has had random introductions after his daughter's soccer matches. He advises *not* sending your business plan without some type of prior contact or request from a partner for it. Booth noted that Atlas has not funded a business that initially came to them via these routes. The take-home message is that qualified referrals usually attract their interest, even if just out of courtesy to the colleague that referred them.

Dana Mead describes a similar sentiment. When asked if any of the deals they invested in came over the "transom" or as cold calls, he indicated that although they receive a lot of investment requests over the "transom," he has not invested in any of those companies. He says that all the ones he has invested in have come through other venture capitalists that he works with and knows, or entrepreneurs or physicians or other people calling him or telling about it. Interestingly, there seems to be a reciprocating obligation as he says, "*never, if I have a recommendation from one of those types of people, will I not take a meeting with the company. So it's just the way it works and a lot of it is just the comfort we have in understanding where the company came from and the people*" [2].

Confidentiality, and Confidentiality Agreements

Realize that VCs review many business plans, pitch decks and executive summaries containing many different technologies. Don't expect a VC to sign a confidentiality agreement just to review your pitch deck or business plan. Understand that anything sent to them should be public information and nonconfidential. For confidential information that is not yet protected by patents, it is best to describe your technology in a nonconfidential manner, but be sure to demonstrate what it can do, and what problem it solves. It is unrealistic to presume that any information sent to a VC will be held in confidence. It is just not possible for anyone to remember what is confidential and what is not confidential when screening the massive amounts of information that they receive. There are some VCs who may actually ask your permission before sending your materials to others. However, you should expect that anything sent to them may be circulated to individuals from whom they may want an opinion.

What You Need to Secure a Meeting With a Venture Capital Firm

A series of interview vignettes with Brook Byers, posted on Stanford's Entrepreneurship Corner, is a valuable resource for understanding how to secure a meeting with a VC. Mr. Byers, a founding partner with Kleiner Perkins, Caufield & Byers, has been in the VC industry since 1972, and a partner with the firm since 1977. He has been closely involved with a myriad of new technology-based ventures, many of which have become public companies. Although the interview was conducted in April 2005, most of the information remains relevant today. He says that all VCs are not the same, and that all VC firms are idiosyncratic based upon the firm, the LPs, and by the individuals who are in each firm. He goes on to say that you want to connect with a person on the VC team who has the same interest and passion as you have, and someone who would become a champion or advocate for you. For those interested in learning more about how to improve your chances of funding from a VC firm, listen to these at the Stanford eCorner.[1]

Most of all VCs are constantly inundated with proposals from companies requesting funding for their product concept. In order to get much further than simply an introduction, you will need a clear, concise, and well-written executive summary, a compelling slide deck and possibly a full business plan, although fewer and fewer VCs are requesting and reading full business plans these days. In addition, you need to understand what a "pitch" is. A pitch is an attention grabber that succinctly describes the technology, the market, and the unmet need, to open the door for future discussions with VC. As VCs are inundated with so many opportunities, it is essential that the entrepreneur presents the most relevant information succinctly so that the VC partner can quickly assess if they want to hear more.

Raising Capital for Biotechnology Companies

In this section, with permission, I have incorporated valuable information from Bruce Booth based upon his website *LifeSciVC* [5], I have also incorporated lessons from my own experience and offer some general guidelines about how to increase your likelihood of successful fundraising.

Know and Understand Your Investor Audience

When approaching any investor audience, it is important to recognize that each investor group has varying investment requirements and motivations. Venture firms have different investing requirements and different capabilities compared with angel investors and angel networks. To begin with, be sure that the VC you are approaching has a focus that matches your product-development stage. Remember, there is a great diversity of VC focuses; some concentrate on seed-stage and early development stages, whereas others concentrate on later-stage-development opportunities. If you are seeking a venture firm to participate in your later-stage opportunity but they focus on early stages, you are unlikely to get their interest. Just be sure that the VC firm interest matches your stage of development and, of course, your product category. In other words, if the VC firm specializes in therapeutics, you are not likely to have much success if you are a diagnostics or medical device company. Pay attention to the VC's portfolio and learn what type of opportunities and at

1. <https://ecorner.stanford.edu/video/looking-for-investors/> [accessed February 16, 2019].

what stage they like to invest. Each individual VC partner specializes in a particular area because of their expertise and background. You can usually find information about a VC's portfolio companies and the backgrounds of their partners on their website.

Make Sure You Have Quality Science and Quality Scientists

Biotechnology products depend on the underlying science and technology in order to develop a successful product and VCs want to invest in opportunities that are based on great science. The quality of the underlying science, the acuteness of the unmet need, and having a breakthrough application will attract the interest of VCs. This is a common theme for many venture firms as these types of opportunities support their expectations of very high returns. VCs also know which are the big markets, so do not spend much time trying to convince investors about the enormous market in cancer, heart disease, or Alzheimer's, rather focus instead on the core issues that impact the investment decision of a science-based biotechnology company. Share the scientific data that supports your claims and avoid too much conjecture, but remain open about what you know and what you do not know. Always focus on data-driven evidence and good assumptions because the quality of the science is a critical component, and all data must be reproducible. As discussed in *Chapter 11: Technology Opportunities: Evaluating the Idea*, great science and great scientists are inseparable. The knowledge and ideas that created the discovery opportunity are inherent within the scientist, physician, engineer, or technology expert. It is important to be sure that the scientist(s) who developed the concepts be in some way associated with the company and its product development.

Be Sure You Have an Experienced and Seasoned Management Team

It is always challenging to recruit great management talent for a development-stage biotechnology company, but it is easier to do so with great science and technology. During the start-up stages, typically the management team is incomplete, yet they should be surrounded by seasoned leaders, expert scientific advisory members, experienced board members, and other quality advisors. As the company grows, there is a need for an experienced and seasoned CEO to lead the organization. The best CEOs in this industry have learned through years of apprenticeship, project leadership, and real-life lessons. Make sure your team members have some of these deep experiences. Moreover, make sure that your leadership, managers, and advisory members have a good blend of experience and enthusiasm for your product and your company. Depending on the type of product being developed, sometimes an early-stage company may not yet require a full-time, high-caliber CEO. However, be honest about the management gaps, and share a time frame in which you intend to fill these positions. One great benefit of having a VC partner is their ability to help recruit top management talent at the appropriate time. Therefore, it is important to get the right group of early executives and leaders when forming a solid management team. It is also important to recognize that different management teams and/or different management styles are often required at different stages of a company's development. For more information about transitioning management styles during different company growth stages, see *Chapter 35: Company Growth Stages and the Value of Corporate Culture.*

Risk Management and Risk Mitigation

The entrepreneur and management team are risk managers of both the business and the science. However, you cannot manage a risk that you don't know or understand. Be sure to honestly evaluate and assess the risks your company will face. Then share with experienced advisors the company and product-development risks, and the manner in which management has steadily reduced these risks relative to its stage of product development. As you identify the risks you are managing, be sure to include a timeline you expect to execute against. Be honest with the risks you perceive because you can be sure that the investor will be looking for them. Having an honest view of these risks and the mitigating milestones that your team is working on, will increase your likelihood of raising money.

Do Not Overvalue Your Company at Any Funding Stage

Most VCs that operate in your product and technology sector will have a good idea what fair valuations are for a company at your particular stage of development. I say most, because there are some what would want to lowball your valuation. Aside from those groups, reputable VCs and partners will know what your current valuation is relative to the current financial markets. Understandably, most entrepreneurs will tend to overvalue their company at the start-up and early development stages. The answer to "how much is your company worth" determines the slice of equity for the founders, employees, and current and future shareholders. However, overvaluing your company is counterproductive and detrimental to attracting institutional and VC during these critical stages. The right company valuation is obviously the market-clearing price at the time. Any entrepreneur who overvalues his or her company will also raise questions about irrational behavior in the future.

There are standard and accepted valuation methods for determining the value of companies *with* product revenue, but these methods cannot be applied accurately to an early or development-stage prerevenue biotechnology company. VCs have a good understanding of the valuation of comparable companies at your stage, in your product sector, and in your target market. This method is analogous to how real estate valuations are determined based upon comparables within a local region and based upon the past sales of comparable properties. Inherent within a VC valuation is an assessment of a return requirement at exit, or an expectation of an investment multiple required to make the investment worthwhile for the venture firm.

Some companies at prerevenue stages may commission a professional valuation assessment by investment bankers or other private equity firms. These firms typically estimate a company valuation using a discounted cash flow (DCF) projection of future revenue streams. This exercise may be helpful, but in reality, no one can predict what actual sales will be in the future, and more importantly, no one can predict the likelihood of the company successfully reaching commercialization. Even if the valuation exercise includes a risk adjustment for achieving each subsequent product-development milestone (risk-adjusted discounted cash flow, rDCF), the risk assigned to any particular development stage is a guess, and someone can make an equally strong argument for a different risk adjustment. Early- and development-stage companies have many financial and scientific uncertainties that weaken the ability to confidently utilize a rDCF method. Moreover, the cost, risk, and time associated with the research and development phase of any particular biotechnology product are uncertain. More importantly, VCs typically do not use rDCF for their valuation of early- or development-stage biotechnology companies, whereas they are the most common investors at this stage of development.

Accurately determining the valuation of a development-stage biotechnology company is important for attracting financing, issuing stock at "fair-market" value, and ensuring that future financing partners are not soured by an unrealistically valued company. Having a realistic valuation for your company will increase the likelihood of financing your enterprise. In reality, never forget that valuation is ultimately determined by the investor who writes the check. You can read more information about the valuation of development-stage biotechnology companies at my website [6] *"How Much is Your Company Really Worth?"*

Estimate the Long-Term Capital Needs and Your Likely Exit

All start-up companies should have a realistic long-term business plan that addresses how much capital is required to reach an exit or liquidity event. Such a plan should include the product-development stages and key milestones that are reached prior to each funding. As we all know, there is a lot of variability in future financing plans, but these must address the amount of capital required to reach each value-enhancing milestone or product-development stage. Moreover, the team should know the total amount of capital needed to reach a liquidity event. For example, does the plan require $5 million, $50 million, or $100 million in equity financing to reach an exit for the investors and shareholders? The VCs like to see capital-efficient organizations that are scaled appropriately for their type of product development and business strategy. The management team must know how to outsource selectively, and how to aggressively leverage nondilutive sources of capital such as grants.

Utilize Experienced Corporate and Patent Counsel

Nothing hurts a start-up company's fundraising momentum more than poor corporate fundamentals, including odd company structures, convoluted capitalization tables, oversized and nonstrategic boards, a poorly drafted license option or license agreement, and a lack of intellectual property or freedom-to-operate. Remember that patents are critical to a biotech company, so make sure you retain seasoned patent counsel, preferably experienced in both prosecution and litigation of patents. Moreover, you must have a biotechnology industry-experienced attorney that has a history of working with start-ups. Obtaining good legal advice is very important for early-stage biotechnology companies (see *"Common Biotech Entrepreneur Mistake #3: Poorly Planned Corporate Documents with Many Hastily Prepared Agreements that Have Conflicting Language" in Chapter 41: Common Biotechnology Entrepreneur Mistakes and How to Avoid Them*).

Be Passionate About Your Company and Vision

Passion is an internal characteristic that is easily recognized by others. It is a requisite for success and for finding interested financial backers of your enterprise. If your product is in the medical field, be sure to share the vision of how your product will impact patients and change medicine for the better. Be excited! Share your infectious passion, because without it, start-ups do not succeed.

Business Plan Contents

Fundraising is never easy, and it never has been. By focusing on the things that are most important you will improve your odds of success for your biotechnology start-up. As you know or will find out, your executive summary and pitch deck are the first documents needed to get the attention of any investor. Here are just a few important topics to be sure that you cover in your executive summary and pitch deck:

- ***Describe the opportunity***—your company mission and its vision.
- ***Explain the problem your product solves***—improvements, cures, treatments, and diagnostic tools.
- ***Describe your target market and the acute unmet need***—who are your target customers, how big is your market, and what are the acute unmet needs.
- ***Explain the technology***—how it works, what it can do, patents, reproducibility, and differentiation.
- ***Share your market strategy***—your business model, market channel, pricing, partnerships, competition, and substitutes.
- ***List the experienced and seasoned team***—how their experience is applicable, background, board members, clinical, and scientific advisors.
- ***Share financial and operating plans***—funding and use of funds, milestones, *pro forma* projections, and risk mitigations.

For more detailed information about what to include in you pitch deck, see *Chapter 23: Investor Presentations: What Do You Need in an Investor Pitch Deck?*.

Your Presentation to Venture Capital Partners

So now you have been invited to give a presentation and give your "pitch" to the VC partners. Here is some brief advice about how to have a great initial meeting with a VC firm:

1. ***Know your audience***—understand to whom you are presenting. Are they scientists, physicians, engineers, business, or marketing professionals? Depending on the audience, be sure to speak to the aspects that are important to those listening. Do not forget to explain the science in terms that everyone can understand. However, if the partners are scientists, do not gloss over the science, but present the relevant data and discuss the risks and implications.
2. ***Share relevant information about the market need***—spend time on any aspect of your target market that may be unique or unappreciated for that particular disease condition or market for your product. Clearly describe the problem that your product will solve. It is not necessary to spend too much time describing general knowledge about markets such as cancer, heart disease, or diabetes. Help your audience know and appreciate key features of your market that make your product ideally suited to meet those needs.
3. ***Point out strengths of team members succinctly***—as mentioned before, a strong management team is critical to the success of any company. Share past accomplishments that are relevant to your current and future needs, but you do not need to go into great detail because all VC firms can recognize great teams when they see them. Point out the strengths that may not be obvious in your founding team members, scientific advisors, and board members—but do not spend more than a few minutes on these.
4. ***Share your vision but be realistic***—share your vision for success, especially how your product will impact and change the lives of those who use them. If you are a biotherapeutic company, share how your patient's lives will be impacted by using your product. If you are a medical device company, share how your device will affect the well-being of those who will use it. Do not overpromote and overpromise. But there needs to be clear scientific evidence supporting the market value of your product and the ability of the technology to deliver these key features and benefits.
5. ***Conclude with realistic exit scenarios***—be prepared to discuss how much equity capital you think it will take to bring this deal to a liquidity event. Most biotechnology companies will have an exit by acquisition. It is important to list some of the likely acquirers and those organizations that acquired similar companies in the past. Unless you are confident that your company has a special story that Wall Street and the public financial market will love, you should not consider including an initial public offering (IPO) in the exit scenario.
6. ***Engage in questions and answers***—be engaging when answering questions from your listeners. Do not become defensive about any question, instead explain the information and data that has led you to your conclusions. If you do not know the answer to a question, share what you do know, then propose to return with an answer later. Do not make up answers when you really do not know them. This is a sure way for your listeners to lose confidence in you. As with all investor presentations, expect to receive some hard questions, but remember, this is beneficial because they are helping you to uncover risks, and you cannot manage a risk that you do not know.
7. ***Manage the meeting's agenda and time***—at the outset, make sure to explicitly ask how much time has been allotted for your meeting. If it is a 1-hour meeting, plan to talk for no more than 30 minutes so you can allow 30 minutes for questions and answers. If it is interesting, the VC partners will easily be pushing for more than an hour. You do not want to find out

that you do not have time to finish your presentation or that you have not managed your allotted time well. Plan to save time for the most important part of the meeting which is the discussion at the end.

Next Steps in the Investment Commitment Process

The Term Sheet

Once the partners at the VC firm have spent considerable time and diligence reviewing your deal, and have collectively concluded that they have interest for investing in your company, they will send you a *"term sheet."* Although this is a "nonbinding" commitment, it is a significant step toward funding, and it indicates that if everything presented holds to be true, the VC firm will make an investment in your company. The term sheet contains a list of terms and conditions under which the VC firm is willing to invest. These terms include the amount of capital that will be invested, the premoney valuation of the company (the value of the company prior to the VC investment), and many addition terms. Some of the more common terms include the following:

- Type of stock to be issued: preferred, junior preferred, common, and warrants
- Liquidation preferences
- Dividend preferences
- Redemption rights and price
- Conversion rights
- Antidilution provisions
- Rights of first refusal
- Price protection
- Voting rights
- Registration rights

This by no means is an exhaustive list of terms but includes some of the most common ones seen in a VC term sheet. Some of these terms may be negotiable and some may not. This is where your attorney can assist by helping you understand the impact of these terms on your company and future fundraising efforts. For more information about the definitions and impact of these terms on a deal, see *Chapter 21: Financial Ramifications of Funding a Biotechnology Venture: What You Need to Know About Valuation and Term Sheets*. You can also find an example of a standard term sheet at the National Venture Capital Association's website, in their Resources Section under "Model Legal Documents" [7].

The Next Step Is Due Diligence

Once a term sheet is received, accepted, and signed, the next step is for the VC firm to perform *due diligence* on the company. Due diligence is a detailed and thorough examination of all the issues and risks of the company including technology issues, intellectual property, market assumptions, and corporate structure and agreements. Completing due diligence requires considerable time and effort from both the company and the interested investment group. This process can consume months for the management team and their corporate counsel depending on the stage of the company and the size of the transaction. Once due diligence is completed, there may be outstanding issues that need to be remedied if they can. If all outstanding issues are successfully resolved, a closing date can be set for funding. Closing is a joyous event and the actual process not too dissimilar to a closing when purchasing a new home—just more paperwork. Upon closing, you will receive a check or wire transfer for the committed funds. This is a significant milestone, and it is a good time to celebrate! However, do not forget that funding simply means the work begins in earnest. Keep in mind that you must reach each successive product-development milestone to ensure continued funding and commercialization success.

Summary

Starting a biotechnology company is a challenge which requires continuous sources of capital over long periods of time. At some stage, most biotechnology companies will need the financial assistance of VC. Finding the right VC partner can assist the entrepreneurial team in successfully overcoming product-development and growth issues. Every VC firm will have a focus on a particular development stage, technology, and market. It is advantageous for the company leaders to understand the interests and motivations of these firms, as it will increase the likelihood of securing funding. Biotechnology product development is a high-risk endeavor, and many product ideas do not always work out as envisioned. However, finding the right VC partnership with expertise in your area can assist you in overcoming development obstacles that previously seemed insurmountable. Spend time researching the best VC partners for your company and work on mitigating the early development risks, which will increase interest from the best VC firms.

Additional information about VC in the United States can be obtained from the National Venture Capital Association (www.nvca.org). VC information in the United Kingdom can be obtained from the British Private Equity and Venture Capital Association (www.bvca.co.uk), in Europe from Invest Europe (www.investeurope.eu), in Canada at Canadian Venture Capital and Private Equity Association (www.cvca.ca), in Japan at the Japan Venture Capital Association (www.jvca.jp), and in China at the China Venture Capital and Private Equity Association (www.cvca.org.cn).

References

[1] Pitchbook.com. <https://files.pitchbook.com/website/files/pdf/4Q_2018_PitchBook_NVCA_Venture_Monitor.pdf> [accessed February 16, 2019].

[2] Stanford University's Entrepreneurship Corner. <http://ecorner.stanford.edu/authorMaterialInfo.html?mid = 2811> [accessed February 16, 2019].

[3] SiliconBeat. <http://www.siliconbeat.com/2013/11/08/elevator-pitch-beth-seidenberg-on-the-shakeup-at-kleiner-perkins/> [accessed February 16, 2019].

[4] Shimasaki CD. Chapter 6: the product development pathway: charting the right course. The business of bioscience: what goes into making a biotechnology product. 1st ed. New York: Springer; 2009. p. 73–92.

[5] LifeSciVC. <http://lifescivc.com/category/general-venture-capital/> [accessed February 16, 2019].

[6] BioSource Consulting Group Bioblog. <http://biosourceconsulting.com/bio-blog/how-much-is-your-company-really-worth/> [accessed February 16, 2019].

[7] National Venture Capital Association. <https://nvca.org/resources/model-legal-documents/> [accessed February 16, 2019].

Chapter 21

Financial Ramifications of Funding a Biotechnology Venture: What You Need to Know About Valuation and Term Sheets

Stephen M. Sammut, MA, MBA, DBA

Health Care Management, Wharton School, University of Pennsylvania, Philadelphia, PA, United States

Chapter Outline

This chapter explores the issues and challenges in the capitalization and valuation of a biotechnology company from several dimensions through the topics listed as follows:

- Why valuation is important to the biotechnology entrepreneur: capital needs analysis, value inflection points, and the 20 questions of value creation in biotechnology
- The valuation exercise: it's not just about what it's worth
- The venture capital (VC) method of valuation and its integration with cap-tables
- Terminal values: from concept to derivation or "back to the future"
- The VC valuation method illustrated
- Cap-tables illustrated
- Relationship of investment terms and valuation
- The great convergence: infection points, capital needs, the VC method, and capitalization tables
- Preparing to negotiate: practical advice for winning what you need
- *Epilog and a few helpful additional resources*

The reader will conclude long before the end of this chapter that valuation in biotechnology is an art form masquerading as a science. It is an ironic twist that enterprises in genetic engineering must be more adept at financial engineering. In short, however, the challenge of valuation should not cause a loss of sleep.

Why Valuation is Important to the Biotechnology Entrepreneur: Capital Needs Analysis, Value Inflection Points, and the 20 Questions of Value Creation in Biotechnology

The creator of a biotechnology company and the management team that has been assembled have a lot on their collective mind. A list of concerns that will unfold over about a decade is as follows:

1. What do we really have in the way of a compound, process or platform in the realm of therapeutics (for acute or chronic care?), vaccines, or diagnostics? In fact, is our Rx distinct from our Dx?

Biotechnology Entrepreneurship. DOI: https://doi.org/10.1016/B978-0-12-815585-1.00021-8

2. What disease indications and molecular targets are suggested by what we have?
3. What are the prevailing clinical contexts for prevention management or interventional strategy for the indications that we appear to address?
4. What is the scope of proprietary protection that we might have, that is, intellectual property rights? Do we own and control all needed rights to go to market? Have we had to rely on licensing the core technology or ancillary technologies necessary for freedom to practice? What are the financial implications of this technology transfer and formation of an intellectual property blockade? Where will it provide protection? Where will it not? How do we manage the implications of that geographic or clinical scope?
5. What do other companies already provide for clinical use? What is in the global development pipeline? What is underway in other commercial laboratories? What is under exploration in academic laboratories?
6. Can we define the unmet medical needs that can be addressed? What is the epidemiologic scope of those needs? How do they translate into total, possible, and realistic available markets? In fact, what do we know about how the natural history of the disease in question and the practices of how physicians segment the market? What does this suggest about clinical end points?
7. What are the prevailing standards of practice or care that govern the interventions that we are considering? How were these derived? What is their flexibility? What resistance to change might exist?
8. What are we putting into the vial? Is it a small molecule, large molecule, other biological? Will it need a companion diagnostic?
9. Who will be interested and why? Are there obvious clinical partners? Are there obvious commercial partners?
10. What are the implications of our product for the prevailing care model? And what does this mean for our business and revenue models? Is it "business as usual" in the biopharmaceutical industry where, as a producer, we simply sell to providers? Or will that relationship diverge from the relationship structures of the last century as producers play a role in engineering the cells and tissues of patients under care at providers?

    Notice, so far, that we have not begun to consider the clinical development cascade. Let's continue.
11. What concerns should we address in preclinical studies beyond the usual toxicology, pharmacokinetics, synthesis, purification, and production challenges? How long will these take? How will we interpret and act upon the results? How do we design and report the studies? What will preclinical work cost? How long will it take? Are we outsourcing?
12. What do the preclinical studies tell us about the indications that we should purse if we have multiple opportunities? What can we now say about desirable clinical endpoints and how will the regulators respond to our views? At what point will we be ready for Phase 1. If we need to look at atypical populations for Phase 1, who are these patients? Do we test domestically or internationally, or both? What are the potential surprises? How long will this phase last? What will it cost? How will we report and interpret the results? Are we outsourcing? What are the odds that our product will survive Phase 1?
13. When will we be ready for Phase 2? Who are the likely clinical partners? What will be their concerns? Can they provide enough patients? In fact, what is the necessary "*n*"? What will this phase cost? How long will it take? How will we report and interpret the results? Will we segment as Phase 2A and 2B? Why? What are the odds that our product will survive Phase 2?
14. As we set the stage for Phase 3, will we undertake a double-blind, randomized clinical trial? Or, will we have an open-label study? In view of the study design, what are the bio-statisticians recommending in the way of the size of the study?
15. Where are the patients? What can we expect in finding patients who qualify? Where will we conduct the trials? Domestically? Internationally? What is a reasonable estimate of duration of trials? What are the likely costs? Per patient? Overall? How will we segment Phase 3A and Phase 3B? Are we outsourcing? In full? In part? What is the role of the clinical research organization vis-à-vis our in-house capability and capacity? Has Phase 2 changed our (and the regulators') views of the clinical end points? How will we interpret and report the clinical findings? What are the odds of surviving Phase 3?
16. How long will it take to prepare the new drug application?
17. How long will it take for the regulators to review and approve our application?
18. How much time will have elapsed? What proprietary life will we have remaining?
19. What other interventions might have emerged during this time period? How might the reimbursement environment change?
20. Who on our current management team will still be around throughout and after this process? What are the implications for continuity? What are the implications for accountability?

What is the purpose of this litany of questions? Each of the above 20 issues challenges us to posit answers and strategies to get from one interval to the next. That is exactly the way that professional investors size-up a biopharmaceutical opportunity, determine the level of capital needed and to be put at risk at any given interval, and determine the interim valuation at that point: the *pre-money value*. Once new capital is invested, the focus is on the *post-money value*, that is, new capital + premoney value.

Depending on the compound or product, clinical target or indication, directness or indirectness of the clinical development, the interlocking answers to the 20 questions define what investors commonly refer to as "value inflection points," that is a landmark or milestone of progress toward the final goal of having a product (or in the current environment a body of products and related services). In the long odyssey of arriving at the market, there may be anywhere from 5 to 10 discernable steps, each lasting 1–3 or more years, each ideally further reducing the overall risk of the project, each better defining the clinical and financial opportunity, and each having—to the experienced team and investor—a predictable budget.

The parade of achieving value inflection points defines the tasks but also the basis on which investors will determine whether to make an investment, the amount of cash to invest at each inflection point, and a guidepost for determining appropriate value of the company at each inflection point.

Some readers may be familiar with the concept of "real options theory." Real options theory is a framework for making investment decisions in the face of present uncertainty and continued uncertainty into the future. We use the term "real" because we refer to tangible assets, not financial instruments. In our case, we are referring to real medicines or diagnostics; however futuristic they may be. In the world of risk investing or "VC" in general, the framework of real options is the organizing principal, whether or not investors actually use that term. Real options mean that at any point along the chain of value inflection points, an investor declines the opportunity or opts-in and makes the investment, thus buying a seat at the table for future rounds of investment where more questions have been answered, risk is reduced, and value, therefore, ramped-up over previous rounds of financing.

Opting in essentially buys an option. At the conclusion of the efforts leading to reaching a value-inflection point, the investors ultimate goal of a realized, handsome return is not yet met, but they then reach a new plateau of insight and—hopefully—reduction of risk, so that they can further invest in the next round of financing, that is, the next attempt at meeting the next value inflection point. In fact, in the VC world, the terms of typical investment agreements guarantee the investor the opportunity to invest again through a provision known as a "preemptive right." This right does not guarantee a level of investment or a predetermined valuation, but it does function as an "option" to continue investing toward the end goal of having a product on the market. In the investment activities associated with biotechnology, in particular, the duration of development and the complex nature of the risks throughout the duration of development, any prudent investor and entrepreneur will put money at risk only to the extent that it is needed to reach the next value inflection point. An investor could make a bold decision to provide all the forecasted capital requirements on Day 1, especially if they could do so at a rock-bottom valuation, for example, 100% ownership for $100 million, but what is the point of that exercise? All the enablers of success—the entrepreneurs, scientists, clinicians—will have no incentive other that the intangible satisfaction of delivering a product that addresses an unmet clinical need. The opportunity cost of a decade's worth of effort, however, sours just about any sense of satisfaction.

The venture capitalists, themselves, are in the business of taking calculated, step-wise risks over time, but even they have their limits when it comes to opportunity costs. The reason is simple in its complexity. Let's say, for example, that a VC general partnership (*the GP or fund manager*) is managing $500 million of other people's money. The other people can be pension funds (yes, the money you will use to retire), high net worth individuals, sovereign wealth funds, and similar others. Collectively, these are the *limited partners* (LPs). The LPs, such as the venture capitalists, want their money used only as needed and only when there is evidence of risk mitigation. For that reason, the funds committed by LPs are only called as needed by the GPs. The GPs are judged and rewarded by the LPs only on the basis of producing returns, and those returns are measured as a function of time, or sometimes as a multiple of what is invested. It should be obvious that the motto of a famous winery, "We serve no wine before its time" can be restated here to, "We take no dime before its time."

The *opportunity cost* concept for the GP has an even deeper level of reasoning that gets back to the value inflection point framework and the associated time and cost it takes to achieve each value inflection point. Back to our GP managing $500 million of LP money. Because of the enormous risk associated with biotechnology, the GP seeks to assemble a portfolio of 20 or so viable companies during the first 5 years of a fund with typically a 10-year life. Some more detail about VC operations will help. From a $500 million fund, the GP will be allowed to take a management fee of 2% a year, or $10 million. It means that only $400 million of the $500 million is actually put into investments. On the strength of that $400 million, the GP is expected to deliver returns on all the investments made. Given the target of 20 portfolio companies, the GP is allocating on average \$20 million per company. Naturally, the GP will invest only a portion of that capital in each round of financing toward accomplishing the value inflection points. The portion held in reserve, usually called *dry powder*, is essentially sequestered for future opportunities.

Putting a finer point on this argument, in the litany of 20 questions asked at the start of this chapter, a common refrain was "How long will it take?" and "What will it cost?". "How long" is key when thinking in a real options framework. A GP is more likely to take a risk with a minimum amount of capital if the answer to a value inflection point will be known sooner rather than later. Why? Because if the company fails to achieve the value inflection point, the GP can then opt-out of future financings and redeploy the sequestered capital to more promising opportunities. For example, let's say that there is an opportunity for a GP to begin investing in a company with a small molecule that would have significant clinical utility. The molecule is ready for preclinical testing. The company claims, and the GP agrees, that preclinical testing will cost \$15 million and take 12 months for completion. This is probably an attractive opportunity for the GP, especially if there are two or three other VC funds willing to *coinvest as a syndication*. In other words, if there are three funds together providing the \$15 million, it means that each fund is putting only \$5 million at risk and will know in 1 year whether they should further invest from their dry powder. If the preclinical studies have a promising outcome, the next step can be prudently taken. If toxicity is discovered in the preclinical testing, the GP knows that the \$15 million kept in reserve for this company can be redeployed elsewhere. If, on the other hand, the GP's stake was \$15 million and preclinical testing was expected to take 2 years, it is likely that the GP would walk away without making the investment. Two years is too long to wait at this stage of development in the real options framework of thinking.

The GPs have learned after 40 years of biotechnology investing that on average it will take a portfolio of 20 companies from which two or three will provide large enough returns to help deliver a total fund return of 200% or 300% over the decade. Put another way, all that work, attention to detail and risk, add up to turning the \$500 million into \$1 or \$1.5 billion. The objective of maximizing use and returns or all available capital should be obvious.

The Valuation Exercise: it's not Just About What it's Worth

It is essential that the biotechnology entrepreneur understand the thought patterns and financial decision frameworks employed by VC investors. The technology due diligence, however promising, is not the final word in making the investment decision. The amount of capital, shared-risk with that capital, time frame for achieving the sought-after value inflection point, the level of risk mitigation represented by that value inflection point, and how these factors merge to suggest a valuation for the next round of financing are the indicators. The entrepreneur and the management team must carefully and thoroughly design the development of the company through the value inflection points, persuasively determine the time frame and the needed capital—documenting and supporting all of these with data—as the pathway to raising capital as needed for every phase of development. Anything less will likely result in disappointment, loss, and missed opportunity.

The valuation process, therefore, achieves more than just a number or index of value. Rather, the exercise produces a series of sign-posts or milestones for the investors, the entrepreneur and the management team, and for other stakeholders such as clinical research organizations, regulators, and strategic partners. Put another way, when done properly, the valuation exercise produces the ultimate project management plan. The reader should easily see how a GANTT chart or similar project management tool emerges from the 20 questions, the allocation of capital in reaching value inflection points, and especially the sensitivity to timing and the duration of achieving answers to questions.

A lesson learned thus far is that if the entrepreneur is obsessing about ownership *dilution* for the founders or the management team, energy and focus are misdirected. Dilution refers to the erosion of an owner's level of ownership that occurs through the issuance of new stock either purchased or issued as incentive shares or stock options for employees. There is a difference between simple stock dilution ("transaction dilution") and dilution in the net tangible book value of the stock ("price dilution"). Simple dilution may be acceptable but dilution in the financial value of stock is not. Put another way, dilution is more acceptable if the new shares are sold at a price greater than the previous share price, because although the percentage of ownership has dropped, the total value of shares owned is greater. Dilution is undesirable if the new shares are sold at a price equal to or less than the previous sale, because the percentage of ownership drops, and the total value of shares owned is the same or less. When the value of shares drops existing shareholders suffer a down round or "smash down." Entrepreneurs and managers want to avoid down rounds at all costs—as do the investors. However, the investors may try to reduce the impact of a down round through antidilution provisions in the investment term sheets. This is a risk mitigation strategy for investors that will be described later.

The best antidilution protection for all concerned, therefore, is intelligent derivation, budgeting, and definition of value inflection points throughout the development process. When that process is managed correctly, everything else will follow.

The Venture Capital Method of Valuation and its Integration With Cap-Tables

The academic field of finance has produced elegant approaches to address the complexities of determining the fair value of an enterprise for the purposes of daily trading of public companies, mergers and acquisitions, private equity investing, and, of course, VC. For all but the last category—VC—the methods can properly rely on performance history and audited financials and forecasts based on the foundation of prior performance and reasonable speculation about changes in the market or underlying technology. The valuation process for VC opportunities, alas, does not have that luxury.

Over the last half-century or so of VC, practicing professionals have relied on their day-to-day experience and knowledge of the markets in which they are active to identify appropriate pre-money and post-money valuations for prospective investments seemingly out of thin-air. While there may be some visceral elements to the VC process, there actually is an algorithm and chain of calculations that are followed. This process is typically referred to as the *VC method.* Some venture capitalists can effectively process that algorithm mentally, but most people need to do research and put pen to paper, or finger tips to Excel. That said, even the most experienced of venture capitalists must forecast the impact of future rounds of financing and dilutive events such as issuance of stock options on the overall ownership or *capital structure* and the underlying value of a company now taking into account a modeled future. That process of modeling the future capital structure is referred to as cap-table analysis. Cap-table analysis is combined with the VC method to produce a present valuation which has some basis in reality, or at least a range of values that can be the basis of negotiation.

Before exploring cap-tables, mastery of the VC method is necessary. A word to the wise, the VC firm will certainly assign one of their young associates to model the future and combine the VC method with cap-table analysis as a joint function of due diligence on the enterprise (VCs ask the same 20 questions in biotechnology ventures) as well as establish a basis for negotiating value and forecasting the amount of capital that will be required now and in the future of the company under review. The entrepreneur should not sit idly by and allow the venture firm to do the work. They might or might not share the results of their efforts in detail. The entrepreneur should bring together the senior management team and through their collective wisdom posit the future inflections points, the timing, and the required capital as well, and prepare their own scaffold for the negotiation of valuation.

The VC method is firmly entrenched, but sometimes it is referred to as the First Chicago Method after the bank that originated and promulgated the method in the very early days of VC. So much for history! The method's approach is a forward look at paid-in capital requirements for a company during its development phases throughout the holding period which is almost always until sale of the company to another company (*trade sale*) or divestment of stock following an initial public offering (IPO). Once again, the 20 questions are a useful foundation, because in addition to identifying the steps and requirements toward building the value inflection points, they can also be used to assign the *a priori* and the *a posteriori* probabilities to outcomes at every stage—factors valuable in construction of a full real options model. This chapter will not elaborate further on incorporating probabilities associated with the steps toward meeting value inflection points.

While there is copious data in the pharmaceutical development literature on the attrition of projects from one development phase to another, when developing biotechnology valuation models, the investors make judgments in terms of their overall portfolios. This is done in full view of particular risk factors for any given portfolio company, but the overall performance expectation of the VC fund is based on a handful of companies delivering the overall return and offsetting the inevitable losses associated with half or more of the portfolio companies. In a sense, when the biotechnology entrepreneur accepts funds from a venture capitalist, they are buying into this milieu of portfolio theory. As the numbers are run below, the reader might conclude that the entrepreneur is paying a severe premium in the form of stock for the cash that flows into the company. This premium is the cost associated with the inherent risk of the individual companies. It derives from the modeling of an "upside case" when all the inflection points are achieved, a "base case" where the inflection points are fully achieved but where macro-conditions or the value of the new medicine was overestimated in clinical terms, or a "worst-case scenario" where the march toward achieving value inflection points fails along the way. Obviously, when failures occur later in the process, the outcome is the most catastrophic.

Once the modelers have established the above cases, there are a series of steps:

1. For each of the three cases, capital needs consistent with the achievement of value inflection points are

established. The resulting capital needs are used to quantify the amount of investment needed at each step of the development process and forecast the likely dilutional effect from one round of funding to the next.

2. A terminal value or a series of terminal values are forecast based on value inflection achievements in light of exit multiples supportable by researching a cross-section of exit events by other companies in the same sector, or with similar products or clinical indications. This can be thought of as "comparables analysis" but differs markedly from the kind of comparables used in real estate.
3. The discrete infusions of cash through rounds of investment (the cash flows) and the terminal values price are then discounted using conventional net present value formulae. There is a difference with typical practice. In strict financial circles the discount rate used in the formulae is derived from other modeling. In the case of the VC method the investor's required rate of return is inserted. This required rate of return is generally reduced from round-to-round of investing. In other words, as value inflection points are achieved, risk is reduced, and the time toward the exit event is closer. Reduced risk lowers the necessary compensation associated with risk.
4. For completeness, there is a final step in general VC practice, although in the case of biotechnology, it is often suspended. For most industrial sectors the values derived for each of the three scenarios are probability adjusted with the value of the investment probability weighted.

The above establishes a basis for the mechanics of employing the VC method and cap-table analysis.

Terminal Values: From Concept to Derivation or "Back to the Future"

This section starts with an example. When the author began writing this chapter, Spark Therapeutics, a specialty gene therapy company, was publicly traded at a market capitalization of $2 billion. That value was serving as a good benchmark for other gene therapy companies as a terminal value in their valuation modeling. However, as of the time of publication of this book, Spark announced that it had accepted a buyout offer from Roche valued at $5 billion. This is just one example of the moving target of terminal values for given sectors within biotechnology. The company and the venture capitalist will inevitably dispute the appropriate benchmark for the terminal value, but both sides should be prepared to argue their positions in the negotiations.

This begs the question, "Is the valuation approach to early-stage biotechnology companies different from the way a company in another technology sector is valued?" Yes and no. The elements and mechanics are the same, but the consideration of the end point or *terminal value* differs. What is terminal value? The terminal value of a company is a determination of what a company will be worth as a whole at the time that the investors can sell their shareholdings to a third party, be that the public or an acquiring company at some arbitrary time in the future. The voodoo essentially starts at this endpoint. First of all, in any technology enterprise how can the future be forecasted with anything approaching certainty? It cannot. In the case of Google, for example, how could its role in the internet be foreseen, let alone how that role would be valued upon the IPO and thereafter? Google, in hindsight, represented a radical approach to search engines upon which a whole series of underlying business and revenue models were built. Likewise, how could the financial and investment destiny of social media companies be forecast when they were still a twinkle in the eyes of the entrepreneurs long before anyone else had thought about the category? The same is true of shared economy enterprises such as Uber, Lyft, and Airbnb. They could not either. In short, the age of unicorns is playing havoc with the terminal value concept and the expectations of both investors and entrepreneurs. If you are reading this book several years after its 2019 publication, take a deep breath when determining terminal value. Carefully observe the then recent activity in company creation, valuation, VC activity, and the response of the capital markets. In addition to disrupting industries, companies also disrupt investment processes. The lessons in this chapter, therefore, must be counter-balanced during the era in which they are read.

The companies that are revolutionary serve the purpose of providing vision and hope, and the fuel for entrepreneurial efforts and investment risk-taking. They are not valuable as benchmarks. Terminal values are determined conservatively and across most industries arbitrarily. In biotechnology, since the exits for investors typically occur postacquisition (and companies are often acquired after they have been traded publicly), the investors will use the prevailing "mood" and values at acquisition as a basis of terminal value, but that value is discounted back to allow for time—5 to 7 years—and risk. The general pattern of these acquisitions, especially once discounted, is somewhat less than inspiring. The history of IPOs does not help the situation. Companies that are traded oftentimes are listed at market capitalizations well below $200 million, and their aftermarket values often fall below that. In the world of biotechnology, IPOs are fund raising events; they generally are not exit events. Hold that thought: Terminal values are estimates based on conservative interpretations of prevailing acquisition activity with discounting for time and risk. For illustrative purposes in this article, we will work with a "universal" biotechnology terminal value of $250 million after discounting for market forces and risk. There is, however, a further discounting, as we will see, when allowing for dilutive events.

Once we have a terminal value, there are other critical considerations. The first is the analysis of capital needs, the process that we undertook in combination with value inflection points at the start of this chapter. There is an aggregate capital need for any company from the time it gets started to the time, once again, that the investors can exit. Capital needs will vary widely for a therapeutics company (and then by therapeutic indication), a diagnostics company, a prosthetics company, a device company, etc. Suffice it to say, the aggregate number is important, but the staged use of capital as driven by scientific, clinical development, and commercial milestones is the critical item to forecast.

The Venture Capital Valuation Method Illustrated

Experienced venture capitalists generally know what these costs should be for any given set of milestones for any given category of company. The challenge for the entrepreneur is to get these milestones and their cost estimates as close to the norm as possible. For illustrative purposes, let's imagine a specialty therapeutics company that will have an aggregate need of $100 million in capital in order to get up to and through Phase 3A of clinical trials. We will also assume that upon completion of Phase 3A, it gets acquired at our previously posited terminal value of $250 million, a figure that has already been discounted.

What happens now? Let's start by integrating value inflection points/milestones and capital needs analysis:

- Financing round "A" is preclinical, intellectual property, core management team build out: $10 million to be spent over a 1-year period.
- Financing round "B" is Phase 1: $10 million to be spent over a 1-year period.
- Financing round "C" is Phase 2A: $10 million to be spent over a 1-year period.
- Financing round "D" is Phase 2B: $20 million to be spent over a 1-year period.
- Financing round "E" is Phase 3A: $30 million to be spent over a 1-year period.

Note that this is a highly oversimplified and unrealistically symmetrical scenario that is crafted for illustration. In the aggregate, this company will use $100 million to get to and through Phase 3A. At this point, we have said, it will be acquired for $250 million. More often than not in the real world, the company would go public at this point, perhaps to raise sufficient capital for Phase 3B, or it might enter a strategic alliance. For simplicity, we will ignore these more likely events and go right to an acquisition or trade sale.

The situation herein is that the reader is a prospective investor in the first round and is planning to lead the first round of hypothetical company DNA Therapeutics, Inc. For the sake of simplicity—and this never happens in reality—you are making your calculations based on the common-stock equivalents of the securities that you plan to purchase. Your task as the prospective investor is to answer this question on behalf of yourself and other venture funds that might also participate in this "A" round of financing: *How much ownership in percentage and shares of DNA Therapeutics do we need to own today in order to meet our return expectations at the time of exit allowing for future dilutive events such as additional capitalization or stock option additions?*

You are working with the following assumptions:

1. The expected rate of return is 50% per year. We are going to use this expected rate of return as our discount rate. Those readers with a background in finance have probably just let out a loud gasp. As described above, in VC the unknowns are so great that traditional methods of deriving a discount rate do not function well. The expected rate of return becomes the proxy.
2. We will sell our shares at year 5. It would be nice in the real world if we had that kind of insight into future liquidity events. Like everything else in this exercise, this is simply an assumption.
3. There will be four additional rounds of financing prior to the sale of the company. Each round of financing will have a dilutive impact of 20% over the previous round. This uniform rate of dilution is irrespective of the amount of money going into the company in those future rounds. We are assuming that the company is on target at the end of each round and has added enough value that the dilutive impact of the new money is a relatively modest 20%. This does not reflect reality all that well but illustrates what must be estimated.
4. The current ownership of the company and a stock option pool (the entrepreneurs and future management) is 2 million shares.

   Let's now apply the VC method using a six-step approach:

   STEP 1: Determine the company's terminal value

   In this case, we are positing $250 million.

STEP 2: Calculate discounted terminal value (DTV)

DNA Therapeutics DTV = terminal value divided by present value of the future income streams over the holding period. The calculations simply put:

$$DTV = \frac{\$250\ \text{million}}{(1\% + 50\%)} + \frac{\$250\ \text{million}}{1.5^5}$$

DTV = \$250 million/7.593

DTV = \$32, 925,000—Yes, that works out to a large discount!

STEP 3: Required ownership at exit assuming no additional financing

To calculate the required final percentage (RFP) ownership at the exit date:

Investment: \$10 million

DTV = \$32,925,000

RFP = investment/DTV

= 0.304% or 30.4%

STEP 4 A: Determine the number of new shares

Existing shares: 2,000,000

RFP = 0.304% or 30.4%

Number of new shares = [2,000,000/(1 − 0.304) − 2,000,000]

= (2,000,000/0.696) − 2,000,000

= 2,873,563 − 2,000,000

= 873,563 new shares

STEP 4B: Allowing for additional rounds

Calculate the retention ratio (the percentage retained after four subsequent rounds each having a dilutive impact; we are assuming 20%).

Retention ratio = 1/(1.2)/(1.2)/(1.2)/(1.2)

= 48.2% or 0.482%

Calculate the required current percent ownership on Day 1. This percentage accounts for how much of the equity is retained, *after* subsequent rounds have been awarded.

The required current percent ownership = 0.304 divided by the retention ratio (0.482):

= 0.631% or 63.1%

STEP 4C: Shares needed allowing for further dilution

The dilutive impact must be translated into a number of shares:

Original shares = 2,000,000

Revised RFP = 63.1%

New shares with dilution

= [2,000,000/(1.00 − 0.631)] − 2,000,000

= 5,420,054 − 2,000,000

= 3,420,054 new shares to be issued

STEP 5A: Share price with no future dilution

For purposes of comparison, let's calculate what the share price would be if there was no dilutive impact of future rounds of financing:

Total amount to be invested = \$10,000,000

Number of new shares with no dilution = 873,563

\$10,000,000/873,563 = *\$11.45 per new share not allowing for future dilution*

STEP 5B: Share price with full dilution

When we allow for the impact of dilution, naturally the share price will fall; in this case, quite dramatically.

Price per share with dilution:

Total amount to be invested = \$10,000,000

Number of new shares with dilution = 3,420,054

Price per share = \$10,000,000/3,420,054

= *\$2.95 per new share allowing for future dilution*

STEP 6A: Pre-money and post-money value of the company allowing for no dilution

The pre-money value is simply the implied value of the company before the new capital is infused. Paradoxically, it is the post-money that is calculated first because as you will read below; it sets the upward bounds of what might be acceptable in the next round of financing.

The pre-money = post-money − new capital

Obviously, the pre-money + new capital = post-money

Existing number of shares outstanding times the price per new share.

= 2,000,000 shares × \$11.45/new share

= 22,900,000 pre-money value, that is, the value of the company before the new funds are invested.

The post-money = \$32,900,000 (the pre-money + the amount invested). This, again, is the value when we do not take dilution into account.

STEP 6B: Pre-money and post-money value of the company allowing for full dilution over subsequent four rounds

Total number of existing shares outstanding times the price per new share:

Pre-money = 2,000,000 shares × 2.95 (fully diluted)

= \$5,900,000

Post-money = \$15,900,000 allowing for full dilution

This is a fourfold drop in the pre-money value; dilution counts.

Comments on Sensitivity

The astute reader—even without a background in finance—probably has an intuitive sense of just how sensitive the calculations will be to the key variables. Terminal value was here set somewhat arbitrarily—but historically supportable—at \$250 million. What would have been the pre-money value of the company had it been \$500 million? It would have doubled preserving for the founders and entrepreneurs tremendous value.

In like manner, the discount rate applied was 50%. Variations in discount rate have a disproportionate impact, all the more when the time period varies; the impact one way or the other is essentially geometric. The numbers put to work are all prospective, and there tends to be little room for negotiation. The venture capitalist will use a lower discount rate in later rounds of financing or in those cases where significant risk has been reduced. If the market, be it M&A or public offerings is frothy, the venture capitalist may run the numbers with a shorter number of years, but the tendency is to be conservative. Similarly, if IPO values are running higher than the historical average for the subsector of the company, the venture fund may be willing to work with a higher terminal value. Here again, investors will tend toward conservative forecasts.

Cap-Tables Illustrated

Capitalization tables or cap-tables are not a mystery. In fact, they are kid stuff. The author has run seminars on entrepreneurial finance for middle-schoolers, and they absorb this concept like a sponge. The best approach to illustration is to walk through a succession of cap-tables for a fictitious company, such as DNA Therapeutics used in illustrating the VC method. First, let's revisit a few foundational concepts and definitions already described. Any infusion of capital from the sale of equity necessarily dilutes the percentage of ownership associated with previously sold shares. The goal of an entrepreneur in selling equity in successive stages is to justify a higher share price by increasing the value of the company. The total pie should grow faster than the number of slices: drive value!

Modeling DNA Therapeutics

These are the facts: three scientists have invented a new vector to be used in gene therapy. They developed the concept in their academic laboratories, disclosed it to their technology transfer office that has filed a US patent but allowed for future international filings under the Patent Cooperation Treaty. The university will be willing to issue a worldwide exclusive license with a right to sublicense to a company. The scientists decide that they should form the company and retain legal counsel to assist them. They are advised to form a State of Delaware C-Corporation using as simple a capital structure as possible. They each purchase 200,000 shares at $0.001 per share. The company's first cap-table looks like Table 21.1.

A few months go by and the founding scientists are starting to get serious about making the company a reality beyond the first cap-table. They are advised by people in the industry as well as by the university that they need a credible biotechnology CEO. In fact, the university will not issue a license to DNA Therapeutics until it has a CEO who will negotiate the license agreement with the university. The founders identify an impressive CEO who agrees to join the company. She praises the progress that they have made and is willing to purchase her shares as CEO at 10 times what they have paid, that is, $0.01. She also feels that on a fully diluted basis that the shares she holds at the conclusion of the round of financing will have to be equal to 30% of the ownership. She also knows that an employee stock option pool of 30% of the capital structure will have to be created in order for her to recruit a top-notch management team. Finally, she has started the process of negotiating with the university. Putting aside the full set of terms demanded by the university, she does want to include the university's expectation of stock ownership of 10% of the company on a fully diluted basis as of the time of her employment and the creation of the stock option pool. She constructs the second cap-table of DNA Therapeutics (Table 21.2).

The company's value is $20,000 because the capital structure is based on 2 million shares priced at the last transactional value that the CEO paid for the shares, that is, $0.01. She has wisely decided to incorporate the option pool into the structure now knowing that VC investors

TABLE 21.1 The first cap-table: creation of DNA therapeutics.

Shareholder	Number of shares	Percent ownership	Value of shares ($)
Founding scientist A	200,000	33.33	200
Founding scientist B	200,000	33.33	200
Founding scientist C	200,000	33.33	200
Total postfinancing valuation	600,000	100	600

Note that the company's value at this point is $600, simply the product of 600,000 shares and the *last transactional value* of $0.001 per share.

TABLE 21.2 The cap-table after the CEO, stock option pool, and university license.

Shareholder	Number of shares	Percent ownership	Value of shares ($)
Founding scientist A	200,000	10	2000
Founding scientist B	200,000	10	2000
Founding scientist C	200,000	10	2000
CEO	600,000	30	6000
Stock option pool	600,000	30	6000
University's shares	200,000	10	2000
Total postfinancing valuation	2000,000	100	20000

TABLE 21.3 The impact of the Series A investors.

Shareholder	Number of shares	Percent ownership	Value of shares ($)
Founding scientist A	200,000	4	666,000
Founding scientist B	200,000	4	666,000
Founding scientist C	200,000	4	666,000
CEO	600,000	12	1998,000
Stock option pool	600,000	12	1998,000
University's shares	200,000	4	666,000
Series A Shareholders	3000,000	60	10,000,000
Total postfinancing valuation	5000,000	100	16,650,000

will want such a pool buried in the pre-money valuation at the time they invest capital. We can also say that the post-money value is $20,000.

Months go by and after intensive promotion and equally intense due diligence, a Series A syndication of VC funds emerges. They have run future cap-table scenarios and have examined the landscape of other gene therapy vector companies and, after looking at publicly traded and acquired companies in the sector, conclude that a terminal value of $250 million is an arguable benchmark. They agree with management that $10 million is an appropriate funding amount for the preclinical studies and the Phase 1 clinical trials. They use the numbers in the sample illustration of the VC method above to determine what percentage of the company they need to own now allowing for dilutive events and further allowing for a projected 5-year holding period with a discount rate—their expected rate of return—of 50%. They conclude that they must receive 60% of the company on a fully diluted basis following completion of the round. This equates to the issuance of 3 million new shares at $3.33 per share. Note that for simplicity, we are rounding the numbers from the calculations above. The cap-table looks like Table 21.3.

The post-money value is $16,650,000. Let's think about that. Given that $10 million of new money went into the company, the implied pre-money value (post-money − invested capital) is $6,650,000. While the dilution for founders and employees looks dramatic, the share price from the previous round increased from $0.01 to $3.33. This is an example of acceptable dilution.

To continue this illustration, we will take one more step before we sell the company for the remarkably prescient $250 million terminal value that the Series A investors posited. In order to do this without creating an additional four capitalization tables, we look back at VC method step 4B when the Series A investors calculated the retention ratio. When they did that, the calculations for four additional dilutive rounds calculated to just under 50%. In other words, they expected that there would be

TABLE 21.4 The Series B–E shareholders.

Shareholder	Number of shares	Percent ownership	Value of shares
Founding scientist A	200,000	2.5	$3000,000
Founding scientist B	200,000	2.5	$3000,000
Founding scientist C	200,000	2.5	$3000,000
CEO	600,000	7.5	$9000,000
Stock option pool	600,000	7.5	$9000,000
University's shares	200,000	2.5	$3000,000
Series A Shareholders	3000,000	37.5	$45,000,000
Series B–E shareholders	3000,000	37.5	$45,000,000
Total postfinancing valuation	8000,000	100	$120,000,000 using $15 per share at the E round

TABLE 21.5 Financial position of shareholders at the time of buyout at $31.25 per share.

Shareholder	Number of shares	Percent ownership	Value of shares
Founding scientist A	200,000	2.5	$6,250,000
Founding scientist B	200,000	2.5	$6,250,000
Founding scientist C	200,000	2.5	$6,250,000
CEO	600,000	7.5	$18,750,000
Stock option pool	600,000	7.5	$18,750,000
University's shares	200,000	2.5	$6,250,000
Series A shareholders	3000,000	37.5	$93,750,000
Series B–E shareholders	3000,000	37.5	$93,750,000
Total postfinancing valuation	8000,000	100	$120,000,000 using $15 per share at the E round.

Series B–E rounds of financing that would have a cumulative dilutional effect of 50% on their holdings. Put in another way, the Series A ownership would be diluted from 60% to 30%, allowing for the future rounds of financing. We will also allow for a share price of $15.00 per share at the Series E round. Let's illustrate Table 21.4.

If 1 year later, another company, let's call it Flash Genomics, offers a buyout of $250 million for DNA Therapeutics, this is how the proceeds would be divided, assuming that 100% of the option pool was issued, vested, and exercised. That works out to $31.25 per share (Table 21.5).

For the Series A investors, this represents a phenomenal return of over nine times the original investment. There are a few takeaways. If the CEO and founders had made more progress with the proceeds of the Series A round, the personal returns would likely have been substantially higher. The earliest rounds are highly sensitive to valuations. You can set up these tables on Excel and then experiment with valuations to determine the degree of sensitivity.

Relationship of Investment Terms and Valuation

The model also does not include other factors that will affect ownership over time. These include investment terms such as the following which are typically required by venture capitalists. Venture funds characteristically structure their investors using the term "Preferred" shares to distinguish the rights associated with their shares from common shares. The preferred terms envelop governance, voting, control, and other matters. There are a few rights, however, that have or could have a direct economic effect, particularly on the founders and other holders of common stock. Here are the key items with economic implications for the founders and other common shareholders:

1. Preferred stockholders get their money back first—a liquidation preference—and thereafter participate in the distribution of proceeds of sale of the company on a pro rata "as converted to common basis" with the other shareholders. This structure is referred to as "participating preferred." *Note*: The liquidation preference refers to the amount that was initially invested by the VC. So, in our cap-table illustration above, the returns of the preferred shareholders would have been further enhanced by the participation provision. In other words, the Series A would have received its initial $10 million investment first, as would the other preferred shareholders. Their aggregated initial investments would come off the top of the $250 million, leaving less to be divided on the common share conversion basis, but nevertheless their returns would be higher at the expense of the common shareholders.
2. It is not unusual for venture capitalists to seek an annual dividend as a condition of their investment. Of course, they generally do not want to extract precious cash from their portfolio companies, but they do like the idea of building in a minimum return for downside protection. Typically, the dividends are administered and represented as common shares on the cap-tables on an on-going basis. The issuance of these common shares is made at the time of exit or conversion of preferred shares. The cap-tables, however, must capture these dividends, so that all parties can track the true dilution underway. The dividends are cumulative, NOT compounded.
3. Investors will typically seek price protection for their shares in the event that a future round of financing prices the shares at less than what they paid. This "antidilution protection" is negotiated in different ways. The most severe is "Full Ratchet," which means that they have absolute price protection. If the share price in any future round is less than the price per share that they paid, they receive additional shares to cover the entire price difference, for example, if they pay $1.00 per share and buy one share, and the price later drops to $0.50, they get one additional share at no additional cost. In this case the shares that they receive in compensation are in the form of common shares (not additional preferred, so none of the special rights described above apply to these new shares) *which are issued at the time of conversion of all shares to common* usually at the time the company is sold. Full ratchet antidilution is rare these days, and the parties will negotiate a weighted-average provision, which is far less severe, but nevertheless affects the returns of all the parties that do not have such protection.

The major lessons here are that the entrepreneur should never zero-in on the pre-money valuation offered by the venture capitalists without taking into full account the impact of the provisions above. These should be added to the cap-tables developed by the company to determine how they will affect the company. Such efforts will better prepare the company for negotiations of valuation.

The Great Convergence: Infection Points, Capital Needs, the Venture Capital Method, and Capitalization Tables

Magically, the bottom line of this exercise with the simplified, hypothetical numbers actually came out to a fairly conventional valuation, at least in the "A" round. A pre-money of $5–$6 million when the company needs $10 million is not far off the mark. Interestingly, the key number in Table 21.3 is the post-money value of $16,650,000. Basically, the company will not be on target unless there is confidence at the end of the depletion of the proceeds of the Series A round that it has achieved this value and then some. If market conditions are good, a "ramp-up" of value such that another $10 million in the "B" round causes only another 20% dilution would be generally considered a good outcome. The venture fund leading the Series B round will repeat the exercise that we have done above with new assumptions, as would the leaders of the subsequent rounds.

There are some caveats here; part of the assumption was that all rounds of financing would be computed with common-stock equivalents. In real life, the venture capitalists would use preferred stock which has many different rights. As described above, be aware that rights such as "participation" and dividends can have profound negative impact on the holdings of the entrepreneurs. For convenience, when we allowed for a 20% dilution, we assumed that the impact of these was built into the pricing. When preparing for a negotiation or in assessing the economics of a term sheet, the entrepreneur should factor these rights into the calculations.

Valuation exercises almost always produce a contentious result. The entrepreneur must bear in mind that the bargain with the venture capitalist is one that buys into a "system" of doing things. The high discount rate of 50% used in the calculations produces a phenomenal return in the face of success, but two-thirds of the investments made are total losses or barely return capital. The take away is that the entrepreneur, for better or for worse, is part of an investment portfolio. The only way to win the game is to stay true to the milestones and projected capital requirements. In such manner, the portion of ownership retained by the entrepreneur will have real value at the end of the game.

Preparing to Negotiate Practical Advice for Winning What You Need

Beyond the caveats in the section immediately above preparation for negotiations is paramount. Term sheets with the accompanying valuation are issued by the venture capitalist. For technical securities reasons, the entrepreneur is not offering to sell securities. The pitch book and the presentation are designed to provoke discussion of the company. It is the venture capitalist who is offering to buy securities. In the course of a life time, an entrepreneur will receive and negotiate only a handful of term sheets. For the venture capitalist, the term sheet is a part of a daily diet. Who has the advantage? The entrepreneur can only take steps to level the playing field and that is accomplished by study and preparation.

Unfortunately, you cannot sit back and let your legal counsel negotiate for you. For reasons of cost and advantage, venture capitalists issue and negotiate their own term sheets. Yes, they are reviewed by counsel, but the investors do not want to have their attorneys in tow. If they bring an attorney, you will as well. That said, your attorneys are part of your preparation. Like the venture capitalists, their daily diets involve term sheets. In addition to knowing the implications of the terms from a legal perspective, they are also the best barometers of what are the actual prevailing practices and provisions that are being accepted and rejected by both parties. Take advantage of that knowledge and always seek suggestions for counter proposals. Term sheet negotiation is a give and take based on the provisions as a whole. Term sheets must be evaluated holistically, and the opportunities for trade-offs and push-back, as well as hidden traps, require a keen eye backed up by knowledge and experience.

While it might seem like an end run around the venture fund, it is not unheard of for entrepreneurs to make discrete inquiries of other entrepreneurs funded by the same venture capitalist as to their style and level of steadfastness. When a conversation is begun with another entrepreneur who has been funded by the venture fund of interest to you, focus on the approach the investor took to due diligence and the issues that were emphasized. That will create the context for a discussion about the term sheet structure and negotiation process. For example, you can ask how the diligence process went, were there any surprises, how is the relationship going, what is the governance and value add style of the venture fund, how the lines of communication work, and other issues that concern you. You are not asking the other entrepreneur to violate confidences. In fact, this is part of your due diligence. Your goal is to make the investment process as smooth as possible and, most importantly, assure success for you and the investors.

Profiling the venture fund in other ways is important. Do a though analysis of their investment history—their winners as well as their losers. This may take some digging, but it is worth the effort. Categorize their investments not only by sector and technology, but also by development stage of the company at the time of the investment. Inquiries will leave you better prepared to qualify the fund as worthy of buying your stock and sitting on your board. Similarly, monitor their due diligence. If you have set up an online data room, track the visits in order to know the pace at which they are proceeding. Check with the references that you provided to learn if conversations took place and what the tone of the discussion was. This, of course, assumes that you have discussed your company with each of your references in advance, given them an update on you personally, and convince them that your concept is great and that you are the best person in the world to take it forward.

Be sure that you carefully observe the quality and depth of the technical due diligence that the investor is conducting. Are they speaking with your advisory board? Who is making the call? A retained expert? How do your advisors feel about that expert? What kind of questions are being asked, and why? Is the caller following through on the responses of your advisors? Are they having a conversation or is the tone more of an inquisition? How can you insert yourself or your resident chief scientist into that dialog? Are they sizing up the opportunity the same way that you see it, or is something else underway? Special attention should be paid to how they are reviewing and evaluating your intellectual property. Typically, a first pass will be made at integrity and enforceability of the patent portfolio. Expensive studies such as "freedom to operate" are usually reserved for the add-on due diligence period following execution of the term sheet. Yes, you don't go from signature to documents without additional study by the venture firm.

Cash is king, and while venture investing is not solely about money, the venture funds focus on how much you need, what you will do with it, and what will be delivered and by when with their money. That is why this chapter opened with the 20 questions related to value creation and meeting value inflection points. While the due diligence is underway, expect to have all your assumptions and plans challenged. If the VC fund is not negotiating your plans to reach value inflections points, there may be a serious problem. You will never know the degree of an investor's understanding of your mission and plans until they can speak with you about your vision on your terms. If there is no dialog about your project plans and the value inflection points, find out why. If you are not satisfied with the reasons, redouble your efforts to find alternative investors. Once you are satisfied that they understand your cash needs and agree with your strategy for reaching your value inflection points, it is your turn to make sure that the venture fund has the human capital and financial resources to meet your needs when you need them. How much capital are they planning to hold in reserve for future rounds of your financing? How engaged will they be on the board? Will you have access to their advisors for technical or commercial reasons? Can they assist you when filling out your management team in supporting the specifications, interviews, and recruitment? What is their network for building strategic alliances? Similarly, what is their exit track record, and what role have they played in IPOs as well as trade sales?

Once agreement is established on the requirements to reach and deliver the value inflection points, how is the investor modeling the future and developing their own cap-table analysis? What is that telling them about valuation now and in the future? Are they transparent with their findings and reasoning? How does this translate into the valuation discussions now? How have they arrived at the bracket or range of the valuation discussions? Is determining valuation a collaborative or adversarial process? Of course, it is always adversarial to a point, but are they trying to reach something grand with you?

When discussing the term sheet, is it in light of the value creation plan? Is the venture fund viewing the plan in the same holistic way that you are, or is the discussion of each point a great siege and seen as a zero-sum game? If the negotiator is the same person who will be on your board of directors, it might be some indicator as to how the relationship will work in the future. In short, are you using the term sheet discussions as a means of maximizing value creation or is the discussion solely about providing downside protection? If the latter, do they truly believe in you and your vision? You do want the money, and you want it now and on reasonable terms, but the bucks aren't worth it if you are sleepless every night for the next few years.

Epilog and a Few Helpful Additional Resources

This chapter was written for entrepreneurs shepherding start-up and early-stage biotechnology companies. It provided a framework useful in building a valuation model based on four major pillars: articulating value inflection points, the VC method, cap-table analysis, and fundamental investment terms. Together these form a tool for aggregating and timing capital needs and establishing a range for the negotiation of valuation with investors. The methods provided here, however, are not tools for securities analysis. Valuation of later stage private companies or publicly traded companies has special requirements that are beyond the purpose and scope of this book.

Readers interested in learning more about securities analysis and the pricing of publicly traded stocks have available several resources. Study is worth the effort, especially in preparing to determine terminal values used in the VC method. As a matter of personal habit, biotechnology entrepreneurs should be chronic observers of developments in the industry through the trade publications such as *BioWorld* and *BioCentury*. *The Journal of Commercial Biotechnology* provides in-depth analysis of trends and developments, as well. Obviously stay close to your own field and keep aware of competition. A weekly view of the biotechnology stock indices is a solid way to stay aware of trends. These include the *NASDAQ Biotechnology Index* and the *S&P Biotechnology Select Industry Index.* Pick a few stocks, ideally in your general field, and follow them regularly as a way of keeping current on the capital market dynamics that will affect your company.

There are two in-depth texts worth noting. *Biotechnology Valuation: An Introductory Guide* by Karl D. Keegan provides a comprehensive review of biotechnology finance in all its elements including valuation of technologies as well as companies as a whole. Similarly, *Valuation in Life Sciences: A Practical Guide* by Boris Bogdan and Ralph Villiger offers applications for several segments of the biotechnology industry illustrated through useful, although somewhat technical, financial modeling techniques. Expansion of your knowledge base of the intricacies of biotechnology valuation will add to your confidence and bring you closer to your capitalization goals.

Chapter 22

Your Business Plan and Presentation: Articulating Your Journey to Commercialization

Lowell W. Busenitz, PhD, MBA

Price College of Business, Center for Entrepreneurship, University of Oklahoma, Norman, OK, United States

Chapter Outline

Pitching to Investors and Partners

Every successful entrepreneur must be able to communicate and sell their venture opportunity to potential stakeholders. The stakeholders such as financial investors, potential partners, industry supporters, suppliers, buyers, and even future employees all have the potential to add value to your venture. Stakeholders want to learn about your venture and its viability before commitments are made. Potential financial investors or strategic partners will probe deeply for information about the market opportunity, the problem solved, the technology, intellectual property, and business model of the venture. A key challenge for entrepreneurs is to get the essence of their underlying technology, market application, and business model communicated clearly and concisely in a way that is enticing to potential stakeholders. Whenever potential stakeholders inquire about the nature, viability, and direction of the venture, the entrepreneur must be ready to respond to these opportunities to offer further information. Having a written business plan is an excellent and frequently expected way for entrepreneurs to signal the depth of their understanding of and commitment to the venture. A written business plan typically has been the most common means used to begin attracting outside stakeholders. While there has been some migration toward the use of a 2–3-page executive summary and a PowerPoint presentation deck, a well-written business plan remains the primary means founders use to think through the issues of their enterprise, and to communicate their vision to others and show venture viability.

Example 1: *Entrepreneur, John Smith (not his real name), was starting a business in the medical device sector and had a couple of different technologies that he was seeking to develop. A new venture forum was offered in his city where a group of entrepreneurs, including John, was asked to give a short presentation about the ventures that they were developing. The audience on that day included a variety of business angels and venture capitalists from the region along with a variety of additional constituents. When it was his time, John gave a 10-minute presentation and then fielded questions from the audience for another 10 minutes. As is typical for these types of meetings, he was asked to respond to a number of probing questions with regard to the nature of his technology (explained in nontechnical language), development time required, how this would this scale, who his target customers were, how he was going to deliver the product, his go-to-market plans, how he was planning to use the*

Biotechnology Entrepreneurship. DOI: https://doi.org/10.1016/B978-0-12-815585-1.00022-X

money that he was hoping to raise, etc. By the end of the Q&A time, John realized that he had not adequately answered the majority of the questions that had been raised. In sensing disappointment from his audience, he offered the following closing statement: "I may not know the direction that this venture is going to take but I invite you to come join me for the ride. I am sure that we will end up someplace good."

Needless to say, John did not attract any investors that day. The investors want to have a strong sense that the entrepreneurial team knows the direction they are going, and that they have a viable venture that they are carving out with an attractive direction. A good way to keep from getting into a situation like John found himself in is to go through the rigorous process of writing a business plan so that you can anticipate these issues and will have already developed a risk-mitigation strategy to offer to stakeholders. There are a couple of reasons for why this is so valuable. First, starting a new venture involves bringing together a team. The team is one of the most critical factors in the determination of the successful outcome of a new venture. Internally, the founding entrepreneur or team will inevitably need to make key hires. Without a clear articulation of the venture, specifications of resources already in place, resources that are yet to be obtained, the proposed direction, and targeted directions for the venture, getting buy-in from key stakeholders becomes increasingly unlikely. A written business plan is a valuable tool to help guide the founders and team members through this process. Building the "team" may also include external stakeholders such as key outsource suppliers, service providers, or consultants. When you set out to raise capital, potential investors will want extensive information about your venture. Moreover, and perhaps most importantly, most financial investors will generally want to be considered part of the team giving meaningful input on the strategic direction and operations of the venture going forward. As more individuals become involved with the venture, the more a business plan becomes a valuable tool for communicating what the venture is really about, and to get the key individuals moving forward in the same direction.

The likelihood of potential investors or other stakeholders asking for a written business plan is what generally motivates entrepreneurs to develop such a document. However, no one will gain more from writing the business plan than the entrepreneur who conducts their own research and puts all the components of the venture together into a concise and coherent plan. It is the building of all the critical components of the enterprise along with the new insights that arise, which make this process valuable to the entrepreneur. As I discuss later, learning and realignment are all integral parts of a quality-evolving business plan and the maturing of the venture.

Feasibility Analysis Versus Business Plans

Foremost in most of the potential stakeholders' mind is whether the proposed venture is likely to be viable and successful. If you are at the concept or inception stage with a technology, and have not done this already, it is important to conduct a feasibility analysis before you start to write your business plan. Is the application of the technology into a business really viable? A feasibility analysis is about a concept that an entrepreneur is interested in pursuing, but he or she does not yet know if it is a viable business opportunity. At its core, feasibility work is most relevant for the earliest stages of concept development and is for internal validation purposes. Although the research and development or discoveries made may be scientifically significant, is this venture concept worth pursuing? A feasibility analysis typically involves determining if the technology is feasible for use in the intended market, if there is a real demand for the product or service, do prospective customers feel a pain that would make the proposed product desirable to them. If so, what is the best way for them to gain access to the product? Some early financial analyses are usually made as well. If the product is a diagnostic or medical device, financial feasibility, such as how much will customers pay, is also important, as opposed to a therapeutic or biologic where that is determined by a pharmaceutical partner. How much will it cost to make the proposed product? How much start-up capital will be required? Doing further research by developing hypotheses about technology, markets, prospective customers, and finances are all part of the feasibility analysis. You must then conduct extensive research to see if the initial hypotheses are substantiated. Some of this work may be done through access to research databases but there are very few substitutes for hitting the pavement to interview industry experts, key opinion leaders, and prospective customers. A feasibility analysis helps the founding team evaluate if this is a potential "go" or "no-go" concept.

Once solid and reasonably objective feasibility has been established, then one is ready to start putting together the various business plans. A business plan should begin once an entrepreneur is reasonably satisfied to know that the venture concept is feasible. The good news then is that a significant proportion of the research and data that was gathered for the feasibility can help create a convincing business plan. A business plan starts with the assumption that the venture concept has significant viability and that the entrepreneur is now in the process of putting the building blocks into place in pursuit of product development and commercialization. Since the research that went into a feasibility analysis is rarely rock solid and airtight, more research is invariably needed to verify various parts of the commercialization process. See Table 22.1 for a summary comparison of the differences

TABLE 22.1 Comparisons of feasibility analysis and business plans.

	Feasibility analysis	Business plan
Central intent	To determine if a business concept has the potential to become a viable business opportunity	To specify the commercialization plan and sell the business concept to prospective investors and stakeholders
Key decisions	Is this venture concept a "go" or "no go?"	What resources are needed to take this concept to the next level? How much capital do we need to raise? From whom will we raise it? What will we give up in return?
For whom	For the nascent entrepreneurs, if it is a "go," then am I the right person to lead this venture?	For prospective investors and potential stakeholders, a form of strategic planning for the entrepreneurs
Data to be gathered	Gathering data from prospective customers to assess market need	Gathering data from experts and prospective customers about how best to launch and implement this venture
Commitment level	Everything is tentative	Fully committed to pressing forward with the venture
Business models	Evaluating different ways that this business could potentially operate	Adopting a specific business model and the specific resources needed to launch the venture

between feasibility analysis and the business plan. The following section addresses the dynamic learning process of putting together various business plans in greater detail.

Example 2: *Wannabe entrepreneur Terrie Schultz (not her real name) wanted to start a business that involved inventing a tool that would allow surgeons to reach into the lung to better operate on human lungs when necessary. To accomplish this, she needed a tool that was agile, could perform multiple procedures at once, and could be easily learned by physicians. With Terrie's early excitement around this product, she thought that she could get this tool designed. With her early feasibility analysis, she was able to get some modest feedback from a doctor that this might indeed be helpful for small subset of patients with lung cancer. Terrie also visited with two lung cancer patients who were all thumbs up about this device. This feedback gave her great excitement for this product, so she now forged ahead with building a business plan. As she got deeper into the business plan along with some additional feedback, she started getting several questions about the economics of the plan and whether hospital administrators would be interested. After all, they are the ones who would be purchasing the device and making sure that it was available for the right doctors and surgeries. It soon became clearer that the best case scenario for this product was that only a very limited subset of lung cancer patients could benefit from this device and surgery. Some further challenges regarding the efficacy of the tool were surfacing as well. It soon became evident that this business concept was not viable. The good thing is that Terrie discovered at this point rather than 6–12 months down the road and after substantially more personal investments. However, a better job with her feasibility analysis would have readily surfaced some of these problems before she ever started investing her time and energies into building the business plan.*

There is clearly a right time to assemble a business plan. If you start it too early, it becomes a glorified feasibility analysis with inevitable dead ends and pivots. Construct it too late in the start-up process, and you do not have the critical building blocks of the venture thought through for discussions with critical stakeholders whom you will be seeking to win over. With that being said, an entrepreneur will never have all the questions answered and all the contingencies nailed down before writing a business plan. Thus a business plan is often referred to as a "living" document that continues to take shape on the basis of learning, time progressions, and further input. Another point to remember is that if the feasibility analysis is not positive for the initial target use as the technology is agnostic to the application, there may be other market applications that could be better choices. The key is to get early feasibility analysis and to be persistent in finding an unmet medical need in which you have a clear future advantage.

The Business Planning Process

Business plans are considered communication tool between the entrepreneur and outside investors such as angel investors and venture capitalists, for example. Although this process can be quite time consuming, and a typical business plan may be of 20–30 pages or more, there are many valuable things that come from putting together a well-crafted business plan as it can be of great assistance in facilitating the support and collaborations of partners and outside investors. Unfortunately, many entrepreneurs find the research and writing process to be challenging. The major resistance to putting together a quality business plan usually comes from the time and effort that it takes to assemble such a document. The research, revisions, reiterations, and time spent are generally substantial.

With the goal of having a viable business plan in hand to help communicate with prospective investors, let's take a closer look at several of the benefits of the process. In preparing for battle, General Dwight Eisenhower once said, "I have always found that plans are useless, but planning is indispensable." Preparing to launch a new venture is a major undertaking that almost always encounters significant obstacles. In response to the risks and unknowns that new ventures face, business plans can be a significant help. Given that, the new venture start-up process typically involves significant adjustments; some have argued that a written business plan quickly becomes out of date and thus is an irrelevant process. However, it is the opposite that is truer. As Eisenhower discovered in preparing for war, the planning process itself is indispensable when preparing for a significant and uncertain road ahead, maybe particularly when it involves uncharted territory.

So what are the real benefits of the business plan process for an entrepreneurial team? First, the process of writing the business plan gives entrepreneurs an enhanced *communication* tool to reach their desired stakeholders. As entrepreneurs move forward with starting to sell their business concept to prospective investors, possible suppliers, and potential customers, they will almost always benefit from having multiple communication tools. As the writing process unfolds, entrepreneurs will develop special communication mediums and terminology and models with some of the unique characteristics of their product. Without this level of articulation that the writing of a plan can help facilitate, outside stakeholders will likely default to thinking that you are just another business much like your competitors. The process of developing special and unique language then becomes a tool for helping entrepreneurs communicate their venture to the needed parties. The writing process facilitates more effective communication.

Second, writing a plan helps entrepreneurs build a *logical whole.* By definition a solid business plan brings together multiple components into one package. It is like a puzzle in which all the pieces need to fit together. A solid plan will effectively include the following components and fit them together in a way that tells a convincing story:

- Identify the technology and the target market for its application
- Analyze competition
- Address the venture's competitive advantage
- Segment the serviceable market and entry points
- Develop a strategy for entering the market
- Cover implementation and operation strategies
- Specify the management team
- Explain the company structure
- Identify the critical risks
- Build the revenue model
- Offer key investment considerations

Without being challenged to integrate all these components into a logical whole, it is unlikely that entrepreneurs would effectively think through the package deal in enough depth. This represents a fairly comprehensive set of issues that are interlinked and build from one to another. It is very easy to lose focus in fitting all the pieces of a venture together. With a well-developed business plan the various pieces fit together like a puzzle integrated nicely into one cohesive package. The process of writing a business plan facilitates this process.

Third, the business plan writing process encourages the development of *creative insights.* The writing and assembling of the business plan into a whole package often entails thought processes that lead to fresh insights into things that previously were not apparent. Most entrepreneurs pursuing a new venture think about it all day, every day. There are many good things to say about that kind of energy and passion. However, with such focus and intensity can also come gaps and tunnel vision. Entrepreneurs need tools that will give them a different perspective on various parts of their venture. The entrepreneurs in this process often come to see and understand their venture in a way they previously had not. Such insights can lead to follow-on opportunities, new ways to deal with potential competitors, or a creative approach to entering the market.

Fourth, the writing process establishes a *foundation* for the ongoing strategic development of the venture. Without actually writing down how you are seeking to build this venture, you can easily end up with an unbalanced view of your venture along with critical gaps. Without actually writing down how you seek to chart this path forward, you can easily end up with an unbalanced view of your venture. However, without established foundations in place, they are in no position for true and meaningful learning about what may be wrong and what needs to be changed. The current paradigm and business plan that are in place for a venture form, in essence, the strategic foundation of the venture. From this paradigm, right or wrong, the venture moves forward. The emerging logic represented in a business plan will almost always need to be adjusted—sometimes substantially. Failure to do so often means a failed venture. Having a logical plan gives entrepreneurs the foundation to evaluate their current logic—where it is strong and where it is flawed. Without this baseline in place the entrepreneurial team will be tossed about like a ship without a rudder. As a written business plan is not set in concrete, it can serve as a great vehicle for strategic thinking. Stated differently, a business plan should always be a working or "living" document.

These four points suggest that writing a business plan can be a very constructive activity on the way to building a viable venture. The thought process needed to build a venture is substantial. Putting together a business plan and continuing to revise it is an amazing process that many thousands of entrepreneurs have found to be beneficial. Most entrepreneurs find putting a business plan together a challenging process but it usually pays dividends many times over. We now move to discuss in a greater detail what actually goes into the making of a quality business plan.

The Contents of the Business Plan

Among prospective stakeholders who consider business concepts and business plans, a relatively clear norm of the key issues that should be covered has emerged. Moreover, and probably to a lesser extent, there are expectations about the order in which the various components should be presented. Sometimes entrepreneurs, being the creative individuals that many of them tend to be, try to change things around to bring some innovation to the business plan. While there is some room for variation, and most business concepts usually call for some tweaking to capture the nuances of that specific venture, business plan order is not the place to get overly creative. On multiple occasions, I have seen entrepreneurs change up the order in what they present. Unfortunately, it invariably comes back to haunt them as the potential stakeholders become confused about the arguments that are being put forward as to why this is a great venture opportunity. I strongly suggest that you largely follow an established outline using the norms for the building of business plans.

The outline and guidelines for building a business plan are found later. The suggested outline offers enough detail to give significant guidance. Moreover, clear distinctions are made between industry, market, and competitive advantage components—issues that are often confused and intermingled. The industry addresses the competitors who are currently in the space now and who are likely to be the key competitors for the venture going forward. The market addresses the prospective customers, the size of the serviceable market, how can the serviceable market be segmented, and where is the sweet spot of all the potential customers. These are clearly quite different from one another, and it will help to maintain the clarity of your presentations to keep these distinct.

As you dig into the details of building a solid and strategic business plan, it is helpful to keep in mind the following bigger picture that most prospective investors want to know about every business they consider:

1. What is the customer pain and is the motivation likely to be strong enough for prospective customers to buy the offered solution?
2. What is the underlying technology and have the critical experiments been completed that would support the likelihood of being efficacious for its intended use?
3. How big is the market and is there significant growth in this space?
4. How will the business make money?
5. What is the reimbursement strategy?
6. Are the regulatory issues sufficiently understood and addressed?
7. Is there intellectual property protection and at what stage?
8. What sets this venture apart from existing competitors and will it be able to build and protect its competitive advantage?
9. Has a quality team been assembled to lead this venture and why are they the right people to lead this concept forward?
10. How much money will you need to reach each value-enhancing milestone? How much money will you need to raise in total before exit?
11. The potential revenue and expenses will need to be shown to be realistic and lead to long-term profitability. Are the potential revenues and profits large enough to adequately reward the type of investors that you will be pitching too?
12. What is the anticipated and likely exit for investors and how long will that take?

With that introduction, I now suggest the following outline. It starts with the executive summary that is a section embedded at the beginning of the complete business plan. This section, while first in the business plan, is usually written last. Remember that in writing your business plan and following the outline, it is important to understand that you are telling a story. Starting with the name of your business, the mission, product name, section titles, and body content, the business plan should communicate a compelling story about a great business venture that is in development and is going to resolve a critical customer pain while

Business Plan Outline

Cover page and table of contents

1. Executive summary (write this section last)

a. The executive summary must make a great *first impression* and tell the complete and comprehensive story in just a few pages.

b. Potential investors should be provided enough relevant information in the executive summary to convince them to inquire further, making clear that they understand such central issues that are as follows:

  i. Your specific product or service offering.

  ii. The underlying technology you are using and proof-of-concept support to demonstrate that it will work in the intended application.

  iii. The reasons a customer would buy this product or service.

  iv. The reasons a customer would buy it from this venture.

  v. The underlying intellectual property and stage at which it is currently in.

  vi. The regulatory hurdles and how they will be addressed.

  vii. Any reimbursement issues that will be experienced and the plan to address them.

  viii. The way the company name, logo, mission, and tag line help to communicate the company's strategy, goals, etc.

c. The executive summary should be brief and should clearly describe the offering to investors. The offering statement should include the type of funding you seek, the amount you want, the use of proceeds, and the key value-enhancing milestones; these funds will help you reach. Also include how much of the company *you are prepared to offer* in exchange for financing and the role you would like a potential investor to have; in other words the pre-money valuation of your company.

2. Venture opportunity (opportunity context)

a. Business description

  i. The company (name/form/logo) and industry category.

  ii. The specific product/service offering.

  iii. The goals, mission (mission), strategy, and objectives.

  iv. What is your business model, or how you will make money (consider using a visual model).

  v. Explain what your interest is in this business concept.

b. The innovation/technology and scientific team working on this product

  i. Identify your technology innovation and all experimental or published data that supports its likely utility in your application. Describe all the proof-of-concept experiments that support its utility.

  ii. Show how it compares to the currently accepted practice.

  iii. Include helpful mechanism-of-action diagrams that inform the investor.

  iv. Emphasize the benefits the end users will experience.

  v. Put together a "product matrix" to show comparisons with currently existing products (see sample worksheet in Table 22.2).

  vi. Any key industry standards or requirements.

  vii. If applicable, put technical specifications in an appendix.

c. Customer value proposition

  i. Remember that in most biotech sectors you will have three customer needs to satisfy: the prescriber, the patient, and the payer.

  ii. What are specific benefits that you will deliver to your principal customers? These will most likely involve financial benefits, but psychological benefits could *also* be noted.

  iii. Develop quantitative numbers comparing and contrasting the way your targeted customer is currently spending time/money with how your new offered product will improve production and/or financial gains for your customer.

d. Financial cost/benefit analysis for the venture

  i. What will be the source(s) for revenue? Provide some meaningful estimations of how much revenue each source will provide for the first 3 years of anticipated revenue.

  ii. What are the main anticipated variable costs required to launch the venture? What are the major anticipated fixed costs required to launch the venture?

  iii. Show that the financial benefits outweigh the costs.

3. Industry examination

a. Macro-factors impacting the overall industry trends: what emerging macro-trends suggest the traditional way of doing business is changing? Substantiate your arguments with changes *starting to appear*, or are projected to appear, in the economic, political, regulatory, demographic, technological, sociocultural, or global arenas. The focus here is on macro-level trends (why the time may be right for your concept).

b. Industry analysis

  i. Description (type, size, segmentation, and major players).

  ii. Demand conditions (life cycle, profitability, history, and trends).

(*Continued*)

(Continued)

iii. Industry attractiveness (Porter's five forces).

c. Current industry models/competitors/trends
   i. Develop a "competitor matrix" (see sample worksheet in Table 22.3).
   ii. What business models are currently used by established firms?
   iii. How are new products typically introduced in this space?
   iv. Provide examples of successful start-ups in this industry.
   v. Provide examples of unsuccessful start-ups in this industry.

4. Market examination

a. Macro-level analysis
   i. Market segmentation of serviceable market.
   ii. Size (must be large enough to sustain a business).
   iii. Demographics (income, habits, personal characteristics, standard of living, etc., for major segments).
   iv. Trends in the various segments.
   v. Psychographic profile (interests, activities, and opinions).

b. Your customers (microlevel analysis)
   i. Identify multiple target segments; compare and evaluate them.
   ii. Identify your initial target customer segment.
   iii. Motivations for target customers to purchase.
   iv. Timing (why is the timing right).
   v. Where is your projected "sweet spot" in the market?
   vi. Scalability—can success in one area lead to success in another?
   vii. Develop a matrix table that summarizes and distinguishes the different customer segments. Conclude with justifying your chosen entry segment and why you think that this is your starting "sweet spot."
   viii. Include customer testimonials that validate your market.

Most top-quality business plans build customer analysis from *primary data* collected by the team. This typically includes structured interviews or survey data (details of data collected are typically included in an appendix). Secondary data can also provide rich sources of customer information.

5. Competitive advantage

a. What resource(s) will be used to seek a competitive advantage?

b. Can the resources to be used be considered "valuable," "rare," and/or hard to "imitate"?
   i. Are there patents, trademarks, and/or copyrights involved?
   ii. Is there intellectual property to be developed?
   iii. What other resources should be considered?

c. For a new venture, it can be very effective to articulate one or two resource-based advantages and by what means you plan to build these competitive advantages down the road assuming that you have a successful launch.

6. Pricing, marketing, and supply chain

7. Implementation and operating strategies

8. Company structure and management

a. Company structure
   i. Legal form of the organization (LLC, LLP, C-Corp., etc.).
   ii. Ownership structure of the business.

b. Management team
   i. Training, academic background, work experience, and the personal capabilities.
   ii. Supporters of the team.
   iii. Profile key future hires needed in the future.

c. The extended team
   i. Advisory board.
   ii. Board of directors.

9. Critical risks

a. Identify three to six of the most critical risk factors. Where might the venture hit obstacles going forward?

b. Possible internal critical risks—technology and the experimental risks, market adoption and acceptance, cost/time over runs, key personnel issues, etc.

c. Possible external critical risks—environmental shifts, market shifts, competitors' actions, etc.

d. For each risk factor, how will you mitigate these risks in the event that they emerge?

10. The revenue model and key investment considerations

a. Specify your financial assumptions (most likely make these explicit in an appendix).

(Continued)

(Continued)

b. An "average unit economic analysis" should show revenue to be received from the first year of sales on a per unit basis, the costs associated with start-up, and ongoing costs in year 1.

c. Summary financials in one table for years 1–5 to include units sold, cost of goods sold (COGS), revenue, and operating income.

  i. Include a "Valley of Death" chart (capital required, breakeven, etc.).

d. Financial analysis schedules (depending on the time to reach market and if your product sector requires revenue generation to reach an exit such as diagnostics and medical devices) (cash flow statement; income statement, balance sheet). The detailed schedules should be monthly for at least 1 year, quarterly for first 2 years, and annually through 5 years. Put in an appendix.

e. Required funding (type of funding and the deal structure).

  i. "Use of funds" statement identifying main expenditures.

  ii. Timing of funds being sought and key milestones.

  iii. Terms to be offered to investors (equity percent).

f. Future growth opportunities (scalability).

  i. Leveraging developed capabilities for further expansion.

  ii. Follow-on products to leverage the customer market opportunities.

g. Key reasons to invest (develop two to four reasons to invest).

  i. Unique product, service, and use of new (existing) technology.

  ii. Any usually qualified individuals, perhaps with linkages?

  iii. Do you have a particularly strong competitive advantage?

h. Likely exit opportunity.

  i. Who are the likely acquirers for your business?

  ii. What was the average or comparative valuations given to similar acquired businesses?

  iii. How long do you anticipate before you would have an exit?

  iv. Realistic assessment of return on investment potential.

Appendix

The appendix is the last section of the business plan. It is used to communicate supplemental and supporting information.

- Detailed financial statements or worksheets.
- Detailed product or technical description and patent grants.
- Published articles and/or technical reports.
- Primary research detailing competitor or customer feedback.
- Business agreements.
- Letters of intent connected to the business.
- Sample of marketing or promotional materials if relevant.
- Accolades/awards/commendations/testimonials.
- Purchase orders for your product/service if relevant.

Miscellaneous information on writing your business plan

- Business plans should be long enough to effectively tell your story. This will most likely be between 20 and 30 pages plus appendices. Longer business plans tend to have too many details that potential investors are unlikely to want to read about here (although they are likely to want to ask you about such details). Moreover, the longer a business plan, the easier it is to repeat information. When repetition is appropriate, at least change the verbiage.

Tables and graphics:

- Never pass up an opportunity to insert some great visuals such as models and tables. They are a welcome sight to most readers and can easily be worth more than a thousand words.
- Overall, pie charts have their place; tables are almost always beneficial; on average, bar charts are the least helpful.

Grammar and miscellaneous details

- Most investors very quickly notice grammar and spelling errors. This presents an image of incompetence and sloppiness. Consider asking other skilled individuals unfamiliar with a business plan to read it.
- Use active voice in your writing.
- Develop structure and hierarchy to your plan. Use first, second, and possibly third-order headings with frequency.
- Intersperse into your written presentation a series of bullet statements, tables, and models wherever possible. Try to have some variations from the typical narrative on every page. Double space between paragraphs.
- Use endnotes to reference your source information.
- Font type should be something common like Times Roman style and probably 12 point.
- Margins are to be at least 1 in.

TABLE 22.2 Product matrix for a new physician office rapid diagnostic test.

	New diagnostic	Rapid strep test	Conventional laboratory
Source of diagnosis	*Saliva*	Throat swab	Blood work
Wait time	*10–15 min*	10–15 min	2–3 days
Cost to produce ($)	*18*	2	None
Price sold to doctors ($)	*45*	3	Outsourced
Insurance reimbursement to doctors ($)	*85*	17	Labs reimbursed

TABLE 22.3 Competitor matrix for new telemedicine dermatology service.

	Telemedicine dermatology	Conventional dermatologist	DermLink.MD	Spot exam
Years in industry	*Start-up*	Decades	5 years	3 years
Service medium	*Mobile*	Face-to-face	Internet	Mobile
Actual consultation	*Yes*	Yes	Yes	No
Consultation time frame	*24 h*	Average 6 weeks	48 h	24 h
Consultation type	*Acne only*	Varies	Follow-up	Mole categorization
Price ($)	*59*	78–139	99	4.99

returning a significant return for your prospective investors. Keep the central theme of your story as a common thread throughout. Always work toward building a compelling *story*.

The previously suggested outline includes the multiple sections that go into making up a plan, and it has been tried and tested many times. However, there are several things, such as the nature of the business, which can alter the outline. For example, if a venture is working on a new drug application with long FDA approvals to obtain, developing an extensive marketing program would not be appropriate. Consequently, flexibility is important, but the completeness of the outline presented is to help the entrepreneur understand all the components that prospective stakeholders are accustomed to seeing and are likely to inquire about sooner or later.

Presenting the Written Business Plan

Having worked through the building of the content of your business plan, we now move to explicitly address the presentation aspects of the plan—first, the written presentation followed by a section on in-person presentations. With the context of today's entrepreneur and investor, expectations can be quite varied. If one was pursuing a new start-up 20 years ago and needed funding, there were venture capitalists on the equity side and banks on the loan side. These are the two very distinct types of financing, and the two rarely, if ever, compete for the same investments. We knew very little about business angels back then other than that they existed in the woodwork of communities. Today, we still have venture capitalists and business angels, but each group seems to be becoming more diverse. The venture capital market seems to be emerging with a limited number of very strong players and many smaller players focused on various niches. In the business angel market, there are those who are still largely hidden in the woodwork of communities. However, angel investors are becoming more networked and organized. For example, many angel investor networks have monthly meetings to hear pitches and to pool their investments (see *Chapter 19: Securing Angel Capital and Understanding How Angel Networks Operate*). Much more recently, we have crowdfunding emerging as a funding source for smaller amounts of capital for tech start-up ventures.

Along with the diversity of the today's investment community comes significant variation in the way that investors get their information delivered. The traditional way is the written business plan that is the ticket that gets you through the door to discuss your concept with a venture capitalist. The written business plan was the first screen, and entrepreneurs could rarely get to first base with a venture capitalist unless they cleared the hurdle with a quality concept and written plan that generated further intrigue and interest. With today's investment community, such preferences still exist but the expectations are much more diverse. Some prospective investors now only want to read an executive summary or slide deck first; others want to hear a shorter pitch deck and then seek to engage a written plan if they are interested in moving their interest to a deeper level. In short, investor expectations vary widely, even when compared to investors in the United States and in Europe. Entrepreneurs must be ready to provide prospective investors whatever they request or need.

We will now address some of the modes and types of presentations, first written and then the in-person presentation.

Types of Written Business Plans

Unless specified otherwise, when someone refers to or asks for a written business plan, they are usually referring to the *standard business plan* that typically consists of 20–30 pages, making up the main document plus appendices. Such written plans generally are able to offer enough depth so that the reader can get familiar with the venture concept and how it is approaching the commercialization process. If the main part of the business plan exceeds 30 pages, most readers will become bogged down and lose interest. For internal planning purposes, some entrepreneurs will continue to expand the business plan and use it as an internal working document. Such documents are referred to here as the *internal business plan* and can reach 60–100 pages in length.

Shorter business plans are also used with some frequency in the marketplace. Two of them are addressed here. The *dehydrated business plan* usually runs from 5 to 10 pages and, as the name suggests, it is a scaled-down version of the standard plan. Essentially, such a document covers the key points of the business plan by bringing particular attention to those issues that represent the heart of the business concept. Even with the dehydrated business plan, remember that you are telling a story of the origins of the business concept; why the founder(s) is the right individual to take this concept forward and the projected path of the venture's development. Such features are attractive in luring prospective stakeholders to the venture.

The final written form addressed here is the *executive summary*. It is the complete business plan in miniature comprising usually 1–2 pages in length; sometimes as a stand-alone document, it can run to 3 pages. The executive summary sets the tone by seeking to capture the pertinent points of the whole plan in a brief synopsis. Stated differently, the executive summary should be a succinct and captivating overview that sells the highlights of your vision and objectives for the investor to garner further interest. The goal is to entice the reader to come seeking additional information. Remember that with both of these shorter versions, the point is to use these as a means to invite the reader to something more, such as the standard business plan or engaging the entrepreneur directly.

Readability and Physical Layout

Most entrepreneurs want prospective investors to read the standard business plan if it is available. However, if there are readability problems with the business plan exist, prospective investors are likely to abandon the read and move away from further inquiry. Far too often a failure to read is because the business plan is put together in a way that makes it too hard to get through. A business plan should be put together in a way that accommodates a 10-, 30-, or 60-minute-plus read. This implies that things like headings, models, tables, and listing of bullet statements are all important in helping to get the message of a business plan communicated. Specifically, I suggest the following:

- Use the company name, logo, and mission to help tell your story. These are similar tools that help a reader more quickly comprehend your business concept. Can someone get a good idea of what your venture is about by just looking at the name, logo, and mission?
- Make the section titles meaningful. How much be communicated if everything but the name, logo, mission, and section titles were deleted. Could the reader get a decent feel for what the venture is about if only these were read? Would they by themselves invite further inquiry?
- Structure the sections using multilevel headings. Take main headings such as industry examination, market examination, and competitive advantage, and beneath them use subheadings. This helps the reader greatly by communicating the structure and overall direction of the business plan and what is being addressed.
- Leave a reasonable amount of "white" space on each page. The norm is single-spaced text with one blank line between paragraphs.
- Each page should look different. Try not to have pages with just straight text in traditional paragraphs. A possible means of breaking up a page includes bullet statement subsections, tables and charts, and meaningful pictures that help tell your story. Meaningful charts and tables can be worth thousands of words; they can also help condense the length of the plan. Most readers would rather read a great summary table than 2–3 pages of typed detail. Your reader will appreciate you for it.

- Beware of repetition. With a document that encompasses as much material as a business plan does with multiple cross-linkages, it is easy to repeat oneself. Where it is appropriate to discuss something that has been discussed earlier, say it differently. Moreover, get someone with fresh eyes to read your business plan and help with things like this.
- Eliminate all grammatical errors. Like it or not, with just a few grammatical errors, most readers start making inferences about the capabilities of the person writing the plan. It is always a good practice to get someone with good writing and grammar skills to make the necessary corrections.

Accommodating Different "Reads"

As mentioned earlier, potential stakeholders have multiple preferences for how they like to become familiar with a new business concept (executive summary, dehydrated or standard business plans, slide decks, in-person presentations, etc.). Now let's assume we have a group of potential stakeholders, all of whom have chosen the standard business plan to first become familiar with a given business concept. There will be a very significant variance in the time and approach they take to read it. As the author of your business plan, you need anticipate these different reads. Some will read the executive summary and then leaf through the rest of the plan in a matter of a few minutes. At the other extreme will be those who give it a very solid read taking 60–90 minutes. In between, there are those who will read little more than the section headings, bulleted statements and tables, and then perhaps supplement it with reading the sections they consider to be their most important section(s). To make things harder, most readers have their unique preferences about what they consider to be the most important sections. As a writer of your business plan, it serves you well to keep the reading style of these various readers in mind and seek to write the plan in a way that accommodates multiple types of reads.

Communicating Your Business Plan

While the focus of this chapter is primarily on the written business plan, they usually go hand-in-hand with the in-person presentation. While there are materials dedicated to make effective pitch deck presentations that are certainly worthy of further study (see *Chapter 23: Investor Presentations: What do You Need in an Investor Pitch Deck*), I will address a few central perspectives specific to business plans to keep in mind for the in-person presentation.

Pitch Deck Presentation Length and Content

Just as prospective stakeholders have varying preferences on the length of the written business plan, they also have a specific length of time for the in-person presentation. Some situations will call for a 5-minute presentation; yet another may allow 15 or even as long as 20 minutes. Again, nothing is set in concrete and rarely does the entrepreneur get to choose. So you have to be ready to adapt. This brings up the central point of any in-person presentation: the goal is to give your audience a meaningful snapshot of your venture and how it addresses an important customer pain, key advantages you have moving forward, and what is in it for prospective investors. Entrepreneurs should *not* try to communicate everything they know about their concept, even if it is a longer presentation (like 20 minutes). Instead, with energy and passion, deliver the most important points that accurately reflect the venture. Think about it in terms of saying enough to bait some interesting questions that will lead to deeper interactions. More in-depth communications commonly come during the question and answer time and particularly within one-on-one conversations.

Preparing slides for a presentation is also very important. First, here are the four most common complaints that I hear about for business plan presentations.

1. The business concept is NOT understood.
2. Too technology focused without an understanding of the target market and application.
3. Too much industry and technology jargon.
4. No clear story; the flow is lost.

With these failures far too common in the presentation of business concepts, let me make the following suggestions:

1. Get the story right.
2. Bring solid energy and confidence to the presentation.
3. Always think about what is in it for your audience.
4. Plan for approximately one slide about every 45 seconds.
5. As much as possible use simple pictures and models. Use variation from slide to slide.
6. No more than 15–20 words per slide.
7. Font size, no less than 28 point.
8. Use contrast—usually dark text on a light background.
9. Be presentable, well dressed, and neat.

Elevator Pitch

The elevator pitch is your first impression and sets the stage for the rest of your in-person presentation. First, never assume that you have your audience's attention. If you miss them with your elevator pitch, in all likelihood, they are gone for the entire presentation. Second, develop a pitch that gets to the heart of the customer pain and the product that you deliver. Here are six different mechanisms around which elevator pitches can be developed:

1. Question—directed straight at the audience to get them involved.
2. A factoid—a striking or little known fact.
3. A physical object or demonstration.
4. An anecdote—a quick human interest story.
5. A quotation—an endorsement from a notable figure.
6. An analogy—a striking comparison.

Conclusion

A business plan is a strategic tool for communicating what your new venture is about and what it seeks to accomplish. Business plans are written with the intent of helping to inform prospective investors and other stakeholders of the opportunities that lie ahead for the proposed venture, how the company will mitigate the risks, and how it plans to achieve attractive outcomes. Although the trend currently in the United States with busy investors is moving toward sharing an executive summary or a PowerPoint pitch deck, business plans serve as an invaluable tool for helping the entrepreneurs to carve out a strategic plan and to think through strategically how all the different pieces of this business puzzle fit together in the venture going forward. In addition, if you are applying for nondilutive grants to support your business and move your project further before securing investor capital, these agencies typically require some form of a business plan to review. The better the strategy of a venture is understood by the entrepreneurs in the context of competition and emerging technologies, the more prepared they will be in leading the venture onward toward a successful outcome. It will also make them more convincing in telling their stories to prospective stakeholders.

Chapter 23

Investor Presentations: What Do You Need in an Investor Pitch Deck?

Craig Shimasaki, PhD, MBA
CEO, BioSource Consulting Group and Moleculera Labs, Oklahoma City, OK, United States

Chapter Outline

Capital is the lifeblood of all developing biotechnology companies because it is vitally needed to continue fueling the engine of innovation for your company. When capital is limited, the pace of a company's product development slows down, or sometimes takes unwise shortcuts, or, worse yet, development completely stops. The entrepreneurial leader and leadership team has the responsibility to continuously raise enough capital to allow the company to reach the next value-enhancing milestones before running out of money. Raising capital in sequential and incremental amounts to make progressive milestones is discussed in *Chapter 17: Sources of Capital and Investor Motivations.* A critical tool required for raising capital in the biotech industry is a PowerPoint slide presentation or "***pitch deck***." In this chapter, we will discuss and review the essential topics to cover in a biotech investor pitch deck and why these topics are important when conveying the company value and readiness for investment. I'll review 18 topics essential to have in your investor pitch deck and discuss the type of information that should be contained within these slides.

What Is a Pitch Deck?

A pitch deck is a collection of PowerPoint slides used to communicate your company and investment opportunity to different groups of potential investors. These slides should contain a complete summary of all the essential topics and risk elements that must be addressed when building a successful biotechnology company. In essence, it is a well-thought-out sequence of critical information about the various aspects of a company's business and commercialization strategy. This information is succinctly outlined in slides with imagery that helps the viewer quickly comprehend and assess the desirability of investing in your company. Today, in the United States the pitch deck has predominately replaced the business plan as the first exchange of information that potential investors request to help them assess their initial investment interest in your company.

In the past, a complete and formal business plan was used to interest prospective investors. Due to the faster pace of investor decisions, the increasing number of

Biotechnology Entrepreneurship. DOI: https://doi.org/10.1016/B978-0-12-815585-1.00023-1

investment opportunities investors must review, and the limited time they possess to evaluate interest in any one deal, the pitch deck has become the preferred communication tool by most investors today. It is not unusual for a typical venture capital firm to screen up to 1000 companies each year and to perform research on about 20–30 companies. Of those companies, they may invite 10 companies for in-depth formal presentations to their entire partner team and then invest in two to three deals annually. Having a well-thought-out pitch deck is an essential requirement for all biotech entrepreneurs and leadership teams who want to obtain funding. This is not to imply that the business plan is not necessary. In fact, a well-thought-out business plan is an essential tool for the company because it is the strategic plan contained within the business plan that makes up the pitch deck. It is vital that the entrepreneurial team think though the strategy required to write a complete business plan. Portions of the formal business plan are still necessary for grant applications, competitive funding opportunities, and sometimes a final due diligence requirement for venture funding. Writing a business plan is an essential exercise for the entrepreneurial team, as it makes them think through the entire business strategy and the underlying assumptions.

The transition toward the pitch deck as the preferred communication tool for investors *unfortunately* allows the entrepreneurial team to bypass the need to carefully think through their entire business and product development strategy. Certain weaknesses can result from this shortcut in that the team may not have carefully thought through portions of the business strategy in detail, and they may have missed key issues that may be obvious to investors. On the other hand, the use of the pitch deck allows the entrepreneurial team to rapidly adjust, pivot, reinvent, or modify their plans based upon uncovering new information. Even though we will walk through the essential topics and slides that biotech investors want to see in a pitch deck, let me encourage you to be sure and spend the time in the beginning, developing a well-thought-out business plan. Writing a business plan requires that the leadership team think through the company business model (see *Chapter 12: Understanding Biotechnology Business Models and Managing Risk*) and assess all the risks inherent within product development, regulatory, reimbursement and intellectual property, market, commercialization, and your exit. You will benefit from this exercise, and it will cause you to strategically think about how you build your business, identify the development risks, and give you and your investors more confidence that you have a well-thought path to commercialization. *Chapter 22: Your Business Plan and Presentation: Articulating Your Journey to Commercialization*, takes you through the steps in creating a solid business plan, and in many ways the business plan is more important for the entrepreneur and leadership team than it is for anyone else. It forces the team to think about all the issues and devise a strategy while developing plans to manage these risks.

Why You Need More Than One Pitch Deck

At the outset, let me emphasize that you will eventually need more than one pitch deck at your disposal. In fact, you will likely have multiple pitch decks directed toward different audiences for a variety of purposes, and in varying lengths. In this chapter, we will start by creating an "*Introductory Pitch Deck*" which is an overview of your complete business, and from this deck, you can create additional presentations later. For instance, will need a more detailed slide deck that elaborates on some of these topics in greater detail based upon the audience and the stage of due diligence they are at. A more detailed presentation is sometimes referred to as a "*Management Presentation*" in contrast to your "*Introductory Pitch Deck*." In addition, you will likely need a shorter slide deck of 10–12 slides for competition presentations that organizations use to showcase many companies within a condensed meeting schedule timeframe. This "*Short Presentation*" may be used for initial investor screens when you may only have as little as 6–10 minutes to present; therefore you must be very succinct and hit the key points investors want to see. In addition, you will likely need additional slides that are made for heavily focused scientific and medical investor audiences, and of course a slide deck for the general public when promoting your company to broader audiences for awareness. If you are at an early development stage, or just creating your enterprise, start by developing this *Introductory Pitch Deck* for initial meetings with potential investors. Later, you can produce other slide decks as the need arises. I recommend as you do this, you create a "*Master Slide Deck*." Within this *Master Slide Deck*, you hold *all* your slides which will comprise more detailed scientific data, key experimental results, publications supporting your product's future utility, in-depth target market data and market sizing information, more detail on likely exits, growth plans, and more specific use of proceeds, to name a few. Having a *Master Slide Deck* makes it easier to pick and choose appropriate slides for a presentation directly tailored to your audience, and later it allows you the ability to select the number and type of slides based upon the time allotted for your presentation.

In this chapter, we will walk through the practical aspects of putting together a compelling biotech pitch deck with the essential elements of interest to a biotech investor. Although you can find a number of good consumer product investor pitch deck recommendations, a biotechnology product vastly differs from other products and so does its development requirements; therefore the topics that biotech investors want to hear are also different. Unlike IT products and other consumer technology products, biotechnology products have longer development timeframes, more exorbitant development costs, much more stringent regulatory requirements, unique reimbursement issues, and a need for diversely skilled individuals. Therefore, one cannot follow a general industry pitch deck when presenting to biotech investors. Although there are some key topics that are universal for all entrepreneurial companies to be successful, the slides we will discuss are specifically directed toward the biotechnology industry and their investors.

18 Topical Slides You Need in a Biotech Investor Pitch Deck

Title slide
Topic 1: Company Purpose, History, and Mission
Topic 2: The Problem or "Pain," Unmet Medical Need and "Why" There Is a Problem
Topic 3: Technology and Product "Solution"
Topic 4: Target Market Opportunity
Topic 5: Competition and/or Substitutes
Topic 6: Describe Your Business Model
Topic 7: Product Development and Regulatory Pathway
Topic 8: Intellectual Property and/or Secret Sauce, and Partnerships
Topic 9: Insurance Reimbursement Strategy
Topic 10: Go-to-Market Strategy
Topic 11: Proforma Projections and Financing "Ask"
Topic 12: Use of Proceeds
Topic 13: Likely Exits and Estimated Timeframe
Topic 14: Leadership Team
Topic 15: Reasons to Invest Summary
Topic 16: Thank You Q&A
Topic 17: Potential Risks and How They Will Be Mitigated
Topic 18: Support and Appendix Slides

The Biotech Pitch Deck

The following 18 topical sections are presented in a logical sequence to assist in telling a "story" that listeners can follow. These topics are essential to cover when making an investor pitch for potential investment in your company. Depending upon the stage of your business and the biotech sector you are in, certain topics will require more than one slide, especially your technology and data section. In my experience, the sequence of topics listed has been most effective in conveying a company story in an understandable manner as subsequent slides build on the logic of previous ones. With the exception of the "Ask slide," depending on the time given to present and the investors you are presenting to, this slide may be presented at the beginning. This is usually necessary if you are in a time-limiting pitch competition or presenting to investors for the very first time and they have not heard anything about you before. The goal of your slide deck and presentation is to interest your investor audience enough that they will ask more questions and want to dig deeper into a process of due diligence. At that time, you will have the opportunity to present more thoroughly these topics, and investors can evaluate all the aspects of your business opportunity and risks in more detail.

Title Slide

This is your title slide that stays up prior to the beginning of your presentation (see Fig. 23.1). You want to use this slide to orient your audience to your company so they have a context of your business. In this slide, you have your company logo, company name, usually the date, location, and occasion of the presentation or name of the event or group you are presenting. It is helpful to have a tag line, vision, or mission-type statement that implies what biotech sector you are in and what condition, disease, problem, service, or need you are filling. This helps to orient the listeners before you begin and it gives them a general idea of what market you are focused on. Later in this chapter, we will discuss helpful tips for giving good presentations and describe things you want to tell your audience, and things do not want to say or do. I'll share with you some things that I have learned over the past 30 years in giving hundreds of investor presentations to a myriad of different types of investors—some successful, some not so successful, and what I learned in the process. Remember, *You only get one chance to make a first impression*; therefore be sure to start confidently, not arrogantly, and look into the eyes of those you are talking to, rather than looking down at your feet.

FIGURE 23.1 Title Slide

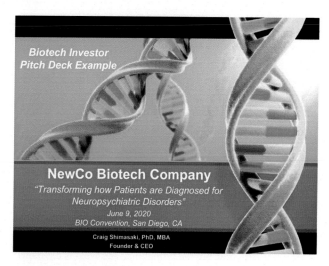

Topic 1: Company Purpose, History, and Mission

This next slide (Fig. 23.2) briefly describes your company background. You want to include any relevant history that has value and lends credibility to the company, such as a license from a prestigious university or work in a well-known research laboratory in a particular field. Be sure to orient the audience to what product sector you are in, and any other information that helps set the stage for what you will be communicating later. For instance, sometimes entrepreneurs begin their presentation without giving the investors a clear understanding if their product is a diagnostic, therapeutic, medical device or service. Are you a start-up, in preclinical testing, or prototype testing? Be sure to succinctly describe your company and its purpose and mission. You should indicate when the company officially started operating as a relevant gauge for what has been accomplished to date. For instance, if you have only been operating for one year and you are already in animal testing for a therapeutic, this is encouraging; whereas if you have been operating for five years and are still in drug discovery mode, this is not. Before you leave your first slide, tell the investors why you are in front of them. For instance, "we are raising $2.5 million in Series A preferred round of capital," or "we are seeking partnership for clinical development," etc.

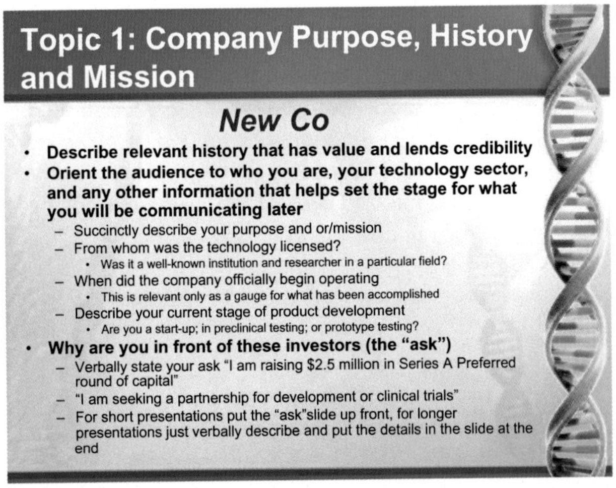

FIGURE 23.2 Company Purpose, History, and Mission Slide

Topic 2: The Problem or "Pain," Unmet Medical Need, and "Why" There Is a Problem

In this slide (Fig. 23.3), you must describe the significance of the problem, how big the problem is, and what is the pain or need in the market. The information on this slide is of

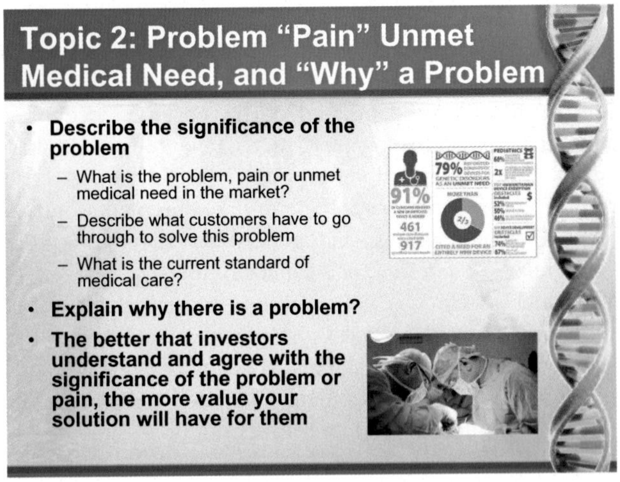

FIGURE 23.3 The Problem or "Pain," Unmet Medical Need, and "Why" There Is a Problem Slide

importance to the technology you will be describing next, as it is the reason your technology solution is needed. Sometimes investors you are pitching to may not be intimately familiar with the problem you are addressing. If you are addressing well-known conditions such as cancer or diabetes or heart disease, don't spend lots of time describing the market for these; whereas you should discuss the particular nuances you are addressing if you are targeting these well-understood markets. Be sure to explain what your customers must go through to solve this problem, and explain why there is a problem, and why it is not solved or addressed yet. As you raise money during your latter development stages, you will be pitching to more sophisticated investors who have heard myriads of pitches and often they are familiar with many of the unmet medical needs. However, no one individual can know all the nuances and problems in every area that biotechnology products can address. Therefore, it is important to make sure that this slide thoroughly addresses the problem. Remember, the bigger, and more significant and critical the problem, an investor can appreciate the importance of the solution. When an investor understands and sees the magnitude of the problem or pain, they will have greater interest in the solution.

Topic 3: Technology and Product "Solution"

This is a key component of your presentation (Fig. 23.4), it represents your strategic advantage and your breakthrough solution to the problem. You want to show how your technology/product application specifically solves the problem or alleviates the "pain" you described in your previous slide. In this section, you must clearly convey the uniqueness of your technology and/or product solution. You want to directly connect your technology solution to the problem you described, and

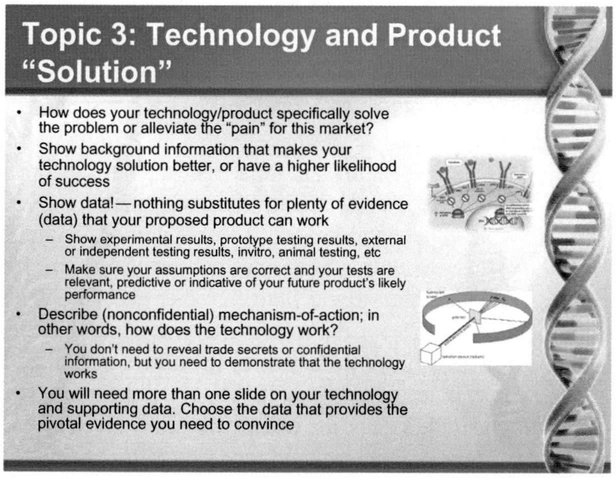

FIGURE 23.4 Technology and Product "Solution" Slide

demonstrate how it is more effective, more efficient, or has strategic advantages such that it will be adopted by your target market. In the biotech industry, nothing is believed without data and there is no substitute for convincing evidence (data) that your proposed product works or has been demonstrated to have a high probability of working when completed. In this section, you will show key experimental results, prototype testing results, and external or independent testing results. Make sure the assumptions and conclusions from your experiments are logical and your tests are relevant, predictive, or indicative of your future product's likely performance. You also need to describe in a nonconfidential manner the mechanism-of-action for your technology or product solution. You don't need to reveal trade secrets or confidential information at this point, but you need to demonstrate that the technology works, is logical, makes sense to extrapolate your conclusions, and you have plenty of supportive data. If the technology is difficult to understand, think about producing a short animation clip to help convey how your technology works. This section will usually require several key experimental or data slides.

If your product is creating a new category, you may need to prove that there is a medical need based upon scientific or medical evidence. Therefore, in some presentations when the investment professionals are scientists, physicians, or engineers, this section may constitute a large number of slides as they may want to see very detailed information. To the extent you can, use data to convince potential investors that the technology you are working on has been proven and that it can perform what you need it to do, and that the down-side risks have been addressed or mitigated. Sometimes, biotech entrepreneurs tend to expound too much on the science and technology without focusing on the pivotal message to take away from the data. As a result, too much technical detail does not help the investor understand your technology differences compared to other solutions, or too much focus on the technology without presenting the rest of the business reveals a traditional scientist, engineer, or physician who may not be perceived as the best leader of the company. However, regardless of the audience, you need to balance talking about the novelty of the technology with the other parts of the business, because you want to convey that you are a *company* developing a commercial *product* rather than an *individual* working on a research *project*.

Topic 4: Your Target Market Opportunity

In this section, you want to show how big the market is people and in dollars—and you want to show how it was calculated (Fig. 23.5). If you used secondary market research, give sources for the market data. Investors want to know if this is a multi-billion dollar market or a niche market. Be sure to describe your target market and drill down to the customer segment that will likely purchase your product. Your objective is to show that there is a large market need. Share information from key opinion leaders in your field and their opinions about this market. Sometimes, testimonials supporting the critical need for your product may help. If there are patient advocacy groups in the field you are targeting, list them and show any support they have for your product.

If the market you are targeting is very well understood, do not spend much time on a detailed description of the market. For instance, if you are targeting cancer, investors know this is big market; however, you should describe the details of the target market your product will focus on, such as subsegments of refractive cancer or second- or third-line therapy, as the size of these markets need elaboration.

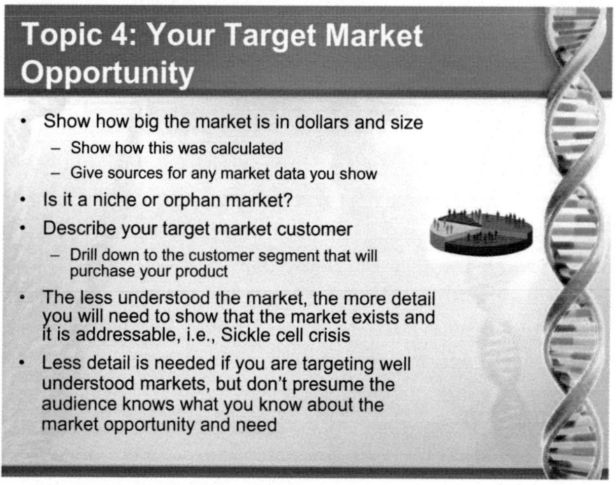

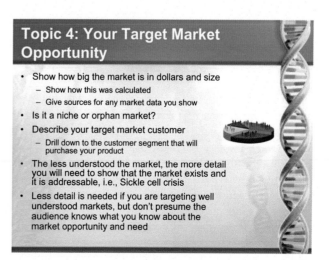

FIGURE 23.5 Your Target Market Opportunity Slide

Topic 5: Your Competition and/or Substitutes

This slide addresses the competition or substitutes that are in the market solving the problem you described (Fig. 23.6). Discuss what is currently being used to alleviate the market "pain;" in other words, what are the substitutes used to attempt to solve the problem. Unless you are in the biosimilar sector, biotechnology products usually do not have much in the way of competition; however, they will all have "*substitutes*." Substitutes are products that individuals use to solve problems in the absence of more direct products or therapies. For instance, in the early days of biotechnology, human insulin was not available, so there was technically no competition for human insulin, whereas porcine and equine insulin was a substitute until genetic engineering was available to produce human insulin. A substitute may be an alternative method for dealing with a medical problem, or a treatment that addresses symptoms rather than treating the underlying etiology. Be sure to think through what are the substitutes for your product, as this will demonstrate that there is an unmet medical need.

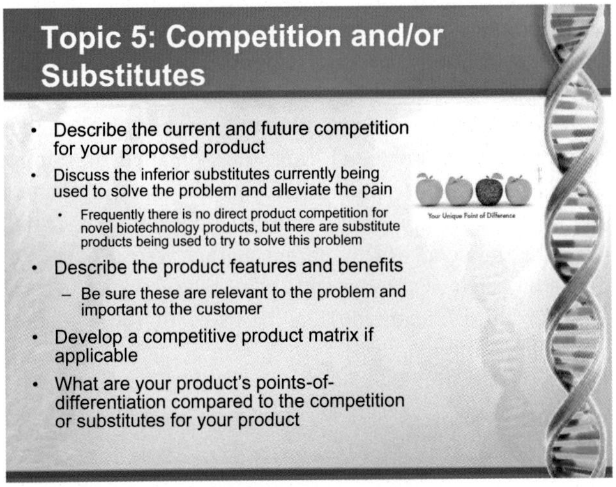

FIGURE 23.6 Your Competition and/or Substitutes Slide

Competition may not always refer to a particular company but more often it is competing technologies capable of addressing the same problem in a different manner. For example, in the past, technologies used for the treatment of viral infections utilized nucleoside analogs. If you are working on antivirals using a different technology, such as stapled peptides that inhibit viral assembly, you can explain how this method would be more effective or have potentially fewer side effects than nucleoside analogs. With new or competitive technologies, you also must address any corresponding issues that new technologies bring. In the antiviral example, you will need to address the ability to orally deliver a peptide that would be resistant to proteases in the gut.

Be sure to describe the current and future competition for your proposed product. You will want to describe your product's features and benefits but be sure these are relevant to the problem and important to the customer. For instance, don't waste much time on the fact that your product is *inexpensive* if there is no product on the market to treat, diagnose, or ameliorate the problem you are addressing. Sometimes in a field that has many competitive technologies, or in the medical device sector that has many substitutes, it may be helpful to show a competitive product matrix to visually help others understand your product advantages over the competition. In this way, you are pointing out your product's *points of differentiation* compared to the competition or substitutes.

Topic 6: Describe Your Business Model

In this slide, you are describing how you will make money (Fig. 23.7). In biotechnology sectors, such as therapeutics, biologics, and even bioagricultural products, it is understood that your model is to partner with a pharmaceutical company at later human clinical stages or a large agriculture company that will advance the product through later stages, regulatory approvals, and commercialization. Unless you are planning to be a vertically integrated pharmaceutical company (which is not something you should tell an investor if you are an early stage company), just list the top pharma companies with an interest in your product market, and show your proposed exit stages and potential valuation. Whereas with most other biotech sectors, you need to describe how you expect to commercialize your product. Do you plan to sell the end product, or are you an intermediary? Show how you will reach your customers and if you will you need

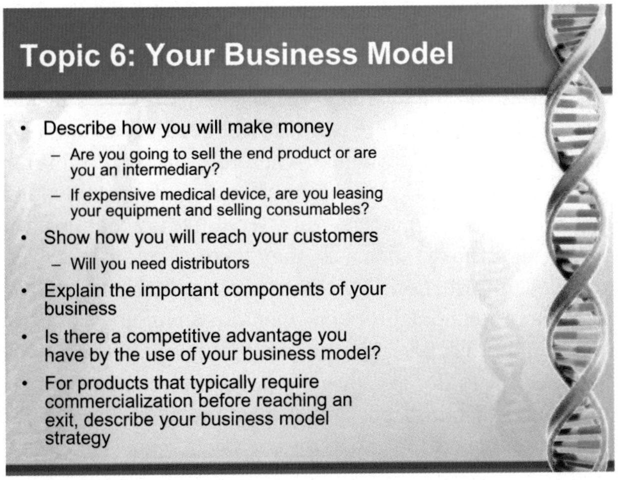

FIGURE 23.7 Describe Your Business Model Slide

distributors. Be sure to explain the important components of your business and if there is a competitive advantage you have by the use of your business model.

Topic 7: Product Development and Regulatory Pathway

In this slide, you will describe your current product development stage and list what has been accomplished to date (Fig. 23.8). Describe the upcoming product development milestones and the timeframe in which you expect to reach these. Make sure you understand which milestones have significant value inflection points for the company, and briefly discuss the regulatory path for approval. Be sure to identify any issues in your regulatory pathway that need to be addressed before you can proceed. If there have been other company failures in the field you are working in, it is important to describe what you are doing differently and why you will not be expected to follow down the same path.

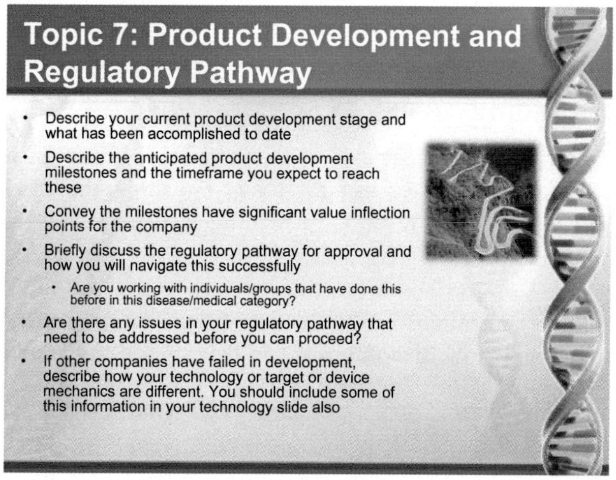

FIGURE 23.8 Product Development and Regulatory Pathway Slide

Topic 8: Intellectual Property and/or Secret Sauce, and Partnerships

In this slide, you want to discuss any issued patents or patent application and list the firm and individuals who are prosecuting your patents (Fig. 23.9). Many times, investors may be familiar with the good IP law firms and if they recognize them, it is helpful reassurance that your IP is being handled properly. In biotechnology, much of the value resides on the IP in the early stages, and it provides the assurance of a future acquiror that they will have a right to the technology developed. If you do not have any issued patents yet, describe the stage of your

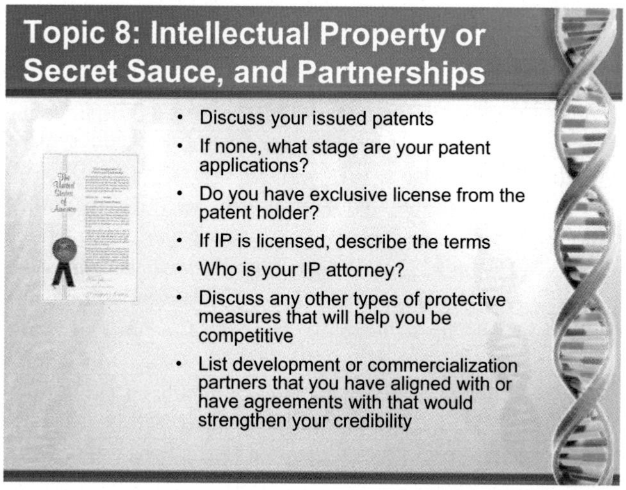

FIGURE 23.9 Insurance Reimbursement Strategy Slide

patent applications and what aspects your pending claims cover. If you licensed the IP, indicate that you have an exclusive license from the institution that owns the IP and describe the terms of the license. Discuss any other types of protective measures that will help you be competitive, such as the use of trade secrets or other knowhow. Although you want to be as clear as possible when discussing your technology, you do not want to share anything that is a trade secret or parts of patent applications that have not yet been issued. If you let the investor know that a part of the technology is a trade secret, or that you have patent applications that have not yet been filed, they will understand and not press for more information. However, you should share as much as you can without revealing confidential information. Investors listen to numerous pitches and it is difficult for them to remember where they have heard something or if it was confidential. As a result, they prefer not to be told anything that is of a confidential nature.

You should discuss any partnerships here or in a subsequent slide. If you have partnerships or are working on partnerships that strengthen your ability to advance your technology or product, describe these and why they are significant. If these partnerships are with organizations that have credible value and are recognized experts, it is important to mention them. The purpose of describing a partnership or collaborative relationship is to convey validation of what you are doing evidenced by the partner's interest. Depending on your stage and sector, these can be early stage relationships with big pharma, a co-development relationship with an enabling technology company, a co-marketing arrangement with a vertical that is in your value chain, or a strategic relationship that could end up as a future acquiror of your company.

Topic 9: Insurance Reimbursement Strategy

The biotech and medical industry have multiple stakeholders that need to be satisfied for these products to be commercially successful, and investors recognize this. The three customers you must provide value to include the physician, the patient, and the payer. You should review *Chapter 32: Biotechnology Products and Their Customers: Developing a Successful Market Strategy*, and *Chapter 33: Biotechnology Product Coverage, Coding, and Reimbursement Strategies*. In this slide, you want to describe the reimbursement environment and strategy for your product, or similar products in a similar category (Fig. 23.10). Address whether or not your product needs to have insurance reimbursement to be accepted by your market. For diagnostics, you want to address whether there are existing Current Procedural Terminology (CPT) codes available for your product category, or if you need to file for a new CPT code to get medical insurance reimbursed. Is there a pharmacoeconomic case for using your product that will save the insurance companies money? Is this a strategy you need to be successful, and if so, how long will that take, and who are the experts that you are working with to get this accomplished?

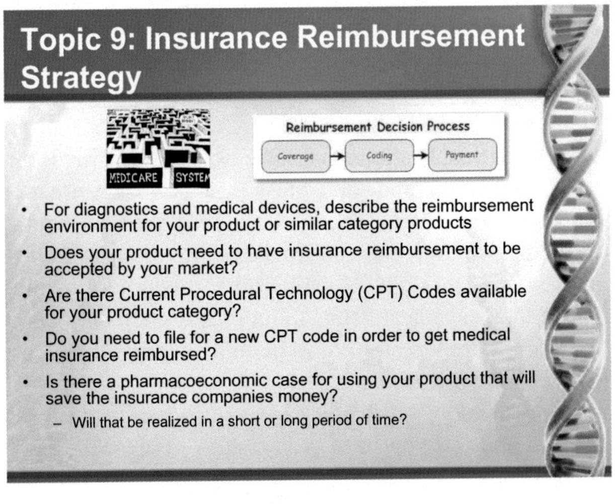

FIGURE 23.10 Go-to-Market Strategy Slide

Topic 10: Go-to-Market Strategy

For products in the sectors of diagnostics, medical devices, research tools, and reagents, your investor exits are most often post-regulatory approval and commercialization. Therefore, you need to describe how you will reach your customers (Fig. 23.11). Are you going to partner for commercialization? Will you need market channel partners?—If so, who and why would they want to work with you? Depending on how difficult or straightforward the marketing is in your sector, you need to explain to your audience that you understand the issues and have a plausible plan to address these.

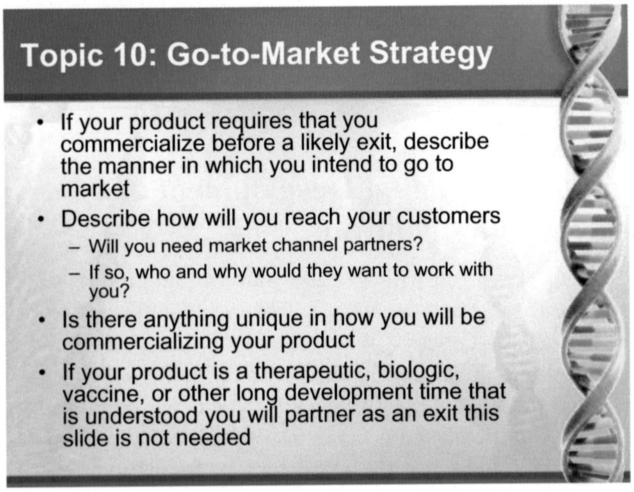

Topic 10: Go-to-Market Strategy
If your product requires that you commercialize before a likely exit, describe the manner in which you intend to go to market
Describe how will you reach your customers
– Will you need market channel partners?
– If so, who and why would they want to work with you?
Is there anything unique in how you will be commercializing your product
If your product is a therapeutic, biologic, vaccine, or other long development time that is understood you will partner as an exit this slide is not needed

FIGURE 23.11 Intellectual Property and/or Secret Sauce, and Partnerships Slide

Topic 11: Proforma Projections and Financing "Ask"

As mentioned earlier, depending on the sector you are in, you may, or may not, need a 5-year pro forma projection of revenue. For biotech sectors in diagnostics or medical device or research reagents or tools, you will need to have revenue projections depending on how close you are to commercialization. In this section (Fig. 23.12), you also want show how much money you have raised to date and tell how much capital you anticipate needing in the next round. It is important to know how many rounds you anticipate needing to reach commercialization or an exit for investors. When you make your revenue projections, you need to start with some assumptions that you can articulate such as growth rate based upon a substitute product, any traction you already have for your product, expectations of published clinical studies or reimbursement decisions, etc. Just projecting revenue based upon a percentage of the market will be an immediate "red flag" to investors on you and your company. Make sure you use a "bottom-up" build of your revenue projections described in *Chapter 32: Biotechnology Products and Their Customers: Developing a Successful Market Strategy*.

The "*ask*" is the amount of money you are requesting and the investment vehicle that you will be using for this round. For instance, are you raising $3 million dollars under a Convertible Note structure or a SAFE investment, or are you raising $15 million dollars in a Series B

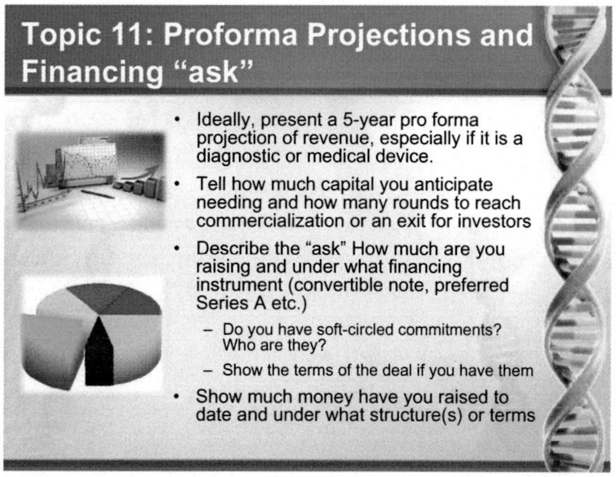

FIGURE 23.12 Proforma Projections and Financing "Ask" Slide

preferred round. The terms will be set by the investor who is interested in your company, but you can determine what investment vehicle you will be using for this round. For more information on the terms of investment vehicles, see *Chapter 21: Financial Ramifications of Funding a Biotechnology Venture: What You Need to Know About Valuation And Term Sheets.*

Topic 12: Use of Proceeds

In this slide, you will have a table or bullet-point list describing your *use of proceeds* for the round you are raising (Fig. 23.13). In broad general categories, you want to show what the money will be used for, and in what categories. For instance, you may have 50% of the funds directed toward product development or prototype development if you are a medical device company. Other categories could include specimen testing, clinical development, software validation, regulatory consultants, reimbursement research, and many others. The point you will need to make clear is that the use of these proceeds will

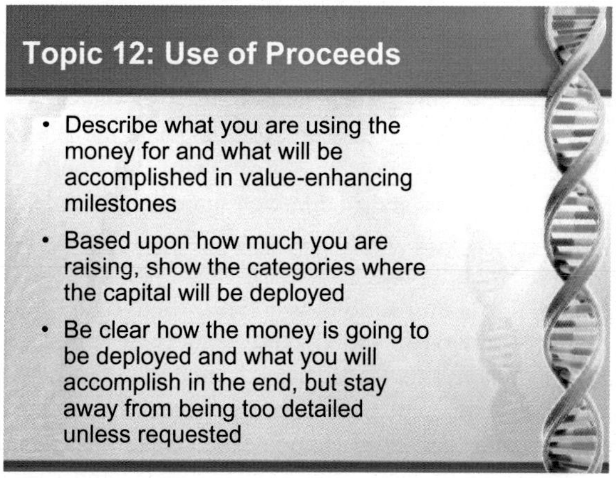

FIGURE 23.13 Use of Proceeds Slide

result in reaching a value-enhancing milestone for the company with the money that is being raised in the current round. You will need to specify what milestone(s) will be accomplished, and their significance in increasing the value of your organization and reducing the risk going forward. Because you will likely be raising another round after these funds are utilized, the investors want to know your plans for the next round, and that their ownership equity or investment will have increased in value.

Topic 13: Likely Exits and Estimated Timeframe

Investors invest for a return on their money. They have an interest in your company's mission but they are investors first. In this slide, you will need to tell them the potential exits and timing based upon the most likely exit scenarios in your sector (Fig. 23.14). If your most likely exit is an acquisition, list the top three most likely acquirers and why. Do you anticipate a potential IPO, and if so in what timeframe? Investors will want to know how long you anticipate it may be before an exit, and how much capital you anticipate needing to raise before then. You will need some help from other sources, but you should provide data on exit valuation or revenue multiples for your sector. Be sure to share any preliminary interest from any potential partners or acquirers if you have them.

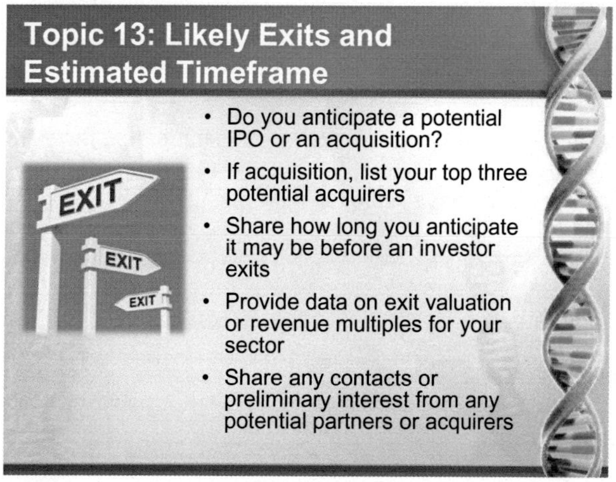

FIGURE 23.14 Likely Exits and Estimated Timeframe Slide

Topic 14: Leadership Team

Investors carefully evaluate the team leading the company because the team and their experience is one of the best predictors of success for a company. Unfortunately, most start-up and development stage companies do not have a

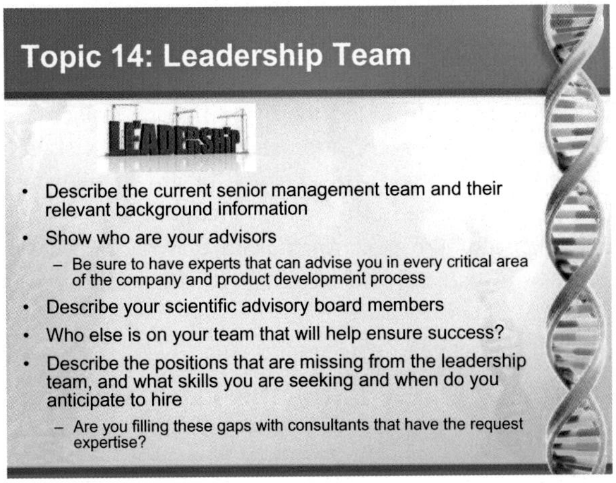

FIGURE 23.15 Leadership Team Slide

full senior management team in place. However, be sure to describe the current management team's relevant background related to your sector and their role (Fig. 23.15). Your leadership team should include a list of your advisors, board members, and consultants which can show you are filling those roles in another way until funds can support a full management team. If you have gaps in your team, be sure to explain when you expect to add that key position. Describe these positions and what skills you are seeking and when you anticipate hiring. Investors want to see a team that has the background and experience to lead the company to be successful. Be sure that you have experts who can advise you in every critical area of the company and product development process.

Topic 15: Reasons to Invest Summary

In this slide, you want to succinctly summarize the points you want the audience to remember when they walk away (Fig. 23.16). These points can include: the novelty of

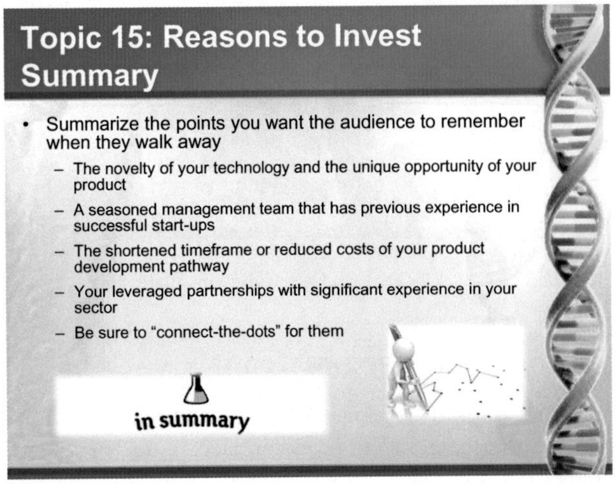

FIGURE 23.16 Reasons to Invest Summary Slide

your technology and the unique opportunity of your product, an untapped medical market, a seasoned management team that has previous experience in successful start-ups, a shortened timeframe or reduced costs of your product development pathway, and your leveraged partnerships with significant experience in your sector. This slide is to "connect-the-dots" for them so investors are reminded of the key points that make your company an attractive investment with a great upside for an exit.

Topic 16: Thank You, Q&A

Verbally thank the audience for the opportunity to present to them and acknowledge any special efforts to give you that opportunity (Fig. 23.17). Be sure to allow plenty of time for Q&A because this is where investors learn what you know and how you respond to issues.

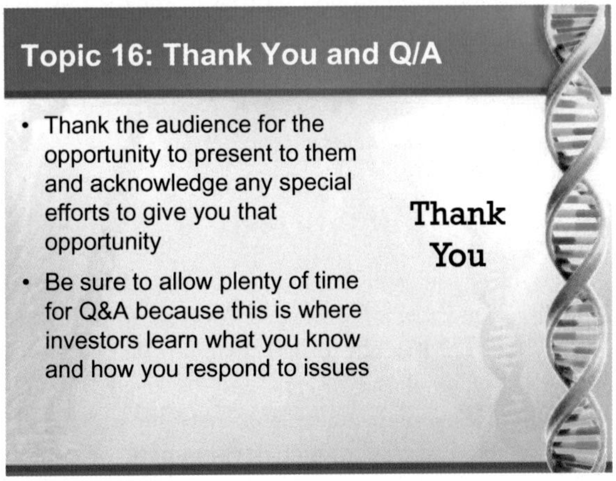

FIGURE 23.17 Thank You, Q&A Slide

Topic 17: Potential Risks and How They Will Be Mitigated

This is a slide that should be reserved for Q&A and should be detailed enough that it answers many of the anticipated questions from the audience. If these risk questions are asked, you can quickly use this slide to share the key risks, and describe how you intend to mitigate these risks (Fig. 23.18). This slide addresses anticipated topics that may be looming in investors' minds based upon issues in the industry or your sector or field you are in. For instance, if you are working in a field where many companies have previously failed, you want to be prepared to show or demonstrate the differences and the evidence why you believe you will be successful where they were not. Examples of other key risks may include critical technology development risks, all regulatory issues and risks for your product, any reimbursement issues, major market

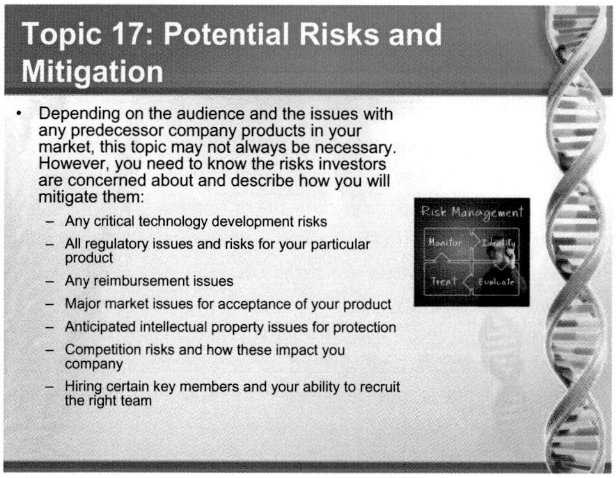

FIGURE 23.18 Potential Risks and How They Will Be Mitigated

issues for acceptance of your product, anticipated intellectual property issues for protection, competition risks and how these impact your company, even hiring certain key members, or your ability to recruit the right team. Depending on the audience and the issues with any predecessor company products in your market, this slide may not always be necessary, but it is a good practice to have these slides available as it demonstrates that you are aware of these risks and are prepared to address them.

Topic 18: Support and Appendix Slides

These slides are of your choosing and are supportive with greater detail on specific topics that you perceive may be needed. Select the slides that help explain the issues you anticipate investors may ask about in more detail (Fig. 23.19). It is likely that you will want additional data slides supporting that your technology and/or product can

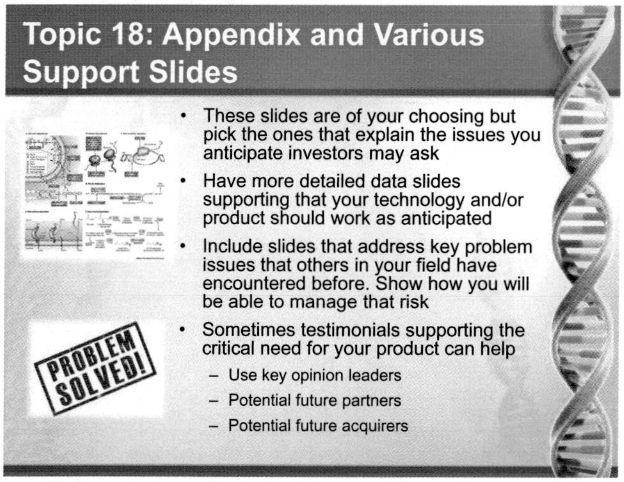

FIGURE 23.19 Support and Appendix Slides

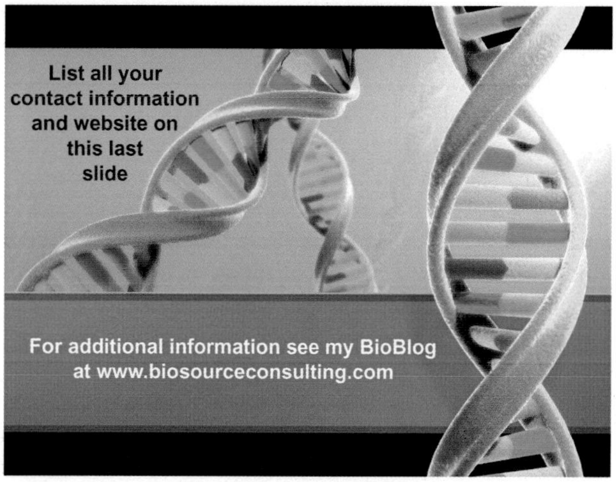

FIGURE 23.20 Contact Information Slide

work as anticipated. You can include slides that address key problems that others in your field have encountered before. For a concluding slide, you can leave up your contact information side so if you have a large audience, some may want to know how to get in contact with you later (Fig. 23.20).

Avoid Technical Problems by Being Prepared

Now, for advice about some problems that you can avoid. On the technical side, always check your slides to be sure they are in proper order, the appropriate number of slides for the time allotted, allowing plenty of time for Q&A. Some investor groups such as angel networks have a coordinator who requests your slide deck ahead of time and has it ready for you when you arrive. Bring a back-up slide deck on a jump drive if you have been asked to send the slides ahead of time, or if you are using your computer for presenting. The back-up jump drive is in case your computer does not work or your computer does not interface with the investors' overhead projection system. Also bring some common connectors for your laptop to plug into their projectors' inputs in case they don't have the right ones. Just be prepared, as an investor's time is limited, and they hear many presentations, therefore you want to avoid the technical problems that could start your meeting off poorly.

Giving Your Presentation

When you get the opportunity to have a face-to-face meeting, this is your chance to personally share your company story. Your pitch deck displays information, but *you* communicate the story to the listening audience in your own personal way. Investing in a company results in a relationship between the company and investors who fund people they like and trust. Be yourself. Don't try to be someone else in your presentation style or conversation. You are the best "*you*," and you are *not* the best at imitating others. Be engaging with your audience. Look them in the eyes and let them see your enthusiasm and passion for what you are doing. Get to know the individuals you are talking to, ask them questions also. Try to find out some information about them and their backgrounds and look for any common interests. Know your material, don't speak as if you memorized, and don't read the slides. Conversationally discuss the information. Always learn from your audience, ask *them* questions, listen to their feedback, and use that information to improve your business. Don't be defensive when a person makes a detracting or offensive comment. Respond in a constructive manner as you can always learn something. After your presentation is over, ask for an opportunity for a follow-up meeting or a day and time when you can come back with more information or answers to questions.

In this chapter, we reviewed 18 topics that are important to put into a biotech investor pitch deck. Depending on your industry sector, there may be additional information that you will need to include. These topics are the basic components of a biotech business and it is important that when presenting to investors, you cover these topics. With practice and a willingness to learn from everyone, you will become more proficient at conveying the key information and knowing how to engage with your audience such that it is an enjoyable experience. Remember that investors are people and they all have personalities. Learn to interact with all individuals in a positive and engaging manner, and you will find that giving presentations may become a gratifying and rewarding experience. As this occurs, you will find that your success rate for getting investors interested in your business will increase.

Section VII

Biotechnology Product Development

Chapter 24

Therapeutic Drug Development and Human Clinical Trials

Donald R. Kirsch, PhD
Harvard Extension School, Cambridge, MA, United States

Chapter Outline

The 1950s can be considered to be the start of the modern drug-discovery era. Although a number of effective medicines were available for clinical use at the end of World War II, most of these were traditional medicines that had been discovered long ago and the vast majority of the medicines that had been discovered in the 19th and the first half of the 20th centuries were basically found by pure chance. Only two medicines discovered during the late 19th and first half of the 20th centuries could be said to have resulted from a pure directed effort to find a new therapy: the discoveries of arsphenamine (Salvarsan) by Ehrlich, the first effective treatment for syphilis [1], and streptomycin by Waksman, the first effective treatment for tuberculosis [2]. In both of these cases the inventors set out with the specific goal to find a new treatment for a specific disease and were successful.

Each of these directed discoveries provided invaluable discovery strategies that were adopted by the drug development industry. The lesson from streptomycin was that although substances with medicinal properties are very rare, medicines, or chemical compounds that could be modified and then turned into medicines, could be found through methodical screening approaches. The lesson from Salvarsan was that a drug could be created through the application of biological assays to guide chemical analog synthesis efforts to identify compounds with therapeutic value.

Small Molecule Drugs

Small molecule drugs are either synthetic chemicals or chemical metabolites produced by plants or microorganisms. (In some cases, these metabolites need to be chemically modified to produce a clinically effective therapeutic.) Synthetic chemicals are custom designed to be drugs, or in rare cases, chemicals that turn out to have

Biotechnology Entrepreneurship. DOI: https://doi.org/10.1016/B978-0-12-815585-1.00024-3

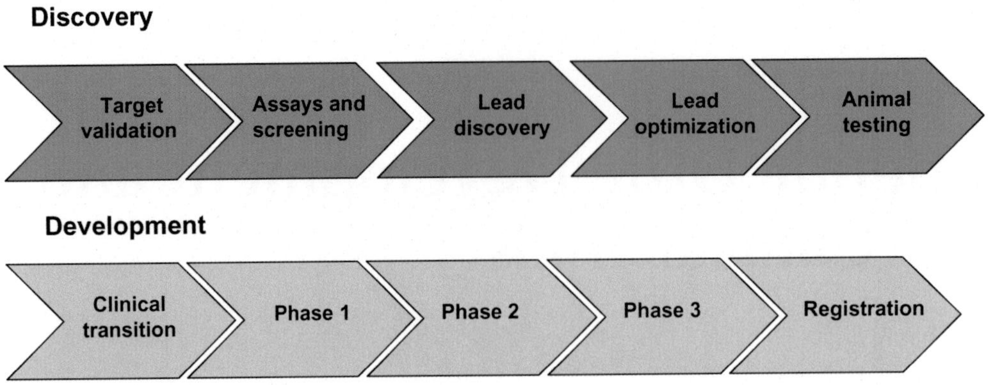

FIGURE 24.1 Drug discovery (therapeutic discovery and preclinical testing) and development (human clinical testing). Standard phases of drug discovery and development. Development processes encompass the preclinical and clinical studies whose results will be used in regulatory submissions (to the FDA in the United States).

drug properties by accident. The clinical utility of naturally occurring small molecule drugs is probably almost certainly due to chance since these compounds are not made by the plant or microorganism with the intended purpose of being drugs. In other words the foxglove plant does not synthesize digitalis in order to treat heart failure. Rather, these naturally occurring metabolites are exploited by humans and repurposed for therapeutic use.

The contemporary approach to small molecule drug discovery was born out of, and is an amalgam of, the abovementioned century-old research strategies. There is now a strong general consensus regarding the standard steps and phases of the drug-discovery process (Fig. 24.1) [3,4]. However, there is no standardized method for drug discovery and every novel drug is discovered in its own unique way. The consensus steps presented later should be taken simply as a broad experience-based, general guide to the drug-discovery process.

Small Molecule Target Identification and Validation

The ultimate success or failure of any drug-discovery project is fundamentally dependent upon the correct selection of the drug target for the chosen disease. As will be discussed in greater detail later, the drug-discovery project will fail if the selected target is not in a pathway driving the underlying basis of the disease, or if the selected target affects other metabolic processes in the body that negatively affects the viability (side effects). The methods currently available to identify and validate effective drug targets are limited and imprecise as is the knowledge of the underlying molecular etiology of many important diseases. These shortcomings are a major factor driving the high failure rate in drug discovery. However, patients need medicines, and biopharmaceutical companies need new products, and therefore the drug-discovery enterprise carries on.

Perhaps the single most important guiding concept in contemporary pharmacology is Paul Ehrlich's receptor theory which states that all drugs work by binding to a specific chemical component or receptor within the cell and that drugs act by modifying the activity of the receptor. Receptors are most commonly (1) enzymes which are proteins that speed up reactions within the organism, (2) cellular switches that are actually called receptors because in many cases they were identified as drug targets before their biological cellular functions became known, and (3) signaling pathway elements that act downstream from receptors (see Fig. 24.2). While traditional drugs were discovered through serendipity, the field has changed so that instead of finding a drug by good fortune and then determining how it acts, receptor targets are now selected based on fundamental scientific principles and drugs are then sought that will act on the chosen receptor target.

All diseases have an underlying cause or molecular mechanism that produces the disease called the disease molecular etiology. This idea can probably be most easily understood for infectious diseases; for instance, the molecular etiology for tuberculosis is infection by the pathogenic bacterium *Mycobacterium tuberculosis*. The bacterium produces damage to the body and leads to the symptoms of the disease. Eliminate the bacterial pathogen and you cure the disease (of course you still need to identify a molecular target within the bacterium that will kill the bacteria without harming the patient). Other disease classes can be similarly understood. Heart disease can be caused by arrhythmia, a condition in which the natural heartbeat or rhythm is disturbed, leading to a weakening of the action of the heart. The rhythm of the heartbeat is produced through the interaction of a number of receptors and ion channels (cell membrane proteins that allow inorganic ions such as sodium, potassium, or

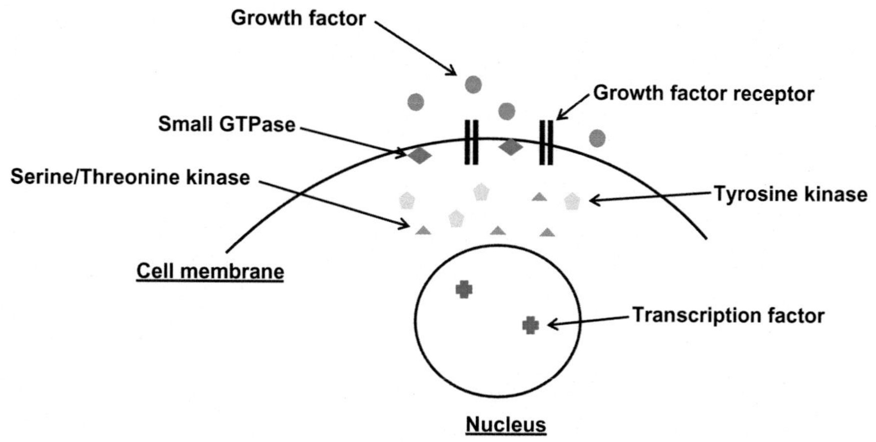

FIGURE 24.2 Drug targeting example. Growth factors are produced by specialized cells to induce the growth and division of target cells, acting through growth factor receptors present on the surface of the cell and spanning the cell membrane. These growth factor receptors, in response to the presence of growth factors, transfer the growth signal into the interior of the cell. The interior of the cell has a variety of components mediating cell growth and division including, in this example, a number of classic enzymes—tyrosine kinases, serine/threonine kinases, and small GTPases. When activated by signaling cascades, transcription factors enter the cell nucleus where they bind to specific DNA sequences and regulate genes that control cell growth and cell division.

calcium to enter or leave the cell) within the heart. Drugs that act on these controllers of the heart rhythm can restore the heartbeat back to normal. Similarly, high-serum cholesterol can lead to heart disease; so, drugs that block the synthesis of cholesterol within the body lower cholesterol levels and thus lower the probability of heart disease.

Since everything that follows depends on the correct selection of the target, much effort is put into providing confidence that the target has been correctly chosen. This is the process called target validation. Target validation is unfortunately far from a precise endeavor. One overarching problem is that for many diseases, the underlying molecular etiology is not known with precision and, not surprisingly, these are the diseases for which new therapies are most desperately needed. The strategies used to validate hypotheses regarding disease etiology are far from definitive because of their inability to precisely model the disease in question (Fig. 24.3). For such diseases, there are commonly a set of competing unproven hypotheses regarding what causes the disease. While the drug developer could initiate a basic research program to identify the cause of the disease with certainty, this is a long and drawn out process with an uncertain outcome. Therefore drug developers will most commonly make a highly educated guess as to which of the competing hypotheses is correct, knowing that successful development of a drug will be one means to provide confirmation of the underlying hypothesis.

As an example, many scientists working on Alzheimer's disease think that Alzheimer's could best be treated by targeting a protein called beta-amyloid protein [5]. Others think the best strategy would be to target a different protein called tau [6]. Perhaps, one group is correct

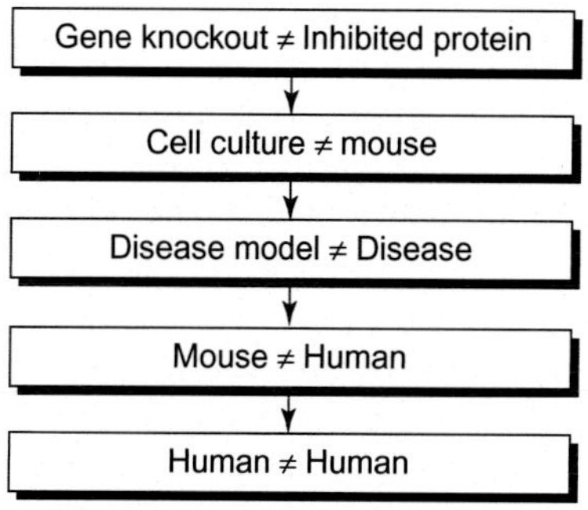

FIGURE 24.3 Five sources of error that can produce discordance between studies to validate a drug target and the effects of a drug acting on that target in a clinical trial. See the text for details.

and the other wrong. Maybe they are both right and the disease is caused by multiple protein dysfunctions or that some cases of the disease are caused by the dysfunction of beta-amyloid protein and other cases are caused by the dysfunction of tau. Another possibility is that both groups are wrong and these protein dysfunctions are actually a result of the disease and that the actual cause is something upstream from beta-amyloid and tau. However, patients and their families (not to mention pharmaceutical corporate management) do not want to wait to find out. They want scientists to work on the development of a treatment despite the risk of failure. Thus the drug developer moves forward while research groups are competing with each other working on beta-amyloid or tau, depending on their best guess.

Once a disease etiology is selected, one still needs to select a drug target to counter the suspected cause of the disease. If you think that beta-amyloid causes

Alzheimer's disease, then you have to come up with an approach to block the destructive actions of beta-amyloid and have good underlying evidence supporting the validity of the approach. Such evidence is commonly accumulated from multiple sources and approaches. One strategy is to start with an existing biochemical reagent that acts on the target in a nonselective fashion and test the reagent in a way that subtracts out the *nonspecific* actions of the chemical to try to predict the activity of a *selective* drug. However, many times, such reagents do not exist.

Another approach is to utilize standard molecular biology techniques. These techniques make it possible to up- or downmodulate a potential protein drug target in cells via reagents that up- or downregulate or even knockout (eliminate) the gene that encodes it. The premise is that simply making more of the protein mimic a drug that stimulates the activity of the protein and making less of the protein mimic a drug that inhibits the activity of the protein. A confounding issue is that many proteins have scaffolding functions in addition to their primary activity as a receptor or enzyme. Proteins commonly appear in complexes with multiple other proteins. Changing the level of a protein can have effects on all the proteins in the complex. Drugs, however, only affect the enzyme or receptor activity while molecular biology techniques affect both the enzyme or receptor activity and any scaffolding activity.

Additional limitations include the fact that testing in cells (in vitro) only approximates a portion of what goes on in an intact animal (in vivo). Alternately, one can use molecular biology techniques to produce gene knockouts or knockins in laboratory mice. This is where the gene encoding the target of interest can be disrupted (knockout) in the genome of a laboratory mouse, or a hyperactive version of the gene can be added (knockin) into a mouse genome. Characterization of the resulting mouse strain will reveal a number of important things about the target. For one, if the target has an essential function, the resulting knockout mouse strain will be dead or have some clear biological defect. Thus the drug developer will be warned away from inhibiting a target that could produce toxic consequences. The knockout/knockin can also be introduced into a mouse disease model to determine whether the genetic modification modifies the course of the disease. Finding that such a genetic change modifies the disease is highly encouraging, although not conclusive because a medicine is given only after the disease is diagnosed. In contrast the gene knockout or knockin is present from the moment of conception and certainly precedes the onset of disease symptoms in the animal model. Therefore one might be validating a target that could only work if the drug was given prior to disease onset, something which is unlikely to happen clinically.

Target Identification and Validation—Areas of Uncertainty

Disease animal models are most commonly used to evaluate the effects of a potential therapeutic. However, disease animal models are imperfect representations of the actual disease because mice are not people and there are biochemical, metabolic, and genetic differences between species. This is a particular concern for diseases of the elderly. For instance, current life expectancy at birth in the United States is approximately 78 years. Mice in contrast can live about a year in the wild and about 2–3 years in a highly protected laboratory environment. Since many diseases of the elderly are thought to be at least in part the result of long-term subtle toxic environmental exposures, mice arguably do not make a good model for such diseases. Even patients with a specific disease are not identical. As a result, patients do not respond in the same way even to well-established drugs. Clinical studies have shown that 10%–30% of the patients will not respond to a selected antihypertensive ACE (angiotensin converting enzyme) inhibitor, 15%–25% of heart failure patients will not respond to a selected beta blocker, 20%–50% of the patients will not respond to a specific SSRI (selective serotonin reuptake inhibitor) antidepressant, etc. Thus even for well-established therapies, the physician will often empirically try different members of a drug class on their patient until they find one that works for them.

Given these limitations, on average, only 30% of the target validation projects are successful, meaning that the tested target appears to provide benefit in treating the disease. A target identification and validation study would typically take a year and cost $500,000–1 million to complete in an industrial laboratory (see Fig. 24.4). If the target is not validated, this is a sunk cost and the research team proceeds to test the next candidate target. However, an even worse outcome is the incorrect validation of the drug target. In this case, work goes forward with mounting costs for a project that is ultimately doomed to failure. (Study costs, timing, and success rates in this and all succeeding sections were established by combining information taken from the following references: Brown and Superti-Furgam [7], Drews [8], Koppal [9], Nwaka and Ridley [3], and Reichert [10].)

Assay Development and High-Throughput Screening

Once a therapeutic target is validated, the next step is to identify chemical compounds that act on the target in the desired way. This requires a screening assay, a biological or biochemical test that can clearly distinguish between active compounds that produce the desired effect, and inactive compounds that do not interact with the target.

Drug-discovery phases and metrics

Exploratory		
	Target validation	**Assays and screening**
Activity	Target ID, characterization	Assay development, HTS implementation
Duration	6–12 months	6–12 months
Success rate	30%	65%
FTE/cost	1–2 FTE	2–3 FTE

Hit-to-lead		
	Lead discovery	**Lead optimization**
Activity	Counterscreens, confirm hits, test analogs	SAR, in vivo testing, exploratory ADME, 2 series; 1 lead each
Duration	12–15 months	12–24 months
Success rate	65%	55%
FTE/cost	3–5 FTE	8–12 FTE

Preclinical studies		
	Animal testing	**Preclinical transition**
Activity	In vivo efficacy, animal ADMET	Process chemistry, scale up, formulation, GLP ADMET, IND
Duration	12 months	12 months
Success rate		55%
FTE/cost	~$500,000	~$5.0 million

FIGURE 24.4 A summary of drug discovery phases with associated costs, staffing, durations, and historical success rates. See text for additional details and references.

The screening assay must have the following characteristics:

1. The assay must be relatively inexpensive since a few hundred thousand compounds are commonly tested in a typical screening campaign. (See later for a discussion of the selection of compounds for screening.) If each assay, fully loaded for reagents, labor, laboratory automation, and overhead, costs 10 cents per assay, expenses for the screening campaign alone will be about $20,000 not counting expenditures for assay design and validation. As a general rule of thumb, the per assay cost needs to be under $1 so that the screening campaign will cost no more than $200,000–300,000.
2. The assay must also be highly sensitive. At this point in the project, the investigator is looking for a chemical lead, not a finished drug. One must expect that the crude chemical lead will have low potency that will be improved by subsequent chemical synthesis. Only a sensitive assay can detect such crude, weak leads.
3. The assay must be selective for the activity of interest. All biological assays are subject to artifacts and identify compounds that are not real hits. If such artifacts are both rare and anticipated ahead of time, they can be easily weeded out through subsequent experimentation. If, however, they are common and confused with real hits, the entire enterprise will fail.

Assay Development and High-Throughput Screening—Screen Implementation

Screening can commence once the assay is designed and validated. The question at this point is what samples and how many of them to screen. Because chemical optimization of a lead compound is a long and expensive process, it makes sense to start with a good lead that will hopefully limit the number of chemical iterations needed to produce the clinical lead compound. The assembly of chemical files for screening is a much-debated process. In the mid-1990s, chemists at Ciba-Geigy, now part of Novartis, calculated the number of possible drug-type compounds that could in theory exist, estimating that there are 3×10^{62} such compounds [11].

Such a large number cannot be handled in practice. Therefore only a tiny subset of all possible compounds will actually be screened. During the 1990s a "more is better" philosophy took hold. Each of the established large pharmaceutical companies had a screening collection of around 50,000–200,000 compounds that had been prepared through their chemical synthesis efforts during the first 150 or so years of their existence. These collections came into being because it was standard practice to retain an aliquot for future screening every time a compound was synthesized at these companies. The 1990s was an era of intense mergers and acquisitions within the biopharmaceutical industry, and as a result many companies were in possession of the combined screening collections from multiple predecessors. American Home Products (later renamed Wyeth) had the chemical collections of Wyeth, Ayerst, Cyanamid/Lederle, and AH Robbins. SmithKline Beecham had collections from Beecham, Smith Kline, and the French, Richard and Company. Glaxo Welcome had the combined collections of Glaxo Laboratories and Burroughs Wellcome. Pharmacia had the combined historical collections of Searle, Upjohn, and Pharmacia. Bristol-Myers Squibb had the combined collections of Bristol-Myers and Squibb. Thus many hundreds of thousands of compounds became available for the screening.

To address this perceived limitation a number of combinatorial chemistry start-up companies were established during the same period. The goal of these companies was to make small-size samples of a large number of different chemical compounds for screening. The companies exploited laboratory robots and simple chemical reactions that could be performed with a wide range of starting materials in a combinatorial fashion. For example, a reaction of 10 starting compounds of type "A" with 10 starting compounds of type "B" in all possible combinations could rapidly yield 100 new compounds for screening. Such companies quickly built up collections of 100,000 or more new compounds for screening.

Unfortunately, the results from the "more is better" approach did not meet expectations. All companies came to roughly the same conclusion following their analysis of the output from multiple screening campaigns:

1. The types of compounds from the combinatorial chemistry companies were constrained by the necessity to run simple reactions in a massively parallel fashion. As a result of this constraint, the output compounds were most often not drug-like, did not result in good screening hits, and were not worth the effort involved to screen the collections.
2. A subset of compounds from both the historical libraries and combinatorial collections was found to be active in a wide variety of assays. These compounds were named "frequent hitters" and their performance was inconsistent with the expectation that screening hits would selectively hit targets like a key fitting into a lock. After extensive follow-up research it was determined that such frequent hitter compounds were artifacts and produced activity because of chemical properties that would not make them useful drugs.
3. Other compounds were consistently inactive over an extremely wide range of targets suggesting that they lacked drug-like properties and were probably not worth screening.
4. Many active compounds were dropped following chemistry review because they lacked good opportunities for further chemical modifications.

This raised the question that if there was no opportunity for follow-up, why were these compounds being screened in the first place? The earlier observations led to a rationalization of the compounds being screened. Today, screening campaigns are typically conducted using smaller rationally assembled chemical libraries, and a campaign including 50,000–200,000 rationally selected compounds is generally considered to be a reasonable test of a good volume of chemical space.

Assay development, validation, and implementation typically in aggregate take about a year and cost $1 million or more in a large biopharmaceutical company. The overall success rate for this research phase is about 65% (see Fig. 24.4). Failures principally come in two areas. First, it can be maddeningly difficult to develop assays for some biological processes, especially when the assay needs to meet the difficult combined criteria of low cost, robustness, ease and speed of operation, high selectivity, and freedom from artifact. Some screening assays are never successfully completed. Second, for reasons that are not completely understood, not all targets are equally "druggable," a term meaning that the target activity can be modified by the action of a drug or drug-like chemical. The only way to know with some confidence that your target is druggable is to test a compound file and see whether any bona fide actives are recovered. There have been many instances when I designed a screen, tested several hundred thousands of compounds, and found no active compounds.

Lead Discovery

Hopefully, at the end of the screening campaign, the drug developer has a hit list—all the compounds that were active in the screen along with their chemical structures. What should a reasonable hit list look like? The first question is "what is the hit rate?" It is the percent of the tested compounds that showed activity. If one is looking for a treatment for an incurable disease, I think it is reasonable to expect that compounds with therapeutic potential will be rare, few, and far between. I have seen cases where investigators report that a few percents of the tested compounds are active. I think this is unreasonable. If such potential treatments were so common—a few per hundred random compounds—it stands to reason that they would have been found previously through pure serendipity and the disease would have been cured.

I believe that most screeners would say that a reasonable hit rate would be no higher than 0.1%. I find that a hit rate of 0.01% is very workable, producing about 20 actives from a screen of 200,000 samples. These actives are then characterized biologically and chemically to produce leads for the chemical optimization process. Artifacts are removed in so far as possible via biological secondary assays and the potency and efficacy of the true hits are determined. Potency indicates how low a concentration of a compound is needed to produce the desired effect, and efficacy means how strong a biological response can ultimately be produced by the compound. In general, it is best to focus work on high potency and efficacy actives since these compounds provide a starting point that is closer to the ultimately desired drug.

Chemical analysis will demonstrate whether similar chemical types are recovered repeatedly or whether all the actives are chemically unrelated. Finding similar compounds repeatedly is generally a good sign that the screen ran well since it would be reasonable to expect that certain chemical structural types will be best able to hit the target of interest. Chemical compounds that are structurally related to the actives are then purchased and tested to crudely identify which chemical features are needed to produce activity. It is a bad sign if the hit compound is active but all related compounds are inactive. This result suggests that it will be very difficult to find chemical analogs with improved activity. Similarly, it is a bad sign if virtually all analogs are active. Drugs fit into their site of action like a key into a lock. As a result, some analogs should work and others should be inactive. If everything works, it suggests that the hit is working indiscriminately, possibly because of its chemical reactive properties rather than because of its selective action on a target.

All the abovementioned information is used to select two to three actives as leads for further work. In many cases the biologists' favorite hits will be different from the chemists' favorite hits. This is because each group looks at the results through the lens of their own scientific discipline and training. Biologists look at the actives for high potency, efficacy, and activity in a variety of relevant biological assays coupled with validation in multiple models with appropriate selectivity and low toxicity. Chemists look at the actives for chemical novelty, drug-like character, ease of chemical synthesis, and opportunities to chemically elaborate the active compound. In addition, chemical intuition is important. The very best medicinal chemists who have repeatedly discovered useful drugs will have intuitive feelings regarding which actives can eventually turn into drugs. Such feelings cannot be rationally described, but they are important and will contribute to the project success. The bottom line is that biologists and chemists have different, *but equally valid*, perspectives on the drug-discovery process. Successful projects incorporate the perspectives from both disciplines.

Lead discovery typically takes over a year, at this point employing expanded staff and at an average cost of over \$1.5−2 million. The success rate is on average 65% (see Fig. 24.4). Failure is typically caused by poor leads or in some cases no leads. Poor leads have weak biological activity suggesting that it will require extreme effort to bring the lead to a point where it will have clinically relevant activity. Poor leads can also be chemically intractable with difficult multistep syntheses and poor potential for analog design. A decision to move forward commits to a lead optimization stage with significantly increased expenses and a longer timeframe.

Lead Optimization

Once a lead is selected, the next step in the process is optimization. With a preliminary knowledge established regarding which chemical features are needed to carry the desired biological activity, it is common to now refer to the lead as a "scaffold." The concept is that while the basic form of the drug has been identified, this basic form, or scaffold, will now be decorated with chemical substituents to produce the final drug molecule. Analogs are made and then tested in multiple biological systems—initially in the test tube and later in cells and laboratory animals. Obviously, analogs will be tested for improved potency and efficacy against the target because highly potent and efficacious compounds can be dosed at low levels reducing the potential for side effects. Testing is also conducted for selectivity to ensure that the compound acts on the target of interest and not on similar proteins. Commonly, assays for the most closely related enzymes or receptors are established and run as counter-screens looking for inactivity or low potency.

However, drugs must act in the body of a living organism and not just in a test tube (in vitro). In traditional drug discoveries, compounds were tested in animals at the very earliest phases of the project. Thus there would be an early assurance that not only did the compound hit the target of interest but that it was also pharmacologically well behaved in animals. In current practice, however, evaluation in animals is deferred until much later stages of development—arguably a major weakness of the current drug-discovery model.

In fact, in recent times, some drug developers have continued to believe that postponing animal testing was completely wrong headed. Probably the most famous of these critics was Dr. Paul Janssen, founder of Janssen Pharmaceuticals. Dr. Janssen's record of productivity speaks for itself [12,13]. Janssen and the scientists at Janssen Pharmaceuticals discovered more than 80 new medicines and 4 of Janssen's medicines are on the World Health Organization's list of essential medicines—an absolute world record. Prior to his retirement, Janssen Pharmaceuticals was screening well over 10,000 chemical compounds annually directly in a group of animal-based assays.

The current discovery model defers animal testing largely because in vitro testing is less expensive, quicker, and higher throughput. However, it is recognized that it will not be effective to simply optimize compounds for effects on the target because issues of whether the drug will work in a living organism are crucial for the ultimate success of the project.

There are five types of pharmacological properties that characterize how a drug behaves in the body. This set of pharmacological properties is referred to as the drug's ADMET, an acronym standing for absorption, distribution, metabolism, elimination, and toxicity. In vitro, test tube-based assays are available to roughly measure each of these properties and such assays are currently employed during the lead optimization at early stages in place of animal testing [14,15].

Drug Absorption and Distribution

Oral activity is desired for most drugs since patients prefer taking a pill to an injection, suppository, or other alternate means of administration. The oral activity requires that the drug is able to survive the acidic environment of the stomach and that it can be absorbed from the digestive tract. Digestive-tract absorption is modeled using a system based on Caco-2 cells, cells derived from the lining of the digestive tract. Compounds that pass a monolayer will commonly, but not always, absorbed through the digestive tract.

Once in the body, various drugs will distribute differently, and where the drug goes is a crucial determinant of efficacy. For example, any drug that works on a neurological disease must enter the brain. However, there is an obstacle called the blood–brain barrier that keeps most compounds out of the brain. This barrier is believed to have evolved so that pharmacologically active substances in the foods we eat will be unable to enter our brains after a meal and disrupt neurological processes. The barrier is very effective although imperfect. For example, caffeine, present in many beverages, is able to enter the brain and disrupt sleep. The existence of this barrier is an important issue for drug developers and much work has gone into the development of test tube models for the blood–brain barrier. Similarly, much work has also gone into producing drugs with appropriate brain distribution profiles.

As an example, histamine receptors in cells of the nasopharynx control the release of cellular metabolites that produce allergy symptoms—stuffiness and runny noses. Antihistamines block these receptors and produce good relief for allergy sufferers, but with one major problem—histamine receptors are also in the brain and antihistamines interact with these receptors causing drowsiness (sleepiness). The earliest antihistamines, for example, diphenhydramine (Benadryl), penetrate well into the brain and cause sleepiness as a major undesired side effect. Diphenhydramine in addition to being effective in relieving allergy symptoms is unfortunately a potent sedative and, although it was originally developed to treat allergy symptoms, it is now commonly used in over-the-counter sleep agents like Tylenol PM. In this case, pharmacologists wanted to block the brain penetration of the antihistamines to produce a superior nonsedating side-effect-free allergy pill. Terfenadine (Seldane) was an early antihistamine compound that was unable to enter the brain and was marketed as the first nonsedating allergy medication [16]. However, the structural changes that blocked brain penetration also enabled the drug to block an ion channel in the heart called the hERG channel. This effect was first discovered only after the drug was on the market and used in a larger population of people. Blocking the hERG channel can produce a heart arrhythmia called QT interval prolongation which in some cases causes a potentially fatal heart arrhythmia called "Torsades de pointes." The Food and Drug Administration (FDA) later banned the drug and required its removal from the market. Subsequent drug development goals became more complex: to block the histamine receptor, to block brain penetration, and to not block the hERG channel. Further work led to the development of loratadine (Claritin), which is currently available as a safe, nonsedating allergy medication, advertised as "Claritin clear" because it leaves you nonsedated and clear headed [17].

Drug Metabolism

The next property that needs to be considered in lead optimization is metabolism. There are well-established test tube-based assays to measure metabolism. Most drugs are metabolized (broken down) by liver enzymes called cytochromes P450. The liver eliminates toxic compounds in the diet and this activity allows us to safely eat many things that would otherwise be poisonous. However, these liver enzymes become a problem if they break down useful medicines too quickly. You can begin to understand how susceptible a drug is to these liver enzymes by examining the dosing information on the label. A drug that must be taken four times a day is most likely broken down quickly by these enzymes while a once-a-day medicine is probably broken down much more slowly. Patients prefer once-a-day dosing, but that can be difficult to achieve while maintaining a variety of other beneficial properties in a medicine. If it were easy, of course all drugs would be dosed once-a-day.

As an extreme example of a drug metabolism issue, cardiac patients will take a tiny pill by placing it under his or her tongue. The drug in this example is nitroglycerin, which is given to treat angina pectoris, pain in the chest that results because of insufficient blood flow through blood vessels within the heart. Nitroglycerin dilates or expands these vessels allowing more blood to flow through and thus relieves the pain. But, why not just swallow the pill instead of sticking it under your tongue? Nitroglycerin is very rapidly broken down by liver enzymes. Materials absorbed from the stomach go directly to the liver and nitroglycerin that is absorbed from the stomach is destroyed immediately and never makes it to the heart. In contrast, drugs placed under the tongue rapidly diffuse through the mucous membranes in the mouth, enter capillaries and the venous circulation, and can then go directly to the heart without first entering the liver and be metabolized. Thus nitroglycerin is effective when placed under the tongue but is ineffective when swallowed [18].

In the current practice, chemists prepare analogs of the lead compound and each lead is tested for activity against the target; potency and efficacy and, using the above-described in vitro assays, for desirable pharmacological properties; oral absorption, distribution to the diseased tissue/organs, and resistance to rapid metabolism. The overall goal is to synthesize at least one compound that can be moved forward into clinical trials. This stage of research employs a greatly expanded staff of about 8–12 scientists working in all disciplines. The greatest staff expansion is in the area of chemistry, with typically four to eight chemists synthesizing compounds full time. On average, and depending on the number of synthetic steps involved and the difficulty of the chemistry, each chemist can synthesize about two custom compounds per week. The synthesis of 1500 or more custom compounds would typically be needed to produce a clinical candidate and thus would take about 2 years with a cost on the order of $4–8 million. Historically, the success rate for lead optimization has been about 55% (see Fig. 24.4).

Clinical Candidate Compound Selection and Characterization in Animal Disease Models

The selection of a clinical candidate compound is not an exact science. Therapeutic products are not designed to meet a certain specification, rather they just need to incorporate a combination of properties that allows them to be both safe and effective. A truck will be designed to carry a certain load, carry a certain number of people, or pull a trailer of a certain weight. A computer will be designed to have a certain amount of memory or to operate specific software programs. In contrast, there is really no clear design specification for a new first-in-class medicine. The new medicine should treat the target disease, but beyond that it is not a matter of hitting a design specification but rather to provide some measurable clinical benefit for patients without burdensome side effects. The exact nature of that benefit is not predesigned but determined in practice. In other words the exact benefit is not known or predicted with any confidence going into the clinical trials but rather is defined as a result of the clinical trials.

An almost imponderable question at any particular point is whether additional chemical synthesis will yield a superior compound or whether it is the right point to halt chemical efforts and move into the clinic. This is a question for hot debate among members of the project team. There is always the possibility that the next compound made will be superior to what is in hand. When do you stop? Commercial issues must be addressed as part of this debate. For instance, drugs need to be patent protected, enabling companies to maintain exclusivity in the market for a period of time to ensure profitability. The patent life clock begins to tick once patents are filed. Expanding development time in analog synthesis decreases profits by compressing the time on the market prior to the introduction of the generic version of the drug. Alternatively, delaying patent filing could provide the opportunity for a competitor to beat you to the patent office. There are also tactical issues. The research team typically is dissolved once the clinical candidate is called. What if a problem is identified during the next step, the clinical transition studies? Who will address the problem if the team has been disbanded and the members are off on a new set of projects? In many companies, this last problem is often addressed by having the team identify a backup compound in addition to the clinical candidate, which will be in hand should the clinical candidate stumble.

Lastly, since costs will escalate at the next steps in the process, the team will carefully characterize the clinical candidate in multiple animal disease models before deciding to move it on into clinical transition studies. You want to be as sure as possible that your molecule merits the resources that will be needed for clinical testing. The strategic goal is if you are going to fail, and most projects do, fail as soon as possible before too much time and too many resources are wasted on a project that will not go forward. A failure at the late stage is a disaster for all involved and is to be avoided whenever possible. Research teams, therefore, constantly try to design and implement what are commonly called killer experiments—studies that would provide a yes/no answer on whether to move the project forward.

Large Molecule Drugs

Elsewhere in this volume, you will see the term "biologics," often used as a synonym for "large molecule drugs." "Biologic" is, however, a more general term than "large molecule drug." The FDA defines a biologic as something manufactured in a living system including a wide range of products including vaccines, blood and blood components, allergenics, somatic cells, gene therapy, tissues, and recombinant therapeutic proteins. Thus large molecule drugs are a subset of the biologic therapeutic category. (Note that in contrast, conventional, small molecule drugs are manufactured without the use of living cells via chemical synthesis.)

Target Identification and Validation

Large molecule drugs are in a separate category from small molecule drugs, which include inorganic and organic polymers (such as proteins) and biochemicals (such as polysaccharides, nucleic acids, and proteins). Large molecule drugs are most commonly proteins already present in humans and animals that have evolved to carry out a specific function. That exact same function is utilized in the desired therapeutic application of the protein. So, while the small molecule drug developer looks outside the body for his or her drug, the large molecule drug developer looks within the body. Once a protein of interest is identified and its therapeutic activity validated, the goal is to manufacture it in quantity for therapeutic use, sometimes with, but commonly without, modification. Large molecule drugs largely fall into four categories: (1) hormones and other replacement proteins, (2) cytokines (signaling molecules employed by the immune system), (3) vaccines, and (4) antibodies.

Hormones

Insulin is the founding member of the large molecule hormone drug group, used to treat type 1 diabetics who are unable to synthesize insulin. Historically, it was extremely fortunate that insulin from animals, specifically cows and pigs, worked well in humans. Pancreas from these species was available in quantity from slaughterhouses to serve as source material for the preparation of therapeutic insulin. In more recent times, true human insulin, made by recombinant DNA methods, is instead given to diabetic patients. Other commonly used replacement therapies include recombinant factor VIII (Recombinate, Kogenate) and factor IX (Benefix), both used to treat hemophiliacs who as the result of genetic mutations are unable to make these proteins and erythropoietin, a hormone that stimulates the production and survival of blood cells. Patients with end-stage renal disease produce little erythropoietin and must be given the hormone as a replacement therapy. Also, patients undergoing cancer chemotherapy commonly become anemic and such patients can better tolerate their chemotherapy when treated with erythropoietin. Relative to small molecule drugs, target identification and validation for these replacement-type proteins is much more straightforward. If it is clear that a missing protein is causing the disease, it obviously makes sense to treat the disease by replacing the protein [19,20].

Cytokines

Cytokines are employed therapeutically mainly because of their ability to modulate the immune system. The modulation could be "stimulating" to treat an infection, or "inhibitory" to treat autoimmune diseases in which the patient's own immune system is inappropriately attacking their body. Examples include human interferon alpha, used to treat hepatitis B and C (viral infections); human interferon beta, used to treat multiple sclerosis (an autoimmune disease); and modified interleukin-II to treat thrombocytopenia (another autoimmune disease). In terms of target identification and validation, when a disease course is known to be driven by the activity of the immune system, the therapeutic goal is to pair a known modifier of the immune system activity with the disease of interest, which is almost always determined via animal model testing [19,20].

Vaccines

Humans have two immune systems—innate immunity and adaptive immunity. The innate immune system defends the host from infections by pathogens in a nonspecific manner. This innate system recognizes pathogens in a generic way, sensing biochemical features of the pathogen that differ from the host. This immune system responds by producing generally toxic substances and as a result will harm the host as well as the pathogen. The innate system is ancient and ubiquitous and appears across the biosphere in plants and insects as well as in animals. The toxic effect of the innate system response is particularly easy to see in plants, where it is common to see an entire limb of a fungus-infected plant wither and die. The innate system sacrifices the limb to save the plant. This evolutionarily ancient defense strategy is the only immune system found in most organisms including plants, fungi, insects, primitive multicellular organisms, and some vertebrate animals. A second system, called adaptive immunity, is believed to have first appeared in jawed vertebrates (vertebrate species without a jaw such as the lamprey eel). Adaptive immunity provides jawed vertebrates with the ability to specifically recognize and remember each pathogen, generating a selective antibody response to a pathogen that can be rapidly mounted later in time if the pathogen is encountered again. The system is adaptive because although the organism is naïve to the first attack and responds slowly and weakly, a rapid robust response will be mounted to subsequent attacks by the same pathogen. Moreover, because the response is selective, collateral damage to the host is minimized. Vaccination is basically a method to prime the adaptive immune system to prepare it for attack by a pathogen that had never previously been encountered.

The traditional vaccine strategy is to prepare a pathogen in an inactivated form, one that is unable to produce the disease, and to then introduce the inactivated pathogen into the patient. Inactivation can be produced via chemical treatment (the Salk polio vaccine is a classic example) or via the isolation of a mutant form of the pathogen that has attenuated virulence (the Sabin live polio vaccine is a good example of an attenuated vaccine). However, with the advent of gene cloning, it has been possible to produce protein subunit vaccines. Subunit vaccines are made by producing viral pathogen surface proteins via recombinant DNA techniques and then utilizing the resulting proteins as a vaccine. An example of a protein subunit vaccine is the Hepatitis B virus in which viral surface proteins are produced by recombinant methods in yeast and then employed to formulate the vaccine protein [19,20].

Therapeutic Antibodies

Antibodies are the primary effector agents of the adaptive immune system. The adaptive immune system is activated by a pathogen and, after a lag, begins to make new antibodies directed against the structural proteins from which the pathogen is constructed. These antibodies physically bind to the pathogen. Antibodies are also very selective. They will bind to the proteins of a specific pathogen and commonly, not to a closely related pathogen. Importantly, antibodies normally do not bind to proteins which are part of the host's own cells. Once bound, the antibodies direct destructive components of the immune system to eliminate the pathogen, and once the disease resolves, memory cells are retained within the immune system to rapidly make this group of antibodies if, and when, the same pathogen strikes again. This is the underlying mechanism by which vaccines work.

The immune system has extremely broad capabilities. It is estimated that humans are capable of generating about 10 billion different antibodies, each able to bind to a distinct feature of a foreign protein. Thousands of new antibodies are produced when a pathogen infects an organism. This made it impossible to purify a specific antibody from this mixture for close study and, as a result, only the most general antibody characteristics were known. Prior to 1975, the only system through which large quantities of pure antibody could be obtained was from a rare cancer called multiple myeloma. In multiple myeloma a single antibody-producing cell becomes cancerous and proliferates in the bone marrow. As the cancer grows, it secretes huge quantities of the single specific antibody made by the cell. In many cases, so many antibodies are produced that they spill out into the urine of the patient. In the mid-19th century, urine-secreted proteins in this disease were called Bence-Jones proteins by physicians who were not yet aware of the nature of the spilled material. As a result, the entire field had to depend on these rare freaks of nature for their investigations. Most limiting was the fact that since multiple myeloma cancers occur at random, there is no way to know what the antibody produced in the disease binds to. As a result, if one has the key but not the lock into which it fits: not a good situation through which to figure out how antibodies work or, for that matter, to turn them into therapeutics. This situation dramatically changed in the late 20th century through the work of Georges Köhler and César Milstein. Milstein developed a technique called the monoclonal antibody method through which pure individual antibodies directed against any protein of interest could be produced in quantity and studied in detail. Köhler and Milstein were awarded the Nobel Prize for Physiology or Medicine in 1984 for this work [21].

Scientists began to think about therapeutic applications for antibodies once it became technically possible to produce quantities of specific antibodies with a desired set of selected characteristics. Like any new idea, this concept was initially met with some negativity within the industry. Since antibodies are proteins, they would thus have to be administered via injection and possibly multiple times a day, a distinct disadvantage relative to traditional small molecule orally active drugs. Second, antibodies are extremely costly to produce when compared with traditional small molecule drugs, potentially reducing profits. Third, manufacturing plants that produce therapeutic proteins are expensive to build and thus require substantial capital investment, another discouraging feature of the approach.

However, with time, the industry began to appreciate the positive features of therapeutic antibodies. Antibodies are hard to make, but they are also hard to copy, discouraging generic manufacturers from taking the market after patent expiration. It could also be possible to enter therapeutic areas where no pharmaceutical options existed and thus where no competing oral alternative was available. Lastly, antibodies can be very long lived in the body. For example, antibodies of the IgG class have in vivo half-lives in the 7–23-day range and thus while antibody dosing is via injection, the injections can be infrequent, on the order of once a week, making the medicine more convenient and desirable to the patient.

With protein hormones and cytokines, the objective is to replace or augment a naturally occurring protein. In contrast, antibodies are developed to inhibit and diminish the activity of a naturally occurring protein. While it can be clear when an important protein is missing and needs to be replaced, for example, in the case of insulin, determining the therapeutic value of inhibiting a protein is much less straightforward. In a sense, this type of target identification closely resembles the target identification for small molecule drugs. As for small molecules, a candidate target is identified based on the scientific literature. The target is validated in cell culture and animals through the use of gene knockout methodology or some preliminarily generated antibodies. If the idea proves out, work commences to identify the clinical candidate antibody [22].

The first therapeutic monoclonal antibody product, muromonab-CD3 (Orthoclone OKT3), was commercialized in 1986 [Liu, Ann Med Surg, 3, 113 (2014)]. This class of biopharmaceutical products has grown significantly since that time. A recent review reported that by the end of 2015, 47 monoclonal antibody products had been approved in the United States or Europe for the treatment of a variety of diseases [Ecker et al., mAbs, 7, 9 (2015)]. The current approval rate is approximately 4 new monoclonal antibody products per year, which predicts that more than 70 monoclonal antibody products will be on the market by 2020 with predicted combined worldwide sales of nearly $125 billion [Ecker et al., mAbs, 7, 9 (2015)].

As more and more monoclonal antibody drugs reach regulatory approval, we now have examples of small molecule and monoclonal antibody drugs acting on the same process and for the same indication. Statin pharmaceuticals, HMG-CoA reductase inhibitors, are the standard of care for hyperlipidemia (high-serum cholesterol levels) [18]. These drugs are generally safe and highly effective oral medications, so there would seem to be little incentive to develop monoclonal antibody therapeutics to treat this condition.

However, a new clinically valuable class of hyperlipidemia treating monoclonal antibody drugs has recently achieved regulatory approval [Latimer et al., J Thromb Thrombolysis, 42, 405 (2016); Reiss et al., Clin Sci, 132, 1135 (2018)]. These drugs inhibit proprotein convertase subtilisin/kexin type 9 (PCSK9), a regulatory protein that decreases the number of LDL (low density lipoprotein) receptors on the plasma membrane. The inhibition of PCSK9 increases the number of plasma membrane LDL receptors and thus reduces plasma LDL levels.

The two clinically approved PSCK9 inhibitors, alirocumab and evolocumab, provide an important new strategy for the control of hypercholesterolemia. While there are drawbacks to PSCK9 inhibitor treatment including administration by subcutaneous injection, adverse events, and high cost, alirocumab and evolocumab provide an important therapeutic alternative for certain patient populations.

These drugs are valuable in patients who cannot tolerate statin drugs and they appear to work synergistically with statins in lowering LDL levels and thus are valuable for patients who cannot achieve desired serum cholesterol levels with statin therapy alone. PCSK9 inhibitors are of particularly great value in certain familial hypercholesterolemia where statin therapy alone has been shown to be inadequate.

Structure Optimization and Identification of a Clinical Candidate

Structure optimization follows two distinct courses for large molecule drugs. In the case of hormones and cytokines, where the goal is to replace or augment a naturally occurring protein, the objective is to precisely mimic and administer the natural protein, therefore no optimization is required. In contrast, therapeutic antibody development strategically resembles small molecule discovery in that a number of desired features must be built into the clinical candidate antibody. The first goal is to find an antibody that binds the target with high efficacy and selectivity. This starting antibody will commonly be a mouse antibody as a consequence of the monoclonal antibody technology employed to identify the antibody of interest. One cannot develop treatments based on mouse antibodies because the patient will recognize the mouse antibody as a foreign protein and mount an immunological attack against it. This problem is overcome by "humanizing" the antibody, basically converting the mouse antibody into the human equivalent. More recently, methods have been developed that make it possible to start with a human rather than a mouse antibody. The next step is to consider the efficacy of the antibody—its ability to block the target. Binding to the target is determined by the Fab (fragment, antigen-binding) region of the antibody—the portion that binds to the antigen. In some cases, however, the efficacy is determined by the Fc region (fragment, constant; the nonbinding portion) of the antibody and variants of this region are made and tested to optimize efficacy. Lastly, the half-life of the antibody will determine how frequently it needs to be administered, and structural variants are made and tested to optimize the half-life and thus optimize the dosing schedule.

Similar to small molecule drugs, making a change in an antibody that beneficially changes one characteristic can concomitantly affect other features negatively. Thus the final clinical candidate molecule can end up being a compromise of the desired target features. Lastly, antibodies are made in cells, not factories. Thus a major consideration in selecting the clinical candidate is the development of a cellular production system that can be employed to make the antibody in an economically viable process for eventual commercialization.

Clinical Transition Studies—Investigational New Drug Approval

The goal of clinical transition studies is to demonstrate the safety of the drug before it is first dosed in humans. From this step forward, every experiment and study that is carried out will be reviewed by regulatory authorities (in the United States, by the FDA). The review of drugs by the FDA is a relatively recent development. The law regulating the safety of new drugs, the Food, Drug and Cosmetic Act of 1938, established the functioning of the FDA as we now know it. Most of the countries have their own regulatory agency that reviews and approves human therapeutics, and many of their requirements for approval are similar.

The FDA currently has over 9000 employees and an annual budget of over $1.25 billion. The FDA Center for Drug Evaluation and Research (CDER) oversees the research, development, manufacture, and marketing of synthetic small molecule drugs. Since 2003, the CDER has also been responsible for the regulation of biologic therapeutic products. CDER's involvement starts with the Phase 1 clinical study via their approval of a manufacturer's Investigational New Drug Application (IND). The IND application consists of the results from a highly defined set of studies designed to demonstrate the safety of new pharmaceutical agents and the consistency of the manufacturing process through which they will be produced. The core set of experiments conducted to support the submission of an IND dossier is commonly called the clinical transition studies.

A battery of specific studies is required to be included in the IND application. Although all scientists are trained to carry out experiments in a carefully designed and executed fashion and to record their observations with high precision, studies intended for submission to a regulatory agency are in addition subject to a system of management controls called Good Laboratory Practice (GLP). GLP was instituted as a standard meant to ensure the quality, integrity, and reliability of safety data following cases of safety and efficacy testing fraud by pharmaceutical and industrial manufacturers. Good Manufacturing Practice (GMP) is a similar parallel system for studies of manufacturing processes and analytical testing of active ingredients.

Regulatory authorities have established a set of requirements that drugs need to meet prior to entering clinical use but have avoided providing a defined checklist of experiments, instead of issuing general guidance notes for the required studies. Despite this, the required studies can easily be described via a checklist (e.g., see next) [19,20].

Acute toxicity—The drug is administered to a laboratory animal, usually a rodent, in increasing doses and the animal is observed for toxic effects following each dose. The dose range is large; from very low doses to the highest well-tolerated level called the "no toxic effect level" and beyond to higher doses that produce obvious toxicity. At the end of the experiment the animals are sacrificed and autopsied to search for any effects the drug may have had on the internal organs.

Test for QT interval prolongation—It is well known that some pharmaceutical targets (human biochemical or metabolic functions) can be very difficult to inhibit while others are easier to inhibit, and some targets are so susceptible that they are sometimes unintentionally inhibited by drugs designed to act elsewhere. One of these easy-to-hit targets is the cardiac hERG channel, an ion channel involved in regulating the rhythmic action of the heart. Inhibition of the hERG channel causes prolongation of QT interval in the heart rhythm which can lead to a potentially fatal heart arrhythmia called Torsades de pointes. Drugs from many different therapeutic classes, including several tricyclic antidepressants, antipsychotic drugs (thioridazine and droperidol), antihistamines (astemizole and terfenadine), and certain antimalarial drugs (halofantrine), will inhibit the hERG channel. hERG channel inhibition, therefore, needs to be measured by what is by now standard in vitro testing prior to the initiation of clinical trials [23].

Genotoxicity—Cancer is caused by gene mutations which can either be inherited or produced during the course of life by exposure to certain viruses, radiation, or mutagenic chemicals. It is, therefore, crucial to avoid producing drugs that have any mutagenic activity, as such drugs could be carcinogenic. Bruce Ames, one of the scientists responsible for our current understanding of the mutagenic nature of carcinogenesis, developed a straightforward bacterial-based test, named the Ames Test in his honor, to detect mutagenic activity and thus carcinogenic potential in a chemical compound. The FDA requires Ames testing as part of the IND application as well as related tests based on rodent cells for chromosomal abnormalities and chromosomal damage [24].

Chronic toxicology—The acute toxicity study described earlier looks for immediate damage produced by a drug. There are also concerns that toxicity can occur, even with low doses of a drug, when the drug is dosed repeatedly over time. This concern is addressed by chronic toxicology studies. Three or more drug doses are administered over a period of time: a dose known to be toxic from the acute toxicity study, a therapeutic dose, and an intermediary dose. This test is carried out using two species: a rodent, usually rats, and a nonrodent, usually dogs, although monkeys and pigs are used in certain circumstances. The duration of the chronic toxicity trial must match the intended clinical use. A 2-week trial is adequate for a compound like an antibiotic that will only be given for a few days. Studies of 6 months or more in duration are required for drugs that will be given chronically, such as high blood pressure medications. Such studies can obviously be extraordinarily expensive because they are conducted over a long period of time, require a large number of animals (100 rats and 20 dogs would be typical for a long-term study), plus the chronic dosing consumes large amounts of drug test article which must be prepared in a costly fashion to meet the FDA standards.

Costs are high to manufacture drug substance used in studies for an FDA submission because they must be prepared under the GMP guidelines. The synthetic process must be clearly defined and described in detail and followed precisely from batch to batch. Analytical procedures must be developed and validated to ensure quality control of the manufactured drug. The purity of the test article must be determined and any impurities present must be defined, characterized, and consistent from batch to batch. Moreover, drugs are not just given straight up but are dosed in a formulation that optimizes the delivery of the drug. The formulation must be optimized and defined at this point and remain set for all further studies. Studies for the IND regulatory submission are carried out in specialized GLP/GMP laboratories operated with close regulatory oversight.

While the cost for a minimal clinical transition study could be as low as $1–2 million, it would be prudent to budget at least $5 million for a clinical transition study on a specific compound. Costs can be significantly higher if long-term chronic studies are needed or if tests need to be modified and repeated. Historically, the success rate for projects going through clinical transition is about 55%. It is clearly very hard to design a drug that is both effective and extremely safe (see Fig. 24.4).

Clinical Trials

Phase 1

Clinical investigations of a new drug candidate start with a group of studies commonly called Phase 1 testing. A series of ethical considerations is involved in the design of all clinical studies since human subjects could potentially be put at risk:

1. ***Social value***—The contemplated study should bring value to society, for example, by improving human health or advancing scientific knowledge.
2. ***Scientific validity***—The clinical trial should be conducted in a scientifically rigorous way and with clear objectives so that the resulting data can be interpreted in a meaningful fashion.
3. ***Fair subject selection***—The subjects for the trial should be selected purely based on scientific criteria and not because they are privileged or vulnerable.
4. ***Informed consent***—The subjects should be well informed about the trial and consent to participate without coercion.
5. ***Favorable risk/benefit ratio***—The risk/benefit ratio for the trial should be analyzed and must be favorable for the study to be conducted.
6. ***Independent review***—An independent, disinterested group of qualified individuals must review the proposed trial to identify any possible conflict of interest issues.
7. ***Respect for human subjects***—As the trial goes on, subjects must be informed without prejudice of any new developments, negative or positive, and any resulting decisions made by the subjects must be honored.

Phase 1 trials involve healthy volunteers, not patients, with the primary aim to assess the safety of the new drug and these volunteers are financially compensated for their participation in a manner consistent with the abovementioned ethical considerations. The Phase 1 study will also produce data on the pharmacokinetics of the drug (absorption, distribution, metabolism, and elimination) and its pharmacodynamic properties (biochemical and physiological effects on the body). These studies are conducted under what is called an "open label" format—everyone is aware of what drugs and doses are being given. There are commonly two components to the Phase 1 trial. First, a rising dose study in which increasingly higher doses of the drug are administered to determine how much drug can be given without producing deleterious effects. This is followed by a multidose study in which one or more selected doses is administered repeatedly over time to determine the long-term effects of the drug. Such studies commonly involve 20–80 subjects and take about 6 months to complete. The cost for such a study is $3 million or more with an overall historical success rate of 70% (see Fig. 24.5).

This high success rate of Phase 1 studies is a tribute to the effectiveness of clinical transition testing in demonstrating the safety of a drug which is then, in the majority

Drug-development phases and metrics

	Phase 1	Phase 2	Phase 3	Registration
	1a/1b	2a/2b		
Activity	First in man, safety, tolerability, PK	Dose range, safety/efficacy profile, proof-of-concept	Large safety efficacy trial	
Size	20–80 subjects	300 patients	1000–3000 patients	
Duration	6 months	12–24 months	24–48 months	
Success rate	70%	50%	65%	95%
Cost	$8000/subject	$10,000/patient	$6,000/patient	

FIGURE 24.5 Summary of drug development phases with associated costs, durations, and historical success rates. See text for additional details and references.

of cases, confirmed in human testing. Even when safety is not confirmed, there is little chance for harm because of the slow and cautious design of the initial human tests. However, like anything in life, mistakes do occur: *Errare humanum est*—to err is human. TGN1412 was a therapeutic antibody-type drug developed by TeGenero Immuno Therapeutics as a potential treatment for B-cell chronic lymphocytic leukemia and rheumatoid arthritis. Phase 1 clinical studies of TGN1412 were initiated in March 2006, conducted by Parexel, an independent clinical trials unit at Northwick Park and St. Mark's Hospital in London. Six volunteers were treated with the drug at a dose of 0.1 mg/ kg, 500 times lower than the dose shown to be safe in animals. All six subjects became extremely ill shortly after the treatment and were hospitalized, with at least four of the men suffering from multiple organ dysfunctions. All of the men were reported to have experienced cytokine-release syndrome resulting in angioedema, a rapid swelling of the skin and underlying tissue. Treating physicians said that the men had suffered from a cytokine storm and that the men's white blood cells had almost completely vanished. It has been suggested that the men may never recover fully and suffer long-term disruption to their immune systems [25].

The reason why TGN1412 was safe in animals and yet highly toxic in humans may never be determined. In a preliminary report the Medicines and Healthcare Products Regulatory Agency (MHRA), the group that oversees clinical trials in the United Kingdom, found no deficiencies in TeGenero's preclinical work, no failure of disclosure, record keeping, or processes and stated that TeGenero's actions did not contribute to the serious adverse events. TeGenero Immuno Therapeutics has, however, entered into insolvency as a result of these events.

Phase 2

The aim of Phase 2 clinical trial is to test the safety and, in a preliminary fashion, the effectiveness of a therapeutic candidate compound in patients with the targeted disease. Phase 2 design most commonly includes a control group that is not given the drug and instead receives a placebo. In many illnesses, especially those in which the measurement of disease severity is difficult to quantify, the placebo can show substantial effects. For example, it is clear from many trials in clinical depression that simply entering into a trial and being repeatedly seen and counseled by a physician will produce significant therapeutic effects. These effects must be subtracted out to determine whether the test drug shows efficacy in its own right. Patients are carefully randomized into the control and drug groups to ensure that average disease severity is the same in the two groups. If, for example, healthier patients were mistakenly placed in the drug group, the study might lead to the false conclusion that an inactive drug was effective. A related common practice is to blind the trial, that is not to inform patients as to whether they are receiving the drug or placebo. In many cases the physician may also not be informed as to whether the test agent or placebo is being administered. This design is called a double-blinded trial. Data from the Phase 2 trial are used to select a dose regimen (amount, frequency, and duration) for expanded, and hopefully conclusive, studies in a larger group of patients in Phase 3.

Because Phase 2 trials have dual and sequential goals, they are commonly divided into two subtrials: Phases 2a and 2b. Phase 2a concentrates on safety and dosing while Phase 2b is an extension of 2a with an increased focus on efficacy. The number of patients in a Phase 2 study can range from 50 to 500 and 1 to 2 years or more depending on the study design. A cost in the $3–4 million range would be typical for an academically led study, with industrial studies typically costing much, much more. The historical success rate for Phase 2 studies has been on the order of 50% (see Fig. 24.5).

Phase 3

The goal of the Phase 3 trial is to unambiguously show whether or not a new compound is effective in treating the target disease. These trials are termed pivotal in the industry because they will make or break the success of the drug. The design of the Phase 3 trial combines scientific and financial considerations. If a drug is highly effective, only a relatively small number of patients may be needed to show a statistically significant positive effect. For example, if every patient who does not take the drug quickly dies and every patient taking the drug survives, you do not have to be a professional statistician to conclude that only a small number of patients will be needed to produce a convincing data set. However, a larger number of patients will be needed if the effect of the drug is small. For example, patients with amyotrophic lateral sclerosis (ALS or Lou Gehrig's disease) typically live 3–5 years postdiagnosis. Riluzole (Rilutek), the only drug clinically approved for the treatment of ALS, extends life on average by 2–3 months. The Phase 3 study to register riluzole included more than 1200 patients who were treated for almost 2 years, a study size which was needed to convincingly demonstrate in a statistically significant fashion that the drug produced this small positive effect [26].

While from a scientific perspective, it is critical to ensure that the Phase 3 study is adequately powered, financial considerations will influence the design of the trial toward the minimum size that effectively meets the desired goal. A consideration that is intimately tied to statistical power is how drug effectiveness will be determined, commonly called "outcome measures." As in Phase 2 trials, this is especially important in cases where there is subjectivity in assessing effectiveness. For example, in neuropsychiatric diseases, effectiveness is determined by the patient's verbal disclosure of his or her symptoms and the simple act of including a patient in a trial can be therapeutic. A clinical effect that can be measured with a simple blood test, such as cholesterol level, will obviously produce clearer and less subjective results. Variation in patient response to a drug is another confounding issue that impacts the power of a clinical trial. Even well-established FDA-approved drugs can vary in their effectiveness in different patients. In extreme cases, 70% of the patients will not respond to a drug that is highly efficacious in 30% of the patients. Since patient response cannot be predicted ahead of time (although new personalized medicine studies are attempting to address this), the size of the Phase 3 trial may have to be increased to provide statistically significant results in a patient population that includes large numbers of nonresponders.

The Pfizer drug torcetrapib is an excellent example of the intersection of science and finance in clinical trials [27]. Torcetrapib inhibits the enzyme cholesteryl ester transfer protein (CETP). Inhibition of CETP would be expected to raise levels of the so-called good high-density lipoprotein (HDL) cholesterol, which would make torcetrapib a highly desirable therapeutic agent for lowering the risk of cardiovascular disease. In 2004 Pfizer initiated its Phase 3 ILLUMINATE trial to demonstrate the clinical efficacy of torcetrapib. However, in December 2006, and after investing $800 million, Pfizer learned that torcetrapib actually *raised* the risk of death and cardiovascular disease and, therefore, the development of torcetrapib was halted. What happened?

Early-stage clinical trials of torcetrapib showed that the drug elevated blood pressure in treated patients. Pfizer experts said that a modest effect on raising blood pressure would be of minor importance relative to the HDL-stimulating effect of the drug and argued that costly Phase 3 trials should be initiated. The Pfizer commercial group also contributed to the decision-making process as Pfizer was anticipating the expiration of the atorvastatin (Lipitor) patent in 2011 with the concomitant loss of greater than $10 billion per year in revenue. Torcetrapib seemed to be just what the doctor, in this case the accountant, ordered with a prediction of $10 billion in good year sales. It was estimated that the FDA approval could be in hand by 2011 if the Phase 3 trial was started in 2004. We can now see the process was rushed for commercial reasons. Roche is now developing its own CETP inhibitor dalcetrapib and Merck has a similar compound called anacetrapib. Neither dalcetrapib nor anacetrapib raise blood pressure showing that torcetrapib's hypertensive activity was neither a class nor mechanistic effect of inhibiting CETP. Roche initiated a 15,600-patient trial with their compound in 2008 and Merck a 30,000-patient trial in 2011. It turns out that torcetrapib, but neither of the other two drugs, increases aldosterone levels, leading to elevated blood pressure. (Increasing aldosterone is definitely not a good thing; in fact, drugs such as spironolactone were developed to act as aldosterone-antagonist diuretics for use in the treatment of hypertension.) With the wisdom of hindsight, Pfizer should have invested more time up front to synthesize a torcetrapib analog lacking hypertensive activity. This course might have been taken in the absence of commercial pressures on the project; but commercial pressures are a fundamental reality in the pharmaceutical industry.

Everyone, myself, the editor of this monograph, and astute readers of the first edition, was expecting to read in this second edition of *Biotechnology Entrepreneurship* how dalcetrapib and/or anacetrapib produced positive clinical trial data and were approved and helping patients in the clinic. But drug discovery does not work that way. The target of these drugs, CETP, was identified based on human genetics [Inazu et al., N Engl J Med, 323, 1234 (1990)]. Humans who carry a genetic deficiency for CETP show markedly elevated levels of HDL cholesterol. It seemed almost certain that drugs that lowered CETP levels would do the exact same thing.

In 2012, investigators studying dalcetrapib in an almost 16,000 patients clinical trial reported that the compound was inactive and terminated the study early on the basis of futility [Schwartz et al., N Engl J Med, 367, (2012)]. The Merck drug, anacetrapib, had only a slightly better outcome. The trial with this drug, including over 30,000 patients, went to completion and was shown to reduce major coronary events [The HPS3/TIMI55−REVEAL Collaborative Group, N Engl J Med, 377, 1217 (2017)]. But Merck ultimately decided not to seek marketing approval for anacetrapib, apparently based on a combination of its disappointingly relatively modest clinical performance, pharmaco-distribution profile, and marketing considerations [Tall, Atherosclerosis, 267, 39 (2018)].

Thus even in the absence of commercial pressure, things can go terribly wrong. A lesson here is that target validation is not an exact science and even the most convincing target validation evidence with a highly selective and potent drug does not assure a successful drug launch.

In general, and including issues such as trial design, defining outcome measures, identifying performance sites, and recruiting patients, Phase 3 trials can be 3−5 years in duration and cost $50−100 million or more. Historically, approximately 65% of Phase 3 trials have been successful (see Fig. 24.5). A new drug application (NDA) is submitted to the FDA following the successful completion of the Phase 3 trial.

New Drug Application Approval and Postlaunch Surveillance

In recent years the FDA has approved 15−20 drugs annually. This is a significant decline from the late 1990s when typically 30 new drugs were approved each year. This decline has occurred despite dramatic increases in research and development spending during this period. A recent paper proposed "Eroom's Law" (Moore's law spelled backwards), which states that the number of new drugs approved per billion US dollars spent on R&D is halved roughly every 9 years, falling around 80-fold in inflation-adjusted terms since 1950 [28]. The reason(s) for the decline in research productivity is not known with certainty but obviously raises great concern regarding the long-term prospects for the pharmaceutical industry. Fortunately, once a drug achieves statistically significant efficacy in treating a disease, the FDA will approve the drug for sale approximately 95% of the time.

Following the NDA approval, the drug goes on sale and will then be used for the first time to treat extremely large numbers of patients. The manufacturer is required to collect safety data on the product while it is on the market and to periodically analyze these data to look for any indication of a safety issue that was not revealed in the Phase 3 trial. It is estimated that up to 20% of new drugs will be recalled from the market as a result of safety issues only identified after the drug is used to treat very large numbers of patients.

A classic example of such a recall is terfenadine, marketed by Hoechst Marion Roussel (now Aventis) under the trade name Seldane as the first nonsedating antihistamine. Terfenadine was approved for marketing in the United States in 1985. By 1990 it had been prescribed for over 100 million patients worldwide and it was becoming clear that terfenadine was causing cardiac toxicity in some patients as the result of hERG inhibition. While terfenadine is not overtly hERG inhibiting at therapeutic doses, the drug will accumulate to high toxic levels if dosed in combination with other drugs such as erythromycin and ketoconazole, drugs that inhibit the cytochrome P450 enzyme CYP3A4 that metabolizes terfenadine. Even more concerning and more difficult to control, one of the ingredients of grapefruit juice also inhibits the same enzyme. In June 1990 the FDA issued a risk report on terfenadine and 2 months later required the manufacturer to send a letter to all physicians alerting them to the problem. A black box warning describing the problem was added to the package inserted in July 1992. (A black box warning indicates that medical studies have shown that the drug carries a significant risk of serious or even life-threatening adverse effects and is the strongest caution that is issued by the FDA.) Terfenadine was removed from the US market by the manufacturer in late 1997 [29].

Areas of Uncertainty

It is difficult to think of any first-in-class pharmaceutical that was discovered using exactly the path described earlier. Moreover, no two first-in-class compounds have been discovered in exactly the same way. The process described earlier is an amalgam of good practices, but each discovery is unique, with each drug campaign diverging from the previous path in various ways. Ivermectin (Mectizan) was discovered using an animal-disease model primary screen of a group of fewer than 100 test samples, and the initial screening active compound possessed almost ideal ADME properties [30].

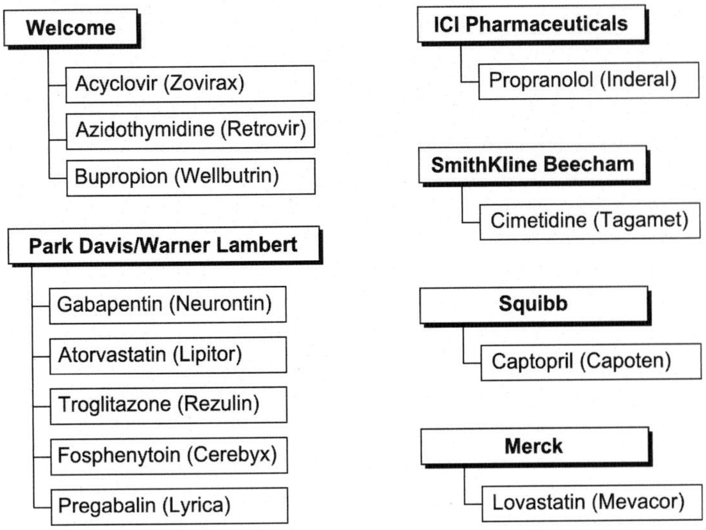

FIGURE 24.6 Drugs almost canceled during development.

Initial clinical testing of imipramine was in schizophrenic patients. When the drug failed, it was empirically dosed in patients suffering from major depression where it showed activity [31]. Lovastatin (Mevacor) was identified following the screening of only a few hundred samples [32]. Only 60 analogs were made in chemical optimization of captopril (Capoten) [33]. The lead upon which the antibiotic aztreonam (Azactam) was based on was virtually devoid of antibacterial activity [34]. Ezetimibe (Zetia) came from a research program to identify cholesterol-lowering acetyl-coenzyme A acetyltransferase (ACAT) inhibitors. Ezetimibe, however, lacks ACAT inhibitory activity and instead inhibits the NPC1L1 cholesterol transporter [35]. Sildenafil (Viagra) was developed to treat hypertension and then angina. The drug came to be used as a treatment for erectile dysfunction only because of side effects that were noted during a failed angina clinical trial [36].

Second, there is rarely, if ever, organizational consensus regarding the future clinical value of a therapeutic under development. It is never clear that a drug will truly be beneficial until the very end of the development process or perhaps even until the drug is introduced into clinical use. Fig. 24.6 provides a list of highly successful compounds that were almost canceled during the development process. The list contains many now-recognized blockbuster drugs including cimetidine (Tagamet), the first billion dollar a year selling a blockbuster drug, and atorvastatin (Lipitor), the best-selling drug of all time with annual sales of over $14 billion per year [37].

The Human Dimension

Alignment of the commercial and R&D sides of any biopharmaceutical company is essential for success. Yet in the pharmaceutical businesses, conflicts between science and business occur commonly and at a pretty fundamental level. Let us imagine two biopharma companies.

NewBio develops a new drug. They are fortunate to find investors to fund the development of the drug through Phase 3 clinical trials and the FDA approves the drug for marketing. However, the patient population receiving the drug is small and payer issues limit reimbursement. Although the drug provides significant clinical value to patients, earnings are limited and ultimately they never repay the R&D costs to discover and develop the drug.

NewPharma also develops a new drug. Their drug shows very positive results in its Phase 2 trial and the drug is then purchased by a large pharmaceutical company for a high upfront payment, greatly more than the costs incurred by NewPharma to bring it through Phase 2. The large pharmaceutical company then takes the drug through Phase 3 trials where it unfortunately does not reach significance in achieving the desired outcome measures. As a result the large pharmaceutical company drops the project.

The scientists at NewBio are pleased that their project was a success while the scientists at NewPharma are disappointed by their failure. On the other side, the business people at NewBio feel that they failed while the business people at NewPharma are delighted by their success. With such a profound disagreement regarding the definition of success and failure, it should be of little surprise that this fundamental difference in perspective leads to conflict between the technical and commercial groups within biopharmaceutical industry. And pressures from each side of the organization can bring the other side into the undesired territory.

One not uncommon source of technical success and financial failure comes from decisions by business management to reject the commercialization of technically successful projects. However, such stories are difficult to access. No one writes up insightful summaries of abandoned projects. And institutional knowledge of such projects is easily lost due to mergers and acquisitions. Yet, every pharmaceutical industry scientist with more than a couple of years of experience knows of promising projects that were discarded by the commercial group despite the enthusiastic support of the scientific team. {See above Fig. 24.6 - About 10 years ago, Pedro Cuatrecasas compiled a list of highly successful drugs whose development had been almost halted by commercial management [37].

Given the enormous cost of drug discovery and development, it's fairly intuitive that many drugs, including some marketed drugs, will not be able to repay their R&D costs [38]. But how could you achieve financial success together with technical failure? How would it be possible to make money from a product that does not work?

Stories of technical failure and financial success, if not common, have been written up in business journals. Sirtris Pharmaceuticals is a good example [39]. Sirtris was founded in August 2004 and funded with $102.9 million in venture investment over five stages. In 2007 less than 3 years after its founding, Sirtis had a successful initial public offering (IPO) and a market capitalization of $278 million. And in 2008 slightly less than 1 year after the IPO, Sirtris was purchased by Glaxo SmithKline for $720 million [40].

But then only 5 years later, Glaxo SmithKline shut down Sirtris [41] and although some Sirtris-based R&D was moved in the house, it now appears that Sirtris science has yielded no new therapy.

So finally, how do you achieve the ideal: technical success along with financial success? About 10 years ago, I had a meeting with Ed Scolnick who at the time was the director of the psychiatric disease program at the Broad Institute's Stanley Center. Prior to joining the Broad Institute, Scolnick had been the head of research at Merck from 1985 until he stepped down in 2002. His productivity as the Merck research leader is legendary. An outstanding series of unique drugs was launched during Scolnick's tenure as the head of Merck R&D, many of which became blockbusters, including Indinavir (Crixivan), alendronate (Fosamax), rizatriptan (Maxalt), lovastatin (Mevacor), finasteride (Proscar/Propecia), montelukast (Singulair), and simvastatin (Zocor).

I had come to meet with Dr. Scolnick to discuss his new drug-discovery program for psychiatric diseases, but we soon digressed into a general discussion of large pharmaceutical R&D. Ed told a story about his relationship with the commercial side of the Merck organization. At one point, he attended a biotechnology conference and appeared on an expert panel discussing the relationship between R&D and marketing. The head of the Merck marketing group was also on the panel.

The moderator asked the panel to discuss the process by which R&D chooses which projects to pursue. Conscious of his need to maintain a good working relationship with the marketing group, Ed told the moderator that he would like to defer this question to his marketing colleague on the panel.

This head of marketing then told the audience "This is how we do it. We tell R&D which products we need to grow the business and they then go out and discover the products we want." As this point, Ed and I both laughed. In fact, whenever I tell this story to drug-discovery scientists, they always laugh.

Drugs aren't engineered products like computer tablets or cell phones or electric cars. Drugs aren't designed. They are discovered, like a new gold mine, and luck plays an enormous role in determining what is discovered. In fact, the marketing head's answer is probably a giant tribute the Ed Scolnick's relationship with his commercial colleagues. He was able to, and comfortable with, making them feel as they did.

Communication is tough. Within their own group, the commercial people speak a language that sounds like Swahili to the scientists while the scientists speak with each other using a language that sounds like Serbo-Croatian to their commercial colleagues. While these groups use English when speaking with each other, this is not the native tongue for either group, so the intergroup communication is rife with inaccuracy and misunderstanding, compounding substantial cultural differences. The best among us work hard at achieving superior intergroup communication.

Conclusion

The abovementioned may seem to be more than a little bit technically daunting. I started my industrial career in 1981. The golden age of antibiotic discovery was 20 years in the past. The ethylamine privileged structure family of drugs (including the antihistamines, neuroleptic antipsychotic drugs, and tricyclic antidepressants) appeared to have been totally mined out as had the benzodiazepine privileged structure tranquilizer drug family. Everyone was saying that all the easy stuff had been done, that all the low hanging fruit had been picked.

At that time, recombinant DNA drugs were a mere hope. The antihypertensive and cholesterol-lowing drugs, which are now all patent expired generics and the mainstay of therapy, had not yet been discovered. Monoclonal antibody therapeutics had not yet been dreamt of. Work on the SSRI antidepressants and proton pump inhibitor gastrointestinal medications was in progress, but these drugs had not yet been proven out. Things looked grim.

So always keep in mind, the challenges of today will be remembered as the good old days, when everything was easy.

Summary

There is no one "correct" way to discover a new drug. Instead, drug developers have a "tool kit" of strategies and methods they can choose from among which, when properly deployed and exploited, will on occasion lead to the discovery of a new medicine. What constitutes a valuable new clinical therapeutic is commonly recognized only in hindsight. Thus there is neither a clear path to drug discovery nor a marker to show that you have gotten there. Not surprisingly, drug discovery is highly inefficient, with less than 2% of project compounds moving from conception to regulatory approval, and frighteningly expensive, with costs of over $1 billion commonly estimated for the discovery of a new drug.

References

[1] Bosch F, Rosich L. Pharmacology 2008;82:171.
[2] Sakula A. Br J Dis Chest 1988;82:23.
[3] Nwaka S, Ridley RG. Nat Rev Drug Discov 2003;2:919.
[4] Federsel H. Nat Rev Drug Discov 2003;2:654.
[5] Tanzi RE, Bertram L. Cellule 2005;120:545.
[6] Gotz J. Brain Res Rev 2001;35:266.
[7] Brown D, Superti-Furgam G. DDT 2003;8:1067.
[8] Drews J. Science 2000;287:1960.
[9] Koppal T. Drug Discov Development 2004;7:24.
[10] Reichert JM. Nat Rev Drug Discov 2003;2:695.
[11] Bohacek RS, McMartin C, Guida WC. Med Res Rev 1996;16:3.
[12] Black JJ. Med Chem 2005;48:1687.
[13] Stanley TH, Egan TD, Van Aken H. Anesth Analg 2008;106:451.
[14] Kerns EH, Di L. Curr Opin Chem Biol 2003;7:402.
[15] Di L, Kerns EH. Curr Top Med Chem 2002;2:87.
[16] Slater JW, Zechnich AD, Haxby DG. Drugs 1999;57:31.
[17] Brown AM. Cell Calcium 2004;35:543.
[18] Brunton LL, Hilal-Dandan R, Björn C, Knollmann BC, editors. Goodman and Gilman's pharmacological basis of therapeutics. 13th ed. McGraw-Hill, 2017
[19] Ng R. Drugs from discovery to approval. 2nd ed. Wiley-Blackwell, 2008
[20] Rang HP, editor. Drug discovery and development—technology in transition. Elsevier, 2006
[21] Nissim A, Chernajovsky Y. Handb Exp Pharmacol, 181. 2008. p. 3.
[22] Reichert JM, Rosebsweug CJ, Faden LB, Dewitz MC. Nat Biotechnol 2005;23:1073.
[23] Hammond TG, Pollard CE. Toxicol Appl Pharmacol 2005;207 (Suppl. 2):446.
[24] McCann J, Ames BN. PNAS Proc Nat Acad Sci 1976;73:950.
[25] Hansel TT, et al. Nat Rev Drug Discov 2010;9:325.
[26] Miller RG, Mitchell JD, Lton M, Moore DH. ALS Other Motor Neuron Dis 2003;4:191.
[27] News and Analysis. Nat Rev Drug Discov 2011;10:163.
[28] Scannell JW, Blackley A, Boldon H, Warrington B. Nat Rev Drug Discov 2012;11:191.
[29] Alfaro CL. Psychopharmacol Bull 2001;35:80.
[30] Omura S, Crump A. Nat Rev Microbiol 2004;2:984.
[31] Fangmann P, Assion H, Juckel G, Gonzalez CA, Lopez-Munoz F. J Clin Psychopharm J Psychopharmacol 2008;28:1.
[32] Vagelos PR. Science 1991;252:1080.
[33] Ondetti MA, Rubin B, Cushman DW. Science 1977;196 (1077):441.
[34] Sykes RB, Bonner DP, Bush K, Georgopapadakou NH, Wells JS. J Antimicrob Chemother 1981;8(Suppl. E):1.
[35] Betters JL, Yu L. Clin Pharmacol Ther 2010;87:117.
[36] Ghofrani HA, Osterloh IH, Grimminger F. Nat Rev Drug Discov 2006;5:689.
[37] Cuatrecasas P. Clin Invest 2006;116:2837.
[38] Garnier. Harvard Business Review May 2008;4.
[39] Stuart T, Kiron D. Harvard Business School case study N9-808-112, March 18, 2008.
[40] Herper M. Why Glaxo Bought Sirtris. https://www.forbes.com/2008/04/23/pharmaceuticals-sirtris-glaxosmithkline-biz-healthcare-cx_mh_0424glaxo.html#5695e7011762, accessed August 8, 2019].
[41] "GSK absorbs controversial 'longevity' company: News blog," http://blogs.nature.com/news/2013/03/gsk-absorbs-controversial-longevity-company.html, accessed August 8, 2018.

Chapter 25

Integrating Diagnostic Products Into the Drug Development Workflow: Applications for Companion Diagnostics*

John F. Beeler, PhD

Translational Medicine, Bristol-Myers Squibb, Cambridge, MA, United States

Chapter Outline

Introduction

The field of clinical diagnostics plays an increasingly important role in today's medical evaluations, clinical decision-making, and disease management (Fig. 25.1). Although accounting for only 2% of overall healthcare spending, clinical diagnostic products can influence 70% of medical decisions, illustrating their dominant role in determining healthcare outcomes ranging from risk assessment to monitoring disease progression [1]. The utility of these diagnostic products to provide actionable information is evident by more than 6.8 billion in vitro diagnostic (IVD) tests performed each year from a menu representing more than 4000 products available for clinical use [2]. Diagnostic applications encompass a broad range of technologies and are utilized in a wide range of facilities, including physician office labs, hospitals, and reference laboratories, comprising a multibillion dollar industry. Together, these diagnostic products contribute to a global diagnostic market valued at approximately $64.48 billion in 2017, which is estimated to reach at $93.61 billion by 2025, registering a compound-adjusted growth rate (CAGR) of 4.8% from 2018 to 2025 [3].

Medical devices encompass the field of in vivo and IVD tests. In vivo diagnostics include imaging tests performed directly on a patient, such as ultrasound scanning, magnetic resonance imaging, and positron emission tomography. In contrast, an IVD test refers to those procedures that process biological samples taken directly from the patient (i.e., salvia, blood, urine, and feces) and are analyzed outside the body to detect and quantify the presence of a specific biological analyte. These biomarkers include pathogens, circulating proteins, and electrolytes, as well as genomic alterations, including gene mutations, chromosomal copy number variations, and messenger RNA transcripts.

IVDs encompass a diverse range of technologies, including clinical chemistry panels, microbiology cultures, immunoassays, and molecular applications, including polymerase chain reaction–based assays and in situ hybridization techniques. IVD products measure a wide range of analytes from the concentration of vital

*The opinions expressed here are those of John Beeler in his personal capacity and not those of Bristol-Myers Squibb.

Biotechnology Entrepreneurship. DOI: https://doi.org/10.1016/B978-0-12-815585-1.00025-5

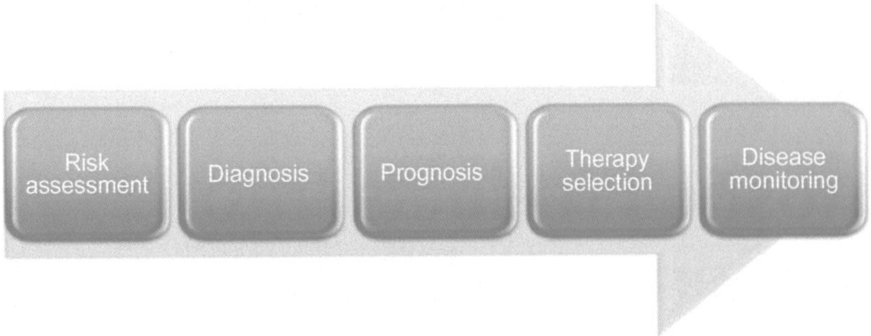

FIGURE 25.1 The application of *in vitro* diagnostic applications across the healthcare spectrum.

electrolytes (i.e., sodium, potassium, magnesium, and calcium) and other vital serum components (glucose, lipids, cholesterol, etc.) to detecting specific biomarkers, such as procalcitonin, prostate-specific antigen (PSA), and troponin as well as specific genetic alterations, such as mutations (BRAF, EGFR, KRAS), amplifications (HER2/neu), translocations (EML4-ALK), and polymorphisms (HLA-B*5701).

The Federal Code of Regulations [21CFR.809.3] defines in vivo diagnostic devices as "those reagents, instruments, and systems intended for use in diagnosis of disease or other conditions, including a determination of the state of health, in order to cure, mitigate, treat, or prevent disease or its sequelae. Such products are intended for use in the collection, preparation, and examination of specimens taken from the human body" [4]. From a regulatory perspective, an IVD product, therefore, refers collectively to the device or kit that is a composite of all the components of the assay, including reagents, ancillary buffers, and software working together on a compatible platform or instrument to deliver a result.

IVDs can be developed either as a distributable product (i.e., kit) or as a laboratory-developed test (LDT). Both offer viable routes to market but have significant differences in how both these products are developed, regulated, and commercialized, each having their own specific advantages and disadvantages (Table 25.1). The differences in their development, regulatory, and commercial characteristics can have a profound impact on development timelines, market adoption, and commercial success. For example, LDTs, also known as "homebrews," are assays developed and validated by individual testing labs for use in that facility only and subject to regulations of the Clinical Laboratory Improvement Act. In contrast, IVD kits are developed under quality system regulations (QSRs) for global distribution and because they are viewed as medical devices are subject to review by regulatory authorities, such as the Food and Drug Administration (FDA).

Regulation of Diagnostic Products

In the United States, the FDA is responsible for administering regulatory oversight, including premarket activities, such as risk classification, review of marketing applications, as well as surveillance of IVD-postmarked performance. Specifically, the Office of in vitro Diagnostics and Radiological Health (OIR) within the Center for Devices and Radiological Health (CDRH) is responsible for administering the federal law pertaining to IVDs and assuring their safe and effective performance. The sponsor of the marketed IVD is required to submit a premarket submission to OIR and receive marketing authorization prior to

TABLE 25.1 Comparison on in vitro diagnostics (IVD) and laboratory-developed tests (LDT).

Requirements	IVDs	LDTs
Marketing authorization	FDA/Section 520 FD&C Act	CMS/CLIA standards
Time to develop	Long (12–24 months)	Short (4–6 months)
Subject to quality systems	Yes	No
• Design controls • Manufacturing controls • Complaint handling		
Establish clinical validation prior to marketing	Yes	No
FDA guidance for use as a companion diagnostic	Yes	No
Global reach/distribution	Yes	No

CLIA, Clinical Laboratory Improvement Act; *CMS*, Centers for Medicare and Medicaid Services; *FD&C*, Federal Food, Drug, and Cosmetic; *FDA*, Food and Drug Administration.

TABLE 25.2 Control guidelines for *in vitro* diagnostics.

General controls	Special controls
• Registering manufacturers and distributers	• Special labeling requirements
• Listing of device with the FDA	• Mandatory performance standards
• Manufacturing the device in accordance with Good Manufacturing Practices	• Postmarket surveillance
• Labeling devices in accordance with labeling regulations in 21 CFR Part 801 or 809	• FDA medical device specific guidance
• Submission of premarket notification [510(k)] prior to marketing device	*Special controls for class III devices*
	• Full report demonstrating the device is safe and effective (i.e., clinical trial)

FDA, Food and Drug Administration.

commercializing the product. To facilitate development of IVD products, CDRH periodically publishes guidance documents to address innovative approaches and the changing diagnostic landscape. Developers of IVDs are encouraged to check the CDRH website for new guidance documents that may provide insights into relevant applications [5].

510(k) Versus Premarket Approval

The FDA considers IVDs as medical devices subject to the premarket controls as defined in the Federal Food, Drug, and Cosmetic (FD&C) Act and contained in the procedural regulations outlined in Title 21 Code of Federal Regulations Part 800−1200 (Table 25.2).

The level of control required to establish safe and effective use of the device is dictated by the FDA's risk-based classification system established for IVD products and categorizes IVD products as Class I, II, or III devices with Class III devices designated as high-risk devices (Fig. 25.2). This classification system outlines the compliance requirements that will guide the development of the IVD product and whether the subsequent regulatory pathway will require a premarket notification [510(k)] or submission of a premarket approval (PMA) application for marketing authorization. The perceived level of risk is a reflection of the intended use of the IVD and there are examples where the FDA has approved assays detecting the same analyte under different regulatory pathways depending on the intended use of the assay. For example, the bioMerieux VIDAS total PSA assay, which is indicated as an aid in the detection of prostate cancer, was approved by the FDA under the PMA pathway due to the perceived high level of risk to the patient for subsequent follow-up and treatment [6]. In contrast, the NADiA ProsVue PSA assay is indicated for use as a prognostic marker in conjunction with clinical evaluation as an aid in identifying those patients at reduced risk for the recurrence of prostate cancer and monitoring the recurrence of prostate cancer [7]. The device is designated as having a lower level of risk to patients due to their already having been treated and therefore received clearance under the 510(k) pathway.

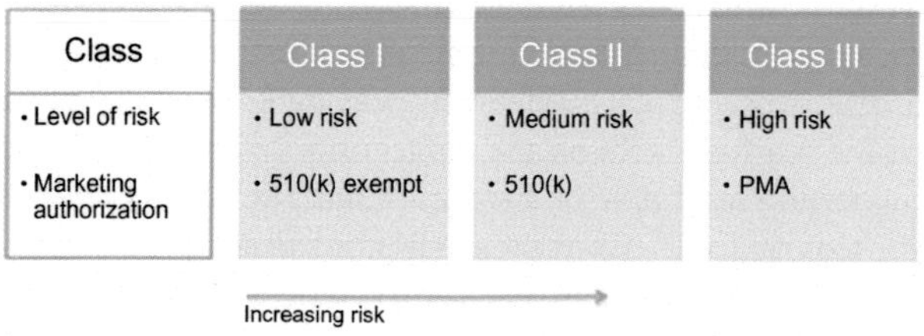

FIGURE 25.2 FDA classification of *in vitro* diagnostic devices.

To facilitate a review of an IVD product, Congress passed the FDA Safety and Improvement Act assigning the FDA with the authority to collect user fees on applications for medical devices that included IVD products. First enacted in 2002, the Medical Device User Fee Act (MDUFA) provides funding to the FDA to support the staff of trained reviewers. The standard rates implemented for 2019 include a user fee of $322,147 for PMA applications and $10,953 for 510(k) notifications [8]. Reduced fees for small businesses are available.

The marketing application process for an IVD is intended to provide sufficient information verifying the product which has been validated to ensure that it is safe and effective for its intended use. In some cases, Class I products with low risk may be exempt from premarket submissions. For IVDs with low to moderate risk, the 510 (k) submission process requires a sponsor to demonstrate that the product is substantially equivalent to a preexisting or predicate device already cleared by the FDA for the same intended use. Establishing substantial equivalence requires the submission of basic data requirements to provide the FDA with a reasonable assurance the product is safe and effective. In addition to demonstrating general controls are in place, the submission of preclinical data on the analytical performance of the assay illustrating accuracy, precision, and limit of detection, linearity, and cross-reactivity is also required. While 510(k) filings do not generally require performing a clinical trial, the need to include clinical data varies on the assay being evaluated and its intended use. If the FDA determines that substantial equivalence has been demonstrated to either a reference method (i.e., gold standard) or a predicate device for the same intended use, the IVD will be cleared for marketing. Other options available to the FDA include requesting additional information or determining the assay is not substantially equivalent (NSE). If the issuance of an NSE is the result of the lack of a predicate device, the sponsor has the option to seek the approval of the device via a de novo 510(k) pathway or by submitting a PMA application. The average time to clear a 510(k) device by the FDA was reported to be approximately 3−6 months with approximately 80% of 510(k)s reviewed determined to be substantially equivalent and cleared for marketing [9].

IVDs designated as high-risk devices (i.e., Class III) are required to submit a PMA application to OIR. These include assays that are used to diagnose a life-threatening disease (i.e., PSA) and assays utilized as companion diagnostics (CDxs) and used to determine a course of treatment (THxID-BRAF). In contrast to a 510(k) application, a PMA filing does not seek to establish substantial equivalence to a preexisting product. While a PMA application will include preclinical data on its analytical performance similar to that included for a 510(k) filing, PMA filings are required to include a more comprehensive demonstration of its safe and effective use. Therefore a sponsor submitting a PMA application is required to demonstrate a clinical validation of the test by performing a clinical trial to generate clinical data illustrating the test that performs according to its intended use, using the designated samples (i.e., blood, tissue, sputum, and urine) from a defined patient population. The testing is required to be performed in a setting representative of where it is intended to be sold (i.e., clinical reference lab and physician lab office). Although prospective studies are encouraged, retrospective analyses of banked samples have been used to support an application's intended use (TheraScreen-KRAS) [10]. In addition to the submission of preclinical and clinical data, PMA applications are also required to include information on design control and manufacturing of the IVD product. Sponsors of PMA applications are subject to inspections prior to approval to assure adherence to QSRs and the implementation of Good Manufacturing Practices to ensure IVDs are safe and effective. A key feature to mitigate regulatory risk is the availability to sponsors to engage feedback from the agency via the pre-investigational device (pre-IDE) meeting. This mechanism allows sponsors to seek advice and clarification from the FDA on such matters pertaining to intended use of the assay, clinical protocol design, validation procedures, and other parameters required for approval. Although not binding on the FDA's part, pre-IDE meetings can provide valuable information and guidance on the FDA's expectations. The FDA has committed to making a determination on a PMA application within 180 days, but typically the process can often take longer. In 2014 the average number of days between filing of a PMA application and the receipt of the MDUFA decision (approval or nonapproval) was 270 [9]. The majority of IVDs reviewed by the FDA are in fact cleared as 510(k) products. In 2017 the FDA cleared 3173 products under the 510(k) process having demonstrated substantial equivalence to existing approved devices [11]. In contrast, only a small percentage (~1%) of device approvals are PMAs. In 2018 a total of 106 novel devices, including original and panel track supplement PMAs, de novos, HDE (Humanitarian Device Exemption), and BreakThrough 510(k)s received FDA approvals [12].

In Europe, market access for a diagnostic product is in a state of transition. The previous IVD Directive 98/79/CE (CE stands for Conformité Européene, or European Conformity) that allowed self-certification of a diagnostic assay to be commercialized is being repealed and replaced with the In Vitro Diagnostic Device Regulation (IVDR) [13]. The IVDR that was approved in May of 2017 will be fully enacted and operational by May 2022. Under the new regulation, significant changes will be implemented compared to the previous directive, including installation of a risk-based classification scheme and new requirements for conformity assessment. The manufacturer of the diagnostic product (either distributable kit or a lab-based service offering) will be required to submit a technical file on the product along with information on their quality-manufacturing (QM) system to a nationally accredited group (i.e., notified body).

The new process requires the preparation of a technical document file (TDF) that includes performance evaluation, clinical evidence, and a postmarketing surveillance plan along with the documentation of having used a QM system. The accredited group will perform an assessment of the TDF prior to granting a conformity mark (CE mark) necessary for sales and distribution to the member states of the European Economic Area (EEA) and the European Free Trade Association. CE marking encompasses 32 member states, including Switzerland and Turkey, which has established mutual recognition agreements with the EEA. It is anticipated that the level of risk a device poses to a patient will determine the involvement of the notified body on the conformity assessment, including requirements for QM systems and premarket review of the technical file. Even preexisting medical devices will be required to go through the certification process as grandfathering of existing assays will not be allowed. Given the uncertainty over what clinical evidence will be sufficient or what will be considered appropriate sample requirements, companies intending to pursue an opportunity in Europe are advised to plan in advance and schedule premeetings with the notified body to review and discuss the intended submission.

The Role of Diagnostics in Delivering on the Promise of Precision Medicine

Technological advances have facilitated the ability to extract information from a patient sample in a rapid and accurate manner and as a result are helping one to transform these diagnostic products into key drivers of a more personalized and cost-efficient healthcare system [14]. An exciting application of devices is their potential to enable the realization of precision medicine, in which healthcare is delivered more efficiently and accurately based on the context of an individual's genetic content or other molecular analysis. This opportunity has captured the attention of the biopharmaceutical industry as employing diagnostic-based approaches across the drug-development process offers the potential to improve the efficiency of drug development and enhance the value proposition of a therapeutic asset. Integrating diagnostic applications into the development process provides an opportunity to utilize biomarkers as real-time pharmacodynamic tools to assess engagement of targets, monitor response, and stratify patients most likely to benefit from a specific therapy. Of particular interest is the integration of biomarkers into the drug-development workflow to guide therapeutic selection and tailor treatments to well-defined patient subgroups via CDx assays. This codevelopment paradigm of pairing a therapeutic with a companion biomarker is fostering a new set of partnerships between pharmaceutical and diagnostic developers. Although most development programs to date have focused on oncology applications, ideal to segmentation because of cancer's heterogeneous nature and low response rates to current therapies, there are increasing trends implanting a drug-biomarker codevelopment approach to other therapeutic areas, including autoimmune diseases, cardiovascular and metabolic disorders, infectious disease, and neurological conditions. It is anticipated that the codevelopment of a therapeutic along with its companion biomarker and the ability to select optimal responders and spare others from ineffective and costly or even unsafe treatments will help one to improve therapeutic development efforts, deliver more efficacious therapies to the market, and improve pharmacoeconomic benefits.

The Current Companion Diagnostic Landscape

The goal of precision or personalized medicine is to direct therapeutic products to those patients most likely to derive a therapeutic benefit and spare others from ineffective treatments. A CDx is defined as an IVD device that can qualitatively and quantitatively measure a specific biomarker and guide the safe and effective use of a corresponding therapeutic product [15]. The use of a CDx with a therapeutic product is referenced in the instructions for use in the labeling of both the CDx and the corresponding therapeutic product. Integrating this companion biomarker strategy for patient selection is proposed to provide numerous benefits (Table 25.3). The codevelopment approach was first illustrated in 1998 with the approval of Genentech's Herceptin and Dako's HercepTest [16]. Since that time, 35 CDx devices supporting the safe and effective use of 31 therapeutics (Table 25.4) have received FDA approval (PMA) or clearance [510(k)]. Although a CDx is essential for the safe and effective use of the companion drug, and is indicated in the drug label, the FDA has implemented a second class of devices referred to as complementary diagnostics. Although not required for the use of the drug, a complementary diagnostic can help inform a physician's decision as to the risk–benefit analysis for its use. As of the end of 2018, three devices have been cleared as complementary assays (Table 25.5).

TABLE 25.3 Therapeutic benefits from companion diagnostic products.

• Improves efficacy
• Reduces toxicity; patients spared exposure to ineffective medicines
• Drug development timeliness shortened
• Lower drug development costs
• Regulatory risk mitigated
• Faster therapeutic adoption
• Improved pharmacoeconomics

Today, the use of biomarkers to guide therapeutic selection is being driven by a paradigm shift in the drug-development process, migrating away from its traditional "blockbuster" model in which every patient is treated with the same therapeutic for a particular condition, in favor of adopting a "targeted" approach in which therapeutics are directed to discreet populations based on the use of a patient's molecular profile. The adoption of this approach is being facilitated by the technological advances in genomic, transcriptomic, and proteomic platforms that are providing insights into the molecular correlates of response. Consequently, there is an increasing number of therapeutics whose use is being guided by a diagnostic assay, thus giving rise to the field of CDxs and creating innovative growth opportunities for IVD products.

TABLE 25.4 Listing of Food and Drug Administration (FDA)–approved companion diagnostic devices since 2013.

Diagnostic CDx *Manufacturer*	Approval date	Disease	Companion Rx
BRACAnalysis CDx *Myriad Genetic Laboratories, Inc.*	12/19/2014	Breast cancer	Lynparza (olaparib)
		Ovarian cancer	Talzenna (talazoparib)
			Lynparza (olaparib)
			Rubraca (rucaparib)
Therascreen EGFR RGQ PCR kit Qiagen Manchester, Ltd.	7/12/2013	Non–small cell lung cancer	Iressa (gefitinib)
			Gilotrif (afatininb)
			Vizimpro (dacomitinib)
Cobas EGFR Mutation Test v2 *Roche Molecular Systems, Inc.*	5/14/2013	Non–small cell lung cancer (tissue and plasma)	Tarceva (erlotinib)
			Tagrisso (osimerininib)
			Iressa (gefitinib)
PD-L1 IHC 22C3 pharmDx *Dako North America, Inc.*	12/2/2015	Non–small cell lung cancer, gastric or gastroesophageal junction adenocarcinoma, cervical cancer, and urothelial carcinoma	Keytruda (pembrolizumab)
PD-L1 (SP142) *Ventana Medical Systems, Inc.*	5/18/2016	Breast cancer	Tecentriq (atzeolizumab)
Abbott RealTime IDH1 *Abbott Molecular, Inc.*	7/20/2018	Acute myeloid leukemia	Tibsova (ivosidenib)
MRDxBCR-ABL Test *MolecularMD Corporation*	12/22/2017	Chronic myeloid leukemia	Tasigna (nilotinib)
FoundationOne CDx *Foundation Medicine, Inc.*	11/30/2017	Non–small cell lung cancer	Gilotrif (afatinib) Iressa (gefitinib) Tarceva (erlotinib) Tagrisso (osimertinib) Alecensa (alectinib) Xalkori (crizotinib) Zykadia (ceritinib) Tafinlar (dabrafenib) in combination with Mekinist (trametinib)
		Melanoma	Tafinlar (dabrafenib) Zelboraf (vemurafenib) Mekinist (trametinib) or Cotellic (cobimetinib)in combination with Zelboraf (vemurafenib)
		Breast cancer	Herceptin (trastuzumab) Perjeta (pertuzumab) Kadcyla (ado-trastuzumab emtansine)
		Colorectal cancer	Erbitux (cetuximab) Vectibix (panitumumab)
		Ovarian cancer	Rubraca (rucaparib)
VENTANA ALK (D5F3) CDx Assay *Ventana Medical Systems, Inc.*	11/6/2017	Non–small cell lung cancer	Zykadia (ceritinib) Xalkori (crizotinib) Alecensa (alectinib)
Abbott RealTime IDH2 *Abbott Molecular, Inc.*	8/1/2017	Acute myeloid leukemia	Idhifa (enasidenib)

(*Continued*)

TABLE 25.4 (Continued)

Diagnostic CDx *Manufacturer*	Approval date	Disease	Companion Rx
Praxis Extended RAS Panel *Illumina, Inc.*	6/29/2017	Colorectal cancer	Vectibix (panitumumab)
Oncomine Dx Target Test *Life Technologies Corporation*	6/22/2017	Non–small cell lung cancer	Tafinlar (dabrafenib) Mekinist (trametinib) Xalkori (crizotinib) Iressa (gefitinib)
LeukoStart CDx FLT3 Mutation Assay *Invivoscribe Technologies, Inc.*	4/28/2017	Acute myelogenous leukemia	Rydapt (midostaurin) Xospata (gilterinib)
FoundationFocus CDx*BRCA* Assay *Foundation Medicine, Inc.*	12/19/2016	Ovarian cancer	Rubraca (rucaparib)
Vysis CLL FISH Probe Kit *Abbott Molecular, Inc.*	4/11/2016	B-cell chronic lymphocytic leukemia	Venclexta (venetoclax)
KIT D816V Mutation Detection by PCR for Gleevec Eligibility in ASM *ARUP Laboratories, Inc.*	12/18/2015	Aggressive systemic mastocytosis	Gleevec (imatinib mesylate)
PDGFRB FISH for Gleevec Eligibility in Myelodysplastic Syndrome/Myeloproliferative Disease (MDS/MPD) *ARUP Laboratories, Inc.*	12/18/2015	Myelodysplastic syndrome/myeloproliferative disease	Gleevec (imatinib mesylate)
cobas KRAS Mutation Test *Roche Molecular Systems, Inc.*	5/7/2015	Colorectal cancer	Erbitux (cetuximab)
			Vectibix (panitumumab)
FerriScan	1/23/2013	Non–transfusion-dependent thalassemia	Exiade (deferasirox)

ASM, Aggressive systemic masto cytosis; *CDx*, companion diagnostic; *PCR*, polymerase chain reaction.
Source: http://www.fda.gov/MedicalDevices/ProductsandMedicalProcedures/InVitriDiagnostics/ucm301431.html.

TABLE 25.5 Listing of Food and Drug Administration (FDA)–approved complimentary diagnostic devices since 2013.

Diagnostic CDx *Manufacturer*	Approval date	Disease	Companion Rx
PD-L2 IHC 28-8 *Dako North America, Inc.*	1/23/2016	Melanoma	Opdivo (nivolumab)
		Non–small cell lung cancer	
Ventana PD-L1 (SP142)Assay *Ventana Medical Systems, Inc.*	7/2/2018	Bladder cancer Non–small cell lung cancer	Tecentriq (atzeolizumab)
Ventana PD-L1 (SP263) Assay *Ventana Medical Systems, Inc.*	5/1/2017	Bladder cancer	Imfinzi (durvalumab)

CDx, Companion diagnostic.
Source: http://www.fda.gov/MedicalDevices/ProductsandMedicalProcedures/InVitriDiagnostics/ucm301431.html.

The clinical utility of employing a CDx strategy has illustrated the exciting and transformative outcomes possible with this approach. Not only do CDx-based programs demonstrate enhanced efficacy and mitigate regulatory risk by helping one to demonstrate meaningful clinical improvement, but the CDx approach has also helped one to complete development programs in record time. For example, the efficacy demonstrated by both Zelboraf and Xalkori in preselected patient populations outperformed the previous standard of care by proportions, not previously seen in metastatic melanoma or non−small cell lung cancer, respectively [17,18]. In addition, a CDx approach has been shown to have a positive impact on development timelines, reducing the average time from IND filing through to regulatory approval for oncology new molecular entities by 40%−60% [19].

The majority of the CDx approved to date have focused on employing a biomarker-guided selection strategy that detects the expression of a particular protein (HER2) or a wide range of measurable genetic alterations, such as mutated forms of KRAS, BRAF, EGFR, and gene-fusion products including EML4-ALK. Today the landscape of oncology drug development is rapidly changing with the introduction of immune-targeting therapies, highlighted by the recent approvals of monoclonal antibodies that target programmed death receptor (PD-1) and programmed death ligand 1 (PD-L1) [20,21]. Enrichment of patient populations via the use of companion or complimentary diagnostics to detect the expression of the PD-L1 ligand has demonstrated durable clinical benefit across a range of tumor indications. Unfortunately, clinical benefit is limited to a fraction of patients highlighting the critical need for predictive biomarkers capable of identifying patients most likely to benefit. It is clear that combination strategies with existing therapeutics and the next wave of immuno-oncology agents will depend on the continued integration of CDxs to guide therapeutic use.

Sales of CDxs are projected to have a CAGR of 20.2% between 2018 and 2024 and achieving sales of $7 billion by 2024 [22]. When used as a CDx, biomarkers carry a strong value proposition as it is anticipated that their ability to select optimal responders and spare other patients from ineffective and costly or even unsafe treatments will enhance the therapeutic value proposition. However, because of the significant costs associated with developing and validating companion assays and the need for access to samples with well-annotated clinical outcomes data, it is envisioned that these requirements will necessitate the need for increased partnerships between assay and therapeutic developers.

Development of Companion Diagnostics Products

Traditionally, an assay is developed as an IVD only when the biomarker it detects has been well characterized at the academic level, documented through a robust series of publications illustrating its clinical utility, and demonstrating the need for a standardized and reproducible detection method [23]. The quality of the diagnostic assay is paramount to delivering optimum results whether to assess therapeutic response or guiding therapeutic selection. When qualifying a new assay to measuring a biomarker of interest, adherence to quality is an absolute requirement to insure that data is robust and reproducible and has been developed accordingly if needed to support a drug registration file. Given the importance to both the diagnostic and the therapeutic developer of integrating a diagnostic into the drug-development pathway, the following provides guidance on factors that need to be taken into consideration for not only development of the diagnostic application but also aligning the workflow with the therapeutic development, specifically as it relates to the development of companion and complimentary diagnostics.

The pathway from development to commercialization for a biomarker assay follows a well-defined process as illustrated in Fig. 25.3. Most assay developers apply a stage gate process that is initiated by the business case and guided by the intended use of the product. CDx assays are intended to provide information that is essential for the safe and effective use of a corresponding therapeutic product have been classified by the FDA as devices, subject to certain premarket controls as defined by the FD&C Act. In order to commercialize CDx assay for clinical use, CDx developers are required to obtain either PMA or clearance [510(k)] of the assay. The regulatory standards necessary for the marketing approval of CDx assays dictate strict adherence to QSRs required to develop well-characterized, robust, and reproducible assays.

These are the regulatory requirements that guide the development and validation activities verifying if the product is safe and effective for its intended use. In addition to demonstrating general controls that are in place, development requirements are focused on demonstrating that the assay's analytical performance reflects the capability of detecting the analyte in an accurate and reproducible manner. The data package therefore consists of performance metrics demonstrating accuracy, precision, limit of detection, linearity, and cross-reactivity. Once confirmed, the assay's clinical performance can be assessed to validate that it performs according to its intended use and in its intended population.

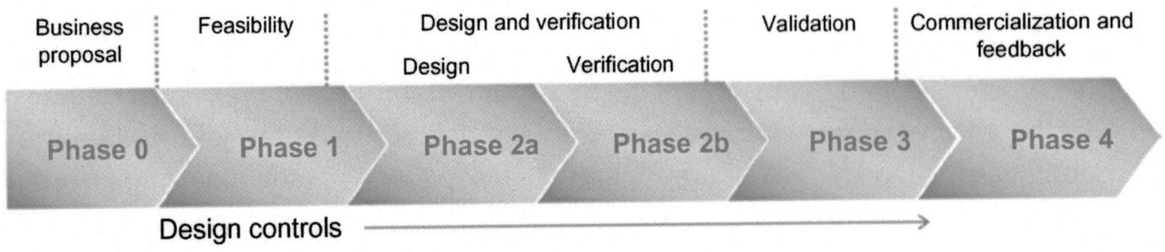

FIGURE 25.3 Development pathway for diagnostic products from discovery to commercialization.

Integrating a Companion Diagnostics Assay Into the Therapeutic Development Workflow

This new paradigm of codevelopment creates significant opportunities for both pharmaceutical and diagnostic developers but challenges as well. Diagnostic developers have a new opportunity to participate in the emerging field of precision medicine, as it will be their assays which help one to alter the standard of care and segment patients into optimal responders and spare those who would not benefit from a particular therapeutic. Opportunity is also created for pharmaceutical companies who adopt this codevelopment approach, as their therapies, guided by the use of a CDx assay, will replace existing therapies and become the new standard of care. However, a successful integration of this approach requires these two distinct business entities collaborate to facilitate the codevelopment process and drive adoption of this new paradigm. Although clear and exciting examples of success have recently been demonstrated, there are still challenges pertaining to partnering, logistical, and economic incentives that need to be addressed in order to drive adoption and allow the CDx field to move forward and achieve its full potential to deliver on the promise of delivering medicine with more precision.

Challenges to Forging Diagnostic and Therapeutic Partnerships

Pharmaceutical companies have traditionally controlled all aspects of the development and marketing of their therapeutic products. Those who have been brought into the development cycle have usually been compensated on a fee-for-service schedule, such as contract manufacturing organizations, clinical research organizations, and marketing and communication firms. In contrast, CDx codevelopment programs require pharmaceutical companies to partner with a diagnostic provider and be dependent on their diagnostic product for the therapeutic to reach the market. In essence, the process requires joining two very unique and complex organizations that are built on different cultures, different business models, and vastly different approaches to developing, commercializing and being reimbursed for their respective products. The shift from the traditional "blockbuster" one-size-fits-all model to a targeted, patient segmentation approach and incorporating biomarkers into the development paradigm is disruptive compared to the way pharmaceutical developers have traditionally operated. This is typically viewed by therapeutic developer as adding complexity and higher development costs and also increasing risks of delays in clinical development timelines. While many partnerships will focus on drafting a codevelopment agreement that addresses roles and responsibilities, intellectual property rights, financial obligations, governance, and termination procedures, it is equally important to focus on mechanisms that will forge strong pharma-diagnostic relationships as a means to overcome the inherent logistical challenges associated with these codevelopment programs. Codevelopment programs are true alliances unlike any other collaboration program pharmaceutical developers that have entered into. Given the very different business models and cultures between pharmaceutical and diagnostic developers, mutual education is essential to ensure a common understanding of each partner's roles and responsibilities. As such, significant alliance management activity is necessary to guide the early and frequent communication required to ensure a collaborative atmosphere between the codevelopment teams.

Time Line Challenges

The most pressing challenge to CDx development is being able to align the respective development timelines required for a biomarker with that of the therapeutic (Fig. 25.4). With the goal of obtaining simultaneous Rx and Dx approval, synchronizing the development process of the paired products and avoiding a situation in which the Dx is delaying the approval of the Rx can be challenging. Ideally, if the biomarker assay is prospectively incorporated into the early clinical development program, the benefit of employing a biomarker strategy can be established early in the therapeutic development life cycle. However, this is rarely the case with the development

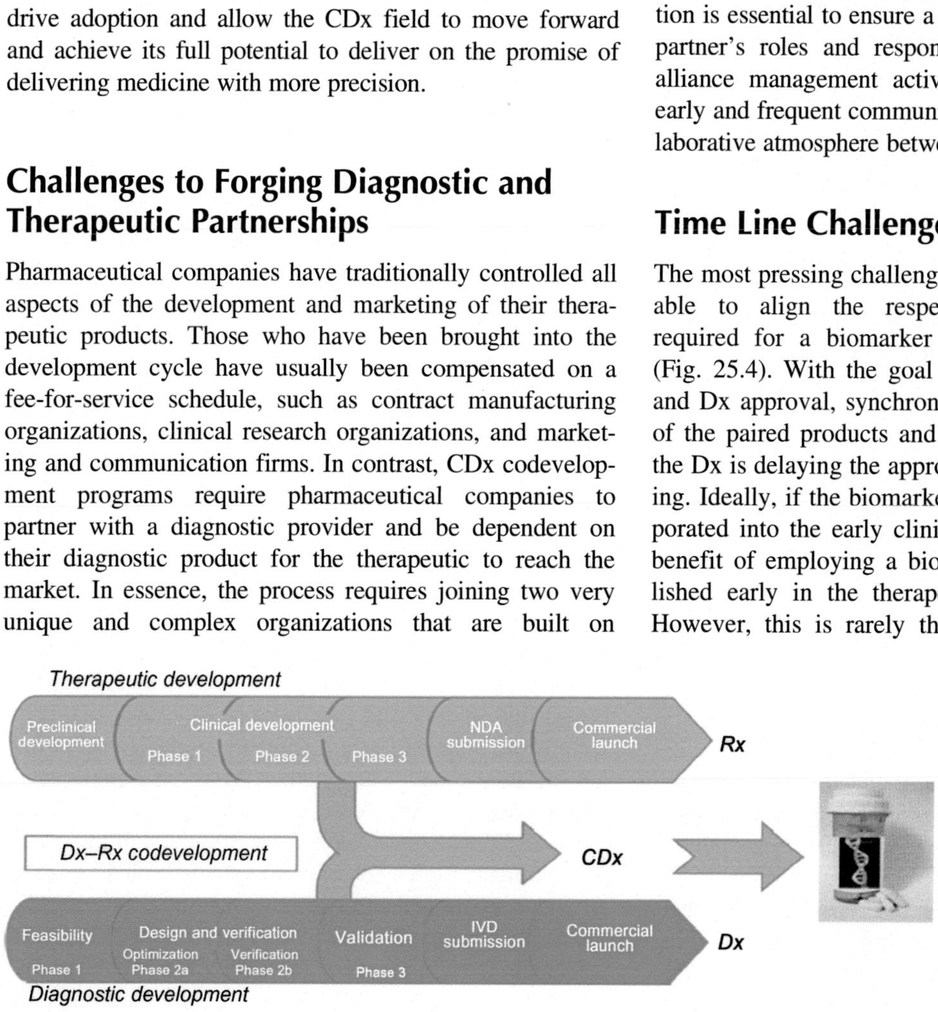

FIGURE 25.4 Aligning the development of a therapeutic and it's companion diagnostic product.

process as a result of the CDx assay adhering to regulatory standards. Only after the quality system requirements have been achieved and the assay "locked" for the validation of its intended use with a specific therapeutic can be integrated into the therapeutic development pathway. The diverse development paths between the therapeutic and diagnostic, with their inherent differences, present risks that could affect the development timelines. This is particularly relevant given the time needed to develop and verify the performance of the assay prior to its availability for use in supporting the clinical trials of the therapeutic.

Regulatory Challenges

Although the paired products are dependent on each other's regulatory approval for market access, there is a universal absence of structure allowing for the simultaneous submission and review of the paired products as one regulatory file. For example, a PMA submission is reviewed by CDRH while in contrast, a new drug application for a therapeutic is submitted and reviewed by a completely separate entity of the FDA, either the Center for Drug Evaluation and Research or the Center for Biological Evaluation and Research. This lack of regulatory harmonization is evident across major markets, including the European Union, where IVD Directive 98/79/CE (CE stands for Conformité Europèene, or European Conformity) stipulates self-certification for the diagnostic assay, while therapeutics are submitted to the European Medical Agency for review by the Committee for Human Medicinal Products. In Japan, a process for the simultaneous review of therapeutic-diagnostic (Rx–Dx) pairs is still lacking, and in emerging markets such as China, a process for CDx development is still being defined. Establishing a uniform process for simultaneous review and approval will create a more efficient system and help one to mitigate risks in these codevelopment programs. In recognizing this challenging landscape of CDx development, the FDA recently updated its draft guidance in December of 2018 [24].

Economic Challenges to Companion Diagnostics Development

For a diagnostic developer, assay development must represent a compelling investment opportunity. The traditional IVD diagnostic business model has been built on the concept that low margins could be offset with high volume tests. However, recent CDx assays have tended to be niche indications representing "orphan-like" diagnostic opportunities that can result in economic misalignment. For example, the annual numbers of metastatic colorectal cancer and metastatic melanoma cases in the United States are approximately 50,000 and 10,000, respectively [25].

Although low volume can typically be offset by higher pricing (i.e., orphan therapeutics), diagnostic developers tend to be prohibited from this approach and are challenged to obtain value-based pricing. In the United States, the reimbursement system dictates a model in which the clinical laboratory fee schedule, managed by the Centers for Medicare and Medicaid Services, assigns analyte-specific codes to an assay via Common Procedural Terminology codes that determine the cost that a lab can submit for the reimbursement of an approved assay. For kit developers, the test must be sold at a fraction of the total cost to ensure profitability of the lab performing the assay. As a result, reimbursement for molecular CDx tests currently fails to exhibit pricing that is reflective of the value they deliver.

In European markets, developers of CDxs often lack sufficient clarity on the appropriate technology assessment and reimbursement pathways needed to ensure adoption and utilization of such tests. The situation is further complicated when authorities consider drugs and diagnostics under separate evaluation and payment processes, with many countries putting drugs through a more well-defined appraisal process that is currently available for CDxs. Furthermore, while mandatory CE marking under the IVD Directive 98/79/CE requirements facilitates the access of diagnostic tests across the European Union, the European market is characterized as a heterogeneous region in terms of assessment and reimbursement approaches, with every country having its own distinct requirements. As a result, potential differences arise across members of the European Union, including the tendency of most of the European nations to review therapeutics at the national level and diagnostic tests at the local level. This local approach to technology assessment and reimbursement of CDxs compared with national-level reviews for most of the drugs can result in substantial delays to reimbursement of a diagnostic product and hence its availability. For example, although Herceptin received approval in France in 2000, funding for HER2 testing was not approved until 2007 [26].

In addition to the challenges of niche market opportunities, low pricing and lags in reimbursement, diagnostic developers who pursue a regulatory-guided route to market are confronted with another set of challenges in the market place in the form of "Home Brews" or LDTs. Once an IVD kit receives regulatory approval, the current environment allows for clinical reference and academic labs to develop and offer their own tests, thus presenting the IVD developer with a competitive market beginning at launch of the assay. The presence of competing LDTs, coupled with low volume, low pricing, and potential delays in reimbursement, presents significant challenges to the traditional IVD business model. Coupled with the risk of a failed drug in development and its associated opportunity cost, there is a risk in attaining a viable business model and therefore it is imperative to address these challenges and find solutions that incentivizes the IVD developer to participate in this emerging field.

Driving Adoption of In Vitro Diagnostics

In addition to obtaining the necessary regulatory clearance or approval to market an IVD product, there are several other market barriers that need to be addressed to drive a wide-spread adoption of an IVD and assure a product's commercial success. In addition to demonstrating robust and reproducible analytical performance, an assay must also demonstrate its validation in a clinical setting and confirm its intended use. While several of these requirements are generated to support regulatory authorization, other market barriers must be addressed postapproval. A key driver in the adoption of an IVD assay into routine clinical testing is demonstrating its clinical utility, in which the assay must deliver clinically actionable data capable of influencing medical decisions. Faruki and Lai-Goldman have presented intriguing data supporting the acceleration of test acceptance for several IVDs once clinical utility is definitively established [27]. The "early development" period that precedes the establishment of clinical utility was reported to last up to 5 years and is characterized by performing clinical studies to support the incorporation of the assay into clinical practice guidelines. Finally, data must be generated illustrating the health economic benefits of a particular assay to establish and obtain value-based reimbursement and aid in the adoption of the assay. Demonstrating these four parameters of analytical performance, clinical validation, clinical utility, and economic benefits are essential for achieving success in the market.

Future Applications for Integrating Diagnostics Into the Drug-Development Pathway

Aside from the current single biomarker CDx model established today for targeted therapies, the complexity of disease will drive future growth opportunities employing a multianalyte approach. The growing appreciation for spatial heterogeneity, the status of immune competency, and the role that the microbiome plays in maintaining homeostasis will all play a role in requiring incorporation of multiple data points to define the appropriate drug responsive phenotype. This composite biomarker approach will be further complexed by the emergence of biomarkers derived from sensors and mobile technologies. The culmination of these advances is that the lack of one entity providing an end-to-end solution and necessitating therapeutic developers establishes multiple partnerships with device developers. Therefore understanding and appreciating the challenges of these partnerships and identifying solutions will be paramount for the successful integration of diagnostic devices into the drug-development workflow and delivering on the promise of precision medicine.

Summary

Diagnostic products are an integral component to the delivery of an optimal healthcare system. A growing application of these products is their use as CDxs to select patients who are most likely to derive benefit from a corresponding therapeutic. Implementing CDxs has reached a "tipping point," in which we have been able to witness a growing number of new chemical entities coming to market with their safe and effective use dependent on an IVD product. By providing optimal selection of patients most likely to benefit, the promise of precision medicine will become a realization. IVD manufacturers with their regulatory expertise and global sales and marketing capabilities can be ideal partners for pharmaceutical companies requiring diagnostic assays to guide therapeutic selection. However, integrating these biomarker approaches into the therapeutic development workflow is disruptive to the traditional development pathway as it represents a paradigm shift in drug development with pharmaceutical companies having to form partnerships with diagnostic companies to codevelop their paired products. While initial results have illustrated transformative effects associated with the codevelopment process, several challenges remain to be addressed that underscore the traditional IVD business model. Value capture remains a major challenge going forward, together with regulatory uncertainty and operational issues between codevelopment partners recognizing the challenges associated with the development and commercialization of these paired products and identifying strategies to address them will allow the field of CDx to successfully advance and facilitate the adoption of precision medicine into routine clinical practice.

References

[1] Aspinall MG, Hamermesh RG. Realizing the promise of personalized medicine. Harv Bus Rev 2007;85(10):108–17.

[2] AdvaMedDx 2019, Innovation and Value. <https://dx.advamed.org/diagnostics-policy/innovation-value> [accessed April 2, 2019].

[3] Report Linker 2019, *In Vitro* Diagnostics Market by Product Type, Technique, Application, and End User: Global Opportunity Analysis and Industry Forecast, 2018–2025. <https://www.reportlinker.com/p05698753> [accessed April 2, 2019].

[4] 21 C.F.R. Part 809. In vito diagnostic products for human use, 2019.
[5] U.S Food and Drug Administration, Center for Devices and Radiological Health, 2019. <https://www.fda.gov/aboutfda/centersoffices/officeofmedicalproductsandtobacco/cdrh/> [accessed April 2, 2019].
[6] Biomerieux, Inc. VIDAS® Total Prostate Specific Antigen (TPSA) [package insert] U.S. Food and Drug Administration website. <https://www.accessdata.fda.gov/cdrh_docs/pdf4/P040008c.pdf> [accessed April 2, 2019].
[7] Iris Molecular Diagnostics. NADiA® ProsVue™ 510(k) Substantial Equivalence Determination Decision Summary US Food and Drug Administration website. <https://www.accessdata.fda.gov/cdrh_docs/reviews/K101185.pdf> [accessed April 2, 2019].
[8] U.S Food and Drug Administration, FDA User Fee Programs. <https://www.fda.gov/industry/fda-user-fee-programs> [accessed April 4, 2020].
[9] MedPac. Chapter 7—An overview of the medical device industry. In: MedPac: report to the congress: medicare and the health care delivery system; 2017. <http://www.medpac.gov/docs/default-source/reports/jun17_ch7.pdf?sfvrsn = 0> [accessed April 2, 2019].
[10] Douillard JY, Oliner KS, Siena S, Tabernero J, Burkes R, Barugel M, et al. Panitumumab-FOLFOX4 treatment and RAS mutations in colorectal cancer. N Engl J Med 2013;369(11):1023–34.
[11] U.S. Food and Drug Administration, Statement from FDA Commissioner Scott Gottlieb, M.D. and Jeff Shuren, M.D., Director of the Center for Devices and Radiological Health, on transformative new steps to modernize FDA's 510(k) program to advance the review of the safety and effectiveness of medical devices. <https://www.fda.gov/newsevents/newsroom/pressAnnouncements/ucm626572.htm> [accessed April 2, 2019].
[12] U.S Food and Drug Administration, Statement from FDA Commissioner Scott Gottlieb, M.D., and Jeff Shuren, M.D., Director of the Center for Devices and Radiological Health, on a record year for device innovation. <https://www.fda.gov/NewsEvents/Newsroom/PressAnnouncements/ucm629917.htm> [accessed April 2, 2019].
[13] Moan B, Rabin N. In vitro medical devices: how businesses can successfully comply with the new European regulation. Ann Biol Clin (Paris) 2018;76(6):716–18.
[14] Topol EJ. Individualized medicine from prewomb to tomb. Cell 2014;157(1):241–53.
[15] Scheerens H, Malong A, Bassett K, Boyd Z, Gupta V, Harris J, et al. Current status of companion and complementary diagnostics: strategic considerations for development and launch. Clin Transl Sci. 2017;10(2):84–92.
[16] Jørgensen JT, Hersom M. Companion diagnostics—a tool to improve pharmacotherapy. Ann Transl Med 2016;4(24):482.
[17] Chapman PB, Hauschild A, Robert C, Haanen JB, Ascierto P, Larkin J, et al. Improved survival with vemurafenib in melanoma with BRAF V600E mutation. N Engl J Med 2011;364(26):2507–16.
[18] Kwak EL, Bang YJ, Camidge DR, Shaw AT, Solomon B, Maki RG, et al. Anaplastic lymphoma kinase inhibition in non–small-cell lung cancer. N Engl J Med 2010;363(18):1693–703.
[19] Beeler J. Integrating companion diagnostic assays into drug development: addressing the challenges from the diagnostic perspective. Drug Dev Res 2013;74(2):148–54.
[20] Borghaei H, Paz-Ares L, Horn L, Spigel DR, Steins M, Ready NE, et al. Nivolumab versus docetaxel in advanced nonsquamous non-small-cell lung cancer. N Engl J Med 2015;373(17):1627–39.
[21] Reck M, Rodriguez-Abreu D, Robinson AG, Hui R, Csöszi T, Fülöp A, et al. Pembrolizumab versus chemotherapy for PD-L1-positive non-small-cell lung cancer. N Engl J Med 2016;375(19):1823–33.
[22] Market Research Engine, Companion Diagnostics Market By Indication; By Technologynand by Regional Analysis - Global Forecast by 2020–2025. <https://www.marketresearchengine.com/companion-diagnostics-market> [accessed April 2, 2019].
[23] Baker M. New-wave diagnostics. Nat Biotechnol 2006;24(8):931–8.
[24] U.S Food and Drug Administration, Guidance Document, *InVitro* Companion Diagnostic Devices. <https://www.fda.gov/regulatory-information/search-fda-guidance-documents/vitro-companion-diagnostic-devices> [accessed April 2, 2019].
[25] Noone AM, Howlader N, Krapcho M, Miller D, Brest A, Yu M, et al., editors. SEER cancer statistics review, 1975–2015. Bethesda, MD: National Cancer Institute; 2017. https://seer.cancer.gov/csr/1975_2015/[accessed April 2, 2019].
[26] Miller I, Ashon-Chess J, Spolders H, Fert V, Ferrara J, Kroll W, et al. Market access challenges in the EU for high medical value diagnostic tests. Pers Med 2011;8(2):137–48.
[27] Faruki H, Lai-Goldman M. Application of a pharamcogenetic test adoption model to six oncology biomarkers. Pers Med 2010;7(4):441–50.

Chapter 26

The Development and Commercialization of Medical Devices

Mark Byrne, MS[1,2]
[1]President, PriMedicus Development, Loveland, OH, United States, [2]Chief Executive Officer, ProteoSense, Columbus, OH, United States

Chapter Outline

Introduction

Medical devices come in many forms, purposes, and degrees of complexity—from mundane and simple items that are used once and discarded—such as a tongue depressor—to devices used for a few days (e.g., contact lenses) to critical life supporting and highly complex systems—such as implantable cardio defibrillators that are surgically implanted and expected to last for the remainder of a patient's life. Because of this extreme variety in complexity, intended use, and resultant risk to patients, the medical device industry is one of the most highly regulated sectors in the world. Most national governments have created legal requirements for medical devices made, used, or sold in their country. These external requirements include specific quality systems (QSs), product development (PD), manufacturing, and regulatory agency (RA) approval rules that must be satisfied, typically before marketing, to ensure that medical devices are safe and effective for their intended purpose. The human and financial costs of failure are extremely high and can range from product marketing delays to patient injury and death.

This chapter covers medical device development primarily in the context of the US legal and regulatory framework established by 21 CFR Chapter 1 Subchapter H [1] and enforced by the Food and Drug Administration (FDA). Additional references to specific European Union (EU) and Canadian requirements are included to highlight relevant differences. The approach is an introductory discussion of QS, PD, manufacturing, and RA considerations for entrepreneurs; it is not a comprehensive review of the all applicable US regulations. All medical device companies from the largest—Johnson & Johnson or Medtronic, for example, to the smallest—your nascent start-up, must comply with the applicable regulations. While all face the same external requirements, not all have the same resources or degree of established processes and systems. Often a medical device entrepreneur has to build a procedural foundation before creating the "house." While some familiarity with quality, product design, manufacturing, and regulatory terminology is expected, this chapter is intended as a starting point for further investigation. It is not a "cookbook" nor does it cover every possible consideration or scenario. Medical device development is an art—there is no one standard process. Nonetheless, there are common phases and issues that the entrepreneur must deal with. Numerous references are cited where the reader can obtain more detail in pursuit of a deeper understanding leading to successful medical device development.

Following the "Introduction" section, the remainder of the chapter is organized by the usual and customary phases of medical device development: planning, requirements definition, design and development, verification and validation, design transfer, and launch.

Biotechnology Entrepreneurship. DOI: https://doi.org/10.1016/B978-0-12-815585-1.00026-7

Medical Device Definition

Whenever a product is labeled, promoted, or used in a manner that meets the legal definition established by Section 201(h) of the Federal Food, Drug and Cosmetic Act (FD&C Act), it will be regulated by the FDA as a medical device, requiring premarketing and postmarketing controls [2]:

... A device is: an instrument, apparatus, implement, machine, contrivance, implant, in vitro reagent, or other similar or related article, including a component part, or accessory which is:

1. recognized in the official National Formulary, or the United States Pharmacopoeia, or any supplement to them,
2. intended for use in the diagnosis of disease or other conditions, or in the cure, mitigation, treatment, or prevention of disease, in man or other animals, or
3. intended to affect the structure or any function of the body of man or other animals, and which does not achieve its primary intended purposes through chemical action within or on the body of man or other animals and

which does not achieve its primary intended purposes through chemical action within or on the body of man or other animals and which is not dependent upon being metabolized for the achievement of its primary intended purposes. The term "device" does not include software functions excluded pursuant to section 520(o).

This definition is very broad and includes most in vitro diagnostic (IVD) products as well.

Industry Trends

Globally, the medical devices industry is quite large with sales of $379 billion in 2017—a new record—and represents about 5% of the $7.7 trillion global health-care economy [3]. While the growth in the global health-care economy is increasing [4], in recent years, growth in the medical device industry has slowed. From 2008 until now, annual medical revenue growth has tended toward 4% versus the average 15% annual revenue growth from 2000 to 2007. Along with the slowdown in revenue growth, the industry has substantially reduced its growth in R&D expenses from a high of 25% in 2002 to a flat year—zero growth—in 2017. Some industry observers attribute this slow growth to tactical product line acquisitions and portfolio optimization strategies rather than major new product releases [5]. Original premarket approvals by the FDA, which represent the newest and most innovative devices, dropped from 46 in 2017 to 31 in 2018 [6].

Nonetheless, the field of medical devices represents an area of advanced technology in which the United States holds a strong competitive advantage over the rest of the world. The United States is the largest medical device market in the world, with a market size of around $156 billion, representing about 40% of the 2017 global medical device market. The US exports of medical devices in key product categories identified by the Department of Commerce exceeded $41 billion that year. The industry is responsible for almost 2 million jobs, including both direct and indirect employment. Medical technology directly accounts for well over 500,000 of these jobs.

Medical devices are one of the few economic sectors that are attractive to angel and venture capital, collectively referred to as "venture," investors. The year 2018 was a record-setting year for venture investment activity in the US economy. Venture investors completed 8948 deals and invested $131 billion. The life sciences sector, which includes pharma, biotech, and medical devices, comprised 1308 deals and $23.2 billion. Of this total, 588 investments totaling $5.87 billion were made in medical device companies. This represents an increase of over $1 billion compared to 2017 and continues an upward trend in both number of deals and dollars invested [7]. This level of investment helps to stimulate a vibrant entrepreneurial ecosystem where more than 80% of the US medical device companies have fewer than 50 employees, and many (e.g., entrepreneurial ventures) have little or no sales revenue [8].

During the planning phase, the entrepreneur has to determine a way to fund their proposed project. Venture finance along with grants and contracts are the most common financing methods for entrepreneurial medical device ventures. In addition to the macroeconomic and investment trends described earlier, there are three major trends the entrepreneur needs to be aware of as follows:

1. ***The end of "me-too" devices***—once upon a time, many medical device entrepreneurs found success building a new and improved "thing" that represented an incremental improvement on a product offered by another company, usually a larger market incumbent. By offering a better product solution within the same category (e.g., a new and improved surgical stapler with a smaller profile to better fit tight anatomical spaces), entrepreneurs could enter the market, find customers, and capture a respectable share. Today, the only incremental improvement that gets customers'

attention is lower price. Offering an otherwise incremental product is not a winning strategy for entrepreneurs and has been increasingly difficult to finance.

2. ***Channel is everything***—the customers for medical devices (e.g., hospitals and health-care providers) are consolidating rapidly into integrated health-care systems. Hospitals are buying one another and forming networks, in turn the networks are vertically integrating to provide everything from primary care to imaging and rehabilitative services. Quality health outcomes, reduced cost, and efficiency are emphasized. Purchasing decisions for medical devices used within a network consolidate to the point where an entrepreneurial start-up has difficulty getting in the door without a very unique product that will allow the network to somehow offer a new or differentiated service or save large sums of money. In this environment, entrepreneurs need a partner and that partner may be a larger established medical device company that has specific access to the channel. For example, Medtronic Inc. invested in Mazor Robotics, Inc. a small Israeli company developing treatment planning and robotic systems for spine surgery 2016. The two companies worked together to integrate various technologies for spine surgery to extend the market reach of Mazor's technology through Medtronic's much larger footprint. Medtronic eventually acquired the smaller company for $1.7 billion in 2018 [9].
3. ***Emphasis on digital information and transformation***—in light of the macro trends and the convergence of advanced software and data communications, there is a new emphasis on data-enabled devices that can measure and report on aspects of the patient in order to improve outcomes and create new revenue opportunities for health-care providers. For example, Philips' "Connected Care Solutions" is an intelligent health-care service that collects patient data (generally related to chronic diseases) and allows providers to monitor and deliver round-the-clock solutions by linking patient data with hospitals [10].

Major Milestones in Medical Device Development

The history of medical devices has many examples of new products and techniques that have profoundly improved and extended countless patients' lives. Table 26.1 contains a few selected major milestones in medical device development. The significance of the inventions on this list should provide the medical device entrepreneur with substantial motivation and encouragement for their chosen path.

Planning Phase

A key to starting and building a successful entrepreneurial business is planning. The objective of the planning phase (sometimes referred to as the concept phase) is to define all aspects of a medical device in sufficient detail and rigor to be able to plan for its financing, development, regulatory approval, production, and selling. In the context of an entrepreneurial venture the output of this phase may be compiled into a detailed business plan or equivalent document used to communicate the opportunity to investors in order to obtain financing. In an established company the output may be a management presentation and accompanying financial analysis, this time to obtain internal prioritization for human and financial resources.

However, a complete business plan is not always required. It's not the only way to create a successful business. In particular, in the early stages of the planning phase, a shorthand or "lean" method may be more appropriate, especially if it enables rapid consideration of several scenarios before selecting the best one and jumpstarting the detailed assessment. One model, described later in this section, is based on the Business Model Canvas, which is a strategic management and lean start-up template for developing new or documenting existing business models [11]. More information about using the Business Model Canvas for biotechnology products can be found in *Chapter 13: Directing Your Technology Toward a Market Problem: What You Need to Know Before Using the Business Model Canvas?*

In either scenario a key activity in this phase is the systematic reduction of uncertainty or risk in each of the major dimensions of the project. Cutting corners in the planning phase will almost always result in expensive surprises, in time, dollars or both, during one of the later development phases.

During the planning phase, there are four major topics areas to be answered

1. ***Product and market***—What is the stakeholder need, how is it solved today? Can we solve it in a better way that is more appealing to stakeholders? What are the stakeholder requirements? Who will pay for it? Is the underlying technology available and ready for commercialization? What is the Intellectual Property (IP) landscape?
2. ***Operational***—How will the organization produce, distribute, sell, and support the proposed solution? How much will it cost to produce?
3. ***Regulatory and clinical***—What is the regulatory strategy to obtain necessary approvals in each major market where stakeholders would purchase the product? Is clinical data needed for market acceptance?

TABLE 26.1 Major medical device milestones.[a]

Year	Inventors	Event	Significance
1958	Forrest M. Bird, Henry L. Pohndorf	Bird Universal Medical Respirator for acute or chronic cardiopulmonary care introduced	First highly reliable, low-cost, mass-produced medical respirator in the world
1953	John Gibbon	First use of the heart-lung machine	Enabled open-heart surgical procedures previously considered too risky
1957	Earl Bakken	External pacemaker development	Bakken founded Medtronic, developing the first external, battery-operated, wearable artificial pacemaker
1960	Wilson Greatbatch	First human implantable pacemaker	Ushered in an era of cardiac rhythm management, saving countless lives. His original pacemaker patent resulted in the first implantable cardiac pacemaker, which led to heart patient survival rates comparable to that of a healthy population of similar age
1960	Paul Terasaki, Dennis Akoi	Tissue Typing for Organ Transplants	He invented a tissue-typing test that became an international standard for matching potential kidney, heart, liver, pancreas, lung, and bone marrow donors and recipients
1969	Thomas Fogarty	Patent issued for balloon embolectomy catheter	Fogarty's catheter revolutionized vascular surgery; it is still the most widely used technique for blood clot removal and encouraged advances for other minimally invasive surgeries, including angioplasty
1956	Alfred H. Free, Helen M. Free	Development of a dip-and-read test, Clinistix, for detecting glucose in urine	Revolutionized urinalysis and advanced diabetes testing with the first one-minute test for blood glucose, leading to the concept of self-testing for diabetics
1957	William P. Murphy	Medical Development Corporation (forerunner of Cordis Medical) founded	Pioneered applying engineering to medicine. His many successful medical devices include disposable medical procedure trays, blood bags, physiologic cardiac pacemakers, angiographic injectors, and hollow fiber artificial kidneys
1975	Robert S. Ledley	Patent issued for the whole-body CT diagnostic X-ray scanner	Set the basic design for modern CT scanners
1982	Willem J. Kolff	Invented the soft shell mushroom shaped heart and the artificial kidney dialysis machine.	There are over 400,000 people in the US with end-stage renal disease that are being kept alive by the kidney dialysis machine
1984	Raymond V. Damadian	FDA approval of the first MRI scanner	Revolutionized the field of diagnostic medicine
1994	Julio C. Palmaz	FDA approval of the Palmaz Stent for coronary use.	Revolutionized cardiac care with an alternative to bypass surgery

CT, Computerized tomographic; *FDA*, Food and Drug Administration; *MRI*, magnetic resonance imaging; *US*, United States.
[a] *www.invent.org/inductees/search [accessed February 22, 2019].*

4. ***Financial***—Considering all the costs of development, regulatory approval, production, sales, and support can the entrepreneur or their organization sell sufficient quantities at a price that will make money? When and how much?

Notice that these questions are centered on "stakeholders" as opposed to users or customers. In today's complex medical device marketplace, there are several stakeholders involved in every purchasing decision. For example, while an implantable hip prosthesis is "used" by an orthopedic surgeon to restore a patient's ability to walk without discomfort, there are several stakeholders in addition to the surgeon: the hospital where the surgical procedure takes place, insurance plans (public or private) that pay for it, and the patient who may have a say in which manufacturer's implant is used as well as the method of implantation (i.e., a traditional vs robotic-assisted surgery). At a minimum, all are involved in the decision to some degree. Furthermore, stakeholders may vary by geographic region due to difference in local regulations or market factors. Using the hip prosthesis example, but now in a market with a single-payer health-care system, such as the

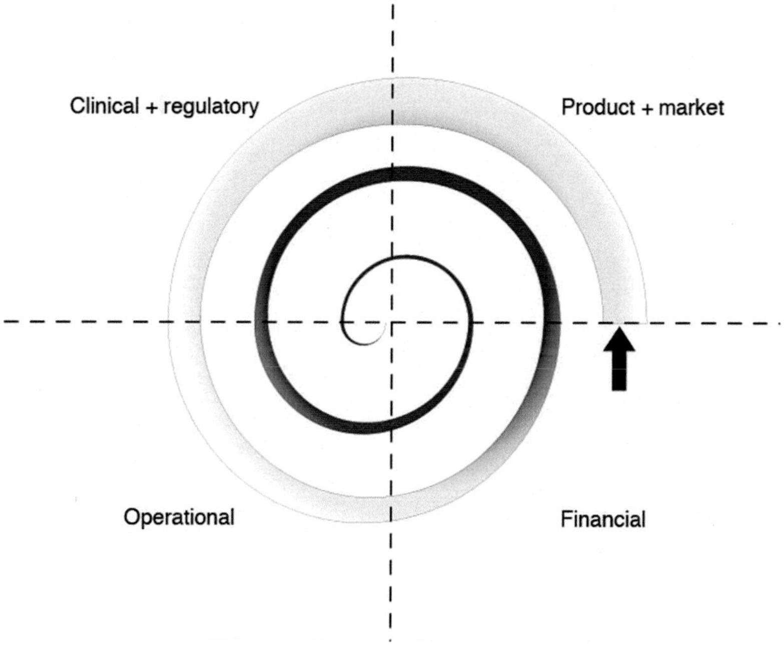

FIGURE 26.1 The planning phase spiral.

United Kingdom, the relative importance of surgeons and patients will be significantly reduced relative to the voice of the public health plan. Understanding who the stakeholders are, their relative importance, motivations, and decision-making criteria on a new device, is an essential activity in the planning phase.

There are various methods to organize and conduct the planning phase. One can visualize the major topics forming quadrants in a chart or as shown in Fig. 26.1. Each quadrant will cover specific groups of questions and be organized to facilitate quick communications. The spiral illustrates the concept of starting with a wide view that becomes tighter with each successive loop around the four quadrants. To help guide an entrepreneur through the planning phase, Table 26.2 expands each quadrant's topic into groups of related subquestions suitable for each successive loop. Remember, these are general example questions. Fig. 26.1 is an illustration intended to show that the planning phase is not a linear process. Each project is unique and will have its own specific planning questions and challenges. There is nothing magic about three loops of levels of questions, it is just an example.

A key to starting and building a successful business is planning. However, a complete business plan is not always required. An alternative (or maybe a precursor?) to the detailed questions of Table 26.2 is a "lean" approach based on the Business Model Canvas or one of its many derivatives. The Business Model Canvas is a strategic management and lean start-up template for developing new or documenting existing business models *Chapter 13: Directing Your Technology Toward a Market Problem: What You Need to Know Before Using the Business Model Canvas?*. It is a visual chart with elements describing a product's value proposition, infrastructure, customers, and finances. It is designed to drive thought processes to evaluate trade-offs, identify information gaps, and formulate plans rapidly.

One derivative form of the Business Model Canvas the author has used is The Lean Canvas. It was created by Ash Maurya in 2010 specifically for entrepreneurial ventures [12]. The Lean Canvas focuses on addressing customer problems, defining solutions, and delivering them through a unique value proposition, creating a "blueprint" of your business. Entrepreneurs may access an online version of the Lean Canvas at www.leanstack.com. Both free and paid accounts are available [13].

Some of the key issues the Lean Canvas will help entrepreneurs uncover are (1) the key categories of starting, testing, and growing your business; (2) target customer identification; (3) recognition of customers' problems and how your product or service will solve them; (4) value proposition communication; (5) financial projections; and (6) develop key metrics.

Each organization will have their preferred approach. In entrepreneurial ventures, it is common for the founder (s) to conduct the planning phase activities as part of the start-up due diligence. The strength of this approach is the focus and passion a founder brings to a new innovation is hard to beat, unfortunately founders may have blind spots too. Thus their planning phase output may overemphasize some factors while overlooking others. To solve this, savvy founders seek out additional points of view during planning. In more established companies a small team

TABLE 26.2 Example medical device planning questions.

Topic	1st Level	2nd Level	3rd Level
Product and market			
	Describe the problem, who has it?	Provide and explicit problem statement, answer: who, what, when, where, now big	Quantify the market opportunity, total addressable market, and segmentation
	How is it solved today?	Identify alternatives	Assess relative strengths and weaknesses of each
	What are the stakeholder's requirements?	Interview stakeholders	Written interview summaries
	Who will pay for it?	Is there existing third-party reimbursement? If not, is it necessary and/or possible?	Detail the reimbursement model
	Can we solve it in a better way that is more appealing to stakeholders? How? When?	Develop/test/refine minimum viable product What is the value proposition?	Prepare marketing specification Understand patent landscape
	Is the underlying technology available and ready for commercialization?	Who can provide key technologies? Suppliers?Partners?Customers?	Prepare risk assessment
Operational			
	How and where will the product be produced? How many?	New or existing supply chain? Needed capacity? Does it fit the organization's capabilities? If not, who can provide	Prepare a production plan
	What is the distribution channel?	Direct to customer, through distributor, third-party private label?	Prepare a channel strategy
	Does the product have training or service requirements?	Who needs to be trained? When? How? What level of service/support is anticipated?	Prepare a customer experience plan
	How much will the product cost to produce?	Estimate material/labor/yield	Prepare a cost of goods forecast
Regulatory and clinical			
	What is the regulatory strategy for each major market?	In the United States: • PMA • 510(k) application • HDE • De novo determination • Class 1 determination Are guidance documents available? Any external standards? Cybersecurity strategy?	Written regulatory strategy
	International regulatory strategy for each major market	What are the requirements and pathway to approval?	Written regulatory strategy for each market
	Is clinical data needed for regulatory approval? Is additional clinical and/or economic data needed for reimbursement or market acceptance?	How many patients, what inclusion/exclusion criteria? Single center/multicenter? Primary endpoints? Secondary endpoints?	Written clinical plan and study design(s)

(*Continued*)

TABLE 26.2 (Continued)

Topic	1st Level	2nd Level	3rd Level
Financial			
	Describe the business model	What are the revenue streams, determine if it's a onetime sale, recurring sale, subscription, license fee, per-use fee, service/parts sale, lease, or a combination thereof	Prepare a 3-year (or more) sales forecast, document all assumptions
	What is the estimated selling price?	What is the pricing strategy for the product? Are there competitors or reimbursement limits that will set the price?	
	What is the estimated development cost?	Product development, clinical, regulatory, manufacturing start-up and commercial launch expenses	Prepare detailed project plan, identify major milestones
	What is the expected gross margin?	Estimate selling and marketing expenses, detail sales cycle	Prepare 3-year (or more) financial model with projections of income, cash flow and project financing needed to reach cash flow break even. Considering all the costs of development, regulatory approval, production, sales, and support can the entrepreneur sell sufficient quantities at a price that will make money?

HDE, Humanitarian device exemption; *PMA*, premarket approval.

with diverse skills and perspectives may tackle the planning. In either scenario, it is important to approach the major questions in a sequential fashion, much like peeling and onion. Start with the outer layers of each question, research, analyze, and process to develop the next set of successively more detailed questions. Rinse and repeat until there is sufficient detail and clarity for each topic area.

Design and Development Phase

The objective of the design and development phase is to translate the outputs of the planning phase into a finished product ready for launch and its associated supply chain in accordance to QS compliant with applicable regulations. Unlike the iterative or spiral planning phase previously discussed, the design and development phase typically follows a waterfall or concurrent engineering processes as described in the US FDA design control guidance document [14].

Quality Systems

QSs are a set of processes and procedures the entrepreneur defines and implements to describe how your venture addresses the current medical device regulations, including design controls. QS will cover the organizational structure, procedures, processes, personnel responsibilities, and resources designed to manage product quality throughout the full product life cycle. In the context of a medical device, product quality means safe and effective for its intended use.

The US, European, and Canadian regulations describe in great detail a series of requirements that a medical device manufacturer's QS must cover. Spanning the product life cycle from design, to production, distribution, servicing, and numerous associated activities, the QS requirements will drive the organizational structure, responsibilities, and processes within a company. For design and development the QS will establish a documentation hierarchy and design control methodology that will guide and sequence all activities. Note that the regulation includes the notion of "appropriateness." A manufacturer/developer of a medical device for life support applications will undoubtedly have a different and more comprehensive QS than one that designs and produces a much simpler (and lower risk) product. Both FDA design controls regulations and ISO 13485 design and development requirements expect you to keep documentation and records throughout the PD process. The design history file (DHF) is a great place to keep all of your design controls "evidence."

In the United States, these requirements are covered in 21 CFR Section 820, Medical devices—quality regulation [1]. This regulation requires each medical device manufacturer (and PD) to establish, maintain, and follow a system that is appropriate for the specific medical device(s) to be produced or designed that is in compliance with the Federal regulation.

Europe requires a QS be established to meet the medical device regulations (and/or IVD regulations). Many medical device companies choose to implement a QS and have it certified to ISO 13485:2016 to satisfy EU needs. Fortunately, FDA 21 CFR Part 820 and ISO 13485 are very similar. ISO 13485:2016 is in one-to-one alignment with FDA 21 CFR Part 820.30 regarding design controls [15]. This means the entrepreneur can establish single QS fulfilling both sets of requirements.

While Canada requires a QS be established, it is somewhat different than the U.S or European approach. Canada requires ISO 13485:2016 certification, the Canadian Medical Devices Conformity Assessment System, and the Medical Device Single Audit Program.

Establishing a complete quality management system according to FDA and/or ISO can be a time-consuming process that may not add value to the efforts of the medical device start-up. Early on, it is not necessary to spend a lot of time implementing a robust system. Focus on the planning phase, focus on PD, and fill in the QS gaps as you get closer commercialization. The common expectation is that a start-up will have all parts and pieces defined and implemented by the time of commercialization. Many start-ups bootstrap their QS. Today, there are several software tools and services one can use to gradually implement the full QS. The need for policies and procedures is dependent upon the types of devices manufactured by the venture and the risks associated with their use. Management with executive responsibility has the responsibility for determining what is needed. Nonetheless, there are parts of the FDA regulations and ISO requirements that do apply in the premarket phase. As shown in Table 26.3, there are least four parts of QS that need to be in place (and followed) for medical device development [16].

In addition to procedures and work instructions necessary for the implementation of design controls, policies, and procedures may also be needed for other determinants of device quality that should be considered during the design process.

Product Development

Effective PD requires that all of the organizational groups involved develop and bring to bear the appropriate specialized capabilities and that the efforts be appropriately integrated. For most young, small organizations,

TABLE 26.3 Essential quality system components medical device development projects.

Section	Description
Design controls	• A systematic framework for capturing key aspects of medical device product development in order to prove the product meets user needs and is safe and effective • Traceability, an industry best practice, shows the relationship and linkages between all of your design controls. A traceability matrix is an invaluable tool to show a high-level view and the flow of product-development medical device from beginning to end. • How do user needs relate to design inputs? How do design outputs relate to design inputs? How do design verifications link to design inputs and design outputs? How do design validations relate to user needs?
Risk management	• The intent behind risk management is to identify, evaluate, analyze, assess, and mitigate potential product issues • Complementary to design control, risk management includes the analysis, documents, and records created during the design process to demonstrate that risks have been considered and steps taken to reduce their impact • Risk management is a key focus area of medical device regulators, thus risk management should be part of the entire product life cycle process
Document control and records management	• Establishing a system for managing your documentation and records is critical, not just for product development but throughout the life of your entrepreneurial venture • Define how documents get approved, how and where (physical or cloud-based services) revisions are maintained. Ensure product-development records are generated and maintained
Supplier management	• Most medical device ventures rely heavily on suppliers for many critical materials and processes. A supplier management process should define how suppliers are qualified, evaluated, monitored, and managed for specific materials and services

Source: Adapted from Wheelright and Clark, Exhibit 2-8, p. 47.

particularly those in the start-up phase, successful PD is an existential issue, with organizational success dependent on effective, efficient new product commercialization. The organization's structure and the role of the project manager are not burning issues. The entire organization is focused on a single major development project, and the CEO or some other senior executive serves as a strong project leader [17].

As part of development, it is important to define what performance measures will be used, why, and to consistently apply them to evaluate performance. Table 26.4 presents the examples of performance measures and their connection to competitiveness and medical devices. Taken together, time, quality, and productivity define the performance of development, and in combination with activities such as sales, manufacturing, advertising, and customer service determine the market impact of the project and its profitability [18].

Source: Adapted from Wheelright and Clark, Exhibit 2-8, p. 47.

Major Development Activities

As discussed earlier, all these development activities take place in a design control environment. Design control refers to a rigorous system of document review, verification, validation, approvals, and revision history maintenance. The specifications, documents, reviews, analysis, and test data produced during from this phase form a core of regulatory submissions, so expect scrutiny from FDA and other agency reviewers.

Fig. 26.2 illustrates the flow and linkage of the major development activities in a design control environment. Each shape represents a defined step. Squares are design-related activities. The triangles represent reviews and rectangles, verification and validation. An organization's QS should contain detailed procedural descriptions defining responsibilities, scope, and deliverables for each activity. Basically, requirements are developed, and a device is designed to meet those requirements. The design is then evaluated, transferred to production, and the device is manufactured. However, in practice, there are feedback paths between each step of the process as well as previous step phases, representing the iterative nature of PD.

In a traditional waterfall development methodology, engineers and designers complete the product design and formally transfer it to production. Subsequently, other groups develop processes to manufacture and service the product, leading to a potential for divergence between the designer's intent and production reality. As an alternative design methodology, concurrent engineering overcomes this deficiency by involving production and supports personnel throughout the design process. While the primary motivations of concurrent engineering are shorter development time and reduced production cost, the practical result is often improved the product quality. There are many PD methodologies, regardless of the approach used, demonstrating design controls as defined by FDA and ISO 13485 are still a requirement.

Design reviews—are snapshot evaluations of the medical device project as it progresses through development. Typically, design reviews occur after each step in the design control process as shown in Fig. 26.2. During design reviews, the project team formally reviews, and agrees to, design controls such as user needs, design inputs, design outputs, design verifications, and design

TABLE 26.4 Performance measures for medical product-development projects.

Dimension	Measures	Competitive impact	Medical device implications
Time-to-market	• Frequency of new product introductions • Time from initial concept to market introduction • Percent of sales coming from new products	• Responsiveness to customers/ competitors • Quality of design • Frequency of projects, model life	• Customer engagement • Innovative reputation
Productivity	• Personnel expense • Cost of materials and capital expenses • Actual versus plan	• Number of products—freshness and breadth of line • Frequency of projects, economics of development	• Operational efficiency
Quality	• Conformance, reliability in use • Design performance and customer satisfaction • Yield	• Reputation, customer loyalty • Relative attractiveness to customers, market share • Profitability, cost of ongoing product and/or service	• Patient safety • Customer satisfaction

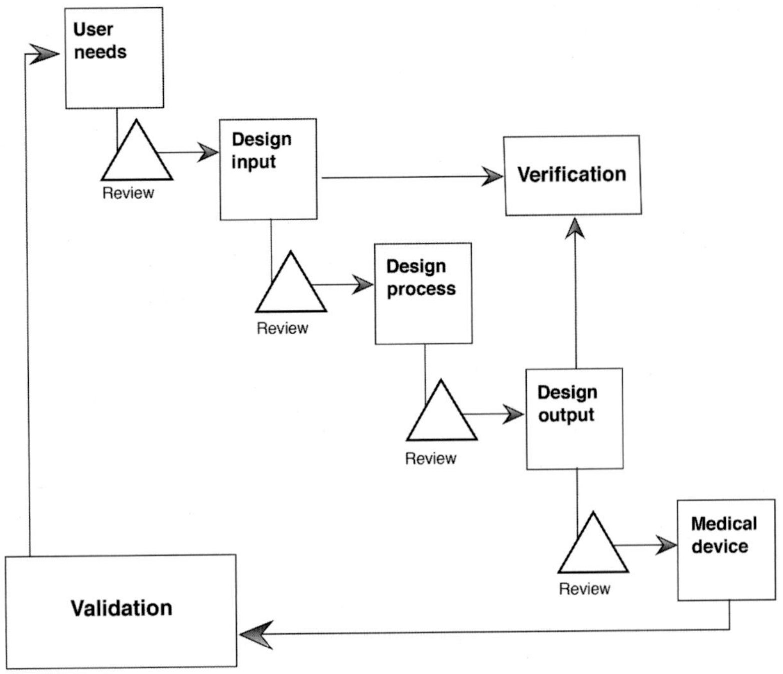

FIGURE 26.2 Design control process schematic. *Adapted from Food and Drug Administration, Center for Devices and Radiological Health. Design control guidance for medical device manufacturers; 1997.*

validations. Design reviews are also a time in a project to bring the team together in order to scrutinize and evaluate the state of the medical device and ensure that what needs to be done has been addressed. Design reviews should include the right functions (engineering, marketing, manufacturing, etc.) as well as an independent resource. For small entrepreneurial ventures, design reviews pose a problem since everyone in the organization is working on the same project and no one is "independent." One way to approach to solving the problem is to loan someone to another company in the same situation in return for them returning the favor. That way each company can have an independent reviewer. There should also be a record to demonstrate that design controls have been included as part of a design review, when it occurred the attendees and any deficiencies noted.

User needs—describe how a medical device is going to be used and helps one establish the framework for medical device design. Incorporating the results of the planning phase, user needs include the "intended use" that describes the clinical issue to be addressed and the device function, as well as the "indications for use" that pertain to clinical applications, diseases or conditions the medical device will diagnose, treat, prevent, or mitigate including a description of the target patient population and end user. They are an abstract description using broad statements about the intended use of a medical device using qualitative descriptions such as easy, better, and faster. User needs follow the vernacular of the end user, not engineering or marketing language. Later, during the verification, the entrepreneur will need to demonstrate that the developed product fulfills the user needs. The traceability matrix described earlier with the user needs that feed into design inputs. User needs is followed by a design review.

Design inputs—define all the performance criteria, requirements, and features of your medical device. This is often considered the foundation of the medical device development process [19]. Its importance to a successful device cannot be understated. There are numerous resources that feed into design inputs. From a design controls perspective the primary resource that feeds design inputs is the user needs that are precursor to design inputs. A traceability matrix should show how these are linked.

Design inputs should be objective and measurable, not qualitative. Crafting design inputs is an iterative process; the early versions may well include abstract terms, which are successively refined and made objective and measurable. Prototyping and bench testing are useful tools to make design inputs clear and objective. Design inputs should capture all functional, performance, safety, relevant industry standards, benchmarks from the previous projects or competitive products, and regulatory requirements (external) to build upon user needs and intended use to make them clear and objective.

The entrepreneur's goal should be to state design inputs in a way that allow them to be proven or disproved during design verification. Considering how to verify will have a profound impact on the content of design inputs. Taking design verification into consideration when defining design inputs will also help the entrepreneur's PD efforts. This approach will also help one plan and understand potential design verification activities, potentially saving time and money. Design inputs are followed by a design review.

Design process—represents the traditional detailed product engineering process and involves all tangible aspects of product design such as industrial and user interface design, definition and design of individual subsystems and components, software architecture and design, sterile or nonsterile packaging design, and user instructions (including multiple languages where needed). During this time, design teams will update the hazard analysis and risk assessment, striving to eliminate risks through a mitigation plan. Various traceability matrices will be prepared to enable top-down flow of requirements and bottom's up verification that each aspect of the design meets a stakeholder need. The design process is followed by a design review.

Design output—is the final stage of the design and development phase and refers to the totality of the work product produced. Design outputs are the complete recipe for making a medical device and should be of sufficient detail for someone to build the product. A final design review should be held to verify fidelity to the original user needs. Design outputs include, where applicable, system architecture, subsystems, components, software, assembly, testing, packaging, and the supply chain. Each of these parts items needs to be defined and documented using drawings, code, specifications, instructions, etc. The design outputs need to relate and link to the design inputs through a traceability matrix. Design outputs form the preliminary device master record. Design output is followed by a design review.

Design verification—is intended to demonstrate, or prove, that the design outputs fulfill the design inputs. It is an exercise to demonstrate correct product design. The traceability matrix plays an important role here as it should accurately show the relationship between your design inputs and design outputs. Design verification should be conducted following a written version-controlled verification plan specific for the medical device, it may incorporate a variety of methods including testing, inspection, and analysis. Once design verification activities are complete, document the results, identify any corrective actions required, and update the traceability matrix. Successful completion of design verification marks the time when the entrepreneur can complete and submit a regulatory submission as required by the path to market clearance. In the US, this submission may be a FDA 510(k) application or an FDA investigational device exemption submission. Outside the United States, regulatory submissions and files, such as CE Mark Technical Files, are provided to regulatory bodies upon completion of design validation. Design verification is followed by a design review.

Design validation—is intended to prove a medical device is correct by demonstrating that it meets user needs and its intended uses (see outer loop in Fig. 26.2) [20]. The end goal of design validation is to have objective, documented evidence that the user needs are met. To accomplish this, first prepare a written, version-controlled design validation plan that identifies how many end users and what type of testing are required. Finished products are needed to complete design validation; therefore design transfer, the process of transferring a medical device from PD to production, begins during design validation. The finished products for design validation should be built using production equivalent materials, documentation, and processes. Thus the design outputs (preliminary DMR) are converted to the production documentation and used by production personnel to assemble finished products for end users to test. Completing design validation is an important step in closing the loop on the traceability matrix that started with user needs and ends with design validation. Once design validation activities are complete, document the results, identify any corrective actions required, and update the traceability matrix. Design validation is followed by a design review.

Design transfer—begins when finished products are built for design validation. Completion of the activity that demonstrates a medical device is ready to exit PD and officially enter into production. This is a significant milestone where the "control" of the medical device shifts from the project team to production resources. After completing design transfer the DHF becomes the ultimate record to prove design controls were satisfied. Design transfer is followed by a design review, whose goal is to make sure everything that is needed for the production is ready and done prior to market launch.

Market launch—after completing a design transfer design review, and verifying that all necessary regulatory clearances are in place, the entrepreneur is ready for market launch. This event is a major milestone for any medical device company, but it is especially critical for entrepreneurial ventures because it marks a major lifecycle transition from premarket to generating sales revenue. How the venture attracts and retains customers, develops pricing strategies, and maintains an efficient supply chain to ensure continuity of production are all important considerations beyond the scope of this chapter.

Resources

Entrepreneurs developing new medical devices can find a wealth of informative resources covering topics ranging from grants and public policy initiatives, to reimbursement and potential injection molding suppliers. This section describes several resources the author has used and found to be helpful.

The Advanced Medical Technology Association (AdvaMed)—is a membership-based global trade association that leads the effort to advance medical technology in order to achieve healthier lives and healthier economies around the world. AdvaMed's membership has over 400 members [21]. Historically, AdvaMed membership comprises established medical device companies. Exploring their website, entrepreneurs will find content relating to the public policy and regulatory aspects of medical devices.

Association for the Advancement of Medical Instrumentation (AAMI)—is a membership-based organization, which is the primary source of consensus standards for the medical device industry, as well as practical information, support, and guidance for health-care technology and sterilization professionals. The AAMI standards program consists of more than 100 technical committees and working groups that produce Standards, Recommended Practices, and Technical Information Reports for medical devices. Many Standards and Recommended Practices have been approved by the American National Standards Institute as American National Standards. AAMI also administers a number of international technical committees of the International Organization for Standardization (ISO) and the International Electrotechnical Commission, as well as the US Technical Advisory Groups [22].

Centers for disease control and prevention (CDC) [23]—is the leading Federal government agency tasked with protecting and improving public health. The CDC website contains a wealth of information and statistics that are helpful to entrepreneurs. For example, one can look up a disease condition and relatively quickly identify key facts: prevalence, incidence, underlying causes, and treatments [24]. The high-quality data provided free by the CDC can help entrepreneurs better assess new product opportunities and provide important references for business plans and investor presentations.

Crunchbase [25]—is an online platform for finding business information about private and public companies, including investments and funding information. Crunchbase offers some free content but users will hit a paywall pretty quickly. Nonetheless, it is a very useful information source on companies that have been financed as well as their investors for the medical device entrepreneur. The author uses this website often to develop lists of target investors for specific business opportunities.

Fierce Biotech [26]—is an online news source focused on the biotech industry, including medical devices. Fierce Biotech covers the business side of the industry with an emphasis on financing, mergers and acquisitions, and public policy.

FDA—the FDA's website contains a wealth of information for medical device developers. Medical devices fall under the Center for Devices and Radiological Health. The trade-off is that information can sometimes be hard to find. Nonetheless, this should be a first and frequent stop for entrepreneurs looking for background information on regulations, fees, guidance documents, webinars, and other industry-related events [27].

Grants.gov [28]—serves as the US Federal clearing house for funding opportunities from its agencies and is the first place to look for possible grant and contract funding news. In addition to a searchable database of sources and opportunities, the site contains significant educational materials covering the relevant topics essential to preparation and submission of grant applications. There is now a corresponding mobile application that allows a user to set up alerts and rapidly screen for opportunities of interest.

MedCity News—is an online news source for the business of health-care innovation [29].

Medical Device Manufacturers Association (MDMA)—was created in 1992 by a group of medical device company executives who believed that the innovative and entrepreneurial sector of the industry needed a strong and independent voice in the nation's capital. Since its inception, MDMA can claim credit for a number of policy achievements, from the defeat of legislative proposals to foist "user fees" upon the industry in 1993 and 1994 to the development and passage of the landmark FDA Modernization Act of 1997 [30].

Medical Device Daily—is a paid subscription newsletter, which has morphed from a print publication to a daily email report and is now published under the name *BioWorld Medtech* [31]. Its focus is on industry news, policy, M&A across major subsectors, for example, cancer, orthopedics, and cardiovascular.

National Institutes of Health (NIH) [32]—is part of the US Department of Health and Human Services. NIH is the largest biomedical research agency in the world and a significant funding source for academic research and entrepreneurial ventures through the Small Business Innovation Research (SBIR) and Small Business Technology Transfer (STTR) set-aside. The NIH is comprised 27 institutes or centers each with a specific research agenda, often focusing on particular diseases or body systems. Each institute and center publishes its research priorities annually. Entrepreneurs should seriously investigate NIH grant and contract opportunities. Many early stage ventures have received NIH funding long before they were ready for venture investors.

National Science Foundation (NSF) [33]—is an independent US Federal agency created to promote the progress of science. NSF has a broad mission that includes many scientific and engineering fields. The website contains an extensive list of funding opportunities by topic area that medical device entrepreneurs should investigate as possible sources. One can also find information about prior awards for each funding topic; this can help to identify collaborators and or competitors for further assessment. In addition to its standard grant and contract mechanisms, NIH participates in the SBIR/STTR programs.

Small Business Administration (SBA) [34]—helps Americans start, build, and grow businesses. The SBA is an independent agency of the Federal government focused on the interests of small business concerns. Among its many program the SBIR and STTR are highly relevant for medical device entrepreneurs [35]. Each year, thousands of small businesses receive SBIR and/or STTR awards from the participating agencies, including the Department of Health and Human Services (which includes CDC, FDA, and NIH), Department of Defense, National Aeronautics and Space Agency, and the NSF. The mission of each agency includes solving problems addressed by medical devices and their underlying technologies.

Szycher's Dictionary of Medical Devices [36]—is a compact reference book, while somewhat dated, provides a useful listing of known medical devices and their regulatory classification. It is a good starting point for further investigation.

References

[1] CFR—Code of Federal Regulations title 21 [Internet]. Accessdata.fda.gov [cited February 10, 2019]. Available from: <https://www.accessdata.fda.gov/scripts/cdrh/cfdocs/cfCFR/CFRSearch.cfm>.

[2] Is the product a medical device? [Internet]. Fda.gov [cited February 10, 2019]. Available from: <https://www.fda.gov/MedicalDevices/DeviceRegulationandGuidance/Overview/ClassifyYourDevice/ucm051512.htm>.

[3] Deloitte. 2019 Global health care outlook; 2019. p. 7.

[4] Deloitte. 2019 Global health care outlook; 2019. p. 4.

[5] Ernst & Young. Pulse of the industry 2018; 2018. p. 13.

[6] Premarket approval (PMA) [Internet]. Accessdata.fda.gov [cited February 10, 2019]. Available from: <https://www.accessdata.fda.gov/scripts/cdrh/cfdocs/cfPMA/pma.cfm>.

[7] Pitchbook Inc. and the National Venture Capital Association. Venture Monitor 4Q 2018 [Internet]; 2019. p. 19–20. Available from: <https://pitchbook.com/news/reports/4q-2018-pitchbook-nvca-venture-monitor>.

[8] Medical technology industry spotlight | SelectUSA.gov [Internet]. Selectusa.gov [cited February 10, 2019]. Available from: <https://www.selectusa.gov/medical-technology-industry-united-states>.

[9] Perriello B. Mazor robotics acquired by Medtronic in $1.7B deal [Internet]. The robot report; 2018 [cited March 19, 2019]. Available from: <https://www.therobotreport.com/medtronic-17b-mazor-robotics/>.

[10] Deloitte. 2019 Global health care outlook; 2019. p. 9.

[11] Barquet Ana Paula B, et al. Business model elements for product-service system. Functional thinking for value creation. Berlin Heidelberg: Springer; 2011. p. 332–7.

[12] Maurya A. Running lean: iterate from plan A to a plan that works. In: The lean series. 2nd ed. Sebastopol, CA: O'Reilly; 2012 [2010]. p. 12.

[13] Pricing Plans | LEANSTACK [Internet]; 2019. Leanstack.com [cited March 18, 2019]. Available from: <https://leanstack.com/pricing>.

[14] Food and Drug Administration, Center for Devices and Radiological Health. Design control guidance for medical device manufacturers; 1997.

[15] Speer J. The ultimate guide to design controls for medical device companies [Internet]; 2018. Greenlight.guru. [cited March 19, 2019]. Available from: <https://www.greenlight.guru/blog/design-controls#quality-system>.

[16] Speer J. 4 QMS musts for medical device startup—Creo Quality [Internet]. Creo Quality; 2015 [cited March 19, 2019]. Available from: <https://creoquality.com/quality-system-2/4-qms-musts-medical-device-startup/>.

[17] Wheelwright S, Clark K. [u.a.] Revolutionizing product development. New York: Free Press; 1992. p. 198.

[18] Wheelwright S, Clark K. [u.a.] Revolutionizing product development. New York: Free Press; 1992. p. 47.

[19] Speer L. The art of medical device design inputs [Internet]; 2015 [cited March 18, 2019]. Available from: <https://www.meddeviceonline.com/doc/the-art-of-medical-device-design-inputs-0001>.

[20] Speer J. The ultimate guide to design controls for medical device companies [Internet]; 2018. Greenlight.guru. [cited March 20, 2019]. Available from: <https://www.greenlight.guru/blog/design-controls#design-transfer>.

[21] AdvaMed | [Internet]; 2018. Advamed.org. [cited February 10, 2019]. Available from: <https://www.advamed.org/>.

[22] Association for the advancement of medical instrumentation [Internet]. Aami.org. [cited February 10, 2019]. Available from: <http://www.aami.org/>.

[23] Centers for Disease Control and Prevention. CDC works 24/7 [Internet]. [cited March 14, 2019]. Available from: <https://www.cdc.gov/>.

[24] Heart disease facts & statistics | cdc.gov [Internet]; 2017. Cdc.gov. [cited March 14, 2019]. Available from: <https://www.cdc.gov/heartdisease/facts.htm>.

[25] Discover innovative companies and the people behind them [Internet]; 2019. Available from: <https://www.crunchbase.com> [cited March 14, 2019].

[26] Biotech industry, biotech news, biotechnology articles—FierceBiotech [Internet]; 2019. Fiercebiotech.com. [cited March 13, 2019]. Available from: <https://www.fiercebiotech.com/>.

[27] Medical devices [Internet]; 2019. Fda.gov. [cited February 10, 2019]. Available from: <https://www.fda.gov/MedicalDevices/default.htm>.

[28] Home | GRANTS.GOV [Internet]. Grants.gov. [cited March 21, 2019]. Available from: <https://www.grants.gov/>.

[29] Parmar A, Baum S, DeArment A, Dietsche E, Truong K. MedCity news—healthcare technology news, life science current events [Internet]. MedCity News 2019 [cited March 6, 2019]. Available from: <https://medcitynews.com/>.

[30] Publications—Medical Device Manufacturers Association (MDMA) [Internet]. Medicaldevices.site-ym.com. [cited February 10, 2019]. Available from: <https://medicaldevices.site-ym.com/page/Publications>.

[31] BioWorld MedTech. The Daily Medical Technology Newspaper [Internet]; 2018. Medicaldevicedaily.com. [cited February 10, 2019]. Available from: <http://www.medicaldevicedaily.com/>.
[32] National Institutes of Health (NIH) [Internet]. [cited March 13, 2019]. Available from: <https://www.nih.gov/>.
[33] NSF—National Science Foundation [Internet]. Nsf.gov. [cited March 13, 2019]. Available from: <https://www.nsf.gov/>.
[34] Small Business Administration [Internet]. [cited March 14, 2019]. Available from: <https://www.sba.gov/>.
[35] SBIR.gov [Internet]. Sbir.gov. [cited March 14, 19]. Available from: https://www.sbir.gov/.
[36] Szycher M. Szycher's dictionary of medical devices. Lancaster, PA: Technomic; 1995.

Chapter 27

Commercialization and Applications of Agricultural Biotechnology

Neal Gutterson, PhD

Corteva Agrisciences, Johnston, Iowa, United States

Chapter Outline

It wasn't long after the early therapeutic biotechnology companies were founded that creative entrepreneurs began to develop agricultural applications of biotechnology. Not dissuaded by the lack of applicable technology, the first companies that developed biotechnology-derived crops were founded, even though methods for delivering stable DNA into plants had yet to be explored. The year 1983 witnessed a major breakthrough when the first patent applications were filed on *Agrobacterium*-mediated delivery of DNA into dicotyledonous plants. *Agrobacterium* is a soil microbe commonly used to transfer DNA into dicotyledonous (a broad-leaved plant such as soybean and cotton) and monocotyledonous plants (a narrow-leaved plant such as corn or wheat). More importantly, broad patent applications for DNA delivery into monocotyledonous plants (such as corn, rice, and grasses) were not filed until the early 1990s.

At that time, I was finishing a postdoc at University of California, Berkeley and was interested in joining this emerging industry that was not yet a popular route for promising Ph.D. students in biochemistry. While I was very engaged with this emerging field and wanted to have an impact on this very practical problem, I would not have considered myself an entrepreneur. I simply wanted to apply science to solving pressing global challenges. I was influenced by the writings of Rachel Carson, whose *Silent Spring* [1] spoke to me, inspiring me to replace agricultural chemistries with biological solutions; whether with microbes that used natural mechanisms for controlling diseases in plants, or plants engineered to resist disease by direct gene introduction. In hindsight, perhaps, I was more entrepreneurial than I realized at first because I later left the safer academic environment of basic research to join this new wave of science that could impact agriculture in ways yet unknown.

I spent the first 5 years of my career working at Advanced Genetic Sciences finding ways to improve microbial fungicides—specifically, fluorescent pseudomonads that colonize plant roots to reduce seedling diseases using genetic engineering. During this time, my company and I ran up against difficult and increasingly complex regulatory systems, as well as public concerns for our products, which killed a promising application for improved microbial fungicides.

From the early 1980s through the mid-1990s, I evolved from a scientist in an industrial environment into a full-blooded entrepreneur who was comfortable with the nexus of business and science, patents and products, basic

Biotechnology Entrepreneurship. DOI: https://doi.org/10.1016/B978-0-12-815585-1.00027-9

research, and applied outcomes. I grew to know the agricultural biotechnology (Ag Biotech) landscape intimately, working in a company that competed with teams at Monsanto and collaborated with teams at DuPont and Rohm and Haas. Those were heady days in which many of us talked about how we could change the world, change global agriculture, and do it quickly. As with any new technology, the world was not as ready as we, the developers, were for our first products. This is because Ag Biotech is a slow and cautious business serving naturally conservative farmers. Nonetheless, biotechnology has put its mark on agriculture and will continue to do so in even more diverse ways. My hope is that at least one reader of this chapter will recognize some intriguing opportunities and challenges and apply themselves to changing the face of global agriculture.

What Is Agricultural Biotechnology?

Throughout the 1980s and 1990s the focus of most Ag Biotech entrepreneurs was the creation of new ways to genetically engineer crops to protect them against insects (insect resistance) and to make them more hardy in the presence of weed-killing chemicals (herbicide tolerance). Throughout much of the later 1990s and the 2000s, this focus continued along with the creation of biotech "traits" such as increased yield, stress tolerance, and increased nitrogen-use efficiency. Many small companies and entrepreneurs were instrumental in the development of these traits, although it was the large chemical and seed companies that brought these new products to the market. Monsanto emerged as the leading developer of Ag Biotech trait products as they quickly recognized and commercialized valuable technologies that enabled them to be a market leader, disrupting the crop-protection market, leading to major shifts in value from crop-protection companies to seed companies.

Biotechnology has many different product applications aside from the creation of new medicines and drugs. When we talk about Ag Biotech, broadly writ, we are speaking of any application that impacts crop production as opposed to processing of the resulting grain or biomass that is the domain of *industrial* biotechnology.

The groups that serve crop production with new products that enhance or preserve the value of the crop include three major sectors (see Fig. 27.1):

1. **The seed sector**
2. **The agrochemical sector**
3. **The fertilizer sector**

The seed, fertilizer, and chemical products commercialized by these companies are purchased by growers to assure maximum value from their land.

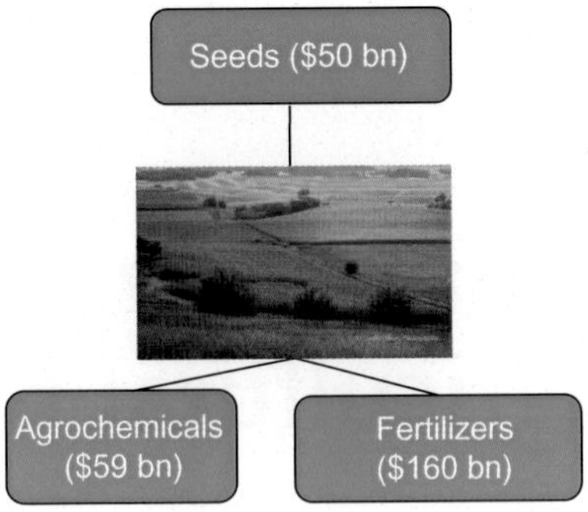

FIGURE 27.1 The estimated size of the three principal Ag Biotech sectors. *Ag Biotech*, Agricultural biotechnology.

The Seed Sector

The seed sector, through differentiation and patent protection, can secure reliable product price premiums, and as a result, it was the first sector to attract investor interest from the very beginning of the Ag Biotech industry in the early 1980s. The companies in this sector focus on producing and selling the seeds of crops such as corn, soybean, canola, and cotton. Conventional varieties are improved regularly through advanced breeding systems enabled by biotechnology tools to combine alleles of small effect for yield and other major traits. Biotech varieties benefit from incorporation of large-effect traits such as insect control and herbicide tolerance, with biotech traits delivered through constructs integrated into the genome of the crop.

The Agrochemical Sector

The agrochemical sector produces value-added products of great interest to growers, but the successful application of biotechnology to the development of novel agrochemical products has been much slower to materialize. Crop Solutions, founded by Erik Ward and Scott Uknes, was one of the few start-up companies that focused on the crop-protection sector. Paradigm Genetics, led by John Ryals, focused on novel herbicide targets in collaboration with Bayer CropScience, a combination of a biotech-trait (herbicide-tolerance traits) and crop-protection strategies, with novel herbicides based on new targets for herbicide screening. With the crossover between pharmaceutical and agricultural applications of technologies for screening novel chemistries, we are seeing increased interest in the application of biotechnology to chemical discovery today, by companies such as Enko Chem and Agrimetis. Applications of technology companies focused more on pharmaceuticals, but expanding to agriculture for drug discovery, Ginkgo Bioworks, Trana Discovery, and Evogene are additional examples.

The Fertilizer Sector

Fertilizers are generally commodity products and receive very little impact from biotechnology. The crop-protection sector has deployed biotechnology methods but without significant change to product categories to date, in contrast to the seed sector with the introduction of biotech traits. The commercial and financial values of these products are determined in part by the regulatory framework for the approval in each sector and the potential for incorporating added value, as opposed to commodity products, which in turn determines the product margins and the entrepreneurial focus.

New Ag Biotech markets are emerging that are likely to rapidly increase entrepreneurial opportunities within the broader agrochemical sector. The potential of effective live biological and natural products is reenergizing this market for the first time since it was explored in the 1980s. Finally, the fertilizer sector is a commodity industry with little application to date of biotechnology and has limited scope for entrepreneurs today. However, there is emerging interest in new ways to make nitrogen available to crops using engineered microbes, which, if successful, could be disruptive to the fertilizer industry and open up a new wave of entrepreneurship. One example is Pivot Bio, a San Francisco Bay Area–based company that is applying pathway engineering to improve the release of nitrogen by microbes that naturally can generate

Regulation of Agricultural Biotechnology

Ag Biotech is possibly a greater challenge for entrepreneurs than medical biotechnology—an entrepreneurial challenge of its own. The time to market for Ag Biotech products in the category of biotech traits is just as long as in medical biotechnology but the payout is not as compelling. Blockbuster products in the Ag Biotech sector are rare and perhaps equate to only 10% the value of blockbuster drugs. However, the inherent competitive advantages of major players in Ag Biotech are stronger than even those of major pharmaceutical companies. This is because biotech traits represent an inherent characteristic of a plant variety, and therefore need to be tested in a company's proprietary *germplasm* and brought to the market by that company as part of its overall product offering. Germplasm refers to a seed or a plant part such as a leaf, a stem, pollen, or even a few cells that can be turned into a whole plant. Germplasm contains the information for a species' genetic makeup and therefore can be a barrier to entry for companies with outstanding germplasm libraries.

In the United States, the regulatory environment for Ag Biotech traits can be challenging to manage, with potentially three following federal agencies involved in the product approval:

1. The Environmental Protection Agency (EPA)
2. The Department of Agriculture (USDA)
3. The Food and Drug Administration (FDA)

In addition to cultivation approvals within a country, export market regulatory processes can be highly variable in different geographies and costly to manage. In addition to these regulatory challenges, the biotech trait path is fraught with risk and uncertainty given the public's adverse perceptions of biotech traits in much of the world, often driven by scientifically misinformed nongovernmental organizations (NGOs), organic growers, marketers, etc. Today, we also see emerging brands that cast a GMO (Genetically Modified Organism) as an undesirable product—such as the butterfly brand of the non-GMO project that labels even water as non-GMO. Unwarranted fears about the safety of Ag Biotech products have made it nearly impossible for small companies to compete in the biotech trait business today. As a result, the Ag Biotech trait entrepreneurial ecosystem is small and fragile compared with the medical biotechnology entrepreneurial ecosystem. For instance, rather than having thousands of small biotech companies (such as in the life sciences sector) working in an ecosystem with 20–30 large pharmaceutical companies able to partner and fund early-stage R&D, we find perhaps 20–30 small Ag Biotech companies with only 5 large integrated agricultural seed and crop-protection companies with the ability to fund early-stage R&D. While there is some outsourcing of discovery for Ag as there is for pharma, the transfer of much discovery to an entrepreneurial ecosystem of small companies that exist today in pharma has not emerged to a similar extent in Ag. As a result, there are fewer investors in the Ag Biotech trait market compared to the life science biotechnology market.

In addition, over the past decade, biotech traits have proven to be ever more complicated to bring to the market, even for large companies. Regulatory uncertainty has increased, and despite the expiration of some seminal patents, the intellectual property (IP) landscape remains very complex. Due to the successes of the past 25 years, a new trait must be combined (stacked) with the previous traits that already have become foundational products, and this trait must be introduced into specialized germplasm, making it much more difficult for a small company to bring a new trait to the market. With the even longer time—as of 2019, compared with 1994—to bring a trait to the market from initial conception and testing—closer to 15 years than 10 years—the opportunity for entrepreneurs to build new companies that focused on the trait market has been diminished. The key bottleneck is access to the proprietary germplasm in which a new trait must be tested and validated. This means that biotech trait development is more and more the province of major seed companies, with limited but interesting impact of small companies. One compelling example is Okanagan Specialty Fruits, founded by Neal Carter, to bring non-browning apples to the market using biotechnology. The Arctic apple is now beginning scaling phase in the market, following the acquisition of Okanagan by Intrexon in 2015.

Does that mean there is little opportunity for Ag Biotech entrepreneurs today? Not at all. There is a tremendous amount of investment in companies deploying biotechnology in agriculture, along with venture investment more broadly in technologies applied to agriculture. Investors and entrepreneurs are focused on ways to use biotechnology and genomics to create new technologies needed by large companies and new products that improve the crop production or crop protection. The financing of the start-up company AgBiome in 2013 demonstrated that biological products, such as live microbes that can colonize plant roots, which can come to the market in less than 5 years with quite limited regulatory requirements compared to Ag biotech traits, offer a new direction for bioentrepreneurs. The recognition of the importance of the human microbiome has triggered increased interest in crop microbiomes—the collection of microbes that stably interact with plant root or leaf surfaces. Pam Marrone was able to bring her company, Marrone Bio Innovations, to the public market in 2013 based on the same basic proposition of a short and low-cost path to the market (4–5 years and less than $10 million) and microbial and plant extracts that provide crop-protection benefits. The application of biotechnology is primarily in tools for the discovery of products that are not then improved through the use of biotechnology, though biotechnology is certainly being applied in some cases such as Pivot Bio. BioConsortia also is applying modern biotechnology to the discovery of new microbial consortia that foster improved crop performance.

One new Ag Biotech opportunity is the identification of natural products that improve crop productivity using high-throughput biotechnology-developed screens based on genomic insights. Delivery of benefits can be through commercialization of microbial extracts containing those natural products, or of purified and even improved versions of the natural products. Mendel Biotechnology's biologicals research business for discovery and development of natural product extracts was acquired by Koch Agronomic Services in 2014. As with biopesticidal products, their development has a short and low-cost path to the market, and testing and launch of these products do not require access to proprietary germplasm or prior generations of biotech traits.

The application of biotechnology, particularly genomics and "synthetic biology," to the discovery of natural products and to the improvement of the production of those natural products has emerged as a well-funded field. This is a very powerful example of the leverage to agriculture of approaches developed initially focused on the more valuable pharmaceuticals opportunity. This can be seen through the partnership struck between Gingko and Bayer, and the work of Zymergen and other pathway engineering companies.

Another example of using biotechnology to create new products is Ag Biotech start-up Kaiima, a company creating polyploid (having more than two copies of each chromosome, such as 4 or 6) versions of crops that have higher yields with more robust growth and development capabilities. Investors have shown favorable interest in the entrepreneurs with these ideas.

So gird your loins those of you who plan to embark on the Ag Biotech entrepreneurial road! Keep a thick skin and a strong heart. Focus on the great opportunity to help feed, fuel, and clothe the 21st century. Be willing to learn. Be highly focused, and yet be highly flexible, especially with the business model needed to generate value from a new technology. Be as willing to experiment with your business model as you are with your technology. More likely than not the original business model pursued will not be your final and successful business model you use. Often, even the best applications of your technology are not the original ones you started out trying to develop.

Ag Biotech already has a dramatic impact on reducing the costs of producing food around the planet. More than half of all growers using biotech products are in the developing world today [2]! With this in mind, let's turn now to a brief review of the Ag Biotech product-development process and associated challenges, the past accomplishments of the industry, and the opportunities that lie ahead for AgBio entrepreneurs.

The Agricultural Biotechnology Trait Commercialization Process

Early in the life of the biopharmaceutical industry, investors acquired an understanding of the stages involved in the development of new biotechnology-based drugs and the risks associated with each stage and process. The Ag Biotech industry consolidated views for a similar product-development process in the early 2000s, in part to help investors understand the risk profile of biotech trait products and the reduction in risk (see Fig. 27.2). Although similar terminology was adopted for Ag Biotech product development, the overall risk profile at each respective phase is not equivalent. This was important both for large companies defining their future product pipeline value as

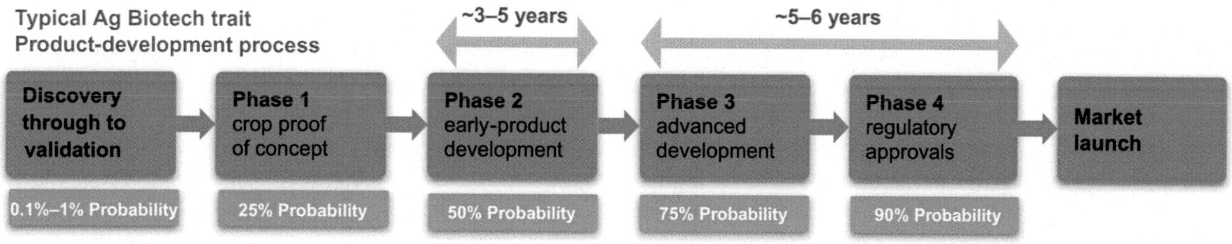

FIGURE 27.2 The typical agricultural biotechnology development cycle for the introduction of a novel biotech trait. *Phillips McDougal.*

well as for small companies seeking investment from either corporate partners or venture investors.

Discovery Through to Validation

Biotech trait development begins with a discovery phase using many different research strategies to drive that process. Genomics applications in the 2000s included the extensive use of *Arabidopsis*, a small weed with a short time required to produce seed and a small genome, adopted broadly as the white rat of plant science. This model plant was used for testing various DNA constructs for positive benefits in first-generation traits such as herbicide tolerance and insect resistance, and particularly for potential second-generation traits such as yield improvement, stress tolerance, nutrient use, and other properties. Many research strategies successfully contributed to the selection of genes to be tested.

Phase 1 Testing

With a positive result during validation, these product ideas (i.e., trait candidates) move on to Phase 1. This involves testing the same or similar construct in a target crop such as corn or soybean, first in the greenhouse then in small field plots. A number of different transgenic events (each a specific location in the genome for the delivered construct) are created in the target crop, and these events are evaluated to determine the likely benefit of the resulting biotech trait. At this stage the likelihood that a particular trait candidate will be commercialized is less than 25%. Once confirmation of that desired trait (e.g., tolerance to drought, herbicide tolerance, or better use of a nutrient) is obtained at small scale, the product moves to Phase 2.

Phase 2 Testing

Phase 2 includes testing a recombinant DNA construct that conferred the trait in the target crop with a much larger number of individual transgenic events in commercial target varieties and with a construct that could pass all regulatory hurdles. With sufficient confidence in commercial performance, regulatory studies would also be initiated to begin to understand if there would be any regulatory impediments to commercial deployment of the trait. At this stage, the likelihood of commercial success increased to 50%. With the initial regulatory studies in hand, and selection of one or a few events that could be commercial based on molecular analysis of the integrated transgene, the product moves to Phase 3.

Phase 3 Testing

Phase 3 includes larger scale field trials in many locations in major target markets such as the United States, and South American locations, allowing two sets of field trials per growing season, as well as the opportunity to explore each attractive market. During the Phase 3 testing, the selected events are also introduced into a wider set of commercial varieties (i.e., a diverse genetic selection of the company's germplasm) for that large-scale testing. Unlike drug development, in which Phase 3 failures are *not unusual*, failure of an Ag Biotech trait in Phase 3 is relatively *uncommon*, with a 75% likelihood of success ascribed to this phase of development.

Ultimately, regulatory approval processes are conducted during the development of Phases 2 and 3 of novel biotech traits. Depending upon the functions of the trait and the crop in which it is deployed, as many as three different agencies may be involved in the United States alone: the EPA, the USDA, and the FDA. In addition, since grain or other products from crops grown in the United States are exported to other countries, and of course major crops are grown in many other countries, regulatory approval in other countries is needed prior to the commercial launch of a new biotech trait for the production in the United States.

Phase 4 Testing

Finally, during Phase 4, regulatory submissions are made in multiple countries, including countries where the crop is grown and those countries that will receive products by importing the resulting grain or oil. The events are introduced into the commercial varieties for launch, and seed is produced in large amounts preparing for the product launch. The probability of success in Phase 4, precommercial testing, is generally estimated at 90%. The benefits of the trait product are communicated to the market broadly and to growers specifically in the Phase 4 run-up to commercial launch.

While the development process as shown in Fig. 27.2 is particularly applicable to a biotech trait itself, a similar process would apply to other Ag Biotech products derived through the use of biotechnology. The application of exogenous RNAi molecules (short duplex RNA molecules of 21–24 nucleotides that trigger gene silencing in eukaryotic organisms) to control pests has been developed by DevGen (acquired in 2012 by Syngenta) and some other companies. Testing of such pest-targeting RNAi requires a related and lengthy development process, with RNAi treatments first conducted with pests directly, then on crops in glasshouse tests prior to testing in crops in small-scale field trials and large-scale trials in diverse environments. The regulatory process required of novel RNAi molecules is still in development globally.

Agricultural Biotechnology Product Commercialization

The wave of investments from strategic investors and some private companies in the late 1990s and early 2000s focused on the earliest phases of the development process, primarily discovery through validation, and then in some cases, proof-of-concept demonstration in relevant target crops. Companies such as Mendel, Ceres, and Paradigm all ran high-throughput processes of genomics-driven discovery, using primarily *Arabidopsis* as a system for testing novel-trait constructs. In most cases, these constructs used one or more different promoter sequences to program expression of a wide range of different gene sequences from *Arabidopsis* or crop plants. The premise during the earliest days of the genomics era was that although all the large companies understood the trait targets (such as increased stress tolerance, increased yield, increased nitrogen-use efficiency), these companies often lacked the correct genes whose expression could be modified in plants to effect these improvements. Rather than applying an academic style research program to dissect the molecular basis for a trait or process and then using that knowledge to engineer crop improvement, an unbiased approach to high-throughput screening was adopted throughout the industry. This was much like a land grab, a rapid phase of investment to secure critical IP positions, much like when the rail industry secured important physical locations for expansion in the mid-1800s.

The value associated with this early-stage validation would ultimately be paid to these companies via milestones and royalties upon product sales in the future. Of course, most genes that pass early-stage validation still failed in later testing. The probability of success slowly increases with additional crop testing in greenhouses, then small-plot field testing, then broad-acre field testing in multiple locations. Similar to the biopharmaceutical-development process, where failure of a promising drug may result from variable performance in different (human) genetic backgrounds, or variable toxicity occurring in different (human) genetic backgrounds, failure of promising leads for biotech traits such as improved yield or stress tolerance would often occur due to either variable performances in different (crop) genetic backgrounds or in different environments or climates. Major companies invested heavily in new biotech trait-testing pipelines with a goal of identifying successful product candidates as quickly as possible, through testing in multiple geographies and crop-variety backgrounds.

The earliest products of the Ag Biotech industry were herbicide-tolerance and insect-resistance traits based on bacterial protein sequences, such as an EPSPS gene (encoding 5-enolpyruvylshikimate-3-phosphate synthase, an early enzyme of aromatic acid synthesis) from *Agrobacterium* and insect toxin genes from *Bacillus thuringiensis*. These products were revolutionary and grower adoption followed very quickly. The EPSPS gene resistant to Monsanto's herbicide glyphosate (RoundUp) enabled the rapid expansion in the use of glyphosate, an herbicide with excellent environmental, and performance properties. Until the introduction of the first RoundUp Ready trait in soybean in 1996 based on the resistant form of the EPSPS gene, glyphosate was a nonselective herbicide that could not be used in the major crops such as soybean or corn. In these major crops, glyphosate replaced older herbicides with less-desirable properties, including environmental persistence. These other herbicides rapidly lost market share after RoundUp Ready products made growers' lives much simpler. A range of different insect toxin genes enabled the replacement of synthetic insecticides applied to a crop with a crop that produced its own highly effective insecticidal activity, and ones with very good safety profiles.

These herbicide-tolerance and insect-resistance trait products performed well in a diverse set of genetic backgrounds and environments, though these traits still required rounds of development to minimize the impact on yields of elite germplasm. This has contrasted with the lower probability of success for yield and stress-tolerance traits, due to required interaction with plant proteins from within an endogenous crop genome for improved crop performance. Herbicide- and insect-resistance traits are not as difficult to engineer as other desirable traits, such as enhanced-yield and stress-tolerance traits, which are analogous to installing a radio in an automobile without one. In comparison, new-yield and stress-tolerance traits require reengineering of existing functional plant systems that govern stress tolerance, analogous to trying to engineer existing automobile systems—such as engines and transmissions. While small entrepreneurial companies have the wherewithal to conduct laboratory and even some greenhouse screening in *Arabidopsis* or a well-studied crop such as rice (e.g., Crop Design did), they do not have the financial resources to conduct the large-scale field trials required in the development of Phases 2 and 3 that parallel the large-scale human drug trials in similar phases of a therapeutic development program. Companies such as Evogene and Arcadia operate in these earlier stages of discovery and early development today, and they adopt diverse business partnership strategies to capture market value. Given the much reduced overall value of even a high-value product (perhaps 10–30-fold less than a blockbuster drug), financial investors have traditionally been less interested in backing such efforts in Ag compared to pharma. As a result, small companies remained largely dependent upon the large seed companies for the financing of field testing; and therefore greater value would accrue to the large seed companies rather than the small companies who initially discovered exciting new leads.

The overall regulatory approval process has become more cumbersome and complex on a global level over the past 20 years than we might have imagined when the industry emerged in the 1980s, or when the first RoundUp Ready soybean product was launched in 1996. As a result, successful entrepreneurs need to have a committed strategic partner, and probably have already been bought by them, before a trait they have initiated can come to the market. This is particularly true for the second-generation biotech traits of yield increase, stress tolerance, and nutrient-use efficiency, which are more complex to test than the earlier traits of herbicide-tolerance or insect-resistance traits. Companies that pioneered such approaches, such as Mendel Biotechnology and Ceres, eventually struggled and failed in these efforts given the difficulty of delivering reliable performance of these traits across environment and germplasm diversity.

There Is a Path!

So now that you have read all the disclaimers, let's get to the excitement, those few of you still wanting to read the rest of this chapter and possibly pursue an AgBio dream. What does success look like? What should your goals be as an entrepreneur? A serious technology entrepreneur will want to change how products are developed for today's markets (e.g., better marker tools for the same types of conventional varieties, a strategy developed by KeyGene in the 1990s). A serious commercial entrepreneur will want to change the face of agriculture, its practice around the planet, and the products that growers need to improve the yield and value of their products. To do, this requires at least three key assets: a compelling vision, talented people, and committed capital. And once early-stage capital has been utilized by your team to demonstrate potential, much larger amounts of capital will be needed to realize the complete vision. In Ag Biotech, company financing has not traditionally come through public financial markets because of the more limited value of agriculture compared with human health in developed countries, but rather through an acquisition by a large Ag Biotech company.

Let's examine some examples of success to understand the path. Athenix is an attractive model of success. Bayer CropScience acquired Athenix in 2009 to gain control of relatively early-stage but well-demonstrated crop-protection traits of insect and nematode resistance. Athenix was developed into a center of excellence within Bayer for these new trait products, with the greater resources of Bayer to realize the vision of the founders, and with a nice return for them and their investors. The founders, people such as Mike Koziel, had both prior entrepreneurial as well as larger company background (people), a clear vision of their product goals (vision), and capital largely from the venture community but also from a number of strategic deals with smaller Ag Biotech companies (capital).

The initial public offering path is not broadly available for Ag Biotech companies today, given the long time-frames to market and more limited value of biotech trait products compared to blockbuster drugs. The primary exit has been through acquisition by a large company wanting to own and control key technologies, IP positions, or emerging products. Rarely, has there been an Ag Biotech company in the public market in the past 20 years until recently, unlike the early phase of the Ag Biotech sector where there were plenty. As of 2019, we now have six companies public on US exchanges: Evogene, an Israeli Ag Biotech company that has been public for about a decade; Arcadia Bioscience, public since 2015; Origin Agritech Limited, a Chinese Ag Biotech company; Yield10 Biosciences, public for a decade now based on its origins in the biofuels industry; and Calyxt more recently based on the emerging opportunities through genome editing. There is much to be learned from these companies, including the challenge of sustaining share price while pursuing the advancement of technologies to the market.

I believe that entrepreneurs need to decide on the appropriate business model given its capabilities and investor interest. One path is to focus on products, and building capabilities that can become part of a larger enterprise, one that has already nucleated new opportunities, but knowing that the goal is to secure greater resources through incorporation into a larger corporate partner. Major venture investments, including those from strategic venture funds of major companies, remain critically important for Ag Biotech entrepreneurship and are perhaps more important than ever before.

Another path is demonstrated in a nice exit for another Ag Biotech, an approach in which capital requirements and company size were minimized. GrassRoots was started through project funding by Monsanto in 2009 and was subsequently acquired by Monsanto in 2013. As a board member for most of the company's life, I worked with the company founders to navigate toward an exit without relying on venture investments of any kind. As a result the company remained largely a financed project serving Monsanto's need for novel gene-expression programs for its biotech trait business. The company's purpose was to be technology-focused, as opposed to commercially focused, working entirely within a conventional biotech trait business model. The company was able to secure additional funding through grants that enabled the development of some critical technology not owned by Monsanto. Consequently, the company developed both technologies that would be owned by Monsanto through commercial agreements, as well as new technologies developed with grant funding. GrassRoots was effectively launched through project funding. This combination drove the acquisition at a relatively early stage, after only 4 years of the strategic alliance. Philip Benfey was the key founder who learned important lessons from other companies, kept his eye on the prize, and recognized the need for technologies other than those defined entirely by the funded partnership to create high financial value in the company. Philip and the leadership team also recognized the difficulty of migrating from a technology to a commercially driven company, as well as migrating from one major partner to other major partners. This success could be an attractive model for entrepreneurial academics, especially in a world with highly focused strategic venture units at most of the major Ag companies. Some strategic investors, as demonstrated by Merck in the pharmaceutical industry, are looking to create project-type venture models that build on this type of success, but which define exit value and timing based on up-front vision and milestones.

What's Been Achieved so Far

The World Food Prize is generally considered the Nobel Prize for food and agriculture, with a global, feed-the-world priority. In 2013 the prize was awarded to three plant scientists each of whom contributed to the fundamental invention for the Ag Biotech industry in the 1980s, agrobacterium-mediated transformation of crops: Robb Fraley, Mary-Dell Chilton, and Marc van Montagu. In fact, each of these individuals are inventors on key patent filings from 1983, the year that bore witness to the first practical means for introducing recombinant DNA into plants. The early 1980s saw the birth and growth of several companies dedicated to creating value using such technology to impact agriculture. The enthusiasm and excitement of the market for this emergent industry was remarkable given that a number of companies were able to go public without significant revenues in the near-term, and with only the first hints of how to create novel plant varieties.

Technologies of the early Ag Biotech companies spanned cell culture-based mutagenesis (somaclonal variation), genetic engineering of microbes that would prevent plant diseases or reduce frost damage when applied to crops, cell culture-based production of plant secondary metabolites, and genetic engineering of crops for a wide range of different benefits. Somaclonal variation and cell cultures proved to be too limited in utility, and consumers were clearly not ready then—nor are they now—to allow genetically engineered bacteria loose in the environment. In fact, my own first foray in the industry was an effort to use microbial genetic engineering to improve microbial colonization of plant roots and the production of antifungal secondary metabolites for effective "microbial fungicides." This effort was shut down in the late 1980s due to public resistance to releasing engineered microbes into the environment. However, biotech crops are much easier to track than microbes, and the public seemed content, initially, with the creation and commercialization of such products. Interestingly, we are seeing a new wave of interest in microbial products that offer pesticidal and growth benefits to plants, but without having to engineer them, given consumer desire for more natural approaches to producing our food.

Many of the early Ag Biotech companies were financed through both private financing from venture investors and through the public markets. They created key enabling tools for the creation of biotech traits in important commercial crops, including corn, soybean, cotton, tomato, and canola. These early companies created the first traits that would later be tested in field trials that were regulated under the Coordinated Framework. Companies such as Calgene, Agracetus, Agrigenetics, Mycogen, AGS, DNAP, and others raised money, went public, and thought they could change the world and create new products and entire new markets.

The science was exciting and thrilling. These new tools enabled both academics and company scientists a glimpse of the behavior of plant gene function in a way never before possible. Some companies invested heavily in the basic understanding of transgene behavior, in the context of conventional gene function in plants. We first came to understand how genes delivered by *Agrobacterium* into the genome of a plant were structured, and how variable structure influenced variable expression outcomes. These fundamental properties needed to be mastered if we were to deliver new products into the market with sufficient understanding of their behavior to give growers, and ultimately consumers, confidence in these new products of biotechnology. We learned ways to shut off gene function as well as activate gene expression. We mastered antisense silencing of gene expression, and then sense gene-mediated silencing of gene expression (cosuppression). The latter was done at DNA Plant Technology where I took on major responsibility for securing patent protection for cosuppression-mediated gene silencing. This led to major insights in plant biology, as cosuppression gave way to RNAi-mediated gene silencing, based on the designed creation of double-stranded RNA molecules (dsRNA) as opposed to incidental dsRNA produced when transgenes integrated in the genome in specific structures such as inverted repeats. The improved ability to silence plant genes for research applications, as well as the ability to silence pest genes essential for viability, has had a major impact on plant science in academia and industry.

In those days, we saw few impediments and a blank canvas to sketch the future on it. Major shifts were anticipated from genetic engineering of crops. New product possibilities such as tomatoes that would not ripen and rot on the vine but would be delivered to consumers in good shape and then ripen. Bananas that would ripen and not rot, because they no longer produced the plant hormone, ethylene, known to induce ripening, but which could be induced to ripen on demand. Crops would be resistant to all types viral diseases. Crops would come in novel colors and with novel flavors. Crops, such as peanuts, failed to produce antigens that are the cause of allergenic responses in foods. A number of such traits and improved crops were developed, but many remain "on the shelf" as opposed to in the market for a range of reasons, including public perception, regulatory and development costs that outstrip potential values.

Herbicide-Tolerance and Insect-Resistance Traits

Herbicide-tolerance and insect-resistance traits were high on the list of companies with a clear-eyed view of the needs of agriculture, as identified by crop-protection companies. An enormous shift in market value was driven by Monsanto's launch of RoundUp Ready soybean in 1996, and RoundUp Ready corn in 1999, as companies selling soybean and corn herbicides lost market share rapidly to Monsanto's RoundUp branded herbicide, glyphosate. Biotechnology offered a novel way to confer selective activity to a nonselective herbicide, such as glyphosate, turning a useful but limited herbicide into the most important herbicide in the world over the past 20 years. Today, herbicide-tolerance and insect-resistance traits represent more than 99% of the market share of the Ag Biotech industry (See Table 27.1). Only a few crops have been successfully targeted for significant biotech trait penetration, with corn and soybean being the predominant crops in both North and South America.

The rate of penetration of insect-resistance and herbicide-tolerance traits (Fig. 27.3) not only demonstrates the success of these biotech trait technologies but also indicates the limitations for entrepreneurs in the biotech trait market, since these crops are dominated by a very few seed companies. In fact, most of the developments in biotech traits have been financed by major companies as strategic investments focused on technologies as opposed to equity value growth. This was the case for Mendel Biotechnology's long-term relationship with Monsanto, which invested substantially over a 15-year period in research and development activities conducted

TABLE 27.1 Biotech traits have penetrated only a few crop-production systems and seed businesses globally, with a focus on corn, soybean, cotton, and canola.

Traits	2017	%
Herbicide tolerance	88.7	47
Insect resistance	23.3	12
Stacked HT/IR	77.7	41

GM market by trait penetration (ha)

Crops	2017	%
Soybean	94.1	50
Maize	59.7	31
Cotton	24.1	13
Canola	10.2	5

GM market by crops penetration globally (ha)

Biotech traits in alfalfa, sugar beet and a few other crops represent small acreage contribution to the total. Only two major trait categories have impacted the market at any substantial level in nearly 25 years, herbicide tolerance and insect resistance, with many varieties having both traits. HT: herbicide tolerance; IR: insect resistance; GM: genetically modified.

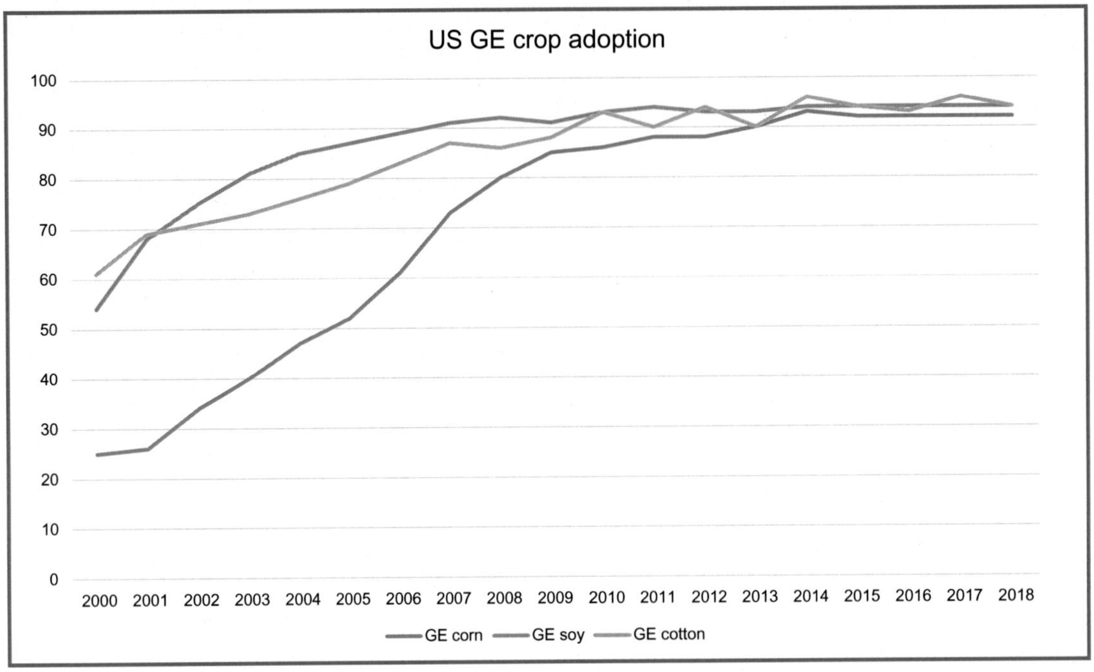

FIGURE 27.3 Three crops represent greater than 98% of the commercialized biotech acres in the United States in 2018.

at Mendel. Athenix is a rare exception to the requirement for major strategic investment, with some venture investors and a solid return in a reasonable period of time.

A few lesser known products have come to the market, with some of these remaining in the market today. Virus-resistant papaya has been a tremendous success in Hawaii, enabling the papaya industry threatened by the devastating *papaya ringspot virus* to survive (well described by Brian Dick in "The Fate of a Fruit: Creating the Transgenic Papaya," *Life Sciences Foundation Magazine*, summer 2013). Virus-resistant squash, brought to the market through the efforts of Asgrow, is still commercialized by Monsanto, who acquired Seminis (which had previously acquired the vegetable seed business of Asgrow in the 1990s). Ripening-delayed tomato products were developed in the mid-1990s by Calgene and DNAP, with Calgene's Flavr Savr tomato reaching the market in 1994, and DNAP's Endless Summer tomato was unable to reach the market in 1995 through lack of obtaining licenses to recently patented technologies. Nontransgenic solutions for delayed ripening in tomatoes became available in the mid-1990s, eliminating the need for the biotech product. Since then, the mainstream produce industry has abandoned biotech traits due to both costs of development as well as consumer resistance to engineered fresh food products.

Perhaps, the best known and most compelling consumer product that has never yet come to the market is Golden Rice, a product developed in the 1990s through the efforts primarily of two academic scientists, Ingo Potrykus and Peter Beyer, funded by the Rockefeller Foundation and the European Union [3]. These scientists engineered rice with genes from both plants and a bacterium to encode proteins needed to produce substantial amounts of beta-carotene (precursor for vitamin A synthesis) in grain, leading to the golden color of the rice. Children without adequate supplies of vitamin A or a precursor such as beta-carotene have a marked incidence of blindness and susceptibility to disease, leading to an increased incidence of premature death of small children, who are most susceptible to the vitamin A deficiency. Syngenta stepped up more than a decade ago to help get that product to the market, but it languishes in a convoluted global process of product approvals and testing. The potential benefit of this vitamin A–enriched rice to prevent childhood blindness and death is recognized, and yet the product languishes. This may still be one of the great humanitarian achievements through biotechnology in agriculture, if and when it finally comes to the market. It represents a systemic failure of regulatory agencies in many countries and a demonstration of the unreasoned fear of a sound technology platform. It is a case study that entrepreneurs interested in Ag Biotech would be well advised to be aware of and to know the pitfalls that they might face.

Recognizing that biotechnology applications could accelerate conventional breeding, with the result generating no biotech trait and no opposition, vegetable seed companies in Europe focused on molecular markers. Several Dutch vegetable seed companies joined together to form a company, Keygene, that they jointly owned and which would generate precompetitive markers. Keygene focused on the continued development of molecular markers and marker technologies with increasingly sophisticated biotechnology tools that would reduce the price of marker discovery and application. Technology innovation was the key to their business model, with the same market outcomes, through the same companies, but with novel and higher value strategies for value creation. The challenges of biotech trait adoption provided an entrepreneurial context for new technologies such as amplified fragment length polymorphism, the key platform technology at Keygene's inception. The critical context for this entrepreneurial company was the lack of competing biotech traits in markets such as vegetable seeds, and particularly in Europe. Keygene continues to innovate and find novel ways to use biotechnology to create improved crop varieties that are not themselves the subject of biotech trait regulation since they are usually based on naturally occurring alleles or alleles derived through mutagenesis and rapidly identified using modern tools of biotechnology.

As with other examples, this demonstrates the value of strategic investment as opposed to financial investment for Ag Biotech entrepreneurs. Keygene's investors were a consortium of major Dutch seed companies whose interest was the technologies to enhance value in their own companies as opposed to growing Keygene's enterprise value as an independent company. This model is fairly similar to the strategy adopted by three forestry companies to develop biotechnology applications for the forestry industry in 2000. Westvaco Corporation, International Paper Company, and Fletcher Challenge came together to form ArborGen, combining R&D assets and financing development of biotech traits, that each would ultimately use in their own plantation forest business. Unlike Keygene, however, which was focused on nonbiotech applications, ArborGen focused largely on a biotech trait development model that has recently foundered due to consumer and NGO opposition to the incorporation of biotech traits into tree species.

How the Landscape Has Changed

Over the past 5 years, many venture funds have increased their interest in Ag broadly, as well as in the Ag Biotech sector. This sector is seen to have long-term, stable demand drivers that attract investment, as well as a number of technology disruptors that attract venture investment. The level of investment to support companies pursuing digital or software applications is the largest segment, perhaps in part based on investment in an adjacent sector for other industries. Given the limitations of Ag Biotech traits from a venture investor's perspective, investors in 2019 and beyond are looking for other entrepreneurial Ag Biotech opportunities, the ones that can lead to products and a realistic exit in only a few years as opposed to more than a decade and the ones that can lead to products that can event be brought to the market directly by the entrepreneurial company, not by a large company licensee of that company. The key challenge is identifying growth sectors in a large, slow-growing industry. Recent trends point to new sectors that interest today's venture investors. Some of these may be developed using biotechnology to differentiate a product or offering; others do not require biotechnology.

One example is in agronomic practices, enabled by artificial intelligence and access to large data sets on farmer practices and outcomes. The initial demonstration of the importance of this opportunity came through Monsanto's acquisition of The Climate Corporation for $930MM in 2013. The acquisition of Precision Planting for more than $200 million spurred further venture capital interest in this sector, with a focus on new information tools coupled with agronomic applications and agricultural equipment. The acquisition of granular Ag by Corteva Agriscience in 2017 was another demonstration of the importance of this emerging opportunity, outside of the realm of biotechnology, but where ultimately biotechnology will likely intersect with farmer practices and better data and operational management. This emphasizes an important theme: the need for very uniform practices on increasingly large acreages managed by large growers and grower groups. The aggregation of land into larger units, as well as larger management units, is a theme seen in all major agricultural regions.

In terms of Ag biotechnology—enabled companies and venture investments, biologicals emerged as one of the most compelling areas of interest. Companies such as Indigo Ag have raised very large sums driving a hefty evaluation, with a combination of microbial products linked to novel business models with direct engagement with the farmer. Evogene has also broadened focus over the past few years to the discovery and development of biologicals, based on the same computational platform used to discovery novel pesticide targets and pesticides, as well as productivity traits in crops.

Another area of increased interest is the application of metabolic engineering, enabled by deep learning, to the improved production of natural products and the improvement of live microbes for a range of applications including a new interest in nitrogen fixation. And a third area of increased interest is the application of biotechnology, genomics, and artificial intelligence to new breeding systems, with today's entrepreneurs recognizing the market need for accelerated improvement of crop performance. Very early-stage companies have entered this field, such as Verinomics, founded by Steve Dellaporta and Albert

Kausch, identified as genomic and computational solutions. Hi Fidelity Genetics is another relatively early-stage company focused on what they call computational breeding. And more established companies have seen opportunity, such as Benson Hill Biosystems, which has focused on breeding systems, crop design platform, designated as CropOS, as well as entering the genome editing field. The underlying theme for these efforts is the combination of biotechnology, genomics, computational power, and artificial intelligence to serve an unmet need for some seed companies that cannot afford the sophisticated breeding systems that these technology companies have created.

A fourth area that emerged almost entirely since the first publication of this chapter is genome editing. Several companies are identifying new engineering tools and applying various editing tools to development of improved varieties. Older technology companies such as Cibus continue to pursue these opportunities, the development, and marketing of new varieties of a few crops, with herbicide-tolerant canola most advanced. Calyxt has pursued the use of TALENS (Transcription activator-like effector nucleases), and the interest in editing has been substantiated by the ability of Calyxt to become a public company, establishing an exit pathway for such venture-backed companies. Pairwise Plants is a more recent entrant with strong backing from Bayer, and a broad focus on applications and technologies that include base editing through licenses to technology developed by David Liu at Harvard.

A final area mentioned briefly early is the application of biotechnology to screening for active ingredients, as well as the production of natural product active ingredients, in the form of herbicides, fungicides, insecticides and nematicides. Biotechnology linked with data analytics, deep learning, is the novel advance in this field over the past several years. We see this from Evogene and its Computational Predictive Biology platform, Ginkgo Bioworks, and their custom organism design in their Foundries, and Zymergen and their combination of automation, machine learning and genomics, where the potential to accelerate screening and discovery of pesticides, and their production, if natural products, is being realized today.

Patently Important Trends

IP broadly, and patents specifically, are the life force for most biotechnology businesses. This is, perhaps, a truism, but for Ag Biotech, the impacts are more dramatic even than for medical biotechnology. Unlike medical biotech, where the capability to bring a drug to the market may rely only on a company's solely-owned patent estate, commercialization of new Ag Biotech traits may require licenses to a broad array of enabling technology patents from others. With the stacking of biotech trait products increasingly seen in major crops, new innovations only realize value in combination with other patented technologies. Therefore a biotech trait cannot come to the market on its own, it can only do so in the context of a commercial seed or plant variety that is subject to patents and other forms of proprietary protection owned by others. This contrasts with the biopharmaceutical industry where a blockbuster drug can often come to the market relying just on its own patents.

The entire collection of varieties in a seed company, some of which are certainly trade-secrets but others the subject of an array of IP protection, provide a compelling barrier to entry that makes it very difficult for an Ag Biotech entrepreneur to capture new value in this market. This collection of varieties, known as the germplasm of a seed company, represents a powerful advantage for companies such as Bayer, Corteva, Syngenta, and other international seed companies. The power lies in the elite performance of the best varieties in the collection, as well as in the diversity of alleles represented in that collection, and the difficulty of recreating that elite performance starting from varieties readily accessible to the public through governmental variety collections, such as those managed by the USDA, for example. For crops such as corn and soybean, cotton, many vegetables, and sugar beet with commercial breeding in the hands of private companies for decades if not generations, new biotech traits can only be realistically tested and evaluated by the private breeding companies. The requirement for testing, particularly for traits such as yield and stress tolerance, results in a major barrier to entry. This is different for crops where the breeding is done largely in the public sector, such as wheat, but even this may change if the promise of hybrid wheat is finally realized, so that value capture for improved varieties is more readily possible. The situation is different for chemistries or biologicals that can be applied to a crop, and which may therefore be much less dependent on specific variety performance. In the case of microbials the ruling by the Supreme Court in Ass'n for Molecular Pathology v. Myriad Genetics, Inc., 133 S. Ct. 2107 (2013) made it clear that naturally occurring genes or microbes cannot be protected through patents. Other means are usually sought, for example, nonnaturally occurring combinations of microbes or specific formulations needed for effectiveness, to secure IP protection. Biotechnology played an important role in a crop such as soybean, enabling a new means of capturing value through traits such as herbicide tolerance and insect resistance, which can be handled through patents and contractual protection. Prior to this new added value, many growers would have preferred to save seed rather than buying seed annually from major seed companies.

This structural shift enabled soybean to join maize as the second most important seed crop globally in terms of value capture. Prior to this change, soybean was a required product sold by companies who made most of their money from their corn hybrids, but one from which these companies generated relatively little profit. The difference was that soybean growers could save seed from year to year, whereas corn growers relying on hybrids produced by corn seed companies, would lose the hybrid genetics in the next, save seed generation. The power of biotech traits for soybean was the ability, finally, of major seed companies to provide buyers of their seed sufficient value that they would agree not to save seed, as otherwise the grower would be infringing on a biotech trait patent incorporated into the seed genetics.

Lessons Learned and Opportunities for a New Entrepreneur

The AgBio entrepreneur developing a new technology faces a challenge that differs along many dimensions from that faced by an AgBio entrepreneur trying to introduce a new product category or building a new market and disrupting existing markets. The critical issues differ for these two types of entrepreneurs, who also may have quite different backgrounds. The needs for Neal Carter, the CEO of Okanagan Specialty Fruits, to bring a browning-resistant apple to the market, were ones that a businessman from the orchard industry could appreciate. They are quite different from the needs for Philip Benfey, founder and CEO of GrassRoots, and a highly regarded plant biologist, to develop a new toolbox of gene-expression tools for classical biotech trait products in major row crops. And the motivations of a commercial entrepreneur and a science entrepreneur are also often very different.

The Ag Biotech trait revolution disrupted value amongst existing crop-protection companies, as noted earlier. Monsanto leapfrogged several other crop-protection companies in herbicide sales and has yet to look back, now as part of Bayer Crop Sciences. This was the most significant shift in industry value capture and market position from the biotech trait revolution, as only two traits continue to dominate value of the Ag Biotech trait market. An entrepreneur in the AgBio sector sees that the era of disruptive impact of biotech traits is over, and that the leading companies have tremendous advantages in continuing incremental gains in this technology.

New and disruptive opportunities will arise in ways that leading companies today do not yet recognize! So don't be dismayed when prominent companies don't jump at the chance to partner with you on a new technology. American Cyanamid didn't see the titanic shift in value toward glyphosate-resistance soybeans, as summarized above, until it was too late. RoundUp Ready traits that enabled displacement of American Cyanamid's leading herbicides by Monsanto's RoundUp were not fully appreciated until growers themselves could test and identify the full range of benefits.

Today's new disruptive technologies and products for crop productivity improvement may lead to entirely new categories, or just be successful applications of current strategies, much as biopesticides have come of age through the work of Agraquest and Marrone Bio Innovations, the former being acquired by Bayer, the latter becoming a public company. The value of science well applied, and biotechnology among them, in overcoming limitations of successful biopesticides was key. New business models have also been key to this recent emergence, for example, by securing increased product life for current synthetic pesticides, or addressing new markets, through microbial products. The combination of technology innovation and business model innovation for entrepreneurial success is a key lesson, as meaningful disruptions are usually technology enabled, but business model driven.

The biopesticide sector successes of the past 5 years or more suggest that the dramatic difference in cost and time to bring "bio" products to the market, now combined with new tools and better product efficacy, provides an entrepreneurial context for a new wave of Ag Biotech-derived products (see Fig. 27.4). With a growing interest in natural solutions in the marketplace driven by consumer demand, as well as improving technology for understanding microbial ecosystems interacting with plants, we are clearly seeing the unfolding of a new chapter of Ag Biotech-enabled businesses, both from live microbial applications as well as the production of natural products derived from microbial sources.

As I reflect on lessons I've learned over the past 35 years, starting with the onset of the Ag Biotech industry, my most important lesson of all is best summarized by these words of Albert Einstein: "Out of clutter, find simplicity. From discord, find harmony. In the middle of difficulty lies opportunity." This has helped me numerous times remain focused despite the many challenges I've faced as a scientist entrepreneur. I offer a corollary that one should have in mind at the outset of any new venture: "When you pursue opportunity, you will often face difficulty...when you do, seek simplicity and harmony." Creative solutions to difficulties can emerge when we allow ourselves time to find the simple and harmonious paths, those that enable the entrepreneur to persevere and succeed.

Ultimately, how do we measure success of our ventures, or success as an entrepreneurial leader? Because failures occur in all industries, success is handling the

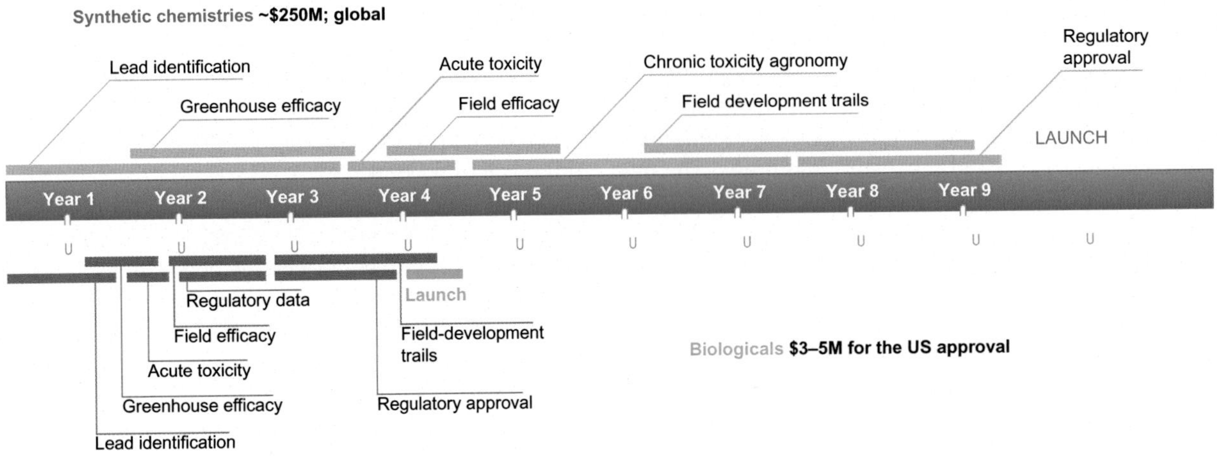

FIGURE 27.4 One driver for a new era of Ag Biotech innovation is the dramatic difference in time requirement and regulatory cost to bring a synthetic chemical versus a biological or natural product to the market. With new technologies to understand and develop biological and natural products and the recent successes of the biopesticide industry, additional new opportunities are likely to be found in the biological and natural product market segments, with biotechnology and genomics as key enablers of new innovation. *Ag Biotech*, Agricultural biotechnology.

process, knowing when to continue and when to stop, knowing how to minimize losses without missing out on big wins, and learning throughout the process. The investors with whom you partner will prize these attributes. David Brooks noted in one of my favorite New York Time op-ed pieces, people "want to find that place, as the novelist Frederick Buechner put it, "where [their] deep gladness and the world's deep hunger meet." If your deep gladness is satisfied by meeting the world's true hunger (for food, energy, and materials, all the key stuff of life in the modern world), then you should be a Bio Ag entrepreneur.

References

[1] Carson, Rachel. *Silent Spring*. Houghton Mifflin Company, 1962.

[2] Data from the International Service for the Acquisition of agri-biotech applications. <http://www.isaaa.org/> (accessed February 20, 2019).

[3] <http://www.goldenrice.org/> (accessed February 20, 2019).

Chapter 28

Artificial Intelligence: Emerging Applications in Biotechnology and Pharma

David Sahner, MD[1,2] and David C. Spellmeyer, PhD[3,4]

[1]*Chief Medical and Chief Scientific Officer, EigenMed, Inc., Santa Rosa, CA, United States,* [2]*Consultant to Biotechnology, Data Science, and Venture Capital companies, Santa Cruz, CA, United States,* [3]*Adjunct Associate Professor, Department of Pharmaceutical Chemistry, University of California, San Francisco and Principal, Interlaken Associates, LLC, San Francisco, CA, United States,* [4]*Principal, Interlaken Associates, LLC, Oakland, CA, United States*

Chapter Outline

Introduction

Artificial intelligence (AI), machine learning (ML), and deep learning (DL) have become phrases that typically inspire a mix of awe, perplexity, and, among some, an unjustified fear of the loss of human relevance. Simply put, however, AI is a branch of computational science that seeks to instill intelligent decision-making or behavior in machines. While computers have accomplished astounding feats in the performance of discrete tasks, "generalized human intelligence" is many decades away, if it ever materializes. The imminent risk of subjugation of humanity by devices of its own making is overstated, even though those decision-making tools may have the ability to simultaneously consider a profusion of variables that would baffle a human mind, learn novel strategies, or search for an answer at lightning speed and, by extension, beat exceptionally adept humans at specific games such as Jeopardy (Watson), Go (AlphaGo), and chess (Deep Blue).

ML, of which DL is an example, is a branch of AI in which intelligent decision-making, classification, or prediction is computationally learned rather than hard-wired (Fig. 28.1). The origin of the differentiation of "DL" (historically used to refer to the capabilities of "deep" neural nets) from more traditional forms of ML resides in the anatomy of deep neural nets, which consist of multiple layers that encode increasingly refined abstractions of input data. The layers may be thought of as strata, hence the choice of the term "deep" when the tiers in the architecture are numerous. ML comes in three major flavors: (1) supervised learning (in which predictive models or "classifiers" are developed with the knowledge of the class to which an example belongs in a "training dataset"), (2) unsupervised learning (in which an algorithm clusters training examples without any such foreknowledge), and (3) reinforcement-based learning (in which the machine is "rewarded" for making an intelligent decision). In this

Biotechnology Entrepreneurship. DOI: https://doi.org/10.1016/B978-0-12-815585-1.00028-0

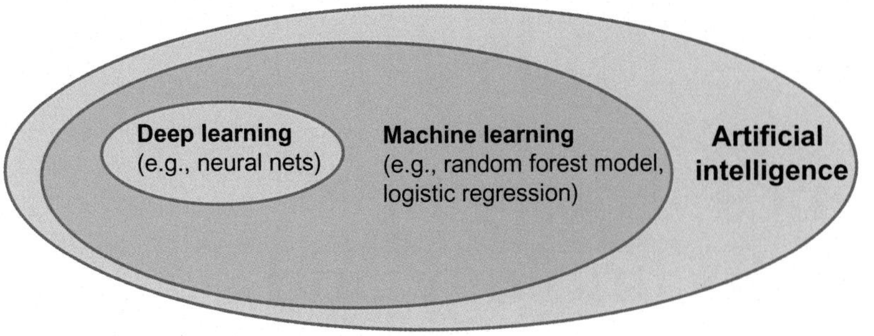

FIGURE 28.1 Machine learning and deep learning as parts of the AI universe. *AI*, Artificial intelligence.

chapter, we will concentrate primarily on "supervised" learning and, to a lesser extent, unsupervised learning.

That AI is transforming the lives of humans is obvious. Smart phones enabled with voice recognition technology, for example, rely upon natural language processing applications. DL also powers computer vision vital to self-driving cars. Clinical decision support tools based on ML (e.g., X-ray interpretation and choice of therapy for cancer) are wending their way into practice. These and other applications of AI, such as navigation systems and increasing automation in the manufacturing sector, are merely several examples of innovations that have changed, or will soon alter, the manner in which we deal with each other, the environment, and the evolving challenges we face as a species.

Within the realm of biotechnology and biopharmaceuticals, computational science and modeling have been regarded by some as a panacea for our imperfect understanding of biological pathways and drug targets, optimal drug design, molecular docking (target engagement of a ligand by a drug), disease classification, and the prediction of clinical outcomes. Others take an unjustifiably dim view of the potential these tools hold. As usual, the truth resides at neither of these extremes. While the implements of ML are sharp and often utilitarian, they are not flawless, and, if used inappropriately, they can lead to grievous mistakes. In the proper hands, however, one can optimize model performance and simulations to useful advantage, while appreciating the limitations of the results. However one prediction can be made with reasonably high certainty. Namely, ML and modeling are likely to transform biological research and the practice of clinical medicine over the ensuing years and decades. We should welcome this, because the amount of knowledge about disease pathogenesis, mechanisms of drug and biologic effects, and biology in general with its vast networks is growing at an enormous pace and has reached the point at which we have exceeded the capacity of any single human intellect to form a detailed, comprehensive, and integrated understanding of the complexity that must be mastered to reliably achieve optimal clinical results.

This chapter provides an overview of basic and strategic principles of ML, high-level descriptions of various methods, means of enhancing the likelihood of success in the application of those methods, and examples whereby ML and modeling may increase the efficiency and fruitfulness of target discovery, drug design, prediction of ligand engagement, and identification of patient populations ideally poised to respond to a particular therapeutic intervention. We will not cover the detailed mathematical underpinnings of specific techniques, each of which would require separate in-depth treatment, but clinicians, biologists, and drug developers who wish to leverage ML in projects should understand the basics outlined in this chapter in order to effectively collaborate with their data scientist colleagues. As emphasized in the next section, it takes a team.

Section I: Machine Learning

Basic Requisites for Success in Machine Learning

Before describing the content of the ML toolshed, we touch on several fundamentals, which may be thought of as warnings on a sign at the entrance that the owner of the shed might post to lessen the risk of liability stemming from unsafe use of, say, a chainsaw. There is a tendency on the part of novices to regard specific ML methods, especially newer ones with impressive-sounding names, such as deep neural nets, as "better" than humbler techniques. While several contemporary methods are extraordinarily powerful, they are not always appropriate in a given case and carry major risks if used when they should be left in the shed in favor of a more suitable implement. We would not use a sledgehammer to place a nail on a wall made of particle board in order to hang a picture. As we will see, much of ML relies upon sound data preprocessing, domain expertise within the field of study, and knowing when, precisely, to use a hammer as opposed to a screwdriver. These tenets or "precautions" are outlined later.

Good Data and Data Processing Are Crucial

Data preprocessing is step number one. Despite its obviousness, it is not possible to overstate the need to respect the "primacy of the data" or, more coarsely, recognize that "trash in = trash out" no matter how refined the algorithm may be. The majority of the data scientist's time generally should be spent selecting, scrubbing, reconciling, and integrating data, addressing missing values, mapping ordinal (e.g., tumor stage) and nominal (e.g., gender) variables, scaling features to mitigate the risk of the undue influence of certain variables, and, if dealing with unstructured text (e.g., medical notes), attempting to extract semantically meaningful information. Consideration needs to be given to the source and integrity of the data. For example, cell lines consist of biological systems and can vary over time. As a result, they may, or may not, be the same across experiments. Furthermore, a dataset might not distinguish among the various cell lines used, a potentially critical feature of the data. Missing values for an assay can be handled in a variety of ways (e.g., by omitting samples for which the data are delinquent or by "imputing" a value such as an average or most common value, a last observation carried forward, or through probabilistic inference). By extension, scientists from other disciplines collaborating with the data scientist should require clear descriptions of the decisions used in preparing datasets for use.

Select the Appropriate Algorithm and Validate Its Fitness to the Task

The type of ML algorithm one selects must be fit-to-task given the extent of the available data. Machine learners navigate a strait between the twin banes of "overfitting" a model (use of an algorithm variety, such as a deep neural net, that is overly powerful) and "underfitting" a model (adoption of a model type that is too feeble to make the necessary discriminations between classes). *Inherently musclebound ML algorithms*, such as complex deep neural nets and polynomial classifiers (both to be discussed later), *generally require larger training datasets*. If the "data clothes" are not ample enough, the model is "overfitted." Such a model may perfectly classify objects in a training set but will fail abjectly when presented with a test dataset to which it has not been exposed before, the litmus test of the value of an algorithm. Similarly, a model which simply considers too many features (including irrelevant features) in learning to discriminate between, say, disease A and disease B, may be overfitted. That is to say, ironically, the piling on of more features (e.g., thousands of transcriptomic, proteomic, and clinical model parameters) may be deleterious to a model's predictive performance (Fig. 28.2).

To best understand the essential concept of overfitting, let's consider a very straightforward toy example. Suppose we have 80 pieces of fruit in a basket, consisting of 40 Scifresh apples (2 examples presented on the left) and 40 Honeycrisp apples (third apple), as shown in Fig. 28.3.

Now, in inspecting these two images, one appreciates some fairly obvious distinctions between the two types of apples that may be used to help differentiate the classes. The Scifresh variety (first two apples) is dual-colored and may be elongate in shape, while the Honeycrisp (third apple) is predominantly red and, in this example at least, squat in appearance. One also sees that the Honeycrisp can have stripes. All is well, we have candidate features for an algorithm that seeks to discriminate between the two types of apples, such as primarily red (Y/N), elongated (Y/N), and striped (Y/N). What types of features do we typically like to include in algorithms? Those that are predictive and that provide what is sometimes referred to as "independent" or "orthogonal" information (i.e., bits of information that are not correlated with each other).

But what if we toss in one or two random monkey wrenches? Suppose, purely by chance, the apple picker at Orchard B (the source of the Honeycrisps) was more prone to collect apples that had fallen to the ground and that were bruised than the picker at Orchard A (the provenance of the Scifresh apples). Let's say, then, that 65% of the Honeycrisp apples he contributes to our basket have bruises, while only 5% of the Scifresh apples from the other orchid have contusions. Or, perhaps, again by fluke, 50% of the apples from Orchid A harbor apple maggots, whereas only 3% of apples from Orchid B play host to these "railroad worms." If we included railroad worms and bruises as additional features in our model (or classifier—we will loosely use those terms interchangeably here), we may have a predictive algorithm that, with 100% accuracy, specifically distinguishes Scifresh apples from Honeycrisp apples in the training set, but which, as one would expect with the inclusion of such "random nonsense" features, fails miserably when applied to other mixed apple baskets containing Scifresh and Honeycrisp apples from a variety of other orchids. The moral of the story is: The merit of a ML algorithm is measured not by its ability to perfectly classify examples in a training dataset, but to correctly make such predictions for novel examples not included in the training dataset (i.e., an independent 'test' set). If the 'the fit is right' (not too tight, not too loose), performance is optimized. An overfitted model, including random nonsense features, has to be avoided even if the model training results seem to be completely on target.

Fortunately, there are ways to reduce the risk of model overfitting, a detailed discussion of which is beyond the scope of this chapter. These include a variety of "model regularization techniques" which exact a cost penalty on models of greater complexity, and "dimensionality reduction" methods (e.g., feature selection to identify "keeper features" that genuinely matter in a model, or feature extraction to identify a limited number of novel feature components). Dimensionality reduction, traditionally reliant upon a relatively limited set of methods (e.g., sequential backward selection, principal component analysis, linear discriminant analysis), have burgeoned in recent years. The size of a dataset can also be "matched" to the appropriate degree of model complexity using a specific metric known as the Vapnik–Chervonenkis dimension.

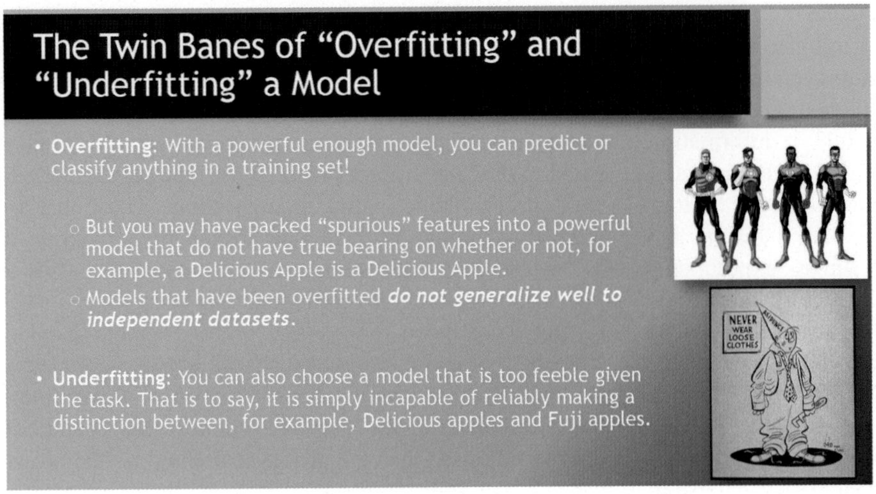

The Twin Banes of "Overfitting" and "Underfitting" a Model
• Overfitting: With a powerful enough model, you can predict or classify anything in a training set!
○ But you may have packed "spurious" features into a powerful model that do not have true bearing on whether or not, for example, a Delicious Apple is a Delicious Apple.
○ Models that have been overfitted do not generalize well to independent datasets.
• Underfitting: You can also choose a model that is too feeble given the task. That is to say, it is simply incapable of reliably making a distinction between, for example, Delicious apples and Fuji apples.
NEVER WEAR LOOSE CLOTHES

FIGURE 28.2 Top: Overfitting of "superhero models" too powerful for the small datasets they wear. Bottom: Underfitting of a model lost in the suit of data it which it is clothed.

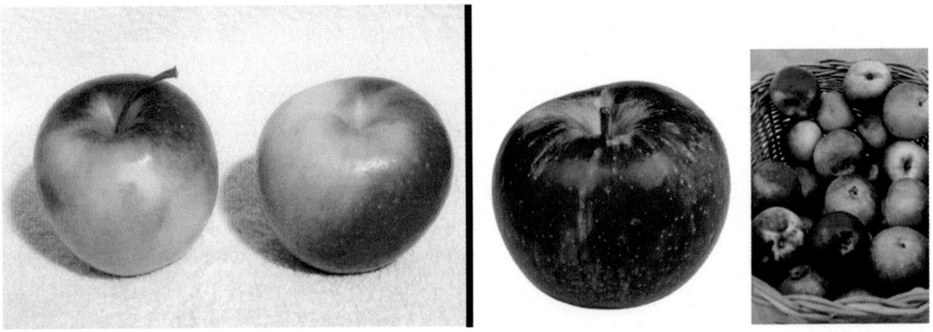

FIGURE 28.3 Apple classification problem.

Dataset augmentation is another technique whereby the dataset is expanded using fictional examples, inspired by real examples, as variations on a theme to increase the size and "challenge level" of a dataset. The training of neural nets for image recognition relies on this last tactic.

So, to prime ourselves for success, it is critical to ensure that the size of the "data suit" fits the body morphology of the model. In this way, we know the model is most likely to perform well in the wild, classifying or making predictions in terra incognita. *What better way to ensure a good fit but a fitting room? In ML, that fitting room is called "cross validation."* The underlying concept is simple. We divide our data into a training set, from which the algorithm learns, and a separate test set (with which it is not trained) to later evaluate how well it generalizes to novel datasets. Then, we revert to a trick. We split the training set still further, creating, in effect, a "mock test set" which is withheld during training, with which we "pretest" the accuracy of the trained model. The mock test set, or "validation set," serves as a fitting room. If performance is unacceptable, we know we need to tweak the model, use a different method, or seek to increase the size of our dataset. In fact, cross validation can be performed repeatedly with many mock test sets using a technique known as *k*-fold cross validation, which produces a more accurate assessment of the expected error rate if the algorithm were to be tested with an independent test set.

In the apple example, we intentionally made a specific choice to only include two types of apples. We must be very careful to apply the algorithm to only those types of apples and not to other closely related types where the results are not valid.

Finally, to succeed in ML, particularly in fields of byzantine complexity, such as biological science and medicine, it is instrumental to ensure that an interdisciplinary team, comprising an amalgam of expertise in biology, medicine, computational science, and statistics, takes the problem on as a group with mutual respect among its members. A clinician or biologist cannot toss data over the fence to a data scientist and expect miracles. And a data scientist, operating in a vacuum without adequate clinical or biological acumen, should not presume that he or she can do it alone without guidance from domain experts on relevant features, data challenges, etc. The cross talk must be abundant and frequent. Extending the fitting room example, everyone on the team needs to provide feedback to ensure the data scientist has selected the right fabric and has produced clothing that fits.

Machine Learning: The Major Members of the Cast and an Illustrative Example

ML can be likened to a theatrical production. There are hits and duds tied, to some degree (but not entirely as we have seen earlier), to the skill of the actors cast in various roles and the chemistry that exists between them. Here then are the roles variably filled by different actors in several major forms of ML, each of whom we will meet in turn in this chapter:

- ***Feature matrix***: A matrix, which resembles a simple spreadsheet, consists of columns and rows with each cell filled by an element of the data. Features are typically placed in columns (e.g., clinical findings, labs, and imaging results) and each row corresponds to a patient, for example. There is one entry for each feature per patient (Table 28.1).
- ***Target vector (or "labels")***: This is like a list which provides the "ground truth answers" that a learning algorithm learns to predict during training. It is composed of one column, with one entry (label) per patient (e.g., a *known* unifying diagnosis such as "pulmonary embolism" or "pneumonia" that the model attempts to infer from a patient's features).
- ***The predictor***: This is the character who makes predictions. That is, what is the likely diagnosis for patient X based on his/her features? Consider this the gray matter of a predictive algorithm, an oracle that makes pronouncements through what is known as an "output function."
- ***Cost or "performance function"***: During training, the algorithm is penalized for wrong answers and then modifies itself (e.g., through "weight" adjustments) to improve its performance ("optimize" itself). The "cost" of an incorrect prophecy by "the predictor" is calculated using a formula, and we will see how that information is used to adjust model parameters (e.g., weights attached to specific variables in the input data).
- ***Algorithm optimizer***: This is the mathematical method by which weights are optimized to reduce cost.

These are the fundamental building blocks of an algorithm. Each "role" is filled by a particular actor. Although the specific actors vary among various types of algorithms, for major forms of ML the parts they play are the same. Let's illustrate the manner in which the members of the cast cooperate during a production using the prototypical, and still quite useful, ML algorithm, logistic regression (Fig. 28.4). Armed with an understanding of logistic regression, we will later see that we are well on our way toward grasping the workings of a basic feedforward neural net.

Core principles of ML are captured by the surprisingly straightforward flowchart in Fig. 28.4. Step-by-step, a feature matrix for a training dataset in the upper left is fed into the algorithm. For a given example (patient), each variable is multiplied by a specific weight and a sum is calculated. This sum, for a given case, is then channeled into a sigmoid output function which converts it to a number between 0 and 1. If the output of the sigmoid function is ≥ 0.5, the algorithm predicts death within 30 days of the onset of septic shock. That prediction is compared with "reality" for each patient in the training set (as captured by the target vector in the lower right). If the answer is wrong, a cost is incurred. The algorithm iteratively adjusts model parameters (weights) to minimize cost and thereby optimize accuracy. It is that simple. At the end of the day, variables with more "predictive heft" will be tethered to larger weights. One of the advantages of linear regression (and other linear classifiers) is that if there is a linear decision boundary between classes, we can find it with certainty.

The cost of wrong decisions during training is how the model learns. There are several means by which cost

TABLE 28.1 Example of a simple feature matrix.

Example	Fever	Leukocytosis (WBC above a threshold)	Increased respiratory rate (> threshold)	Hypoxemia (O_2 saturation <threshold)	D-Dimer elevation (> threshold)
Patient 1	Y	N	Y	Y	Y
Patient 2	Y	N	Y	N	N
Patient 3	N	Y	Y	Y	N
Patient 4	Y	Y	Y	N	N
Patient N	Y	N	Y	Y	Y

The feature variables in this case are dichotomous (they are either present or absent). Each row encapsulates data from a single example (patient) in the algorithm training set.
Source: Modified from Sahner D. Machine learning, modeling and predictive analytics: key principles for the clinical scientist. Appl Clin Trials 2017 (published online). Available from: <http://www.appliedclinicaltrialsonline.com/machine-learning-modeling-and-predictive-analytics-key-principles-clinical-scientist> [1].

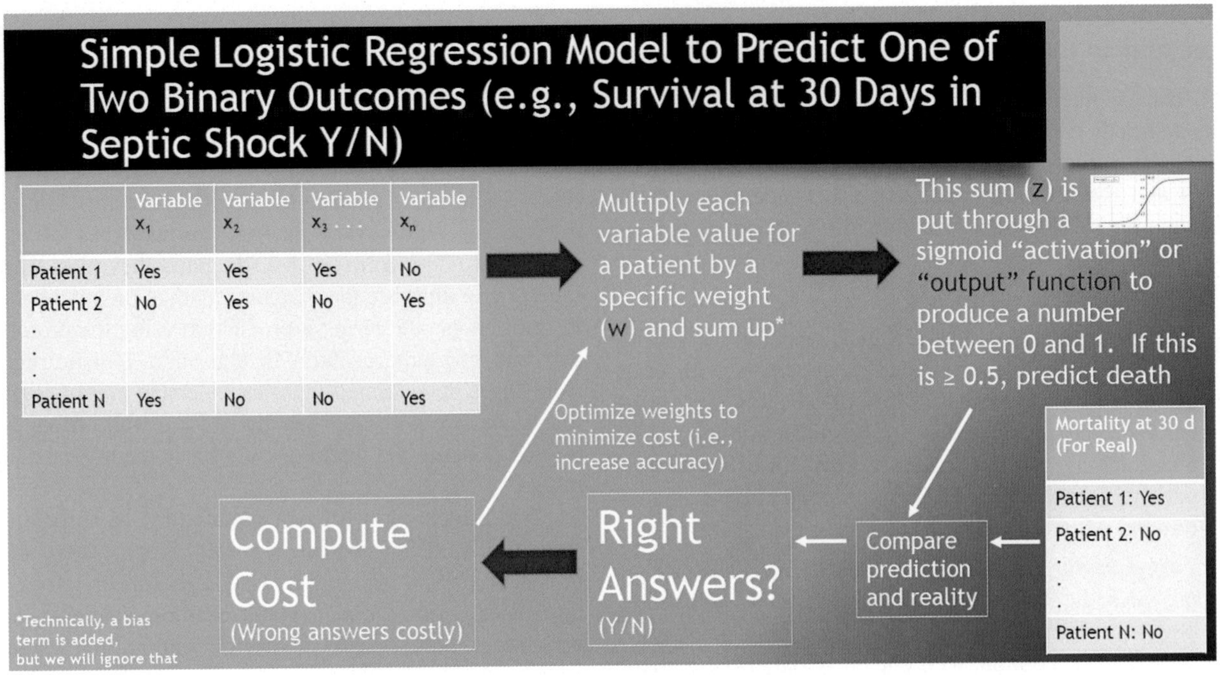

FIGURE 28.4 Hypothetical logistic regression classifier for predicted septic shock outcome at 30 days.

can be calculated for all or a subset of the training examples, including mean squared error and negative log likelihood, and, although we will eschew the detailed mathematics, suffice it to say that this choice is not made willy-nilly, as we shall learn. With knowledge of cost in hand, the learning algorithm iteratively modifies its weights to minimize this cost, classically using an optimization technique called gradient descent. The (evolving) model churns through the dataset many times in search of parsimony, essentially skiing down a gradient to a minimum cost. In essence, gradient descent relies upon the rate of change of the cost with respect to a given weight (i.e., a partial derivative for those familiar with calculus) to decide how that weight should be changed for the next training "go around." If the cost is increasing with respect to a weight, that weight is decreased. Conversely, if the cost is diminishing, the weight is augmented. Again, no legerdemain.

One of the challenges in ML is preservation of this crucial gradient during learning. To maintain the skiing metaphor, if there is no gradient, the skier does not move down the slope and learn. Alternatively, if the gradient is too steep, the skier overshoots the base of the mountain (i.e., the lowest cost), which sacrifices learning efficiency. A glance at the S-shaped sigmoid output function in Fig. 28.4 provides an intuition. That output (the y value) does not change a great deal near the tail or the tip of the "S." This translates into a loss of the gradient toward those extremes (and inefficient learning). Fortunately, prudent pairing of that output function with a specific cost function based on maximum likelihood "undoes" that gradient loss, saving the day (for the mathematically inclined, a log value and an exponent "cancel each other out" in this happy wedding).

Although all of this may sound straightforward, there is no dearth of unanswered questions in ML, some of which are shockingly vital. For one, if the "topology" of the cost landscape is complex (envision multiple hills, moguls, and hollows), there is no guarantee that the algorithm will converge to minimum cost. The skier may become stranded in a "local minimum" rather than making his way to the true "global minimum" at the foot of the mountain. In fact, the likelihood of reaching the base of the mountain (rather than getting stuck in a local minimum) may be influenced by how weights are initialized at the outset of training. A more sophisticated technique can be employed, which evaluates the "rate of change of the rate of change" of cost with respect to a weight to preferentially favor routes of downward curvature, but this has its own liabilities. Furthermore, models require "hyperparameters" (such as the critical weight "learning rate" or the number of neurons in a layer of a neural net) that are chosen heuristically, often based on trial and error. Oftentimes, it is not practical to assess all potential permutations of these hyperparameters. Ultimately, then, ML entails an element of art as well as science.

Summary of Major Types of Machine Learning

Now that the basics are under our belt, we can look at a menu of specific ML techniques. Many would merit standalone chapters in and of themselves, but, knowing the major categories might guide further reading for those who are interested in these specific methods. We focus chiefly on supervised learning. Broadly, these techniques tend to fall into three subcategories: (1) linear models such as logistic regression, which, in a sense, provide a "line" that best separates classes based on weighted features, (2) nonlinear models (such as neural nets and less commonly used polynomial classifiers) which accommodate nonlinear decision boundaries, and (3) models that exploit probability or "information content" (Bayesian classifiers, graphical models, and decision trees). As one would expect, nonlinear models are more flexible and mightier than linear techniques, but more prone to overfitting. Polynomial classifiers, for example, include supplementary features that represent the "product" of two individual features, or a feature raised to an exponent. More features implies greater model complexity, with an attendant increase in the danger of overfitting, as exemplified by the polynomial classifier that "strains" to separate rheumatoid arthritis patients with different outcomes using a counter-intuitive, serpentine, nonlinear boundary (Fig. 28.5). One notable model class [support vector machines (SVMs)], formerly relied upon heavily but less frequently now with the advent of deep neural nets, cleverly embraces nonlinearity under the guise of linearity.

Various ML methods are briefly described in Table 28.2. This is followed by somewhat more detail on selected techniques. Logistic regression and polynomial classifiers (covered above) have been omitted from the table.

One major genus of modeling that is not discussed in Table 28.2, but which may be helpful clinically and biologically, is probabilistic graphical models. The unifying features of these models are nodes and edges (links). Graphs may be "undirected," for example, Markov Random Fields that capture probabilistic relationships among nodes (in effect, correlations) in networks (Fig. 28.7), or "directed" (e.g., Bayesian graphs) in which an arrow points from one node (parent) to another (child) whose truth value (T or F) is conditionally dependent upon the parent's value (i.e., there is a conditional probability that may reflect a causal relationship between parent and offspring).

Graphical models are "parameterized" with "potential functions" or conditional probabilities that capture the probabilistic relationships between and among variables. These can be learned or estimated, through algorithms, from data. Once those parameters are known, one can infer an "unknown node value" (e.g., is X likely to happen within 6 months?) in a given case using specific techniques. Graphical models, especially large and densely connected models, although appealing, may suffer, however, from practical limitations that are mathematically and computationally too complex to cover here. For details on graphical modeling techniques, see Sucar [2].

Since neural nets are so topical, powerful, utilitarian, *and* simultaneously susceptible to abuse, we now elaborate on them here. What makes deep neural nets deep? Hidden layers. Think of each hidden layer as housing a new abstract representation of the input data within a hierarchical learning structure. The most homespun (pun intended) type of neural net is a "feedforward" net in which information flows in one direction, from input to output. An example is provided in Fig. 28.9.

Varieties of more sophisticated neural nets, capable of astonishing accomplishments, have burgeoned in recent years, forming a substrate for exciting and endless innovation, the pace of which is now rapid. For example, in "adversarial training," one neural net attempts to hoodwink another by producing "perturbed" ambiguous examples that are difficult to classify. The second net learns how to avoid being fooled. Recurrent and recursive neural nets can be used to model sequences of events. "Long short-term memory" (LSTM), a recent tactic, promotes the retention of information regarding long-term dependencies in time-series data. In supervised pretraining, short squat neural nets (wide but not deep) teach more

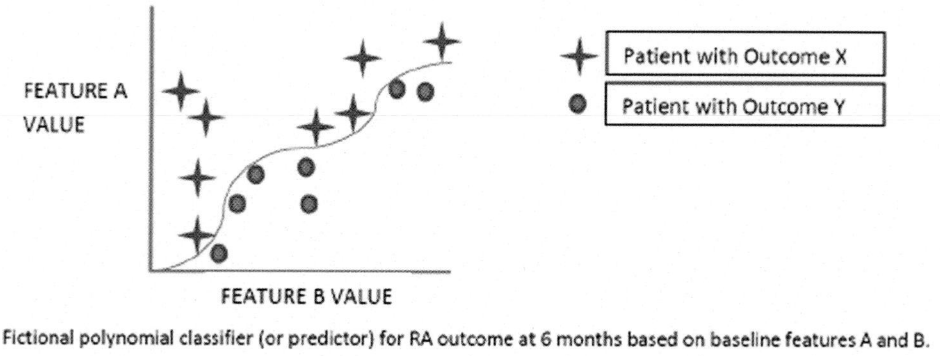

FIGURE 28.5 Fictional polynomial classifier. *From Sahner D. Machine learning, modeling and predictive analytics: key principles for the clinical scientist. Appl Clin Trials 2017 (published online). Available from: <http://www.appliedclinicaltrialsonline.com/machine-learning-modeling-and-predictive-analytics-key-principles-clinical-scientist>.*

TABLE 28.2 Types of machine-learning algorithms.

Method type	Basic concept/advantages	Disadvantages	Comments
Bayesian classifiers	Probabilistic reasoning. Can leverage both prior expectations and observed data. Intuitive	"Naïve Bayes" assumes feature independence. "Ideal Bayes" requires complete knowledge of probabilities which is often not realistic	When feature independence is not justifiable, data preprocessing can be of help
***k*-Nearest neighbor**	Labels a new example based on the classes of an arbitrary number (i.e., *k*) of its nearest neighbors in a multidimensional feature space. See Fig. 28.6. Intuitive	Sensitive to irrelevant attributes. Choice of *k* value affects risk of overfitting. Computational cost (but this can be reduced by creating a specific type of subset of the training set)	Generally inferior to Ideal Bayes. Must address feature scaling issues (not unique to *k*-NN). Can improve performance with data preprocessing
Neural nets	Extremely powerful classifiers, particularly deep neural nets. See Fig. 28.7. Many important varieties (see text)	Risk of overfitting. Potentially high computational load "Black box"—no intuitive understanding of the abstractions used to separate classes	Technique can be deployed to minimize risk of "getting stuck" in local minima and not finding global minimum for cost function (i.e., optimal weight assignments)
Decision tree; random forest	Intuitive interpretability of a decision tree. Basically begin with a root and progressively divide into branches that "arborize" based on features. The terminal "leaves" represent classes (see Fig. 28.8)	Single larger trees can overfit but can be pruned to improve performance. Random forest mitigates risk of overfitting. Forest with numerous trees is computationally expensive	Generally favor smaller trees (less irrelevant or redundant information). Must deal with missing edges (branches) between features
Voting assemblies (ensemble learning)	Tap into collective wisdom of multiple classifiers to improve performance. "Votes" can be weighted or unweighted. Schapire's "boosting" *specifically* seeks out complementary classifiers (in contrast to "bagging"). Random forest method is a type of bagging (multiple decision trees)	May need numerous training examples for Schapire's boosting whereas AdaBoost is more practical (see comments)	AdaBoost *probabilistically* favors selection of misclassified training set examples for next classifier in ensemble, concentrating effort on examples the prior classifier stumbled upon

Source: Modified from Sahner D. Machine learning, modeling and predictive analytics: key principles for the clinical scientist. Appl Clin Trials 2017 (published online). Available from: <http://www.appliedclinicaltrialsonline.com/machine-learning-modeling-and-predictive-analytics-key-principles-clinical-scientist>.

"difficult-to-train" (i.e., deep) neural nets. Convolutional neural nets (CNNs) are used extensively in computer vision and have also been applied to the analysis of molecular docking. The convolution operation permits sparse connectivity among neurons in the net and "parameter sharing," which increases computational efficiency. In essence, a single feature detector can be drawn across an entire image. Goodfellow, Bengio, and Courville [3] provide excellent overviews of the details concerning neural nets mentioned above. Experimental "capsule nets" may prove to offer advantages over convolutional nets since they are, by their nature, "equivariant" (i.e., effectively immunized against the effects of) image rotation, so that smaller datasets may be used to train an algorithm. Neural nets have also been built to mimic the bidirectional flow of information thought to occur in the human brain during perception [4]. Tensor-factorized neural networks enable data representation as a multidimensional array, which may better capture the spatiotemporal structure of data [5]. Finally, newer optimization techniques, exploiting adaptive learning rates during training, may offer significant advantages/efficiencies over classical gradient descent. Innovation, as can be seen, is rife is this field (Fig. 28.10).

Ensemble learning methods extract and tally votes from a "legislature" or caucus of discrete learners, which, individually, may not be sharp enough to ably draw distinctions among classes. The group consensus wins. Votes may be weighted, such that some learners have more of an influence on the election outcome than others. These techniques, of which AdaBoost (Table 28.2) is an example, can be extremely powerful, winning ML competitions, but they may be prone to overfitting of noisy data. An innovative twist on AdaBoost, incorporating label confidence (i.e., a sense of the trustworthiness of classifications) and a conditional risk loss function, may help one to overcome this particular drawback [6].

Space limitations do not allow the treatment of a variety of other tools and models, including pathway activation scores and pathway signatures [7–9], traditional systems biology mass action stoichiometric simulations based on linear algebra and ordinary differential equations (ODE) (which, although promising, may be limited by the curse of data dimensionality and lack of consistently reliable in vivo enzymatic rate constant data) as described extensively by Palsson [10,11], more abstract biological models leveraging declarative programming such as MAUDE, and agent-based models.

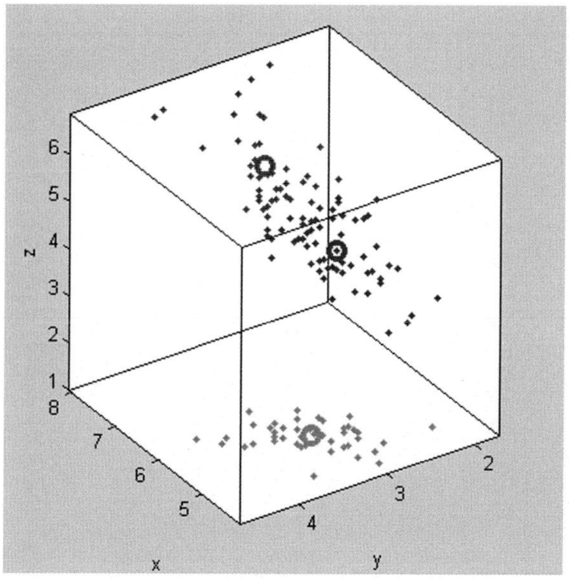

FIGURE 28.6 *k*-Nearest neighbor. Each axis corresponds to a feature, thus an example (e.g., patient) can be plotted in multidimensional space. The class of a new (unclassified) example is inferred from that of its neighbors.

Section II: How Might Machine Learning Help in Drug Discovery?

Discovering new therapeutics is an expensive, challenging endeavor with an extremely high failure rate. Practitioners are confronted by the complex tasks of finding and validating novel biological targets, and intervening at the right time with the right dose of new chemical matter that has appropriate properties and activities, yet lacks unacceptable toxicities. Although technology has advanced substantially in the last decades, the process still involves a great deal of art along with trial and error. Any potential innovation that reduces costs or increases the chances of success is likely to be explored. Only those new technologies that prove to be applicable across many drug discovery projects are likely to be adopted quickly and widely.

Classical ML methods have had a significant impact on the field and adoption of new AI and DL methods in drug discovery is accelerating rapidly. Fig. 28.11 provides an overview of steps in the process. Covering all potential applications is beyond the scope of this chapter. We offer glimpses into a few areas where ML/AI have been applied. In many cases, it is too early to proclaim success, but the promise is real. Personalized medicine is becoming more prevalent as algorithms improve our ability to identify biomarkers that mark patient

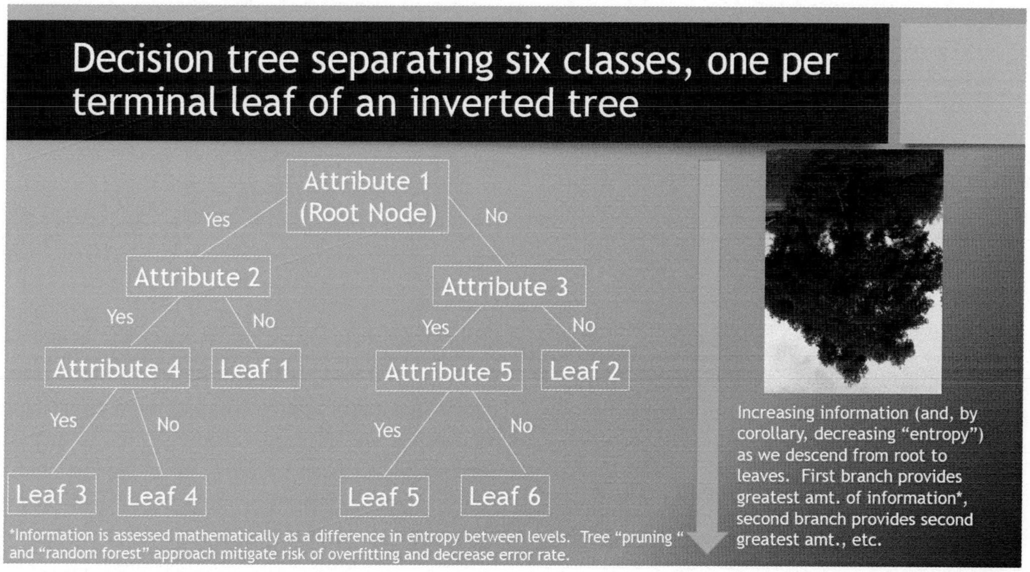

FIGURE 28.7 Decision tree (which actually resembles an inverted tree).

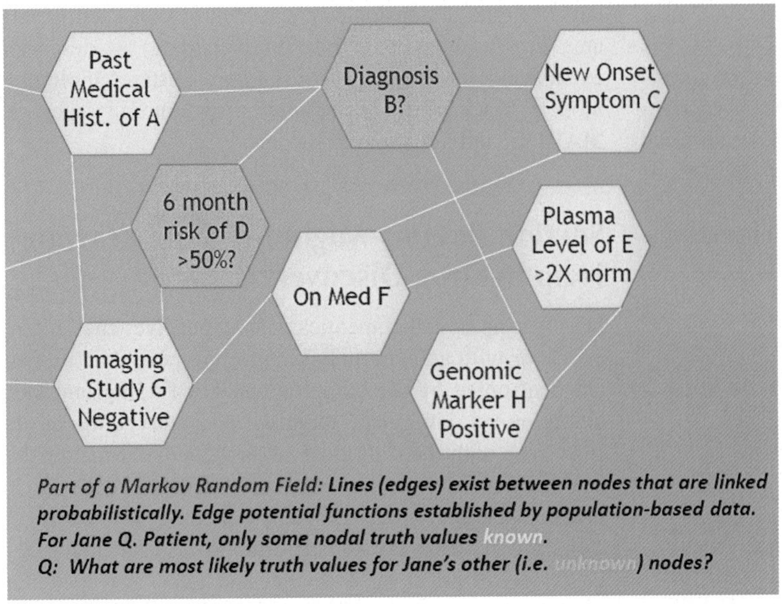

FIGURE 28.8 Example of an undirected graphical model (a Markov random field). With knowledge of the model parameters, we can solve for the values of"unknown nodes" in a given case using an inference technique.

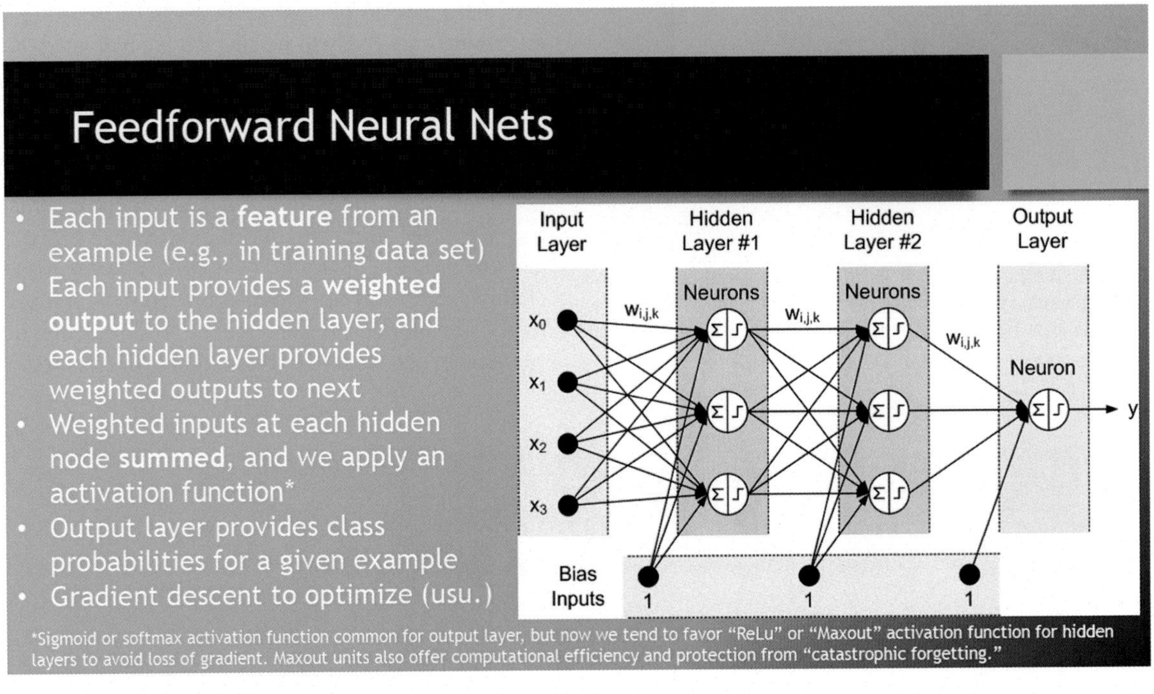

FIGURE 28.9 Architecture of a plain feedforward neural net.

subpopulations. Those can be used sometimes to search for elusive biological targets within a more well-defined clinical indication.

Interpreting and Integrating Omics Data for Target Identification

Target identification is the essential first step in the drug discovery process. We select a specific target that is well characterized as causally related to a relevant biological process and a specific clinical outcome. It can be very difficult to tease apart association with an outcome from causation in biology, although, in theory, probabilistic graphical causal models may be of help [2]. High throughput technologies have been used to generate large amounts of "omics" data in the form of DNA, levels of mRNA, proteins, and metabolites, and epigenetics. A good deal of these data is publicly available. Historically,

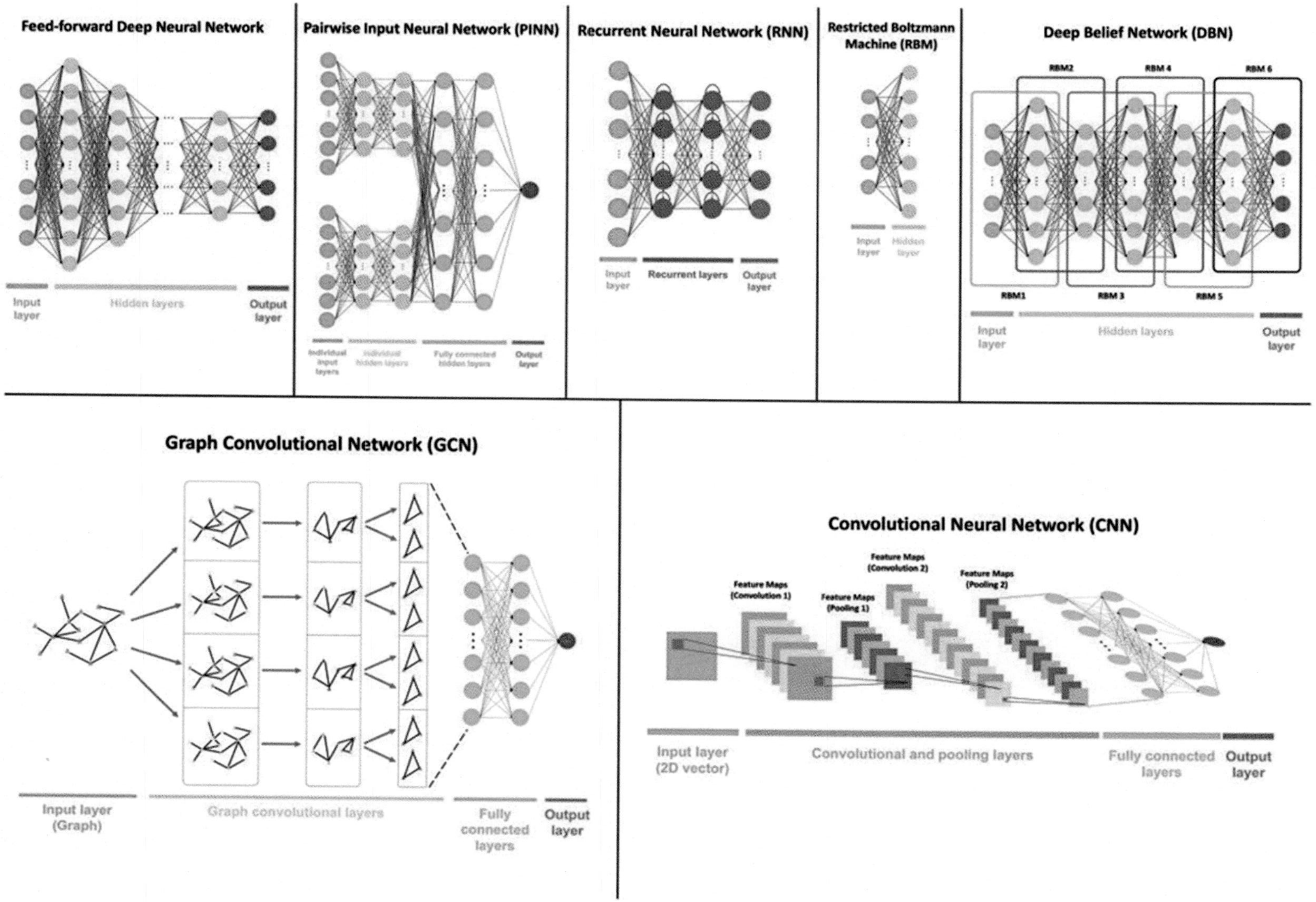

FIGURE 28.10 Several varieties of neural net architectures. *From Rifaioglu AS, Atas H, Martin MJ, Cetin-Atalay R, Atalay V, Doğan T. Recent applications of deep learning and machine intelligence on in silico drug discovery: methods, tools and databases. Brief Bioinf [Internet] 2018. Available from: <https://academic.oup.com/bib/advance-article/doi/10.1093/bib/bby061/5062947> [cited October 22, 2018].*

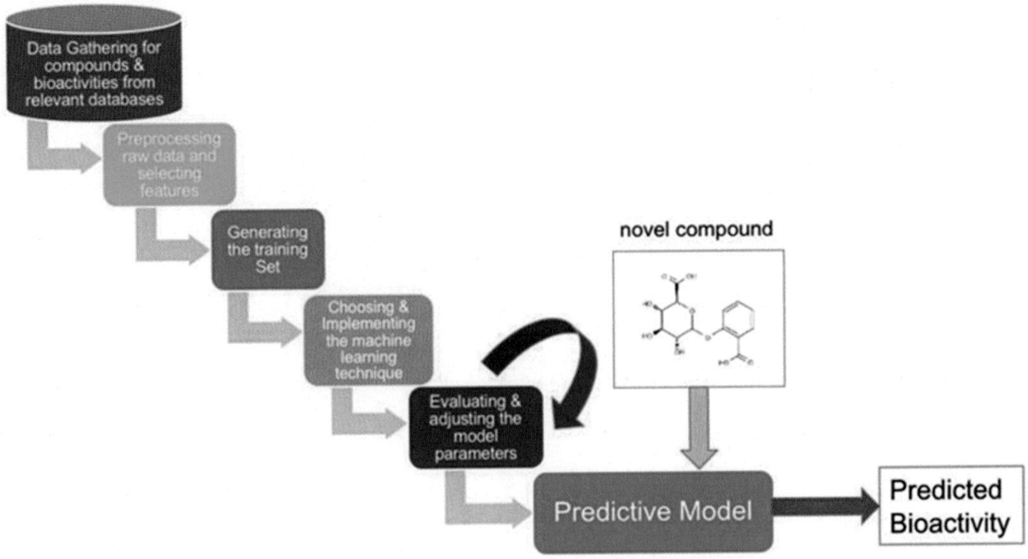

FIGURE 28.11 Machine learning steps in drug discovery. *From Rifaioglu AS, Atas H, Martin MJ, Cetin-Atalay R, Atalay V, Doğan T. Recent applications of deep learning and machine intelligence on in silico drug discovery: methods, tools and databases. Brief Bioinf [Internet] 2018. Available from: <https://academic.oup.com/bib/advance-article/doi/10.1093/bib/bby061/5062947> [cited October 22, 2018].*

methods for evaluating the possible significance of single nucleotide polymorphisms (SNPs) or gene expression signatures have relied heavily on classical ML, both supervised and unsupervised [12]. Analysis, however, of this rapidly-increasing trove of information can be difficult due to technical variability involved in sample collection or preparation, instrumentation, and data collection. The number and types of biomarkers have increased significantly in the past two decades as these technologies and algorithms have improved and these may be classified as diagnostic, mechanistic, prognostic, and/or "response" biomarkers, the last of which may augur a favorable clinical course on treatment. In some cases, these biomarkers also represent biological targets of interest for therapeutic development.

The transcriptome has proved a valuable source of biological information, as it reflects, of course, DNA expression. Sequencing increasingly employs Next Generation Sequencing(NGS)-based RNA-seq, which provides a richer dataset across the transcriptome, well-suited for DL methods which are now being applied to these datasets to model biological systems [13]. The ability to sequence and profile single cells will extend this and other types of analysis further as we seek to uncover the rare cell subpopulations that might be associated with disease outcome or severity. Technical hurdles can be substantial in single-cell sequence analysis due to the ever-changing temporal nature of intracellular processes superimposed on variation in sample handling and preparation. Significant advances have been made very recently, and it is likely those will continue. Importantly, these methods will impact the ability to understand gene regulatory networks (GRNs) as single-cell methods enable modeling the behavior of networks at a very granular level, rather than inferences derived from bulk properties [14].

The spliceosome has also attracted considerable interest in recent years in drug discovery. Identification of potential splicing variants has traditionally employed Bayesian approaches and, more recently, DL, which can incorporate higher dimensions. This can lead to potentially new insights into diseases which derive from single mutations [13]. DL has been shown to be accurate in the identification of transcription factor binding motifs, an essential step in understanding underlying causal disease variants [15]. In genomics data analysis, predictions of splice junctions are used to assemble long sequences computationally, which can be a very difficult task.

Of course, biological systems are incredibly complex and dynamically changing. It is important to understand how intervention at a specific point might or might not affect the cell and/or the whole organism. The availability of genomics data in the late 1990s and early 2000s combined with computational efficiencies launched the development of GRN models to capture the dynamic processes at the cellular level and estimate the effects of feedback loops and interacting biological and chemical entities. A recent review of the field provides an excellent overview of the intricacies of data selection, curation, and model types with assumptions and utility [16]. To summarize, we have seen significant advances in high throughput instrumentation and robust applications of systems to gather huge amounts of data from DNA, RNA, proteins, epigenetics, metabolism, and more. These data can be collected with the introduction of some perturbation at a given time point to assess how the dynamics of the network change temporally. Several computational approaches can be applied once sufficient data has been collected. Boolean networks can model cellular processes using categorical approximations of the network in a method like electronic circuits to model propagation of interventions over time. ODE have been used to model the changes in gene networks over time. These methods require encoding constraints based on prior knowledge of biological systems. They evaluate the rate of change in systems using complex models. Bayesian networks have been used extensively in GRNs. They combine probability and graph theory with conditional dependencies in directed acyclic graphs to describe how changes propagate from parent nodes to children. Finally, neural networks are also being applied to GRNs. These models are all complex and require careful selection of the parameters, network structure and the biological data needed for validation [16]. At present, such models remain at some remove from complex creatures such as humans, although, at least in theory, with all requisite pan-omic data in hand, accurate enzymatic rate constants, and unlimited compute power, holistic models might one day be constructed, which enable us to reliably predict biological responses to therapeutic intervention at an organism-level in man. Given the enormous complexity, this would represent a gargantuan task. Early efforts are underway, however, to lift the "curse of dimensionality" of genetic regulatory networks [17]. More abstract models may also be of help, and other more circumscribed efforts have focused on estimations of individual pathway activation scores in predicting the likelihood that a given drug will exert a favorable effect (selected references provided in the first section of this chapter).

Generation of Novel Chemical Matter

Classical ML methods have been used extensively in the drug discovery process for decades as part of hit identification and lead optimization, the process by which we identify and then iteratively improve the affinity of a compound for a given biological target and reduce the likelihood of toxicities. The foundations of quantitative structure–activity relationship (QSAR) were described in the early 1960s and continue to be used and developed today. In a QSAR model, a set of molecular descriptors (features) is used to describe and optimize the biological activity (the target vector) of a related series of compounds using a multiple linear regression approach (the predictor). The molecular descriptors include molecular charge, shape, electronic characteristics, atom counts (donors, acceptors), 2D fingerprints and 3D properties such as shape, polar surface area, and pharmacophores. These approaches have been successful and have been expanded significantly. However, the successes have been accompanied by criticisms that the methods often lack reliability or extensibility. A recent perspective highlights the importance of careful selection of the descriptors, the curation of the biological data to be modeled, and the importance of an integrated interdisciplinary approach as keys to success [18].

The limitations of QSAR's underlying reliance on linear methods led to applications of artificial neural networks starting in the 1990s. These and subsequent AI methods showed an improved ability to predict binding affinity but are often limited by lack of interpretability, as the abstractions encoded by progressive layers of a neural net typically defy intuitive human understanding. That remains true today. Interdisciplinary drug discovery teams should require that any computational method must provide a spotlight to the medicinal chemists illuminating changes that can be made to improve the biological effect. Otherwise, the model is not actionable or useful [19].

Virtual library (VL) screening methods are derived from the structure- and ligand-based design methods developed in the 1980s and 1990s as reviewed recently [20]. Generally, VL screening involves calculating the predicted binding properties of very large numbers of known or theoretical compounds, based on chemical features, vis-à-vis a protein or biological target of interest. The model(s) is/are typically trained on the experimentally determined activities/properties of known compounds first. The many methods now available can rank order a very large number (often millions) of compounds based on their predicted activities relative to other similar or diverse molecules. Traditional methods have been physics-based or use some variant of linear methods. They are being supplemented with new AI/ML methods inspired by the advent of deep neural networks (DNNs) in image analysis. A thorough review of the VL screening tools and approaches has recently been published [21]. Recent studies include the application of several DL approaches, including feedforward DNNs, pairwise input neural nets (NNs), recurrent NNs, CNNs, and graph convolutional networks (CNs). They highlight that DL methods have advantages over traditional methods because of their ability to identify and build relationships that are not directly encoded by the traditional methods.

Recall, though, that there are many tools in the ML toolshed and the utility of a given tool is highly dependent upon its intended use. It is important to evaluate tools with the appropriate performance metrics before claims are made about their superiority for a specific task. Unfortunately, a direct head-to-head comparison of methodologies is logistically difficult, despite the availability of many compound and protein datasets. Each model or approach has unique underlying assumptions in how the molecules and proteins are treated (atom types, conformational approaches, charge models, and other parameters) and in the type of biological data used for training and testing. The tolerance to confounding variables, errors in the descriptors, missing or insufficient data, and redundancy in the dataset must also be considered. It is extremely difficult to ensure that all molecules and proteins are treated similarly across methods. When methods have been shown to be somewhat comparable, the DL methods tend to outperform the more traditional ML methods [21,22]. The exact reasons behind this improved performance have not been fully understood. Recent publications suggest that such comparisons are dependent upon the careful curation and removal of very similar protein sequences and closely related 3D structures of cocrystals with the small molecules used to train and test the models [23,24]. Intuitively, if a model is tested on examples largely identical to those on which it has been trained, it will perform better.

Recent success has been encountered in the de novo generation of novel chemical matter with desired chemical properties using AI. In one case, a generic recurrent neural net (RNN) was fed into a specifically trained deep RNN with LSTM cells to identify compounds for synthesis. In an important experimental test, compounds were shown to be active against therapeutically relevant targets in cellular systems [25]. The ability to generate novel compounds with one or more desired properties and binding has been demonstrated with RNN/LSTMs, reinforcement learning, and conditional adversarial autoencoders. These methods can generate compound libraries for diverse screening and refine libraries around a group of known actives [26–28].

In efforts to discover novel chemical matter of potential therapeutic value, the definition of "success" can be quite varied among the members of an interdisciplinary team, particularly those building the models and the discovery and research scientists who are asked to rely upon their output. While successful rank ordering of compounds for binding activity may be considered a success by computational scientists, most experienced medicinal chemists rightly focus on both the experimental activity levels and an estimate of how likely those hits are to progress towards the clinic, which is influenced by many factors. Lead compounds, regardless of how they are found, must clear significant additional hurdles to establish appropriate profiles using in vitro and in vivo models. Critical steps include demonstration of on-target engagement in vivo and avoidance of off-target toxicities. These are more expensive studies. Fewer compounds can be tested, which means less "where the rubber hits the road data" of these critical varieties is available to inform ML/AI model building.

Predicting Absorption, Distribution, Metabolism, and Excretion Properties of Therapeutics

Goh et al. [29] have recently developed a DNN-based approach to calculate chemical properties such as toxicity, activity, solubility, and solvation energy which outperforms traditional methods. They have also identified a method to explain the results in an interpretable manner, addressing one of the key issues for NN. Li et al. [30] have employed multitask DNNs to develop predictive models of the effect on cytochrome P450 (CYP450) enzymes, a critical step in reducing adverse drug–drug interactions. In contrast, Hop and team [31] have recently applied two DNNs and a random forest (RF) algorithm to commonly used ADME (absorption, distribution, metabolism, and excretion)/pharmacokinetic (PK) datasets and found that none of the methods performed well; the variability in their own models raises questions about the comparability of the methods applied to these datasets.

Automating Tools Used in the Drug Discovery Process

The number of tools available to discovery researchers is astounding. Historically, these techniques and methods, such as image analysis, peptide sequencing, and prediction of secondary protein structure, can be cumbersome, tedious, or difficult, making them good candidates for automation or improvement through adoption of AI/ML methods. Although the immediate impact on the overall cost to develop a drug may be small, the ability to generate and interpret significantly more data in shorter time and with higher quality can be substantial, suggesting potential downstream benefits. A thorough review of the tools in use is beyond the remit of this chapter, so we limit ourselves to a scant few examples.

Image analysis in cellular biology leverages the tremendous advances made in image analysis in general as applied to difficult problems. Examples include cell and tissue analysis, subcellular localization analysis and advanced microscopy [22]. DL and visualization using imaging flow cytometry provides a reconstruction of the cell cycle in cell lines [32]. Ultra-high throughput optical microscopy combined with ML has shown promise in classification of cell heterogeneity. The CNN methods do as well as classical methods do, such as SVMs [33]. Rapid adoption of DNNs for preclinical image analysis is likely to follow clinical adoption, which is already underway. CNNs have also shown promise in using image analysis to free scientists from the tedium of counting cells in wells for single-cell studies [34]. Various types of DNNs and LSTM networks can use protein sequence data to identify subcellular localization of proteins and to successfully predict protein secondary structures [35]. As in other cases, careful selection of data, algorithms and parameter tuning are needed for successful predictions. The application of DL to de novo peptide sequencing, used in the characterization of monoclonal antibodies, can outperform classical methods [36]. Prediction of protein structure contact maps remains a formidable problem despite significant effort. RNNs and DNNs have recently shown promise at improving the success rate to about 35%. Recently, NNs have improved the prediction of secondary structure to just over 80% [37].

Chemical Synthesis Planning Software

Synthetic chemists spend a great deal of their time and effort considering the synthetic pathways to their desired final product. This is a daunting task and requires thorough knowledge of hundreds of possible reactions with their known limitations. Not surprisingly, considerable energy has been invested in making that undertaking easier. Relevant software can be broken into two broad groups, each addressing one of two basic questions: (1) given a set of reactants and reaction conditions, predict all the products and yields (forward synthetic planning); (2) given a desired product, provide the chemist with possible routes from commercially available reactants (retrosynthetic planning). ML methods directed at these goals date back to the 1960s, but recent applications have resulted in substantial improvements in both areas. Retrosynthesis using carefully constructed and extensive rule-based heuristics can provide straightforward reaction pathways and commercially available materials that can be used to synthesize compounds in the laboratory [38]. DNNs and symbolic AI have also been shown to outperform classical retrosynthetic methods [39]. Rapid progress is being made; still there are significant limitations to the practical utility of both approaches. Until those are addressed adequately, the adoption of the methods by the synthetic chemistry community remains uncertain.

Conformational Analysis of Small Molecules

A key step in calculating the physical properties and binding ability of any molecule is the conformational profile of the compound. Molecular mechanics (MM) methods are used extensively in the field, despite their inherent limitations. MM is a classical physics-based model in which the atoms, bonds, and rotations are described by a force-field capturing different bond constants, dihedral angles, van der Waals, and charge−charge interaction terms. We incorporate these features in models that are trained to best fit known structures and chemical properties. Calculating the atomic partial charges for any given molecule can be hard. Recently, atomic partial charges were predicted using an RF regression model and incorporated into force-field calculations, potentially improving the ability to accurately model compounds [40]. A much-improved approach would be to replace traditional MM methods by more detailed quantum mechanical (QM) descriptions of molecules which should yield better insights, but the high computational costs of such a tactic can make this impractical. Recently, however, the work by Smith et al. [41] has shown that a DNN can be trained to produce these QM energies at speeds competitive with those of molecular mechanical methods, with the added benefit of providing energetics for nonequilibrium structures. Investigation of the utility of this approach in refining structure-based design predictions and conformational analyses has quickly commenced, with the promise of increasing the accuracy of the calculations of the physical and binding properties of small molecules.

Do We Need All These New Classifier Methods in Drug Discovery?

As was mentioned earlier, new and elaborately named methods do not always imply they are better methods. It is critical to use the right tool for the problem of interest. Again, direct comparison of methods is often difficult. In one attempt, researchers compared the performance of 179 classifiers in 17 classifier families using 121 publicly available datasets. Overall, they found that the "best" classifier methods were RF, SVMs, neural networks, and boosting ensembles, though any one performed as well as another (Fernandez-Delgado) [42]. The study also highlights several common criticisms and limitations of ML methods: the selection of the dataset on which to apply the method might impact the overall performance of that method; the maximum attainable accuracy for a given dataset is not determined; understanding whether classification errors are due to limitations in the learner or in the dataset; and the lack of standards for data partitioning for cross-validation approaches. Another effort to make direct head-to-head comparisons using known datasets applied older ML methods and several DNN to several important physicochemical and biological datasets. Prediction of physicochemical properties, such as solubility, was comparable between the methods, but predictions of compound activities against clinical strains of bubonic plague were poor across the techniques. These authors cautioned that users should carefully consider all performance characteristics of the model [43].

Section III: How Might Machine Learning Help in Drug and Biologic Development?

ML is not new, of course. Although logistic regression has been used to identify variables predictive of clinical outcome for decades, it is only recently that more advanced techniques of ML and modeling have been applied to clinical data. In contrast to drug discovery, where many companies, as outlined in the previous section, are forging ahead quickly with innovative applications of ML, the use of the latter in clinical drug development is still largely embryonic. *Yet ML is poised to transform the practice of clinical medicine in the not-too-distant future, and that which alters the face of medicine also changes the profile of clinical drug development.* Healthcare analytics studies, focused most frequently on clinical decision support and administrative tools, increased by more than sixfold between the middle of the last decade and the early part of this decade according to a recent comprehensive review spanning the years 2005–16 [44]. Classification was, by far, the most common data mining tool, although clustering and association studies were also relatively well represented. Neural nets, decision trees, SVMs, and logistic regression ranked among the most common classification techniques used. Therapeutic areas for decision support tools varied, with a prominence in oncology, cardiovascular disease, Intensive Care Unit(ICU)/Emergency Room (ER), and diabetes with accuracy rates that generally ranged widely from the mid-50s to well over 90%.

More granular insights into a patient's condition and the possible perils he or she faces in the future, based on a swath of clinical and–omics data, will have implications for target product profiles in drug or biologic development programs, engendering better, safer, and more precise interventions in a given clinical case. In this vein, ML classifiers and "precision medicine" are conjoined twins. Ultimately, with finer parsing of patient populations into more refined diagnostic categories, each tethered to specific risks and therapeutic outcomes, we will be in a better position to more precisely intervene, both preemptively and therapeutically, with an eye toward enhancing human health. Otherwise stated, if we can confirm that the group of patients with an overarching diagnosis of "X" actually consists of multiple subsets (e.g., X_1, X_2, and X_3), each attended by greater or lesser degrees of risk for pathological processes that eventuate in certain disease complications, we can surgically tailor interventions to the specific patient with disease X_1 rather than intervene on the basis of the "averaged knowledge" of future risks for the entire group (i.e., X) as a whole. As has been said, no individual patient is "average." It is of interest that Zarkoob et al. [45] were able to slightly enhance prediction of the development of type 2 diabetes mellitus in a Swedish cohort by feeding both genomic (SNP data) and environmental factors into a risk assessment engine. Genetic data were more helpful in patients at lower environmental risk. In the clinic, individual mutations and polymorphisms may be used to predict the rate of drug metabolism (CYP polymorphisms), drug hypersensitivity (abacavir), and tumor responsiveness (various mutations), but this is the lower lying fruit of genomic studies. In contrast, polygenic inheritance in type 2 diabetes is highly complex and incompletely understood, so it is notable that model predictions did improve at least minimally when genetic data were considered by Zarkoob et al. Transcriptomic data have also been used in many thousands of human and preclinical ML models [46]. We must now consider the potential strength of models that partition patients into response groups based on variables that span the –omics.

Traditionally, our efforts to discern differences between patient groups and outcomes that can be predicted based on patient features or biomarkers have relied upon clinical trials, meta-analyses, or epidemiologic databases using, quite often, simple post-hoc statistics. Sometimes, small underpowered studies of rare patient groups/subgroups or case reports are relied upon by clinicians, despite the inherent limitations of these data sources. But future access to extremely large, anonymized, integrated, multidimensional, longitudinal clinical datasets, spanning electronic health records, medical claims data, and anonymized clinical trial data, will provide unprecedented substrate for insights into biomarkers through potent ML methods with a lower risk of overfitting given the volume of data. In fact, the data integration effort has already begun with companies specifically devoting themselves to attaining this goal. And modern computational firepower will enable us to plumb the canyons of these oceans of integrated data, rather than restrict ourselves to shallow scattered data lakes.

Most of this chapter has thus far been devoted to supervised learning algorithms, in which we choose a panoply of candidate features that are used by the algorithm to predict a class label (e.g., "likely to respond to Drug X"). Feature selection techniques can narrow the playing field to mitigate the risk of overfitting supervised algorithms, thereby increasing the likelihood of teasing out relevant biomarkers. Yet it should be noted that *unsupervised* learning, in which machines create their own categories or clusters based on features, can also be illuminating. This may grant insights into heretofore unknown or undefined patient subsets with particular pathophysiological characteristics that may render them more or less likely to respond to a given intervention. Different techniques can be used. For example, partitional clustering seeks to maximize distances between a preset number of clusters, while hierarchical clustering creates a richly informative nested hierarchy of clusters that can be cut at any desired level of granularity. Unfortunately, hierarchical clustering methods generally exact a high computational load due to time complexity, which can hinder scalability to large data sets. DL and other methods may be of particular use in unsupervised learning. For example, Li et al. [47] identified subtypes of diabetes mellitus patients at risk for certain diseases and complications using (unsupervised) topographical data analysis of high-dimensional electronic medical record and genotypic data. Graphic models, in a manner analogous to unsupervised learning, may also cast light in unseen quarters if the *structure* of the model is learned from data. Surprising risk factors for disease and/or insights into biomarker profiles might derive from such an exercise.

Apart from splintering patients into more refined subsets, novel in silico models of *individual* clinical diseases may also be useful in R&D. Hayete et al. [48] developed a Bayesian model of outcomes in Parkinson's disease. IBM has performed much work in the field of oncology, too extensive to describe in detail here. By using a label propagation method, effectively spreading information over a graph, Zhang et al. [49] showed that combined analysis of patient and drug similarity can predict response to a statin. Tangentially, a recent study has suggested that in silico drug trials might aid in prediction of proarrhythmic cardiotoxicity in the clinic [50].

Drug development is infamously expensive and risk-laden. Risk–benefit ratio optimization in drug development, enabled by insights into biomarkers afforded by ML, would streamline development efforts and minimize cost, as the enhancement of the treatment effect (delta) may permit use of smaller sample sizes to demonstrate clinical benefit, thereby lessening cost. This would also reduce the risk of "gold-plated Phase 2 failures" through the enrichment of study populations better suited to a particular intervention.

Operational efficiencies may also be realized. Classification and search algorithms might be used to match patients to clinical trials. Envision a world in which patients, who own their own data, anonymously and securely share their primary condition and health data with algorithm that returns a ranked list of clinical trials for which they are most likely to be eligible and from which they may derive clinical benefit.

The safety of research subjects and the public might also be better safeguarded by ML. For example, tight ambulatory monitoring of selected patients receiving experimental drugs, thorough the use of mobile medical devices and DL algorithms that lend themselves to the analysis of intensive time-series data, may detect the early portion of a subject's trajectory toward deterioration related to an adverse event, potentially allowing for earlier intervention that would spare morbidity and mortality. ML in the era of big data may also radically alter the practice of post–marketing surveillance, as numerous strands of virtual data are incorporated into the fabric of safety monitoring.

Overall Conclusions

ML in drug and biologic R&D promises abundance in a wide swath of settings, but this relatively young field must be tended carefully by teams of experts with relevant cross-disciplinary expertise. Such cultivators will, through their innovative practices, ultimately transform drug and biologic R&D over ensuing years and decades.

Appropriately choosing a specific ML tool and set of candidate predictive features is not an arbitrary selection process based, for example, on how cutting-edge, complex and powerful that implement might be, or the availability of an enormous array of data features one might happen to have in the form of genomic, transcriptomic, proteomic, and metabolomic databases. As a means of underscoring this point, it is worth noting that data from a multi-site study evaluating >30,000 human and preclinical models of transcriptomic data used by 36 separate teams revealed that the choice of a particular ML algorithm was of less importance than other factors in determining success, such as team proficiency and the manner in which model algorithms are specifically implemented [46].

Some of the other take-home points from the current review are listed as follows:

- Although a truism, we must respect the primacy of data, as a sow's ear is a sow's ear no matter how talented the seamstress. Scrub, reconcile, format, integrate, and address missing values. When dealing with disparate datasets of patient records, for example, accurate linking is indispensable.
- Carefully negotiate the trade-off between overfitting at one pole and impoverished models (i.e., underfitting) at the other. *The goal is to maximize model generalizability to independent datasets on which the model was not trained.*
- Cross validation of a model is your friend and can help one to better assess the generalizability of a model and the need for modifications.
- An assembly of models that complement each other may synergistically achieve, through voting, more accurate predictions than any single constituent model in the assembly. That is, the whole of parliament may be greater than the sum of the individuals.

Biotechnology and pharmaceutical companies have begun to take a genuine interest in the application of AI/ML techniques to their own data repositories, where extensive compound information and experimental data provide rich multidimensional input that is not available in full externally. Negative proprietary data can also be leveraged well in this capacity. Access to electronic lab notebook data on reaction conditions and yields can also be quite helpful [51]. Training models for predicting binding affinity or ADME or toxicology properties could incorporate both public datasets and internally developed data. One key hurdle to surmount, however, is the compartmentalization of data in silos at biopharmaceutical companies. Integration and reconciliation of disparate data sources, even under a single roof may be a complicated ordeal, but the potential payoff is real. Several early stage startup companies are using ML methods to create their own platforms to rapidly identify validated targets, discover novel chemical matter, and elucidate preclinical biology. As noted, newer DL methods may offer some advantages within the realm of drug discovery, although these preliminary findings must be confirmed. ML can also be deployed to gain insights into potential clinical biomarkers that aid in drug development.

Despite the excitement spurred by a treasure trove of new -omics data and powerful ML methods, we must emphasize that the final validation of a hypothesis of therapeutic utility is only achieved once a compound successfully passes through clinical trials and meets with the approval of regulatory agencies. Timelines are long in this industry, and promising drug/target combinations continue to fail with discouraging frequency. This is not for the lack of trying novel ideas. One can reasonably hope that contemporary ML and modeling approaches might reduce timelines and enhance the likelihood of success, but much of the sand that knows whether this hypothesis is true still resides above the waist of the hourglass.

References

[1] Sahner D. Machine learning, modeling and predictive analytics: key principles for the clinical scientist. Appl Clin Trials 2017; (published online). Available from: <http://www.appliedclinicaltrialsonline.com/machine-learning-modeling-and-predictive-analytics-key-principles-clinical-scientist>.

[2] Sucar LE. Probabilistic graphical models principles and applications. London, Heidelberg, New York, Dordrecht: Springer; 2015.

[3] Goodfellow I, Bengio Y, Courville A. Deep learning. Cambridge, MA, and London: The MIT Press; 2016.

[4] Xu D, Clappison A, Seth C, Orchard J. Symmetric predictive estimator for biologically plausible neural learning. IEEE Trans Neural Networks Learn Syst 2018;29(9):4140–51.

[5] Chien J-T, Bao Y-T. Tensor-factorized neural networks. IEEE Trans Neural Networks Learn Syst 2018;29(5):1998–2011.

[6] Xiao Z, Luo Z, Zhong B, Dang X. Robust and efficient boosting method using the conditional risk. IEEE Trans Neural Networks Learn Syst 2018;29(7):3069–83.

[7] Makarev E, Cantor C, Zhavoronkov A, Buzdin A, Aliper A, Csoka AB. Pathway activation profiling reveals new insights into age-related macular degeneration and provides avenues for therapeutic interventions. Aging 2014;6(12):1064–75.

[8] Ozerov IV, Lezhnina KV, Izumchenko E, Artemov A, Medintsev S, et al. *In silico* pathway activation network decomposition analysis (iPANDA) as a method for biomarker development. Nat Commun 2016;. Available from: https://doi.org/10.1038/ncomms13427.

[9] Artemov A, Aliper A, Korzinkin M, Lezhnina K, Jellen L, et al. A method for predicting target drug efficiency in cancer based on the analysis of signaling pathway activation. Oncotarget 2015;6 (30):29347–56.

[10] Palsson BO. Systems biology constraint-based reconstruction and analysis. Cambridge University Press; 2015.

[11] Palsson BO. Systems biology simulation of dynamic network states. New York: Cambridge University Press; 2011.

[12] Hu Z-Z, Huang H, Wu CH, Jung M, Dritschilo A, Riegel AT, et al. Omics-based molecular target and biomarker identification. In: Mayer B, editor. Bioinformatics for omics data [Internet]. Totowa, NJ: Humana Press; 2011. p. 547–71. Available from: <http://link.springer.com/10.1007/978-1-61779-027-0_26> [cited November 14, 2018].

[13] Ching T, Himmelstein DS, Beaulieu-Jones BK, Kalinin AA, Do BT, Way GP, et al. Opportunities and obstacles for deep learning in biology and medicine; 2018. Available from: <http://biorxiv.org/lookup/doi/10.1101/142760> [cited June 30, 2018].

[14] Hwang B, Lee JH, Bang D. Single-cell RNA sequencing technologies and bioinformatics pipelines. Exp Mol Med [Internet] 2018;50(8). Available from: <http://www.nature.com/articles/s12276-018-0071-8> [cited October 31, 2018].

[15] Alipanahi B, Delong A, Weirauch MT, Frey BJ. Predicting the sequence specificities of DNA- and RNA-binding proteins by deep learning. Nat Biotechnol 2015;33(8):831–8.

[16] Delgado FM, Gómez-Vela F. Computational methods for gene regulatory networks reconstruction and analysis: a review. Artif Intell Med [Internet] 2018;. Available from: <https://linkinghub.elsevier.com/retrieve/pii/S0933365718303865> [cited November 16, 2018].

[17] Xue M, Tang Y, Wu L, Qian F. Model approximation for switched genetic regulatory networks. IEEE Trans Neural Networks Learn Syst 2018;29(8):3404–17.

[18] Cherkasov A, Muratov EN, Fourches D, Varnek A, Baskin II, Cronin M, et al. QSAR modeling: where have you been? Where are you going to? J Med Chem 2014;57(12):4977–5010.

[19] Zhavoronkov A. Artificial intelligence for drug discovery, biomarker development, and generation of novel chemistry. Mol Pharm 2018;15(10):4311–13.

[20] Lo Y-C, Rensi SE, Torng W, Altman RB. Machine learning in chemoinformatics and drug discovery. Drug Discov Today 2018;23(8):1538–46.

[21] Rifaioglu AS, Atas H, Martin MJ, Cetin-Atalay R, Atalay V, Doğan T. Recent applications of deep learning and machine intelligence on in silico drug discovery: methods, tools and databases. *Brief Bioinf* [Internet] 2018. Available from: <https://academic.oup.com/bib/advance-article/doi/10.1093/bib/bby061/5062947> [cited October 22, 2018].

[22] Mahmud M, Kaiser MS, Hussain A, Vassanelli S. Applications of deep learning and reinforcement learning to biological data. IEEE Trans Neural Networks Learn Syst 2018;29(6):2063–79.

[23] Li Y, Yang J. Structural and sequence similarity makes a significant impact on machine-learning-based scoring functions for protein–ligand interactions. J Chem Inf Model 2017;57(4) 1007–12.

[24] Wallach I, Heifets A. Most ligand-based classification benchmarks reward memorization rather than generalization. J Chem Inf Model 2018;58(5):916–32.

[25] Merk D, Friedrich L, Grisoni F, Schneider G. De novo design of bioactive small molecules by artificial intelligence. Mol Inf 2018;37(1–2):1700153.

[26] Kadurin A, Aliper A, Kazennov A, Mamoshina P, Vanhaelen Q, Khrabrov K, et al. The cornucopia of meaningful leads: applying deep adversarial autoencoders for new molecule development in oncology. Oncotarget [Internet] 2017;8(7). Available from: <http://www.oncotarget.com/fulltext/14073> [cited October 27, 2018].

[27] Popova M, Isayev O, Tropsha A. Deep reinforcement learning for de novo drug design. Sci Adv 2018;4(7):eaap7885.

[28] Segler MHS, Kogej T, Tyrchan C, Waller MP. Generating focused molecule libraries for drug discovery with recurrent neural networks. ACS Cent Sci 2018;4(1):120–31.

[29] Goh GB, Hodas NO, Siegel C, Vishnu A. SMILES2Vec: an interpretable general-purpose deep neural network for predicting chemical properties. arXiv:171202034 [cs, stat] [Internet] 2017. Available from: <http://arxiv.org/abs/1712.02034> [cited November 5, 2018].

[30] Li X, Xu Y, Lai L, Pei J. Prediction of human cytochrome p450 inhibition using a multitask deep autoencoder neural network. Mol Pharm 2018;15(10):4336–45.

[31] Hop Patrick, Allgood B, Yu J. Geometric deep learning autonomously learns chemical features that outperform those engineered by domain experts. Mol Pharm [Internet] 2018;. Available from: <http://pubs.acs.org/doi/10.1021/acs.molpharmaceut.7b01144> [cited June 30, 2018].

[32] Eulenberg P, Köhler N, Blasi T, Filby A, Carpenter AE, Rees P, et al. Reconstructing cell cycle and disease progression using deep learning. Nat Commun [Internet] 2017;8(1). Available from: <http://www.nature.com/articles/s41467-017-00623-3> [cited November 6, 2018].

[33] Meng N, Lam E, Tsia KKM, So HK-H. Large-scale multi-class image-based cell classification with deep learning. IEEE J Biomed Health Inf 2018;1.

[34] Kamatani T, Fukunaga K, Miyata K, Shirasaki Y, Tanaka J, Baba R, et al. Construction of a system using a deep learning algorithm to count cell numbers in nanoliter wells for viable single-cell experiments. Sci Rep [Internet] 2017;7(1). Available from: <http://www.nature.com/articles/s41598-017-17012-x> [cited November 6, 2018].

[35] Jurtz VI, Johansen AR, Nielsen M, Almagro Armenteros JJ, Nielsen H, Sønderby CK, et al. An introduction to deep learning on biological sequence data: examples and solutions. Bioinformatics 2017;33(22):3685–90.

[36] Tran NH, Zhang X, Xin L, Shan B, Li M. De novo peptide sequencing by deep learning. Proc Natl Acad Sci USA 2017;114 (31):8247–52.

[37] Goh GB, Hodas NO, Vishnu A. Deep learning for computational chemistry. J Comput Chem 2017;38(16):1291–307.

[38] Klucznik T, Mikulak-Klucznik B, McCormack MP, Lima H, Szymkuć S, Bhowmick M, et al. Efficient syntheses of diverse, medicinally relevant targets planned by computer and executed in the laboratory. Chem 2018;(3):522–32.

[39] Segler MHS, Preuss M, Waller MP. Planning chemical syntheses with deep neural networks and symbolic AI. Nature 2018;555 (7698):604–10.

[40] Bleiziffer P, Schaller K, Riniker S. Machine learning of partial charges derived from high-quality quantum-mechanical calculations. J Chem Inf Model 2018;58(3):579–90.

[41] Smith JS, Isayev O, Roitberg AE. ANI-1: an extensible neural network potential with DFT accuracy at force field computational cost. Chem Sci 2017;8(4):3192–203.

[42] Fernandez-Delgado M, Cernadas E, Barro S, Amorim D. Do we need hundreds of classifiers to solve real world classification problems? J Mach Learn Res 2014;15(1):3133–81.

[43] Korotcov A, Tkachenko V, Russo DP, Ekins S. Comparison of deep learning with multiple machine learning methods and metrics using diverse drug discovery data sets. Mol Pharm 2017;14 (12):4462–75.

[44] Islam MS, Hasan MM, Wang X, Germack HD, Noor-E-Alam M. A systematic review on healthcare analytics: application and theoretical perspective of data mining. Healthcare 2018;6(54). Available from: https://doi.org/10.3390/healthcare6020054.

[45] Zarkoob H, Lewinsky S, Almgren P, Melander O, Fakhrai-Rad H. Utilization of genetic data can improve the prediction of type 2 diabetes incidence in a Swedish cohort. PLoS One 2017;12(7):e0180180. Available from: https://doi.org/10.1371/journal.pone.0180180.

[46] MAQC Consortium. The microarray quality control (MAQC)-II study of common practices for the development and validation of microarray-based predictive models. Nat Biotechnol 2010;28 (8):827–38.

[47] Li L, Cheng W-Y, Glicksberg BS, Gottesman O, Tamler R, et al. Identification of type 2 diabetes subgroups through topological analysis of patient similarity. Sci Transl Med 2015;7 (311):311ra174. Available from: https://doi.org/10.1126/scitranslmed.aaa9364. Available from.

[48] Hayete B, Wuest D, Laramie J, McDonagh P, Church B, et al. A Bayesian mathematical model of motor and cognitive outcomes in Parkinson's disease. PLoS One 2017;12(6):e0178982. Available from: https://doi.org/10.1371/journal.pone.0178982. Available from.

[49] Zhang P, Wang F, Hu J, Sorrentino R. Towards personalized medicine: leveraging patient similarity and drug similarity analytics. In: AMIA Joint Summits on Translational Science Proceedings; 2014. p. 132–136.

[50] Passini E, Britton OJ, Lu HR, Rohrbacher J, Hermans AN, et al. Human in silico drug trials demonstrate higher accuracy than animal models in predicting clinical pro-arrhythmic cardiotoxicity. Front Physiol 2017;8:668. Available from: https://doi.org/10.3389/fphys2017.00668. Available from.

[51] Engkvist O, Norrby P-O, Selmi N, Lam Y, Peng Z, Sherer EC, et al. Computational prediction of chemical reactions: current status and outlook. Drug Discov Today 2018;23(6):1203–18.

Chapter 29

Artificial Intelligence in Biotechnology: A Framework for Commercialization[1]

Robert E. Wanerman, JD, MPH*, Gail H. Javitt, JD, MPH* and Alaap B. Shah, JD, MPH*

Partners at Epstein Becker Green, PC, United States

Chapter Outline

The growth of biotechnology research and development has been occurring alongside the development of new and more sophisticated artificial intelligence (AI) tools. The ability to apply AI to health care can already be seen in studies comparing physicians' diagnoses of skin cancer, lung cancer, seizures, and diabetic retinopathy to those made by computer algorithms [1]. A report published by the Pew Research Center estimates that approximately 79% of Americans surveyed believe that within the next 20 years, physicians will use computers to diagnose illnesses and determine plans of care [2]. The incentives for the adoption of AI in health care include reduced health-care costs and improved the quality of care. For example, one estimate of the potential savings to the US health-care system runs as high as $150 billion through 2026 [3]. In parallel, investment in health-care AI is also rising; from approximately $4.3 billion in 2013 to a projected $6.6 billion by 2026 [4]. Recognizing this potential, large pharmaceutical companies have begun to invest in AI through acquisition of or collaboration with software and data analytics companies [5]. As the two strands of technology progress, multiple questions will arise as to how these advances fit within a health-care system. Although long-range predictions are difficult, a framework for analysis is a useful tool. In this chapter we will review some principles to help provide a framework for the biotech entrepreneur to consider, as products from AI and their resulting regulatory guidance evolves.

Background and Context

AI is an umbrella term that incorporates several distinct applications of computer science. Briefly, these applications can be broken down into three general categories. Machine learning (ML) relies on algorithms that apply statistical methods to analyze patterns in data and to identify inferences with specific degrees of certainty. As the available database grows and the algorithm is refined over time, the inferences and their accuracy can grow as well. Currently, machine learning methods can take one of the following three forms:

- **Supervised leaning**, which relies on algorithms set by a human programmer and intended to analyze specific known data for a specific outcome.
- **Unsupervised learning**, which refers to the analysis of unidentified data by an algorithm with the objective of identifying patterns in the database that have not been preset by the programmer.
- **Reinforcement learning**, which can be thought of as a hybrid of supervised and unsupervised learning and is intended to be a test of the underlying algorithm itself to evaluate its predictive accuracy [6].

---

*Robert E. Wanerman, Gail H. Javitt and Alaap B. Shah are partners in the Washington, DC office of Epstein Becker Green, P.C. United States. The discussion in the chapter does not constitute legal advice, as the facts and circumstances of a particular matter may involve questions of law that are not addressed here.

1. The authors gratefully acknowledge the assistance of Brian Hedgeman, J.D., Dr. P.H. in preparing this chapter.

Biotechnology Entrepreneurship. DOI: https://doi.org/10.1016/B978-0-12-815585-1.00029-2

The second form of AI is known as deep learning. This refers to the development of algorithms called artificial neural networks, which attempts to replicate the way that a human brain processes information and makes a decision. The networks act like layers that mimic the structure and functioning of the brain to recognize known or unknown patterns. For example, each layer may analyze a particular feature in an object; once its work is complete, the analysis then moves to another layer to either refine the analysis or add to it by analyzing other features or characteristics of the object. This continues until the object can be identified or classified with a known level of confidence. One familiar example of the application of deep learning is the development of facial recognition programs used by some popular websites.

The third general category of AI is cognitive computing; this integrates multiple forms of machine learning to solve problems without the prompt of a human programmer. One characteristic is their ability to interact directly with humans and to learn from their experiences with humans. An example of cognitive computing in use is IBM Watson ([6]; *see also* https://www.ibm.com/blogs/internet-of-things/iot-cognitive-computing-watson/).

Use of Artificial Intelligence in Health Care: Privacy and Security Risks and Rules

Applications of AI in health care for research, development, or treatment require large amounts of data to produce the results that either complement or replace work done by humans. In the United States and in many other nations the access to that data and its use are regulated. Understanding how the regulatory framework operates in a specific context may be difficult not only due to the diverse segments of the health-care sector, such as research, development, manufacturing, and treatment, but also due to the diversity of settings for each category.[2] Adding to the complexity is the variability among types of AI as discussed previously.[3] Moreover, many AI technologies are designed and function as "black boxes" with opaque processes,[4] often with the capacity to operate in unforeseeable ways.[5]

The current regulation of AI in health care is a patchwork of laws and regulations. This patchwork comprises multiple federal laws and regulations addressing different aspects of risk, international law, and common law. Although few laws explicitly address AI, examining these laws may inform the development of further regulation. Likewise, examining regulation in other areas related to transparency, reliability, fairness, and safety may offer insights that inform how AI regulation ought to be developed. The general outlines of those regulations are discussed in the next subsections, and compliance with those rules should be an integral part of any application of AI for research, diagnosis, or treatment.

Patient Privacy and Data Security Risks

A preliminary issue for researchers and developers is ensuring that they have adequate data rights that permit sharing and using patient data for purposes of development. Even if adequate rights exist, data security should be considered when permitting collection, storage, and processing data through development (i.e., nonproduction) systems.[6]

In the United States the use and disclosure of individually identifiable patient information are governed by the Health Insurance Portability and Accountability Act and regulations, better known as HIPAA. Briefly, a covered entity, which includes health-care providers and plans,

2. Some scholars have argued that lawmakers generally struggle with *ex ante* regulation of technology, and that such attempts have largely resulted in failure. *See generally*, Reed, C. How to make bad law: lessons from cyberspace. Mod. Law Rev. 2010;73:903.

3. *See generally* Giuffrida I, et al. *A legal perspective on the trials and tribulations of AI: how artificial intelligence, the internet of things, smart contracts, and other technologies will affect the law*, 68 Case W. Res. L. Rev. 2018;747:751–59; *See also* Stone P, et al., *Artificial intelligence and life in 2030." One hundred year study on artificial intelligence*: *report of the 2015–2016 study panel.* Stanford, CA: Stanford University at 48 (September 2016). Available at <http://ai100.stanford.edu/2016-report> [last accessed Jan. 30, 2019] (noting that "The Study Panel's consensus is that attempts to regulate 'AI' in general would be misguided, since there is no clear definition of AI (it isn't any one thing), and the risks and considerations are very different in different domains. Instead, policymakers should recognize that to varying degrees and over time, various industries will need distinct, appropriate, regulations that touch on software built using AI or incorporating AI in some way. The government will need the expertise to scrutinize standards and technology developed by the private and public sector, and to craft regulations where necessary.")

4. *See* V. Mayer-schönberger and K. cukier. Big Data: A revolution that will transform how we live, work, and think (2013) at 179 (noting that "we can see the risk that big-data predictions, and the algorithms and datasets behind the, will become black boxes that offer us no accountability, traceability, or confidence. To prevent this, big data will require monitoring and transparency, which in turn will require new types of expertise and institutions).

5. *See* R. Calo, *Robotics and the Lessons of Cyberlaw*, 103 calif. L. Rev. 513, 539 (2015) (discussing the concept of "emergence" whereby a "system learns from previous behavior" and "improve at a task over time", but also noting that "emergent behavior can lead to solutions no human would have come to on her own"); *See also* M. Scherer, *Regulating Artificial Intelligence Systems: Risks, Challenges, Competencies, and Strategies.* 29(2) Harvard J. Law & Tech. 354, 366 (2016) (arguing that "a learning AI's designer will not be able to foresee how it will act after it is sent out into the world . . ." (citing J. Balkin, *The Path of Robotics Law*, 6 calif. L. Rev. circuit 45, 52 (2015)).

6. *See, for example*, SANS Institute. Making Database Security an IT Security Priority (Nov. 2009) at 11–12. Available at: <https://software-security.sans.org/resources/paper/reading-room/making-database-security-security-priority>; (Informatica. Best Practices for Ensuring Data Privacy in Production and Nonproduction Systems (2011). Available at: <https://www.informatica.com/downloads/6993_Data_Privacy_BestPractices_wp.pdf>.

may not use or disclose protected health information (PHI) unless the patient provides a written authorization to do so or a specific exception to the authorization requirement applies. There are exceptions for the covered entity's own treatment, payment, and health-care operations functions, but these do not apply to research and development of new drugs or treatments using that patient data. Although some research organizations are not covered by the regulations because they are not covered entities, they may come into contact with covered entities that store PHI that can be used in a database.

PHI that is used as part of an AI database can be obtained in several ways. First, as noted previously, if the covered entity uses the data in an AI application that is limited to its treatment of its patients or its operations, no authorization is necessary.[7] Second, the covered entity may disclose the PHI for use in an AI database by a business associate that performs certain work for the covered entity and has entered into an agreement that addresses the privacy and security of the PHI it receives.[8] Researchers can obtain patient data through several methods. Under the general HIPAA rule, researchers can obtain an authorization for the release of PHI along with obtaining informed consent. An alternative is to request approval from an institutional review board or a privacy board to approve the release of PHI without an individual's authorization provided that several prerequisites addressing the security of the PHI are met.[9] Third, the covered entity may release PHI in a limited data set for research or public health objectives that partially deidentifies the PHI. In this situation the recipient of the limited data set must execute a data use agreement before the covered entity can release the data.[10] Finally, deidentified data is no longer considered to be PHI and may be released freely by the covered entity.[11]

Once a system is in place, patient data can continue to flow through AI systems; this creates a potential secondary risk that requires including AI in privacy and security risk assessments and mitigation activities.[12] Risks may also arise due to deep learning in neural networks that can result in an AI algorithm acting in unanticipated and perhaps undesirable ways. Therefore it is conceivable that an AI system designed to process patients' data in one manner may, over time, process such data in other unforeseen ways. Even after an AI technology is decommissioned, residual risk to privacy and data security must be addressed through secure transfer of data out of such technologies and secure sanitization or the disposal of physical devices housing patient data.

Patient Safety Risks

Patient harm may occur if AI supplants clinical judgment such that a clinician is not making any clinical judgment. For example, a radiological imaging technology powered by AI could adversely affect patient safety if it were vulnerable to a cybersecurity compromise that would allow tampering with scan results.[13] A breach that allows unauthorized access could result in tampering with data integrity or the proper functioning of the item, which can result in patient harm. Likewise, clinical decision support tools,[14] the automation of surgical intervention,[15] radiological imaging review [7], and medical consults through chatbots[16] could pose patient safety risks if these technologies fail to function with sufficient accuracy, precision, and accountability.

Risks Arising from Bias and Unfairness

Improper design and application of AI in health care may generate risks associated with patient discrimination due to insufficient training of an AI algorithm. Further, there may be a risk of violating fraud and abuse laws arising from unreliability, inaccuracy, or bias associated with outputs.[17] For example, inaccuracy in AI algorithm outputs

7. 45 C.F.R. § 164.506.
8. 45 C.F.R. § 164.502.
9. 45 C.F.R. § 164.512(i).
10. 45 C.F.R. § 164.514(e)(1).
11. 45 C.F.R. § 164.514(a).
12. *See generally*, Shah A. Death by a thousand cuts: cybersecurity risk in the health care internet of things. AHLA Wkly May 19, 2018.
13. *See, for example*, Zetter K. Hospital viruses: fake cancerous nodes in CT scans, created by malware, trick radiologists. N.Y. Times Apr. 3, 2019. Available at: <https://www.washingtonpost.com/technology/2019/04/03/hospital-viruses-fake-cancerous-nodes-ct-scans-created-by-malware-trick-radiologists/?utm_term = .83f8487873b8> [last accessed Apr. 17, 2019].
14. *See generally*, Daniel G, et al. Current state and near-term priorities for AI-enabled diagnostic support software in health care. Duke Margolis Center for Health Policy; 2018. Available at: <https://healthpolicy.duke.edu/sites/default/files/atoms/files/dukemargolisaienableddxss.pdf>.
15. A preliminary study on robot surgery involving suturing a portion of human intestine showed promise with results indicating the Smart Tissue Autonomous Robot could perform the surgery without human intervention 60% of the time with higher quality stitches as compared to humans; however, 40% of the time a human did need to intervene to assist the robot from making an error.
16. *See, for example*, Fadhil A. A conversational interface to improve medication adherence: towards AI support in patient's treatment. U. Trento; 2018. Available at: <https://arxiv.org/ftp/arxiv/papers/1803/1803.09844.pdf>.
17. *See, for example*, A.I. could worsen health disparities, N.Y. Times Jan. 31, 2019. Available at: <https://www.nytimes.com/2019/01/31/opinion/ai-bias-healthcare.html> [last accessed Jan. 31, 2019].

could produce discriminatory coverage decisions by payors, adverse treatment determinations by providers, drive patients to seek inappropriate care, or even reduce access to health-care altogether [8]. As with other areas of risk, the use of AI technologies without sufficiently robust training of underlying AI algorithms with high-quality data and implementing mechanisms to verify the accuracy and precision of outputs could pose significant risks.[18]

Regulatory Oversight of Data Collection

In the United States a variety of federal authorities have jurisdiction over the regulatory schemes applicable to AI. These include, but are not limited to the Department of Health and Human Services (HHS), HHS's Office for Civil Rights, the Office of the National Coordinator for Health Information Technology, the Food and Drug Administration (FDA), and the Federal Trade Commission (FTC).

Federal Trade Commission Authority and Oversight

The FTC has enforcement authority under Section 5(a) of the FTC Act, which regulates unfair and deceptive trade practices. The FTC has also used its authority to expand the reach of HIPAA standards. In particular, the FTC has leveraged its broad authority under the FTC Act to start enforcement actions against entities that may have engaged in deceptive or unfair acts (that violate HIPAA and/or industry best practices). The FTC has pursued investigation and cases involving companies based on allegations related to failures to (1) sufficiently notify consumers about privacy practices, (2) adhere to representations made in privacy policies, and (3) implement reasonable security safeguards to protect consumer health information.

Food and Drug Administration Authority and Oversight

Like the FTC, the FDA has expressed keen interest related to privacy and security issues related to the medical device regulation. The FDA's regulatory authority generally relates to evaluating the safety and efficacy of drugs and devices in both the premarket and postmarket contexts. As a result of innovation in the digital and connect health arena, the FDA recognized the importance of managing privacy and security risks by releasing two sets of guidance. First, the FDA issued voluntary postmarket guidance addressing cybersecurity for connected medical devices [9]. Second, the FDA issued draft guidance on premarket submission related to medical device cybersecurity management.[19] In addition, the FDA collaborated with the MITRE Corporation to develop a cybersecurity playbook to guide the health-care community in managing risks associated with medical devices [10]. Collectively, through these publications, the FDA aims to establish a more robust trust framework predicated on transparency, accountability, and reliability of medical devices, including AI technologies that may power such devices.

European Union—General Data Protection Regulation

Entities that use AI to process the personal data of European Union (EU) residents will likely be subject to the EU's General Data Protection Regulation (GDPR). The GDPR is one of the first privacy regimes to directly address the automated processing of personal data. Specifically, GDPR Article 22 states that "[t]he data subject shall have the right not to be subject to a decision based solely on automated processing, including profiling, which produces legal effects concerning him or her or similarly significantly affects him or her." Limited exceptions to this rule exist if certain conditions are present, such as if processing "is based on the data subject's explicit consent."[20]

In addition, under GDPR Article 15, a "data subject shall have the right to obtain from the controller confirmation as to whether or not personal data concerning him or her are being processed, and, where that is the case, access to the personal data and the following information: the existence of automated decision-making, including profiling, referred to in Article 22(1) and (4) and, at least in those cases, meaningful information about the logic involved, as well as the significance and the envisaged consequences of such processing for the data subject."[21] Although certain US-based health-care entities may not be subject to these requirements, the GDPR is informative

18. Note that as a general matter, the quality of data used to train an AI algorithm is crucial to the reliability of its outputs. Accordingly, great risk of error and bias in results may occur if data of insufficient quality or volume is used for training.

19. *See* FDA. Content of premarket submissions for management of cybersecurity in medical devices – draft guidance for industry and Food and Drug Administration Staff. Oct. 18, 2018. Available at <https://www.fda.gov/downloads/MedicalDevices/DeviceRegulationandGuidance/GuidanceDocuments/UCM623529.pdf>. Interestingly, consistent with emerging consensus regarding AI and IoT regulation, the FDA employs a sliding scale approach by tiering medical device cybersecurity requirements based on whether patients may be directly harmed or not.

20. *See* <http://www.privacy-regulation.eu/en/article-22-automated-individual-decision-making-including-profiling-GDPR.htm>.

21. *See* <http://www.privacy-regulation.eu/en/article-15-right-of-access-by-the-data-subject-GDPR.htm>.

regarding the need for transparency in the processing of personal data by AI technology.

Regulatory Approval and Clearance of Artificial Intelligence Applications

Former FDA Commissioner Scott Gottlieb on several occasions noted the transformative potential of AI and ML technologies for health care and acknowledged the need for FDA to modernize its approach to evaluating these new innovations [11]. Consequently, FDA has begun to examine whether and to what extent the agency's existing regulatory authorities are appropriately tailored to the regulation of new AI and machine learning technologies. While a handful of AI and machine learning-based medical devices have already entered the market following FDA review, FDA's regulatory approach will continue to evolve, and it will be critical for FDA to engage with stakeholders to understand the particular challenges of regulating these technologies and to develop an approach that both ensure patient safety while fostering innovation on this promising new field.

FDA's ability to regulate AI depends on whether or not a specific application falls within the agency's statutory jurisdiction, which includes medical devices. The Federal Food, Drug, and Cosmetic Act defines devices to include instruments, machines, and similar or related articles that are "intended for use in the diagnosis of disease or other conditions, or in the cure, mitigation, treatment, or prevention of disease," but unlike drugs do not achieve their intended use through chemical action on or within the body and that are not dependent on being metabolized to achieve their intended purpose.[22] Based on this high-level distinction, AI applications are viewed by the FDA as medical devices.

Medical devices are subject to varying degrees of regulatory control according to their risk classification. Class I (low risk) devices comprise those products whose safety can adequately be assured through the application of "general controls," such as registration and listing, recordkeeping, adverse event reporting, and the implementation of a quality system. Class I devices generally do not require FDA premarket review. Class II (moderate risk) devices are those for which both general and "special" controls—such as adherence to product standards or specified labeling—are necessary to ensure safety. Manufacturers of Class II devices generally must submit a "510(k) premarket notification" submission to FDA and demonstrate "substantial equivalence" (i.e., equivalent safety and effectiveness) to a previously marketed (predicate) device for the same intended use. Where there is no applicable predicate device, a manufacturer of a moderate risk device can request "de novo" authorization, which means that FDA will establish a new classification for the product. Finally, Class III (high risk) devices are those whose safety and effectiveness cannot be assured through the application of general and special controls, and for which the manufacturer must obtain FDA approval of an application for premarket approval that includes clinical evidence sufficient to establish the safety and effectiveness of the device.

FDA has defined AI as "[a] device or product that can imitate intelligent behavior or mimics human learning and reasoning."[23] Machine learning, which FDA describes as a "rapidly growing area" of AI, is "used to design an algorithm or model without explicit programming ... through the use of automated training with data" (see footnote 23). As a result, the threshold question in considering FDA regulation of AI and machine learning technologies is what the regulated "article" would be and whether, and under what circumstances, such article would meet the medical device definition. FDA's historical position on the regulation of software is directly relevant to answering this question, as AI algorithms are embedded in software. FDA historically has taken the position that software may be regulated as a medical device if it has the requisite intended use (i.e., intended for diagnosis and treatment). Where software is integrated into an instrument or machine that has a medical device intended use, the software is necessarily regulated as a component of such instrument or machine, and the degree of FDA regulation of the software depends on the classification of the device in which it resides.[24]

In contrast, FDA's approach to regulating stand-alone software has been less straightforward. FDA has historically exercised enforcement discretion with respect to (i.e., has not regulated) a number of software applications used as part of health care. FDA's ad hoc enforcement discretion approach was codified by Congress in 2016 pursuant to the 21st Century Cures Act,[25] which excluded a newly defined category of products known as medical software from the FDA's jurisdiction. This category includes software intended for (1) administrative support of health-care facility; (2) maintaining or encouraging a healthy lifestyle; or (3) transferring, storing, converting formats, or displaying electronic patient records, clinical

22. 21 U.S.C. § 321 (h)(3).

23. US Food & Drug Administration. Digital health criteria. <https://www.fda.gov/medicaldevices/digitalhealth/ucm575766.htm>.

24. IMDRF SaMD Working Group. Software as a Medical Device (SaMD): key definitions. Dec. 9, 2013. <http://www.imdrf.org/docs/imdrf/final/technical/imdrf-tech-131209-samd-key-definitions-140901.pdf>.

25. 21st Century Cures Act, Pub. L. 114-25 (2016).

laboratory tests, or other device data and results. The medical software category also includes certain types of clinical decision support software that are intended to assist physicians in making clinical diagnosis and treatment decisions.

This exception is limited and does not include clinical decision support software that is intended to "acquire, process, or analyze a medical image or a signal from an in vitro diagnostic device or a pattern or signal from a signal-acquisition system." Rather, such software is subject to regulation by FDA pursuant to the agency's "software as a medical device" (SaMD) policy. FDA defines SaMD as "software intended to be used for one or more medical purposes that perform these purposes without being part of a hardware medical device."[26] Such software "utilizes an algorithm (logic, set of rules, or model) that operates on data input (digitized content) to produce an output for a medical use specified by the manufacturer."[27] FDA's SaMD definition is consistent with that proposed by the International Medical Device Regulators Forum (IMDRF), of which FDA is a member, and which seeks to provide harmonized principles for individual jurisdictions to incorporate into their own regulatory framework.

In December 2017, FDA issued final guidance that the IMDRF principles for "clinical evaluation" of SaMD, that is, a "set of ongoing activities conducted in the assessment and analysis of a SaMD's clinical safety, effectiveness and performed as intended by the manufacturer in the SaMD's definition statement" (see footnote 27). The SaMD guidance builds on previous IMDRF SaMD documents, which addressed SaMD terminology, risk categorization, and quality-management system principles, respectively. The guidance identifies the following three pillars of clinical evaluation:

- Establishing a valid clinical association between the SaMD output and the targeted clinical condition;
- Demonstrating that the SaMD is analytically valid, meaning that it correctly processes input data to generate accurate, reliable, and precise output data; and
- Demonstrating that the SaMD is clinically valid, meaning that the output data achieves the intended purpose in the target population in the context of clinical care (see footnote 27).

The SaMD guidance explains that clinical evaluation should be a systematic and planned process that continues through the device life cycle as part of the quality-management system. Further, the guidance states that the "level of evaluation and independent review" of a particular SaMD should be commensurate with its risk (see footnote 27). The guidance encourages manufacturers to leverage the connectivity inherent in SaMD to modify software based on "real-world" performance.

Finally, the SaMD guidance addressed, at a high level, how to satisfy the three pillars of clinical evaluation. According to the guidance, evidence of a valid clinical association may be demonstrated through existing evidence derived from literature searches, professional society guidelines, or clinical research or by generating new evidence from secondary data analysis or clinical trials. Evidence of analytical validation may be generated during verification and validation activities as part of a manufacturer's quality-management system or as part of its good software engineering practices, or by generating new evidence through the use of curated databases or previously collected patient data. Evidence of clinical validation similarly may be generated as part of a quality-management system or good software engineering practices, as well as by referencing existing data sources from studies conducted for the same intended use. In some cases, generation of new clinical data may be required.

If AI and machine learning software is integrated into another regulated product (e.g., a continuous glucose monitor that uses AI to predict hypoglycemic events), then it is regulated as part of the broader product (i.e., as a component of or accessory to the underlying device). If the software is freestanding, however, it is subject to regulation as SaMD, although the SaMD guidance does not specifically address requirements for AI and machine learning SaMD. Nevertheless, several manufacturers of AI and machine learning algorithms have successfully navigated the FDA premarket review process in the past few years, and their experience provides some insight into the regulatory pathway and evidentiary support that the FDA will require for these technologies. These devices include, namely, AI contact, which uses an AI algorithm to analyze CT images of the brain and send a text notification to a neurovascular specialist if a suspected large vessel blockage has been identified[28]; IDX-DR, which uses an AI algorithm to analyze images of the eye taken with a retinal camera for more than mild diabetic retinopathy and makes recommendation to refer to eye care

26. IMDRF SaMD Working Group. Software as a Medical Device (SaMD): key definitions. Dec. 9, 2013. <http://www.imdrf.org/docs/imdrf/final/technical/imdrf-tech-131209-samd-key-definitions-140901.pdf>.

27. US Food & Drug Administration. Software as a Medical Device (SAMD): clinical evaluation. Dec. 8, 2017. <https://www.fda.gov/downloads/medicaldevices/deviceregulationandguidance/guidancedocuments/ucm524904.pdf>.

28. US Food & Drug Administration. FDA permits marketing of clinical decision support software for alerting providers of a potential stroke in patients. Feb. 13, 2018. <https://www.fda.gov/newsevents/newsroom/pressannouncements/ucm596575.htm>.

professional or rescreen in 12 months[29]; and Osteodetect, which uses machine learning to analyze wrist radiographs and highlight distal radius fractures during the review of posterior–anterior and lateral radiographs of adult wrists.[30] Due to the novelty of the intended use proposed for each of these devices, there was no predicate device to which they could demonstrate substantial equivalence. Consequently, each manufacturer was required to submit a de novo request seeking that FDA classifies the device. In granting de novo authorization, FDA also established a new classification regulation defining the generic device category, assigning a risk classification (in each case Class II) and establishing special controls to assure a safe use of the device. Subsequent manufacturers may seek 510(k) clearance for devices that fall within the newly created classification by establishing substantial equivalence to the de novo-authorized device. Thus, for example, FDA granted 510(k) clearance to AccipioIX[31], which is intended to aid in prioritizing clinical assessment of adult noncontrast head CT cases that may suggest an acute intracranial hemorrhage using an AI algorithm, based on the manufacturer's demonstration of substantial equivalence to, namely, AI.

The proof of concept for AI and machine learning SaMD has generally been based on data from retrospective studies demonstrating the software's ability to accurately detect the condition of interest. For example, the de novo submission for AI contact included data from a retrospective study of 300 CT images that assessed the independent performance of the image analysis and notification functionality of the device against the performance of two trained neuroradiologists for the detection of large vessel blockages in the brain.[32] The submission also included data demonstrating that the elapsed time between CT and notification of a specialist of a potential large vessel occlusion was lower when using the device than with the standard of care treatment.

A significant potential benefit of AI and machine learning technologies for health-care delivery lies in the potential of the software to "learn" from real-world use and experience and thereby improve its performance (what FDA terms "adaptive AI"). However, this unique characteristic raises FDA regulatory challenges, since, under existing FDA guidance, manufacturers must prospectively evaluate every postmarket modification to software and assess whether, based on the impact of the modification on functionality or performance, a new submission to the FDA is required. To date, all of the FDA cleared or approved AI/ML-based SaMDs have included locked algorithms (i.e., algorithms that apply a fixed function to a given set of inputs, and where changes to the function require manual input), thus enabling FDA review of changes to software. Adaptive AI and machine learning SaMD, in contrast, will use a defined learning process to make changes autonomously over time, which challenges the existing regulatory paradigm.

In April 2019, FDA issued a proposed regulatory framework to govern changed to AI and machine learning-based SaMD, with the goal of allowing FDA oversight that both "embrace[s] the iterative improvement power of AI and machine learning SaMD while assuring that patient safety is maintained."[33] FDA emphasized that the proposed framework is intended for discussion purposes only and does not reflect the agency's current regulatory expectations. The document poses a number of specific questions for stakeholder feedback, which the agency plans to use to develop a draft guidance.

While noting that AI and machine learning-based SaMD exists on a "spectrum from locked to continuously adaptive algorithms," the discussion draft identifies a "common set of considerations" for data management, retraining, and performance evaluation that can be applied across the spectrum. Furthermore, FDA stresses the importance of a total product life cycle (TPLC) regulatory approach to AI and machine learning-based SaMD, which would enable the "evaluation and monitoring of a software product from its premarket development to postmarket performance, along with continued demonstration of [a manufacturer's] excellence" (see footnote 33). The TPLC approach is based on the following four general principles: (1) establishing clear expectations on quality systems and good ML practices; (2) conducting premarket review where needed and establishing clear expectations for manufacturers to continually manage patient risks throughout the life cycle; (3) expecting manufacturers to monitor AI and machine learning devices and incorporate

29. US Food & Drug Administration. FDA permits marketing of artificial intelligence-based device to detect certain diabetes-related eye problems. Apr. 11, 2018. <https://www.fda.gov/newsevents/newsroom/pressannouncements/ucm604357.htm>.

30. US Food & Drug Administration. FDA permits marketing of artificial intelligence algorithm for aiding providers in detecting wrist fractures. May 24, 2018. <https://www.fda.gov/newsevents/newsroom/pressannouncements/ucm608833.htm>.

31. Dave Muoio, MaxQ AI wins FDA 510(k) clearance for acute intracranial hemorrhage triage algorithm. Nov. 8, 2018. <https://www.mobihealthnews.com/content/maxq-ai-wins-fda-510k-clearance-acute-intracranial-hemorrhage-triage-algorithm>.

32. US Food & Drug Administration. FDA permits marketing of clinical decision support software for alerting providers of a potential stroke in patients. Feb. 13, 2018. <https://www.fda.gov/newsevents/newsroom/pressannouncements/ucm596575.htm>.

33. US Food & Drug Administration. Proposed regulatory framework for modifications to artificial intelligence/machine learning (AI/ML)—based Software as a Medical Device (SaMD). <www.fda.gov>.

a risk management approach to algorithm changes; and (4) enabling increased transparency to users and FDA using postmarket real-world performance reporting for maintain continued assurance of safety and effectiveness (see footnote 33).

To deal with the issue of adaptive algorithms specifically, FDA proposes a framework for modification that relies on the principle of a "predetermined change control plan" that would be included in an initial submission to FDA, which would address the types of changes a manufacturer anticipates making (the "SaMD Pre-Specification") and the processes that will be used to make these changes (the "Algorithm Change Protocol"). This framework would avoid the need for a new submission for certain types of changes, such as improvements in performance and changes in data inputs, but would still require new submissions for some changes, such as significant changes to intended use.

In issuing the proposed framework, former Commissioner Gottlieb acknowledged that it was only a "first step" of many that will be needed for FDA to develop a regulatory approach that fosters the development of safe, beneficial, and innovative AI and machine learning SaMD. Given the rapid pace at which manufacturers are developing new AI and machine learning SaMD for the health-care market, future steps by the agency to articulate its regulatory approach almost certainly will be taken concurrently with the agency's review and authorization of new devices.

Artificial Intelligence Coverage and Reimbursement

The next major hurdle for AI applications in biotechnology is that the AI itself is neither an item (such as a drug or device) nor a service (such as an inpatient hospital admission or care by a professional). Rather, most applications of AI are intended to enhance an item or service. For example, an application of AI may make a diagnostic more reliable at an earlier stage of an illness, may allow for more rapid diagnosis, or make the diagnosis more accurate and consistent. Several promising applications have been reported in studies comparing diagnoses by physicians to computer-generated diagnoses (*see* footnote 1). The challenge here is to determine how to capture the application of AI within current coverage and reimbursement systems.[34]

One potential model for putting AI (machine learning) applications into practice as an enhancement of an existing procedure is the adoption of computer-aided detection (CAD) of breast lesions. At the beginning of 2007 the CPT code set for professional services included two codes for CAD of lesions that could be reported along with screening and diagnostic mammograms. In 2017 the CPT Editorial Panel deleted these codes and replaced them with the following three new CPT codes for screening and diagnostic mammography using CAD:

> 77065 Diagnostic mammography, including CAD when performed unilateral
> 77066 Diagnostic mammography, including CAD when performed bilateral
> 77067 Screening mammography, bilateral (2-view study of each breast), including CAD when performed

The CPT Editorial Panel explained that the new codes were being created to bundle the use of AI into a single procedure. The bundling did not result in a decrease in reimbursement; during 2016 the last full year for the separate codes, the Medicare fee schedule amount for a computer-aided diagnostic bilateral mammogram combining two codes was $124.24, of which $8.23 was attributable to the AI code.[35] For 2019 the bundled Medicare fee schedule rate for a computer-aided diagnostic bilateral mammogram is $ 171.91.[36]

Notwithstanding the incorporation of AI into existing procedures, taking the next step of replacing health-care professionals with an AI-equipped system faces significant hurdles. For example, in the case of breast cancer detection discussed previously, the Medicare statute and regulations require that a screening or diagnostic mammogram be interpreted by a physician in order to be covered and paid.[37] Therefore any major changes to these programs will require revisions to accepted professional practices as well as changes in the laws that govern the programs.

Summary

The potential for applying AI to health-care services, and to biotechnology in particular, lies in the ability to provide items and services that are more precise, faster, and are more efficient. Yet, in order to do so, researchers and developers must have a reliable source of data and be able to use that data ethically. The current safeguards within the US health-care system address many of these concerns, but as the scope of AI applications grows, additional protections may become necessary. Researchers and entrepreneurs should recognize that the current

---

34. For additional background on coverage, coding, and reimbursement, see Chapter 17, *supra*.
35. CMS 2016 Medicare physician fee schedule. Available at: <https://www.cms.gov/apps/physician-fee-schedule/search/search-criteria.aspx>.
36. CMS 2019 Medicare physician fee schedule. Available at: <https://www.cms.gov/apps/physician-fee-schedule/search/search-criteria.aspx>.
37. 42 U.S.C. § 1395x(jj); 42 C.F.R. § 410.34(a).

structures for marketing new items and services that incorporate AI will include regulation by entities, such as the FDA, and since AI is neither an item nor a service, for the foreseeable future it will likely supplement an item or service but will not be a stand-alone product. As a result, the opportunity lies in the ability to provide more efficient care and to expand access to care within the global health-care system. For more information on the expanding applications of AI, see *Chapter 28: Artificial Intelligence: Emerging Applications in Biotechnology and Pharma.*

References

[1] Estava A, Kuprel B, Novoa R, Ko J, Swetter SM, Blau HM, et al. Dermatologist-level classification of skin cancer with deep neural networks. Nature 2017;542:115–18.
Liang M, Tang W, Xu DM, Jirapatnakul AC, Reeves AP, Henschke CI, et al. Low-dose CT screening for lung cancer: computer-aided detection of missed lung cancers. Radiology 2016;281:279–88.
Fergus P, Hussain A, Hignett D, Al-Jumeily D, Abdel-Aziz K, Hamdan H. A machine learning system for automated whole-brain seizure detection. Appl. Comput. Inf. 2016;12:70–89.
Gulshan V, Peng L, Coram M. Development and validation of a deep learning algorithm for detection of diabetic retinopathy in retinal fundus photographs. JAMA 2016;316(22):2402–10.

[2] Smith A, Anderson M. Automation in Everyday Life. Pew Research Center. Oct. 2017. p. 10, 28. Available at: <http://www.pewinternet.org/2017/10/04/americans-attitudes-toward-a-future-in-which-robots-and-computers-can-do-many-human-jobs/> [last accessed Jan. 30, 2019].

[3] Accenture. Artificial Intelligence: Healthcare's New Nervous System. p. 3. Available at: <https://www.accenture.com/t20171215T032059Z__w__/us-en/_acnmedia/PDF-49/Accenture-Health-Artificial-Intelligence.pdf#zoom = 50> [last accessed Jan. 31, 2019], 2017.

[4] CBInsights. Top Healthcare AI Trends to Watch. p. ii. Available at: <https://www.cbinsights.com/research/report/ai-trends-health-care/> [last accessed Jan. 14, 2019], 2018.

[5] Bulgaru I. Pharma Industry in the Age of Artificial Intelligence: The Future is Bright. <https://healthcareweekly.com/artificial-intelligence-in-pharmacology/>, 2019.

[6] Krittanawong C, Zhang H, Wang Z, Aydar M, Kitai T. Artificial intelligence in precision cardiovascular medicine. J Am Coll Cardiol 2017;69:2657–64.

[7] See Al-shamasneh A, Obaidellah U. Artificial intelligence techniques for cancer detection and classification: review study. Eur. Sci. J 2017;13:1857–7881.

[8] Caruana R, et al., Intelligible models for healthcare: predicting pneumonia risk and hospital 30-day readmission. In: Proc. 21th ACM SIGKDD Int. Conf. on Knowledge Discovery and Data Mining. August 10–13, 2015, Sydney, Australia, pp. 1721–1730. Available at: <http://people.dbmi.columbia.edu/noemie/papers/15kdd.pdf>.

[9] See FDA. Postmarket Management of Cybersecurity in Medical Devices—Guidance for Industry and Food and Drug Administration Staff. Jan. 22, 2016. Available at: <https://www.fda.gov/downloads/MedicalDevices/DeviceRegulationandGuidance/ GuidanceDocuments/ucm482022.pdf>.

[10] MITRE. Medical Device Cybersecurity: Regional Incident Preparedness and Response Playbook. Oct. 2018. Available at: <https://www.mitre.org/sites/default/files/publications/pr-18-1550-Medical-Device-Cybersecurity-Playbook.pdf>.

[11] Kent J. FDA sets goals for big data, clinical trials, artificial intelligence. Health IT Analytics Sept. 4, 2018. <https://healthitanalytics.com/news/fda-sets-goals-for-big-data-clinical-trials-artificial-intelligence>.

Chapter 30

Regulatory Approval and Compliances for Biotechnology Products

Norman W. Baylor, PhD[1] and Donna-Bea Tillman, PhD[2]

[1]*President & CEO, Biologics Consulting Group, Inc., Alexandria, VA, United States,* [2]*Team Lead, Devices, Biologics Consulting Group, Inc., Alexandria, VA, United States*

Chapter Outline

Introduction

Biomedical products are regulated by National Regulatory Authorities (NRAs) to ensure that patients and consumers have access to high quality, safe and effective products, and restrict access to those products that are unsafe or have limited clinical use. When appropriately implemented, regulation ensures public health benefit and the safety of patients, health-care workers, and the broader community. Before new technologies can be used, they must be evaluated and approved by authorized regulatory agencies. Detailed safety review during research and development stages, regulatory approval, and legal registration are necessary stages of product development.

Biomedical products must be reviewed and licensed or cleared by the NRA of the country in which they will be marketed and distributed. These authorities evaluate whether a product is safe for widespread use and whether manufacturers can consistently produce high-quality products. Among the issues that regulatory authorities considered are as follows: (1) whether the design for clinical testing is safe enough to warrant human participation, (2) whether there is sufficient data to ascertain risks and benefits, (3) whether the benefits from any given product outweigh the risks that may be associated with its use, and (4) whether data collected in one country can be applied to the use of a product in another country. After a product is approved, licensed, and marketed, it must be monitored throughout its life cycle to ensure that its benefit continues to match expectations of safety and effectiveness. National and regional regulatory authorities throughout the world such as the US Food and Drug Administration (FDA) are responsible for overseeing and managing the regulatory review and approval process in their respective countries. The approval process for biomedical products is similar in most countries; however, there are some aspects that differ based on specific laws and regulations in each country. In all countries, information submitted to regulatory authorities regarding the quality, safety, and efficacy of the product is similar; however, the review process for clinical trials and marketing authorization applications may differ. The chapter will primarily cover the US FDA approval process for biomedical products including drugs, biologics, devices, and *in vitro* diagnostics. These principles are generally applicable to other NRAs, but for specific differences, you will need to refer to the regulations of each specific country's NRA.

Regulatory procedures impact all stages of biomedical product development. Therefore it is critical that developers of biomedical products (drugs, biologics, devices,

Biotechnology Entrepreneurship. DOI: https://doi.org/10.1016/B978-0-12-815585-1.00030-9

in vitro diagnostics, or some combination) possess the knowledge and awareness of the regulatory challenges and opportunities to expedite the development of safe and effective products in a cost-effective manner. The pathway from discovery to marketing of a new biomedical product can be long, complex, and costly. A clear understanding of the FDA regulatory process, regulations, and policies is essential when developing an effective product life cycle management strategy, seeking product approval or clearance, and assuring that products are marketed in compliance with federal requirements. To minimize the risks and costs involved in the biomedical product–development process, it is imperative that clear planning is performed during the early stages of product development, with regular assessment of chemistry, manufacturing, and control (CMC); nonclinical and clinical data; and design controls for medical devices as it is generated. The aim of this chapter is to provide an overview of the FDA regulatory product approval process and discuss considerations for successfully developing a regulatory strategy that leads to product-marketing authorization, or clearance for devices, from NRA.

Food and Drug Administration Historical Background

The FDA is responsible for ensuring the safety of an array of consumer products. The FDA is part of the Executive Branch of the US federal government located in the Department of Health and Human Services (DHHS). The US Department of Agriculture Bureau of Chemistry was the predecessor of the FDA. Prior to 1902, the manufacture of vaccines, antitoxins, and other biologicals was unregulated by the federal government. In response to the tragic deaths of 14 children due to contaminated diphtheria antitoxin, Congress enacted the Biologics Control Act of 1902 that gave the federal government the authority to grant premarket approval for every biological drug and for the process and facility producing such drugs [1]. This legislation contained the initial concepts for the regulation of biologics. In 1906 Congress passed the Federal Food and Drugs Act, to address increasing consumer concern about the safety of foods and drugs in the United States. The FDA was one of the first agencies established by the US government dedicated to consumer protections [2]. In 1927 the regulatory functions of the Bureau of Chemistry were reorganized to become the Food, Drug, and Insecticide Administration, which in 1930 changed its name to the FDA. In 1938 the FDA was overhauled with the passage of the Pure Food, Drug, and Cosmetics Act.

Oversight of medical devices was the responsibility of the US Post Office Department and the Federal Trade Commission to a limited extent prior to 1938 and came under the authority of the FDA after 1938. Although premarket approval did not apply to devices, the Pure Food, Drug, and Cosmetics Act equated some medical devices to drugs for regulatory purposes.[1] With the proliferation of medical technology and an increase in the development of various types of medical devices, Congress considered passing laws for the regulation of devices, which would be comparable to the 1962 Drug Amendments Act. This legislation failed, and the Secretary of the Department of Health Education and Welfare commissioned the Study Group on Medical Devices, which recommended in 1970 that medical devices be classified according to their comparative risk and regulated accordingly. In the early 1970s a government report documented thousands of injuries resulting from medical devices [3]. Soon after, the Dalkon Shield intrauterine device was withdrawn from the market after more than 200 second-trimester septic abortions and 11 maternal deaths occurred. In response to these adverse events, Congress enacted the 1976 Medical Device Amendments to enhance FDA's ability to establish the safety and effectiveness of medical devices.

FDA's authority for regulating laboratory tests, that is, *in vitro* diagnostic devices or IVDs was also established as a result of passage of the Medical Device Amendments of 1976. Under this law, all medical devices, including IVDs, are subject to a variety of controls, including the requirement for manufacturers to register with the FDA and list their products, comply with current good manufacturing practices (cGMPs), and report serious device failures. This law provided the FDA, for the first time in the late 1970s, with an inventory of tests already in the marketplace, tools to require that manufacturing practices be sound, and a system to ensure that serious problems are identified and remedied. Further, the law established requirements for premarket review of medical devices entering the market for the first time [4].

Additional refinements to the function, organization, and authority of the FDA continue as new public health threats and issues emerge. There are several different departments within the FDA that handle issues such as drug development, food safety, cosmetics, blood products, medical devices, vaccines, veterinary medicine, and radiation-emitting products. Under current law, every human medical product is classifiable as a drug, device, biologic, or combination product. The classification of the product determines the review and approval/clearance processes that the FDA may use in assessing the safety and efficacy of the product for human use. In addition to

1. The History of FDA Regulation of Biotechnology in the Twentieth Century (1999 Third Year Paper) http://nrs.harvard.edu/urn-3:HUL.InstRepos:8965554.

evaluating new products before they are released into the market to determine their safety and effectiveness, the FDA also routinely inspects existing products and the facilities in which they are manufactured and evaluates labeling, advertising, and other claims made about the products for which it regulates.

The US FDA's organization includes, among other units, the Office of the Commissioner and three directorates (Medical Products and Tobacco, Foods and Veterinary Medicine, and Global Regulatory Operations and Policy) overseeing the core functions of the agency. The Office of Medical Products and Tobacco provides high-level coordination and leadership across the Center for Drug Evaluation and Research (CDER), the Center for Biologics Evaluation and Research (CBER), the Center for Devices and Radiological Health (CDRH), and the Center for Tobacco Products (Fig. 30.1). The agency responsible for the regulation of biological products previously resided under the National Institutes of Health; this authority was transferred to the FDA in 1972. Currently, both CBER and CDER are responsible for regulating therapeutic biological products, including premarket review and oversight.

FDA's CBER regulates a wide range of biological products, including allergenic extracts, blood and blood components, gene therapy products, devices and test kits, human tissue and cellular products used in transplantation, and vaccines. FDA's CDER, in addition to regulating pharmaceuticals, regulates other categories of biological products mostly produced by biotechnology methods. These include monoclonal antibodies designed as targeted therapies in cancer and other diseases, cytokines, growth factors, and enzymes (e.g., thrombolytics and immunomodulators). The CDRH within the FDA not only regulates traditional medical devices but also is involved in the regulatory assessment of combination products such as device–drug and device–biologics.

Biological products (biologics) are distinguished from chemical pharmaceuticals primarily due to their derivation from living organisms with an innate molecular complexity that cannot be simply defined by physical or chemical means alone. Further, the intrinsic variability of living organisms and the potential for contamination of materials from adventitious agents, which may come from starting materials or from the environment, require special quality control and quality assurance mechanisms. Moreover, biologics are composed of complex molecules such as nucleic acids, proteins, carbohydrates, or a combination thereof that replicate natural substances such as enzymes, antibodies, or hormones in humans. Thus, biologics are inherently more difficult to develop, characterize, and manufacture than most pharmaceutical products.

In contrast, small molecule drugs are typically manufactured through chemical synthesis, which means that they are made by combining specific chemical ingredients in an ordered process. Drugs generally have well-defined chemical structures, and a finished drug can usually be analyzed to determine all its various components. Biologics, on the other hand, are difficult and sometimes impossible to fully characterize by laboratory testing alone because some of the product components of a finished biologic may be unknown. Therefore, it is the manufacturing process that defines a biological product. Because the finished product cannot be fully characterized in the laboratory, manufacturers must ensure product

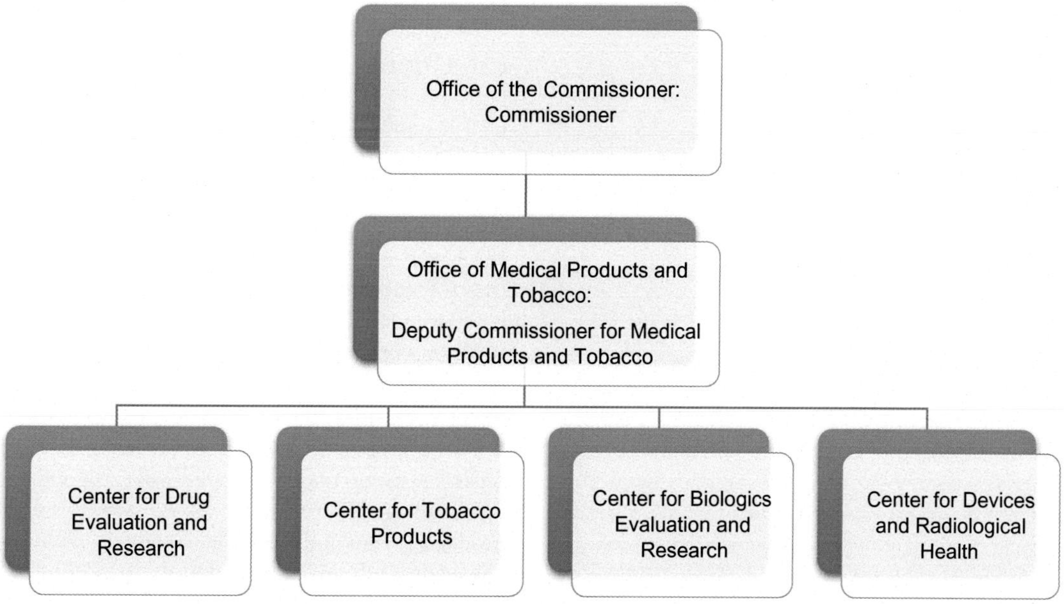

FIGURE 30.1 Organization chart of US FDA. *FDA*, Food and Drug Administration.

consistency, quality, and purity by ensuring that the manufacturing process remains substantially the same over time.

The living systems used to produce biologics can be sensitive to very minor changes in the manufacturing process. Small process differences can significantly affect the nature of the finished biologic and, most importantly, the way it functions in the body. To ensure that a manufacturing process remains the same over time, biologics manufacturers must tightly control the source and nature of starting materials and consistently employ hundreds of process controls that assure predictable manufacturing outcomes. Process controls for biologics are established separately for each unique manufacturing process/product and are not applicable to a manufacturing process/product created by another manufacturer.

FDA's regulatory authority for the approval of biologics resides in the Public Health Service Act (PHS). However, biologics are also subject to regulation under the Federal Food, Drug, and Cosmetic Act (FD&C Act) because most biological products also meet the definition of "drugs" cited within this Act. Thus, CBER and CDER regulate biological products for human use under both the PHS Act and the FD&C Act (Table 30.1). New biologics are required to go through a premarket approval process similar to that for drugs. However, the PHS Act provides that marketing approval for a biologic shall be obtained through the submission and approval of a Biologics License Application (BLA). CBER also regulates medical devices related to licensed blood and cellular products under the FD&C Act's Medical Device Amendments of 1976 [5]. Moreover, premarket review of IVDs for infectious agents that involve the blood supply and for retroviral testing is usually done within CBER.

TABLE 30.1 Acts and regulations pertinent to the development and licensure of biomedical products.

Congressional Acts
Public Health Service Act (42 USC 262-63) Section 351
Food, Drug & Cosmetic Act (21 USC 301-392)
Food and Drug Administration Modernization Act, 1997
Food and Drug Administration Amendments Act, 2007
Title 21 Code of Federal Regulations (CFR)
Subchapter A: General
21 CFR 58 Good Laboratory Practices
21 CFR 56 Institutional Review Boards
21 CFR 50 Protection of Human Subjects
Subchapter C: Drugs—General
21 CFR 201
21 CFR 210-211 Good Manufacturing Practices
Subchapter D: Drugs for human use
21 CFR 314.126 Adequate and well-controlled trials
21 CFR 312 Investigational New Drug Application
Subchapter F: Biologics
21 CFR 600-680 Biological Product Standards
Subchapter devices
21 CFR 800-1299

The PHS Act requires individuals or companies who manufacture biologics for introduction into interstate commerce to hold a license for the products. FDA issues these licenses. Some responsibilities of a licensed biologics manufacturer include complying with the appropriate laws and regulations relevant to their biologics license and identifying any changes needed to help ensure product quality, reporting certain problems to FDA's Biological Product Deviation Reporting System, reporting and correcting product problems within established timeframes, and recalling or stopping the manufacture of a product if a significant problem is detected.

CDER regulates over-the-counter and prescription drugs, including biological therapeutics and generic drugs. CDER has different requirements for the three main types of drug products: new drugs, generic drugs, and over-the-counter drugs. The FD&C Act requires a sponsor to submit a New Drug Application (NDA) for FDA's evaluation to market a drug. The biological therapeutics regulated by CDER require the submission of a BLA and include monoclonal antibodies for *in vivo* use designed as targeted therapies in cancer and other diseases; proteins intended for therapeutic use, including cytokines (interferons), and enzymes (e.g., thrombolytics); immunomodulators (nonvaccine and nonallergenic products) intended to treat disease by inhibiting or modifying a preexisting immune response; and growth factors intended to mobilize, stimulate, decrease, or otherwise alter the production of hematopoietic cells *in vivo*.

Product types continue to merge because of technological advances and blur the historical lines of separation between FDA's medical product centers, that is, CBER, CDER, and CDRH. Combination products are medical and diagnostic products that involve combining a medical device with a drug and/or a biologic. A combination product is classified, assigned to a specific Center within the FDA, and may be regulated as a drug, device, or biologic depending upon its primary mode of action as determined by FDA (see Table 30.2). Because combination products involve components that would normally be regulated under different types of regulatory authorities, and frequently by different FDA centers, they raise challenging regulatory, policy, and review management challenges. Differences in regulatory pathways for each component can impact the regulatory processes for all aspects of product development and management, including preclinical testing, clinical investigation, marketing applications, manufacturing and quality control, adverse event

TABLE 30.2 Medical device and combination products classifications by the Food and Drug Administration.

Classification	Comments
Class I	Low risk of harm to user; registration only unless 510(k) clearance required; compliance with general controls
Class II	Moderate risk of harm to user; 510(k) clearance unless waived; compliance with general controls and special controls
Class III	High risk of harm to user; often requires premarket approval (PMA); compliance with general controls and PMA
Combination product	Depending on the primary mode-of-action, may be reviewed by multiple interagency divisions (see text for more details)

reporting, promotion and advertising, and post-approval modifications.

Regulations Pertinent to Biomedical Product Development

A single set of basic regulatory approval criteria apply to biomedical products, regardless of the technology used to produce them. The current legal authority for the regulation of biologics derives primarily from Section 351 of the PHS Act and from certain sections of the US Food, Drug, and Cosmetic Act.[2,3] The statutes of the PHS Act are implemented through regulations codified in Title 21 of the Code of Federal Regulations, parts 600–680, which contains regulations specifically applicable to biologics. The PHS Act requires individuals or companies who manufacture biologics for introduction into interstate commerce to hold a license for these products. FDA issues these licenses. In addition, because biologics meet the legal definition of a drug under the FD&C Act, manufacturers must comply with the drug cGMPs regulations (parts 210 and 211). Regulations applicable to biomedical products and devices are summarized in Table 30.1. These regulations include the minimum requirements for the manufacturing of biologics, drugs, devices, and combinations thereof, as well as the requirements for performing clinical trials.

The FDA periodically publishes various guidelines and guidance documents to assist developers of new biomedical products in regard to the manufacture and clinical evaluation of these products (see Tables 30.3–30.5). In addition, international guidelines developed and published by the International Conference on Harmonization have been adopted by the FDA. Guidance documents do not have the force of law but are intended to provide useful and timely recommendations and represent the Agency's current thinking on particular topics. These documents are particularly useful in rapidly progressing areas of science and for specifying a degree of detail beyond what is included in the regulations.

To understand how FDA regulates biomedical products, it is important to understand some of the more pertinent operational definitions contained in the statutes and regulations. Section 351 of the PHS Act defines a biological product as any virus, therapeutic serum, toxin, antitoxin, vaccine, blood, blood component or derivative, allergenic product, or analogous product applicable to the prevention, treatment, or cure of diseases or conditions of human beings.[4]

The regulations regarding biological products define effectiveness as the reasonable expectation that, in a significant proportion of the target population, pharmacologic, or other effects of the biological product, when administered under adequate directions for use and warnings against unsafe use, will serve a clinically significant function in the diagnosis, cure, mitigation, treatment, or prevention of disease in humans.

cGMPs define a quality system that manufacturers use as they build quality into their products. The regulations outline the minimum manufacturing, quality control, and quality assurance requirements for the preparation of a drug or biological product for commercial distribution. For example, approved products developed and produced according to cGMPs are safe, properly identified, of the correct strength, pure, and of high quality.

Current Regulatory Pathways

The regulatory pathways for evaluation and approval of biomedical products are outlined in Table 30.6. The regulatory requirements for biomedical products cover both

2. Federal Food, Drug and Cosmetic Act. 21 United States Code, Sec 321.
3. Public Health Service Act. Chap. 373, Title III, Sec. 351, 58: Stat. 702, 42 United States Code, Sec. 262; 1944.
4. US Code of Federal Regulations. Title 21, Part 600.3(h). *Definitions*. Washington, DC: Office of the Federal Register, National Archives and Records Administration; 2012.

TABLE 30.3 Combination products guidance documents.

Guidance documents
10/2018 Selection of the Appropriate Package Type Terms and Recommendations for Labeling Injectable Medical Products Packaged in Multiple-Dose, Single-Dose, and Single-Patient-Use Containers for Human Use (PDF—167 kB)
03/2018 Compliance Policy for Combination Product Postmarketing Safety Reporting
03/2018 Postmarketing Safety Reporting for Combination Products
02/2018 How to Prepare a Pre-Request for Designation (Pre-RFD)
09/2017 Classification of Products as Drugs and Devices and Additional Product Classification Issues
01/2017 Current Good Manufacturing Practice Requirements for Combination Products
02/2016 Human Factors Studies and Related Clinical Study Considerations in Combination Product Design and Development (PDF—336 kB)
06/2013 Technical Considerations for Pen, Jet, and Related Injectors Intended for Use with Drugs and Biological Products (PDF—153 kB)
04/2013 Glass Syringes for Delivering Drug and Biological Products: Technical Information to Supplement International Organization for Standardization (ISO) Standard 11040-4
01/2013 Submissions for Postapproval Modifications to a Combination Product Approved Under a BLA, NDA, or PMA (PDF—101 kB)
04/2011 How to Write a Request for Designation (RFD)
12/2009 New Contrast Imaging Indication Considerations for Devices and Approved Drug and Biological Products (PDF—159 kB)
07/2007 Devices Used to Process Human Cells, Tissues, and Cellular and Tissue-Based Products (HCT/Ps)
09/2006 Early Development Considerations for Innovative Combination Products
04/2005 Application User Fees for Combination Products
05/2004 Submission and Resolution of Formal Disputes Regarding the Timeliness of Premarket Review of a Combination Product

Source: http://www.fda.gov/regulatoryinformation/guidances/ucm122047.htm.

TABLE 30.4 Key medical device premarket submission guidance documents.

510(k)
- Format for Traditional and Abbreviated 510(k)s (August 12, 2005)
- The 510(k) Program: Evaluating Substantial Equivalence in Premarket Notifications (510(k)) (July 28, 2014)
- Refuse to Accept Policy for 510(k)s (January 30, 2018)
- Deciding When to Submit a 510(k) for a Change to an Existing Device (October 25, 2017)

De novo
- De Novo Classification Process (Evaluation of Automatic Class III Designation) (October 30, 2017)

PMA
- Quality System Information for Certain Premarket Application Reviews (February 3, 2003)
- Acceptance and Filing Reviews of Premarket Approval Applications (January 30, 2018)
- Modifications to Devices Subject to Premarket Approval (PMA)—The PMA Supplement Decision-Making Process (December 11, 2008)

IVD
- Select Updates for Recommendations for Clinical Laboratory Improvement Amendments of 1988 (CLIA) Waiver Applications for Manufacturers of In Vitro Diagnostic Devices; Draft Guidance for Industry and FDA Staff (Draft)
- Recommendations for Dual 510(k) and CLIA Waiver by Application Studies; Draft Guidance for Industry and FDA Staff (Draft)

IVD, In vitro diagnostic device; *PMA*, premarket approval.

the premarketing phase, consisting of the investigational and licensing phases, and the postmarketing phase. These requirements can be found in the Investigational New Drug (IND) or the Investigational Device Exemption (IDE) regulations.[5] The first step, prior to evaluating a new product in human clinical trials, is the

5. US Code of Federal Regulations. Title 21, Part 312 and Part 800.

TABLE 30.5 Biosimilarity guidances.

Biosimilarity	Scientific Considerations in Demonstrating Biosimilarity to a Reference Product (PDF—169 kB)	Final guidance	04/28/15
Biosimilarity	Quality Considerations in Demonstrating Biosimilarity of a Therapeutic Protein Product to a Reference Product (PDF—144 kB)	Final guidance	04/28/15
Biosimilarity	Clinical Pharmacology Data to Support a Demonstration of Biosimilarity to a Reference Product (PDF—150 kB)	Final guidance	12/28/16
Procedural; Biosimilarity	Reference Product Exclusivity for Biological Products Filed Under (PDF—99 kB)	Draft guidance	08/04/14
Biosimilarity	Biosimilars: Additional Questions and Answers Regarding Implementation of the Biologics Price Competition and Innovation Act of 2009 (PDF—104 kB)	Draft guidance	05/12/15
Biosimilars	Biosimilars: Questions and Answers Regarding Implementation of the Biologics Price Competition and Innovation Act of 2009 Guidance for Industry (PDF—107 kB)	Final guidance	04/28/15
Biosimilars	Considerations in Demonstrating Interchangeability with a Reference Product Guidance for Industry (PDF—229 kB)	Draft guidance	01/17/17
Biosimilars and Procedural	Formal Meetings Between the FDA and Sponsors or Applicants of BsUFA Products Guidance for Industry (PDF—184 kB)	Draft guidance	06/04/18

Source: https://wayback.archive-it.org/7993/20180125144335/https://www.fda.gov/AboutFDA/WhatWeDo/History/FOrgsHistory/EvolvingPowers/ucm056044.htm.

TABLE 30.6 Current US Food and Drug Administration regulatory pathways.

Biologic products
IND—Investigational New Drug Application
BLA—Biologics License Application

Drugs
IND Application
NDA—New Drug Application

Medical devices
IDE—Investigational Device Exemption
510(k)—Premarket notification
IDE
PMA—Premarket Application
De novo

preclinical phase. The FDA requires that certain animal tests be conducted before humans are exposed to a new molecular entity. The objectives of early *in vivo* testing are to demonstrate the safety of the proposed product. For example, tests should prove that the product is not toxic at the doses that would most likely be effective in humans. The results of these tests are used to support the IND application that is filed with the FDA. Sponsors are encouraged to request a pre-IND (or pre-Sub for devices) meeting with the FDA to discuss preclinical studies, clinical study design, and data requirements that may need to be agreed upon prior to initiation of human clinical studies.

Expedited Regulatory Pathways

There are several expedited review mechanisms available to the US FDA to advance the review and/or licensure of biomedical products against severe and life-threatening conditions, including accelerated approval, fast track, priority review, breakthrough therapy, and emergency use authorization (EUA) (see Table 30.7). Designation of a biomedical product under these mechanisms does not lower the required scientific/medical standards, the quality of data necessary for approval, or the length of the clinical trial period.

The fast-track mechanism is designed to facilitate the development and expedite the review of new drugs that are intended to treat serious or life-threatening conditions and that demonstrate the potential to address unmet medical needs (e.g., providing a therapy when none exists) [6]. Most products that are eligible for fast-track designation are likely to be considered appropriate to receive a priority review designation. A priority review designation is given to products that offer major advances in treatment or provide the same when no adequate therapy exists. A priority review reduces the FDA review time. The time for completing a priority review is 6 months as opposed to 10 months for standard review.

Breakthrough therapy is described in Section 506(a) of the FD&C Act. Breakthrough therapy provides for the designation of a drug as a breakthrough therapy "... if the drug is intended, alone or in combination with one or more other drugs, to treat a serious or life-threatening

TABLE 30.7 US Food and Drug Administration (FDA) expedited regulatory pathways.

Pathway	Description of pathway[a]	Criteria	Attributes
Fast track	Program designation	Drug intended to treat a serious condition, and nonclinical or clinical data demonstrate the potential to address an unmet medical need or a product designated as a qualifying infectious disease product[b]	Actions to expedite development and review; rolling review
Breakthrough therapy	Program designation	Drug intended to treat a serious condition and *preliminary* clinical evidence indicating the drug may demonstrate substantial improvement on a clinically significant end point(s) over existing therapies	Intensive guidance on efficient drug development; FDA organizational commitment; rolling review
Priority review	Program designation	An application or efficacy supplement for a drug that treats a serious condition and if approved would provide a significant improvement in safety or effectiveness[c]	Shorter review clock (6 months review time vs 10 months for standard review)
Accelerated approval	Approval pathway	A drug that treats a serious condition and generally provides a meaningful advantage over available therapies and demonstrates an effect on a surrogate end point that is reasonably likely to predict clinical benefit	Approval based on an effect on surrogate end points or intermediate clinical end points
EUA	Approval Pathway	Authorization of the use of an unapproved product or the unapproved use of an approved product when an emergency or a potential emergency exists	Allows introduction of drug, device or biological into interstate commerce by the Section of DHHS for use in an actual or potential emergency

DHHS, Department of Health and Human Services; *EUA*, Emergency use authorization.
[a]*Description of regulatory pathways includes regulatory programs such as fast track, breakthrough therapy and priority review. Emergency use authorization and accelerated approval are mechanisms whereby products may be approved for introduction into interstate commerce.*
[b]*Title V111 of FDASIA,* Generating Antibiotic Incentive Now (GAIN), *provides incentives for the development of antibacterial and antifungal drugs for human use.*
[c]*Priority review also applies to any supplement that proposes a labeling change pursuant to 505 of the FD&C Act on a pediatric study under this section or an application for a drug that has been designated as a qualified infectious disease product or an application or supplement for a drug submitted with a priority review voucher.*
Adapted from the FDA Guidance for Industry: Expedited Programs for Serious Conditions—Drugs and Biologics.

disease or condition and preliminary clinical evidence indicates that the drug may demonstrate substantial improvement over existing therapies on one or more clinically significant end points, such as substantial treatment effects observed early in clinical development." [7]. The clinical evidence needed to support breakthrough designation is preliminary. In contrast to the data needed to support approval, as is the case for all drugs, FDA will review the full data submitted to support the approval of drugs designated as breakthrough therapies to determine whether the drugs are safe and effective for their intended use before they are approved for marketing.

The accelerated approval regulation allows approval on the basis of a surrogate end point for drugs intended to treat serious diseases and that fill an unmet medical need. A surrogate end point is a marker (e.g., a laboratory measurement or physical sign) used in clinical trials as an indirect or substitute measurement that represents a clinically meaningful outcome, such as survival or symptom improvement.[6] The use of surrogate end points may shorten the FDA approval time. Approval of a drug on the basis of such end points is given on the condition that postmarketing clinical trials verify the anticipated clinical benefit.

EUA is another regulatory mechanism by which the US FDA can accelerate the availability of vaccines and other pharmaceutical products.[7] Under EUA the FDA can authorize the use of an unapproved product or the unapproved use of an approved product when an emergency or a potential emergency exists. Section 564(b)(1) of the FD&C Act allows the Secretary of the US DHHS to authorize the introduction into interstate commerce of a

6. US Code of Federal Regulations. Title 21, Part 312.
7. Emergency Use Authorization of Medical Products. Guidance – emergency use authorization of medical products. Available at: http://www.fda.gov/RegulatoryInformation/Guidances/ucm125127.htm.

drug, device, or biological product intended for use in an actual or potential emergency. Once the Secretary of DHHS declares an emergency, the FDA may authorize the emergency use of a particular product, if other statutory criteria and conditions are met.

The assessment of efficacy for some biomedical products cannot be ethically conducted under human clinical trials, such as those for certain bioterrorism agents. In 2002 the FDA amended the biological products regulations to incorporate 21 CFR 601.90, Approval of Biological Products When Human Efficacy Studies Are Not Ethical or Feasible.[8] This rule, referred to as the "animal rule," provides that approval of certain new drug and biological products can be based on animal data when adequate and well-controlled efficacy studies in humans cannot be ethically conducted because the studies would involve administering a potentially lethal or permanently disabling toxic substance or organism to healthy human subjects. In these situations, certain new drug and biological products can be approved for marketing on the basis of evidence of effectiveness derived from appropriate studies in animals without adequate and well-controlled efficacy studies in humans. When assessing the sufficiency of animal data, FDA may take into account other data, including human data that may be available to the agency. Safety must be evaluated in humans as a prerequisite for approval.

Translational Development

Industry's goals are to develop a commercially viable product and make a meaningful contribution to available therapeutic options, while satisfying a myriad of regulatory requirements. The introduction of new biomedical products typically involves a long and expensive process that may begin with a relatively simple initial discovery but includes an extended period of development, which addresses formulation and manufacturing, preclinical evaluation, safety, efficacy, and commercial potential. Table 30.8 includes a list of the phases in product development from discovery through postlicensure. In order to understand the timeframe required for a product to become commercially available, one must understand how the product development stages are intertwined with the stages of the regulatory process.

Translational development involves the process of transitioning from the basic research and discovery phase to a regulated product development phase beginning with the preclinical stage (Fig. 30.2). The research and discovery phase may be empirical and based on trial and error and occurs in an unregulated environment, whereas the impact of regulatory affairs on clinical development is significant and expands the IND phases through licensure and beyond. Although there is no FDA regulatory oversight in the basic research and discovery phase as described at the beginning of this chapter, each of the product development stages beginning with the preclinical stage is impacted by the regulatory process (Fig. 30.3). Failure to understand and appreciate the regulatory impact for future product development can result in significant delays when attempting to transition a product from the research lab to the clinic. A discovery process that is focused on the development of a drug for one purpose may lead to its use in another, unanticipated, disease indication. Once a potential candidate drug is identified, it must be evaluated in the structured highly regulated environment as previously described.

TABLE 30.8 Product development phases.

Discovery/Basic research—(pre-IND)
Process and analytical development (pre- and post-IND)
Process—development and optimization
Manufacturing consistency
Assays—development and specifications
Identity, purity, and potency
Stability indicating
Drug substance (bulk substance) and drug product
Characterization
Product development phases
Preclinical animal studies (pre-IND)
Proof of concept
Toxicology
Safety pharmacology
IND submission
Clinical trials
Phases 0, 1, 2, and 3
Product approval/licensure
Postmarket studies (Phase 4)

IND, Investigational new drug.

Once product development enters the regulated environment, there are challenges that must be overcome. Preclinical studies must be done under good laboratory practices, CMC procedures must be done under cGMP, and clinical studies must be done under good clinical practices. It is highly recommended that a gap analysis of all development areas be done as part of a product development plan. Comprehensive product-development planning should be based on a clear understanding of the FDA regulations and expectations. This includes effective communication with the FDA to assure concurrence with the development plan. A project-management expert should oversee the execution of the PDP. Product development requires a team effort, and success is highly dependent on

8. US Code of Federal Regulations. 21 CFR part 601.90; 2009.

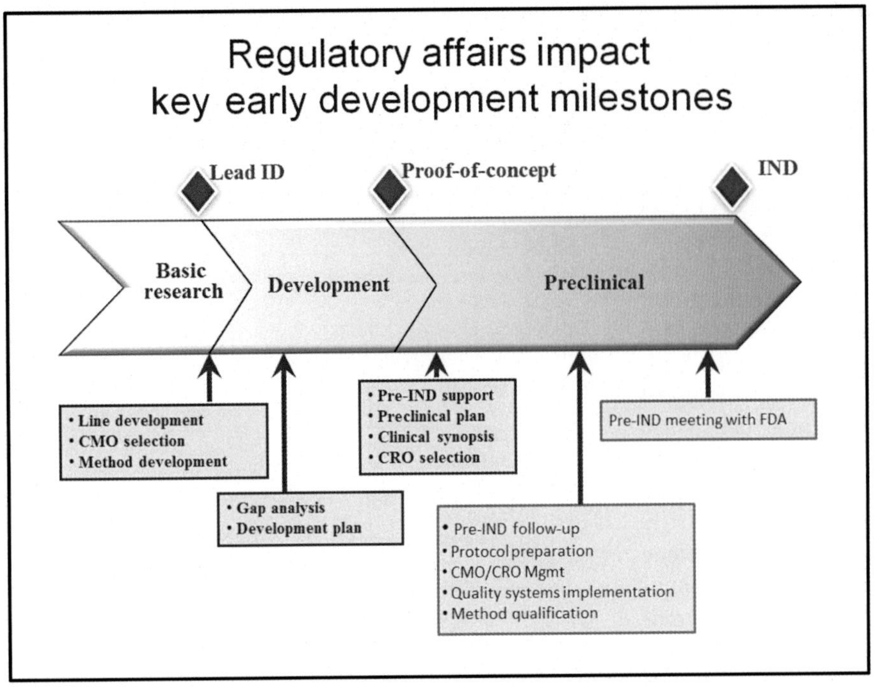

FIGURE 30.2 Impact of the regulatory process on key early development milestones.

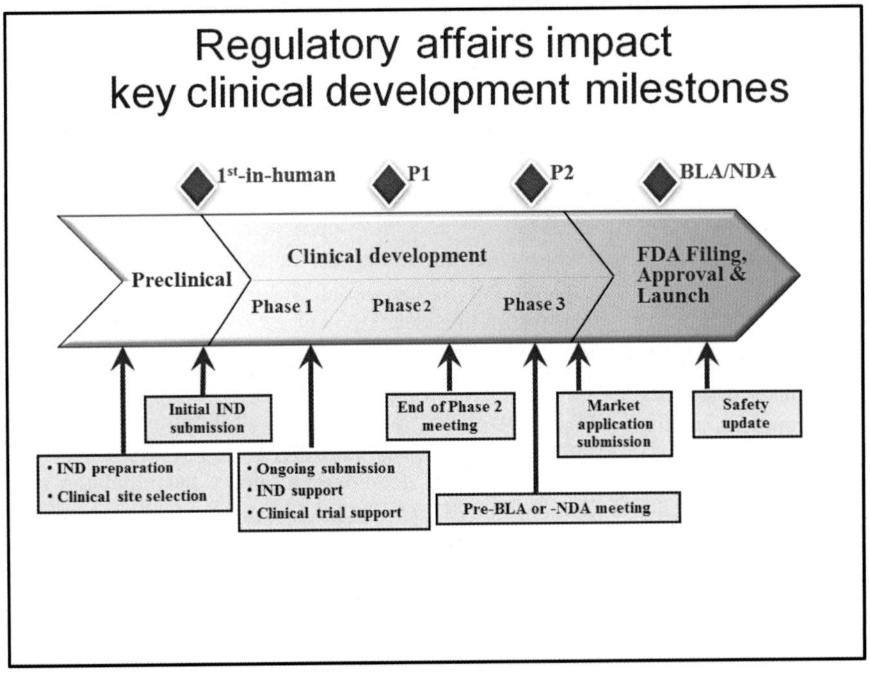

FIGURE 30.3 Impact of the regulatory process on key clinical development milestones.

support from upper management and availability of appropriate resources. Product development regulatory goals should include (1) developing a reproducible process that can yield a consistent product and that can be manufactured under cGMPs; (2) developing analytical procedures that can reliably measure product parameters that are stability indicating and can demonstrate product comparability following changes to manufacturing, facilities, or equipment; (3) develop animal models that can demonstrate proof of concept and safety; and (4) demonstrate safety and efficacy in clinical trials.

After the completion of appropriate preclinical studies the FDA requires that sponsors of regulated products first obtain preliminary permission for conducting clinical trials in humans. The clinical development of a new drug in the United States usually begins with a sponsor approaching the FDA for permission to conduct a clinical study with an investigational product through submission of an IND application form. Clinical trials in support of a premarket approval may be conducted only after the FDA has issued an IDE. In the application the sponsor (1) describes the composition, source, and method of manufacture of the product and the methods used in testing its safety, purity, and potency; (2) provides a summary of all laboratory and preclinical animal testing; and (3) provides a description of the proposed clinical study and the names and qualifications of each clinical investigator. The FDA has a maximum of 30 days to review the original IND application and determine whether study participants will be exposed to any unacceptable risks. As part of the IND process, each clinical investigator files information describing his or her qualifications for performing clinical trials, details of the proposed study, and assurance that a number of conditions specified by the regulations will be met. A signed informed consent must be obtained from each study participant.[9] Approval for the study must be obtained in advance from a local institutional review board. Once the FDA is satisfied with the documentation, the Phase 1 clinical trial can begin. If the documentation is inadequate, the FDA can place the IND on clinical hold.[10]

Premarketing Investigational Phase

Only licensed or approved biomedical products may be shipped from one state to another; however, during the premarketing phase, interstate shipment of products for investigational use is allowed under the law and regulations.[11] There are generally three separate phases (Phases 1, 2, and 3) in the clinical evaluation of experimental biomedical products at the premarketing stage (Fig. 30.4). These phases may overlap, and the clinical testing may be highly iterative because multiple Phase 1 or 2 trials may be performed as new data are obtained. The respective responsibilities of the regulatory authority, that is, FDA and the sponsor are also outlined in Fig. 30.4. One should note that the FDA is not responsible for completing the appropriate studies in support of the safety and efficacy of the product. This is solely the responsibility of the sponsor.

In a *Phase 1 trial*, generally, 20–100 volunteers are enrolled depending on the product, available alternatives, and indications for use. The Phase 1 trial is primarily focused on an assessment of safety of the product. During this stage low doses of the product are administered to healthy volunteers who are closely supervised. During the *Phase 2 trials* the drug may be administered to 100–300 volunteers with the disease or condition to be treated, diagnosed, or prevented to determine the drug's effective dose, the method of delivery, and the dosing interval, as well as reconfirm product safety. Moreover, the Phase 2 clinical trial stage may be divided into Phase 2a (safety and proof of concept) and Phase 2b (clinical efficacy and dose finding). On exception, Phase 2b studies may be used as pivotal trials if the drug is intended to treat life-threatening or severely debilitating illnesses such as cancer. Product efficacy is generally studied in Phase 3 clinical trials; however, in an effort to reduce costs during

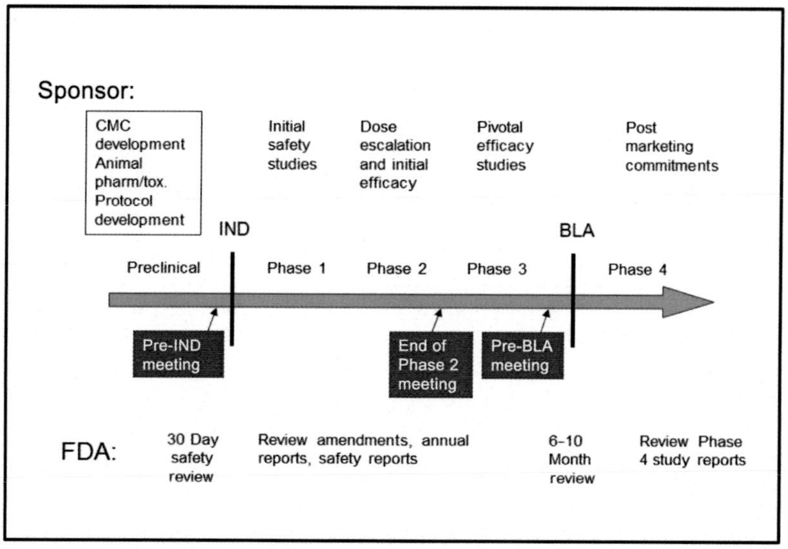

FIGURE 30.4 Product-development phases.

9. US Code of Federal Regulations. Title 21, Part 312.
10. US Code of Federal Regulations. Title 21, Part 312.
11. US Code of Federal Regulations. Title 21, Part 312.

clinical development, the usage of Phase 2b trials has increased to generate earlier data on how effective a product will be at treating certain conditions in patients.

Pre-IND meetings are particularly important for new sponsors and for products that incorporate novel features. Other meetings are also encouraged at critical points throughout the IND review, including "end-of-Phase 2" meetings. The purpose of an end-of-Phase 2 meeting is to assess the adequacy of the Phase 2 safety and effectiveness data that support advancement to Phase 3, to evaluate the Phase 3 plan and draft protocols, and to identify any additional information necessary to support a marketing application for the uses under investigation. The end-of-Phase 2 meeting is generally held before major commitments of effort and resources to specific Phase 3 studies are made.

A *Phase 3 trial* may involve anywhere from 1000 or more volunteers across multiple study sites and is considered the pivotal efficacy trial. These studies are used to demonstrate further safety and effectiveness and to determine the best dosage. As far as efficacy evaluation, efficacy is demonstrated ideally in randomized, double-blind, well-controlled trials. The end points will be product specific. Additional controlled safety studies are often requested when the numbers of subjects included in the efficacy studies is deemed insufficient to provide adequate safety data. The studies need to be designed in such a way that statistical methods may be applied to their evaluation. Safety studies may be unblinded if the number of injections, route of administration, or schedule differs between groups, in particular when infants and young children are involved. Phase 3 trials are the final step before seeking FDA approval.

Licensing Phase

Biological products require FDA approval through a BLA as opposed to new molecular entities, which are approved through a NDA, or new devices, which are approved through the 510(k) procedures or PMA. Types of products requiring a BLA include vaccines, blood and blood by-products, some types of monoclonal antibodies, and tissue and cellular products. Once all three phases of the clinical trials are complete, the sponsoring company analyzes all of the data. If the findings demonstrate that the investigational product is both safe and effective for its intended use, the company may file a BLA with the FDA requesting approval to market and distribute the product commercially. FDA experts review all the information included in the BLA to determine if the data demonstrates that the product is safe and effective enough to be approved. Following rigorous review, the FDA can either (1) approve the BLA, (2) send the company a "complete response" letter requesting more information or studies before approval can be granted, or (3) deny approval.

Review of a BLA usually includes an evaluation by an advisory committee—an independent, external panel of FDA-appointed experts who consider data presented by company representatives and FDA reviewers. The advisory committee then votes on whether the data support the safety and effectiveness of the product in order for the FDA to consider approval of the BLA, and under what conditions. The FDA is not required to follow the recommendations of the advisory committees but often does.

Prior to the submission of a BLA, a pre-BLA meeting with the agency is strongly encouraged to discuss the sponsor's product developmental plan. The FDA has determined that delays associated with the initial review of a BLA may be reduced by exchanges of information about a proposed marketing application.[12] The primary purpose of a pre-BLA meeting is to discuss any major unresolved issues, to identify those studies that the sponsor is relying on as adequate and well controlled to establish the product's effectiveness, to identify the status of ongoing studies, to acquaint FDA reviewers with the general information to be submitted in the BLA (including technical information), to review methods used in the statistical analysis of the data, and to discuss the best approach for the presentation and formatting of data in the application.

The BLA should contain details of the manufacturing facility and equipment as well as data derived from nonclinical laboratory and clinical studies that demonstrate that the manufactured product meets prescribed requirements for safety, purity, and potency. Information should be submitted in the BLA that confirms that there is compliance with standards addressing requirements for (1) organization and personnel; (2) buildings and facilities; (3) equipment; (4) control of components, containers, and closures; (5) production and process controls; (6) packaging and labeling controls; (7) holding and distribution; (8) laboratory controls; and (9) records to be maintained. Furthermore, a full description of manufacturing methods; data establishing stability of the product through the dating period; sample(s) representative of the product for introduction or delivery for introduction into interstate commerce; summaries of test results performed on the lot(s) represented by the submitted sample(s); specimens of the labels, enclosures, and containers; and the address of each location involved in the manufacture of the biological product should be included in the BLA. The manufacturing facility must also be inspection-ready at the time the BLA is

12. Findings: issues and communication: independent evaluation of FDA's first cycle review performance – final report. https://www.accessdata.fda.gov/scripts/cdrh/cfdocs/cfcfr/CFRSearch.cfm?fr = 312.47.

submitted. If the information provided meets FDA requirements, the application is approved, and a license is issued allowing the firm to market the product. Issuance of a biologics license is the final determination that the product, the manufacturing process, and facilities meet applicable requirements to ensure the continued safety, purity, and potency of the product.

Regulatory oversight continues after licensure. Phase 4 studies are required to assess the safety of the product in larger populations. Additionally, any changes to the manufacturing process or change in therapeutic indications must be reported to the FDA for approval in the form of a BLA supplement.

Regulation of Medical Devices

CDRH regulates all medical devices under the FD&C Act, inclusive of radiation-related devices, that are not assigned categorically or specifically to CBER. The FDA has divided devices into three classes to identify the level of regulatory control applicable to them (see Table 30.2).

Class I devices are the lowest risk devices, for which "general controls" are adequate to provide a reasonable assurance of safety and effectiveness. General controls include prohibition against adulteration or misbranding, good manufacturing practices (as implemented in the quality system regulation), registration of device manufacturing facilities, listing of the device types, record keeping, repair, replacement and refund, and provisions regarding banned devices.

Class II devices are moderate risk devices, for which general and "special controls" are adequate to provide a reasonable assurance of safety and effectiveness. They are generally subject to FDA review and clearance of a "premarket notification" (commonly referred to as a 510(k)).

Class III devices are the highest risk or most novel device types, for which general and special controls are not adequate to provide a reasonable assurance of safety and effectiveness. They are generally subject to FDA review and approval of a premarket approval (PMA) application, which requires a demonstration of a reasonable assurance of safety and effectiveness, based on valid scientific evidence.

FDA has established classifications for approximately 1700 different generic types of devices and grouped them into 16 medical specialties referred to as panels. Each of these generic types of devices is assigned to one of the three regulatory classes based on the level of control necessary to assure the safety and effectiveness of the device. FDA also organizes information about device types using product codes or "procodes," assigning a unique three-letter product code for each generic type of device.

In vitro diagnostic products are medical devices as defined in section 210(h) of the FD&C Act and may also be biological products subject to section 351 of the PHS. Like other medical devices, IVDs are subject to premarket and postmarket controls. IVDs are also subject to the Clinical Laboratory Improvement Amendments of 1988 (CLIA '88). Diagnostic testing helps health-care providers screen for or monitor specific diseases or conditions and also helps assess patient health to make clinical decisions for patient care. Three federal agencies are responsible for CLIA: the FDA, the Center for Medicaid Services, and the Centers for Disease Control. Each agency has a unique role in assuring quality laboratory testing.

The FDA categorizes diagnostic tests by their complexity—from the least to the most complex: waived tests, moderate complexity tests, and high complexity tests. Tests that are waived by regulation under 42 CFR 493.15 (c), or cleared or approved for home use or for over-the-counter use, are automatically categorized as waived following clearance or approval. Otherwise, following clearance or approval, tests may be categorized either as moderate or as high complexity according to the CLIA categorization criteria listed in 42 CFR 493.17.

Diagnostic tests are categorized as waived based on the premise that they are simple to use, and there is little chance the test will provide incorrect information or cause harm if it is done incorrectly. Tests that are cleared by the FDA for home or over-the-counter use are automatically assigned a waived categorization. CLIA categorization is determined after the FDA has cleared or approved a marketing submission. The FDA determines the test's complexity by reviewing the package insert test instructions and using a criteria scorecard to categorize a test as moderate or high complexity. Each test is graded for level of complexity by assigning scores of 1, 2, or 3 for each of the seven criteria on the scorecard. A score of 1 indicates the lowest level of complexity, and the score of 3 indicates the highest. The 7 scores are added together and the tests with a score of 12 or less are categorized as moderate complexity, and those with a score above 12 are categorized as high complexity.

Medical Devices: Design Controls

FDA's cGMPs for medical devices were first authorized by section 520(f) of the Act and codified under 21 CFR 820 in 1978. However, FDA determined that lack of design controls in these early cGMP regulations was one of the major causes of medical device recalls, and stated the following:

> *The intrinsic quality of devices, including their safety and effectiveness, is established during the design phase. Thus FDA believes that unless appropriate design controls are observed during preproduction stages of development, a*

finished device may be neither safe nor effective for its intended use.[13]

The 1990 Safe Medical Devices Act authorized FDA to add design controls to its cGMP regulation, and in 1996 FDA published the final rule for the new Quality System Regulation, which implemented the design control regulations that are still in effect today. The current Quality System Regulation (21 CFR 820) requires that device manufacturers implement a quality system for the design and production of medical devices intended for commercial distribution in the United States. The regulation requires the establishment of various specifications and controls for devices; that devices are designed under a quality system to meet these specifications; that devices are manufactured under a quality system; that finished devices meet these specifications; that devices are correctly installed, checked and serviced; that quality data are analyzed to identify and correct quality problems; and that complaints are processed.

The design controls provisions of the Quality System Regulation provide a systematic approach to medical device design to ensure that the finished device meets its stated requirements and performs in accordance with user needs and intended uses. It is a total systems approach that extends from the development of device requirements through design, production, distribution, use, maintenance, and, eventually, obsolescence. By establishing and implementing design control processes, medical-device manufacturers increase the likelihood that the finished device will meet requirements, perform according to user needs and intended uses, and is safe and effective.

Medical Devices: Premarketing Investigational Phase

The premarket investigational phase for medical devices involves determining how the device will likely be classified, determining what information and data will be necessary to support the premarket submission, and collecting that data. Devices that are subject to the premarket notification (510(k)) requirements (usually Class II devices) cannot be legally marketed in the United States until FDA has issued an order finding that the device is substantially equivalent (SE) to a "predicate" device. A predicate device is a device that was legally marketed prior to May 28, 1976 (the enactment date of the Medical Device amendments), for which a PMA is not required, or a device which has been reclassified from Class III to Class II or I, or a device which has been found SE through the 510(k) process.[14]

If the device requires a premarket notification (510(k)), the first part of this phase is identifying an appropriate device to use as a predicate for substantial equivalence. In general, it is best to choose a predicate device whose indications for use are as similar as possible to the proposed new device.

In order for FDA to determine that a new device is SE to a predicate device, FDA must determine the following:

1. The device has the same intended use as the predicate device.
2. The device either has the same technological characteristics as the predicate device, or if it has new technological characteristics:
   a. The differences do not raise different questions of safety and effectiveness.
   b. Performance data demonstrates that the new device is as safe and effective as the predicate device.[15]

At the present time, very few 510(k)s are submitted to FDA for devices that have the same technological characteristics as the predicate device, and most 510(k) submissions include some combination of bench and animal data demonstrating that the performance of the new device is equivalent to that of the predicate.

If the device is Class III and requires a premarket approval, the investigational phase is similar to what is required for a new drug or biologic. The process usually begins with submission of a presubmission to obtain FDA feedback on key preclinical and clinical studies. If the clinical study will be conducted in the United States (and most such studies have at least some US sites), once the basic safety of the device has been established, an IDE is submitted to obtain FDA approval to begin the clinical study. This usually includes an initial feasibility study to demonstrate proof of concept, and then a pivotal study to demonstrate a reasonable assurance of safety and effectiveness.

Medical Devices: Premarket Submission Phase

The key elements of a 510(k) submission are a detailed description of the device and its principle of operation, a comparison of the new device to the predicate, the results of performance testing, and device labeling (see the FDA guidance "Format for Traditional and Abbreviated 510(k)s," August 12, 2005). FDA's performance goals for the 510(k) program require FDA to review most 510(k)s in 90 days. After receiving the 510(k), FDA conducts an

13. Federal Register Notice. Medical devices; current good manufacturing practice (CGMP) final rule; quality system regulation. October 7, 1996.
14. 21 CFR 807.92(a)(3).
15. 21 USC 360c (i)(1)(A).

initial review to determine if it meets the "Refuse-To-Accept" criteria, and if it does, begins its substantive review process. If FDA has significant questions for the submitter, these are communicated in a formal request for additional information by day 60 of the review process. The submitter then has 180 days to respond. Any remaining issues that FDA has must be resolved during the final interactive review period. The review process ends with FDA issuing a SE or Not SE (NSE) letter. A device that FDA has found to be SE is said to have been "cleared," not approved. Any modifications to a 510(k)-cleared device must be assessed to determine if a new 510(k) is required (see FDA guidance documents).

If there is no predicate device and FDA determines that the new device is low risk and appropriate for classification into Class I or Class II, then the device can be marketed through the "de novo" classification process. A de novo submission needs to provide the risks to health presented by the device, how these risks have been mitigated, and the results of testing demonstrating the successful implementation of the risk mitigations.

A PMA application must include the necessary elements specified in 21 CFR 814.20. This includes administrative items, preclinical and clinical data needed to demonstrate a reasonable assurance of safety and effectiveness, draft labeling, and manufacturing information demonstrating compliance with the Quality System regulation (21 CFR 820).

Although the manufacturer may submit any form of evidence to the FDA to substantiate the safety and effectiveness of a device, the agency relies upon only "valid scientific evidence" to determine whether there is reasonable assurance that the device is safe and effective. Valid scientific evidence is defined as[16]

> *... evidence from well-controlled investigations, partially controlled studies, studies and objective trials without matched controls, well-documented case histories conducted by qualified experts, and reports of significant human experience with a marketed device, from which it can fairly and responsibly be concluded by qualified experts that there is reasonable assurance of the safety and effectiveness of a device under its conditions of use.*

The FDA review of a PMA proceeds along two related but largely independent tracks that address: (1) the safety and effectiveness of the device and (2) the Quality System. The process for an IVD is somewhat different and will be discussed later in the chapter.

A multidisciplinary team headed by a lead reviewer who is usually a scientist or engineer conducts the safety and effectiveness review process. After FDA receives the PMA application a filing review is conducted to determine if the submission is administratively complete. If the PMA is accepted for review, FDA generally completes its initial substantive review of the PMA within 90 days of receipt of the PMA. If this review identifies significant issues, FDA will issue a Major Deficiency letter, requesting additional information from the sponsor. If the device is novel, or the review process identifies complex issues, FDA may decide to convene an Advisory Committee to provide review and recommendation regarding the PMA, similar to the process for a biologic.

In order for FDA to approve a PMA, they must also determine that the manufacturing facilities, methods, and controls for the device comply with the Quality System regulations in 21 CFR 820. Each original PMA submission is required to include a separate section that identifies the facilities involved in the manufacturing of the device and that provides detailed information regarding the design controls procedures implemented by the manufacturer. If significant quality system issues are identified, they are communicated to the submitter in Major Deficiency Letters, similar to the process used by the safety and effectiveness review team. FDA will also conduct an inspection of the sponsor's manufacturing facilities.

The PMA can only be approved once both the safety and effectiveness and the quality system reviews (including the inspection) are successfully completed. Most PMA approvals also include requirements for conducting post-approval studies. Following issuance of the approval order, any changes to the device or its manufacturing process must be assessed to determine if a PMA supplement is required (see the FDA guidance "Modifications to Devices Subject to Premarket Approval (PMA) – The PMA Supplement Decision-Making Process," December 11, 2008).

Regulation of Biosimilars

Congress enacted an abbreviated FDA licensure pathway through the Biologics Price Competition and Innovation Act (BPCIA) of 2009 for biological products that are demonstrated to be biosimilar to or interchangeable with an FDA-approved biological product.[17] Section 351(k) of the PHS defines an abbreviated licensure pathway as less than a full complement of product-specific preclinical and clinical data. This licensure pathway was established with the intent to provide increased treatment options, more

16. 21 CFR 860.7.

17. Implementation of the Biologics Price Competition and Innovation Act of 2009. https://www.fda.gov/Drugs/GuidanceComplianceRegulatoryInformation/ucm215089.htm.

access to lifesaving medications, and potentially lower health-care costs through competition.

An interchangeable product is a biosimilar product that meets additional requirements outlined by the BPCIA. As part of fulfilling these additional requirements, data must be submitted that demonstrates that an interchangeable product elicits the same clinical result as the reference product in any given patient. Additionally, for products that are indicated to be administered to a patient multiple times, an assessment of the risk in terms of safety and reduced efficacy of alternating between an interchangeable product and a reference product must be completed.

Biosimilars must be highly analogous to FDA-approved reference products and have no clinically meaningful differences in safety, purity, and potency from the reference product. Further, there is no regulatory requirement to independently establish the safety and effectiveness of the proposed biosimilar. A reference product is an FDA-approved single biological product, against which a proposed biosimilar product is compared. The reference product is approved in a stand-alone application that must contain the requisite relevant data necessary to demonstrate its safety and effectiveness. Generally, the data and information necessary to demonstrate the safety and effectiveness of a reference product will include clinical trials for the disease indication(s) being sought by the manufacturer.

A manufacturer of a proposed biosimilar product must develop comparative data between the proposed product and the FDA-approved reference product to demonstrate biosimilarity. To support biosimilarity to an existing FDA-approved reference product, the FDA has established a stepwise approach that supports a totality of evidence for approval, instead of a one-size-fits-all assessment for manufacturers [8]. In this stepwise approach, data from each phase of development are evaluated to determine differences observed between the tested product and its reference product, and any potential impact of these differences. The accumulation of comparative data begins with a detailed analytical characterization and comparison of the products, followed by animal studies, including assessment of toxicity, if necessary, and adequate comparative clinical studies to demonstrate safety, purity, and potency of the proposed biosimilar product. This typically includes assessing immunogenicity, pharmacokinetics (PK), and, in some cases, pharmacodynamics (PD) and may also include a comparative clinical study (see Table 30.9 and Fig. 30.5).

The abbreviated licensure pathway should not be interpreted as having a lower approval standard for biosimilar or interchangeable products. Just the opposite, that is, the data package required for approval of a biosimilar or interchangeable product is extensive. If a biosimilar manufacturer can demonstrate that its product is biosimilar to the reference product, then it is scientifically acceptable to rely on certain existing scientific evidence about the safety and effectiveness of the reference product to support approval.

A biosimilar product may be approved for an indication without direct studies of the biosimilar in that indication. If the total evidence in the biosimilar application supports a demonstration of biosimilarity for at least one of the reference product's indications, then it is possible for the biosimilar manufacturer to use data and information to scientifically justify approval for other indications that were not directly studied by the biosimilar manufacturer. This concept is called "extrapolation" and is critical to the goals of an abbreviated pathway, that is, improving access and options at a potentially lower cost [9].

Extrapolation is based on (1) all available data and information in the biosimilar application, (2) FDA's previous finding of safety and efficacy for other approved indications for the reference product, and (3) knowledge and consideration of various scientific factors for each indication. Extrapolation is not an assumption that the data from one directly studied indication or population alone are sufficient to support approval in a different non-studied indication or population. The biosimilar manufacturer must provide scientific justification to support extrapolation. These scientific justification factors include knowledge of the mechanism(s) of action, PK, PD, efficacy, safety, and immunogenicity of the reference product in each of its approved indications. FDA evaluates all the biosimilar product data to assess whether there are differences between the biosimilar and the reference product that may affect these scientific factors in any of the indications or populations not directly studied by the biosimilar manufacturer. If no such differences are identified, approval of the biosimilar for other nonstudied indications or populations is generally supported.

FDA works with biosimilar manufacturers during product development to determine what data are needed to support extrapolation. Manufacturers must demonstrate that products are safe and effective for each indication for which approval is sought, most often through indication-specific clinical trials. Since the goals of a biosimilar development program are different from those of a reference product development program, it is generally unnecessary from a scientific perspective to require a biosimilar manufacturer to conduct clinical trials in all the same disease indications for which the reference product was studied and approved.

Summary

Development of biomedical products is an expensive and long process that requires significant advanced planning. In planning a biomedical product–development program, it is important to determine whether the proposed CMC as

TABLE 30.9 Stepwise approach to support evidence for Food and Drug Administration approval of a biosimilar.

Key steps		Purpose
Analytical (foundation)	Extensive structural and functional characterization	Demonstration that the biologic is highly similar to the reference product in clinically inactive components
Nonclinical research	Animal studies and assessment of toxicity	Determination of any remaining uncertainties concerning safety of the proposed biologic prior to initiating human clinical studies
Clinical pharmacology	Human clinical studies including at least one study of immunogenicity and pharmacokinetics and pharmacodynamics if relevant	Determination of whether there are residual uncertainties between the proposed and reference products
Additional human clinical studies	Human clinical studies to further investigate if there are clinically meaningful differences in safety and efficacy between biosimilar and reference product	Demonstration of safety, purity, and potency in one or more appropriate conditions of use for which the reference product is licensed and licensure is sought for the biosimilar

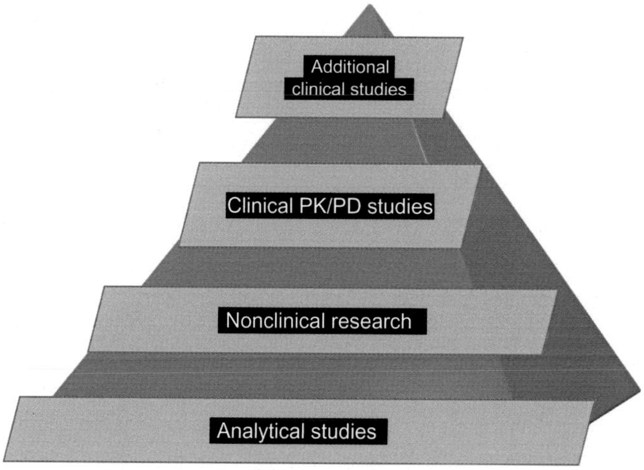

FIGURE 30.5 Stepwise evidence development to demonstrate biosimilarity.

well as preclinical and clinical studies will satisfy regulatory requirements to support safety and efficacy which will lead to approval of the new product. Developers must work interactively with regulatory officials to produce a plan that will support their proposed mechanism and satisfy regulatory needs. Once a biomedical product is approved, it must be consistently manufactured according to high standards of purity and stability as prescribed by regulatory authorities. Although manufacturing is oftentimes not a concern for R&D scientists, the process of manufacturing a new product can be complex and expensive, particularly for biological products. The complexity of manufacturing may play a role in determining the financial viability of investment in a specific biological target.

Regulatory procedures impact all stages of the biomedical product–development process. The rapid development of new technologies in human medical products blur the line between what is a device versus a biologic or drug, and ultimately the final product(s) made from many of these new technologies will be regulated as combination medical products. It is critical in today's evolving regulatory landscape for product developers to have a working knowledge and understanding of the FDA regulatory process across all medical product centers, that is, CBER, CDER, and CDRH. Rapid advances in technology and our understanding of disease may challenge current regulatory paradigms. In order to successfully develop a marketable product it is critical that developers are not only aware of but have an understanding of regulatory obligations and opportunities. Moreover, clear regulatory planning during the early stages of product development is essential to develop a focused regulatory strategy that can be presented to the regulatory authorities.

References

[1] Kondratas RA. Death helped write the biologics law. FDA Consum 1982;16:23–5.

[2] Regulatory Information. Other laws affecting FDA. Legislation, The Story of the Laws Behind the Labels. FDA Consumer.

June 1981. <https://wayback.archive-it.org/7993/20180125144335/https://www.fda.gov/AboutFDA/WhatWeDo/History/FOrgsHistory/EvolvingPowers/ucm056044.htm>. Retrieved March 2013.

[3] Maisel WH. Medical device regulation: an introduction for the practicing physician. Ann Intern Med 2004;140:296–302.

[4] Gutman S, Richter K, Alpert S. Update on FDA regulation of in vitro diagnostic devices. JAMA 1998;280(2):190–2.

[5] FDA, 1991. <http://www.fda.gov/biologicsbloodvaccines/developmentapprovalprocess/510kprocess/default.htm> Retrieved February 2013.

[6] Center for Biologics Evaluation and Research and Center for Drug Evaluation and Research. Guidance for industry: fast track drug development programs - designation, development, and application review. US Department of Health and Human Services; Food and Drug Administration, 2013. Available at: <https://www.fda.gov/downloads/Drugs/Guidances/UCM358301.pdf>.

[7] Sherman RE, Li J, Shapley S, Robb M, Woodcock J. Breakthrough therapy: expediting drug development – the FDA's new "breakthrough therapy" designation. NEJM 2013;369:1877–80.

[8] Christl L; US Food and Drug Administration. FDA's overview of the regulatory guidance for the development and approval of biosimilar products in the US, 2015. <https://www.fda.gov/Drugs/DevelopmentApprovalProcess/HowDrugsareDevelopedandApproved/ApprovalApplications/TherapeuticBiologicApplications/Biosimilars/ucm428730.htm>.

[9] Lim S; US Food and Drug Administration. Overview of the regulatory framework and FDA's guidance for the development and approval of biosimilar and interchangeable products in the US. <https://www.fda.gov/downloads/Drugs/DevelopmentApprovalProcess/HowDrugsareDevelopedandApproved/ApprovalApplications/TherapeuticBiologicApplications/Biosimilars/UCM610804.pdf>; 2013.

Chapter 31

The Biomanufacturing of Biotechnology Products

John Conner, MS[1], Don Wuchterl[2], Maria Lopez[3], Bill Minshall, MS[4], Rabi Prusti, PhD[5], Dave Boclair[6], Jay Peterson[7] and Chris Allen, MS[8]

[1]*Chief Manufacturing Officer, Paragon Bioservices, Inc., Baltimore, MD, United States,* [2]*Senior Vice President, Technical Operations and Quality, Audentes Therapeutics, San Francisco, CA, United States,* [3]*Vice President, Quality and Regulatory Affairs, SIWA Biotech Corp., Oklahoma City, OK, United States,* [4]*Owner, ASL Consulting, Ocala, FL, United States,* [5]*Executive Director, Quality Control, Cytovance Biologics Inc., Oklahoma City, OK, United States,* [6]*Director, Operational Excellence, Paragon Bioservices Inc., Baltimore, MD, United States,* [7]*Manager, Manufacturing, Cytovance Biologics Inc., Oklahoma City, OK, United States,* [8]*Director, Capital Projects, Paragon Bioservices Inc., Baltimore, MD, United States*

Chapter Outline

What is biologics manufacturing? How is it different from small molecule pharmaceutical manufacturing? Biologics manufacturing, or biomanufacturing for short, is a complex process that produces a product largely derived from discoveries using recombinant DNA technology to develop processes and analytics to manufacture biotherapeutic products. These recombinant products were developed from several platforms, such as whole *multicellular* systems encompassing transgenic plants, animals, and *unicellular* microbials (bacteria and yeast), and insect and

Biotechnology Entrepreneurship. DOI: https://doi.org/10.1016/B978-0-12-815585-1.00031-0

mammalian cell cultures. The discovery and "proof-of-concept" from the research bench are transferred to a process and analytical group that will use science and engineering as well as regulatory experience to scale up the product efficiently with sufficient product yield to support the clinical program and a quality product expressing the quality attributes of the product as well as profile any product-associated impurities. The process for different biologic platforms is complex and unlike traditional chemical synthesis, the biologic product resulting from a living system is not as an exact science as chemistry.

The long-existing paradigm for biologics was "the process is the product" and any variation in the process could impart a change in the product's safety and efficacy, although today's raw materials, process, and analytics are better defined and allow a lot more flexibility in the design and development of the process. Changes in the process or materials could severely alter the product's safety and characteristics, thus one may end up with a product with a different profile. Changes in the manufacturing process can alter the "impurity profile" of a biologic, thus imparting changes in the product's purity can have an adverse effect on safety. It has been demonstrated that endogenous adventitious viruses may result from processing changes or the extension of the production process. Therefore end-of-production processes and genotypic studies on the cell line have been required to understand the implications of changes in the production process that can affect the product's quality attributes and impurity profiles that could impact the safety of the therapeutic. Today's biologic manufacturing facilities incorporate analytical (AD) and process development (PD) capabilities to develop and test the scale up of the process to deliver sufficient productivity of a quality product. The development will support a Phase 1 clinical study focusing on the safety and efficacy of the product. If the product can demonstrate safety and efficacy the product with a regulatory agency and business-positive feedback will continue the manufacturing of the biologics until reaching final approval and licensing.

A Typical Biomanufacturing Process

Figs. 31.1 and 31.2 show typical biomanufacturing processes for upstream processes, and regulatory milestones from preclinical, clinical, Biologics License Application (BLA), and New Drug Application (NDA) submissions.

A Typical Biologic Product Development Diagram and Regulatory Milestones From Preclinical, Clinical, BLA, and NDA Submission

There are various regulatory opinions in the United States, European, Japanese pharmaceutical industries, and

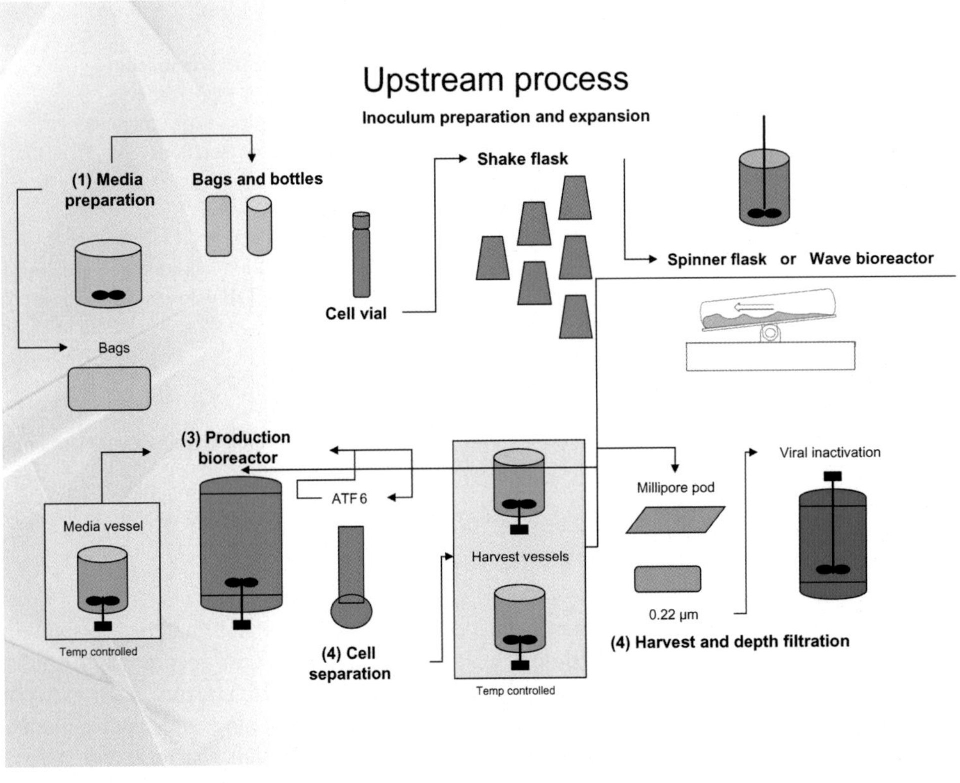

FIGURE 31.1 A typical biomanufacturing diagram of an upstream process. *Cytovance Biologics Inc., John Conner, 2013.*

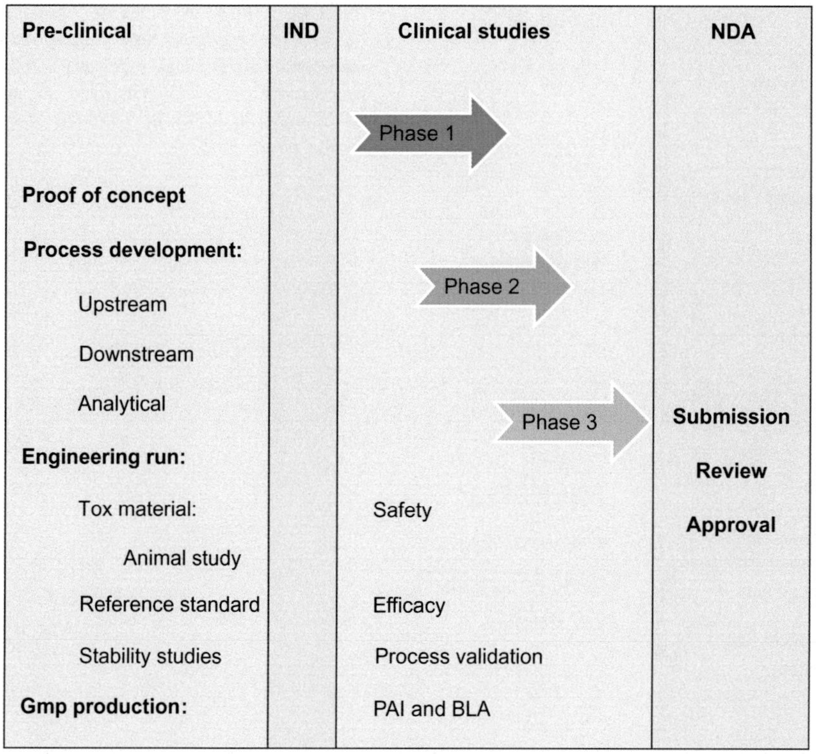

FIGURE 31.2 A typical biologic product development diagram and regulatory milestones from a preclinical, clinical, BLA, and NDA submission. *BLA*, Biologics License Application; *NDA*, New Drug Application. *Cytovance Biologics Inc., John Conner, 2013.*

other countries that regulate biologics. It is quite confusing and overlaps in opinions and redundancies. In order to bring together these regulatory authorities the International Conference on Harmonization (ICH) of Technical Requirements for Registration of Pharmaceuticals for Human Use was formed in 1990. This organization brings together these regulatory authorities to discuss scientific and technical aspects of drug registration. Since 1990 the increase in drug development has grown globally and at an incredible pace. The ICH has harmonized regulatory guidance documents to help biopharmaceutical entities to register and develop safe, quality, and effective drugs. There are guidances covering quality, safety, and efficacy guidelines. A list of ICH guidances that are relevant to the manufacture of a common biologic, a "therapeutic protein" (TP) known as a monoclonal antibody (mAb), is given later. The following slides list the pertinent ICH guidance document for a mAb biomanufacturing process and the diagram illustrates the typical biomanufacturing process flow for a mAb (see Fig. 31.3).

Biotechnology products are derived from the manipulation of various cells and their subsequent products these engineered cell systems produce. These biologic products are produced from various biomanufacturing platforms. One platform produces TPs, such as mAbs, cytokines, fusion proteins, and a number of therapeutic and process enzymes. There are also vaccines, whole cell, and gene therapy products being developed and biomanufactured.

A biologic therapeutic product, also known as a biologic, is a therapeutic product developed to treat a variety of diseases. This biologic product can be a mAb, a vaccine, a tissue, or various proteins, such as cytokines, enzymes, fusion proteins, whole cells, and viral and nonviral gene therapies. Biologic products are derived from living systems that may or may not be altered. Recombinant DNA technology has produced many biological products and has allowed research an avenue to discover many more. The paradigm for biologics "the process is the product" still is viable today. Biologics are also known as large molecules (nucleic acid and protein platforms). It is generally known that a therapeutic biologic is a product derived from or part of a cell or tissue, while the term biologic is used more often when the medical product consists of a cellular or tissue.

There are several classes of biologic products. Some are naturally occurring biologics, such as whole blood and blood components, organ and tissue transplantations, vaccines, and recently stem cell therapy. Those therapeutic biologics that are derived via recombinant DNA technology have developed a large number of therapeutics and have replaced older naturally derived drugs with recombinant DNA technology, such as "insulin" that was originally derived up until the 1980s from insulin extracted from cattle and pig pancreas (when comparing nonrecombinant insulin, there are only three amino acid differences between cattle and human insulin. There is also only one amino acid difference between human and

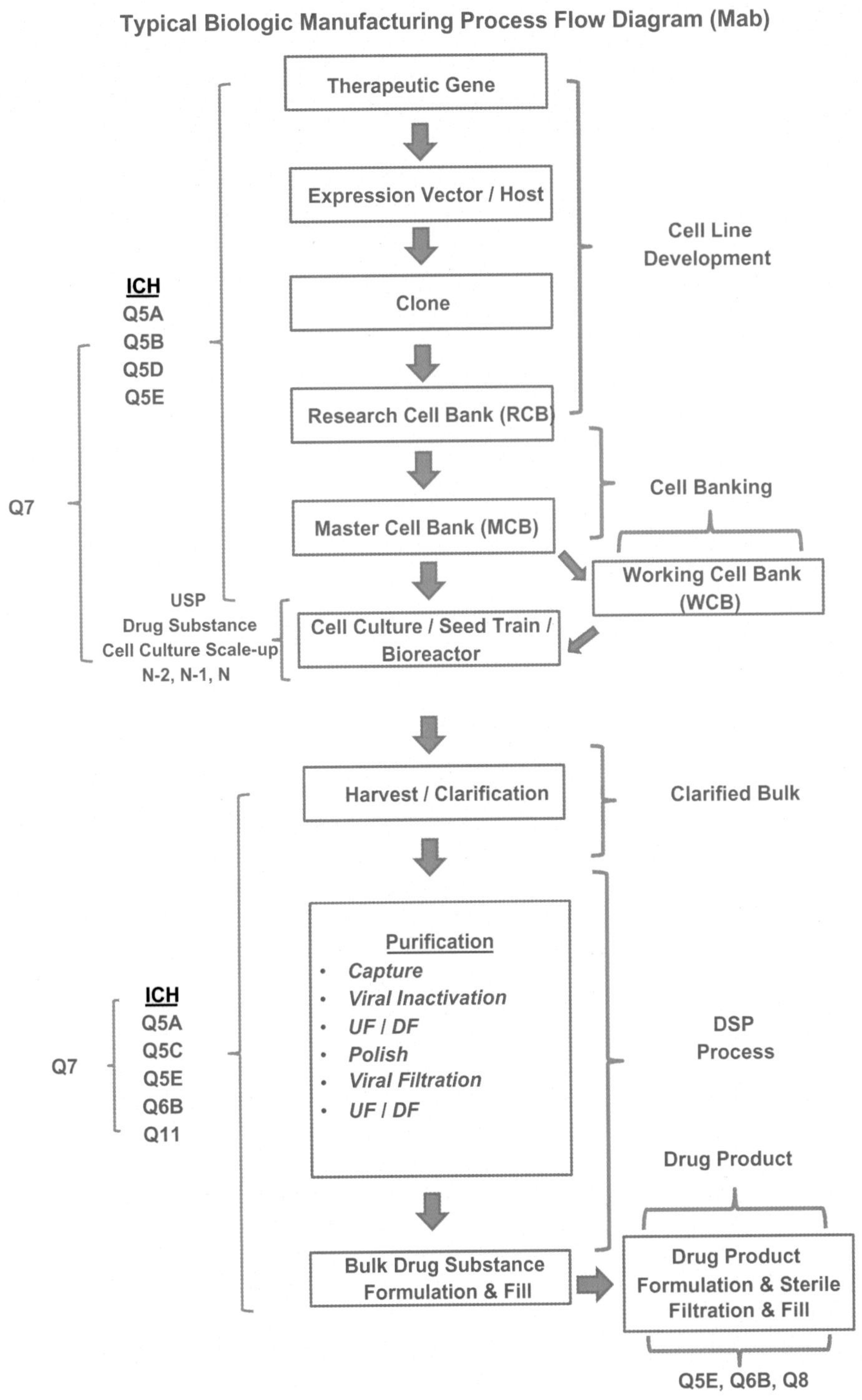

FIGURE 31.3 A typical biologic manufacturing process flow diagram with appropriate ICH guidance per steps. *ICH*, International Conference on Harmonization. *Cytovance Biologics Inc., John Conner, 2013.*

pig insulin). Today, most insulin is biomanufactured via recombinant DNA technology or "genetic engineering."

Recombinant DNA technology products are wide ranging and include proteins derived that are mAbs, signaling-type proteins, and receptor-type proteins.

In general, following are a number of types of biologics derived from recombinant DNA technology:

- Article I. mAbs
- Article II. Cytokines
- Article III. Process or intermediates used in manufacturing
- Article IV. Recombinant proteins
- Article V. Therapeutic vaccines

- Article VI. Growth hormones
- Article VII. Blood production-stimulating proteins
- Article VIII. Insulin and analogs
- Article IX. Therapeutic enzymes
- Article X. Fusion proteins
- Article XI. Therapeutic peptides
- Article XII. Therapeutic oligos
- Article XIII. Vaccines
- Article XIV. Gene therapy
- Article XV. Whole cells
- Article XVI. Tissues
- Article XVII. Biosimilars

A biologic can be defined as a large complex molecule produced from or extracted from a biological or living system. The biomanufacturing process, process controls, and the complete physiochemical and biological testing all together characterize the biologic product. For example, in regard to the biomanufacturing process, a biologic can be derived from biotechnology or it may be prepared using more conventional methods as is the case for blood- or plasma-derived products and a number of vaccines. In regard to the nature of a biologic's active substance, it may consist entirely of microorganisms or mammalian cells, nucleic acids (DNA or RNA), be a protein (antibody, cytokine, enzyme, protein-like, etc.) all originating from either a microbial, animal, human, or plant sources.

A biologics mode of action may describe a biologic platform, such as an immunotherapeutic, gene therapy, or a cellular therapeutic (see Table 31.1).

Biosimilars

What is a biosimilar? How is it different than a generic? Generic is the designation for (off-patent) small-molecule drugs that are exactly identical to the properties and the process to manufacture is the same and reproducible. In essence, chemically synthesized drugs are pretty much add component $A + B = C$ (product) almost all of the time. Biosimilars are much more complex and larger molecules can be influenced by the manufacturing process. Because of the biologics complexity, biosimilar manufacturers cannot guarantee that their biosimilar is exactly identical to the original manufacturer's version, but rather it is similar to the original biologic. The biosimilar manufacturer's manufacturing process may be slightly different. This may produce significantly different effects which may impact product quality, have no effect, or in some cases elicit additional quality attributes—now

TABLE 31.1 A variety of biologics.

Designation	Name	Indication	Technology	Mechanism of action
Abatacept	Orencia	Rheumatoid arthritis	Immunoglobin CTLA-4 fusion protein	T-cell deactivation
Adalimumab	Humira	Rheumatoid arthritis, ankylosing spondylitis, psoriatic arthritis, psoriasis, Crohn's disease	Monoclonal antibody	TNF antagonist
Alefacept	Amevive	Chronic plaque psoriasis	Immunoglobin G1 fusion protein	Incompletely characterized
Erythropoietin	Epogen	Anemia arising from cancer chemotherapy, chronic renal failure, etc.	Recombinant protein	Stimulation of red blood cell production
Etanercept	Enbrel	Rheumatoid arthritis, ankylosing spondylitis, psoriatic arthritis, psoriasis	Recombinant human TNF-receptor fusion protein	TNF antagonist
Infliximab	Remicade	Rheumatoid arthritis, ankylosing spondylitis, psoriatic arthritis, psoriasis, Crohn's disease	Monoclonal antibody	TNF antagonist
Trastuzumab	Herceptin	Breast cancer	Humanized monoclonal antibody	HER2/neu (erbB2) antagonist
Ustekinumab	Stelara	Psoriasis	Humanized monoclonal antibody	IL-12 and IL-23 antagonist
Denileukin Diftitox	Ontak	Cutaneous T cell Lymphoma (CTCL)	Diphtheria toxin Engineered protein combining Interleukin-2 and Diphtheria toxin	Interleukin-2 Receptor binder

Source: http://en.wikipedia.org/wiki/Monoclonal_antibody_therapy#FDA_approved_therapeutic_antibodies [accessed March 16, 2019].

you have a biobetter, thus requiring clinical development. A disadvantage of the biosimilar developer is that in developing the innovator's process to produce the biosimilar, the innovator's starting material, that is, the recombinant cell line or clone, is not available to the developer unlike generics where raw materials and process chemicals are known or can be derived. Finally, the impurity profiles may impart a variety of similar impurities or degradation products that may elicit harmful side effects.

Thus biosimilar manufacturers produce products that are slightly different from the innovator's and cannot guarantee that their biosimilar is as safe and effective as the innovator's product. So, unlike generics, biosimilars were not authorized in the United States or the European Union through the procedures that allowed generic approvals. So as a result, to date, all biosimilar drugs have targeted well-known approved and coming off-patent biologic drugs. The regulatory agencies have required biosimilar therapeutics to undergo a very detailed comparability review and testing. In 2012 the United States Federal Drug Agency (USFDA) published a guidance as part of the "Patient Protection and Affordable Care Act of 2010" part of the Public Health Service Act (PHS Act) which was created to provide an approval pathway known as the Biologics Price Competition and Innovation Act (BPCI Act). This approach or law allows for a potential approval of biological products that can demonstrate "biosimilar" properties that are "very similar" to the original biologic or one that "closely resembles" the FDA-licensed biological product.

The European regulatory authority [European Medicines Agency (EMA)] has provided an approach and coined their biosimilar as "similar biological medicinal products." Their document guides biosimilar companies in the manufacture and approval of these complex biologics to demonstrate comprehensive comparability of the biosimilar to the innovator's product. The EMA accomplished this well before the FDA. Thus the EU has been further ahead of the United States in biosimilars with the EMA approving the first biosimilar "Omnitrope" in 2006. In June 2010 a biosimilar copy of Amgen's Neupogen was approved and since then, a total of 12 biosimilars have been approved between 2006 and 2012. In July 2013, two mAb biosimilars (Remsima-Celltrion and Inflectra-Hospira) were approved by the EMA. These mAbs were very similar to the innovator molecule known as Remicade (infliximab) originally approved in 1999 for rheumatoid arthritis, Crohn's disease, ulcerative colitis, psoriatic arthritis, and psoriasis. All of these diseases are classified as autoimmune diseases.

Therefore a biosimilar product is similar to a biologic reference or innovator product, has the same mechanism of action for the intended use, preapproved label use, has the same route of administration, dose formulation, and has similar potency or strength as the reference or innovator product. The biosimilar also should show no clinical differences between the biosimilar and the innovator product in terms of the safety, purity, and potency.

Therefore the regulatory theme for the manufacture and approval is midway between testing and comparability for a new therapeutic biologic and more than the testing of a generic drug. Comprehensive comparability is the key. Following is a list of classes of biologics that are in the current biologic development or have been approved:

- epoetins,
- filgrastims,
- insulins,
- growth hormones,
- mAbs,
- low molecular weight heparins, and
- beta interferons.

Key Phases of Biologics Development

The biologic product to be developed and manufactured starts with the discovery and proof-of-concept studies characterizing the product as well as defining the actual molecule and its mode of action. The study and knowledge of the molecule's characteristics will be important in designing cell culture and bioreactor parameters in order to scale up and produce a sufficient yield of product to satisfy early experiments and AD. This crude product will also be used for early clarification, downstream process (DSP) development, and formulation studies. During the discovery phase, in vitro and in vivo (small animal) studies will be performed. Once the product proof-of-concept is achieved, a decision to move forward with PD and the eventual investigational new drug (IND) finally is agreed upon. In today's drug development world, the next step is to secure funding to continue developing the therapeutic. This usually involves forming a company and securing funding from private sources, venture capital, or government grants. Most of these companies do not have sufficient funding to build development, manufacturing, and quality laboratories nor the time it takes to build this infrastructure. These companies partner with contract manufacturing organizations (CMOs) to help develop and manufacture the drug and offer quality and regulatory support.

Discovery

Target identification (ID) of a therapeutic biologic molecule involves choosing a disease with an unmet need or an improvement of a current therapeutic, and usually the group or person may have a personal or scientific interest in studying and developing a drug candidate. These biologic drugs are usually discovered in academic and biotech research labs. Once a molecule is chosen, the biochemical mechanism and other biological characteristics are tested for their interaction with the drug or disease target. There are thousands of biologic molecules studied and they go through a very arduous process to profile and characterize the molecule and its potential drug or disease target. Proof-of-concept in vitro and in vivo (small animals such as rodents) must be validated before any drug can move from discovery and into a clinical development program. Once a promising therapeutic candidate or several leading candidates are validated, the company or group will set up and budget a preclinical development program.

Process Development

All biologic products transition from bench scale research and proof-of-concept to the next stage of product development called PD and AD. The TP candidate's characteristics, purification strategies, analytical methods for in-process and final product characterization, and any stability data are supplied to the PD and AD groups. This is typically called the technology transfer or "tech transfer." The tech transfer is the most important phase of product development as it is the hand-off to the scale-up team (PD and AD, respectively), manufacturing science and technology (MST), manufacturing and quality assurance (QA), and quality control (QC) teams. A thorough understanding of the product's characteristics and the process at bench scale is necessary in order to facilitate the transfer of all of the critical parameters.

Once the tech transfer is initiated from the client, the upstream process (USP) development, or cell culture group, embarks on accessing the media and cell culture conditions relative to the correct ID of the cell line, the growth and viability of the cell line is robust, and the productivity of the cell line's product (TP) titer (yield) is adequate to scale up. Once, the cell line and growth conditions are confirmed, the PD group will make a development cell bank from the research cell bank (RCB) and will use this to develop a scale-up process and optimize the media and supplements used in the cell culture. The USP development will also make material to be used in the DSP development which is the purification and formulation development group. This group will also work on the postharvest clarification (removal of the cells and other large molecules as well as some large protein and DNA aggregates) prior to the first chromatography or purification steps. The first steps postclarification is usually a capture- or affinity-binding step. In essence the TP is bound to a chromatographic resin's [e.g., Protein A mAbSelect Sure from General Electric (GE) packed in a column allowing for impurities to flow through the column]. The bound TP is then pulled off or eluted from the resin and collected for the purification steps that take the TP through various chromatographic column steps to remove impurities and aggregates, such as host-cell proteins and host DNA. All of these chromatographic purification and polishing steps are designed based on the protein properties and characteristics described during the discovery bench scale or preclinical phase of the product development. The DSP also will include viral clearance studies to reduce the risk of viral contaminants. Several resins or filters significantly reduce viral load or give "*x* amount of Log reduction of virus." The DSP team also develops the formulation steps for bulk drug substance (BDS) and the final formulation of the drug product (DP) and excipients (other materials in the formulation that impart a property such as providing stability to the DP). During the DSP process, the development and optimization of the DSP team will provide the AD team process/ product material to work on designing, confirming, qualifying, or validating analytical methods needed for in-process and release testing.

As the PD phase of the product development proceeds the MST, the group will work with the PD and AD teams to capture and work on the tech transfer from the development groups into the manufacturing and quality groups.

Clinical Manufacturing

Preclinical Trials

In the preclinical phase the product is further characterized. The biologic molecule's phenotypic, genotypic, and biochemical profiles must be determined. Attributes and parameters useful in determining its strengths and weaknesses, such as shape, amino acid sequence, isoelectric point, drug candidates mechanism of action, its potential bioactivity or availability, and any possible toxicity issues, are some of the characterizations that will need to be studied or elucidated. These will be the building blocks of information that will be transferred to other groups responsible for PD and AD.

How are we going to manufacture the novel therapeutic biologic? During this phase, a process is developed to scale up the process to manufacture a quality product that can be used in a Phase 1 clinical trial. Typically, a master cell bank (MCB) will be produced from an RCB or a pre-MCB. A working cell bank (WCB) may be produced from an MCB that has been fully tested for biosafety and has also been fully characterized. If a WCB is produced, it too will be tested as the MCB was tested for biosafety and characterized as defined per the Q7 ICH Guidance. These cells will be used in PD DEMO (demonstration) runs and the data from the PD work will be transferred (tech transfer) to manufacturing. Concurrently, AD will be working on developing and qualifying in-process and release analytics which will then be transferred into QC.

Manufacturing scientists and engineers will then take the process and design a scale-up plan and tech transfer into manufacturing. The first run will be a non-GMP (good manufacturing practice) engineering run that will lead to a GMP run. Typically, the engineering run is a process dress rehearsal for the GMP run. This run will manufacture products for the following:

- toxicology-primate study;
- viral clearance/validation;
- reference standard;
- stability studies;
- storage;
- shipping;
- container closure BDS and DP;
- AD (e.g., bioassays);
- other analytical methods work;
- compendial; and
- method qualification/validation work.

The GMP run will be prepared by reviewing the engineering run outcome based on the process review, in-process data, and final testing of the product. The engineering run will be deemed successful and ready for GMP production if there are no major process or testing issues and the product has met all of its quality parameters allowing for the release of the drug substance (DS) and if the DP is formulated to pass all of the acceptance criteria which would allow for the product to be released. The documents would be revised and updated from the engineering run redlined batch records. The final production records would be reviewed and approved for GMP production. The GMP run would provide material to support the following needed for IND filing and the start of the Phase 1 clinical trial:

- clinical trial material,
- stability,
- reference standard,
- end-of-production cell bank, and
- genetic stability.

The GMP clinical trial material is held in quarantine at the biomanufacturing site and when it passes all of the release testing and document review, the GMP lot will be released to the in-house clinical distribution group for clinical studies once the IND is approved. The clinical trials are usually managed by the in-house clinical group or outsourced to companies, such as Almac, Quintiles, or Covance.

Another important part of the preclinical phase of the product development is drug formulation and drug delivery. How are we going to present this drug to the patient's biologic system? Formulation, delivery, and container/closure development must be studied at this early stage. If you cannot develop a stable formulation matrix and do not know the delivery path, the drug candidate development will be delayed or stopped. Formulation and the product's delivery parameter development is a critical element that must be developed and understood. The key is stability (biosafety and product maintain its quality attributes) of the drug candidate's formulation, safety as determined initially by biosafety testing of the bulk, and final product. It must also be noted that this formulation and drug delivery system may be revised during the development of the product.

Once formulated, several other important studies are important to develop and understand the formulated biologic drug. Pharmacokinetic (PK) studies look at absorption, drug distribution, metabolism of the drug, and the excretion or elimination of the biologic drug. Why is this important? PK data from animal toxicity (TOX) studies (product produced from non-GMP scale up or engineering run) will be used to compare to the eventual early-phase studies. These preclinical TOX studies are typically dosing studies (acute and chronic dosing that help determine the specific dose and range in the animal TOX and first in the human Phase I clinical study). Other toxicity studies look at carcinogenic, mutagenic, and reproductive toxicity. This should give an idea of the potential degree of safety and efficacy of the formulated drug candidate as well as a foundation to support the PD, AD, and the IND application filing. Once filed and approved, the preclinical and discovery information will help support the clinical development of the biologic drug. *Note*: All of the proposed preclinical toxicity studies are actual guidances from various regulatory agencies.

In order to understand and support the product characteristics and quality attributes and support preclinical and clinical in-process and release testing, bioanalytical testing must be developed in the preclinical phase of the biologics development. Thus the AD group will support methods for cell culture, fermentation, assay to determine titers or process yields as well as bioassays, and other assays to elicit the identity, potency, purity, and safety of the product (e.g., in mAbs) to use size-exclusion chromatography to determine the percent of purity by evaluating the amount of aggregation and other product impurities. It is important to understand the impurity profile of the product and the final formulated product.

Clinical Trials

Clinical studies are grouped according to their objective into three types or phases (Phases 1, 2, and 3). How does biomanufacturing activities correlate to the different phases of a clinical trial leading up to the commercialization of a biologic product? Manufacturing of the therapeutic biologic will continue through the preclinical and clinical phase of the trial to supply the clinic with the trial product to the patients enrolled in the clinical study, stability programs, additional reference standards, additional process-optimization studies, and additional studies as needed to support investigations.

Phase 1 Clinical Development

Thirty days after a "biotech" company has filed its IND, it may begin a small-scale Phase 1 clinical trial to demonstrate human pharmacology and safety. Phase 1 parameters, such as PK and tolerance in healthy recruited volunteers, will be studied. These studies include acute and chronic dosing studies including initial single-dose, a dose escalation, and repeated-dose studies.

Phase 2 Clinical Development

Phase 2 clinical studies are small-scale trials to continue to evaluate the safety and PK of the biologic and also to evaluate the efficacy and possible side effects in a small set of patients (commonly 100–200). Typical Phase 2 objectives are as follows:

- safety;
- efficacy;
- risk assessment;
- process review;
- raw materials;
- analytical methods;
- BDS container closure;
- DP container closure;
- storage;
- shipping; and
- Phase 2b (Phase 2a and b review and requirements to move to Phase 3).

Phase 3 Clinical Development

Phase 3 studies are large-scale clinical trials for continued safety and efficacy in a larger patient population. While Phase 3 studies are in progress, there are several interim analyses available to show continued safety and efficacy. During this phase, the final process is determined and "locked down." A gap analysis of the process to support process validation is conducted and any gaps or risks are addressed. Process validation commences, and if all goes well, the company will commence manufacturing of the three registration or conformance lots prior to the filing of a BLA or a NDA. Typical Phase 3 objectives are as follows:

- safety,
- efficacy,
- risk assessment,
- lockdown process,
- process and analytical gap analysis (FMEA),
- process validation,
- minimum three conformance or registration lots,
- BLA submission,
- PAI facility and quality assessment inspection,
- BLA approval,
- secondary labeling and packaging approval, and
- inventory build.

Phase 4 Marketing

Prepare for Commercial Launch and Commercial Manufacturing

Once a BLA and NDA have been approved, the biotech company will be seeking to launch the released DP in the approved market. The inventory to launch may be the three conformance lots or other released lots manufactured in anticipation of an approved license to manufacture, distribute, and market the new drug.

Good Manufacturing Practices

Requirements

Biologics manufacturing requires the use of GMP or current good manufacturing practices (cGMP) to ensure that adequate history is maintained for each product run. As the product manufacturing process is developed and defined and as it matures from the lab bench development through Phases 1, 2, and 3, the regulatory expectation is that appropriate GMP will be applied to help ensure subject safety. This is especially critical at Phase 1 where the clinical trial focus is safety and efficacy.

In order to support clinical trial drugs, manufacturers are expected to implement manufacturing controls that reflect product and manufacturing considerations, evolving process and product knowledge, and manufacturing experience. As the process becomes better defined, critical control points are identified, and experience in the process increases, increased GMP documentation must be implemented and maintained. This means that information that is gained from the lab development bench scale all the way through Phase 3 trials must be translated into compliant GMP documents that house product production history.

Code of Federal Regulations and European Regulations

The USFDA and the European Union provide regulations for the manufacture of DPs. These are the laws that biologics manufacturers are required to follow.

The FDA regulations are defined in 21 CFR 210, "Current Good Manufacturing Practice in Manufacturing, Processing, Packaging, or Holding of Drugs; General," and 21 CFR 211, "Current Good Manufacturing Practices for Finished Pharmaceuticals." EU regulations are defined in the EudraLex, Volume 4, "EU Guidelines to Good Manufacturing Practice Medicinal Products for Human and Veterinary Use."

In addition, the United States publishes guidance documents that provide the agencies current thinking on topics. These guidance documents provide valuable details into how the agencies expect manufacturers to show compliance to the regulations. The most used guidance documents can be found at http://www.fda.gov/Drugs/GuidanceComplianceRegulatoryInformation/Guidances/ucm065005.htm (accessed March 16, 2019). Here is a list of the ICH Guidances specifically related to Quality and Manufacturing of Biologics:

FDA Guidance for Industry—Q7A Good Manufacturing Practice Guidance for Active Pharmaceutical Ingredients, August 2001

FDA Guidance for Industry—Q8 (R2) Pharmaceutical Development

FDA Guidance for Industry—Q9 Quality Risk Management

FDA Guidance for Industry—Q10 Pharmaceutical Quality System

FDA Guidance for Industry—Q11 Development and Manufacture of Drug Substances

FDA Guidance for Industry—Sterile Drug Products Produced by Aseptic Processing—Current Good Manufacturing Practices

FDA Guidance for Industry—CGMP for Phase 1 Investigational Drugs

FDA Guidance for Industry—Investigating Out-of-Specification (OOS) Test Results for Pharmaceutical Production

FDA Guidance for Industry—Process Validation: General Principles and Practices

EU Guidelines to Good Manufacturing Practice—Annex 1, Manufacture of Sterile Medicinal Products

EU Guidelines to Good Manufacturing Practice—Annex 12, Investigational Medicinal Products

Oversight and Compliance

Regulatory compliance in biologics manufacturing requires that the implemented quality unit and system be robust enough to support the product production throughout its clinical phase maturation.

The quality unit is expected to be independent of the operations/manufacturing unit and that it fulfills both the QA and QC responsibilities. Their roles and responsibilities should be defined and documented. Critical roles of the quality unit are the review and approval of all quality-related documents; disposition of raw materials, intermediates, packaging, labeling materials, and the final product; conduct internal and supplier audits; review completed batch production and laboratory control records before determining disposition; approve changes that could potentially affect the intermediate and final product; and ensure the complete investigation and resolution into deviations and complaints.

In biologics manufacturing, especially with Phase 1 material, not all critical parameters, control points, and at times raw material may all be defined or identified. Knowing this and knowing that the process will continue to grow through its clinical phases, oversight from the quality unit must ensure that the manufacturing process adheres to the foundational components of GMPs. These foundational components are those that ensure full support of the product production and are maintained within the quality system. All components of the quality system are controlled through written and approved policies and procedures.

Documentation

Change control—A system established to evaluate all changes that could affect the production and control of the product.

Personnel—A system for maintaining and evaluating personnel qualifications and training for job-related functions.

Building and facilities—Systems that provide evidence of the adequacy of the facility. These systems include at minimum, design, qualification, calibration, cleaning, maintenance, and monitoring.

Laboratory control records—Systems that ensure records include complete data derived from all tests conducted to ensure compliance with established specification and standards.

Batch records and specifications—A system that ensures that documents related to the manufacture of intermediates and product be prepared, reviewed, approved, and distributed according to written procedures.

Materials management—A system for the receipt, ID, quarantine, storage, handling, sampling, testing, and disposition of material.

Production and process controls—A system for the control of critical steps, such as weight and measurement, time limits, in-process sample testing, and contamination control.

Facility Requirements

The facility and the utility requirements are the fundamental backbones of the process flow and production effectiveness. In facility design, it is important to consider the regulatory nature of the industry and seeking some in-depth knowledge of the requirements will pay big dividends in the long run. Let us briefly look at a few of these systems and their importance to the overall health of the business platform (see Fig. 31.4A and B).

Air-Handling Equipment

Large volumes of air are required to properly satisfy the international standards for clean room air. This is an area where many people may underestimate their current and future needs. This can be a costly upfront mistake and can further restrict a company's ability to grow additional revenue streams. Industry airflow standards are dictated by international standards. Airflows dictate clean room classifications. Current classifications and room air changes per hour are found in Table 31.2.

These clean air room classifications must be considered as they dictate the allowable operations in each area. Due to the large volumes of air flows, building chilling capacity must be a strategic part of the facility design as well.

Process Water (Purified Water and Water for Injection)

Another crucial element in the success of your production processes is the demand and need for ultrapure water, which cannot be overstated. Purified water (PW) is to be used for the production of USP products. PW and sterile PW may be obtained by any suitable process (see Fig. 31.5). Water for injection is water purified by distillation or reverse osmosis (see Fig. 31.6). As cost is an important factor in the implementation of these systems, at a minimum, a healthy Reverse Osmosis Deionized water or distillation system should be utilized. Attention should be given to the design and installation of this critical system. Details, such as storage, sanitization, number of water loops (ambient and hot), and the number of water drops, need to be carefully planned in advance. In addition, the maintenance of the PW systems is the most important element of continuously producing USP-acceptable water to support the facility's biological manufacturing processes.

Building Automation and Alarm Systems

Proper building automation and alarming is paramount to effective and efficient operations. Clients and auditors will want to see if you have control of the critical facility and process-related parameters, such as differential pressures, temperatures, humidity, pressure, flows, and more. There are many off-the-shelf systems that provide control and capture of important and useful information. Skillful use of automation and alarms can quickly pay dividends in facility utility costs. In addition, these automation software packages provide tools for trending, tracking, and troubleshooting various production-related applications. Building automation and alarm systems is an essential part of a cGMP enterprise.

Additional Facility Requirements

In addition to the earlier referenced critical systems, there are many areas of consideration when designing or operating a compliant good manufacturing facility and organization. Topics noteworthy of additional study are included, but not limited to, cleanliness, validation and commissioning, process-material personnel and airflows, cold storage, dry storage, emergency procedures, safety, security, pest control, environmental monitoring (EM), preventive maintenance and calibrations, and all possible redundancies that may be required to support utility and processes.

The Biomanufacturing Team—Their Typical Roles and Responsibilities in a Biologics Manufacturing Facility

Manufacturing-Related Functions

Manufacturing-related positions typically make up the majority of positions in a biologics manufacturing facility. These can be classified as positions that directly interact with the manufacturing process. Typical functions include upstream manufacturing, downstream manufacturing (purification), fill/finish operations, a manufacturing support team, and a manufacturing technical support (MTS) function.

Upstream Manufacturing

Upstream manufacturing responsibilities routinely include operations related to cell expansion steps starting with a single vial of frozen cells and growing these exponentially

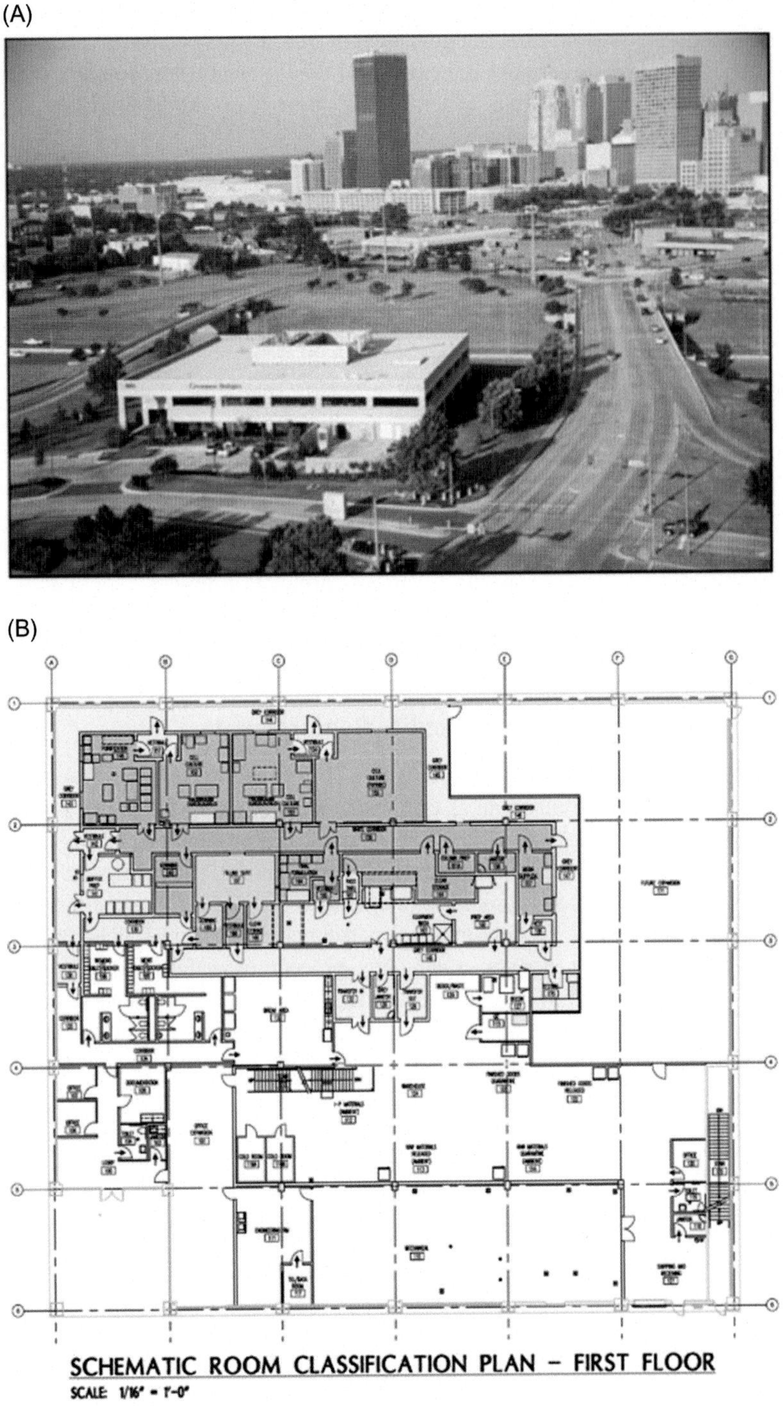

FIGURE 31.4 A typical biomanufacturing facility. (A) Outside the facility. (B) A schematic of the first floor. *Cytovance Biologics Inc., 2013.*

into larger and larger systems eventually reaching your large-scale terminal reactor where the targeted protein is expressed. These operations require highly skilled specialists trained in microbiological processes, GMPs, fermenter and bioreactor systems, automation systems, and in-process analysis instruments. While not always required, typical employees will have a bachelor's degree in biology, microbiology, or a similar science (see Fig. 31.7).

Downstream Manufacturing

Downstream manufacturing, or commonly referred to as purification, is focused on the capture and isolation of a targeted molecule and the removal of impurities. This is accomplished through several different processes to include filtration, column chromatography, and tangential flow filtration (TFF). These operations also require highly skilled specialists trained in chemical properties,

TABLE 31.2 International airflow standards for clean rooms: current classifications and room air changes.

FS cleanroom class	ISO equivalent class	Air change rate (per hour)
1	ISO 3	360–540
10	ISO 4	300–540
100	ISO 5	240–480
1000	ISO 6	150–240
10,000	ISO 7	60–90
100,000	ISO 8	5–48

Source: Figure reprinted from the "IEST. Energy efficient low operating cost cleanroom airflow design. In: IEST 2003 ESTECH proceedings" with permission from the Institute of Environmental Sciences and Technology. © 2003 by IEST, www.iest.org (847):981-0100.

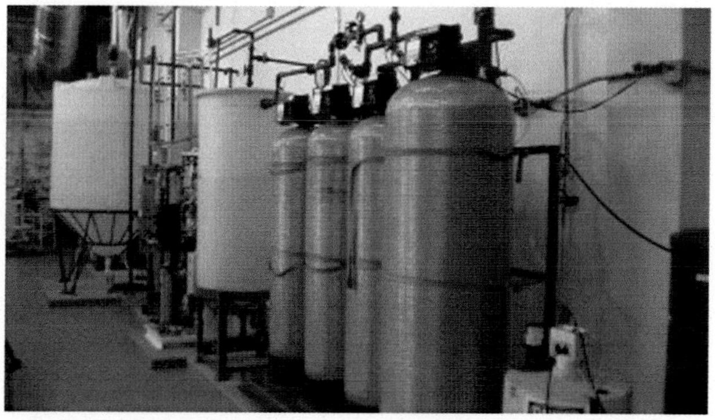

FIGURE 31.5 A typical purified water system. *Cytovance Biologics Inc., 2013.*

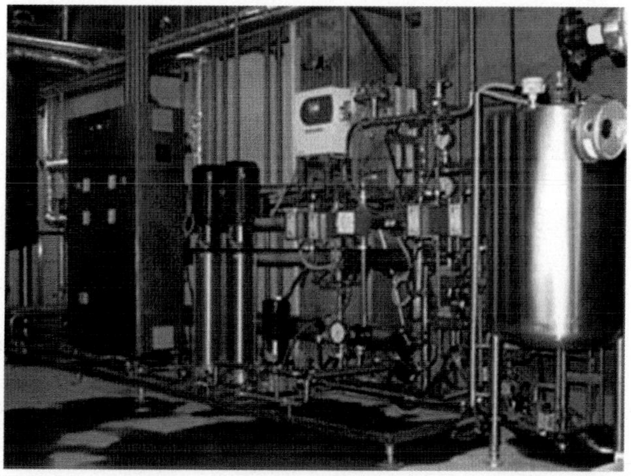

FIGURE 31.6 Typical water for injection system. *Water Sciences. <http://www.watersciences.biz/Purified_Water_Generation_Plant.html> [accessed March 16, 2019].*

chromatography, TFF, filtration systems, GMPs, automation systems, and in-process analysis instruments. Typical employees will have a bachelor's degree in chemistry,

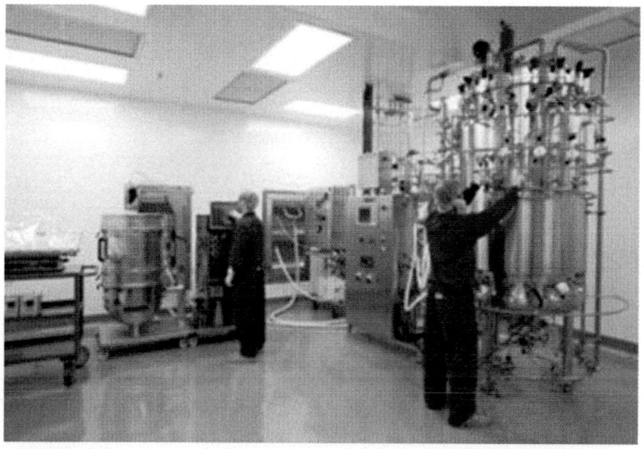

FIGURE 31.7 Upstream manufacturing: bioreactor operations. *Cytovance Biologics Inc., 2013.*

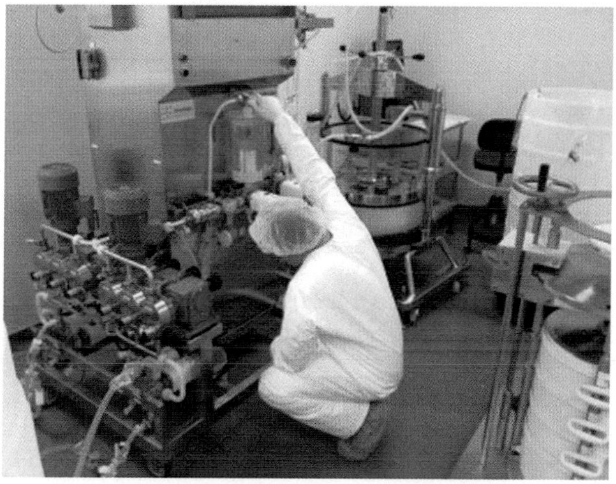

FIGURE 31.8 Downstream manufacturing: chromatography operations. *Cytovance Biologics Inc., 2013.*

chemical engineering, biology, or a similar science (see Fig. 31.8).

Production Support

The production support function is commonly utilized in biologics manufacturing facilities. While these functions can be performed by the upstream and downstream functions, the amount of coordination and activity in these areas would usually warrant a separate team. These functions perform a variety of supporting tasks to include media and buffer preparation, equipment and component preparation, chemical dispensing, equipment and environmental cleaning, and some in-process testing. Associates on this team are trained in the use of glass washers, autoclaves, solution prep equipment, and GMPs. Typical employees will have a bachelor's degree in science or engineering (see Fig. 31.9).

Fill/finish Operations

The fill/finish team is a specialized function within the manufacturing team dedicated to the manufacture of the DP. A DP refers to the final formulated product in its delivery container. In most cases for biologic products, these will be traditional glass vials. Other systems include prefilled syringes or intravenous bags. As these steps in the process are the last manufacturing steps, they must be performed in highly contained environments. Typically, these areas will be the cleanest areas in the facility with the highest levels of control (see Fig. 31.10A and B).

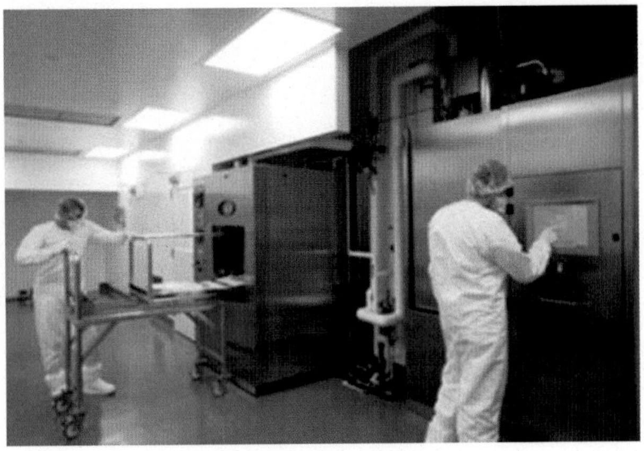

FIGURE 31.9 Manufacturing support: glass washer, autoclave (steam sterilizer), and prep area. *Cytovance Biologics Inc., 2013.*

(A)

(B)

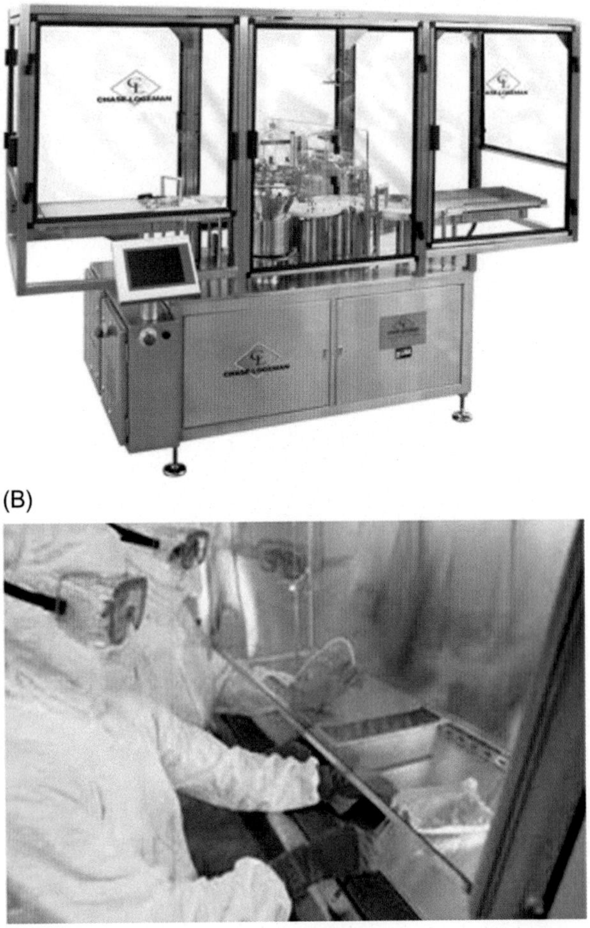

FIGURE 31.10 (A) Chase Logeman automated vial fill machine. (B) Fill/Finish operations. *(A) Cytovance Biologics Inc. and Chase Logeman, 2013. (B) Cytovance Biologics Inc., 2013.*

Manufacturing Technical Support

The MTS function provides scientific support to the manufacturing team. Their roles include tech transfer activities from the PD group, new equipment ID and qualification, on the floor support for complex process steps, troubleshooting complex process–related issues, and support technical investigations. Skilled specialists and engineers on this team are familiar with the scientific principles related to one or more areas of a traditional process. They are also skilled and knowledgeable on the process equipment utilized throughout the process train. Specialists on this team will typically have many years of relevant experience as well as bachelor's level degrees in a scientific discipline (many have advanced degrees) (see Fig. 31.11).

Quality Assurance

One of the most important functions in a biologics manufacturing facility is the quality unit. As this is a heavily regulated industry, a robust internal quality system is required to ensure adherence to all regulations and patient safety. QA provides a fully independent look at all documentation, production areas, and supply chain functions to ensure compliance. Quality is responsible for ensuring all raw materials, procedures, and areas are released for production. They will also perform reviews of all documentation, QC samples, and final release

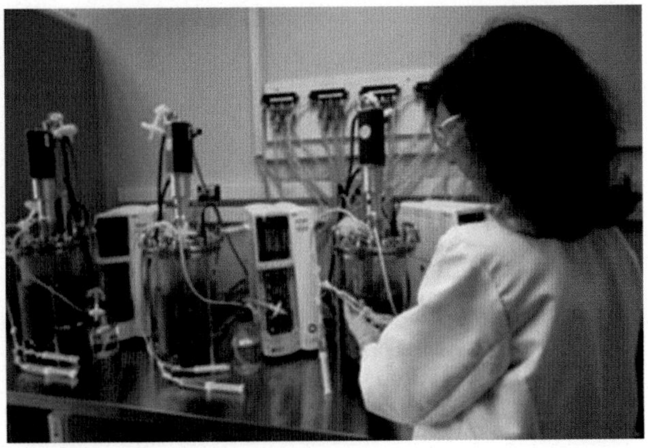

FIGURE 31.11 Manufacturing technical support. *Cytovance Biologics Inc., 2013.*

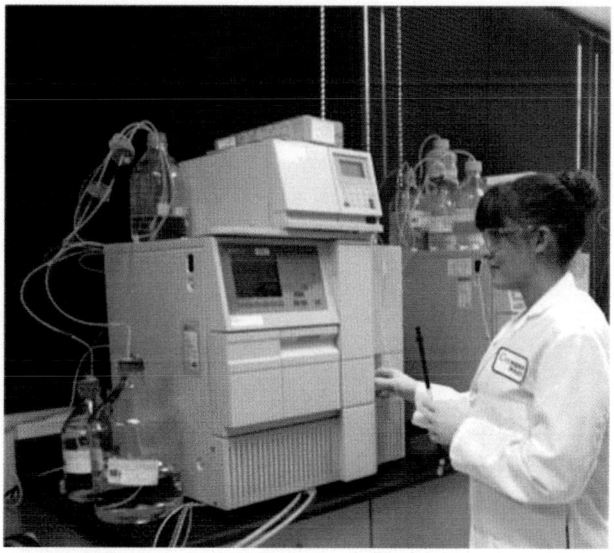

FIGURE 31.12 A quality control laboratory. *Cytovance Biologics Inc., 2013.*

specifications before approving a batch for release. Typically, the quality unit will be the second largest function in the facility behind the manufacturing staff. Specialists on this team will typically have bachelor's degrees in a scientific discipline.

Quality Control

The QC unit is responsible for performing testing on raw materials, in-process and final product testing, and EM activities in a biologics facility. Analysts on this team will typically have bachelor's or master's degrees in chemistry, biology, microbiology, or engineering (see Fig. 31.12).

Facilities and Engineering

The facilities and engineering teams oversee all of the key systems required to keep the manufacturing plant operational. This includes base building systems, process equipment, utilities, building automation, and heating, ventilation, and air-conditioning (HVAC). They also perform routine and nonroutine maintenance activities on the aforementioned systems. These teams are staffed with skilled trade's people, plant and process engineers, and calibration (metrology) professionals (see Fig. 31.13).

Supply Chain

The supply chain function is responsible for the procurement, warehousing, delivery, and management of all materials used in the process. This includes all shipping and receiving activities for raw materials as well as finished products.

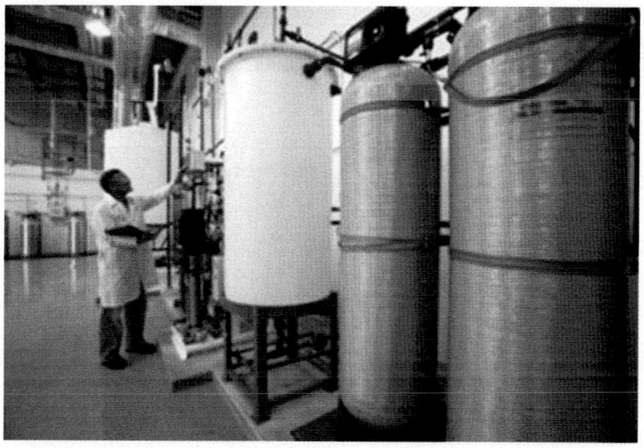

FIGURE 31.13 Facilities and engineering. *Cytovance Biologics Inc., 2013.*

Material Management

Materials utilized in the production of biological manufacturing are required to be controlled through documented systems that ensure adequate controls beginning from vendor selection through receipt, inspection, and release for use.

All raw materials should be acquired from a reputable source that has been audited and approved by QA. The raw materials should be animal-component free. An audit of all product contact materials should be performed and animal-component free statements acquired from the manufacturer. All materials should have manufacturer specifications and certificates-of-acceptance (COAs) when received. Material specifications are required to be established for all materials utilized in the manufacture of the product. These specifications should include COAs, certificates-of-sterility, and requirements for any testing and release of the material. The specifications will be used by manufacturing and the supply chain or purchasing department to acquire the appropriate material for GMP manufacturing. Once the material is ordered, the receiving department will use the purchase order and the material specifications to review the receipt of the material and ensure that it meets all material specifications.

It is important that the quality system that governs material management include controls to determine sampling requirements and quantities required per the vendor lot. These requirements can be found in the US and the EU regulations and guidance documents. Raw material sampling and testing is required for all phases of clinical trials and the expectation is that a robust sampling

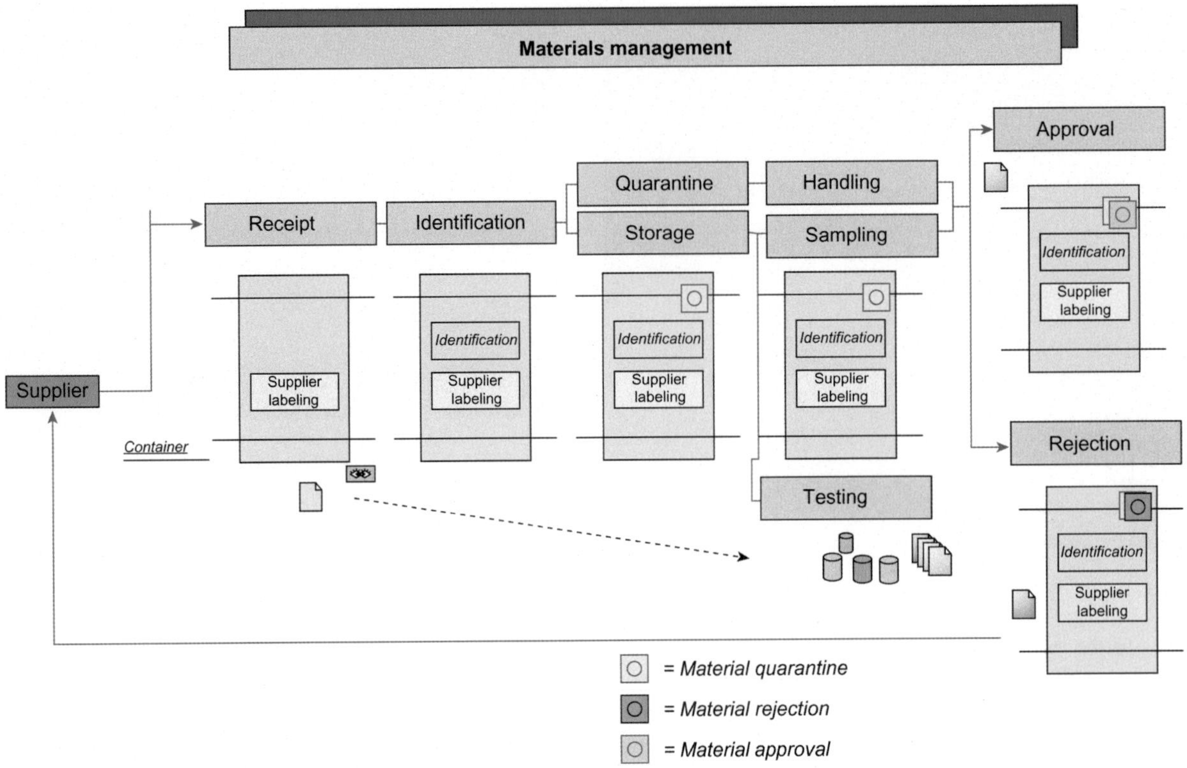

FIGURE 31.14 Materials management flowchart. *http://2.bp.blogspot.com/-HLm1RlaWsN8/UArpSsteZII/AAAAAAAABJk/xLZIA9oulow/s1600/MATERIAL + MANAGEMENT.JPG [accessed March 16, 2019].*

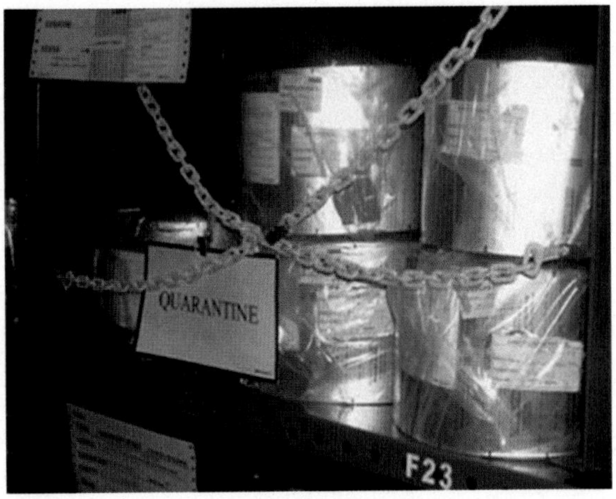

FIGURE 31.15 Materials quarantine. *Essential Medicines and Health Products Information Portal: A World Health Organization resource.*

program be implemented prior to commercialization of the product.

Raw material specifications will spell out the incoming sampling for ID testing and the storage conditions and will require a COA from the vendor. All raw materials should be sampled and tested per the material specifications. The impact of a raw material that is not ID tested or any quality attribute could have a significant impact on the production of the product or its release. Not vetting the raw material ID or quality will impact Phase 2 and 3 clinical trials. Any issues during these late phase trials could have a significant setback to the development of the DP (see Figs. 31.14 and 31.15).

Biologics Drug Substance Manufacturing

An example of a typical biologics manufacturing process is shown in Fig. 31.16.

Upstream Biologics Manufacturing

Cell Banking

Biotechnology requires the creation of a cell that has the capabilities to produce the mAbs or proteins desired for use. These cells are created by transfecting the required genes with a marker into a host cell. Once this transfection has been completed, cells that exhibit the traits of the marker that was introduced are isolated and cloned. These clones are then frozen in small quantities and therefore producing an RCB. RCBs are evaluated for production capabilities and normally one RCB will be selected to move forward with testing and/or production.

Once a specific RCB has been selected, a two-tiered cell banking system is utilized (see Fig. 31.17A and B).

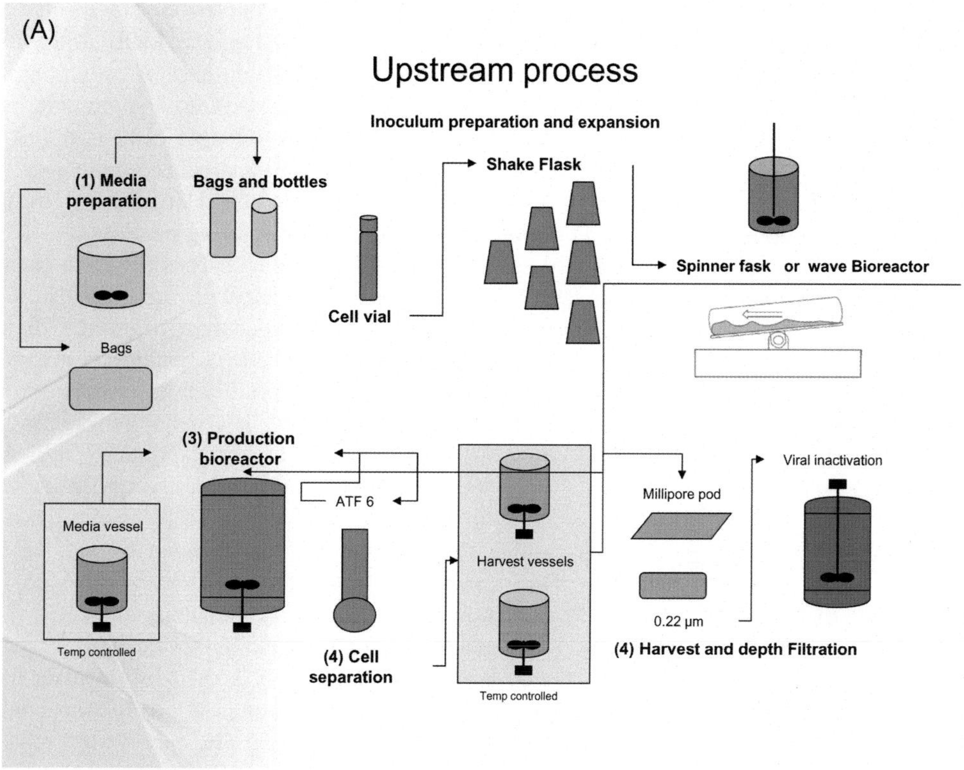

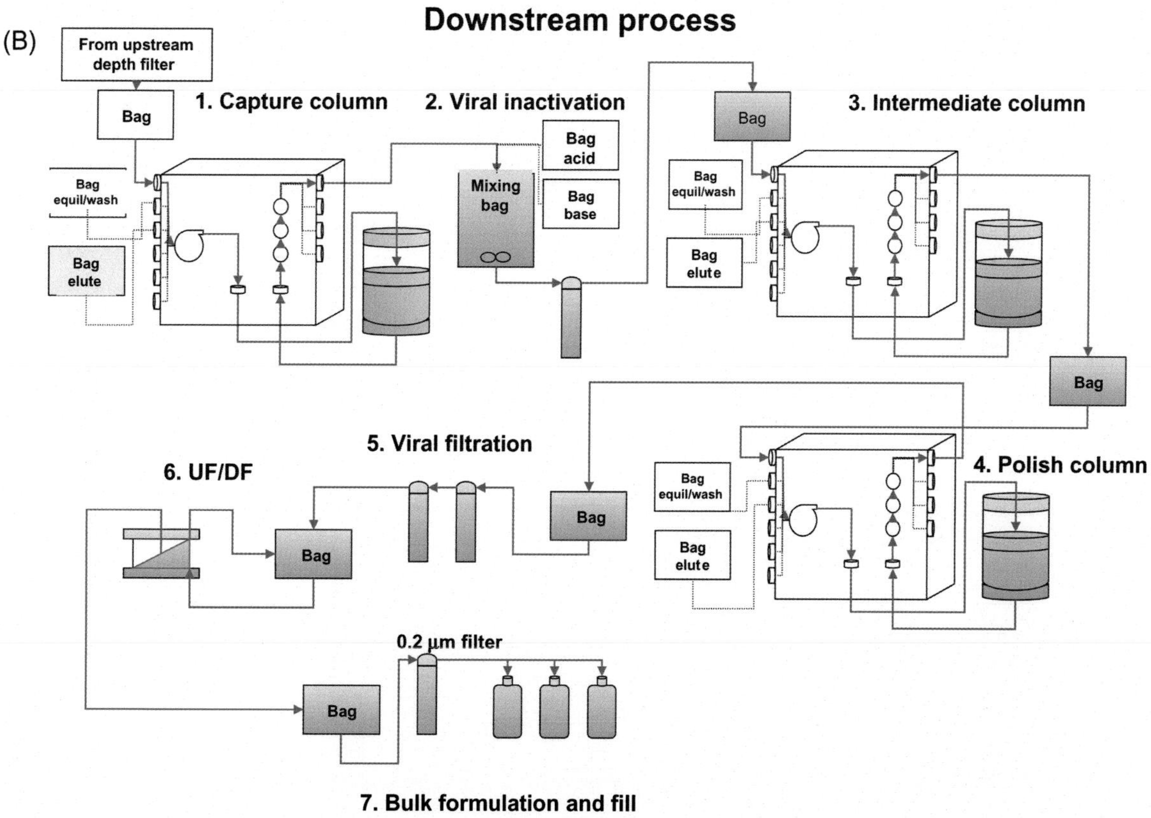

FIGURE 31.16 Biologics manufacturing process: (A) upstream process, (B) downstream processes, and (C) fill finish processes. *Cytovance Biologics Inc., John Conner, 2013.*

The first tier is referred to as a MCB. This cell bank is manufactured from the selected RCB. One vial of the RCB is thawed and expanded until a required number of cells are available for the creation of the cell bank. These cells are then aliquoted into small-volume cryopreservation vessels and frozen using dimethyl sulfoxide (DMSO) (5%–10%) at less than −130°C. These conditions limit the cellular activity which allows for long-term storage. Once produced, the MCB is tested for cell growth, cell viability, characterization, sterility, and various other tests as deemed necessary.

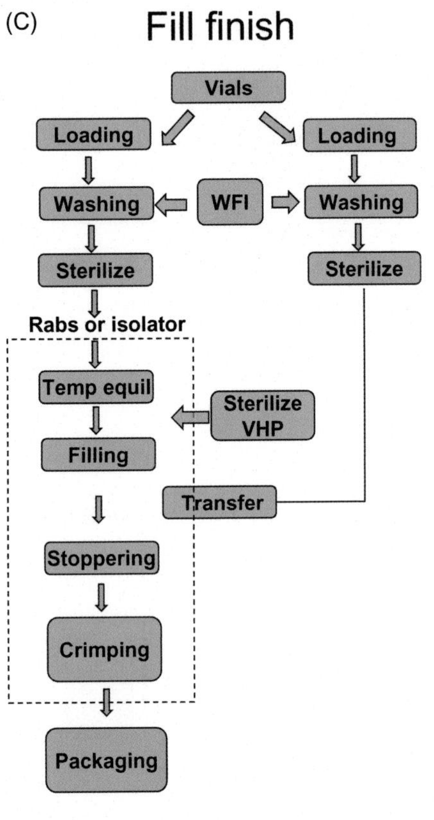

FIGURE 31.16 Continued.

Once the MCB has been tested, the second tier or WCB is initiated. One vial of the MCB is thawed and expanded until the required number of cells is available. These cells are again aliquoted into cryopreservation vessels for storage in DMSO (5%–10%) at less than −130°C. Each WCB that is produced undergoes testing (cell growth, cell viability, characterization, sterility, etc.) before using further manufacturing processes.

Production of the targeted substance (mAb or protein) begins by preparing the inoculum to be used in the production bioreactor. This inoculum begins by thawing a vial of the tested WCB. The WCB culture is suspended in a specialized growth medium within a shake flask. The culture is then maintained in a monitored incubator that controls temperature, CO_2 concentration, and shaking rate. As the initial culture grows, it proceeds through scale-up increasing the volume of the shake flasks. This allows the inoculum volume to increase with each step. The scale-up process might use any number of vessels that allow for increasing the inoculum volume.

Once the inoculum culture has reached a sufficient cell density and volume, it is used to inoculate the production bioreactor. Bioreactors allow for the control of various conditions, including pH, dissolved oxygen (DO), gas flow, and temperature. The controlled conditions allow for the creation of an ideal environment for the cell culture to produce the targeted substance.

Bioreactors

There are two main types of bioreactors: multiple-use (stainless steel) and single-use bioreactors (SUBs) (disposable).

Multiple-use bioreactors are made of stainless steel and currently are the predominant version of bioreactors used in production settings. Multiuse bioreactors generally require a large capital investment for purchase and installation. They also require validated processes for cleaning, and sterilization increases cost and time of maintenance and a skilled staff for operation. For this reason, in

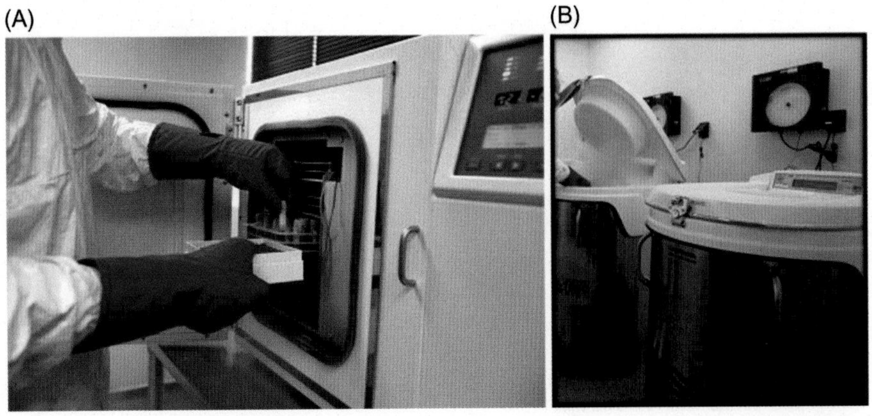

FIGURE 31.17 (A) Manufacturing cell bank production. (B) Cryopreservation and cryostorage. *Cytovance Biologics Inc., 2013.*

smaller volume operations, disposable bioreactors are being used increasingly (see Figs. 31.18 and 31.19).

Disposable bioreactors utilize a disposable sterilized cell chamber in which the cell culture is maintained. This cell chamber minimizes the risks of cross contamination as it is only used for one growth operation. The use of disposable bioreactors decreases the amount of validation, cleaning, sterilization, and maintenance needed per bioreactor run. For this reason, disposable bioreactor runs are able to be scheduled closer together allowing for an increase in plant production.

After the bioreactor has been inoculated, there are three main types of bioreactor processes that are used: batch, continuous, and fed-batch. Batch bioreactor processes consist of filling the bioreactor with medium and inoculum and operating the bioreactor without additions of nutrients or medium until the growth profile is finished. Continuous bioreactor processes continually feed nutrients and medium into the bioreactor while also continually harvesting material from the bioreactor. Since material is continuously being harvested, these processes can result in larger amounts of harvested material and longer bioreactor campaigns. Unfortunately, the longer bioreactor campaigns greatly increase the chance for contamination. Fed-batch bioreactor processes are the most common bioreactor processes used. This process starts with a lower starting volume and feeds nutrients and medium on a set schedule without a contentious removal of harvest material. Once the process has finished, the material is harvested for downstream processing.

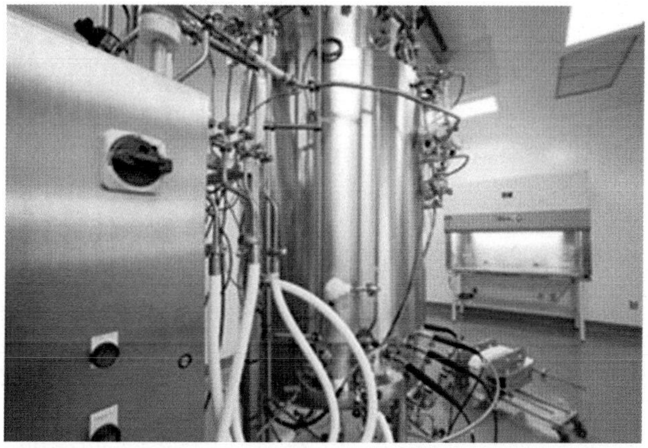

FIGURE 31.18 Mammalian upstream bioreactor operations. *Cytovance Biologics Inc., 2013.*

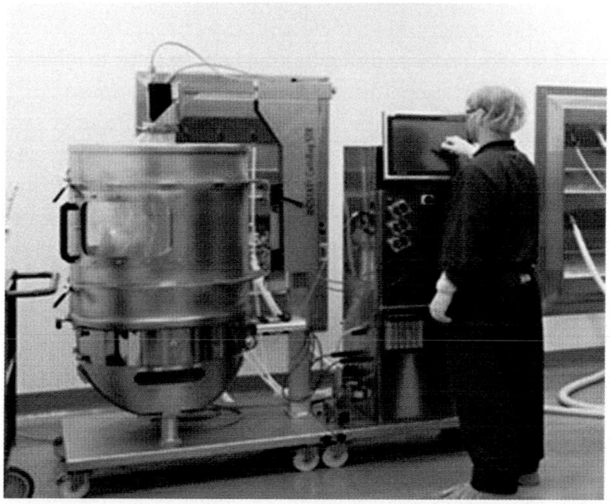

FIGURE 31.19 Mammalian upstream SUB operations. *SUB*, Single-use bioreactor. *Cytovance Biologics Inc., 2013.*

Microbial Upstream Operations

Microbial fermentation involves the growth of a specific microorganism that has been programed to produce a specific protein. An example of a host organism used for this purpose is *Escherichia coli.* The production of the target substance begins with the thawing of the microbial cell bank. This cell bank is resuspended in growth medium and incubated within an incubator/shaker that controls the temperature and agitation rate of the culture. The culture is incubated to allow growth to the proper optical density for inoculation of the production fermenter. The production fermenter is designed to control parameters including DO, pH, temperature, and gas flows. This control allows for an optimized environment to be created for the growth of the microorganism. The fermentation process usually utilizes a fed-batch process which allows for feeding of additional specialized medium and supplements designed to support the growth of the microorganism (Fig. 31.20).

Once the fermentation process is completed (approximately 48 hours), the microorganisms are harvested by centrifugation. This is important as the targeted substances are intracellular (inside the host cell). The centrifugation step allows for the removal of the growth medium. Being as the targeted substance is intracellular, the host cells must be disrupted to allow the extraction of the product. A common practice to accomplish this is the use of a high-pressure homogenizer. Once the targeted substance has been released for the cell, the resulting lysate must be centrifuged. This last centrifugation step results in the separation of the inclusion bodies from the remaining cell debris (a result of the homogenization process). The isolated inclusion bodies may then be frozen and stored before further downstream purification.

Downstream Bioprocessing Operations

Downstream processing, as it applies to biomanufacturing, refers to the separation, purification, and modification

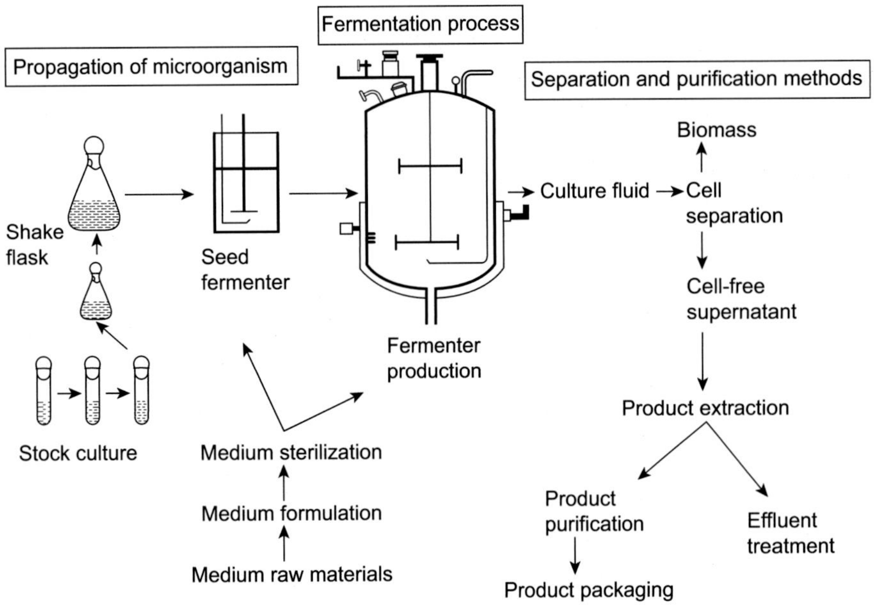

FIGURE 31.20 Microbial fermentation operations. *Intech. <http://www.intechopen.com/books/biomass-now-sustainable-growth-and-use/continuous-agave-juice-fermentation-for-producing-bioethanol> [accessed March 16, 2019].*

of macromolecules from complex biological feedstocks. Most commonly the feedstock is a cell suspension containing billions of "host cells" that synthesized the macromolecule of interest. The ultimate goal of a pharmaceutical downstream processing operation is to prepare a DP for safe and effective delivery into humans or animals. The delivery method is a primary focus of fill/finish operations and can be parenteral, oral, or topical.

Pharmaceutical macromolecules are used in a vast array of applications including the following:

1. cancer therapy,
2. enzyme replacement for enzyme-deficiency syndromes,
3. immune system suppression for autoimmune disorders,
4. elimination of infectious agents,
5. anemia,
6. diabetes, and
7. gene therapy.

Downstream processing has undergone drastic advances in the last 30 years as new strategies have emerged to increase throughput, purity, and process yield. The recent technological advances in downstream processing have driven operating margins upward and have broken down costly barriers to entry into the biologics market. Start-up companies who are mindful of the recent cost-saving and process-optimization technologies in downstream processing are now more able than ever to bring life-saving biologic therapies to market, often tapping into the expertise of contract manufacturers and clinical research firms. Furthermore, regulatory agencies around the globe have established robust guidelines to ensure the new strategies being implemented in downstream processing keep the safety of the patient as a top priority. Due to the close proximity of downstream process operations to the final DP, patient safety considerations are absolutely critical.

Downstream Process Flow

A downstream unit operation, a single step in the downstream process, can be categorized into a mechanical separation, chemical separation, or dual mechanical/chemical separation step. In other words the molecule of interest is separated from the remaining impurities mechanically, by its dimensional (size, shape) characteristics, or, chemically, by its biochemical (electrical charge, interaction with other macromolecules, oiliness) properties. Several downstream processing techniques apply both mechanical and chemical separations simultaneously and can be highly selective for the molecule of interest. Product separation and purification is accomplished through a series of process steps including, but not limited to, filtration, chromatography, precipitation, and centrifugation. As a general rule of thumb, product purity increases and volume decreases through each unit operation of the downstream process (see Fig. 31.21).

In addition to the separation and purification of the target drug molecule, downstream processes modify the drug molecule and its environment. These modifications can be minor or extensive, depending on the ability of the expression system to produce the molecule. Some examples of product modification in downstream processing include the following:

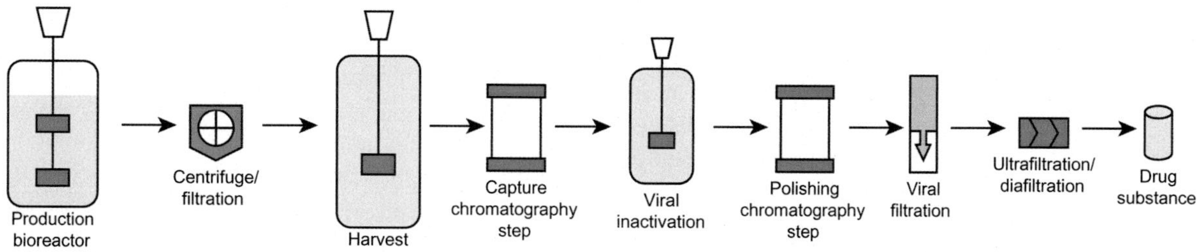

FIGURE 31.21 Typical downstream processing flow of an mAb. The arrows represent the flow of the antibody product between unit operations. Each unit operation mechanically or chemically separates the antibody from host-cell contaminants. *mAb*, Monoclonal antibody. *Figure modified from Ahmed I, Kaspar B, Sharma U. Biosimilars: impact of biologic product life cycle and European experience on the regulatory trajectory in the United States. Clin Ther 2012;34(2):400–19.*

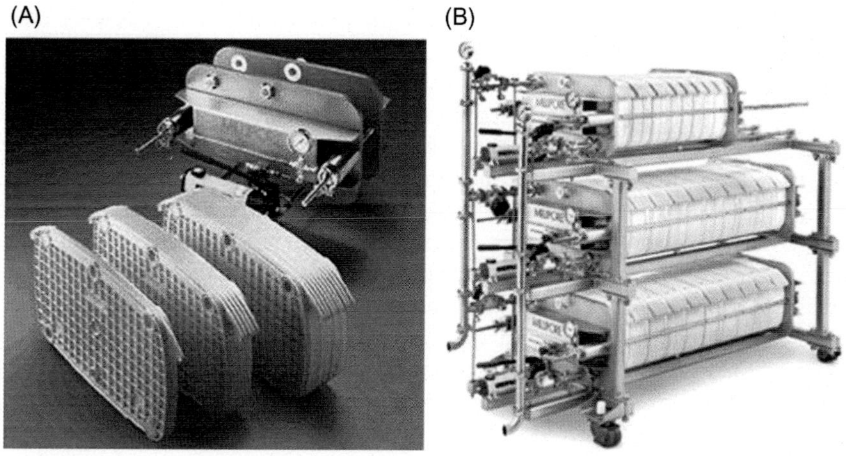

FIGURE 31.22 Typical depth filtration used in cell culture harvest clarification. Example of a small (A) and large (B) production-scale disposable depth filtration system. These units are Millipore Millistak + POD disposable depth filters manufactured by EMD Millipore. *www.millipore.com [accessed March 16, 2019].*

1. complete reconstruction of the product in solution (protein refolding);
2. increasing the concentration of product in solution;
3. attaching synthetic molecules to the product to enhance immune response or product stability;
4. splitting of the product into multiple subunits; and
5. adding excipients (salts, amino acids, detergents, emulsifiers) to enhance product stability.

Harvest and Clarification

Downstream processing begins with the separation of large insoluble contaminants from the feedstock or "harvest" solution, usually whole cells and cell debris. This mechanical separation process is referred to as clarification. For expression systems in which the molecule of interest is secreted out of the cell into the surrounding solution (mammalian cell culture) and a relatively low density of cell debris is present, depth filtration is a common clarification technique. Depth filtration is a 3D filter matrix that serves to remove the bulk of large particulates from the feedstock, analogous to a sand bank at the foot of a river. Water and very small particles pass through the sand while large debris cannot.

The advantage of depth filtration is low equipment cost and seamless transfer from bench scale to production scale. Several varieties of depth filters are readily available with some acting as both mechanical and chemical separators that bind charged contaminants from the host cell, such as DNA and proteins (see Fig. 31.22A and B).

Certain feedstocks with a high density of cell debris (microbial fermentation broth) require a primary clarification with a centrifuge prior to, or in lieu of, depth filtration. In contrast to traditional laboratory centrifuges that require multiple batches to process large volumes, continuous flow centrifuges mechanically separate the product from the feedstock in a single batch, taking advantage of density differences between liquids and solids. The feedstock is split into two or more portions: product stream(s) and a waste stream. The waste stream is discarded and the product stream(s) captured for further downstream processing (see Fig. 31.23).

After the large insoluble particulates have been removed via depth filtration and/or continuous flow centrifugation, the harvest solution is passed through a fine filter that ensures all living cells are removed. This final filtration step ensures that further downstream processing steps are protected from unwanted contaminants and debris.

Chromatography

Chromatography is a general term that refers to the separation of molecules that exist together in a solution. Chromatography is the primary tool used in downstream processing, enabling biologics manufacturers to separate a product molecule from thousands of others in solution. Column chromatography is by far the most common form of chromatography in biomanufacturing, in which a liquid "mobile phase" containing the molecule of interest passes through a solid "stationary phase." Columns are essentially hollow tubes made of glass, plastic, or steel with nets on both ends that contain the stationary phase within the column. A pump system with an array of monitoring device pushes the mobile phase through the column and directs the product stream away from the waste stream. Based on the scale of the operation, columns can vary in size from 1 cm in diameter to 200 cm in diameter and greater. Regardless of size, the principle of column chromatography remains the same (see Fig. 31.24A and B).

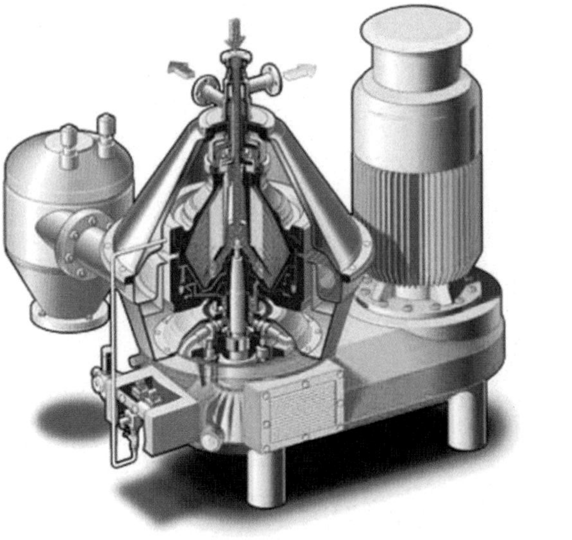

FIGURE 31.23 A typical centrifuge used in downstream operations to separate product from feedstock. A specialized centrifuge from GEA/Westfalia for the separation of a feedstock into low-density liquid, high-density liquid, and solid components. *GEA Westfalia Separator Group. https://www.gea.com/en/productgroups/centrifuges-separation_equipment/index.jsp. Accessed March 16, 2019. Copyright GEA.*

The stationary phase, commonly referred to as chromatography resin or media, contains immobilized chemicals called "ligands" and can operate in different ways depending on the downstream process operation. The ligands can bind to the product molecule, allowing other unwanted molecules to pass through the column and be discarded. This strategy is referred to as "bind-and-elute" chromatography. The exact opposite occurs in "flow through" chromatography, in which the product molecule passes through the column and is captured while impurities bind to the ligands. Lastly, all molecules pass through the column in size-exclusion chromatography, with separation being achieved because molecules travel at different speeds through the column (see Fig. 31.25).

Only a small portion of a chromatography column is actually ligand, with most of the column volume consisting of a polymer that holds the ligands upright and typically does not interact with macromolecules in solution. The polymer backbone is a highly porous spherical bead in column chromatography, or in a 3D matrix in the case of membrane chromatography. In both cases the goal is to maximize the exposure of ligands to the surrounding solution so that chromatographic separation can occur (see Fig. 31.26).

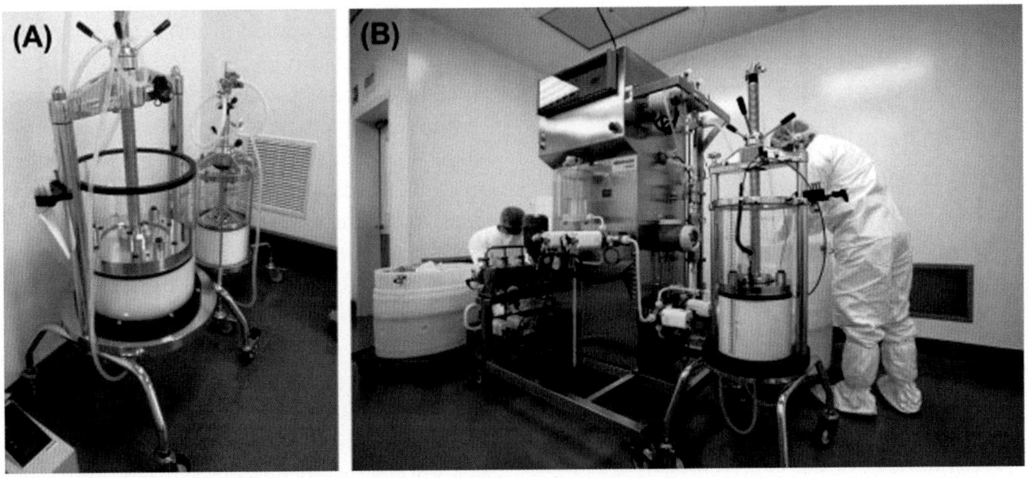

FIGURE 31.24 (A) Typical chromatography columns packed with various chromatography resins. (B) Downstream purification technician using a chromatography skid connected to buffer and chromatography column to purify protein therapeutics. Note the white resin matrix used to separate the macromolecules in solution. *Cytovance Biologics Inc., 2013.*

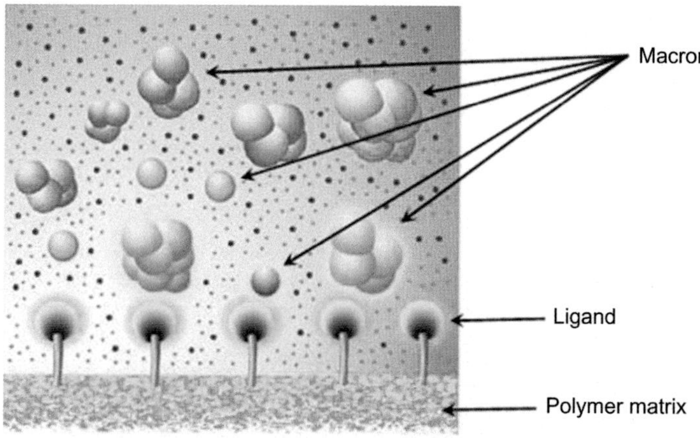

FIGURE 31.25 Chromatography resin in action: highly magnified artist's model of a chromatography resin in action. Blue and green macromolecules do not interact with the ligands, while the orange and red macromolecules are bound to the ligands. *http://microsite.sartorius.com/sartobind-phenyl/hic.html [accessed March 16, 2019].*

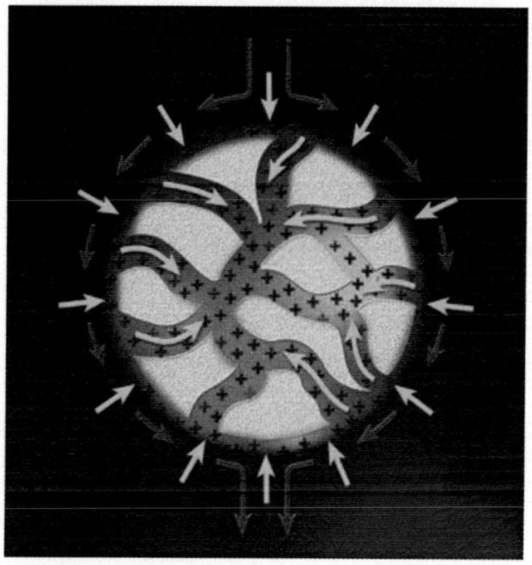

FIGURE 31.26 Positively charged chromatography resin bead. Note the porous nature of the bead, with channels throughout to allow access to the surrounding solution. Light gray arrows represent macromolecules that pass through the interior of the bead, while dark gray arrows represent macromolecules that are excluded from the resin bead. Plus signs (+) represent ligands affixed to the polymer matrix. *Pall Corporation. <www.pall.com> [accessed March 16, 2019].*

Column packing refers to the various strategies used to optimally place chromatography media within a column tube. A delicate balance exists with packing a column with media: chromatography. Media should be installed into a column tube to ensure it remains stationary (hence the "stationary phase") but does not become damaged or compressed to the extent that ligands cannot be accessed by the molecules in solution. A variety of strategies exist to pack columns and the appropriate method should be selected based on the resin's properties and the type of column hardware used in the manufacturing facility. In recent years, automated column packing methods (GE AxiChrom) have been developed to improve the reproducibility and robustness of column chromatography unit operations.

Capture Chromatography

The capture chromatography step is the first chromatography step of a downstream process and is the "workhorse" of the entire process. Imagine a gold prospector on an average day in the field who pans for several hours, ending up with a few small gold flakes at the end of the day. Hundreds of pounds of silt, water, and microscopic gold dust pass through the pan for every visible gold flake. Even the visible gold flakes are compounded with other metal impurities. The gold gathered is not the final product yet, but the prospector is much closer to the end result than he or she was several hours ago. Capture chromatography follows the same principle as gold panning; a relatively small loss of product yields huge dividends with at least a 100-fold increase in purity. Capture chromatography is typically the most efficient downstream process step.

Capture chromatography usually involves the use of an affinity ligand, a molecule that strongly attracts the product's macromolecule. A common affinity ligand is Protein A, a naturally occurring bacterial protein that "locks on" to human antibodies. Protein A–based resins are widely used in biomanufacturing to separate mAb products from mammalian host-cell impurities. For nonantibody products, most chromatography resins can be used as the initial capture step. Fine tuning is often required to capture nonantibody products from a feedstock solution, and precise conditions must exist to bind the macromolecule product and allow others to pass through.

Polishing Chromatography

Polishing chromatography is the general term that refers to additional chromatography unit operations after the capture step. Polishing chromatography further enhances the purity of the target macromolecule to greater than 95%, in preparation for delivery of the drug to the patient. If applied to the gold panning analogy, polishing chromatography is the metallurgist that transforms the dull gold flakes into pure 24K gold bars. Hundreds of resin types for polishing chromatography are available in varying bead sizes, ligand types, and polymer matrices. The vast diversity of biological macromolecules is a reflection of the numerous types of polishing chromatography resins and strategies which contract manufacturers can expect to work with.

Membrane Chromatography

Membrane chromatography is an alternative to traditional column chromatography, as ligands are attached to a 3D matrix rather than a spherical bead. Membrane chromatography exists in most of the same ligand types as traditional resin. The use of membrane chromatography is advantageous for some downstream processes as higher flow rates through the chromatography matrix can be achieved as compared to most traditional resin types, and capital costs are lower without the need for expensive column hardware. However, membrane chromatography can be cumbersome to use at commercial production scales, where the material costs of the membranes can outweigh the capital cost savings of opting out of column chromatography.

A small subset of membrane chromatography systems combines the flow rate advantages of membrane chromatography with the reusability of traditional column chromatography (see Fig. 31.27). BIA separations have developed a membrane chromatography column for the production use. The steel cylinder contains a 3D matrix with bound ligands rather than spherical beads.

Buffer Preparation

While choosing the proper stationary phase is critical to a downstream processing operation, selecting the right mobile phase is equally important. The salt solutions passed through chromatography media that establish the proper mobile phase conditions are called buffers. A great deal of attention is directed at buffer preparation to ensure the chemical components meet rigorous regulatory standards for pharmaceutical use and the buffers are prepared correctly. A buffer that does not meet the requirements for its downstream unit operation can mean the difference between the product macromolecule binding to the resin or being discarded to waste. Advances in disposable technology are particularly applicable to the buffer preparation process. A capital cost to store large volumes of buffer solutions in stainless steel tanks is not feasible for most biomanufacturers, so disposable plastic bags are preferred.

Tangential Flow Filtration

TFF is a technique widely adopted in downstream processing and is similar in principle to dialysis. TFF is used to remove the buffer surrounding the macromolecule product and add another buffer to the product that is more suitable for the next process step. The pores in a tangential flow filter are small enough that the DP does not pass through—it moves parallel to the filter surface. Impurities, salts, and water pass through the filter and are discarded. TFF can be utilized as a preparative step between chromatography steps or to formulate the product of interest with the optimal salts and excipients. The exact formulation delivered by a TFF system varies greatly from product-to-product. Salts, amino acids, sugars, and surfactants are common additives (see Fig. 31.28A and B).

Viral Reduction Techniques

Several mammalian expression systems contain viruses that are intentionally present to manufacture the drug macromolecule. Foreign viruses can also contaminate the cell culture and can be difficult to detect. To protect patients from harmful viral agents, downstream processes have built-in safeguards to eliminate viral contamination, known as "viral clearance."

The primary viral clearance operation in most downstream processes is known as viral filtration. Many types of viral filters are available, they are all highly specialized filters with precise pore sizes that allow the product molecule to pass through but trap viruses. The challenge with viral filtration is some viruses, especially parvoviruses, are incredibly small and similar in size to product

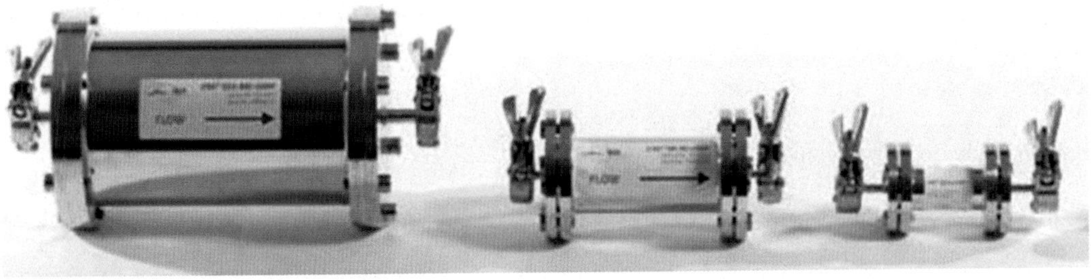

FIGURE 31.27 A membrane chromatography column. The steel cylinder contains a 3D matrix with bound ligands rather than spherical beads. (Family of CIM Monolithic Columns from BIA Separations.) *BIA Separations.* *<http://www.biaseparations.com> [accessed March 16, 2019].*

molecules. The precision to which these filters are made is critical for patient safety. To ensure the filter performs properly, an air test is performed to detect microscopic leaks that could have allowed a virus through.

Viruses are often susceptible to acid and detergents, while many biologic drugs are not as sensitive. Acid treatment is a common tactic for viral reduction in a mAb downstream process, while detergent treatment is sometimes used to reduce viral contamination for enzyme products. Chromatography often doubles as a viral clearance tool. Electrically charged chromatography resins are particularly effective at removing viral contaminants as the ligands attract viruses like a magnet.

Bulk Filtration and Fill

Bulk fill is the final step in the downstream process after the product has been formulated appropriately. A sterile filter is used to ensure any potential contaminants that may have been inadvertently introduced into the product are removed. Downstream processing specialists that perform a bulk fill operation must be highly trained and are monitored for contaminants throughout the process. Once the formulated DP passes through the filter, it is delivered into sterile containers that are stored in highly controlled areas.

Equipment Cleaning

All equipment that has direct contact with products in downstream processing must be vigorously cleaned between uses to remove soilants that remain bound to the equipment surface. The cleaning agents used are either acidic or alkaline, often contain detergents, and can be heated to increase cleaning potency. Applications with difficult-to-clean soilants or applications using large equipment often necessitate automated clean-in-place systems that distribute cleaning solutions to the equipment surfaces. Whether automated clean-in-place or manual cleaning is performed, all cleaning solution residues must be rinsed away with medical-grade water before using the equipment again. Highly sensitive analytical assays, such as the total organic carbon (TOC) assay, are industry standard for the detection of residual soilants and cleaning agents (see Fig. 31.29).

Drug-Product Manufacturing

For biological DPs, having a stability and robust final product formulation buffer is critical to the DP manufacturing process. Developing a DP formulation involves the characterization of a drug's physical, chemical, and biological properties in order to identify those ingredients that can be used in the drug manufacturing process to aid in the processing, storage, and handling of the DP. Evaluating the DS under a variety of stress conditions, such as freeze/thaw, temperature, and shear stress to identify mechanisms of degradation, is extremely important.

Formulation studies should consider such factors as particle size, polymorphism, pH, and solubility that can influence the bioavailability and the activity of a drug. The drug in combination with inactive additives must ensure that the quality of the drug is consistent in each dosage unit throughout the manufacture, storage, and handling to the point of use. It is essential that these initial studies be conducted using drug samples of known purity. The presence of impurities can lead to erroneous conclusions. Stability testing during each stage of drug development is a critical facet to ensuring product quality. Drug stability testing is important during preclinical testing and

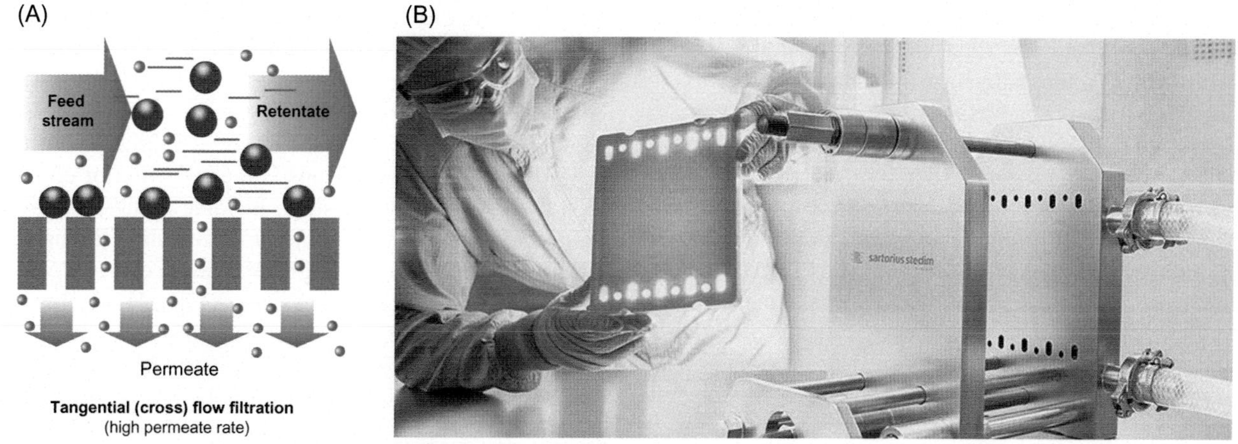

FIGURE 31.28 (A) Tangential flow filtration model. The feed stream containing the product molecule, travels in parallel to the filter surface. Only impurities such as salts and smaller molecules pass through the filter. (B) An example of a production-scale tangential flow filtration system. The stainless steel plates on the right are used to hold the tangential flow filters (held by the technician) in place. *(A) Spectrum Labs. <www.spectrumlabs.com> [accessed March 16, 2019]. (B) Sartorius. <www.sartorius.com> [accessed March 16, 2019].*

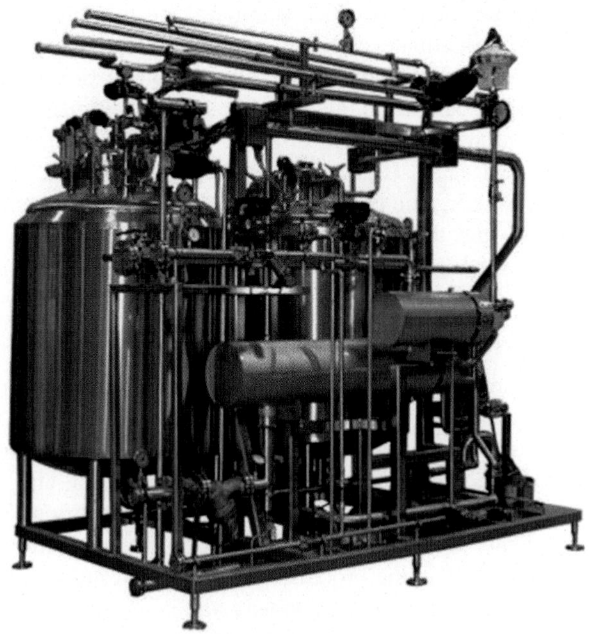

FIGURE 31.29 A typical clean-in-place system used to clean upstream and downstream process equipment. The tanks in the background are used to mix and heat up the cleaning solutions before the delivery of the cleaning solutions to the downstream process equipment through a network of piping. *Turn-Key Modular Systems. <http://www.tkmodular.com/StandardProducts/CIPSystems.aspx> [accessed March 16, 2019].*

clinical trials to establish an accurate assessment of the product being evaluated. Stability data are required at each of the various stages of development to demonstrate and document the product's stability profile. A product's stability must be assessed with regard to its formulation; the influence of its pharmaceutical ingredients; the influence of the container and closure; the manufacturing and processing conditions; packaging components; storage conditions; anticipated conditions of shipping, temperature, light, and humidity; and the anticipated duration and conditions of pharmacy shelf life and patient use. Holding process bulk intermediates or product components for long periods before processing into finished DPs can also affect the stability of both the intermediate component and the finished product. Therefore in-process stability testing, including testing of intermediate components, is essential. The following harmonized guidelines provide an outline of the regulatory requirements for DS and DP stability testing to aid in formulation development:

1. stability testing of new DSs and products;
2. quality of biotechnological products: stability testing of biotechnology/biological;
3. DPs;
4. photostability testing of new DSs and products; and
5. stability testing of new dosage forms.

A drug's kinetic and shelf life stability profile is the extent to which a product remains within specification limits through its period of storage and use while maintaining the same properties and characteristics that it possessed at the time of manufacture. Stability studies should address several key drug stability concerns:

1. active ingredients retain their chemical integrity within the specified limits,
2. drug physical properties are retained,
3. sterility and/or container integrity is maintained,
4. potency/therapeutic effect of the drug remains unchanged, and
5. no increase in toxicity occurs.

DPs should be subjected to long-term stability studies under the conditions of transport and storage expected during product distribution. In conducting these studies the different climate zones to which the product may be subjected must be evaluated for expected variances in conditions of temperature and humidity. A DP may encounter more than a single zone of temperature and humidity variations during its production and shelf life. In general, long-term testing of new drug entities should be conducted at $25°C \pm 2°C$ and at a relative humidity of $60\% \pm 5\%$.

There are many agents and ingredients that can be used to prepare the final formulation buffer of a DS to enhance the stability profile of the drug. These ingredients may be used to achieve the desired physical and chemical characteristics of the product or to enhance the stability of the DS, particularly against hydrolysis and oxidation. In each instance the added agent or ingredient must be compatible with and must not detract from the stability or potency of the DS.

Hydrolysis is the most important cause of drug decomposition primarily because of the number of active agents that are susceptible to the hydrolytic process. Hydrolysis is a process in which drug molecules interact with water molecules to yield breakdown byproducts. There are several approaches to the stabilization of drugs subject to hydrolysis. The most obvious is the reduction or elimination of water from the system. In some liquid DPs, water can be replaced or reduced in the formulation through the use of glycerin, propylene glycol, and alcohol. In certain injectable products, anhydrous vegetable oils may be used as the drug's solvent to reduce the chance of hydrolytic decomposition. Decomposition by hydrolysis may also be prevented in other liquid drug formulations by suspending them in a nonaqueous vehicle. For certain unstable active agents, when an aqueous preparation is desired, the drug may be supplied in a dry form for reconstitution by adding a specified volume of PW just before dispensing to a patient. Refrigeration is generally required for most drugs subject to hydrolysis. In addition to temperature, pH is also a factor that affects the stability of a drug prone to hydrolytic decomposition. Drug stability can frequently be improved through the use of buffering agents between pH 5 and 6.

Oxidation is another destructive process that produces instability in DPs. Oxidation is the loss of electrons from an atom or a molecule. Each electron lost is accepted by some other molecule, reducing the recipient. Oxidation frequently involves free chemical radicals, which are molecules containing one or more unpaired electrons, such as oxygen and free hydroxyl. These radicals tend to take electrons from other chemicals, thereby oxidizing the donor. Oxidation of a DS is most likely to occur when it is not kept dry in the presence of oxygen, when it is exposed to light, or combined with other chemical agents. Oxidation of a chemical in a DS is usually accompanied by an alteration in the color of that drug and may also result in precipitation or a change in odor. The oxidative process can be controlled with the use of antioxidants that react with one or more compounds in the drug to prevent the oxidation progress. Antioxidants act by providing electrons and hydrogen atoms that are accepted more readily by the free radicals rather than those present in the drug. Among those most frequently used in aqueous preparations are sodium sulfite, sodium bisulfite, sodium metabisulfite, hypophosphorous acid, and ascorbic acid. The FDA labeling regulations require a warning about possible allergic-type reactions, including anaphylaxis, in the package insert for prescription drugs that contain sulfites in the final dosage form.

Because oxygen can adversely affect their stability, certain drugs require an oxygen-free atmosphere during processing and storage. Oxygen is present in the airspace within the storage container or may be dissolved in the liquid vehicle. Oxygen-sensitive drugs must be prepared in the dry state and packaged in sealed containers with the air replaced by an inert gas, such as nitrogen. Light can also act as a catalyst to oxidation reactions by transferring energy to drug molecules making them more reactive. As a precaution against light-induced oxidation, sensitive drugs must be packaged in light-resistant or opaque containers. Because most drug degradations proceed more rapidly as the temperature increases, it is also advisable to store oxidizable drugs under refrigerated temperatures. Another factor that can affect the stability of an oxidizable drug in solution is the pH of the formulation buffer. Each drug must be maintained in solution at the pH most favorable to its stability. This varies from preparation-to-preparation and must be determined on an individual basis for the drug.

Formulated DSs and DPs are stored in container closure systems for extended periods of time. For biological drugs, container closures typically include plastic bags/containers, bottles, vials, and syringes. The containers are typically made from glass or plastic. It is important to determine that there no interactions between the drug and the container. When a plastic container is used, tests should be conducted to determine if any of the ingredients become adsorbed by the plastic or whether any plasticizers, lubricants, pigments, or stabilizers leach out of the plastic into the drug. The adhesives for the container label need to be tested to ensure they do not leach through the plastic container into the drug. Trace metals originating from the chemical in the drug, solvent, container, or stopper may also be a source of concern in preparing stable solutions of oxidizable drugs.

Freezing and thawing of bulk protein solutions are common practices in bulk intermediate, DS, and drug-product manufacturing. Freezing-induced aggregation and denaturation caused by cryopreservation or a pH shift due to crystallization of buffer components can lead to a significant loss in the biological activity of the drug. Formulation development and analysis of the impact of freezing on proteins are a significant part of optimizing biological drug storage systems involving cryoprotectants, stabilizing excipients, freezing process parameters, and cryocontainers. Cryoprotectants function by lowering the glass transition temperature of a solution. The cryoprotectant prevents freezing, and the solution maintains some flexibility during the freezing process. Some cryoprotectants also function by forming hydrogen bonds with biological molecules displacing water molecules. Hydrogen bonding in aqueous solutions is important for proper protein and DNA function. As the cryoprotectant replaces the water molecules, the biological material retains its native physiological structure and function. Conventional cryoprotectants, such as glycerol and DMSO, have been used to reduce ice formation in biological material stored in liquid nitrogen. For some biological material, mixtures of cryoprotectants have less toxicity and are more effective than single-agent cryoprotectants. Cryoprotectant mixtures have also been used for vitrification (solidification without crystal ice formation). Vitrification has important applications in preserving embryos, biological tissues, and organs for transplantation.

Similar to cryoprotectants, lyoprotectants are molecules that protect material during lyophilization. Lyoprotectants are typically polyhydroxy compounds, such as sugars (mono-, di-, and polysaccharides), polyalcohols, and their derivatives. Lyophilization is frequently used for biological drugs to increase the shelf life of products, such as vaccines and other injectables that are subject to hydrolysis degradation. By removing the water from the material and sealing the material in a vial, the material can be easily stored, shipped, and later reconstituted to its original form for injection. The development of freeze-dried formulations involves selecting a suitable lyoprotectant that stabilizes the drug within a defined amorphous matrix and control key drug process parameters: freeze concentration, solution-phase concentration, product appearance, minimizing reactive products, increasing the surface area, and decreasing vapor pressure of solvents. During the lyophilization process, the freezing phases are the most critical. Amorphous materials do not have a eutectic point but instead have a critical temperature typically between −50°C and −80°C, below which the product must be maintained to prevent melt back or the collapse of the biological material during the lyophilization primary and secondary drying steps.

During the primary freeze–drying phase, the pressure is lowered to the range of a few millibars and the temperature controlled based on the molecule's latent heat of sublimation. It is important to cool the material below its triple point, the lowest temperature at which the solid and liquid phases of the material can coexist. During this initial drying phase, approximately 95% of the water in the form of ice is removed from the product by sublimation. This phase is typically a slow process to avoid altering the molecular structure of the biological material. During this phase, pressure is controlled through the application of partial vacuum. The vacuum speeds up the sublimation during the drying process.

The secondary drying phase removes the remaining unfrozen water molecules from the primary phase. This part of the freeze–drying process is governed by the material's adsorption isotherms. In this phase the temperature is raised higher than in the primary drying phase and can even be above 0°C to break any physicochemical interactions that have formed between the water molecules and the frozen material. Usually, the pressure is also lowered in this stage, typically in the range of microbars or fractions of a Pascal, to encourage desorption. After the freeze–drying process is complete, the vacuum is broken with an inert gas, such as nitrogen, before the container is sealed. At the end of the lyophilization process the final residual water content in the DP is typically around 1%–4%.

The lyophilization process includes the transfer of aseptically filled product in partially sealed containers. To prevent contamination of a partially closed sterile product, an aseptic process must be designed to minimize the exposure of sterile articles to the potential contamination hazards of the manufacturing operation. Limiting the duration of exposure of sterile product components, providing the highest possible environmental control, optimizing process flow, and designing equipment to prevent the introduction of lower quality air into the Class 100 (ISO 5) clean area are essential to achieving a high assurance of final product sterility. In an aseptic process the DP, container, and closure are first subjected to separate sterilization methods before being assembled. Because there is not a terminal sterilization process for biological DPs, it is critical that containers be filled and sealed in an extremely high-quality environment. Before the aseptic assembly of a final product, the individual parts of the final DP are sterilized by separate processes: glass containers by dry heat, rubber closures by moist heat, and liquid dosage forms are subjected to filtration. Each of these manufacturing processes requires validation and control to eliminate the risk of product contamination. Both personnel and material flow must also be optimized to prevent unnecessary activities that could increase the potential for introducing contaminants to the exposed product, container closures, or the surrounding environment. The number of personnel in an aseptic processing room should be minimized. The flow of personnel should be designed to limit the frequency of entries and exits into and from an aseptic processing room. The number of transfers into the critical area of a cleanroom, or an isolator, must be minimized, and movement adjacent to the critical area should be restricted. Any intervention or stoppage during an aseptic process can increase the risk of contamination. The design of equipment used in aseptic processing should limit the number and complexity of aseptic interventions by personnel. Personnel interventions should be reduced by integrating an online weight check device that eliminates a repetitive manual activity within the critical area, sterilizing preassembled connections using sterilize-in-place technology eliminating significant aseptic manipulations, and the use of automation technologies, such as robotics, to further reduce contamination risks to the product (see Fig. 31.30A and B).

Product transfers should occur under appropriate cleanroom conditions. Carefully designed curtains, rigid plastic shields, and the use of isolator systems can be used to achieve segregation of the aseptic processing line. If stoppered, vials exit an aseptic processing zone prior to capping, appropriate controls should be in place to safeguard the product until completion of the crimping step. Use of online detection devices to identify improperly seated stoppers provides additional sterility assurance. Aseptic processing operations must be validated using microbiological growth media fill process simulations. Media fill process simulations should incorporate risk factors that occur during normal product manufacturing, such as exposure to product contact surfaces of equipment, container closure systems, critical environments, and process manipulations. Media fills should closely simulate aseptic manufacturing operations incorporating worst case activities and conditions that may occur during aseptic operations.

Manufacturing Support Functions

Quality Assurance

GMPs require that all persons involved in manufacturing be responsible for quality and that the manufacturers

(A)

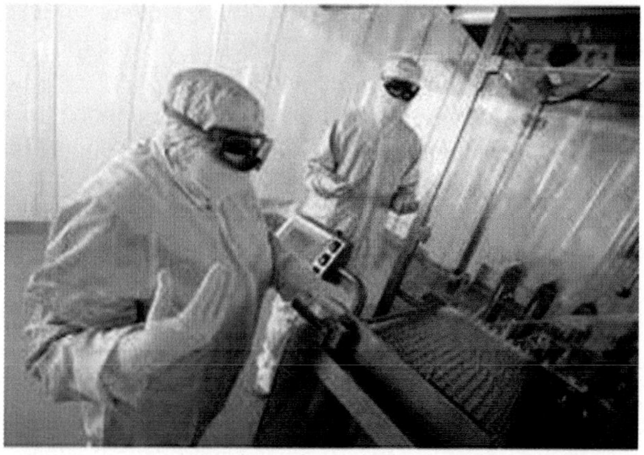

(B)

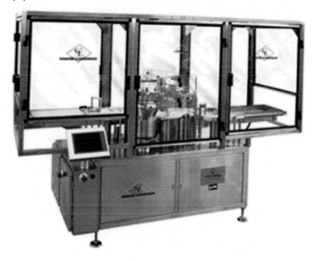

FIGURE 31.30 (A) Drug-product manufacturing: formulation and final container fill finish. An example of a typical glass vial filling operations. (B) Cytovance biologics Chase Logeman Vial Fill Finish System. *(A) Google Images and (B) Cytovance Biologics Inc., 2013.*

implement an effective system for managing quality. This system should require that the quality unit be independent of the manufacturing unit and that the quality unit be involved in all quality-related matters.

Most manufacturers establish the quality unit by developing subteams that support the various manufacturing functions.

Incoming Quality Control/Quality Assurance

This group performs functions related to assessment, testing, and disposition of materials that are designated to be utilized in the manufacture of intermediates and final products. They ensure that proper storage, labeling, and segregation of materials are maintained and also document disposition of incoming material.

Operations Quality Assurance

This group performs functions throughout the actual manufacture of intermediates and final product. They are the independent "eyes" on the floor that provides quality oversight to the manufacturing activities. Their specific activities include but are not limited to verification of critical process steps, line releases, the audit of production areas and perform in-process inspections.

Document Control

This group performs functions related to the control of all quality records. They ensure that revision history is maintained for documents, that processes for the distribution and reconciliation are maintained, and that change notifications are processed and maintained. Some of the types of quality records that are maintained are as follows:

1. *Standard operating procedures (SOPs)*—Contain written instructions on how to perform manufacturing processes and support functions.
2. *Batch records*—Provide a record of actual executed manufacturing steps.
3. *Material specs*—Contain requirements for materials utilized in the manufacture of intermediates and final products.
4. *Training documents*—Provide objective evidence of personnel qualifications and completed training on required processes that are part of or support the manufacture of intermediates and final products.

Quality Assurance for Batch Disposition

This group performs an independent review of product batch records, associated investigations, and test results to verify that all production and testing requirements have been met and/or resolved before determining the final disposition. This group has the authority to determine whether a product will be accepted or rejected.

Quality Compliance

This group provides an oversight of the entire quality system and manufacturing functions. They ensure that internal and external audits are conducted, establish and implement systems that govern quality system monitoring, and are the hosts to inspections and audits from regulatory agencies, customers, and clients.

Qualification/Validation

GMPs require that manufacturers establish systems to ensure that their facilities, equipment, processes, test methods, and automated systems are adequate for the support of intermediate and final product manufacture. This system requires that critical product and process attributes be identified and measures implemented to control, test, and monitor these attributes. These systems require that documented qualifications and validations be executed and documented in order to provide evidence of suitability. These systems are driven and overseen by personnel not involved in the manufacture of the product and are made up of personnel with engineering, facility, and quality backgrounds. These personnel perform multiple yet segregated roles in writing, executing, reviewing, and approving the documents that are utilized in qualifications and validations.

Facility and Equipment

When new facilities are built or reconfigured, building utilities (water, electrical, and HVAC) must be qualified to ensure that the facility can meet the requirements of the manufacturing process.

Process

As manufacturing processes are defined and critical parameters that include ranges and boundaries are established, objective evidence through validation protocols must be executed to ensure that the manufacturing process is robust and controlled at a level that can repeatedly produce the same product that meets the same specifications.

Analytical Methods

During the manufacture of intermediates and products, the verification of critical steps can be determined through sample testing. The test utilized must be qualified or validated. The qualification and/or validation of test methods ensure that the defined method can detect the required component or product ingredient. Depending on the test material, standard pharmacopoeia methods can be implemented or new methods can be developed. These methods must meet the requirements of analytical method validation and show specificity, accuracy, precision, detection limits, quantitation limits, linearity, range, and robustness.

Quality Control

Analytical Methods

Suitable analytical test methods are extremely critical components for establishing identity, quality, purity, and strength/potency of a DP. The cGMP regulations [21 CFR 211.194 (a)] require that test methods used for assessing compliance of pharmaceutical products with established specifications must meet proper standards of accuracy and reliability. All test methods are established as SOP in the QC laboratory. While it is not necessary to have analytical methods being qualified for testing PD demonstration run materials or scale-up engineering run material, all test methods need to be at least qualified for any GMP lot material during early stages of the drug development and manufacturing program. The need and scope of analytical method qualification/validation should be defined under the master validation plan for the organization. This should be established in the form of an approved SOP.

It is necessary to perform qualification/validation of the test methods according to the ICH Tripartite Guideline "Validation of Analytical Procedures: Text and Methodology, Q2 (R1)." Based on the ICH guideline, certain key parameters from the full assay validation program are addressed during the assay qualification. The analytical methods qualification/validation package should include (1) SOP, (2) assay qualification/validation protocol, (3) assay qualification/validation report, and (4) relevant analytical data. Method qualification and validation can be performed in a QC laboratory and/or analytical science laboratory (under R&D unit) of the organization. However, the release tests for the GMP manufactured products must be performed in the QC laboratory. Analytical method qualification/validation needs to be performed with qualified and calibrated instruments/equipment including the material storage units. While noncompendial test methods need to be qualified/validated based on ICH guidelines, according to the regulations [21 CFR 211.194 (a) (2)] all compendial methods as described in the United States Pharmacopeia and the National Formulary are not required to validate the accuracy and reliability of these methods. These methods merely need to be verified for their suitability under actual conditions of use.

Quality Control Laboratory

The QC laboratory is set up to support the manufacturing department for the production of DSs and DPs. As defined in 21 CFR Part 211.22 the responsibility and authority of the QC unit include testing and approval (or rejection) of all components, DP containers, closures, in-process materials, packaging material, labeling, and DPs. According to the regulations, a QC unit also has the responsibility for approving or rejecting all procedures or specifications impacting on the identity, strength, quality, and purity of the DP. It also requires that the responsibilities and procedures applicable to the QC unit shall be in writing and such written procedures shall be followed.

A Description of In-Process and Release Tests Performed in a Quality Control Laboratory for the Product Manufactory Process

The scope of this section is to provide a list of tests generally performed for protein-based drug manufacturing platforms. For nonprotein-based (biologics) drug development program testing, requirements can be different which are highly dependent on the nature and characteristics of the product. The production process of protein drugs (e.g., antibody and other proteins) is a two-stage process. The first stage is a growth and production phase which begins with different protein expression platforms, such as a mammalian expression system (e.g., Chinese hamster ovary cell lines) or a microbial expression system (e.g., *E. coli*). The second stage is a downstream purification and formulation process. In general the required in-process tests while manufacturing a product is defined by the product development phase of the project. All the specifications are developed and established during the process validation in order to define various process control steps. This activity is in turn guided by the PD activities of product development. Release tests for a DS and DP are established based on the DS and DP in question in addition to certain regulatory guidelines, and the tests should demonstrate/establish identity, strength/potency, quality, and purity of a DP. Several of the release test methods also serve as stability-indicating test methods during the required stability study program for DS and DP.

Microbiology

In-Process Tests

For unprocessed bulk harvest common in-process tests are as follows (see Fig. 31.31):

- bioburden,
- mycoplasma detection with mycoplasmastasis,
- in vitro assay for nonendogenous or adventitious viruses,
- detection of mouse minute virus DNA by quantitative polymerase chain reaction, and

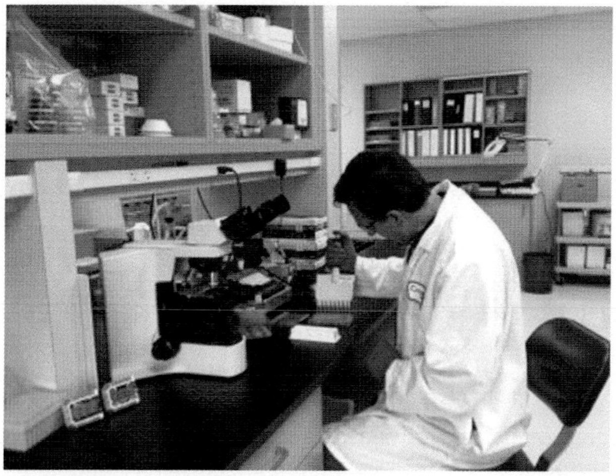

FIGURE 31.31 Quality control microbiology. *Cytovance Biologics Inc., 2013.*

- transmission electron microscopy of supernatant.

Endotoxin testing is performed on the clarified bulk harvest.

Release Tests for Drug Substance

- Bioburden
- Endotoxin

Chemistry

In-Process Tests

- pH.
- Conductivity.
- Protein content by UV A280.
- Titer analysis [e.g., protein A-HPLC (high-performance liquid chromatography) for antibody, or enzyme-linked immunosorbent assay–based test method for other protein products].
- Sometimes, size-exclusion HPLC, reverse-phase HPLC, and sodium dodecyl sulfate polyacrylamide gel electrophoresis (reduced/nonreduced) methods are also used as in-process tests to monitor the efficiency of purification steps, state of aggregation of the product, and stepwise improvement in the product quality. Occasionally, suitable potency or activity assay is also performed as an in-process test to monitor product quality as one moves through the manufacturing process (see Fig. 31.32 and Table 31.3).

Environmental Tests

For a compliant biomanufacturing facility, it is essential to develop a contamination control program. This program needs to address three basic tasks:

1. control (minimization) of bioburden throughout the process of product manufacturing;

FIGURE 31.32 Quality control analytics. *Cytovance Biologics Inc., 2013.*

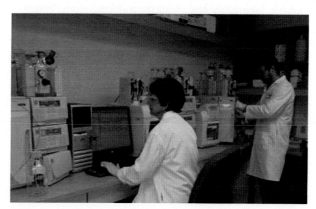

TABLE 31.3 Quality control release tests for drug substance.

Attribute	Drug substance	Drug product
Safety	Endotoxin	Endotoxin
Safety	Bioburden	Sterility
Impurities	HCP	N/A
Impurities	Residual DNA	N/A
Impurities	Tween 20 or Tween 80 or Triton X 100 or any other excipient (if added during formulation)	N/A
Impurities	Residual Protein A (if Protein A was used during purification process, e.g., for antibody product)	N/A
Quality	pH	pH
Quality	Osmolality	Osmolality
Quality	Appearance (color, visible particulate matter)	Appearance (color, visible particulate matter)
Quality	N/A	Subvisible particulate matter (10 and 25 μm) (2, 5, and 8 μm for information only)
Quality	N/A	Volume in container
Quality	N/A	Container closure integrity
Strength/Content	Protein concentration by A280 (or any other assay such as Bradford, BCA)	Protein concentration by A280 (or any other assay such as Bradford, BCA)
Purity	SE-HPLC	
Purity	SDS-PAGE (reduced and nonreduced), CE-SDS	SDS-PAGE (reduced and nonreduced), CE-SDS
Purity	RP-HPLC	RP-HPLC
Identity and charge heterogeneity	IEF, cIEF	IEF, cIEF
Identity and charge heterogeneity	CEX, CZE	CEX, CZE
Identity	Peptide map	Peptide map
Potency	Binding ELISA	Binding ELISA
Potency	Bioassay	Bioassay

ELISA, Enzyme-linked immunosorbent assay; *HCP*, host-cell protein; *RP-HPLC*, reverse-phase-HPLC; *SDS-PAGE*, sodium dodecyl sulfate polyacrylamide gel electrophoresis; *SE-HPLC*, size-exclusion-HPLC.
Source: Cytovance Biologics Inc., 2013.

2. control (minimization) of cross-over contamination of residuals from batch-to-batch production; and
3. control (minimization) of cross-over contamination of residuals from cleaning materials during the production period.

In order to achieve these goals it is critical to establish suitable laboratory test methods and operational practices. Appropriate gowning procedures, personnel monitoring, EM, air quality monitoring with settling plates, facility surface cleaning and disinfection monitoring, and PW monitoring (by TOC analysis) are key programs that need to be established in the form of SOPs and implemented for a compliant biomanufacturing facility which is engaged in the production of quality DPs (see Fig. 31.33A and B).

Contract (Contract Manufacturing Organization) Versus In-House Manufacturing

Traditionally in the pharmaceutical industry the paradigm was to build small molecule manufacturing facilities that could manufacture large quantities of product reproducibly. These plants had enormous amounts of stainless steel and required a large facility footprint as well as a large workforce. With the discovery of therapeutic biologics or (large molecules), biopharmaceutical and biomanufacturing facilities were both newly constructed and others were converted into biomanufacturing facilities. These early in-house facilities were expensive to construct and at times retrofits were not right for the technology or difficult to scale and reproduce. Thus many companies outsourced development and manufacturing of their biologic products to contract development organizations or CMOs or contract development and manufacturing organizations. Most CMO facilities were designed to have a scaled process to support preclinical through Phases 1, 2, and 3 and some that could support the commercial launch of complex biologic products.

Academic facilities, small biotech companies, medium seasoned biotech companies, large biopharmaceutical companies, and virtual companies have varying abilities to financially support and build a facility for multiple biologic platforms in-house. Most CMOs have already built manufacturing capabilities to produce and purify biologic drugs at a certain scale to accommodate their scale or

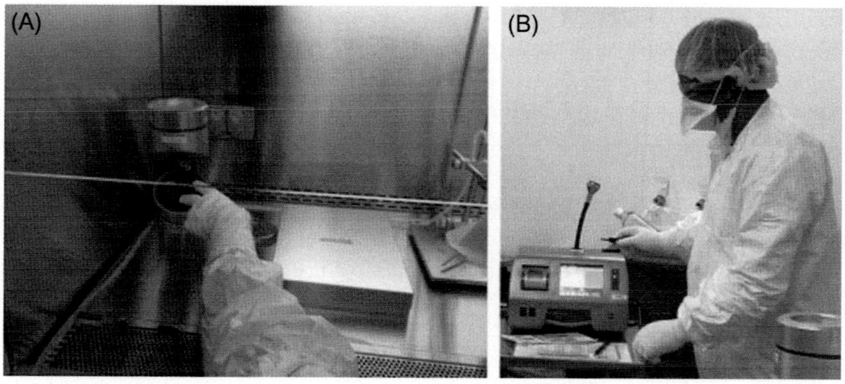

FIGURE 31.33 (A) EM technician setting up test equipment to monitor viable air particles (microbials) during processing. (B) The EM technician setting up a particle counter to monitor particles in the air of the production suite. Quality control environmental microbiology/environmental monitoring. *EM*, Environmental monitoring. *Cytovance Biologics Inc., 2013.*

"niche" market. These capabilities are large capital expenditures, such as stainless steel bioreactors, fermentors, mixing tanks, water systems, chromatography skids, chromatography columns, clean rooms, QC labs, EM Labs, PD labs, and quality systems. The advantage of a CMO facility is that it is ready for manufacturing the developed product. Although today there are a variety of disposable options in the small-scale manufacture of biologics which would allow a small company to consider biomanufacturing in-house, there are SUBs that range from a 25-L to a 2000-L scale as well as single-use mixing units (SUMs) in the same scale. Some biotech companies are using disposables to perform small-scale studies to support some preclinical or pilot-scale work and then transfer the process and further scale-up to a CMO. This allows the biotech company more control and hands on during early-PD.

A major disadvantage for the in-house model is the capital outlay for an in-house facility. In terms of time and equipment, an in-house facility would be very costly in respect to supporting in-house expertise to manage the design, fabrication, installation and qualification of the facility, process, and support equipment. There are other considerations, such as cleaning and maintenance of all product contact surfaces, such as bioreactors and mixing tanks. These require studies and validation of the cleaning processes. Samples would have to be taken and tested creating additional in-house expertise, time, and resources and this would be contingent on suite availability to develop and manufacture the product, whereas outsourcing these activities to a CMO would shorten the timeline significantly because the CMO would already have the expertise, process, and facility equipment in place to support the development and manufacturing activities. Other aspects that need to be considered are the support for biomanufacturing with QA and QC groups that are necessary for the GMP documentation, in-process testing, and release testing. The chemistry, manufacturing, and control section of a company's IND could be completed by the CMO and would be support for the biotech company as one of the CMO's regulatory offerings.

The availability of reliable and functional disposable equipment at small scales, such as SUBs and SUMs, mentioned previously might be reasonable for some small companies that may have a modular (factory-built panels delivered and assembled on-site with a factory-impervious finish) or stick-built (on-site piece-by-piece construction, such as framing, sheet rock, and epoxy-type finishes) facility with proper cleaning and HVAC (that can deliver a classified or controlled environment) to bring in a SUB or SUM. The disposables or single-use equipment offers quick installation, flexibility, and no cleaning validation as compared to its stainless steel bioreactor, buffer tanks, and mixer predecessors. However, a company would still have to invest in clean rooms and infrastructure to support biologic GMP production. At the end of the day it would be more cost and timeline effective to enlist a CMO to carry the "heavy lifting" of the drug development process. As a result, many biotechnology and biopharmaceutical companies are more commonly outsourcing some or all of their biomanufacturing needs. Outsourcing allows a company to remain focused on the crucial components in-house while taking advantage of a CMO to supply their resources for PD, AD, manufacturing, quality, and regulatory support. Utilizing a CMO for outsourcing can help reduce or eliminate the need to build, manage, and maintain a facility, or it allows a company time to grow until it can justify a permanent facility.

Summary

The incredible amount of recent biologic therapeutic discoveries has led to an increased need for scientific and engineering knowledge available to characterize and biomanufacture these large and complex molecules. In this chapter, we have followed what role biomanufacturing has in the development of a biotherapeutic product. We have followed the biologic product's development from "proof-of-concept," examined the history of these large molecules, and developed a knowledge-base that we would use in developing a scaled process that would be tech-transferred into manufacturing. Within this chapter, we also discussed key partners in the biomanufacturing process, such as raw material suppliers, outsource testing vendors, and key support teams, such as facilities, engineering, PD, QA, QC, EM, manufacturing, and MST teams required to fully develop and manufacture a biologic that can meet all of the critical safety, quality, and regulatory parameters.

It is essential that the biomanufacturing process be able to deliver and demonstrate a safe therapeutic drug at each step of the clinical trial, be economically able to reproducibly manufacture sufficient inventory with a stable shelf life, and to successfully traverse the regulatory and efficacy hurdles in order to obtain regulatory approval. In biomanufacturing "the process is the product" is an old paradigm, but it is still relevant in the development and manufacture of a biotherapeutic.

Chapter 32

Biotechnology Products and Their Customers: Developing a Successful Market Strategy

Craig Shimasaki, PhD, MBA
CEO, BioSource Consulting Group and Moleculera Labs, Oklahoma City, OK, United States

Chapter Outline

In most industries a company will discover, develop, manufacture, and then sell their products to one customer who is both the decision-maker and the end user. In those industries the decision-maker *decides* to purchase, then *purchases* the product, and *uses* the product directly. For instance, when Apple Computer creates and sells the latest version of the iPhone, the customer is the same individual who makes a decision to purchase the iPhone, and is the same person who pays for the product, and is the same person who uses the product. This buying decision continuum is *not* how product decisions, purchasing, and utilization occurs in the biotechnology and medical industry. In this industry, there are ***three*** customers, each making independent decisions for selection, purchasing, and utilization of most biotechnology products. One customer is the decision-maker (usually a *physician*) who decides which product should be used, another customer makes an independent decision whether or not to pay for the product, and how much to pay for the product (the *payer*), and a totally different customer uses the product (the *patient*). This separation of customer decisions is an aspect that can hamper the success of many biotechnology company products if not recognized early during development. It is vital to have a clear understanding of these three independent customers, and to understand their motivations and responsibilities if a company expects to experience product-marketing success (see Fig. 32.1). There are some sectors of biotechnology where products

Biotechnology Entrepreneurship. DOI: https://doi.org/10.1016/B978-0-12-815585-1.00032-2

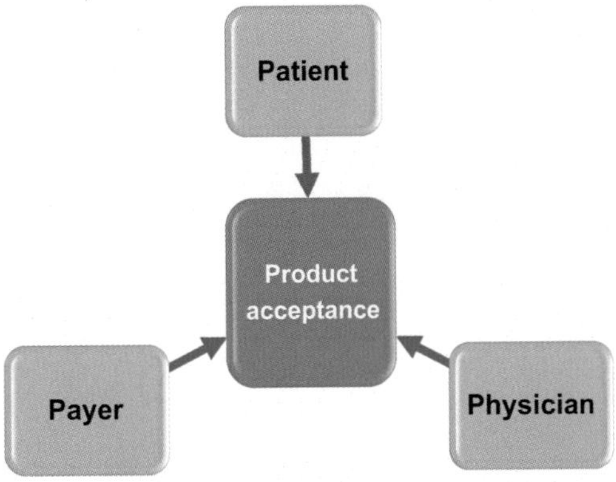

FIGURE 32.1 Medical biotechnology products have three customers.

have only one or two customers, such as agricultural biotechnology, industrial biotechnology, and research tools. and it is important to recognize who the customers are, and what they need.

For medical products in the biotechnology industry, the individual who makes the decision about which product to use is typically the ***physician***. This individual makes a prescribing decision based upon medical standard of care, formulary restrictions, practice guidelines set by their organization and other factors. The entity that makes the decision on how much to pay, or whether to pay, is called the ***payer*** who makes decisions based upon cost/benefit, availability of cost-effective alternatives, pharmacoeconomics, literature support and their own internal protocols. The end user of the product is typically the ***patient*** who is the one impacted by these decisions, who may have some influence on the physician, but usually limited influence on the payer. The physician, payer, and patient each have some input into the decision regarding the product, and each evaluates a product's value differently for determining their respective decision. Successful biotechnology company leaders and managers must make sure their product is offering a compelling value proposition for each of these three customer segments. Unfortunately, young start-up companies may not consider the impact of these three different customer segments responsible for a decision on their product. In countries where the government provides medical services and coverage, such as the United Kingdom and Canada, the payer and the physician are more closely aligned in their decision on the product use because the physician will be paid by the government and they know what is accepted and not accepted for usage by their government. Whereas in the United States, many of the physicians are independent of the payers of medical biotechnology products. The payers are a mix of sources, including numerous private insurance carriers, in addition to the US government that pays through Medicare and the state providers that pay through Medicaid. Private insurance carriers also have customers and attempt to balance the acquisition and retention of customers (the insured) who pay monthly medical insurance premiums, with the ability to offer the best medical care and still make a profit.

Clearly Identify the Patient Segment for Your Product

The patient for a biotechnology product is usually easy to define. They are identified based upon the product's indication-for-use that you are providing. You will have a *target market* and a *broader market* of patients. The *target market* patients are those with the most *acute need* for your product, and they are the customers who have the greatest likelihood of wanting or needing your product. For example, if your product is a drug-eluting stent, your *target market* patient-customer is an individual with coronary artery disease wanting to avoid bypass surgery. If your product is a new statin drug, your *target market* patient-customer is an individual diagnosed with high cholesterol who fits the indications for use of this drug. If your product is used for the diagnosis for respiratory syncytial virus, your *target market* patient-customer is a child presenting to a clinic, hospital, or doctor's office with the disease symptoms. The *broader market* patients are those who could benefit from your product or service, but they may not be the first group that your product will be prescribed for when it first becomes available. The *broader market* patients may have an interest or could receive value from your product but their situation is managed, albeit to a lesser degree than if they used your product.

Identify the Physician Specialty or Health-Care Provider

Determining the target market physician specialty can be a bit more complex than identifying the patient because there are multiple physician specialties and multiple service provider options. There are also *target market* physician groups and *broader market* physician groups just as there is for patients. In the case of the drug-eluting stent product the *target market* physician–customer would be an interventional cardiologist who will be inserting the stent into the appropriate patient-customer. For the statin drug product the *target market* physician–customer would initially be a cardiologist, but the *broader market* physician–customer could be a family practice physician, a geriatrician, or even a physician's assistant. For the infectious disease diagnostic the *target market* physician–customer would be a primary care physician, or any physician, but generally there will be a core group of them that may see more cases of this particular disease than others. For instance, if your test is for respiratory syncytial virus, this disease primarily occurs in children less than two-years old, then the *target market* physician–customer would most likely be a pediatrician or hospital emergency room physician.

Identify the Most Likely Payers Early in Commercialization

Often payers make coverage and payment decisions based upon precedent set by other larger and well-established payers. It is important to understand the issues that influence and guide payment decisions by payers. For more information on this subject, see *Chapter 33: Biotechnology Product Coverage, Coding, and Reimbursement Strategies.* There are multiple payer sources, such as private insurance (large, small, regional, and national), Health Maintenance Organizations (HMOs), Medicare, Medicaid, and each have certain requirements in order to reach a reimbursement coverage decision. In the United States, when it comes to medical care, we tend to have a sense of entitlement and usually do not expect to be paying much out-of-pocket for health-care services. This means that in order to get your products or services adopted, your company needs to secure medical reimbursement. In order to get payer coverage, your product must provide a significant benefit to the patient and the payer. Many private insurances rely upon medical reimbursement evaluation groups for assessing reimbursement decisions—identifying and targeting these groups can save you time and money without having to deal with each payer individually. You will need to spend sufficient time examining medical reimbursement strategy issues in order to get widespread adoption of your product as this is a critical component of success for biotechnology products. Realize that these issues are not ones you should deal with *after* your product is developed. Smart investors will not fund companies that have no reasonable chance of getting medical reimbursement coverage, so be sure to have a good understanding of this before you raise the capital.

Having three customers makes biotech product market research and development more complex than for industries where there is only one customer. You will need to understand the motivations and needs of each of these customers because you cannot market your product successfully without acceptance from all three. For instance, I know of a very innovative prosthetics company that created some amazing prosthetic devices for individuals with physical limitations. One medical device they created was an innovative bionic ankle that had capabilities near to a human ankle. The product was received extremely well by the patient and the physician. However, at a cost of about $15,000, the challenge for the successful adoption of this product was getting insurance reimbursement for such a device. Because there is a less-sophisticated ankles that still functioned adequately for about $3000, the insurance companies did not cover this device. Without the payer having a value benefit, your product will not be widely accepted. For biotechnology products, all three customers must be provided with a significant value proposition in order for your product to be successful.

Develop a Marketing Strategy for Your Future Product

Biotechnology companies that are successful, have a great product idea, they bring together an experienced team to develop their product, and raise enough money to fund a product through development, testing, and regulatory approval. But even if a company navigates through these obstacles and overcomes these hurdles, unless there is good market strategy and their product meets an unmet medical need, there will not be commercial success of their product.

Before funding can be obtained for product development the entrepreneur must prove to investors that the future product will be received by their target audience, and that the company has a marketing strategy that will accomplish this goal. It is not unusual to see that good product technology ideas do not get funded when they are directed at the wrong target market and are coupled to a poor marketing strategy. A market strategy identifies the target market customers, creates a value proposition for each of the three customer groups, and identifies the optimal market channels to successfully provide the product or service to the target market.

Your company's marketing strategy has an impact well before commercialization as it inhibits or increases the company's ability to raise the needed capital to complete product development. Your market strategy is the plan of how your company will provide value to the target market and make money delivering on that promise. Therefore, it is not enough to just develop your product—although it may seem like it should be because of the difficulty accomplishing this in the biotech industry.

If you cannot develop a good marketing strategy before commercialization, then possibly that product application may not be deliverable by the underlying technology, or that product application may not be the best to undertake. Or worse, you may not know who your target market really is, and therefore you will not understand what their ultimate needs are. All entrepreneurs usually have an "idea" of a marketing strategy such that they believe they have knowledge of who the target market is and that they need. However, without identifying a plausible marketing strategy prior to undertaking product

FIGURE 32.2 Product development pathway without first understanding your target market needs through market research.

development, and conducting good market research, you may end up with a product that does *not* meet your target market customer needs (see Fig. 32.2).

When I say "marketing strategy," I am not referring to the detail of how much you will pay the sales and marketing persons, or the product packaging color and who will package it. Sometimes, details such as these are referred to as a "go-to-market plan" where all details are spelled out including the timing for each aspect and the responsible persons for executing that portion of the plan. What I am referring to is a strategy that includes such things as what channels will be used to get your product to the customer; what are the value drivers; and what features you must minimally deliver in order to obtain acceptance. Other factors include your pricing strategy, a cost/benefit analysis for the stakeholders that influence the purchase, prescribing, and product use.

I would encourage you to pick up and read some marketing strategy books to help you gain a better understanding of these concepts. Even though biotechnology products are much more complex and have greater consequences for their choices, similar marketing principles apply for most all products that are purchased and used—even medical products.

In this next section, I want to share a few marketing concepts to help you understand why a well-thought-out marketing strategy is critical even before product development has begun. Sometimes marketing concepts can be abstract and difficult to understand, so in these examples, I will discuss familiar consumer products; later we will apply them to biotechnology products.

What Is Marketing?

Marketing is an art and a science. However, most people view marketing as simply an art, yet there are sound principles that guide the development of competitive marketing strategies for any product, including biotechnology products. Merriam-Webster defines marketing as "*the act or process of selling or purchasing in a market; the process or technique of promoting, selling, and distributing a product or service; an aggregate of functions involved in moving goods from producer to consumer.*" In reality, marketing is not the same as "*sales*" which are the functions that follow good marketing.

I like to think of marketing as "*meeting the acute needs of a select group of people profitably.*" In order to understand what marketing is, let's first discuss what market is not. Below are a few common misconceptions.

Marketing Misconception 1: Marketing Is Not Difficult Because You Just Make It and Sell It!

Although we all know the line from the *Field of Dreams* movie "*build it and they will come,*" it is not a reality in business. However, most biotechnology entrepreneurs subconsciously believe their product is so revolutionary that, at some level, multitudes will clamor to get it because of its awesome technology and the great things it will do. This cannot be further from the truth. Just because a product can do many "great things," it will not be successful unless those "great things" are the *exact* things your target market wants and needs.

To illustrate this point in the consumer market, most people may not know that Apple Computer was the first to invent a type of personal digital assistant (PDA) called the Newton. This PDA-type device was intended to keep your calendar, store your contacts, save your notes, and help keep you organized, all at our fingertips. It had a touch screen with handwriting recognition, but was almost one inch thick, too large and heavy (almost 1 lb) to be considered pocket size. The Newton was manufactured from 1993 to 1998 but discontinued because of lack of consumer interest.

Shortly before the Newton was discontinued, an unknown competitor, Palm, Inc., launched its Palm Pilot developed by first researching the needs of their customers. Palm, Inc. successfully captured a broad market with a second-generation product that was initially introduced by an unsuccessful competitor. Palm developed their product using the marketing concept which we discuss below. The rapid adoption of the PDA was often associated with Palm Pilot and the successful company Palm, Inc. These handheld devices enjoyed widespread market acceptance until these features were combined and incorporated into "smart phones," when the need for a separate PDA device became obsolete.

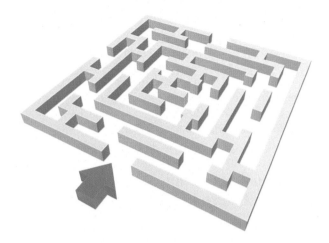

Marketing Misconception 2: If Your Technology Is Better Than the Competition, More People Will Buy Your Product

This is another fallacy, and definitely a slippery slope for biotechnology entrepreneurs who are captivated by their technology. A consumer example is an old one in the video recorder industry where two competitors, Sony and JVC, both had their own technologies for home video recording and playing devices. The first home video recorder was developed and introduced by Sony in 1975 called the Betamax format. One year later, JVC introduced their competitive VHS format. The Betamax and VHS formats were incompatible with each other, and the consumer was left to choose video formats. VHS and Betamax camera recorders were marketed, and the movie industry needed to produce recorded movies in both the VHS and Betamax formats. However, JVC quickly understood the need to license their VHS format to other companies in order to gain broader market acceptance and customer adoption. Sony did not follow suit.

Consumer demand grew for video recorders and companies that manufactured the VHS video recorders served the growing consumer demand, and more studios produced movies in the VHS format. By 1987 the VHS format held 95% of the video recorder market share. As would be expected, movie studios discontinued producing movies in the Betamax format and Sony ultimately discontinued manufacturing its Betamax video recorders. Even though Sony was the first mover in the home video market and their format could be considered superior to the competitor's format, the video tape format battle was won by JVC. This was because of the difference in market strategy, Sony lost the opportunity to be the dominant player in home video recording for the video recorder market. It is estimated that hundreds of millions of dollars were spent in development and manufacturing of the Betamax format including many companies that had products supporting this format.

Between 2006 and 2008 another format war emerged for the high-definition optical disk. In early 2006, Toshiba was the first mover to introduce the HD-DVD format and the first HD-DVD player. Sony followed suit with its own Blu-ray format disk player. Sony quickly secured more commitments from movie studios to offer titles in their Bluray format than Toshiba. In early 2008, Toshiba announced that it would discontinue its HD-DVD player. Although technology enthusiasts say that Toshiba's HD-DVD was a superior format, Sony won the DVD battle. Likely, Sony had a good memory of their previous marketing strategy, and they did not want to repeat a painful marketing lesson previously learned. They recognized that the customer is not as enamored with the technology as much as they want their needs met by the products they purchase.

Marketing Misconception 3: It Is Too Early to Have a Market Strategy Because It Will Get Done Once the Product Is Developed

This sounds logical on the surface, but fundamentally this is disastrous. Remember, a marketing strategy is not the details such as the amount of commission you pay to a sales force, but it is more about how you will reach your target customer and deliver the value that they want and need, and how you will do that strategically, competitively, and profitably. Also, understand that you will not be able to attract knowledgeable investors to fund your company unless you can demonstrate there is a significant unmet market need for your product, and that you have a market strategy that will get your product adopted profitably. Many business plans are turned down by investors simply because the entrepreneur did not prove there was a real market need for their product. Or if the market need was evident, the entrepreneur could not show how to profitably capture this market. Investors do not want to invest in your company just so they can fix a poor marketing strategy for your business. If you do not understand the market needs for your own product, investors conclude you will not make wise decisions in other facets of your business either. As the sophistication level of your investors increase, the more your marketing plan will be scrutinized for flaws. It is vital that you understand the market issues surrounding your product and then develop a well-thought-out market strategy to address these issues. Investors will not get excited about a biotechnology product that does not have a great marketing strategy to reach their customers. A good exercise for entrepreneurs is to ask venture capital fund managers (VCs) to name the three critical elements they need to see in a biotech company before they will invest. You can be sure that demonstrating a real market need coupled to a sensible market strategy will be high on their top-three list.

Understanding the Marketing Concept

The marketing concept is the philosophy that a company first analyzes the needs and wants of their customers ***before*** making their product development decisions. It is the premise that successful products are developed to satisfy the needs of the customer, and this directs the product development so that they can satisfy these needs better than their competitors. These features and benefits provide the best solutions to the customer's problem, and they direct the product development objectives. The marketing concept provides the foundation for a competitive advantage by first knowing who your customers are, then understanding their unique needs because it helps you to develop products that satisfy these needs better than the competition.

The marketing concept evolved as a result of the need for companies to find competitive advantages over other companies in the same market. Understanding how this concept evolved will help entrepreneurs appreciate the value of the marketing concept in business. There were at least three major commercialization concepts that evolved during the development of products and services in the United States which came about because of a need for companies to be more profitable, more competitive and to separate themselves from their competitors. These three concepts are briefly reviewed in the following sections.

The Production Concept

Prior to the Industrial Revolution, there was a limitation of products being made efficiently and in sufficient quantity to make them affordable for everyone. The production concept is the philosophy that companies just needed to produce products at a reasonable price and in sufficient quantities, and these products would sell themselves. During the Industrial Revolution, there was an acute need for basic necessities at affordable prices and the production concept worked well. As better manufacturing processes were developed and became cost-effective, these "affordable" products did indeed sell themselves. As essential consumer products were produced in larger quantities and manufacturing efficiencies continued to improve, products that were previously unattainable by consumers, suddenly became affordable to almost everyone.

A good summary of the production concept is embodied in Henry Ford's statement about selling his Model T automobiles: "*You can have it in any color you want, as long as it is black.*" In other words, products were mass produced and manufactured in sufficient quantities and at affordable prices without regard for specific customer's needs. Eventually, production capabilities for all companies improved, and soon cost-effective manufacturing became the standard. By the late 1940s and early 1950s, most of the basic needs of the average US consumer were being met.

The Sales Concept

Once mass-production manufacturing capabilities became commonplace, there arose competition among companies to sell basic necessity products, and the *sales concept* was born. This philosophy focused on how to persuade consumers to buy *your* product irrespective of whether your product was needed by the customer. Companies began to adopt different methods for "*selling*" their products to customers before their competitors could reach them. This became the era of the "*hard-sell*" and the door-to-door salesmen. As consumers became wiser, these hard-sell tactics no longer produced the type of revenue that organizations required. It was then that clever companies searched for ways to be more competitive.

The Marketing Concept

As competition continued to increase, companies looked for more strategic ways to increase their revenue and maintain an advantage over their competitors. Companies began figuring out their customer's needs *before* they developed their products, and then they created the products that satisfied them. More and more success came to the companies that better understood their customer's wants and needs and delivered the precise products they desired. This was the essence of the *marketing concept.*

The marketing concept is about understanding your customer's needs even if they do not, or cannot express them to you. Proctor & Gamble (P&G) is a very successful marketing concept company. A large part of their target market is women aged 30–45 who purchase household goods and supplies. P&G seeks to better understand the needs of their target market in various ways, even if their customers do not clearly express these needs. P&G asks their customers questions about their household needs, but they also compensate them to visit their homes and follow them throughout their daily activities. Based upon observation and asking their target market segment about their household needs, the company then develops products to meet these needs better than their competitors.

A well-known product developed from this type of market research is the Swiffer. The Swiffer met the target market needs so well that during the first year of introduction, sales were over $200 million. Although the target market customers did not tell the P&G engineers that they needed something like a "Swiffer," the engineers created a product to specifically meet the needs of their customers. This solution was neither a broom nor a mop but accomplished those same functions, which was to capture dirt and clean, but was easier to use, less messy, did not require water, and could be stored in a small space.

The Swiffer example has a parallel for biotechnology companies in which this product created a brand-new category that did not exist before, but was successful because it filled an unmet need that was not satisfied by any other product available. Even though the marketing concept is the most effective marketing strategy, many companies neglect to first define their target market, and they fail to understand their target market's specific needs. Often this is because they become enamored with the technology and captivated by its sophistication and capabilities, whereas customers don't necessarily care about the sophistication of the technology, just that it satisfies their needs.

Market Research and Assessment Tools

When developing a market strategy, it is important to first start with market research because this will be the foundation from which you will later base your assumptions. Market research is the process of gathering information to answer these questions:

1. Is there a general *market opportunity* for your product?
2. Who is your potential *target market* and what is the *total market size*?
3. What are your *target market demographics* and what are their *needs*?
4. What are your *competition's* strengths and weaknesses?

Conducting market research allows you to acquire information and gain insight about the potential market for your product and the needs of your potential customers. Market research may be gathered from medical providers, specialty physicians, insurance companies, researchers, or patients with a particular disease or condition. This information can be obtained through internet searches, literature, publications, or from direct surveys and interviews.

Be sure to conduct thorough market research, gathering as much data as possible, and from as many different sources as possible. When doing market research, it is important to know and understand that there can be source bias. Be sure to guard against selectively hearing information that only confirms a bias for market acceptance of your product. Be critical of your own assumptions and think of reasons why your target market may not want your product and why it may not receive medical reimbursement if it is a human health product. If you are thorough and honest with your questions you will also find the answers that investors will ask when questioning you about the market. All bias is not bad as it may help you know who your best customers may be since they may be biased in their interest of your product. A bias is bad when it is a conclusion about competition or about the risks that you will face in the market. These biases need to be uncovered as you do not want to learn something about your market after you begin commercialization. Once you obtain market research information, you can then form conclusions about the product potential, the target market needs and demographics, the market size, and the competition strengths and weaknesses. Later, we will use this market research to formulate a market strategy. At the end of this chapter, I have provided a template for formulating a market strategy, and it will incorporate much of this information and other information such as market channels and competition.

Primary and Secondary Market Research

Market research is typically categorized as "primary" and "secondary" market research. Primary market research is the information that comes firsthand and directly to you such as interviewing customers and their responses to your questions, conducting focus groups, or commissioning a study by a market research group. Secondary market research is any information that is gathered by and from others, and usually refers to published studies or competitive market information that is commercially available. Since all market research has some bias, it is good to know something about polling and population statistics.

Is There a General Market Opportunity for Your Product?

In order to determine this the entrepreneur must first consider something they may not believe—that potential customers may not be as enthused about their product as they think. One of the purposes of this exercise is to determine if a strong enough market exists for your product before you develop it. Most entrepreneurs have a tendency to underestimate the market risk for their product because they view marketing too simplistically. You need to conduct a "sanity check" because we tend to focus on identifying bits of data to confirm the things that we already believe. There are many ways to do this, and everyone has different ways of validating if there is a real market opportunity. Suffice it to say that it would be advantageous to first start with the hypothesis that individuals would *not* want to purchase or use your product, then identify information that may support that premise. Check out how prevalent the information is about the negative aspects of using your proposed product and see if this may prevent future widespread adoption. No doubt you will find some negativity, and this is helpful at the early stages as it can assist you in directing the technology to deliver the best set of features to overcome most of these issues. In the end, your goal is to be sure that there is a true market opportunity for your future product and that the subsequent steps you take will not be in vain. This information is important to know because often you will run into this information when you talk with potential investors. By understanding this information ahead of time, you can continue your research to find out whether this is a prevailing belief, or it is just the normal arguments that arise with any product.

Who Is Your Target Market and What Is the Potential Total Market Size?

Your *total market* is different from your *target market* in which the total market is always much larger. Total market is the market potential for the ideal product, with no competitors, and everyone that should, would want your product (see Fig. 32.3). The total market is not an expectation of your future sales potential, but it does give a reference to how big a market is, and how much commercial activity exists in that space. Whereas, your target market is a segment of the total market, and it is identified by using various criteria discussed in the following section. For instance, let's say your total market for your product is 15 million individuals, and based upon your pricing model of $1000 per use, your total market size would be $15 billion. Market potential or market opportunity is considered to be all *potential* customers for a product. All companies and their investors would like to have the largest possible market for their product or service. Venture capital likes to see large market potentials for a biotechnology product, usually in the range of a billion dollars.

What Are Your Target Market Demographics and What Are Their Needs?

Your target market will be the most homogeneous population of individuals who have the highest likelihood of initially purchasing and using your product. In order to find this information, we must review some additional tools used when defining a target market and their demographics. For the purposes of assessing who our target market would be, we need to understand the concept of segmentation.

Segmentation

We must somehow divide the universe of people into homogeneous groups that can be reached economically with a similar message. This is because no company can successfully market their product to every individual in the entire world, and every individual is not interested in purchasing your product. Segmentation is how we approach and figure that out. Segmentation is dividing a large population into smaller customer groups based on similar needs, wants, desires, location, demographics, and purchasing habits. Segmentation allows you to identify groups of individuals that can be reasonably reached effectively because the more homogeneous their needs, wants, desires, and purchasing habits, the more likely that segment will respond in a similar manner.

One of the best ways to utilize segmentation is to first know who the potential customers are for your product. This population of interested customers is rarely homogeneous but rather a conglomeration of individuals and groups that you know have an interest in using your product. You begin segmenting this population to reduce them to the most homogeneous target market group of customers who would be the earliest and fastest adopters of your product. Your target market is the potential users of your product with the highest motivation of all individuals to purchase or use your product. Without segmentation, it is impossible to target them appropriately. We segment populations of individuals by using at least three filters: (1) geography, (2) demographics, and (3) behavior/usage. All of these filters may not be applicable to customers of every product because all segmentation factors may not be relevant.

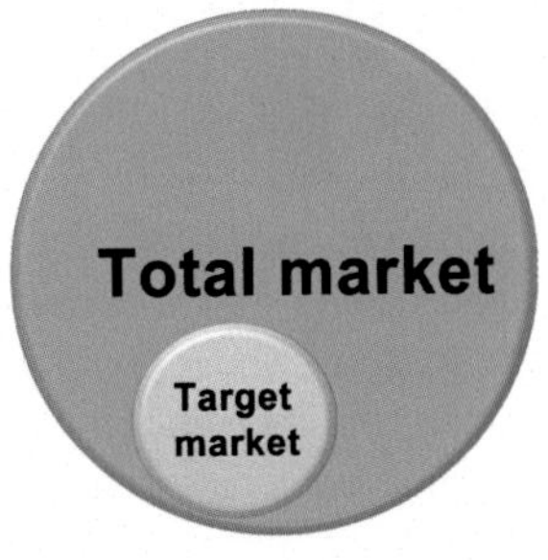

FIGURE 32.3 Total market versus target market.

Segmentation by Geographic Location

Segmentation by geography may or may not be applicable to your biotechnology product, but this is important to determine in the beginning. Some possible geographic segmentation issues could arise for services such as specialty infusion clinics. In this case the customer base would be segmented by using some radius distance of the surrounding geography around all available infusion clinics. Other geographic segmentation applications might include transplantation services if an organ can only be transplanted at specific hospitals and if the recipients must be there within hours limiting the population of potential recipients. For the most part, usage of biotechnology products is less likely to be segmented by geography unless there are issues with worldwide markets and between countries based upon locations for manufacture, testing, or usage of a labile product or service. However, it is important to determine this at the outset.

Segmentation by Demographics

Demographic characteristics are easy to identify. These include qualities such as age, gender, family status, education level, income, occupation, and race, to name a few. Biotechnology products targeting certain physician group practices may include demographic characteristics such as the practice specialty, the number of physicians in a practice, the number of patients seen per day/week/month/year, and the age of the practice and of the physicians. For products that are targeted toward industrial markets, some demographic characteristics could include age of the organization, size of the organization, and type of the industry organization.

Segmentation by Behavior and Usage

This is the most effective and the most successful means of market segmentation, but these can be the most difficult characteristics to identify. Segmenting populations by demographics alone may not be specific enough and too broad since all customers of a particular age and gender do not have the same needs, desires, and wants. For instance, all women aged 25–45 do not have allergies, whereas segmenting populations by behavior *and* by demographics can target individuals with similar needs. For instance, when you segment by geography (areas with higher frequencies of pollen and mold) and include segmentation by family history of allergies *and* include segmentation by age (say children between the ages of 6 and 12), you have specifically identified a more homogeneous population of individuals with similar needs.

Patients can also be segmented by their preference for the usage of a type of medication and amount of expenditures in a particular medical category. There are many ways to use behavior and usage segmentation; it just requires that you find a method that is readily measured. Or sometimes a surrogate category is used if the real behavior pattern cannot be measured. Physicians can also be segmented by prescribing and referral characteristics such as how frequently they prescribe a class of drugs, the frequency of ordering a diagnostic test, the frequency of using certain practice protocols for a particular disease, and how often and to whom they send referrals. Segmentation by behavior and usage is very powerful when coupled to other demographic criteria; however, just remember that the more detailed the segmentation, the smaller the population, because there are opposing forces that expand or refine the segment.

What Are Your Competition's Strengths and Weaknesses?

The first step is to identify who they are. If you are developing or considering developing a product where there are no direct competitors, such as is the case with many biotechnology products, don't forget to include "substitutes." Substitutes are products used by your target market customers that are a "substitute" for the product they really want and need. You can be sure that if there are no direct competitors, there *will* be inferior substitutes that are used. If there are no substitutes, you seriously should reconsider if there really is a market need for your product. Because the greater the market need, in the absence of products that meet that need, there will be efforts by customers to use a variety of substitutes to satisfy their need. In addition, customers will give up their substitutes when your product is available, and that is the essence of "competition." Also, do not forget to identify companies and basic research programs that are developing future products for your target market. Biotechnology product development is lengthy; therefore you must include these emerging activities in your assessment of future competition. Often these future competitors can be found in research literature, news publications and through a company's press releases and their websites.

There are many aspects to consider about your competitors' strengths and weaknesses, but we will only discuss one in this chapter, and that is *their product's features and benefits compared to yours and how much any of these align with the customer's needs.* Most biotechnology products are product innovations in some respects and generally are not commodities; therefore the features and benefits that alignment with the customer's needs are most significant. However, in the bioagricultural sector, many of these food products are commodities, but the features and benefits provided by AgBio are novel. For instance, soybeans are commodities. But soybeans that are resistant to roundup allow weed killer to be sprayed on all the crops, yet it does not damage these soybean crops. Therefore the value lies in the product's features and benefits and its alignment with the customer's needs. However, there is still pricing pressures because commodities cannot be priced too much higher than their competitors.

A helpful exercise is to begin with a matrix list of features and benefits that your product provides and that of your current or future competition, and substitutes. For example, if your product is a novel nonnarcotic pain medication, your matrix may look something like Table 32.1. Although you can add many other competitive values such as delivery, pricing, and technical support, I would encourage you to initially list only the features and benefits that most effectively meet the needs of the customer, and how it is better than your competitors and substitutes. Then rank these benefits on a scale of 1–5 with 1 being the worst and 5 being the best. This will help you determine how much superior your future product may be to the competition.

One note of caution: Do not build this matrix list based upon your *own* products features and benefits. Build this matrix list based upon the *needs of the customers* you are targeting. It is tempting to produce a list where your product has high rankings and the competition is inferior; but this is of no value if the features and benefits you describe have limited or no value to the customer.

TABLE 32.1 Product features and benefits matrix for a novel non-narcotic pain treatment

Feature and benefit	Your product	Competitor 1	Competitor 2	Substitute 1
Relieves pain effectively at rating scale used	5	2	3	1
Requires only one dose daily	5	1	1	0
Fast acting within 1 h	3	3	2	5
Long-term benefit after 2 weeks of use	5	3	3	1
No side effect—headache	4	1	3	5
No side effect—diarrhea	5	5	2	1

For instance, you may list as one feature and benefit as a "10-year stability" and competitors may score poorly. However, if there is no benefit to the *customer* for a 10-year shelf life, this is not a feature that has value to the customer. You can certainly include this "benefit" in an expanded matrix listing all values, as that could provide a financial value to the company in reducing the number of manufacturing runs. However, if it provides no value to the target market customer, omit it from this exercise.

Other Market Tools and Concepts

There are many other market tools that are essential for developing a sound market strategy, and some we want to discuss that are useful for the biotechnology entrepreneur and management team are described below. These include targeting, positioning, branding and developing future sales projections, or a pro forma.

Targeting

Targeting is everything that you do to narrow down the profile for the ideal customer. It is the next step after segmentation, and it is the process of selecting *which* segment to target out of all these market segments that have been previously defined. Targeting allows you to focus and tailor your product values to the specific preferences of the best customer segment. Targeting is the rationale for choosing what market segment will be your best customers for purchasing and using your product. Targeting leads to the next step which is product positioning.

Positioning

Positioning is everything a company does to convey their product's value to the customer and the things that separate it from competitors. Positioning is the way in which a company wants its target segment customers to view their product, and it is the way that their product solves the customer's problem that is different from its competition. Positioning requires that you differentiate your product from other products in the market; otherwise, all products will be grouped together if there is no difference in positioning. In order for potential customers to recognize your product, you have to position it in a way customer can differentiate it from all others. The more effective your product positioning, the easier it is for customers to understand your product's value to them. Positioning has a lot to do with perception in the mind of the customer that is different from your competitors—you are positioning an image of value associated with your product. This is how a company creates a "brand," which we will discuss next.

Branding

Branding is often thought of as a logo, a company and product name, or a catchy phrase. However, that is not branding, but it is how companies *associate* a brand to themselves. Branding includes all the intangible attributes and thoughts in a person's mind that are associated with the company's logo, products, and other tangible aspects. Branding is more than just a product trade name and its recognizable product packaging—it is all the information evoked in the mind of the consumer when they encounter your product. Companies spend many years carefully creating a brand that suggests value in the minds of their customers. Companies sell products, but they are really marketing brands.

Although branding includes attributes of status, image, and the experiential benefit that goes along with a product, biotechnology product branding is strongly associated with the tangible medical benefit a product provides to the patient or physician or medical researcher. There are other factors that help create the brand value, and these can be enhanced if there is a tangible medical benefit from the product. Brands also convey messages about new products that an existing company develops, so it is important to determine what you want your brand to be and to manage that carefully as you can see what can happen with the example below.

Example of the Effect of a Brand

Although all companies have true capabilities to develop many types of products logically, it is important to be consistent with the brand you desire to create, and the one you have already created in the minds of customers. For instance, Colgate has a strong and recognized brand in oral hygiene products, and decided to use its name on a number of food products called Colgate Kitchen Entrees. Unfortunately, the product did not take off. One may be able to guess what the images in the customer's minds may have been about the taste of these food items. The take-home message is that a brand is a powerful competitive strength, and it is important to know the message it evokes in the minds of your customers.

Sales Projections Pro Forma or Management's Projections

Although this is not a tool, it is an essential component of a market strategy when building a biotechnology company, and these projections will become a part of your business plan. By now you will have defined your total market potential in terms of customers and dollars, and identified your target market segment. Now you also need to project what portion of this market you anticipate your product will capture over the first 5 years of marketing. You may wonder, "Why is this important now if I am 3–5 years away from completing product development?" It is important because it makes you evaluate how significantly you can (or you think you can) penetrate the market with your product. And, it is what your investors want to know to determine if they are interested in investing in your company. For biotech products that typically need to reach commercialization before finding an exit such as diagnostics, medical devices, health-care IT, and research reagents, the 5-year projections are expected. In cases such as a biotherapeutic in discovery stages that may be 10–15 years away from potential commercialization, this exercise may not be essential yet, but irrespective, you should still have an appreciation for this process and understand the manner in which it is determined.

This financial projection is referred to as a "pro forma" or "sales projections." These projections are used to show the impact of your market strategy and the attractiveness of your product to your target market. There are two ways to develop a sales forecast, the first is the *top-down* approach and the other is a *bottom-up* approach. The top-down approach is a first approximation of potential market penetration. It is arrived at by taking the market potential and estimating a market penetration percentage based upon various assumptions including penetration rates by other companies in adjacent markets. For instance, let's say you estimate your total market potential to be $15 billion and you estimate a 6% penetration rate by the fifth year. That means that you project to generate $900 million by the fifth year. The top-down approach is occasionally used to provide a general estimate of potential product revenue, but it is rarely taken too seriously because it is not built by the real drivers of demand. The bottom-up approach takes your key assumptions that are supported by data and builds a model based upon these and other quantified factors to estimate a resulting revenue stream.

For a bottom-up example, let's say that your company is developing a diagnostic test for the rapid detection of ovarian cancer in women. Your market research demonstrates that the target market physicians for ordering your test would be obstetrician-gynecologists (OB/GYNs). There is more information that can refine your target market segment as discussed in the segmentation section, but for now, let's use all OB/GYNs as our target market. In this case, to develop a bottom-up financial pro forma, you start with the total number of OB/GYNs in the country or geographic region you will be targeting. Let's say it is the United States, and you find there are approximately 43,000 practicing OB/GYNs in the country. From your market research, you find the average number of patients that one OB/GYN sees per day, per week, per month, per year. Your research can also inform you about the age ranges of women who would likely be screened for ovarian cancer. Based upon your market strategy, you estimate the number of OB/GYNs that your technical sales or market strategy can reach each year based upon an estimate of your conversion rate per sales person per number of visits. This variable is continuously adjusted by the number of sales persons your company plans to hire in years 1–5.

From this type of information and other key assumptions, you can arrive at a plausible predictive model for your sales projections. By using this bottom-up approach, everyone can see the key assumptions, and they can agree or disagree with any of them, whereas this allows you to make adjustments in your projections based upon these changes. The great benefit of this method is that much of this information can be proven and demonstrated, such as the number of OB/GYNs in the United States, or the average number of patients they see in a day, week, month, or year. You should produce your revenue projections by both the bottom-up and the top-down method to arrive at the best estimates of projected revenue generation.

However, you should be aware and forewarned, an entrepreneur's revenue projections are viewed cautiously by investors because they likely have encountered instances in which other entrepreneurs have shown extremely unrealistic projections. As a result, investors rightly discount the sales projections in a business plan until they are comfortable with your assumptions. Because there is no way ahead of time to overcome this bias from potential investors, the best approach is to provide your key assumption with support, then show that the projections are supported with solid data and logic. Sometimes there is no data available to support one particular assumption. In this situation, you should draw parallels from other markets or products; just be sure to acknowledge that these are limitations and then provide the reasons you believe that the estimates are reasonable. Do not make unrealistic assumptions or provide unsupported conclusions—poor assumptions undermine your credibility in the eyes of investors.

Lastly, when building a pro forma, it is a good idea to also produce a worst case scenario for your internal use—one in which some of the key assumptions are not met for one reason or another. If you are in a biotech sector where exits typically occur after commercialization and revenue generation such as diagnostics, medical devices and health-care IT, and you do not build in a worst case scenario, if you are off in your projections you may run out of money or be forced to raise capital under a reduced valuation. Build your pro forma projections using the bottom-up approach and run an additional worst case scenario, you will then have the best estimates for your sales projections and your investors will have more confidence in your judgment.

Steps to Developing a Market Strategy

In this section, I have listed five steps to help you by using an example on formulating your marketing strategy. There are obviously more aspects to building a marketing strategy than just these, but this will help you get started on your own marketing plan. During this process, you will utilize the market research information you previously gathered and include other important aspects such as market channels.

Determine Your Potential Market Size

The potential market for your product is the largest group of customers that could conceivably purchase or use your product at some time. As previously discussed, we calculate the total market opportunity for your product in terms of customers or patients (if it is in health care) and also in dollars. The total market size represents your total market potential, but it is not your sales projections. Rarely does any company's product sales approach the entire market due to many limitations, including your competition.

For example, if your product is a new influenza nasal spray vaccine, since influenza is a disease that potentially affects all individuals, we would take the US population of 327 million people and multiply that number by the price of the vaccine. Let's presume a similar but slightly higher price of $40 per vaccination compared to the regular injectable pricing—this would be a $13.1 billion market in the United States. If we calculated a UK market, we would use 66 million people times $40 per person or a $2.4 billion market. For a worldwide total market, we would do the same. Refinements can be made easily as needed. For instance, since we do not vaccinate infants and children under 6 months of age, we can easily exclude that population from the total market size.

For another example, if you are estimating the total market for a monoclonal antibody therapeutic that increases blood flow to an ischemic artery immediately after cardiac arrest, you find that the total number of heart attack victims per year is about 1.5 million (in the United States) multiplied by the estimated price of your product (presume for now at $2000); therefore the total US market size would be $3 billion annually. For some products, determining potential total market size is not that easy, but there are other ways arrive at these numbers such as evaluating a competitors' potential market if you have competition. If you do not have competition, you can calculate the potential total market size based upon substitutes. An important point when you do this is that you do not use actual sales of competitors or substitute products because this is not the total market potential. You are estimating the *potential* market that could be reached with an ideal product without any competition.

Most total market potential estimates are determined using demographic data such as we did in these examples. Other factors may need to be included when estimating a total potential market, such as the frequency of use. If your product is a diagnostic test for upper respiratory infections, and your market research shows that individuals get an average of 1.7 upper respiratory infections each year, you will multiply the applicable population by the infection frequency of 1.7, then multiply this by the product price to arrive at the total potential market.

A key reason we estimate the total potential market is because investors want to know whether your market is large enough to support their investment and provide them the type of return they desire. Most VC investors like to see total market potentials that exceed $1 billion annually. For instance, it would be foolish for a VC investor to invest $30 million into a company if the total market potential for that product was $25 million annually.

Identify and Define Your Target Market Segment

Next you want to determine who is your best customer. This is a subpopulation of your total market potential. It represents the initial group you will be targeting with the highest likelihood of purchasing or using your product. To identify your target market segment, you will use the segmentation filters we previously described, such as geography, demographics, behavior, and usage. We are seeking to identify homogeneous groups that have similar wants and needs regarding your product. This is the group with the greatest need and desire for your product, and it represents the population that you must capture first in order to reach more of your potential market later.

When you properly segment and identify your target market, you will find that they are easier to reach than the entire potential market because they have many similarities and common behaviors. Products must be able to capture their target market segment first before targeting other market segments as this is the group from which you build your market base.

As an example, let's say your product is a genetic test used to determine a woman's predisposition to breast cancer, and you initially require the patient pay a $500 portion until you can obtain insurance reimbursement coverage. You will segment your market through demographic and behavior characteristics to identify the most homogeneous group with similar motivations and behaviors resulting in the highest likelihood that they will want their physician to prescribe your test. In this example the target market segmentation for this genetic predisposition test may look like this:

- Women (this is segmentation by demographics—gender);
- Ages 40–69 (this is further segmentation by demographics—age);
- With household incomes greater than $75,000 annually (this is further demographic segmentation—income);
- Seeking mammography services annually (this is segmentation by behavior and usage); and
- Family history of breast cancer (this is segmentation by demographics).

This would be an example of a target market with similar wants, needs, and desires as it pertains to your product.

Describe Your Product's Value Proposition for Your Target Market and Identify Your Competitor's

Now that you have identified your target market segment, you must articulate what your value proposition is to these customers. This is what we previously described as positioning and branding. A value proposition is the reason that your product is so valuable to the customer that it makes them want to purchase and use your product. In order to identify your value proposition, you start out by first listing your product's benefits to your target market. Some helpful questions include the following:

- How does your target market customer benefit by using your product?
- What are the compelling points of difference between your product and your competition?
- What needs will be met by your target market customer when they use your product?
- What are the features and benefits of your product that are of great value to your target market customer?

Simultaneously, you must also examine what value your competition or substitute products provide your target market customers. Substitute products are a form of inferior competition, but you still need to determine how, in whatever way, they are meeting the needs of your customers. Compare and contrast your product to these competitors and substitutes. Determine what are the valuable points of differentiation between your product and competitive or substitute products.

Do not forget that for biotechnology products you have three customers and you will need a specific value proposition for each one. For the patient, some of the benefits may be related to values such as less pain, faster acting, and improved health. For the physician, some benefits may be related to values such as lower risk of adverse events and fewer complications. For the payer, some benefits may be related to pharmacoeconomic or cost benefit, quality of life, and survival benefit.

One example of a possible value proposition statement for the genetic predisposition test for breast cancer could be: "*genetic testing, when coupled to an actionable plan can prevent breast cancer or identify it at the earliest possible stages where long-term survival is the greatest.*"

Identify the Best Market Channel(s) to Reach Your Target Market Segment

Although we did not discuss how to identify potential market channels in the previous section, it is an important component of an overall market strategy for reaching your target market segment. Market channels are the methods you will use to gain access to your target market segment customers and the way they will gain access to your product. It is the path that the product takes to reach your customers. There are "direct market channels" where the company sells products directly to customers. There are "intermediary market channels," or third parties, that sell and deliver your products to customers. There are "dual-distribution market channels" where you have more than one distribution method to get products to your customers. Then there are "reverse channels" that go from consumer to intermediary and then to the customer. Reverse channels are used in human blood products such as blood, plasma, platelets, and passive immunoglobulin.

All biotech products will reach their customers via some market channel, and depending on what sector of biotechnology your product is in, you may not sell your product directly to the end user. Find what your best, most effective, and strategic market channel is for your product to reach your customers. Having an effective market channel is a competitive strength for your product.

Do not propose to build a new market channel as part of your market strategy, although this has been done by some biotechnology companies such as Amgen, Genentech, Genzyme, and Genomic Health. Start out by finding ways to leverage existing market channels. There are usually good market channels available to reach your target market, so pursue these first rather than developing your own. Consider collateral and alternative usages of existing market channels that are mutually beneficial to you and your partners. Ideally, you will want to leverage existing market channels because it will take time for the development of a new market channel, which is also a new market risk.

Validate and Refine Your Market Strategy

All marketing plans are intriguing theories, but they are only good if they work for your product. Therefore, you will want to test your market strategy and your market assumptions in some way to see if they are viable and accurate.

There are endless ways you can validate your market strategy. You can hire a consultant to help, you can interview option leaders in this market, or you can hire a contract research organization to conduct independent primary market research to see if it supports each of the assumptions you have made in your market strategy. Another way to validate the market is to test the market receptivity for your product. Market tests can be difficult and expensive to conduct, but they can provide good information and feedback to validate or refine your original market strategy. Your goal is to find some way to validate whether or not your assumptions that your target market wants your product are correct.

The market strategy you develop will be incorporated into your business plan and strategy, and it will be modified over time as refinements will be made when you encounter obstacles and receive new information. This exercise will help you get started developing your own market strategy for your product using established market methods and tools.

Identify Your Market Development Milestones

Market development milestones are important to your company for demonstrating the market progress. Just as you will have value-enhancing *product development milestones*, you need to identify your *market development milestones*. There is great diversity in marketing strategy so formulate your market development milestones with your specific product in mind. These milestones serve the same purpose as your product development milestones—when they are reached, they reduce the risk of your organization and they most likely will improve your company value.

Some examples of market development milestones could include:

- Target market segment defined and tested
- Target market segment needs, wants and points of differentiation from competitors and substitutes defined
- Completed primary research study to validate your target market segment needs
- Value proposition for your product to your target market customers defined and tested
- Completed develop and implementation of a branding strategy for your product and company
- Product pricing model determined and tested
- Pharmacoeconomic assessment of your product used in your target market completed
- Primary research on reimbursement codes and private insurance likelihood of reimbursement completed
- Distribution channels for your product identified and secured and
- International marketing partners identified and secured.

Biotechnology Product Adoption Curve

Market adoption of biotechnology products can have many challenges because of the complexity, limited understanding of the technology, uncertainty of utility, high costs, and other factors. For those interested in understanding more about issues with technology adoption, I highly recommend *Crossing the Chasm: Marketing and Selling Disruptive Products to Mainstream Customers* by Geoffrey Moore [1]. Although his book mostly references the computer and IT industry, the adoption curve is virtually the same for biotechnology products. The adoption stages of a target market can be divided into groups of individuals based upon their speed of adopting new technology. These subcategories of individuals are labeled as innovators, early adopters, early majority, late majority, and laggards. The first to adopt are considered innovators, followed by early adopters and then there is a chasm you must cross in order to reach the early majority and the mainstream market. Recognize that even with the best and most ideal market strategy, widespread product adoption will still require persistence, creativity, and adaptability in order to penetrate a market with even the best of biotechnology products.

Summary

A marketing strategy is a carefully thought-out plan for how your product will bring value to, and reach its best customers. This strategy is based upon both primary and secondary market research and a segmentation analysis defining your target market which is the most homogeneous group of individuals having the highest likelihood of purchasing or using your product.

A marketing strategy must be developed long before you are able to sell your product, and it is a vital component of your business and funding strategy. Be sure that your market plan is well-thought-out and built upon solid data and logical with supported assumptions, not presumptions. Spend plenty of time and effort developing a solid market plan. Understand the market issues, your competitors, and substitutes; know your value proposition to your target market and refine your market strategy as you learn new information. Unless the entrepreneur is an experienced marketing executive from a successful biotechnology or pharmaceutical company, you will likely need help in developing a marketing strategy. This is not an area of business in which you should pinch pennies because developing a good marketing strategy will pay for itself over time. Venture capital partners will quickly recognize a poorly developed and unsupported marketing strategy.

A young biotechnology company that can show a solid marketing plan for their product helps when raising capital and it also demonstrates that the entrepreneur understands the key market issues. A good market development plan with milestones is equally valuable for overall company success as are your product development milestones. Don't forget that biotechnology products must meet the needs of all three of its customers in order to be successful; therefore you will need a value proposition for each of these stakeholders. Successful entrepreneurs demonstrate to their investors that they understand their market risks and embrace a plan to manage these risks. Your marketing strategy is an essential component of your business plan, and it is a key factor in raising capital for your company. In *Chapter 13: Directing Your Technology Toward a Market Problem: What You Need to Know Before Using the Business Model Canvas?*, I describe a helpful tool for building your business model and optimizing your market strategy. In that chapter we walk through what you need to know first before embarking on the Business Model Canvas optimization process.

Reference

[1] Moore GA. Crossing the chasm: marketing and selling disruptive products to mainstream customers. 3rd ed. New York: Collins Business Essentials; 2014.

Section VIII

Biotechnology Market Development

Chapter 33

Biotechnology Product Coverage, Coding, and Reimbursement Strategies

Robert E. Wanerman, JD, MPH[1,*] **and Susan Garfield, DrPH**[2]

[1]*Partner at Epstein Becker Green, P.C., Washington, DC, United States,* [2]*Global Advisory Principal and Life Sciences Sector Commercial Lead, EY, Cambridge, MA, United States*

Chapter Outline

Bringing a new drug, biological, medical device, or diagnostic to market is an arduous process that can take years, cost tens of millions of dollars, and requires compliance with multiple regulatory processes. Even though inventors, investigators, manufacturers, and investors are focused on the clearance or the approval of a new product by the Food and Drug Administration (FDA) or other National Regulatory Authorities outside the United States, a successful strategy for commercializing those new products must also look beyond these regulatory agencies. Even at an early stage of development, overlooking the reimbursement processes that come into play after FDA or other national authority approval can mean the difference between ultimate success and failure. For smaller companies a failure to develop a strategy for obtaining coverage, coding, and reimbursement can mean the difference between attracting investors and not obtaining funding at all. For a large company the lack of a strategy can diminish or eliminate the expected return on investment. This chapter will explain these reimbursement processes. Although the challenges for each product may be different, understanding the mechanics of coverage, coding, and reimbursement is essential for identifying the issues and evaluating any potential options.

Understanding Coverage, Coding, and Reimbursement of Biotechnology Products in the United States[1]

At the outset, a commercialization strategy must recognize the distinctions between the FDA regulatory framework and the regulatory processes that come into play once a product is cleared or approved for sale. Under the Federal Food, Drug, and Cosmetic Act (FDCA) the FDA's authority covers the manufacture and marketing of drugs, biologicals, medical devices, and diagnostics [1]. Since it only regulates the actions of manufacturers, its actions do not dictate the practice of medicine and do not, on their own, regulate the actions of third-party payers such as health plans and government programs including Medicare and Medicaid. As a result, the fact of FDA

*Robert E. Wanerman is a partner in the Washington, DC office of Epstein Becker Green, P.C. United States. The discussion in the chapter does not constitute legal advice, as the facts and circumstances of a particular matter may involve questions of law that are not addressed here.

1. The first part of this chapter is written by Robert Wanerman.

Biotechnology Entrepreneurship. DOI: https://doi.org/10.1016/B978-0-12-815585-1.00033-4

approval or clearance is a first step, with the next being coverage, coding, and reimbursement decisions made by third-party payers [2]. Accordingly, developing a commercialization strategy that takes into account the nuances and challenges of coverage and access should be a part of the initial planning phases to avoid significant delays in bringing the product to market [3].

A commercialization strategy in the United States is complicated by the fact that the entities that develop a new technology and commercialize it are often not the entities that file reimbursement claims with health plans or programs. Instead, manufacturers sell products to providers or suppliers who then submit claims to health plans or programs in accordance with the reimbursement methodology that applies to the particular site of service. This problem can be illustrated in Fig. 33.1.

In order to navigate through this post-FDA regulatory landscape, three fundamental concepts must be defined and understood to avoid costly errors once the organization has developed an idea. Coverage refers to terms and conditions under which a private or public health plan will pay for an item or service [4]. Coverage is not guaranteed once the FDA approves or clears a product, and a favorable coverage determination does not guarantee a particular level of reimbursement [5]. The coverage analysis typically involves the following three-part inquiry:

1. Does the new technology fit into an existing benefit category?
2. Is the new technology excluded by law or by the plan's express terms?
3. Does the new technology satisfy the plan's "reasonable and necessary" or "medically necessary" criteria?

Each element of this inquiry can involve significant barriers. The threshold benefit category question can usually be answered by looking into the law establishing the health benefit in the case of government-funded programs, or to a private plan's contract. For example, under the original Medicare program, screening tests such as those for colorectal cancer or glaucoma did not fit into a defined benefit category and only became covered after Congress amended the statute to create a new screening benefit [6]. Some items such as traditional hearing aids or some forms of cosmetic surgery may be excluded by law or contract [7]. In a small number of cases, state law may mandate coverage for specific items and services in private plan offerings in their state. This is the case with 38 states and the District of Columbia that require coverage for patient costs associated with cancer clinical trials [8]. Finally, even if there is no express inclusion or exclusion, all items and services are subject to the general rule that they must meet a test for medical necessity, sometimes stated as the "reasonable and necessary" standard [9]. The conundrum for developers or investors is that this residual criterion is often undefined or vaguely defined, leaving it a moving target [10]. The converse is that it gives plans a high degree of discretion. Sometimes this discretion is exercised in a measured form. For example, some plans may initially approve coverage for a new technology or treatment only after conventional treatments have been tried and failed; in other situations, the item or service might not be covered unless quantifiable diagnostic prerequisites have been met [11]. In other cases, coverage determinations may turn on data showing improved outcomes using well-defined metrics [12].

The definition of coverage may also be subject to geographic variation. Although some large health plans may operate in multiple states, it should not be presumed that the plan's coverage will be uniform nationwide. Even the Medicare program, which was established by federal law and is administered by a federal agency, may have

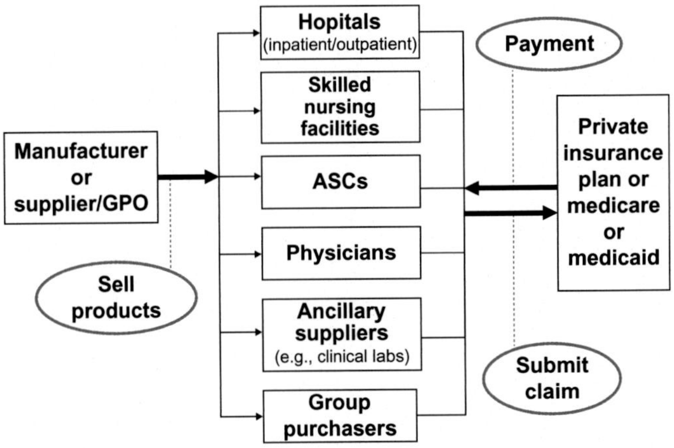

FIGURE 33.1 The US medical reimbursement system.

conflicting coverage policies in different jurisdictions due to the authority delegated to individual contractors to develop local coverage determinations for those items and services where there is neither a statutory mandate nor a national coverage determination [13].

The second basic concept is coding. Codes and code sets are the way that the delivery of health care is identified, monitored, and ultimately paid by third-party plans. Code sets exist for, among other things, diagnoses, procedures, medical devices and supplies, and bundles of direct and indirect costs incurred in furnishing treatment. A code on its own does not guarantee either coverage or a desired reimbursement rate. The control of the relevant code sets in the United States is decentralized, as shown in Fig. 33.2.

For example, the Current Procedural Terminology (CPT) code set that defines work done by physicians and other health professionals is controlled by the American Medical Association's (AMA's) CPT Editorial Panel with input from specialty societies, while a second AMA panel, the AMA/Specialty Society Relative Value Scale Update Committee develops relative value recommendations to the Centers for Medicare and Medicaid Services (CMS) that, if adopted, set the reimbursement rate under the Medicare program for new CPT codes. For supplies and equipment used by physicians and, other health professionals, the relevant code set is the Healthcare Common Procedure Coding System (HCPCS), which is controlled by CMS with input from health plans. The process for obtaining a new code can differ among the various code sets, as does the timing of coding decisions—while the CPT process spans 2 years, the HCPCS codes are updated on an annual cycle.

Due to the importance of codes to a commercialization strategy, stakeholders need to define the codes that apply to a new product or service using that product as well as

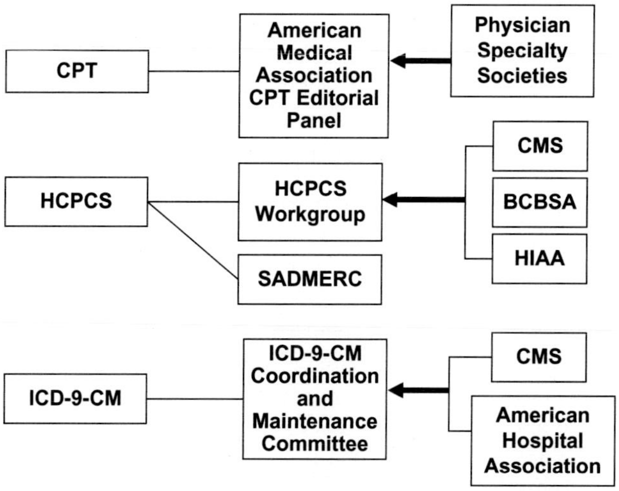

FIGURE 33.2 Process for codes used for procedures, items, and diagnoses.

technology in the site(s) of service where it will be used. For example, while an office-based procedure may be defined by a single diagnosis code and a single CPT code or family of CPT codes, an inpatient procedure such as a joint replacement may involve coordinating diagnosis codes, CPT codes for physician services, and diagnosis-related group (DRG) codes for the hospital's services. Regardless of the number of codes involved in furnishing care to an individual patient, a code is, by itself, not a guarantee of coverage or payment [14]. The process of determining the correct code(s) for a new technology often includes an analysis of whether or not existing codes are sufficient to capture all of the features of that technology. If the existing codes are inadequate, the stakeholders may have to consider the case for creating a new code based on clinical and resource distinctions, as well as the time and effort needed to petition the coding authorities to add a new code.

The third fundamental concept is understanding the payment methodologies that apply to a particular item or service in a specific site of service. Starting from a historical model in which all items and services were paid individually on a piecework basis, health plans and government agencies have developed multiple methodologies tailored to the site of service. Depending on the site of service and the individual plan policies, payment may be made for an item or service individually, or as part of a larger bundle. Even when the payment is bundled, certain items or services may be excluded from the bundle and are separately billable; this is the case with many physicians' services that are furnished to inpatients or outpatients. In addition, the amount of payment for the same service can vary among different sites of service due to factors such as indirect costs and overhead. For example, the Medicare program assumes that when the same service is performed in an ambulatory surgical center and a hospital outpatient department, the latter will have higher overhead and labor costs and sets a higher reimbursement rate for the hospital [15]. As a result, if an existing code fits the technology, stakeholders will want to know if the resulting reimbursement associated with that code under relevant fee schedules makes it economically feasible for professionals and other users to adopt that new technology. If existing codes do not fit and a new code is warranted, the analysis shifts to a consideration of whether the data supports establishing a desirable reimbursement rate for that new code that will lead to the adoption of the technology.

The type and amount of payment a provider or supplier receives may be subject to additional thresholds or limitations, including the use of relative value scales, payment caps or ceilings, and existing payment methods and rates for comparable items and services. Depending on the facts and circumstances, one option is to fit a new technology or product into the existing coverage, coding, and reimbursement terms for a product in the same class. However, if the new technology can be considered a breakthrough or a complementary product that improves overall outcomes or results in other improvements in patient care, accepting the status quo may not be an optimal business decision. For those new technologies that substantially alter the overall cost of care, the health plan may not be able to redefine immediately or revalue a bundled payment to allow the adoption of that new technology. In these limited cases, payers such as the Medicare program can approve payment for the new technology as an "add-on" cost or as a pass-through payment while data on the new technology is compiled and the bundled payment can be reviewed [16].

The Analytical Framework for New Technologies

Regardless of the type of product or technology or the path followed by a developer of a new medical technology, once the new product is ready for testing in a clinical trial, there should be a companion strategy for commercializing the product focusing on coverage, coding, and reimbursement. If the funding for the basic research and proof of the concept through a clinical trial comes from private sources, the approval of that funding (or future funding) may turn on the ability of the new product to generate a return on that investment through the three fundamental concepts described previously. Therefore, the process of designing a clinical trial to prove a concept may have to be broader than just obtaining the information necessary to meet the FDA's criteria for approval or clearance. By integrating the types of outcome data that payers rely on into the trial a sponsor can save the considerable time, effort, and cost of conducting a second trial to obtain the type of information that payers will demand in order to make coverage and reimbursement determinations. This section will focus on the variables that need to be considered in crafting a commercialization strategy that is tailored to a particular item or service.

Defining the Terms of Coverage

As discussed previously, due to absence of a precise statutory or contract directive most health plans have wide discretion in determining which items and services will be covered. The Medicare statute states that items and services will be covered if they are "reasonable and necessary for the diagnosis or treatment of illness or injury" but does not explain the meaning of this term in more detail [17]. Some commercial plans rely on a general notion of medical necessity and accepted standards of practice, but they do not elaborate further [18]. In selected cases, items and services may be subject to a more rigorous evaluation process that examines improvements in outcomes and the relative benefits when compared to existing treatments [19].

Unless the terms of coverage (or an exclusion from coverage) are unambiguously defined by law or by binding policies, the threshold inquiry in developing a coverage, coding, and reimbursement strategy is to identify the type and quality of information and data that may be needed to obtain a favorable coverage determination. This analysis can be broken down to a set of the following basic questions:

- Does the item or service meet a plan's benefit categories or inclusion criteria?
- If professional practice guidelines exist, is the item or service consistent with those guidelines?
- Does the item or service fill an unmet clinical need?
- Who will be benefited from the item or service; is it primarily one group (children or seniors), or is the benefit widely distributed?
- What is the anticipated site of service (e.g., inpatient, outpatient, office, or clinic)?
- What is (are) the expected clinical outcome(s)?
- If there are comparable covered items or services, does the new technology result in better outcomes?
- If the new technology is complex or is expected to be expensive, can it be positioned as a second-line therapy?
- Have relevant professional societies adopted the new technology as a part of their practice guidelines or other formal statements?
- Is there a potential for coverage for "off-label" indications?
- Are there any existing limits on the frequency of service(s)?
- What is the expected financial impact for the payer/consumer (e.g., will adoption of the new item or service raise or lower the aggregate cost of care)?
- Are there other immediate or long-term benefits?

In answering these questions, innovators and other stakeholders should understand the existing scope of coverage for comparable items and services. While the natural tendency is to seek coverage for any and all applications, the coverage for other competing items and services may be limited to specific clinical conditions, specific locations or may be covered only if an existing first-line treatment has been tried but failed to produce results.

After these basic questions are answered, the next phase in the analysis involves a closer look at the existing environment. This may have been done in order to understand whether or not there are any potential competitors, but assuming that competitors exist, the next step is to determine if the new item or service is distinguishable and whether or not that will have any impact on coverage. One critical factor in defining the relevant coverage standard is how the item or service can be compared to other treatments for a given condition. Depending on the nature and scope of the innovation, it may be classified as (1) a breakthrough for patient health that fills a gap in treatment options or offers a treatment where none previously existed; (2) something that replaces an existing item or service; or (3) a product that adds or extends an existing technology or procedure.

Another practical consideration in developing a coverage strategy is the pace of adoption of the new technology. In a paper published in 2000, it was estimated that the average time for published clinical trial data to be translated into general medical practice was 17 years; since that time, the lag time has not changed significantly [20]. While that lag time may be shorter today for innovators and other stakeholders in new technologies, the rate of adoption of new items and services can be a significant factor in planning market entry. That rate can be highly variable from one health plan to another; in the case of an assay used to assist in the treatment of breast cancer, the earliest adopters agreed to provide coverage approximately 1 year after the product's launch while the last adopters took up to an additional 6 years to approve coverage; the median time here was 3 years [21].

Identifying the Type and Quality of Data to Support Coverage

In the current health-care environment, regardless of the pace of adoption, outcomes evidence is a paramount concern for health plans and other payers [22]. For investigators, manufacturers, and other stakeholders identifying the type of data needed to make the strongest case for coverage can be a conundrum given the ambiguity and discretion given to health plans to make coverage determinations. The burden is usually placed on the applicant, and the type of data needed to support coverage differs from the data submitted to the FDA to meet the safe and effective standard under the FDCA. The shift toward evidence-based medical policy therefore relies on published, peer-reviewed studies with sufficient statistical power to establish a given treatment hypothesis, commonly over a long term [23]. While this would call for large randomized, double-blinded studies in all circumstances, this ideal may have to be tempered by practical or ethical considerations that make other acceptable study designs feasible for their intended purpose. As a result, while it may be appropriate to conduct a drug trial involving one arm where a subject receives a placebo, in a device trial involving an implant or an invasive procedure there may be unacceptable and unethical risks if the subjects with the control arm are subjected to a sham surgical procedure; moreover, even if these hurdles could be overcome, a significant number of prospective subjects may refuse to participate under those terms, thwarting any attempt to enroll a sufficient number of subjects to ensure adequate statistical power after an expected number of dropouts. In these cases, other acceptable study designs such as case–control studies may be necessary in order to obtain any useful information at all.

Once a decision about the type of optimal study design has been made, the next step will likely involve defining the population to be studied. The Medicare program and some private payers may demand that the study population match their beneficiaries or covered lives so that the outcomes data are more accurate. This issue was central to the Medicare National Coverage Determination denying coverage for virtual colonoscopies using CT imaging [24]. Although many private health plans did offer limited coverage for CT colonographies, CMS focused its evidence review on how CT colonography compared to optical colonoscopy in the Medicare population, of whom the majority are over the age of 65. It concluded that the available evidence was deficient in part because the published studies contained only a few subjects which were eligible for Medicare, and because CMS could not determine if the results of CT colonography in younger subjects could be applied to the Medicare population [25].

A separate but related coverage issue that should be addressed arises when a new technology has multiple applications, but either the available data or the data that is anticipated is weaker for some potential applications. In these cases, the sponsor or stakeholders will need to make a business decision to focus on the one indication with the best chances for success rather than risk rejection of a request for broader coverage.

Regardless of the type of clinical data that is available or that can be obtained in a clinical trial, the presentation of that data can be enhanced through the participation of professional organizations or thought leaders in a particular specialty who can help bridge the gap between an entity seeking to commercialize an innovation and the health plans that may rely solely on the data before them. The assistance from such organizations and physician-champions can assist in educating payers and explain the reasons why a new technology should be adopted from a clinician's point of view.

The evolution of coverage into a detailed evidence-driven process begs an important question, that is, what if this pathway will not work in an individual case? In other words, is there any middle ground between coverage and noncoverage? In a small number of cases, the new technology or a related service may have promising outcomes and hold out the prospect of cost savings but may lack the quantity or quality of data that would otherwise support a fully favorable determination. In these cases, CMS and some other payers may approve coverage on a temporary basis, typically conditioned on a manufacturer or other stakeholder agreeing to conduct additional acceptable clinical trials or establish a registry and furnish the data to be collected to the payer or plan. After a set time period, the plan can make a permanent coverage decision. In the Medicare program, this has been known as coverage with evidence development [26].

Defining the Coding to Define the Innovation

The introduction of a new technology can have disruptive effects on the delivery of a particular treatment or therapy. One aspect of that disruption is how a provider or supplier captures the use of that technology and attempts to obtain payment. In the absence of a defined code or reimbursement rate, several interim solutions are possible, albeit with varying degrees of risk. First, a provider or supplier may submit claims using a miscellaneous code for procedures or items not otherwise defined in the relevant code set. This allows the provider, supplier, or manufacturer to negotiate a reimbursement rate. In the short run, it allows for some form of payment until a new code and a defined reimbursement rate can be established. There are several key drawbacks to this approach: claims may have to be submitted manually, reimbursement rates can vary significantly among payers, and establishing a database of payments for future use if a new code is approved may be complicated. A second option that has been used for some diagnostics is to break down the steps of the new technology and where possibly assign an existing code to each step, resulting in a sequence of multiple codes in a single claim—often referred to as a "stack"—that when assembled capture all of the resources that went into the service. Once again, the benefit in the short run is that there is a positive cash flow, at the expense of an imperfect claims database to establish a reimbursement rate in the long term. In more egregious cases involving claims submitted to government-funded programs, there is always a risk that unbundling a procedure for any reason could trigger investigations and potential liability under health-care fraud laws, particularly the False Claims Act [27].

What if the new technology, or a service using that technology, cannot be defined using an existing code? Once again, although there are well-defined processes for obtaining new codes, they can be cumbersome and time-consuming, and the standards for approval of a new code can be vague. For example, although the HCPCS Workgroup has developed a decision tree for code requests, the criteria applied for each step are not always transparent [28]. Similarly, while the CPT Editorial Panel has published criteria for new procedure codes, there is a wide degree of latitude in applying those criteria [29]. In general, the entities that control code sets will rely on technological distinctions, clinical improvement, and whether or not the new item or service requires a different or more intense mix of resources to deliver a service. If this is the best option for a manufacturer or stakeholder, the strategy must also factor in the lag period between a coding application and any new code; new CPT codes are assigned on a 2-year cycle and HCPCS codes follow a 1-year cycle.

Positioning the Product for Favorable Reimbursement

All of the work to obtain a favorable coverage determination and a fair coding assignment leads to the last and crucial step in commercializing any new product or service using that new product: what will health plans pay for the item or service? As with coverage and coding, this portion of the analysis does not exist in a vacuum without relevant information as a guide. As with the earlier parts of determining a commercialization strategy, several basic questions should be considered as follows:

- What are the code(s) for similar items or services?
- What is the reimbursement methodology for the relevant site(s) of service for the new item or service?
- What is the range of reimbursement for those existing codes?
- Is that range acceptable, or are there quantitative or qualitative distinctions between the current standard of care and the new technology that may justify a higher reimbursement rate?

As previously discussed, the term "reimbursement" does not refer to a single concept. Depending on the site of service, reimbursement may refer to a payment amount for the new item or service on a stand-alone basis or may refer to the same item or service as part of a bundled payment to the provider or supplier of services to an individual patient. These bundles can have different names such as a DRG for inpatient hospital services and an ambulatory payment classification for outpatient or ambulatory surgical center services, but they typically include all items and services needed to treat a particular condition (as designated by procedure code(s) or a discharge diagnosis code) except for professional fees that are claimed separately. The actual rate for a particular condition is commonly determined based on historical claims data that is trended forward, with adjustments for variables such as case-mix intensity and relative labor costs [30]. Therefore once all these questions have been answered, a reimbursement strategy can begin to take shape. One potential risk for manufacturers of medical devices and diagnostics is that if FDA clearance is based on substantial equivalence under Section 501(k) of the FDCA, some health plans may attempt to apply the same code and reimbursement rate for the predicate product to the new technology. If this threatens the commercialization of the product, the rebuttal to any such proposal would have to be based on data that may be outside the scope of the FDA's review, such as data showing superior clinical outcomes or a different cost basis. Regardless of the setting, if payment is made on a bundled basis, the manufacturer or other stakeholder must examine both its cost of doing business and the economic constraints placed on the provider or supplier purchasing the new product. For the prospective purchaser, the switch to a new technology may involve a trade-off between the higher cost of adopting a new technology and the expected relative efficiencies or improved outcomes that are expected. If the new technology lowers costs and improves outcomes, adoption is easy; however, if the provider's or supplier's overall costs rise too dramatically, then it may not be able to adopt the new technology without incurring losses on each patient treated. The strategy may become more complicated if the shift to the new technology also affects any related professional fee, as may be the case with implanted medical devices. In these cases, the total service must make economic sense to the facility and to the physician, who is likely to be sensitive to changes in the time and effort required to perform procedures using the new technology and how that is reflected in the applicable CPT code for that service.

Putting the Pieces of the Puzzle Together

Developing a successful commercialization strategy for a new technology, or for services using that technology requires that the coverage, coding, and reimbursement pieces fall into place. Due to the number of variables discussed in this chapter, innovators and stakeholders should anticipate some challenges and should expect that the path will be different for each new product. Coordinating and executing each part of a commercialization strategy takes patience, perseverance, excellent information, help from others, and good timing. Although these processes are difficult, thoughtful planning can be an essential tool for meeting these challenges.

European Reimbursement Systems Overview[2]

In Europe, reimbursement and pricing is determined on a country-by-country basis, leading to significant variations in system design, cost, and coverage. In addition, each country has the ability to control reimbursement at the national, regional, or local level. As can be seen in Fig. 33.3, significant variation in pricing, health technology assessment (HTA), and reimbursement negotiation processes exist across countries in Europe.

Regulatory Backdrop

The European Medicines Agency (EMA) is responsible for reviewing and approving all drug products sold in Europe through a centralized process. Operating as a decentralized scientific agency of the European Union, the agency is responsible for coordinating the EU's safety-monitoring or "pharmacovigilance" system for medicines. Specifically, it coordinates the evaluation and monitoring of centrally authorized products and national referrals, develops technical guidance, and provides scientific advice to sponsors [31].

	National price negotiation	Price referencing	IPR	National HE evaluation	Regional HE evaluation	Local price negotiation
France	■	■	■	■	■	■
Germany	■	■	■	■		■
Italy	■	■	■	■	■	■
Spain	■	■	■	■	■	■
England	■			■	■	■
Scotland				■	■	■
Wales				■		■

FIGURE 33.3 Variability in pricing, HTA and reimbursement in Europe. *HTA*, Health technology assessment.

2. The second part of this chapter is written by Susan Garfield.

While drugs must go through the EMA to receive market authorization, diagnostics and devices go through a different process. These types of technologies require a CE-mark from the European Commission, though many tests can be used prior to or without regulatory approval through a laboratory-developed test pathway. In the case of medical technologies, the CE-mark denotes a product's compliance with relevant EU legislation and directives and enables commercialization of the product within the European Union.

Health Technology Assessment

Once a product has received marketing authorization, the reimbursement process begins. In many countries, prior to pricing and coverage, a product must go through a formal HTA process. HTAs systematically examine the short- and long-term health and cost consequences of using a specific technology or set of technologies [32]. The consequences that are considered within an HTA include the direct medical, organizational, economic, and societal impact of use to a given health system. Individuals involved in HTAs in Europe include clinical specialists, economists, policy makers, and statisticians. HTA groups use a variety of methods to consider the comparative impact use that a technology will have to affected populations. HTA analyses typically reflect a specific country's or region's perspective, including disease burden, demographics, and costs.

Elements of a national or regional HTA analysis may include considerations of equity across the population, cost-impact, cost-effectiveness, time horizon of expected benefit, and pure clinical health outcomes. HTA decision-makers are usually considering the comparative effect of a new product against the existing standard of care in that country or region.

The National Institute of Clinical Excellence (NICE) in the United Kingdom and the Institut für Qualität und Wirtschaftlichkeit im Gesundheitswesen in Germany are examples of national HTA groups. The Catalan Agency for Health Information, Assessment and Quality is an example of a regional HTA body in Spain. In many countries, affiliated institutions and academic groups conduct assessments on behalf of decision-making bodies. Italy provides a good example of this where strong regional governments allow regional HTAs to be conducted through universities or other locally founded groups. One of the more active regions, Veneto, conducts HTA assessments through the pharmacy service group, UVEF (Unita di Valutazione dell'Efficacia del Farmaco) at the University of Veneto.

Pricing

Each country in Europe has country-specific pricing and reimbursement systems. Pricing for novel pharmaceutical products is largely based on benefit (or value) assessments by payers or on comparator products and prices in other markets [international price referencing (IPR)]. IPR in most markets leads to a cascade effect of pricing outcomes. When one country sets a price, other countries which reference that country's prices are automatically impacted. As a result, any market that is referenced by other markets has both a significant in-country and external effect—or reference—when a price is established. Fig. 33.4 depicts the complexity and the interrelated nature of the IPR system whereby countries set their own drug prices based on the prices established in other markets.

In several countries, such as Italy and Spain, pricing decisions are made at the national level, while access is determined at the regional level. For many years, the United Kingdom and Germany were the only two European countries with free pricing for pharmaceuticals, meaning the manufacturer could set the price of the product rather than the government setting the price through price negotiation or referencing. Germany, however, recently instituted a series of reform laws that changed the pricing structure for pharmaceuticals, creating a system of initial free pricing which is then subjected to a benefits assessment by the government. Such assessments of medical and relative economic benefit are commonplace in the French market and not too dissimilar from the framework in Germany. The results of this process have significantly impacted pricing outcomes for new products in Germany. The United Kingdom is currently undergoing increasing adoption of "value-based pricing (VBP)" process into routine assessment of new medical technologies.

Pricing decisions for therapies have historically been conducted separately from those related to diagnostics. While pricing for diagnostics may be related to fee schedules, tied to specific codes, or established at the hospital or laboratory level, drug pricing is usually product-specific and can have cross-border implications as a result of international referencing. Currently, no countries have an established VBP pathway for novel diagnostics. Instead, companies with high-value products attempt to work with payers and other decision-makers to enable access on a country-by-country, region-by-region, and in some cases hospital-by-hospital level.

Cost containment is a major priority for health systems in Europe and pharmaceuticals have been a target for budget reductions in many settings. Reforms to health

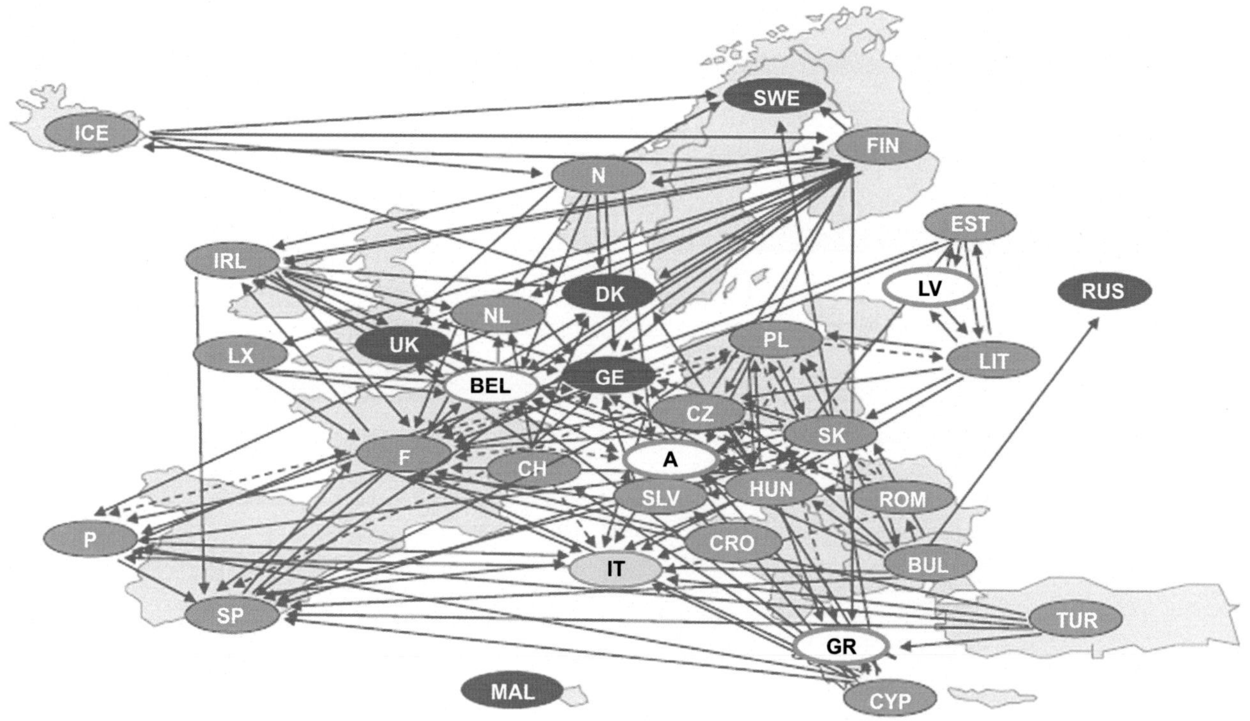

FIGURE 33.4 Complexity of the international pricing reference system.

systems have arisen as the result of a variety of reasons but none more visible than the drive toward austerity, judicious use of resources, and social rebalancing that is impacting many European markets. This impact has been acutely felt by manufacturers of innovative health technologies and will continue to be a factor in most European markets. It is expected that ongoing price pressures will be applied by European health systems as they attempt to manage escalating costs associated with an aging population. (See Figs. 33.5 and 33.6.)

Reimbursement Mechanisms

Most countries in Europe have different mechanisms to reimburse for health-related goods and services. Across countries, most hospital-related costs are reimbursed using a DRG-based system. DRGs are global payments that provide lump sum payment to hospitals to cover all goods and services provided during the course of that stay. In most settings the DRG is based on a patient's primary diagnosis or primary procedure and has the ability to be classified by severity to differentiate routine from complex cases. DRGs allow hospitals to manage care and purchasing decisions and offer little opportunity for separate, or product-specific reimbursement. In many markets, there are routes to funding outside of the DRG for "expensive" or innovative drugs that would significantly disrupt the DRG. This includes exclusion from the Tarification à l'Activité (T2A) list (France), application for a Neue Untersuchungs- und Behandlungsmethoden (Germany).

For outpatient care, there is a mix of fee-for-service, global payment, capitated, and self-pay structures throughout Europe. In countries, such as France and the United Kingdom, where socialized health systems guarantee citizens a minimum level of care paid for by government health insurance, there is very little out-of-pocket cost associated with routine care. Patients do have the option to purchase noncovered services, such as advanced diagnostics, though practices vary by market as does access to private supplemental insurance. Diagnostics are predominantly paid for out-of-hospital and/or laboratory budgets or in some cases based on code-specific fee schedules. Surprisingly, the diagnostic reimbursement pathways in many European countries are not as clearly defined or sophisticated as those for drugs. Consequently, most diagnostic procedures are reimbursed in whole or in part by the national payer directly to hospitals, pharmacies, clinicians, or via patient reimbursement from the drugs budget.

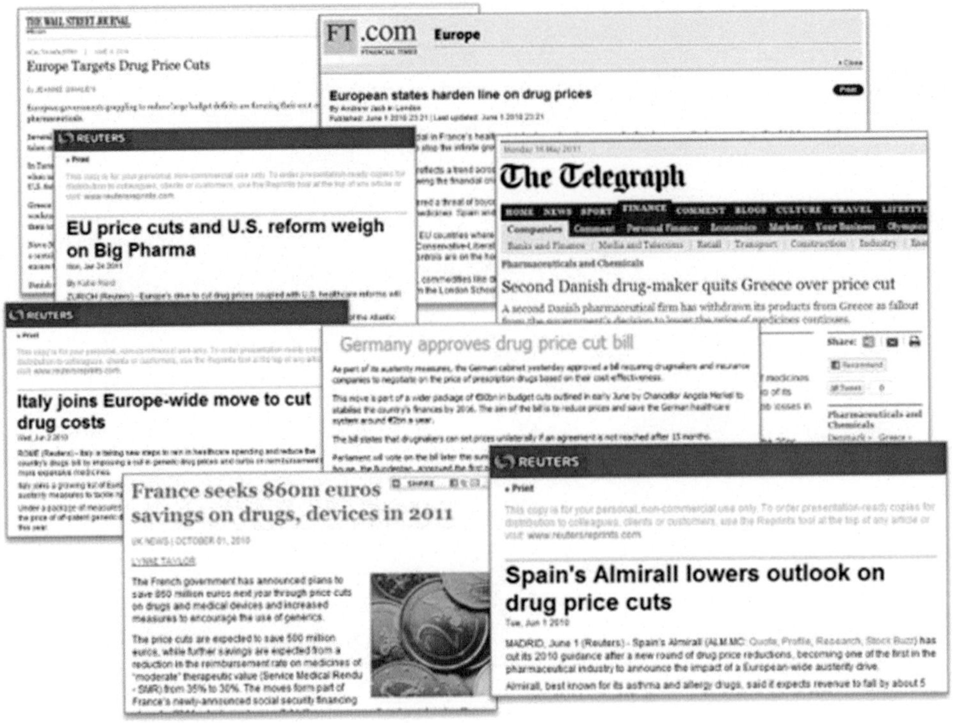

FIGURE 33.5 Illustrative examples of European initiatives to target cost control measures for pharmaceuticals.

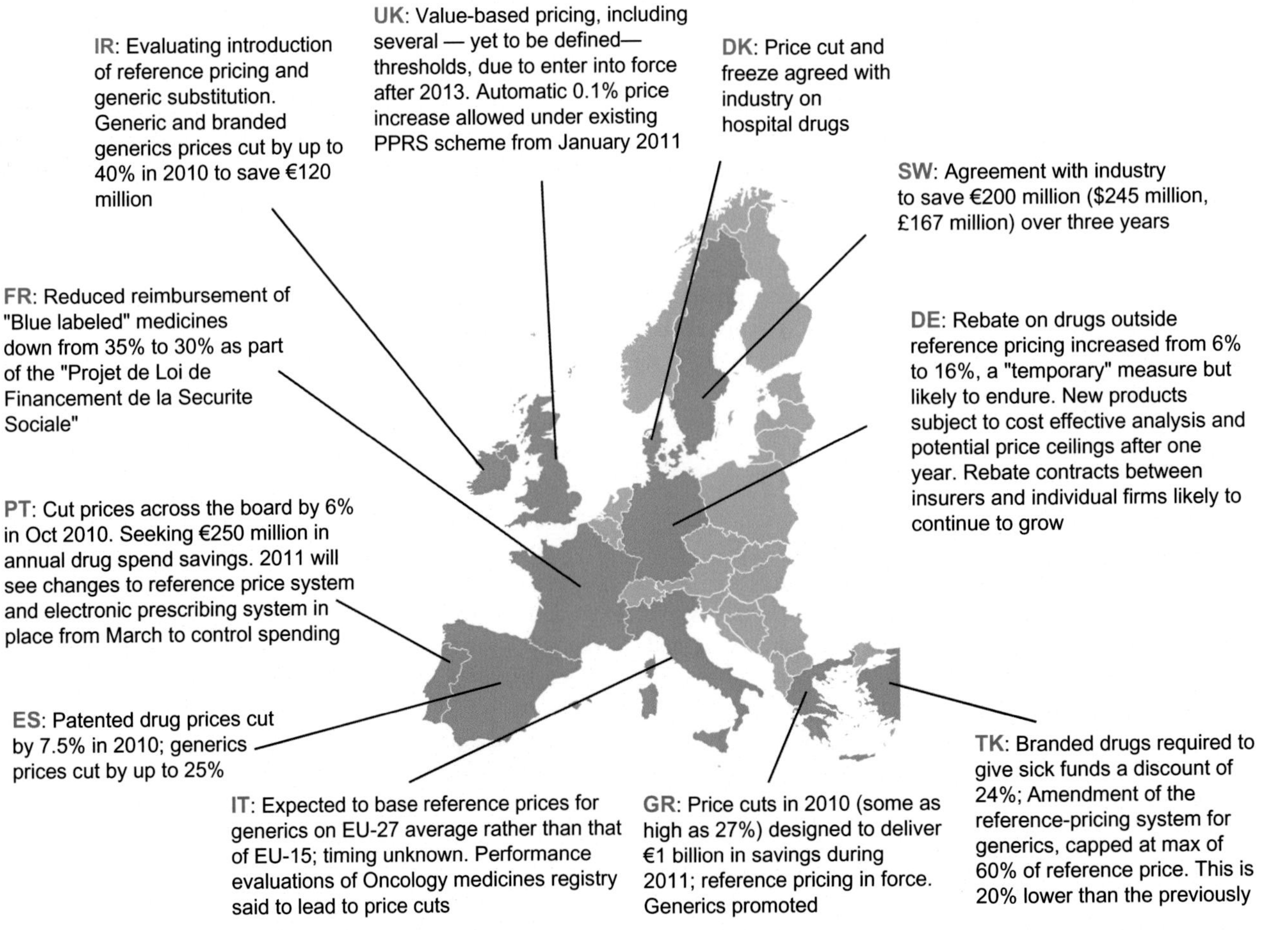

UK: Value-based pricing, including several — yet to be defined— thresholds, due to enter into force after 2013. Automatic 0.1% price increase allowed under existing PPRS scheme from January 2011
IR: Evaluating introduction of reference pricing and generic substitution. Generic and branded generics prices cut by up to 40% in 2010 to save €120 million
DK: Price cut and freeze agreed with industry on hospital drugs
SW: Agreement with industry to save €200 million ($245 million, £167 million) over three years
FR: Reduced reimbursement of "Blue labeled" medicines down from 35% to 30% as part of the "Projet de Loi de Financement de la Securite Sociale"
DE: Rebate on drugs outside reference pricing increased from 6% to 16%, a "temporary" measure but likely to endure. New products subject to cost effective analysis and potential price ceilings after one year. Rebate contracts between insurers and individual firms likely to continue to grow
PT: Cut prices across the board by 6% in Oct 2010. Seeking €250 million in annual drug spend savings. 2011 will see changes to reference price system and electronic prescribing system in place from March to control spending
ES: Patented drug prices cut by 7.5% in 2010; generics prices cut by up to 25%
IT: Expected to base reference prices for generics on EU-27 average rather than that of EU-15; timing unknown. Performance evaluations of Oncology medicines registry said to lead to price cuts
GR: Price cuts in 2010 (some as high as 27%) designed to deliver €1 billion in savings during 2011; reference pricing in force. Generics promoted
TK: Branded drugs required to give sick funds a discount of 24%; Amendment of the reference-pricing system for generics, capped at max of 60% of reference price. This is 20% lower than the previously

FIGURE 33.6 Examples of European pricing and reimbursement cost containment initiatives.

Reimbursement Outcomes

While each European country acts independently when it comes to reimbursement decision-making, there are cross-border implications. For example, in the United Kingdom, NICE makes public their HTA decisions. It is broadly considered that NICE review standards are sophisticated and thorough and, as a result, payers and HTA organizations in other countries often refer to NICE guidance—officially and unofficially—as they develop their own perspectives and assessments. Countries are continuously evolving their reimbursement systems to meet the needs of a rapidly changing health-care landscape. This includes health-care technologies based on complex genetic information, products that provide remote monitoring of patients, advanced biotechnology–based therapies that require specific handling and administration, advanced imaging modalities, and other innovations. Each of these unique innovations and paradigm-shifting new technologies challenges the health-care system's existing framework for evaluation, pricing, and payment pathways. Cell and gene therapies are the latest major therapeutic opportunity with significant reimbursement challenges given high upfront costs.

A Closer Look at Reimbursement in Five Key European Markets

In the United Kingdom, the National Health Service (NHS) provides health care and coverage to all citizens [33]. Individuals can purchase private insurance to supplement NHS care or for payment for noncovered treatments and services. In England, Clinical Commissioning Groups (CCGs) receive around 60% of the NHS budget and are responsible for the commissioning of a wide range of services, including hospital and community care for the local population they serve. The commissioning of services outside the remit of CCGs, such as specialized hospital services and primary care, remains the responsibility of NHS England. However, as part of the NHS Five Year Forward View, NHS England is supporting cocommissioning and delegated commissioning of GP services to CCGs in order to support the development of integrated, high quality, and out-of-hospital care.

In the United Kingdom, there is currently a system of free pricing managed through the Pharmaceutical Price Regulation Scheme system. VBP supplanted the system in 2014 and applies to all innovative medicines brought to market after the initiation of the program. "Innovative" applies any "new chemical entity." The process emphasizes cost-effectiveness, as measured by cost per quality-adjusted life year, reflecting a base case and additional factors (therapeutic innovation, burden of illness, therapeutic improvement, and wider societal benefit). Within the system, there are opportunities for products addressing significant unmet need to move through streamlined processes. VBP at the national level does not remove the need for local negotiation for access and uptake.

Today, many products are reviewed for inclusion within the NHS system by NICE, a system that is regarded as challenging, with a high burden of clinical, economic, and substantiation required to demonstrate successful outcomes. Thresholds are, increasingly, becoming more strict and data requirements more onerous according to many companies. Due to the rigor required to substantiate value in the eyes of NICE, advanced analysis, adept foresight, and a more than marginal clinical benefit is often required to successfully navigate HTA assessment in the United Kingdom.

The vast majority of the German population is covered by a "Bismarck" insurance fund-based system. Statutory health insurance funds (SHIs) are responsible for the costs of health-care provision to their insured population. Private insurance coverage can only be used to supplement improved services or if an individual's yearly income exceeds a predefined level (49,950 EUR in 2010). Traditionally, hospitals are publicly funded institutions, providing only inpatient care, while ambulatory care is supplied by private practices which are paid by SHIs and private insurance. Reimbursement for diagnostics and drugs is dependent on the site of care. In the inpatient system, both are predominantly covered under a DRG global payment system. In the outpatient environment, reimbursement for drugs and diagnostics is provided based on contracted charges (drugs) and a code-based fee schedule (diagnostics). Under the Arzneimittelmarkt-Neuordnungsgesetz (AMNOG) drug pricing legislation previously mentioned, Germany has moved from free pricing to a system of benefit assessment. The Act on the Reform of the Market for Medical Products (AMNOG) process enables drugs that are deemed to have additional clinical benefit to achieve premium pricing through a series of negotiation and arbitration processes. Fig. 33.7 illustrates the process that provides opportunity to assess clinical and cost benefit against a government-chosen standard.

In Italy the national health-care system (Servizio Sanitario Nazionale—SSN) provides health-care coverage to the population through public financing and a mixture of public and private provision of care. The Italian system is largely decentralized and can be broken down into the following three levels: national, regional, and local. The responsibility for delivering hospital and community services falls to the regional level. Local health units (Azienda Sanitaria Locale) coordinate all nonemergency care and are funded by the SSN through a per capita

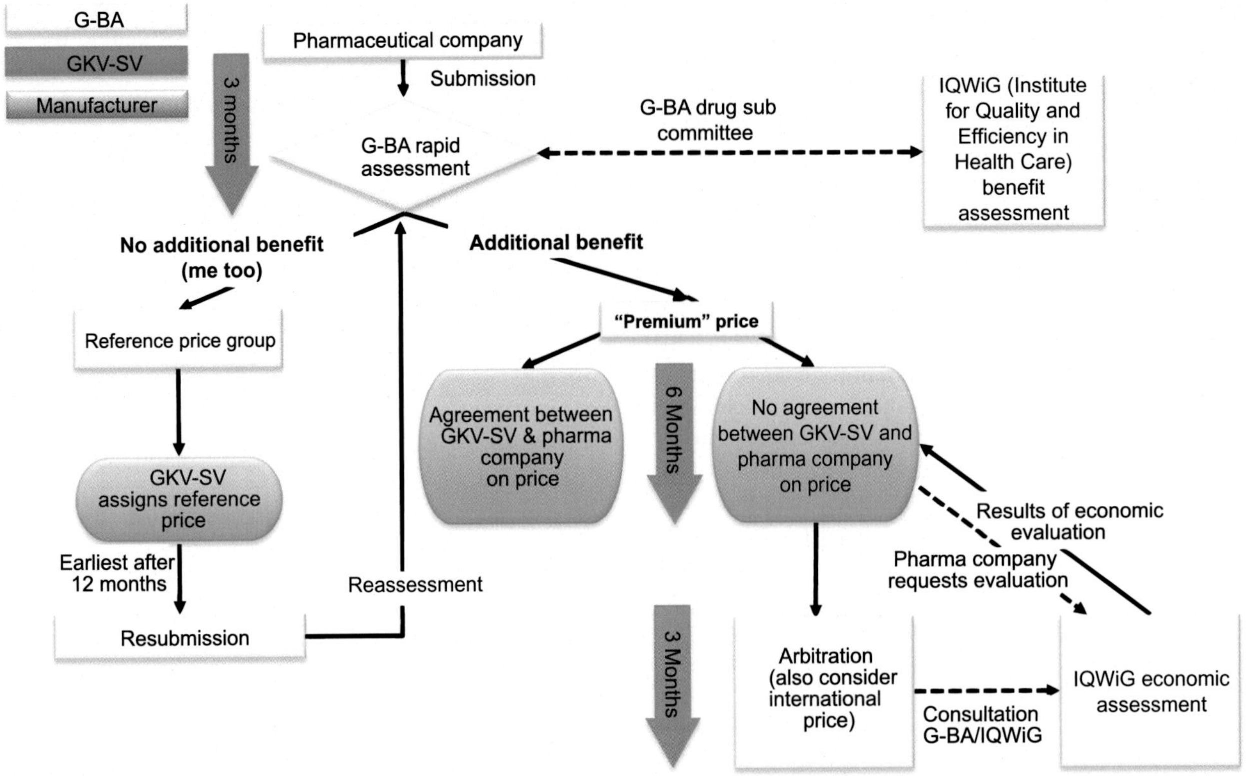

FIGURE 33.7 AMNOG process for assessing clinical and cost benefit against a government chosen standard. *AMNOG*, Arzneimittelmarkt-Neuordnungsgesetz. *Adapted from Skavron R. Germany: latest developments in pricing and reimbursement policy. G-BA 23 March 2011.*

budget. Public and private health-care providers (whether they provide in-patient and/or out-patient care) are remunerated through a fee-for-service system based on two formulary lists, with different tariff levels. Both lists are based on the ICD-10-CM WHO Classification of Diseases and Procedures. The Italian Medicines Agency is the national authority responsible for drug regulation, pricing, and evaluation in Italy.

The French population is almost universally covered (99% of the population) by statutory health insurance (assurance-maladie), managed by the Haute Autorité de Santé (HAS). HAS is in charge of evaluating drugs, devices, diagnostics, and other products. The Commission d'Evaluation des Médicaments (Transparency Commission), within HAS, is used to assess the clinical value provided by a new product and the improvement it will provide subsequent to its use. The opinion is based on a value analysis or SMR (Service Medical Rendu)—that considers whether the product should be reimbursed and what could be the reimbursement rate, comparative assessment of clinical benefit assessment or Amelioration du SMR—the grading that provides a basis for price fixing in comparison with alternatives, and what the target population eligible for treatment should be. The Agence Française de Securité Sanitaire des Produits de Santé carries out scientific and medico-economic evaluation as part of this system. Drugs used in the outpatient setting have patient cost-sharing associated with them in most cases. This cost sharing, however, is often covered by private insurance "mutuelles," under which the vast majority of the French population is covered [34]. Since 2004, hospitals have been funded through DRGs, with most drugs and diagnostics included in the global payment system (although some high-priced drugs are funded separately).

The Spanish health-care system (Sistema Nacional de la Salud) is compulsory and publicly funded, with administration performed at the regional level through regional health authorities (RHA). Roughly, 15% of the population has supplemental private insurance to augment the statutory coverage, which the entire population enjoys. The RHAs fund hospitals within their regions through prospective budgets. The basis for budget allocation is largely derived from the population within the hospital area. Outpatient services are covered based on regional decision-making, largely through a fee-for-service mechanism. A national HTA agency (Instituto de Salud Carlos III-ISCIII) and several regional HTA organizations coexist in the country. Reimbursement is considered at the national level through the Spanish Ministry of Health, while pricing is determined by the Inter-Ministerial Pricing Commission CIPM (La Comisión Interministerial de Precios de los Medicamentos).

European Pricing and Reimbursement Summary

Tensions continue to grow as European payers attempt to manage costs and continue to improve the quality of healthcare for their constituents. Payers are increasingly relying on methods for cost containment, including the following:

- Increasing the role of HTAs
- Price cuts
- Comparative effectiveness requirements
- VBP
- Risk-sharing schemes
- Access with evidence development
- IPR

Because of this trend, innovators must plan for different approaches to product evaluation and in order to meet the needs of HTA organizations. This means that evidence-development planning must be considered early in the product development life cycle to support product value propositions and evaluation by HTAs. In addition, the varying information requirements of regulatory agencies, HTAs, and payers across Europe must be taken into account. This can include requirements for country-specific data, varying types of health economic analyses, or analysis against a specific comparator considered the standard of care in a given context. Industry can then work with payers in each country to establish product value using the various mechanisms available.

While reimbursement systems have strict processes in place to ensure rationale use of resources, opportunities for innovation exist. Funding pathways for unmet needs and high-value treatments persist, with some preferential treatment of drugs for orphan conditions, for example, still in place. In the new world of comparative effectiveness and strict HTA-based evaluations, products most at risk for noncoverage are "me-too" treatments that cannot demonstrate significant incremental value or are significantly more expensive (and similarly or less effective) than the current standard of care.

Across markets, companies are recognizing the additional risk related to pricing and reimbursement beyond regulatory approval. This is impacting early product planning and "go" and "no go" decisions to advance products in development. The uncertainty in terms of reimbursement and pricing has impacted the valuations of many medical technologies, especially those with a significant focus on Europe. Moving forward, EU countries are expected to provide greater clarity in terms of evidence requirements and pricing expectations, which should hopefully, lead to more innovative and impactful health technologies reaching the European markets.

References

[1] 21 U.S.C. §§ 301 et seq.; 21 C.F.R. §§ 200–299 (Drug Regulations); 21 C.F.R. §§ 300–499 (human drug regulations); 21 C.F.R. §§ 600–799 (biological regulations); and 21 C.F.R. §§ 800–1299 (medical device regulations); see also Riegel v. Medtronic, 552 U.S. 352 (2008).

[2] Goodman v. Sullivan, 891 F.2d 449, 451 (2d Cir. 1989) (The Medicare program was not obligated to cover a diagnostic test based only on the FDA's approval of the test.).

[3] CMS and FDA have started a pilot parallel review program under which a limited number of medical products would be considered by each agency simultaneously. 75 Fed. Reg. 57045 (2010) and 76 Fed. Reg. 62808 (2011).

[4] See, for example, Hays v. Sebelius, 589 F.3d 1229 (D.C. Cir. 2009).

[5] See Goodman, note 4, supra.

[6] 42 U.S.C. § 1395y(a).

[7] 42 U.S.C. § 1395y(a).

[8] These state laws have been supplemented by Section 10103(c) of the Patient Protection and Affordable Care Act, Pub. L. No. 111–148. <https://www.asco.org/research-progress/clinical-trials/insurance-coverage-clinical-trials#statelaws>; 2010 [accessed March 27, 2019].

[9] See, for example, 42 U.S.C. § 1395y(a)(1)(A).

[10] See, for example, Neumann P, Chambers J. Medicare's enduring struggle to define 'reasonable and necessary' care. N Engl J Med 2012;367:1775–7.

[11] See, for example, Medicare National Coverage Determinations Manual, § 20.4 (coverage of implantable defibrillators).

[12] Id., §110.8.1 (coverage of stem cell transplantation); see also Neumann P, Tunis S. Medicare and medical technology—the growing demand for relevant outcomes. N Engl J Med 2010;362:377–9.

[13] 42 U.S.C. §§ 1395y(l), 1395w–22, and 1395 mm; 42 C.F.R. § 400.202.

[14] See, for example, Centers for Medicare and Medicaid Services, Innovator's Guide to Navigating Medicare, Version 3.0 (2015) at 16. Available from: <https://www.cms.gov/Medicare/Coverage/CouncilonTechInnov/Downloads/Innovators-Guide-Master-7-23-15.pdf> [accessed March 27, 2019].

[15] See, for example, Centers for Medicare and Medicaid Services, Innovator's Guide to Navigating Medicare, Version 3.0 (2015) at 31–55. Available from: <https://www.cms.gov/Medicare/Coverage/CouncilonTechInnov/Downloads/Innovators-Guide-Master-7-23-15.pdf> [accessed March 27, 2019].

[16] 42 U.S.C. § 1395ww(d)(5)(K-L) and 42 C.F.R. § 412.87(b) (inpatient); 42 U.S.C. § 13951 (t)(6) and 42 C.F.R. §§ 419.62–419.66 (outpatient).

[17] 42 U.S.C. § 1395y(a)(1)(A).

[18] See, for example, Regence Blue Cross and Blue Shield, medical policy development and review process. Available from: <http://blue.regence.com/trgmedpol/intro/> [accessed March 27, 2019].

[19] An example of this is the Blue Cross Blue Shield Evidence Street. <https://app.evidencestreet.com/> [accessed March 27, 2019].

[20] Morris Z, Wooding S, Grant J. The answer is 17 years, what is the question: understanding time lags in translational research. J R Soc Med 2011;104:510–20.

[21] Health Advances. The reimbursement landscape for novel diagnostics 11. Available from: <https://healthadvances.com/admin/resources/noveldiagreimbursement.pdf?ok> [accessed March 27, 2019].

[22] See Neumann P, et al., note 12, supra.

[23] See, for example Eddy D. Evidence-based medicine: a unified approach. Health Aff 2005;24(1):9–17.

[24] Centers for Medicare and Medicaid Services, Decision Memo for Screening Computed Tomography Colonography for Colorectal Cancer. Available from: <https://www.cms.gov/medicare-coverage-database/details/nca-decision-memo.aspx?NCAId = 220&ver = 19&NcaName = Screening + Computed + Tomography + Colonography + (CTC) + for + Colorectal + Cancer&CoverageSelection = Both&ArticleType = All&PolicyType = Final&s = All&KeyWord = colonography&KeyWordLookUp = Title&KeyWordLookUp = Title&KeyWordLookUp = Title&KeyWordSearchType = And&KeyWordSearchType = And&KeyWordSearchType = And&bc = gAAAABAAIAAA&>; 2009 [accessed March 27, 2019].

[25] In addition, CMS was concerned that the data in the available studies found that the CT colonographies showed a lower sensitivity and specificity for polyps smaller than 6 mm when compared to optical colonoscopy.

[26] Centers for Medicare and Medicaid Services. Guidance for the public, industry, and CMS staff: coverage with evidence development. Available from: <https://www.cms.gov/medicare-coverage-database/details/medicare-coverage-document-details.aspx?MCDId = 27>; November 2014 [accessed March 27, 2019].

[27] See, for example, Government Accountability Office. Medicare laboratory tests: implementation of new rates may lead to billions in excess payments. Available from: <https://www.gao.gov/assets/700/695756.pdf>; November 2018 [accessed March 27, 2019]; HHS Office of Inspector General. Questionable billing for Medicare Part B Clinical Laboratory Services at 2. Available from: <https://oig.hhs.gov/oei/reports/oei-03-11-00730.asp>; 2014 [accessed March 27, 2019].

[28] <https://www.cms.gov/Medicare/Coding/MedHCPCSGenInfo/Downloads/HCPCS_Decision_Tree_and_Definitions.pdf> [accessed March 27, 2019].

[29] American Medical Association, CPT 2018 Professional Edition at xii–xvii (2018). The difficulty in selecting the correct code and documenting the basis for selecting a code has been recognized to a limited extent by the Medicare program, which set a uniform reimbursement rate effective January 1, 2019 for a group of office-based evaluation and management services. 83 Fed. Reg. 59452, 59625–59653 (November 23, 2018).

[30] See Medicare Payment Advisory Commission. Payment basics: hospital acute inpatient services. <http://medpac.gov/docs/default-source/payment-basics/medpac_payment_basics_18_hospital_final_v2_sec.pdf?sfvrsn = 0>; 2018 [accessed March 27, 2019].

[31] <https://www.ema.europa.eu/en> [accessed March 30, 2019].

[32] Henshall C, et al. Priority setting for health technology assessment: theoretical considerations and practical approaches. Int J Tech Assess Health Care 1997;13:144–85.

[33] Scotland, Wales, and Northern Ireland have separate systems for evaluation and payment for health services.

[34] Buchmueller T., Couffinhal A. Private health insurance in France. OECD; 2004.

Chapter 34

Getting the Word Out: Public Relations Strategies to Support Biotechnology Business Goals

Joan E. Kureczka, MSEM

Senior Vice President and Stacey Shackford, Director, Social Media. Bioscribe, Inc., California

Chapter Outline

Let's say you just formed your new company. You've got a great idea, gained rights to the intellectual property around your technology or potential product, and assembled your start-up team. You've raised a small amount of money to move things forward using your own capital along with a few "friends and family" investors. Perhaps you even obtained a "seed" round of financing from some angel investors or a venture capital firm. Your research is going well. Now it's time to take things to the next level. However, you are finding that it is very competitive "out there." According to a 2018 report from Techonomy Partners LLC, the Biotechnology Innovation Organization, and Public Affairs Consultants, there were over 85,000 US bioscience establishments as of 2016, which included agricultural and industrial biotech firms; therapeutics and diagnostics developers; medical device companies; research, testing, and medical laboratories; and bioscience-related distribution companies. The vast majority of these companies are private. While each year we see some of these organizations leave the field through mergers or for various other reasons, each year also brings a new crop of start-up companies. All of these businesses are constantly competing with you for investment dollars and funding, corporate partnerships or customers, research collaborators and patients, and for great employees and contractors.

Early-stage biotechnology companies face communication challenges specific to their industry. If you are working in a healthcare-related field, such as therapeutics, diagnostics, or medical technology, you need to consider how regulators view your technology and products, as well as the doctors and patients who will use them. Future payers, including governmental organizations like Medicare and other large healthcare providers and insurance companies, must also be convinced of the value of your technology in order to smooth the path toward coverage and reimbursement. If your business is in a field, such as agricultural biotechnology, or you are introducing new technology with potential environmental or social

Biotechnology Entrepreneurship. DOI: https://doi.org/10.1016/B978-0-12-815585-1.00034-6

impact, you have a special challenge of educating people about the value of your science and products to their lives. Policy makers, potential consumers, and other members of the general public—including highly vocal opposition groups—are going to need to understand the benefits of what you are doing so as not to throw up roadblocks to your ultimate success.

Moreover, no matter what business you are in, good relations with your local community, including city planners, regulators, and neighbors, are needed to smooth the path for growth. Trying to grow your business in an area hostile to your work can be costly as well as frustrating. In every case, your success will depend on reaching and clearly communicating the value of your company, products, and services to a variety of audiences. Public relations (PR) is the most cost-effective method to reach each of those audiences and to create and maintain positive relationships with them.

What is Public Relations and How can it Support Your Business Objectives?

PR is the art of creating and maintaining a positive image of your company, technology, or products in the opinions of each of your target audiences. These include investors, corporate partners, customers, current and potential employees, thought leaders, patients and physicians, the media, and others. A good PR effort will help you stand out from the crowd and give you a competitive edge by creating familiarity with your company and an understanding of your products/services and their value to target audiences. PR can help you build scientific and business credibility, especially by calling attention to, and extending the reach of, peer-reviewed research publications and presentations, as well as business milestones, that validate your science and technology. PR can also help you manage your public reputation and build good relationships with those whom you do business.

Used strategically, PR can support a wide variety of business objectives, including the following:

- Finding funding from investors or foundations
- Securing contracts for corporate alliances
- Attracting potential acquirers
- Creating and maintaining demand for a stock offering
- Supporting sales of products or services
- Educating or influencing policy makers
- Finding top employees, consultants, and other service providers
- Creating community support for your business activities and operations

From its formation, every start-up biotech company should be thinking about PR and when to begin applying its strategies and tactics to support your business goals.

Get Ready: What's Your Story?

People love stories. For example, if you talk to members of the investment community, they will tell you that they invest in good people with good stories. Good stories are engaging and help the entrepreneur break through the competing noise to capture audience's attention. They go beyond your product or technology platform to convey a message that resonates with your target audience and motivates them in some way. Ultimately, PR works by connecting your business with people through a story.

The first step in defining your story is to understand your audience in terms of how you want them to think about you, and what you want them to do. What information may predispose them toward you, your technology, your products, or your services? Different messages have greater or lesser importance to a given audience, so it is useful to understand what motivates the people you are trying to reach with your message. Next, you will need to clearly define the key elements of your story—that is, develop a positioning statement (often alternatively described as your "elevator pitch") and the key message points that explicitly differentiate you from your competition and peers. Your positioning statement is a short paragraph—typically one to three sentences—that clearly and succinctly defines your business and says what makes it unique and why it has value. Table 34.1 gives some examples.

Your key message points are supporting statements that provide specific detail to backup your positioning. The message you define can address a specific audience's needs and wants, providing the opportunity to tailor what you want to emphasize in your communications to them.

A SWOT analysis (strengths, weaknesses, opportunities, and threats analysis) can be a useful exercise when thinking about positioning, as it helps you take a hard look at the elements that define your business and the environment in which it operates. This exercise also helps you list specific differentiators that form the basis of your key message points. Strengths and weaknesses represent internal characteristics of your company, while opportunities and threats represent those of the overall business landscape and how they affect your business or your product sales. Performing a SWOT analysis also helps you identify individual message points that elaborate upon your positioning statement and further differentiate your company from others in the field. What are your most important business and scientific attributes? What market opportunities do you address? What will you deliver to customers, partners, or patients? Why should they care?

TABLE 34.1 Examples of positioning statements.[a]

Transcriptic has developed the *first robotic cloud laboratory platform* for *on-demand life science research*. The TCLE integrates laboratory processes, protocols, and instruments together with IoT technologies through a *single user interface*. Top 10 pharmaceutical and growing biotech companies are using the power of the *Transcriptic software platform*, either in their own labs through the on-premises deployment of TCLE or externally through *Transcriptic's Bioassay Services*. The transcriptic platform allows researchers to carry out *efficient, reproducible, and rapid experimentation remotely* so they can focus on accelerating discoveries instead of labor-intensive bench work
Azitra, Inc. is a preclinical stage biotechnology company *combining the power of the microbiome with cutting-edge genetic engineering* to treat *skin disease*. The company was founded in 2014 by scientists from Yale University and works with world-leading scientists in dermatology, microbiology, and genetic engineering to advance its *consumer health* and *pharmaceutical* programs to treat atopic dermatitis, dry skin, and targeted orphan indications
Sema4 is a *patient-centered predictive health company* founded on the idea that more data, deeper analysis, and increased engagement will improve the diagnosis, treatment, and prevention of disease. According to Mount Sinai Health System venture based in Stamford, Connecticut, Sema4 is *enabling physicians and consumers to more seamlessly engage the digital universe of health data*, from genome test results and clinical records to wearable sensor metrics and more. The company currently offers *advanced genome-based diagnostics* for *reproductive health* and *oncology* and is building *predictive models of complex disease*. Sema4 believes that patients should be treated as partners and that data should be shared for the benefit of all

TCLE, Transcriptic Common Lab Environment.
[a]*The italic text in each example shows how each company has used important attributes and business objectives to create a well-differentiated statement of identity.*

You should take the time to critically understand what sets you apart from others and how best to convey that difference to each of your targeted audiences in a clear, concise way—but without hype. The effective formulation of your positioning statement and key messages can go a long way toward building a strong brand and consistent communications as you move forward with the next step in your PR effort—preparing the various elements of your communications toolbox.

Get Set: Creating *Your* Communications Tools

Communication tools can take many forms. The basic elements for any start-up company include a website with compelling information about your company, technology or research focus, and products or services; a company presentation usually aimed at an investor audience or a potential corporate partner and, ideally, some basic graphics in a high-resolution format (including photos of key executives) suitable for a variety of uses.

Your Corporate Website

Your website should make a great first impression—viewers may not know if you are a Fortune 500 company or a tiny start-up if your site is well designed and professional looking. A good initial website need not be complex or lengthy, but it should look clean, attractive, and be easy to read. The text should also be relatively brief so it can be read quickly. The average person reads only about 20% of the words on a webpage so you need to make sure they efficiently and effectively convey the message you want to get across. The home page should give the visitor a brief idea of what your business is about—a version of your positioning statement will usually work well here. You may choose to include pages about your technology or products that should incorporate appropriate key messages. You also want to include brief biographies of senior management, your board of directors, and, if applicable, your scientific advisors.

A contact page is also essential. Many companies like to use electronic contact forms as part of the website to cut down on unwanted phone calls and to have a record of specific contacts. However, exclusive reliance on such forms can also work against you, especially if a reporter or editor on deadline is trying to reach you. Too often, inquiries sent via website contact forms can languish for long periods of time, thus causing urgent messages to be overlooked and opportunities to be missed. Make sure that there is another way for people to reach you, even if it is just by a phone call or email to a general, but monitored, number or email.

Fact Sheets and Backgrounders

As you begin to talk to potential investors, corporate partners, media, and others, you may be asked to "Send me something about your company." A two-page fact sheet provides essential, nonconfidential information about your company in basic terms and conveys what makes you unique. If you've done your positioning work ahead of writing this document, you've already created much of the useful language that can be tailored further for this use and for other specific audiences, if desired. At a minimum, a corporate fact sheet needs to briefly describe the basis of your company, its business goals, and what makes it noteworthy. You should also include a list of key management and directors, and a financing history if you have one. Don't forget to include contact information and your logo. You may additionally benefit from creating fact sheets on your platform technology or specific products under development. Remember that these documents are intended for a general audience who may not have the scientific background that you do. To ensure that your message is heard and understood, keep your language simple and nontechnical, as well as free of overstatement and hype. If graphics can more simply explain your technology than words, use them.

The Corporate Presentation

Another key element in your communications toolbox is a corporate presentation. Start-up companies will benefit from a basic set of slides that can then be further customized to address the information needs of specific audiences. Good presentations are simple, concise, and compelling. Forget the adjectives, buzzwords, and business clichés—but do use active verbs and be concise. The best presentations are also highly visual. Audiences remember more of your message when key points are conveyed through images and charts rather than through words on a screen. In fact, research shows that we read and retain visualized messages up to 30% better than text because 50% of our brain is involved in visual processing. So, if you must use words, limit their number to make the text as scannable as possible. Overcrowded slides become unreadable in the average large-scale meeting room.

Keep your audience's specific needs and interests in mind. In these days of busy schedules and ever-shortening attention spans, you need to make an impact quickly. If you have not demonstrated to your audience why they should want to learn more in the first few minutes of your presentation, you have probably lost their interest. Describe your business idea, what makes it new and exciting, and how it will deliver what your audience wants—whether that is a great product, or strong, timely investment returns. Then elaborate on that overview with the details of your science, the market opportunity, the work you've accomplished to date, and the backgrounds of your team members. If you are seeking financing, how much do you want to raise and how will you use those funds? How will you create real value out of your idea? And how will an investment in your firm or the licensing of your product bring financial returns to your listeners, and in what timeframe?

Finally, once you have your basic presentation and plenty of backup slides to respond to anticipated questions, practice your delivery. Even for the best companies with great people and stories, an under-rehearsed, ill-prepared presentation can spoil a potential financing or collaboration. One venture capital investor tells of a highly anticipated company presentation that turned into a disaster for the presenting firm. The presenters were unpolished, had inadequate slides, were unprepared for questions, and offered no financial information. As a result, the potential investors were not impressed, and the presenting company was unable to regain their interest.

Graphic Resources

Good graphics are always useful. With the rise of the Internet as a primary medium for communications, graphics have become an essential part of the communications toolbox. Not only are they useful for your website, presentation, and fact sheet, but the availability of photos and other images will open the door to better Web visibility and media coverage. At a minimum, have high-resolution photos (minimum 300 dpi) available of your management and corporate logo. Visual or video representations of how your product or technology works, including animations and product photos where relevant, are also a plus. All these elements have multiple potential uses, including to provide additional visibility and internet pick up for press releases.

Designing and Implementing a Strategic Communications Program

Now that you have the story you want to tell with the communications tools to help you tell it, it's time to think about strategy and tactics. Your aim will be to highlight key events and use a variety of communication channels to tell your story, build visibility, and develop ongoing relationships with target audiences over time.

A low-key strategy that is consistent and persistent can be more effective (and affordable in both time and dollars) than a one-time big splash—which if not followed up with additional near-term activity will soon be forgotten. Your business objectives help prioritize your target audiences, as well as the activities you undertake and the communication channels you use to reach them. What are your business objectives for the next 8–12 months? Is your primary goal to raise financing? Are you looking for development partners? Or are you already seeking customers for your services or products? Generally, the time to get serious about a strategic, ongoing PR program is when you can foresee a stream of potential corporate milestones building. A good starting point is to map these expected business events and important scientific communications, such as peer-reviewed publications or meeting presentations, against your near-term goals. This exercise will help identify important communications opportunities as well as consideration of the timing of news releases and other activities.

News Releases

News releases are a basic currency of a PR program but their intent has changed in recent years. Also known as "press releases," news releases were originally directed chiefly to the media who acted as the gatekeepers over what news was reported. Today, Internet dissemination via newswire services and email enables you to quickly, easily, and cost-efficiently reach your intended audiences directly, without a media filter—thus making a well written, informative news release more important than ever. Effectively distributed for optimum visibility, news releases can help a company achieve several communications objectives. They offer a company-controlled channel to disseminate key messages, reinforce branding, and build thought leadership. They can build visibility with target audiences, especially online. They also can help drive traffic to the company website where viewers can learn more.

Many different events can be suitable as the subject of a news release. Examples include the following:

- Successful financings
- Forming corporate partnerships or major customer relationships
- Senior management, board of directors, or scientific advisory board appointments
- Clinical or other major product development milestones, including the start of major trials as well as trial results
- Product approvals, launches, or new service offerings
- Important scientific publications and presentations
- Important patent issuances or research grants
- Awards and recognitions

A well-written news release should answer the standard journalistic questions: who, what, when, where, and why? They should avoid jargon, meaningless or over-used buzzwords (e.g., do not use "solutions" or "solutions provider" to describe your business or technology without a stated problem unless you are talking about chemical reagents), and technical language and acronyms that go over the heads of most readers. A news release should be crafted with your readers in mind and the information they will be most interested in knowing. Quotes from company spokespersons or others relevant to your news are useful, especially when you can include the perspective of an outside thought leader. Quotes give the news context and emphasis, allowing you to reflect on its importance to the company or target audience, or offer a brief look ahead at your business prospects. Avoid using too many quotes or tired expressions of "pleasure" (i.e., "We are pleased...." or "We are delighted....") that lack real content because they can detract from the overall impact of your news release as well as consume an unnecessary word count in the price of dissemination. Those in industry sectors overseen by the US Food and Drug Administration or other regulatory agencies must also give special consideration to the rules set out by those agencies regarding communications. It is important to get the input of your regulatory and legal counsel in such cases to ensure your release remains within what is allowed. You should especially avoid making overt claims of efficacy or safety for unapproved products.

Once you have a final version of your news release and are ready to make your announcement, you have several options for its dissemination. Full-service, commercial news release distribution businesses (i.e., BusinessWire, PR Newswire, or GlobeNewswire) offer the advantages of fast, efficient, and simultaneous distribution of releases (as well as photos and other multimedia files) to media and throughout the Web. Using such services for release distribution can increase traffic to your website through search engines and can enhance your credibility as your news will appear alongside that of larger, more established companies. These services will also allow you to easily see where your release has appeared through the tracking reports they provide. However, good, effective service comes at a price, and while there are lower cost providers for news release distribution, the quality of your results, including credibility, reach, visibility, and security, is usually reflected in the price you pay.

When determining how you want to disseminate your release, you should consider the likely interest level and value of the overall news to potential readers. If it is relatively low or highly targeted (e.g., a new scientific advisory board member or patent issuance), you may want to spend less money and use a much narrower newswire distribution that national or international, or just send the release via email to relevant publications directly. In some cases (e.g., opening a new facility), you can just post a release to your website. For releases with greater news value, you can still limit the cost of release dissemination by restricting your wire service distribution to certain geographical areas or industry sectors. Doing so will still guarantee the release populates the Web in a comprehensive manner and reaches the industry publications most relevant to your news. For news of potential interest to general audiences, particularly scientific publications and presentations, there are two additional services that can be useful: EurekAlert (www.eurekalert.com) and Newswise (www.newswise.com). Both of these sites are designed specifically to meet the needs and interests of science and health/medical journalists, although they are also read by many of the science-interested public.

Media Relations—Why it Still Matters

While the true audience for your press release is not the press, media coverage of your company remains an important part of any communications program. The media are still important information gatekeepers and their coverage of your company and products is influential. They can provide context, help validate what you say about your company, and extend the reach of your communications to more people for a longer period of time. Media remains a powerful force. They bring third-party credibility by independently reporting about your business or products in newspapers, magazines, and their Internet-based counterparts, wire services, broadcast outlets, and the many other varieties of Internet-based content. Media coverage is an important tool for building recognition and reputation for a new company facing daunting competition from better known firms for funding, partners, and employees. While some start-ups are hesitant to engage with the media, a young company can benefit from a certain amount of outreach even in the early stages of its existence. There are certain audiences and publications that want to know and write about you at that formative stage. In fact, there are a few opportunities in the trade media for company profiles that are especially available to early-stage private companies, most notably with such media outlets as *MedTech Insight*, *BioCentury*, and *Life Science Leader*.

Different types of media have different audiences and, thus, different information needs, as well as different views of what makes a story. The perspective of a pharmaceutical trade journalist will differ from that of a major news outlet like the *New York Times* or *Wall Street Journal*. A locally focused publication will differ from a national or international one and what makes a good story for a science writer may differ significantly from what serves a business reporter's audience, even if both consider the life sciences their beat. It is important to understand the target audience for each type of media outlet, and how their reporters and editors may perceive what their readers or viewers want to read or see. By doing so, you can better choose the media outlets and journalists whose interests most closely serve your own communication purposes and frame your story and key messages in a way that those media will be most receptive to hearing it. You will want to consider the following:

- What is new, exciting, or different about your company, product, or technology?
- What makes the story emotionally compelling?
- Why does your story have importance outside of the small circle of your immediate scientific team?
- If you are looking for mainstream coverage, why should the broader public care about you and what you've accomplished?

You are likely to get the best reception from reporters and editors if you can identify something unique in the story you want to tell and then tell it in a simple, straightforward, and compelling manner. On the flip side, few things are more frustrating and time-wasting to a reporter—and detrimental to building a good working relationship with them—than a wildly off-topic pitch. You will benefit from being well prepared before embarking on a media relations effort. Your company spokespersons should be able to talk knowledgably, comfortably, and understandably about your business, technology, and products. What makes your company different, and why your products are needed? Your spokespersons should be able to communicate your positioning and key messages in a consistent fashion and tell the story in language that is understandable to a nonscientific audience.

Anticipating potential questions about your business and formulating appropriate responses is a valuable exercise before talking with the media (or indeed, all your audiences). The development of a Q&A document for internal use can be particularly helpful when you do not want to disclose all the details of a particular piece of news due to partner constraints, strategic considerations, or intellectual property reasons. Not all stories require detailed disclosure. You can work with your patent counsel, financial disclosure advisor, and other legal counsel in advance to determine the level of detail and timing of what you are willing to disclose or language that provides a simple, polite reason why you aren't going to answer a given question. Consider potential questions in advance, especially "difficult" ones where other factors affect what you might want to say. This can help ensure a smooth interview and make it easier for multiple spokespersons to communicate in a single, consistent voice.

Your news may be the sort, such as the publication of potentially exciting research, where you may want to consider briefing key opinion leaders (KOLs) about your work in advance of your news. Media often look for independent experts to comment on new research, and so educating some of these KOLs about your work allows them to comment knowledgably if they are called upon to do so.

Working with Reporters and Editors

Developing and nurturing positive ongoing relationships with reporters require that you understand and respect their needs throughout your interactions with them. A reporter may not really be your friend, but neither are they your enemy. Most just want to do their job quickly and well to provide to their readers the information important to that particular audience. Your goal is to help them do it in a way that results in fair and accurate coverage of your company. Honoring reporters' deadlines is particularly important, and those deadlines will vary with the type of publication or media outlet. With the rise of Internet journalism, much more news is reported "as it happens" on a daily basis than ever before, often requiring rapid responses within a few hours at most. Other publications maintain weekly or monthly schedules, providing a greater window for response. The bottom line is if you have announced news, make sure that a company spokesperson is available to respond in a timely fashion. If you are contacted by a journalist, one of your first questions should be "What's your deadline?" That reply will tell you how quickly you need to respond—whether in hours or days.

A word about "embargos." An *embargo* is an agreement between you and a journalist that they will not publish or otherwise make public a piece of information until a certain date and time, or until certain conditions are met. The intent of an embargo is to give journalists more time to research and write about the news, so that their published report can coincide with the announcement date and, in theory, those reports should be more accurate. Life science companies have often employed embargoes around peer-reviewed publications or scientific meeting presentations, where the embargo date and time is mandated by the journal or meeting organizers. Embargoes have sometimes been used around major corporate or product announcements. While embargoes may be useful for helping to bring significant attention to your news, it is important to get agreement from specific media that they will honor the embargo, or you will risk having your news get out too soon. Even with such an agreement, embargoes carry significant risks. In today's world where getting a story into print or on the air first is the holy grail, embargos mean very little to some mainstream journalists. One journalist breaking your embargo and getting the news out early can anger other journalists, even though *you* did nothing wrong. Embargos may also be broken unintentionally (usually due to miscommunications in the media outlet's newsroom). As a result, the use of embargos should be considered carefully, especially by public companies where such early "leaks" can have serious investor relation consequences.

When you are speaking with a reporter, do not say anything that you would not want to see in print. Nothing is ever really "off the record," even if you think you have an agreement with your interviewer. You are the expert on your company, technology, and products, so learn to talk comfortably and enthusiastically about them, making sure to clearly deliver the key messages you want your interviewer to take away and echo in their reporting. A good rule of thumb is to deliver your key message first, and then elaborate with the detail, before reinforcing that key message again to complete your response.

It's best to refrain from discussing your competition in any way but the most general terms (and try to redirect any questions about those companies back to your own story)—you don't want the interview to turn into a story about your competition or your feelings about them. If you don't know the answer to a question, just say so and offer to get back to the reporter with an answer later.

Obviously, you may be concerned about the ultimate accuracy of any article that appears. While journalistic etiquette precludes you from asking to review and approve an article before publication (and indeed, writers for many major newspapers and magazines would be in trouble if they complied with such a request), you should offer to fact check or otherwise make yourself available for follow-up calls. You can also help the reporter by sending additional information resources, such as your fact sheet, biographies, and introductions, to industry contacts who can comment knowledgably and positively about your business. Your goal should be to make it as easy as possible for the reporter to write accurately about you and your company. However, even if you have experienced a very positive interview and your reporter is enthusiastic about your story, media coverage is not guaranteed until you see it in print. Many things can affect getting a particular article published, including decisions by senior editors, competing news, and similar pieces in other publications.

Hopefully, if an article about you and your company does appear, it will be positive and accurate. If you don't like the title, in most cases, you should not blame the reporter, who probably didn't write it. If you don't agree with the coverage, before you act, consider why you don't and how best to respond. If there are factual mistakes, you should certainly contact the reporter to correct them in a friendly, straightforward manner. Reporters want to be accurate, and even if you are unable to get an immediate correction, you have educated them for their future coverage. If you disagree for other reasons with the coverage and seriously feel the need to respond, there may be better ways to do so than just contacting the reporter or their editor. For example, a "Letter to the Editor" or other editorial

TABLE 34.2 Six myths of media relations.

Perception	Reality
If I issue a press release, my news will be covered by the media	Your news will only have a chance of coverage if it's understandable and relevant to a publication's particular audience. Internet feeds will pick up news releases, but edited publications choose from hundreds of news releases and story ideas every day
A good PR agency can get me the coverage I want, any place I want	Personal relationships may get your story a hearing. But to gain coverage, your story must fit what a publication's editors or a broadcast outlet's producers perceive as appropriate and of interest to its audience
Every interview leads to coverage	Many factors go into what ultimately sees print or is broadcast, even after the interview, including competing news, editorial preferences, or available space
If I get a writer interested in my story, coverage will come quickly	There is much competition for limited print space or broadcast capacity. Even if a reporter is interested, it can be many months before a story appears, depending on the particular publication
If I ask for the conversation to be "off the record," then nothing I say will be printed	Nothing is ever really off the record. Be careful when saying things or discussing topics that you do not want to appear in print
If I give a journalist information that is embargoed for a certain date and time, nothing will appear in print until then	Like giving "off the record" information, embargoes can be a questionable proposition and should probably be used only when necessitated by the constraints of peer-reviewed journals or major medical meetings. Even then, be prepared for possible embargo breakers to release your news before the agreed time in the heat of competition or sometimes inadvertently

A version of this table previously appeared in *Nature Biotechnology* ("Why Media Relations Matter," by Joan Kureczka, Published online: 20 March 2006, doi:10.1038/bioent906) and appears here with permission of that publication. *PR*, Public relations.

contributions to their publication will enable you to tell your own story and reinforce key message points while rebutting the points you don't agree with in the original piece.

Ultimately, your goal in working with reporters is to build positive working relationships over the long term that lead to repeated coverage in their current publication or other media outlets as well as with media outlets that employ them in the future. To that end, it helps to position yourself as a resource for the reporter: being on-topic, interesting to talk with, and quick to respond whether or not you and your company are the focus of the phone call or interview. Taking the time to meet with reporters where there is no expectation of immediate coverage is also a good way to educate them about your company in advance of news or in anticipation of future coverage (see Table 34.2).

Building Visibility When You Don't Have News

Even when you don't expect to have news for many months, good opportunities exist for building visibility in the media or through other communications activities. You may be able to tap into larger news stories or business trends by showing reporters how your company fits or provides a unique and different view of the situation. There may be a strong human-interest component to your story or a particular local angle that can attract editorial interest. Your experience could serve as a successful case study for other entrepreneurs or businesses. Round-up articles—which discuss multiple companies as part of an overview of a new field of research, technology, or therapeutic focus—provide especially good opportunities for coverage that can put you in the spotlight alongside much more prominent firms. Many trade publications publish annual editorial calendars that reveal general topics for coverage in upcoming issues that could include your company, technology, or products. You can also generate your own coverage through the contribution of articles, such as opinion editorials, white papers, bylined technical articles, or commentaries, on a particular topic. Such articles not only raise your company's visibility and position you as a thought leader but also allow you to differentiate your company from others or establish your emerging business as a peer to much bigger, more established ones. Many of these ideas for building visibility also hold beyond media relations to activities like speaking engagements on conference panels, which can often generate their own media interest, or other visibility with audiences beyond those in attendance.

Case Study—Strategic Use of Public Relations to Support both Financing and Partnering

Here is a real-world example of how one start-up biotechnology company, Resolve Therapeutics of Seattle, Washington, used PR strategies from the time of its formation to support efforts to find both investors and a corporate partner. In the Fall of 2010, financing for most early-stage companies was near its low. Resolve Therapeutics, whose aim was to advance research on a promising potential drug for lupus, was founded with a then-unique LLC business structure aimed at giving investors a realistic chance at significant investment returns within 3 years. The company's objective was to raise a small amount of investment capital and sign a partnership deal as soon as possible that could pay for costly advanced clinical studies and give its founders and initial investors a substantial, relatively fast return on their investment.

Resolve used PR strategies to generate ongoing publicity for its efforts that would help create awareness and generate interest for the company's product, business strategy, and potential value as an investment. These activities included the following:

1. Scheduling interviews with publications targeting both the life sciences investment community and potential corporate partners that could lead within weeks to published emerging company profiles, even in the absence of specific news.
2. Using news of the company formation and initial financings to build significant business and trade media coverage of the company and its business.
3. Positioning and seeking interviews and other opportunities for Resolve's CEO to comment as a thought leader and present a successful case study on alternative financing models for start-up life sciences companies.

The company utilized the news of its formation along with the research and product lead licensed from the University of Washington, as well as information about the Resolve's unique business structure and capitalization strategy, to interest the regional business publication *Xconomy* in writing about Resolve and the company's plans. Resolve also issued a press release and spoke with other trade publications with readership representing the company's principal audiences of corporate executives and life science investors. Additional profiles were also sought and obtained in trade publications willing to write about emerging companies.

This initial PR effort was followed up by subsequent news announcements around the company's two small financings 6 and 13 months later and again when Resolve signed its desired corporate partnership. In between news announcements, the company continued to generate a low level of coverage that helped to keep the Resolve name in the news by positioning and pitching Resolve's CEO as a thought leader on alternative financing strategies—an effort that led to multiple interviews and inclusion in several round-up articles pertaining to financing strategies.

Results: Over a period of less than 3 years, Resolve was able to generate a stream of positive press on its product and business strategy in publications that were widely read by its intended target audiences, thus supporting the company's objectives of finding a small number of new investors and signing a corporate partnership at an early stage of product development.

What About Social Media?

The media landscape has changed enormously over the last 20 years. The rise of the Internet as a channel for providing content at any time, in any place, has been accompanied by a shrinking or transformation of what were previously print and broadcast communications. The result has been both an explosion of new outlets of various qualities and reach as well as the means for interactive communications. For companies, this change means many more ways of reaching your intended audiences, interacting directly with them, and further amplifying what is said about you and your technology or products. To a great extent, this can be accomplished through the various channels that make up social media.

A successful social media strategy involves much more than opening accounts on popular social sites. It requires a solid understanding of your business. You need to set practical goals, engage your target audience(s), and monitor your results. When properly executed, a social media strategy can deliver substantial benefits to your communications efforts:

- *It can help build reputation and relationships*: A well-rounded online reputation means that people can see your business as credible when they do a search on you and your company. Inbound inquiries will flow to firms with a strong reputation. These may include interested contacts from new members of your corporate and financial target audiences, as well as from physicians, patients, and potential employees. Building a credible reputation online can also attract thought leadership opportunities, such as speaking engagements and press coverage: such opportunities come chiefly to people who are easy to find and consistently appear credible online.

- *It can help you track potential impacts on your business*: sentiment, industry news, and activities of your target audiences.
- *It can drive traffic to your website and aid search engine optimization (SEO).*
- *It can aid your networking efforts.*

Setting Goals

The goals of social media marketing are often taken for granted. Most people aim to get as many followers as possible. But that's not all there is to it.

You should identify a range of goals and determine what metrics would define success against those goals. Examples of social media goals for a start-up company might include the following:

- Reaching new audiences
- Driving traffic to your website
- Building your reputation among industry peers; becoming thought leaders
- Increasing brand recognition
- Attracting media attention
- Selling a product

Depending on your particular business and social media goals, measurements of success might include the following:

- Numbers of followers
- Numbers of visitors to your social media profiles
- Number of "impressions" (the number of times a tweet has been delivered to a Twitter account's timeline) and the level of "engagement" (retweets, replies, likes, etc.) with you
- Link clicks and website traffic
- Number of conversions to customers or inquiries by patients/ physicians about trials

Who Do You Want to Reach?

You may be trying to reach one or more different audiences. Who are they? For example, a small private company may want to reach potential investors and corporate partners, attract potential clinical trial participants, and interest the media. Which outlet reaches each audience best? What sort of content would appeal to each of these groups and ideally motivate them to engage in the manner you would like them to?

Select the outlets most suitable to your goals and audiences. Don't spread yourself too thin—effective social media engagement requires time and consistency, and you can always expand your efforts over time. Tailor your content and level of engagement to the medium and to your targeted audience.

Set a Social Media Strategy and Policies—In Writing

How do you plan to engage, how often, and what will be the targeted goals? Who will be responsible and what sort of content will be pursued on the company's behalf? Creating a simple written statement of mission and strategy can help to crystalize your plans, strategic objectives, and tactical goals.

Who will need to approve content before it's posted? FDA or Securities and Exchange Commission (SEC) mandated constraints should be considered in setting your company's social media policy. What regulatory restrictions or legal considerations will you need to consider in your participation? (For example, FDA constraints on discussions of specific drugs rather than talking about the disease indicating such products address.) Drafting a more formal social media policy can help you consider such questions and achieve consistency, something that is especially important if more than one employee will be taking the reins.

Sample mission statement:

We will use Twitter to share news and views from ourselves and the industry in order to help strengthen our brand, engage existing and potential clients, and reach the media.

Sample strategy statement:

For Twitter, we will share links to relevant news, blog posts, publications, and other updates to our site. We will do this by posting at least three tweets per week. Posts will be reviewed and approved prior to posting by designated person or department with insight and authority into appropriate regulatory, legal, or other constraints on corporate commentary. We will also engage followers by retweeting others' posts—including our clients—and responding to direct messages in a professional manner. The target for each tweet is at least five link clicks, three profile visits, and/or three retweets.

Logistics

A number of potential platforms for social media exist—see Table 34.3. Once you decide which of these to use, spend some time looking and listening to the voices there to get a feel for the landscape into which you will be wading. See how your competitors and target audiences are already navigating the space. Learn from their successes and mistakes. Where will you fit in? How could you stand out from the crowd?

How will you manage your social media efforts? Will you use a tool, like Buffer or Hootsuite? Who will be handling social media posts? When will those posts be made and how? Consistency and frequency are important, as is engaging with the crowd. You should be prepared to

TABLE 34.3 Social media platforms.

Facebook The most popular social media website, boasting more than 1.5 billion active monthly users, Facebook has great potential for reaching wide audiences, and people are likely to pay attention to the content shared by their friends. Unfortunately, with shifting algorithms and "pay to play" strategies, it is getting increasingly difficult to get organic reach. So creating funny, informational, or unique content, and/or spending even a small amount on targeted ads and post "boosts," is key
Twitter Twitter can be a great way to reach very targeted and engaged audiences, including investors, industry leaders, clients, and the media. Regular, relevant content will gain you followers, and real value can be realized when posts go viral. Be sure to research and use hashtags to get the widest possible reach, and look out for any opportunities to participate in trending topics or community campaigns, such as disease awareness days
LinkedIn This should be considered your online resume, with business history, core objectives and skills, HR and company news, and recommendations from customers
Instagram This platform provides a great way to showcase your products and services in a very visual way. It should also be used to convey your company's personality, through snapshots of charity events, travel, parties, and so on
YouTube The second largest search engine, and important for search engine optimization, as the site is also owned by Google. YouTube videos are also easy and widely shared on other social media platform
Pinterest Pinterest is another interesting visual sharing platform. Pin clickable images that lead back to your website. While it has a reputation for appealing mostly to mothers, cooks, and crafters, for project, design, and recipe ideas, more than 100 million people use the platform for bookmarking information, and health is an increasingly popular topic of interest

PR, Public relations.

invest at least 5–6 hours per week in these activities in order to be effective.

Track your progress against your stated goals and adjust your strategy based on what works and what doesn't. Most of the major social media sites provide their own free analytic services, of varying degrees of insight. Additional free or low-cost tools are also available, such as Twitonomy, Quintly, and Sprout Social. One of the major advantages of social media engagement, as opposed to other communications activities, is the ability to get instant feedback based on what you post.

Types of Content

Many different types of content can be part of your social media effort, varying with the specific platform on which you choose to engage or sometimes used across two or more platforms. Graphics, videos, and stories are all suitable, especially if they represent an equal mix of communications that promote the company, share interesting or important information, and encourage interaction with your audiences. You can participate in discussions of trending topics and news. Sharing of information that can be used by others, such as best practices, can also promote engagement and interaction.

A number of platforms, including LinkedIn, Facebook, and YouTube, are ideal for sharing original content, including articles, video, or events, such as Facebook Live broadcasts that provide a larger opportunity for promoting your company, product, or idea. Targeted social media advertising, if relevant, can also be effective for meeting defined goals, such as clinical trial recruitment.

Case Studies

Social Media Supports Clinical Trial Recruitment

Tetra Discovery Partners used social media advertising to help quickly enroll a Phase 1 clinical trial targeting healthy volunteers ages 60 and older. The company conducted and monitored an Institutional Review Board–approved Facebook advertising campaign. The advertising directed interested respondents to a trial-specific landing page controlled by the Contract Research Organization (CRO) for the study. The CRO provided all follow-up patient screening and enrollment procedures.

A total of 621 people responded to the Facebook advertisement and the clinical trial fully enrolled 45 individuals within 8 weeks. In comparison, the study's traditional enrollment outreach received only 178 inquiries over 11 weeks of effort (Cowie JM, Gurney ME, JMIR Res Protoc 2018;7(1):e20. The use of Facebook advertising to recruit healthy elderly people for a clinical trial).

Supporting a Community Through Social Media

Like many firms, rare diseases pharmaceutical company BioMarin, a pharmaceutical company specializing in rare genetic diseases, maintains a LinkedIn page to showcase its news. But when it comes to other social media platforms, BioMarin has focused its efforts on the diseases and populations it serves. One of these is phenylketonuria, a rare genetic condition affecting about 16,500 people in the United States. BioMarin hosts an informational website about the disease, as well as Twitter, Facebook, and YouTube accounts geared toward public education and patient/caregiver support.

Reaching the Right Audiences via Social Media

Mt. Sinai Hospital spin-off Sema4, a predictive health and diagnostic testing company, has its toes in several social media waters. Since many of its services are related to the most photogenic products possible—babies—and its primary audience is one of the most trigger happy when it comes to "likes" and "shares"—new parents—it's not surprising that Instagram and Facebook are the company's most successful platforms. Sema4 uses Facebook to showcase news reports, share customer stories, promote new products, and broadcast live events or Q&A sessions with its scientists and physician leaders. Instagram is used to share advertisements, event and staff photos, and educational infographics. The company also uses Twitter and LinkedIn, but for different objectives and audiences, mainly as platforms to build company awareness and reputation among the public, peers, and media. The content reflects this: educational facts, internal news, and other news relevant to the industry.

Summary

PR is an important tool for any company seeking to reach key audiences and support their business objectives, whether those include finding investors, collaborators, customers, acquirers, or employees. A critical step in reaching your target audience is to understand the story you want to tell and relate it to your audiences' needs and interests. Spend time analyzing and defining what makes you different and unique and understand where the opportunities lie in your business for creating value, then frame those attributes in a way that addresses your intended audiences' needs and interests. Utilize the language and key messages you have developed throughout all company communications, including your website, fact sheets, and corporate presentations. Once you understand and craft the story you want to tell, you can design a PR strategy to support many objectives, such as raising capital, finding partners, building a customer base, or any other business goal. This campaign should not be limited to an announcement of major business milestones but can employ a range of strategies. These can include the announcement of other important events for your company, such as major scientific publications and presentations and seeking media coverage in round-up and trend stories as well as through contributed articles of various kinds. Social media provides a unique opportunity to both promote your company and engage with others to meet a variety of communication objectives. Development-stage life science companies need to know the various media and available communication channels, how they reach your desired audience, and how best to work with them. This will help you create an effective communications program that builds broad visibility and credibility for your company over time.

Additional Resources

Each of the three main full-service newswire distribution companies offers a variety of basic instructional resources on their sites including guides for writing press releases and white papers and other articles with more information on SEO, using multimedia in press releases, and working with reporters:

1. PR Newswire: http://www.prnewswire.com/knowledge-center/
2. BusinessWire: http://www.businesswire.com/portal/site/home/education
3. GlobeNewswire: www.globenewswire.com/home/learning-support/

Section IX

The Latter-Stage Biotechnology Company

Chapter 35

Company Growth Stages and the Value of Corporate Culture

Craig Shimasaki, PhD, MBA
CEO, BioSource Consulting Group and Moleculera Labs, Oklahoma City, OK, United States

Chapter Outline

All companies transition through several discrete growth stages along the path to commercialization and maturity. Certain characteristics distinguish each stage of growth, and the transition from one stage to the next is a tangible process but it occurs very subtly over time. Companies *effectively* or *ineffectively* transition through these stages, and their ability to do so impacts the growth and success of their organization. Recognizing and understanding this transition process, and the factors that influence it, will help the entrepreneurial team manage their corporate culture and lead their company through each growth stage in a positive manner. Successful transition through these stages is also influenced by the leader's ability to implement appropriate process changes. For instance, every company adopts certain procedures and policies, and what may have worked for 5 employees do not optimally work for a company of 50 employees, or for 500 employees. Throughout these stages of growth a corporate culture is established, which is initially formed by the core values of the founders. As new employees are hired, the founders consciously or unconsciously select individuals that are either congruent or incongruent with their core values. Over time, the sum of all the core values of the new hires becomes the established culture of the company.

The purpose of this chapter is to help the entrepreneur and leadership team be more effective in managing a highly dynamic scientific business that is dependent on working effectively with knowledgeable and highly motivated individuals. In this chapter, we will cover a variety of topics related to the growth, transition, and management of a company during its evolution. We will not be focusing on the product development in this chapter but on the development of the company culture that occurs in

Biotechnology Entrepreneurship. DOI: https://doi.org/10.1016/B978-0-12-815585-1.00035-8

parallel to the product development and often without realizing it. In addition to an overview of the company transition stages, I'll share with you some changes that management must make and risks that must be managed by the leadership, and a method for evaluating new hires who fit with your culture. As companies transition through these discrete development stages, it is accompanied by changes in communication methods, process changes for making corporate decisions, and a different management level at which certain decisions are made. Being aware of company development stages is vital because problems can occur when an entrepreneurial company transitions to the next development stage, but their leaders *do not*. As an organization makes a transition, its leaders must also make a transition, particularly in their management and communication style if they hope to effectively lead their company in accomplishing their goals.

During the early stages of corporate development the leadership of the organization is usually one individual. As the company grows, leadership responsibilities are shared with other key individuals. As the company continues to mature, leadership responsibilities expand to a greater number of key managers and employees. Throughout this chapter the term "*leadership*" may refer to one or more individuals, yet it always refers to the individuals empowered with the authority and responsibility to make final decisions.

As a company accomplishes each successive milestone toward creating a valuable product or service, it adds staff, expands activities, establishes corporate relationships, and their business practices evolve. Changes and adjustments also occur in the process of how a company makes decisions at all levels. A company that is comprised of 10,000 employees in five geographic locations, that manufactures and markets products worldwide, makes decisions differently than a start-up organization with a handful of employees and one product in development. The optimal methods and decision-making processes for an early-stage company do not work well for a mature company, and vice versa.

Corporate Development and Transition Stages

The corporate-development stages of an organization are outlined in Table 35.1, whereas these stages represent a continuum in which organizations transition through as they grow. Realize that every organization is dynamic and by recognizing these transition stages and understanding the characteristics of different corporate-development stages, the leader can improve their ability to effectively manage their organization for long-term success. It is not necessary to understand everything

TABLE 35.1 Corporate-development stages and focuses.

Corporate-development phases		Key management focuses	Work environment characterization
Start-up phase	**Establishment**	Proper corporate structure, license agreement, key consultants, product-development milestones, creating a business plan, raising start-up capital	Newness, excitement
Development phase	**Early**	Investors and future funding, outside collaborators and contract organizations, meeting product-development milestones, hiring key employees	Anticipation, discovery
	Middle	Major funding, hiring employees, significant product-development milestones, developing market strategy	Expansion, gaining strength, milestone successes, growth
	Late	Additional funding, additional employees, key management, regulatory milestones, prototypes and clinical trials, product launch	Navigating challenges, critical decisions
Expansion phase	**Early**	Corporate partnerships, expanding Market and channels, Reimbursement	Market entry and success
	Late	Additional management, additional market applications, developing new products and expanding applications of existing products	Growing market share
Decline phase	**Decline**	Dealing with competitor products, internal and external challenges, decreasing sales revenue	Internal and external issues, employee concerns

about each corporate-development stage, it is only important to recognize *when* it occurs and *what* changes and adjustments the leader must make so that your organization continues forward momentum and increases in strength as you move toward your corporate goals.

All companies will eventually transition through each of these corporate-development stages, whereas the *time spent* at each stage varies by company and their rate of growth. The following section contains a discussion of the characteristics of each corporate-development stage along with some of the likely key activities you will find to recognize that stage. These key activities may slightly differ in each organization as it will be based upon the type of product being developed and the biotechnology sector in which the company operates. I also share with you some aspects of the leader's management style during these phases.

The Start-Up Phase

For those who are founders, the start-up phase is an exciting experience, and yet at times it can seem frightening because it feels as if you are staring into a vast unknown. When establishing a new company, there is excitement, anticipation, and expectation of the future. There is a sense of newness. In reality, the start-up phase is the most fragile growth stage of the company, and many organizations do not proceed past this stage for a multitude of reasons. A good analogy to the start-up phase is that of the first pioneer settlers who colonized and established the providences in America. They had no roadmap or best practices to guide them, and the opportunity was unlimited. However, success was dependent upon the creative ideas and inherent ability of the founders to create and build something of great value over time.

Start-Up Phase Key Activities

In all start-ups, there are usually one or more founders, and occasionally, a very small team of individuals who may be working part-time or operating in a consulting capacity at the newly formed company. If the technology is owned by a research or academic institution, some key activities may include negotiating and securing a license, securing or filing patents, setting up the proper corporate structure, and formalizing agreements between the company and its founders, and issuing stock and creating an investor pitch deck and business plan. In addition to these corporate activities, there will be a multitude of product-development activities required to move the product forward to achieve milestones and raise start-up or seed capital.

During this stage the biotech entrepreneur will be accomplishing or overseeing almost everything. There will be a myriad of activities, and all of them will be deemed important — and all must somehow get done. While trying to get the company properly established, the entrepreneur sometimes may be transitioning from another full-time job which means working long hours, nights, and weekends. The biotech entrepreneur quickly learns that regardless of what their expertise is, they must adapt and become a jack-of-all trades, and be teachable.

Start-Up Phase Management and Decision-Making

During this phase, the entrepreneur-leader will be shaping the future and the direction in which the organization will be headed. Because the entrepreneur may be the only individual having the completeness of vision for the organization and the product, he or she will be leading the organization with a *command-and-control* management style during this phase. *Command-and-control* simply refers to the fact that all decisions are being made by one individual who then directs the work of others and evaluates the outcomes. This individual makes decisions about outcomes as to their appropriateness, compared to what is required to reach their ultimate goals. This management style can also be called the *entrepreneurial* management style. During the start-up stage, this style of management is essential because the team members are counting on the leader to communicate the company's direction and objectives and to tell them what success looks like. This style of management is *not* the same as micromanaging, nevertheless *all* tasks must be directed toward making incremental advancements with the desired outcome. Micromanaging at its root is an inherent distrust of the capabilities of others (irrespective of their experience) to make decisions, and a personal insecurity and misconception about their loss of control.

An *inappropriate* connotation of the *command-and-control* management style is that of a military boot camp where a demanding leader is ordering recruits around. The correct interpretation of this *command-and-control* management style is interactive, information- and opinion-gathering, yet the ultimate decisions are still made by the leader who is aligning each decision to result in progressive movement toward their envisioned goals. During this time, all team members are depending on the leader for direction and to make quality decisions. Therefore, the leader cannot be tentative or be someone who vacillates in their decisions. The leader must know their goals and how the team will achieve them, even if some of these goals are still being determined along the way. The absence of a strong visionary leader and/or poor strategy and poor execution will result in the demise of a start-up before it has a chance to transition to the next development stage.

The Development Phase

Early-Development Phase

During this phase an organization has made a significant transition from a start-up to a development-stage company. At this stage, there may still only be a handful of individuals who are responsible for accomplishing the company goals. These individuals may be comprised of a full-time employee or two, some working part- time or operating in a consulting capacity depending on the funding situation. At this phase, an initial funding event will have occurred, and the company will possess some capital to advance their product further along in development.

Early-Development Phase Key Activities

The company is most often operating as a virtual organization where most of the activities are contracted to outside organizations, which may include the laboratory of the original inventors. A major focus is on achieving critical product-development milestones utilizing the early capital raised. Other activities include finding key employees and raising additional capital for the next stage of product development. Plans are being made for future regulatory milestones and refining the market strategy.

Early-Development Phase Management and Decision-Making

This early-development phase requires a strong leader with a clear vision and a strategic plan because all activities are essential and need to be completed, and everything seems equally important. Still, without clear priorities and laser focus, little will be accomplished in a timely manner. The leader must continually communicate the corporate plans and the product value to internal and external stakeholders. If the leader is unsure, unclear, or inconsistent in priorities, goals, and objectives, the company's growth becomes stunted and their limited resources are yielding minimal value. During this stage, the leader must still lead with a command-and-control management style and ensure that company growth and progress moves in the right direction and that all activities are directed toward the correct goals. Although, at this stage, there should be team members whom the leader can trust to share a portion of the leadership responsibilities. These individuals must share the same vision as the leader, possess similar core values, and be in agreement with the goals and objectives of the company and the envisioned product being developed. Consistency and perseverence are essential characteristics for companies at this early-development phase. Some organizations never make it past this stage because of unforeseen external or internal challenges, an inability to raise capital, or lack of clear leadership. In order to move to the next phase, the company must persist in accomplishing what it set out to do, being resourceful, and often making some course corrections that improve the value of the developing product or improve its market value and interest.

Mid-Development Phase

During this phase, the organization continues to grow with steady and consistent progress made toward its corporate- and product-development objectives. Major funding has been secured to advance product development to the next significant milestone, and greater value is being attributed to the organization. The employees are content about the organization and its future, and they feel informed about the company and its progress, and they enjoy their work. There is early public or external interest in the product being developed and anticipation that it will meet some important need.

Mid-Development Phase Key Activities

The company has been building internal capabilities, but it still outsources most activities, however, more of these are being integrated and supported within the organization. Major funding has provided ample working capital for additional hires to expand internal functions. Product-development progress has reached key milestones, and the company is overcoming many challenges encountered during its growth and product development. Preliminary meetings are occurring with potential partners and public relations is resulting in some recognition for the company.

Mid-Development Phase Management and Decision-Making

At this phase, the leader must begin transitioning from managing through a *command-and-control* style to a *delegate-and-inspect* management style. If the leader does not adjust their management style during this transition stage, they can become an impediment to the company and its product-development progress. Management-style transition is as much a change for the employees as it is for the leader who in the past made all the decisions. At this stage, there should be other key management who possess leadership skills that can be trusted to make many of the decisions within a particular function, and they should be vested with that responsibility. This transition will not occur instantly, but it occurs gradually over time as the leader begins entrusting more responsibility to other key management. The leader must still communicate a clear vision for the company and must constantly convey, internally and externally, the company's development progress. In spite of this management-style transition, employees must still believe that they can go to the leader for solutions to major problems if necessary, and be confident that the leader is approachable. The leader must create an expanding leadership team and operate within the company's unique strengths. They must not forget that one of their key strengths is their quickness and agility in creatively responding to problems and external challenges.

Late-Development Phase

Because of the lengthy product-development process for all biotechnology products, many companies may spend a great deal of time at this development phase. This is also the stage where large amounts of capital are consumed as companies move through lengthy clinical trials and regulatory processes. By now the company has secured several large rounds of funding. And often at this stage, the company encounters product-development challenges, product-testing issues, and possibly regulatory issues, which all must be overcome. During this phase, there may be tensions developing as to the future of the company, or there may be questions about how the company will overcome these challenges.

Late-Development Phase Key Activities

Key activities include product and field testing, such as human or prototype testing, meeting with regulatory agencies, examining and implementing scale-up options, and finding and forming key external partnerships. Other activities include sourcing and meeting with potential marketing partners or those interested in late-stage clinical trial development and possibly potential acquirers of the company. The leadership staff and the number of employees are increasing, and there usually is an additional layer of management incorporated within the organization.

Late-Development Phase Management and Decision-Making

By this stage the leader must have made a complete transition to a *delegate-and-inspect* management style. By now the hired managers and employees have sufficient expertise and possess untapped capabilities that will be underutilized if the leader does not make a management-style transition by this stage. The leader should be focused on articulating the important and strategic business goals to the senior management and provide the team with measurable goals to evaluate progress. The management team should comprise seasoned individuals having vast but deep experience, but all must support the same goals for the product, the market, and the organization. These senior management individuals may include a chief scientific officer (CSO), chief medical officer (CMO), chief financial officer (CFO), business development executive, regulatory executive, to name a few. If the company is relatively small, then sometimes these individuals or these roles may not be filled with full-time persons, but through consultants as a company will need someone to function within these disciplines. By this phase, it is critical that the leader fully completes the management-style transition and the rest of the management is effectively functioning as a unified leadership team. If this has not occurred by now, other managers and employees will experience growing frustration with the lack of opportunity for themselves and their own career.

Another reason for this management-style transition is that by now the individuals a leader manages may possess more knowledge and understanding about a problem or situation in their area than the leader does. Therefore these individuals are the best ones to make certain decisions, and this may be true at various levels of employees. If the leader's management style does not transition, employees become ineffective and usually find nonproductive activities to occupy their unused capacity, or most often, they will leave to find more motivating positions of employment. A leader who still directs task-oriented work deprives capable employees of the opportunity to step-up and contribute at a greater responsibility level.

Expansion Phase

Early-Expansion Phase

Organizations that reach this stage have successfully passed the hurdles of product development and have received regulatory approval for their new product (if required), and they are manufacturing their product and expanding the market for their product. Reaching this phase means that there is tremendous potential for the company, and staff is being added and capabilities are being expanded. By now the company will have made some mistakes along the way, but none have been beyond repair and they have been quickly corrected. Management must maintain a start-up *mentality and culture*, and not set up a bureaucracy that impedes the company's agility and its ability to respond quickly. Management's challenge will be that of balancing a more process-based infrastructure while maintaining the flexibility and creativity that was a strength at their previous development stage.

Early-Expansion Phase Key Activities

At this stage the company's product is in the market and much activity is concentrated around executing the market strategy, managing market channels, manufacturing activities, and reimbursement challenges (for medical products). Companies now must execute their plan and monitor their external environment for changes that impact them and their products.

Early-Expansion Phase Management and Decision-Making

At this phase the management style has become more similar to that of larger corporate entities, yet there still should be a relatively flat organization, meaning that there are as few layers of management as absolutely necessary. The company should still have the ability to make decisions in a way that takes advantage of a smaller company's strengths. Management focus should include training more leaders at new levels of the organization rather than just better managing tasks because these new leaders can impact greater portions of the organization. The leadership and management are quite capable of handling development and growth needs, but they still experience a few crises every now and then. Communication is vital within the organization and senior leadership should ensure that all employees feel that they are informed about the progress of the company.

Late-Expansion Phase

Companies that reach this phase are successful in their own right. They have developed great capabilities and are efficient producers, manufacturers, and marketers of their products, and they are increasing their market share. Companies such as Gilead Sciences, Amgen, Genentech (acquired by Roche), Biogen, and Genzyme (acquired by Sanofi) are examples of some successful biotechnology enterprises. Of course, each of these organizations has encountered challenges, and some of their early employees may have moved on, some to start companies of their own. It is interesting to note that employees who were there during the early days remember a different company and believe that the company had become "institutionalized." No doubt a few "bureaucratic processes" may have been adopted, but a good percentage of individuals still adhere to the importance of just getting the job done rather than creating additional processes. By now, some of these companies will have been acquired or merged with a larger organization.

Late-Expansion Phase Key Activities

At this phase, the company is focused on market strategy, reimbursement (if medical products), manufacturing, improving quality, and new-product development. If the company is not acquired or the first product is not licensed to a marketing partner, there may be financing activities such as securing mezzanine rounds of capital for expansion.

Late-Expansion Phase Management and Decision-Making

One key characteristic of successful companies at this corporate stage is the implementation of genuine, clear, and frequent communication from management to staff and employees. As organizational structures enlarge, communication channels tend to break down across different functions of the company. When this occurs, misunderstanding and internal problems increase. The absence of information can cause employees to think and presume information that may or may not be true. Several things that can help a company make a successful transition through this stage include frequent and meaningful communications between the leadership, the senior staff, and all levels of the organization about the goals, the plans, and the *reasons* for these choices. Employees want to know "*why*" the organization is taking certain actions or engaging in certain activities. When employees understand why, they will not spend much time being concerned about the company direction because they understand. Employees also want to know what is going on outside of their own discipline or functional area. Cross disciplinary communication increases problem-solving and allows employees to work more knowledgeably. Management must be sure to communicate progress about all aspects of the business to employees, even if it changes frequently. The leadership must continue to share with employees the vision for the future and demonstrate that there is purpose and value in what everyone is doing.

Decline Phase

This is not a planned stage of corporate development, and it is one that must be avoided. Reaching this stage is not a milestone, but it is an indication that either the company and/or its products have become irrelevant to the market, or that their products are nearing the end of their life cycle. Recognizing that a company is at this stage can also mean that the organization has stopped innovating and had relied on a single product for their growth. Arriving at this stage is much less frequent in the biotech industry, but it still happens when their products become commodities, and the company fails to continue product innovation and only focuses on sales and marketing.

Decline Phase Management and Decision-Making

We will not elaborate much on this phase except that it is management's responsibility to lead and guide their organization through each corporate-development stage and avoid entering into this one. Biotech companies are known for innovation and product leadership, and as such it would be unusual to find many biotech companies that reach this stage very often, although it has happened, and it is unfortunate.

The CEO's Role in the Transition of Development Stages

It is the responsibility of the leadership, particularly the CEO, to lead change and to guide their company and employees successfully through each development stage. The CEO needs to recognize these transition phases and respond by managing in an appropriate manner during that corporate-development stage. A *command-and-control* management style is essential for a start-up company with one part-time administrative assistant, a scientist, and a technician. However, this management style will not be effective for 50 employees and a senior management team consisting of a CSO, CFO, CMO, and a business development executive. The CEO's management style must transition as the organization transitions, or the CEO may not be leading the company for long.

Sometimes, the CEO does not know how to change, or they may have difficulty adapting to change and resort to managing as in the start-up stage rather than making a management-style transition. Often the CEO does not want to change, and for a time they can do that, but to the detriment of the organization and its progress. Resistance to change is not uncommon for a first-time entrepreneur who founded a start-up organization then becomes CEO and grows the company to the next level and receives a major round of funding. Although, when a company has received venture capital, a VC general partner will likely be on the company's board. The VC will have limited patience with a CEO who is resistant to change for the betterment of the company, but most often will give the entrepreneur CEO an opportunity to make changes. If the entrepreneur CEO cannot make appropriate changes, the VC will typically replace the CEO and bring on a seasoned and experienced individual who understands how to manage a growth company. Venture capitalists may be seen as only interested in their investment, but they also desire to see the company succeed or they will not have many future investment opportunities themselves. Seasoned and experienced VCs can quickly recognize the signs of an unhealthy organization, and they will do what they need to in order to correct the situation so that the organization can thrive. Founding entrepreneurs should know that there are significant challenges in building a successful biotech company, but ***they*** should not become one of those challenges, as it is counterproductive and can be prematurely fatal to the company.

Leadership Skill Sets

The CEO is the *leader*, but the company *leadership* includes all individuals given responsibility and authority for making decisions for the company. As the organization grows, the leadership will include other individuals who are responsible for scientific, corporate, marketing, regulatory, legal and manufacturing functions. Unfortunately, not everyone who is given responsibility for a function is endowed with great management skills. There are an abundance of helpful books available for improving leadership and management skills, and a young company should invest time and energy in training and equipping their managers and leaders. For brevity, the following is a list of characteristics that are important to be present in all leaders and managers. If a leader or manager does not possess these traits, the first thing they should do is to work on improving their own leadership and management skills so they can help teach and instill them in others.

Five Qualities of Successful Leaders and Managers

1. ***They identify***—Successful leaders and managers have or acquire the ability to recognize the right people for the right positions based upon needs at that time.
2. ***They lead and inspire***—They have knowledge of how to inspire and motivate individuals to achieve their goals, objectives, and tasks and see the vision set before them.
3. ***They teach***—They possess the ability to teach and instruct individuals to accomplish the objectives that align with the vision the company has created.
4. ***They inspect***—They have the ability to appropriately monitor and inspect the progress and results from the efforts of these individuals, and can make necessary adjustments to continue progress toward those goals.
5. ***They reward***—They understand the value of praise, appreciation, increased responsibility, incentives, and remuneration. They know that a different mix of rewards is required for different individuals.

Corporate Culture and Core Values in a Biotechnology Company

Every company is unique in its culture, its employee mix, and the manner in which it conducts its business. One can say that each company has a personality all its own. Typically, the collective characteristics of a company are referred to a *corporate culture*. A company's culture is tangible in that those outside the organization and its customers can sense a real difference between one company's employees and those of another organization. For instance, one company may have a culture that is characterized by innovation, excitement, and collaboration, motivating employees to ignore the traditional work hours and do whatever is necessary to get a job done regardless of the time of day. Conversely, another company may have a minimalist culture with clock-watching employees, doing only what is required and only if it is written in their job description.

Your corporate culture will be a strength or a weakness. Every company encounters problems and challenges, and it seems like biotechnology companies have more than their fair share of them. But the corporate culture of a company is a good predictor of their ability to overcome a crisis, and it is an inherent strength or an inherent weakness.

Example of the Tylenol Scare of 1982

A disaster situation that has been analyzed as a case study in business schools around the world is an example of how to successfully respond to crisis. In 1982, seven consumer deaths occurred when these individuals in the Chicago Metropolitan area ingested tainted Tylenol Extra Strength capsules laced with cyanide. Ortho McNeil's employees (a Johnson & Johnson company) quickly and collectively responded according to their corporate culture of putting first the well-being and needs of the people they serve. Once it was quickly determined that the Tylenol capsules were tampered with *after* they left the manufacturer, and the contamination was not the company's fault, Ortho McNeil executives made the decision to immediately recall 31 million bottles of Tylenol at a cost of over $100 million. To further protect the public, the company nationally advertised not to consume any products containing Tylenol. Most interesting is that this type of crisis management was not really "taught" to the Ortho McNeil employees, nor was it a rehearsed response. It was later recognized that these actions were based upon their organization's core values [1] established by their founder, and this is what guided the employee's decision-making. Ortho McNeil possessed a company culture and core values that were an asset, but these values only became visible to the public as a result of this crisis. As a result of this crisis, Ortho McNeil subsequently created many of the commonly used over-the-counter (OTC) product manufacturing safety measures that are in use today. This crisis, which could have taken a company down, demonstrated that the core values of this company improved their reputation and demonstrated their commitment to the public safety, and resulted in the implementation of tamper-resistant safety features used in OTC products today.

Development of a Corporate Culture

For a biotechnology start-up company, developing a corporate culture may not seem like a high priority compared to the need of raising money, hiring a team, and quickly making product-development progress. Yet, it is critical to pay close attention to the development of your corporate culture because at some point the company reaches a critical mass, and like concrete, the culture of the organization becomes set. A company may temporarily ignore the development of a corporate culture without much consequence, but at some point, this will impact your company's ability to effectively accomplish objectives. One thing is certain, you will have a company culture whether it is by design or default. Every company's corporate culture is somehow different and there is no universal culture that is optimal for everyone. For instance, an organization operating in a highly ordered industry such as accounting may not be best suited to have a culture based upon creativity, but rather one of constancy; yet there are other beneficial qualities that are valuable to all organizations.

If your company has a fully developed culture that is counterproductive to progress, now is time to do something to change your culture. As previously discussed, all companies transition through distinct growth phases, and things do not always work out exactly as planned. Internal and external changes and adjustments are inevitable as a company grows. Whereas your corporate culture will be a facilitator or an obstructor in overcoming these challenges in product development and organizational growth. In order to make change, you must first choose to purposefully create a culture that adds strength, rather than one that is divisive or detrimental to progress. Fortunately, most start-up biotechnology companies begin with an entrepreneurial culture that is energetic, creative, and persevering. When founding team members and management hold themselves to a clear set of core values, the organization operates in a consistent manner, and the employees have confidence as to how problems and issues will be resolved.

Every Individual Defines the Corporate Culture and Core Values

An organization's strength is the sum total of all its individual strengths. Each employee makes decisions based upon their own knowledge and core values. An employee with a core value of "*mutual respect for others*" does not think about how they may leave an unfinished task for another employee to complete. Someone with a core value of "*acceptance of responsibility for ones actions*" will readily admit a mistake rather than cover it up or blame someone else. These examples may seem minor by themselves, but add these up amongst 15, 150, or 1500 employees, and this becomes the prevailing culture of the organization. Individuals who do not share the same core values arrive at different conclusions based upon the same information, and this causes internal conflicts that would have been disastrous for Ortho McNeal during their Tylenol crisis. Your corporate culture does not always impact whether or not things get done, but rather it is the biggest influencer of *how* and *when* things get done.

For stability, organizations need foundational values that are clear and unwavering. Core values that are only framed and hung on a wall and do not penetrate the hearts and minds of the leadership and employees, are eventually resisted or resented by all. The leadership must demonstrate that they operate and make decisions in accordance with their core values in their daily activities. Values that are shown to apply to senior management will be reinforced, embraced, and even expected of all employees throughout the organization. A company without a clear set of quality core values is equivalent to a ship without a compass— there may be progress but it is directionless and haphazard.

Core Value Examples

There are a multitude of core values that great companies espouse, and these values can be different for each company. The key is that an organization has certain core values that all employees embrace and live by. Core values can be thought of as the seeds of an organization's future. The selection and incorporation of a particular set of core values will ultimately bear the fruit that is characteristic of those values. Just as a farmer planting orange trees would not expect to harvest tomatoes, likewise the selection of certain core values predicts that the type of culture a company will yield as it matures (see Fig. 35.1). The following are a set of core values from one of my companies. As a clinical laboratory, testing for autoimmune based neuropsychiatric disorders, these fit with our mission and purpose. These are not the only core values nor are they necessarily the ideal ones for every company, but they are examples of those that are associated with significance to our group.

Corporate Core Value Examples

- ***We give hope***—We impart hope and show compassion to those whom we serve.
- ***We are a cohesive team***—We do not work as individuals in isolation. We are part of a greater purpose. We help each other grow within and across functions.
- ***We have open communications***—We are transparent. We listen and communicate openly with everyone because we value their ideas, thoughts, and concerns.
- ***We honor each other***—We respect and value one another, and it is exemplified by our actions. We honor each other's time and contributions.
- ***We are continuous learners***—We are a unique organization like no other. We are eager to learn and improve our skills and abilities.
- ***We hold ourselves to higher standards***—We strive for excellence in all we do whether anyone sees or notices. We take ownership for our actions whether right or wrong.
- ***We celebrate our successes and gain value from our mistakes***—We rejoice with our team's successes and learn something of value when we make mistakes. We are creative problem solvers.
- ***We are empowered***—We are empowered to perform our tasks and objectives. We understand the value we contribute to the overall mission of our company.

A company that truly embraces their core values and lives to fulfill their mission is a company that will accomplish great things. In order to fully establish your corporate culture, the core values should also be translated into more tangible and practical "*guiding principles*."

Guiding Principle Examples Based Upon Core Values

Core values must be translated into practical guiding principles in order to help individuals better understand how the organization desires its employee to make decisions and operate. A set of guiding principles can be defined, or they can be just understood. The following are some examples of guiding principles that are based upon various core values.

- We are a diverse group of individuals with differing backgrounds who share the same core values and encourage each other, and also remind each other if we don't live up to our own values.
- We highly value our partners and patients and are loyal to them and their needs. Our partners are our physicians, employees, vendors, and suppliers. Our patients are our mission.
- We are a relationship-oriented company. We incorporate into all our business, market, and science endeavors a relationship orientation with our "partners" in achieving common goals that benefit each other. We will seek relationships with partners who share common or mutually beneficial goals.
- We will differ from our competitors by incorporating innovation into all of our products. In addition, the products that we develop will not be an end in themselves but tools to improve healthcare in the broadest sense.

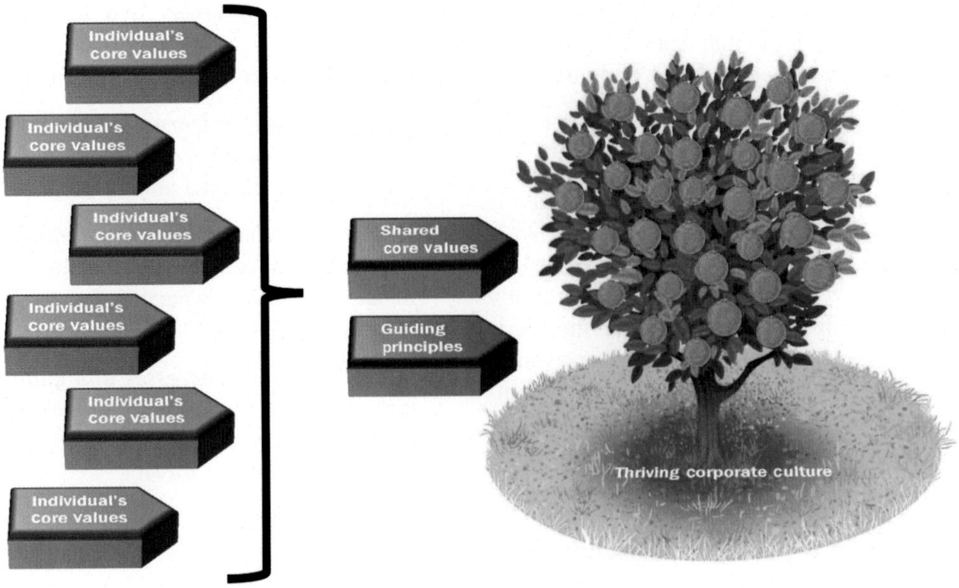

FIGURE 35.1 Illustration of the Development of a Corporate Culture

- Our profitable differences will be seen in our product innovation value and not in the commoditization of products. Our product positioning will be "best-in-class" where there are competitors. This will be accomplished through our products themselves and the collateral services and programs provided that create more value to the customer than the product alone.
- When our products are launched, we will work to improve outcome measurements such that the true long-term benefit of our products will be understood.

Your Mission Statement Summarizes Your Company's Purpose

From these core values and their practical guiding principles, a company then develops and adopts a mission statement. Although core values are inherent within the company's employees, a mission statement is the aspiration of the company as a whole. The Mission Statement of Moleculera Labs is:

> *"We will effect change in the way medicine is practiced forever. We are building a unique company that is different from any other. We are a part of a greater purpose; it is not just a job. Our core values come first, and our products and services are a natural expression of who we are."*

The Impact of Core Values

If the leader respects and keeps their core values, so will the organization. Leaders exemplify the core values that the company will espouse, such as the Credo developed by Robert Wood Johnson in 1943 for the Johnson & Johnson Company. Core values can be thought of as a belief system and a set of nonnegotiable behaviors that a group of individuals embraces as standard practice. Having core values does not automatically guarantee business success, but by consistently operating within a set of worthy values, it will provide the organization with the highest likelihood of success. Once a company is successful, strong core values ensure the likelihood of sustaining success. If your desire is to build an organization with lasting value, establishing a set of key core values should not be ignored. Possessing strong core values are beneficial not only in business but they apply to family life and relationships. A good book with simple truths about core values written by an ex-school teacher is titled *Life's Greatest Lessons: 20 Things that Matter* [2].

Select Partners and Service Providers Based Upon Common Core Values

The selection of suppliers and service providers should be evaluated similarly to the hiring of a senior or executive staff member of the organization. The same care, scrutiny, and examination of common goals should be evaluated prior to forming a relationship because as the organization begins to grow and make progress, the company will become interdependent on the quality and reliability of these external relationships. Since start-up organizations outsource many activities during early development, it is vital that these suppliers and service providers share similar core values. The last thing a growing biotech company needs is to experience problems such as the breakdown of trust and confidence with critical partners. The 80/20 rule is true in external relationships, meaning that 80% of the company's time is spent working on 20% of the worst relationships. These are simply manifestations of inconsistencies in core values between the two parties. These incompatible relationships divert management attention away from building the business and reaching their goals.

The best time to evaluate a relationship is before it is consummated. When choosing a partner, service provider, or supplier, do not make choices based upon pricing alone. You must evaluate all aspects of the partnership including communication, strategic direction, corporate values, and their interest in a long-term synergy rather than just pricing a transaction. We all know that relationships will face difficulties at some time, but these challenges should be opportunities to alter a process, improve a communication channel, or modify a working relationship, rather than a suboptimal way of doing business. When substandard behavior becomes tolerated as the norm, working with these relationships becomes weary and burdensome. Great suppliers and service providers should be willing to concede short-term financial gain to work through issues if your interest is in a long-term relationship, and you have a partnership orientation. Be sure to communicate a long-term partnership goal, and it will reduce the time spent on any one particular issue, and both parties can work toward equitable solutions. Also, do not neglect to give feedback to suppliers and service providers. Let them know how they are doing, and give them recognition for their effort.

Guidance for Hiring Team Members

Before an organization can build a desired corporate culture the company needs a hiring process that carefully identifies ideal members to add to your team. During growth phases a company must ensure their desired culture is maintained, or it will unknowingly transition to the common denominator of the majority of new employees. Recognize that a rapidly growing organization will hire the equivalent of its entire company many times over until it reaches a critical mass. If a company indiscriminately hires individuals who do not share common company core values, divisions occur and new employees may be driven by motivations not shared by the majority of the company.

No biotechnology enterprise can successfully accomplish its goals without the help of a myriad of individuals and external resources. Seasoned entrepreneurs and executives all reach a point in their career where they recognize that their success is no longer determined by what they can do by themselves—but by what they can accomplish with and through the help of others. Building a successful biotech company requires an ever-expanding team. Therefore it is important to find the right mix of individuals with complementary expertise having the leadership characteristics necessary to establish and direct a growing organization to a common goal.

The careful selection of team members is important because (1) these individuals provide the expertise required to reach your corporate and product-development goals and (2) these individuals are evaluated by investors, and they influence the likelihood of securing investment capital. Choose your team wisely, as their credentials, backgrounds, and experience are viewed as indicators of future success. For more information about an interviewing and hiring process, who to hire first, compensation and benefits in the biotechnology industry, see "*Chapter 11: Hiring a Biotech Dream Team*" in *The Business of Bioscience: What Goes Into Making a Biotechnology Product* [3].

When considering someone for a full-time position, the company must first narrow the applicants down to a small group of "*ideal candidates*" for the position. Multiple candidates are screened and interviewed for this position in the hope of finding the right person for the job. How do you determine who is the right person for the position? All companies know the importance of finding individuals who possess "*related experience*" for a position. However, there are two other characteristics that are rarely considered but are equally important as *related experience*. When interviewing individuals to find the ideal candidates at least three characteristics should be examined for fitness: (1) having ***related experience***, (2) having the ***ability to execute***, and (3) possessing ***shared core values***. The Venn diagram in Fig. 35.2 depicts these characteristics as distinct but intersecting, showing their interdependence. The opacity indicates the ability to see these characteristics during a typical interview process.

Having Related Experience

When considering a candidate to hire, all companies look for ***related experience***. Without question, related experience is vital to the position, and it is the easiest quality to identify and evaluate, unfortunately all too often it is the only factor examined. Just because an individual has related experience, this quality alone should not make them "an ideal candidate" for the job. Related experience should be only one of the three required qualities examined before considering an individual as an ideal candidate for a position. Related experience qualifications include depth and breadth of experience, academic credentials, and the type of work experience and length of time in a position. These are all well understood and easy to assess, therefore we will not elaborate on this quality much further.

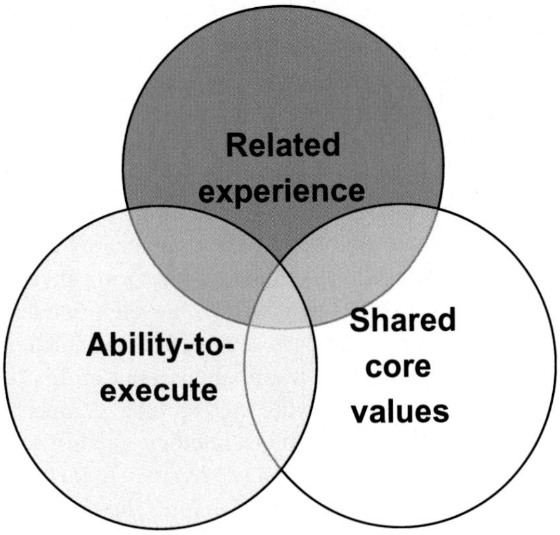

FIGURE 35.2 The "Ideal Candidate" Characteristics

Having the Ability to Execute

Having the ***ability to execute*** is a quality that characterizes "doing" rather than talking or thinking about something. Character qualities, such as "finishing a job started" and "always coming through," are qualities that exemplify having the ability to execute. Individuals that lack this quality usually can talk the language but cannot complete or finish even the simplest of tasks. Those without this quality think they are making progress because they can talk the talk, but upon examination they come up empty-handed time and time again. These individuals are time consumers for management because they divert attention from other work and require constant monitoring and maintenance to keep their project from being in jeopardy. The ability to execute is difficult to teach on the job, and management certainly cannot help them complete all of their tasks. In most organizations, finding out if the new hire has the ability to execute is often realized several months after hiring.

Ideal candidates should have related experience *and* possess the ability to execute. Possessing the combination of these two qualities ensures that an individual can think of ideas, form a strategy, and execute a plan. Although the ability to execute quality is difficult to recognize, a good interview process will help identify individuals possessing these characteristics. The ability to execute *and* related experience are two important qualities, which ensures that a person is able to deliver what is needed in the position. However, having these two characteristics still does not constitute and ideal candidate for employment.

Having Shared Core Values

An individual who possesses *relevant experience*, the *ability to execute*, *and shared core values*, makes an ideal candidate for a position. Without shared core values, two people cannot work together effectively for a sustained period of time nor can they work to their full potential. We previously elaborated on some core values, but core values are as diverse as people. They can include qualities such as "a good work ethic," "responsibility to get the job done," "honesty in all situations," "reliability," and "loyalty to the company."

Everyone possesses core values. No team can be effective without sharing some of the same core values—even street gang members, although their core values are negative ones. Interestingly, even negative core values unite individuals together. The most effective teams are comprised individuals who share a maximum of common core values and influence each other to accept additional core values that are important to the rest of the team. Core values become our personal "well of conscience" from which we draw when we face difficult situations, problems, or crisis, and when we do not know what to do. To become an effective team, all individuals must draw from similar wells, especially when problems are encountered, as all responses need to be consistent with company values. This is how the Ortho McNeil team responded rapidly and in unity to the Tylenol tampering crisis. The most successful leaders are individuals with the ability to recognize good character qualities and great core values that match those that they espouse. Great companies learn to identify shared core values in people before they hire them.

Recognizing When to Let Some People Go

One of the most difficult decisions for a leader is the decision to let an employee or team member go. This can be more difficult if the employee was hired at the beginning or if they are a cofounder. Often these individuals are not unruly or contentious, they may simply be underperformers or difficult to work with and lack the skills needed to perform at that level. This situation can arise if an individual performs adequately during the company's early-development stage but later cannot contribute to the growing or changing needs of the organization. Occasionally, these individuals were set up for failure because they were given exaggerated senior level titles such as vice president or C-level positions just because they were cofounders or early hires.

Because the entrepreneurial leader has many pressing matters to deal with, personnel issues may be sidestepped because these are difficult to deal with or there is uncertainty about what to do. Entrepreneurs should not be afraid of making tough decisions. Once it becomes clear that an individual is not a good fit, and ample effort has been made to deal with the situation to correct it, the situation must be handled swiftly and decisively. If the leader procrastinates in dealing with personnel problems, someone else must make up for that person's shortcomings or other employees must double-check their work because of the lack of confidence in their capabilities. If the problem is with an individual in a senior leadership position, you must weigh the significance of management time, damage to employee morale, and the likelihood of the individual's future contribution to the organization. Ask yourself, "*would this individual, be a great asset for the organization as it continues to grow?*" If the answer is clearly "*no*," then you are setting up the organization for extended and expanded problems by not dealing with this now.

Sometimes, there can be good alternatives to this situation, but these depend on the type of problem and the inherent capabilities of the problem individual. If the problem stems from their abilities being misaligned with their job description, possibly they can be given alternate job responsibilities that are consistent with their skills. For instance, if the individual is a great strategic thinker but is a terrible manager, then consider a role as a nonmanaging member of the organization. If the individual is creative and provides ideas but cannot carry out or manage projects, then possibly a consultant role to the organization will work. However, if the problem stems from the individual's inability to work with others, a misalignment with the company's core values, or the absence of one or more of the three characteristics of an ideal candidate for the position, then termination is usually the only alternative.

Recognize that human relations (HR) issues should be documented throughout this correction process. Some of these activities include performance reviews, corrective actions with clear details about their performance and expectations, documentation of the problems, assistance in helping to remediate the problems, as well as warnings that the lack of correction or improvement can result in termination. These solutions should have been tried prior to reaching a termination decision. Most of the states in the United States acknowledge what is called "at-will" employment, meaning there is an understanding that employees can be terminated "at-will" provided there is no discrimination against any member of a protected group of individuals, such as the aged, handicapped, minorities, and various others. In issues where termination is involved, it is always advisable to consult with an HR attorney or if the company has a shared-employer professional employer organization (PEO), they can provide guidance during this process.

If the leader ignores personnel problem issues, this diminishes the effectiveness of the organization and over time damages trust with other employees, especially if this individual holds a key role in the senior management. Ultimately, these decisions should result in what is best for the organization rather than what is best for one individual. In rescue missions and stories of heroics "the good of the one outweighs the good of the many." However, in start-up and development-stage companies the good of the one cannot outweigh the good of the many. It is not uncommon that in a rapidly growing biotechnology company, the responsibilities and the organization's needs surpass the capability of the founding CEO or other founding employees. Unfortunately, the "one" may even be the founding CEO. There are times when the founding CEO needs to depart for the good of the company. Sometimes, this may be hostile, but in the best of situations, this should be a planned succession.

Summary

Having the ability to recognize the different development stages of an organization is key for an entrepreneurial leader. All companies transition through these development stages, but the time spent within each stage is dependent upon the type of product being developed. At the start-up stage the leader will manage the team with what is called the "entrepreneurial" or "command-and-control" management style. This management style is characterized by centralized decision-making with strong controls. During the corporate-development phase, as the experience level and number of employees increase, the leader must make a management-style change. The leader must successfully transition to a "professional management style," or what is known as "delegate-and-inspect" management style. The professional management style is characterized by a delegation of decision-making responsibilities and formal control mechanisms. Unfortunately, some entrepreneurial leaders do not know how to change, or may not want to change. Failure to make this management-style transition will become detrimental to the company and it will impact the future success of the organization.

A company's new hires are key to getting a strong start on product development and expanding your internal expertise. These individuals also have an impact on your ability to raise capital because a biotech start-up organization must have experienced and qualified individuals in all functions where the company professes expertise. In order to hire the best, develop an interview process that permits the examination of the three important qualities for an ideal candidate such as having related experience, having the ability to execute, and possessing shared core values. Make sure that you have a well-thought-out strategy for hiring individuals at an appropriate level within the organization. As the company grows, be sure to address employee and personnel issues quickly, as these can rapidly destroy a team's motivation and restrict a company's ability to make important product-development progress. Each member of the team will either be an asset or a detriment to progress, so it is critical to identify the best ones and continually help them to become better employees, managers and leaders.

References

[1] Johnson & Johnson. Our Credo Values. Available from: <https://www.jnj.com/credo/> [accessed January 17, 2019].

[2] Urban H. *Life's greatest lessons: 20 things that matter*. 4th ed. New York: Simon & Schuster; 2003.

[3] Shimasaki CD. Hiring a biotech dream team. The business of bioscience: what goes into making a biotechnology product. 1st ed. New York: Springer; 2009. p. 179–95. Chapter 11.

Chapter 36

Biotechnology Business Development: The Art of the Deal

Jack M. Anthony[1], Philip Haworth, PhD[2] and Gayle M. Mills, MBA[2]

[1]*Founder and Former Principal, BioMentorz, Inc., Healdsburg, CA, United States,* [2]*Principal, BioMentorz, Inc., Santa Fe, NM, United States*

Chapter Outline

Introduction

In the biotechnology industry the need for cash is constant. Few, if any, biotech companies can raise enough capital to cover the cost to advance its ideas to commercialization or to execute on all the potential applications of its technology. In this chapter, we describe the functions of a business development (BD) professional and the process of deal making. During the early days of the industry, the need to find capital for human clinical trials opened a door for a new breed of individuals who could integrate the skills of a salesperson, strategic planner, financial forecaster, telemarketer, paralegal, and effective science-friendly presenter, to name a few important traits. BD executives are typically assigned the responsibility to find and negotiate partnerships to provide funding. In a typical partnership, the biotech company may receive upfront payments, equity, milestone payments, fee-for-service payments, and, eventually, royalties on sales; in exchange, the partner receives a license or option to development and marketing rights to the biotechnology company's product. BD executives need a diverse set of traits and skills. Mastering these skills has become more complex. The goal of this chapter is to offer insight into the function responsible for achieving these partnerships focusing on how to organize your efforts, keep the momentum moving, and to reach a successful outcome for your business. This information will be helpful whatever stage of product development your company is at, and it will help you be more aware of the steps involved in this process. Every biotechnology company's survival is dependent on not only its success in the laboratory and the clinic but also by the nature of the transactions it completes—whether they be licensing transactions, merger and acquisition (M&A) transactions or investment transactions, and the biotech's ability to successfully manage the alliances it establishes. Without the occurrence of one or more of these events, there will be limited clinical development pipelines and fewer therapeutic and medical device

Biotechnology Entrepreneurship. DOI: https://doi.org/10.1016/B978-0-12-815585-1.00036-X

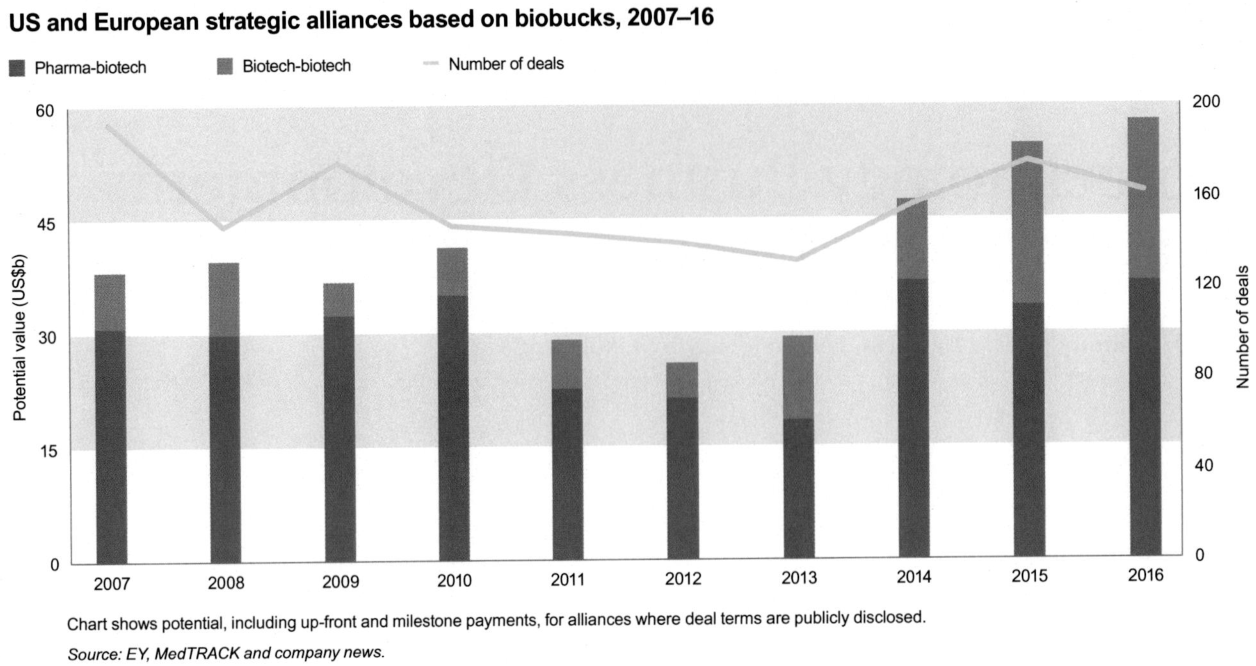

FIGURE 36.1 Average potential deal size.

products reaching the marketplace. A key to the success and future growth of any biotechnology company is creating an environment for deal making through BD.

Background of Biotechnology Licensing and Partnering Deals

To get an idea of the magnitude and significance of these types of biotechnology deals, we look at completed deals over a 10-year period from 2007 to 2016. The components of deals and associated values are constantly evolving; however, it is clear that although the number of deals has remained relatively stable, the expected deal value has continually increased since 2014 (Fig. 36.1).

Even though the volume of deals decreased slightly in 2016, the total value of strategic alliance payments rose in 2016, reaching an all-time high of $57.7 billion. The average potential deal value (for deals with disclosed financials) also rose to $358 million per deal, well above the 10 years average deal value. While the appetite for deals within the drug discovery/development sector remains robust, the variables of a deal in terms of dollars, milestones, and staging have shifted somewhat. In our experience discussions with potential partners it is suggested that obtaining large upfront payments and early milestones versus downstream milestones and even royalties remain challenging as "buyers" are applying more pressure and knowledge on the biotech company to produce and be successful before paying significant milestones or license fees. Countering that trend, however, are newer option-deal structures driven by the financial accounting requirements of pharmaceutical companies, notably Celgene. These deal structures have created the opportunity for some biotechs to negotiate very large upfront payments in exchange for future options to license or buy a product, products, or even the company itself. Examples of deals with the large upfront payments in 2016 are shown in the figure (Fig. 36.2).

Expectations for future deal biotech deal making are dependent on many factors which are difficult, if not impossible, to predict. These factors include but are not limited to the strength of the biotech IPO market, the financial situation of the pharmaceutical industry (e.g., changes in the tax law and repatriation of international income), and the attractiveness of new product candidates available for partnership.

The International Climate for Biotechnology Deal Making—The European Case

Given the substantially smaller number of European biotechnology firms, the number of deals consummated is relatively lower than that by US-based firms. The deal value for EU deals is also smaller, approximately one-half of US-based deals. The figures later illustrate the differences in the deal values between the regions.

In spite of these data, it is possible to consummate a significant transaction as a European biotech. The basic fundamentals on the BD process described in this article are the same, regardless of your company's location.

Alliances with big up-front payments, 2016

Company	Country	Partner	Country	Up-front payment (US$m)
Otsuka Pharmaceutical	Japan	Akebia Therapeutics	US	265
Celgene	US	Jounce Therapeutics	US	261
Teva	Israel	Regeneron Therapeutics	US	250
Celgene	US	Agios Pharmaceuticals	US	200
Incyte	US	Merus	Netherlands	200
Merck & Co.	US	ModeRNA Therapeutics	US	200
Baxalta	US	Symphogen	Denmark	175
Novartis	Switzerland	Xencor	US	150
Allergan	Ireland	Heptares Therapeutics	UK	125
Regeneron Pharmaceuticals	US	Intellia Therapeutics	US	125
Nestle Health Science	Switzerland	Seres Therapeutics Inc.	US	120
Vifor Pharma	Switzerland	ChemoCentryx	US	105
Baxalta	US	Precision BioSciences	US	105
Janssen Biotech	US	MacroGenics	US	75

Source: EY, Capital IQ, Medtrack and company news.

FIGURE 36.2 Potential upfront payments for deal alliances.

In the experience of the authors working with and in some cases for European biotechnology firms, the greatest single difference between smaller biotech firms located in Europe is the lower number of senior employees from pharmaceutical or large biotech companies in these smaller European biotechs. This gap should not be an impediment to executing deals, however. European biotechs can easily surmount this potential problem by employing consultants with experience in the US pharmaceutical industry—whether it be in the BD, commercial, or clinical arenas. Other success factors in European BD are the willingness of the BD leader to attend industry meetings, make phone calls outside of normal working hours to companies located in other time zones (rather than relying entirely on email communication), and ability to forge relationships with pharmaceutical company BD executives.

In Japan, pharma companies are well versed in the business of doing deals. The Japanese market is considered one of the seven major pharmaceutical markets in the world and many of the Japanese companies also have operations outside of Japan. The key difference in negotiating such deals is that rather being "lawyered-up" as many US and European deal meetings may be, the Japanese usually have very wise and experienced BD people in the room to do the dealing, rarely are any lawyers present. The pace may be somewhat slower due to language issues and customs, but in general they are totally focused on the best deal for themselves so being steadfast is important. And then finally—we cannot stress this enough—deals in Japan take longer than they do in the United States. It's not going to happen overnight unless you are very lucky or if one of the senior biotech executives has a close, personal relationship with senior management at the Japanese Pharma.

What Is a Business Development "Deal?"

A deal involves the exchange of goods or assets between two parties. The parties may be two companies or alternatively, the parties may be one company and a group of shareholders in which technology is sold or rented for present or future cash. The deal is a transaction in which, hopefully, both parties realize essential gain in the interest of their respective organizations. In our world the deal includes all forms of licensing transactions, M&A, and the sale of equity to investors.

Let us be clear at the outset, deal making is a form of selling; however, biotech deal making differs from "sales" in one very important aspect. In traditional sales a transaction can be completed by an individual salesperson skilled in the art of presenting product benefits and appropriate closing techniques. But in biotechnology, creating a deal requires the inclusion, cooperation, and coordination of a group of people across multiple company functions. The successful completion of a deal requires a choreographed performance involving scientists, clinicians, manufacturing experts, consultants, and other contributors. It can be a challenging job to sell what are essentially "futures" on today's projects.

We believe that the most important predictor of success in executing a biotech deal is the ability of the BD professional to fully understand the unique needs and individual concerns of the potential partner firm. Without this full understanding, your potential partner will continually identify "red flags" without your company being able to anticipate or fully address their concerns. Key to your ability to gain this understanding is to identify a champion in the potential partner firm and to use all your interpersonal skills to forge a strong relationship based on honesty and transparency. Intensive research into the potential partner firm and discussions with fellow BD colleagues who have already executed deals with the company are also essential.

Starting the Process

Before you start the "deal" process, there are four questions that must be asked and answered by you and your company:

1. What is being "sold?"
2. Why are you selling it?
3. What value can realistically be realized?
4. Who might want to buy "it?"

What Is Being Sold?

Typically, there are three broad categories of products for sale, these are as follows:

1. ***The entire company and its vision.*** Notable recent examples include Gilead's nearly $12 billion acquisition of Kite Pharma and Johnson & Johnson's $30 billion acquisition of Swiss biotech Actelion.
2. ***A specific technology with multiple potential applications.*** For example, in February 2018, Gilead partnered for the use of Sangamo's zinc finger technology in Gilead's CAR-T programs for an upfront of $150 million.
3. ***A single product or products.*** For example, in September 2016, Pfizer acquired a preclinical anti-CTLA4 antibody from OncoImmune with a reported deal value of $250 million.

Reaching an internal agreement on what your company is about to sell can be more difficult than you might expect. Until you have defined what you have to sell, it is difficult to identify those who might want to buy it, and it is impossible to calculate or agree upon what it might be worth.

Why Are You Selling It?

Next, you need to agree on why you want to complete a transaction? The most obvious answers to this question are either (1) you need the money and resources and/or (2) you need the[1] "validation" that a partner would bring to your company. Any deal should have a purpose that is greater than simply a short-term cash payment. Many times, deals are transacted to access resources that in the long term will generate more value for the company if you sell it now, than if you did not. For example, it is very hard for a small biotechnology company to ultimately sell, distribute, and market a chronic use of cardiovascular drug due to the extremely large Phase 3 clinical trials required to obtain regulatory approval. Alternatively, the real purpose of the deal might not be an immediate need. Sometimes, another reason for doing a deal is to unload an asset that no longer fits with the company's focus. Whatever the reason, it is important to reach agreement on the deal rationale among the board of directors and the management team of the company. Without a clear rationale for why this deal is important to the company, frustration from the time and resources spent on the deal process may inevitably focus upon the BD executive tasked with this transaction.

Providing early clarity about why the deal should be done will also help the BD person to recognize when to abandon or substantially modify a proposed transaction. Unless you are simply doing transactions for the sake of doing transactions, it is entirely possible that the deal you have spent months working on is no longer important either because the circumstances have changed or the proposed deal terms no longer meet the reason for doing the deal in the first place. Part of the BD executive's job is to know when to say "no" to a deal. Open, constant, and clear communications up and down the company chain-of-command are critical in the deal-making process. An astute BD executive understands this even if others do not. They understand that part of their job is to be in the front of any discussion no matter which direction it takes.

How Much Is It Worth?

Assuming that at this point, the team has agreed on what it is going to sell and why they want to sell it. Now comes the hard part. How much is it worth? This can be a very delicate discussion both internally and externally. The person charged with leading the deal process has to employ a credible and acceptable valuation process.

There are basically two methods commonly utilized to value a precommercial stage asset. The best method is to use some form of discounted cash-flow model, such as a Net Present Value (NPV) calculation or a Monte Carlo Analysis [1]. There are now readily available product and technology-based NPV models available from a variety of sources. Difficulties may arise in populating your model if an organization is unwilling or unable to effectively assess the risk, cost, and time associated with commercializing a particular asset. Sound, supportable discounted cash-flow calculations can and do occur but require the biotech to embark on a critical internal analysis of the asset that requires a level of detached objectivity. To aid in this the BD professional may find it extremely valuable to bring in experts in the field of research and development in your therapeutic area to provide external input and planning.

Another approach is to base the valuation of your product on comparable deals—deals that have been completed on similar products or assets. This method of evaluating the "comps" is a similar methodology to that used when determining home value in the housing market.

Searchable biotechnology deal databases can be accessed at a cost through organization, such as Recap by Cortellis,[2] BioScience Advisors, or EvaluatePharma.[3] Typically, these databases can be searched on selectable criteria, for instance, "Phase I antibody for solid tumor oncology in Japan." The database will return a selection of transactions meeting these criteria which will include the name of the parties, the date, and subject matter of the transaction and (to greater or lesser extent) information on the deal terms. It is unlikely that the search will turn up a deal involving an asset that is identical to yours but there should be some that are close enough to provide a range of values related to licensing a Phase I antibody to treat solid tumor cancers in Japan. The best part about this approach is that it is driven by objective external data that can be presented to everyone on both sides of the transaction.

One last comment on valuation—the techniques that do not work are "We need $5 million for next year's budget—go get a deal", or "We spent $15 million on this program therefore it must be worth twice that. . .."

Who Will Want to Buy It?

The fourth and final step in preparing your partnering campaign is to determine who may be likely to sign up to pay for your asset. In classical business school terms the Venn diagram methodology for selecting a corporate partner is a strategic modeling approach called the 3C elements of success. The 3C term was originally coined by Kenichi Ohmae, a business and corporate strategist,[4] who referenced the three elements of success as the customer, the competitors, and the corporation. In the context of biotechnology partnering and deals the 3Cs have evolved into the cash, the competency, and the commitment. In short, this translates into can they pay for it, can they develop it, and who will develop it (Fig. 36.3).

In a perfect world, one would begin a partnering campaign with a certainty about who has the cash, competency,

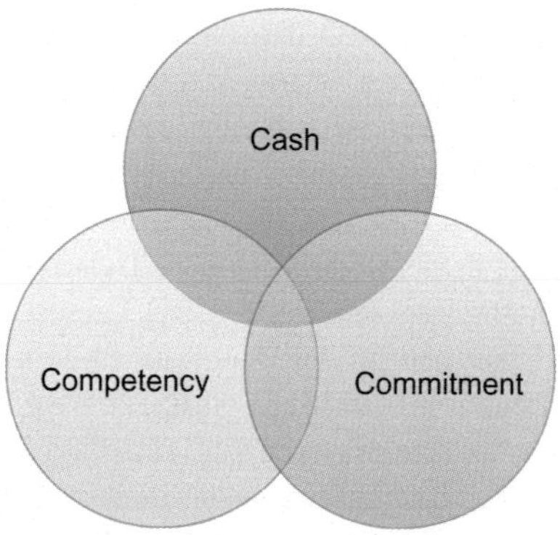

FIGURE 36.3 Three Cs of finding the best deal partner.

and commitment to develop your product. Alas, we do not live in a perfect world. We know that large pharma has "cash" but that does not mean they are willing to spend it, we know what has developed which drugs and presumably, therefore, has competency to develop more but knowing who might be willing to make the commitment is much harder. While the process for identifying potential partners is not perfect, it won't be hard to develop an "A List" of the most likely partner to meet your needs in the deal, but if you begin to reach out to the B List, just make sure they don't know they are the B List.

The Deal Requires a Plan

It is likely that every BD executive accepts the axiom, "it is better to be lucky than smart" but every experienced BD person also knows that in all likelihood, getting a deal done will require something more than luck: a solid plan. The plan will need to encompass every aspect of the deal process from identifying the company contacts to selecting the lawyer for the final contract negotiation. In the following is a template of the plan, the first four steps of which should now be familiar to you:

1. What do you want sell? ✓
2. Why do you want to sell it? ✓
3. What can you expect to get for it? ✓
4. Who can you expect to buy it? ✓

The essential nature of these first four elements should be obvious by now and hopefully getting that far in the process has created a forum for developing the rest of the plan.

Who Is Going to Be Responsible for the Deal Process?

The process needs to have a leader and the likely candidates include the CEO, the CFO, the General Counsel (GC), or the head of BD. The authors of this chapter have a strong bias toward having the leader be the senior BD person, assuming they have the ability and the experience. In most instances the GC or CFO will approach a deal based upon their individual technical expertise, whether it be law or finance. While the expertise of a GC and/or CFO can be invaluable in the deal-making process, simply viewing the deal through just one lens can be annoying to the other party and destructive to the deal. While your CEO may have the necessary experience and knowledge to carry out the deal, they will almost certainly be too busy to be engaged in every element of the process. Most importantly, there can be a very real advantage in not having the final decision maker in the room during key parts of the negotiation. There is a sound academic basis for using a phrase that is heard from every car salesperson in America, "I need to take that to my manager." [2]. It actually works in a negotiation. It works because it allows time for a more thoughtful response and it works because it tells the buyer that they are pushing close to the limits of the deal.

Who Is on the Deal Team?

Initially, everyone may want to play a role in the deal (this enthusiasm will decrease over time) but it is essential to define and limit the core membership of the team. Recruitment to the team should be based partially on the skills and experience of individuals, but the leader will also need to make some decisions based on an individual's personality. Who would you want to spend a rainy, gray weekend in a foreign country with? If the thought of this concerns you when you think about any particular individual, they may not be the best person to include on your deal team. Not everyone in your organization has the skill and temperament to do this work; so, while your chief scientific officer might be the best scientist in your company, he or she may not have the patience or time to schlep around the world visiting potential partners. Pick your team wisely and keep them happy. Often, potential partners may be located in a country other than yours and for a number of months you may end up spending more time with these folks then your spouse and your children. As the deal team leader, you need to recognize that in addition to working on the deal, your team members have a regular day job and you need to reward and encourage your team: a good meal in a fun restaurant goes a long way, take them to a sporting event in some new city, or try a museum in a new city. If this kind of expense doesn't work with your company policies, you may have to pay it out of your own pocket, but that just binds the team to you more closely.

The essential elements of any deal team will be BD, R&D (clinical), and legal, although it is less likely that legal will be required on the traveling squad at least at the beginning stages of the process. Other occasional team members might include members from finance, commercial, manufacturing, and regulatory. It is important to recognize that some of the team may view the intended transaction as a threat to their role in the company and the larger the size of the deal team, the more likely it is to include members of the "resistance" and managing, this tension will be a test of leadership skills. If you have time to read it, there is a great book that can help with these issues called "Thinking Fast and Slow" by Daniel Kahneman [3].

Establish the Role of Each Member of the Deal Team at the Outset

There are a number of serious conversations that will need to occur between you and your team members. Defining each team member's role in the deal process and making sure each member understands their role is vital.

Of crucial importance is that your scientific team member must be an excellent presenter who answers questions thoughtfully, is able to forge a relationship with the other side's scientist, and most importantly is able to establish her/his credibility and expertise. For instance, a scientist and or a clinician will at some point start to speculate on data that have yet to be generated or yet to be shared with your potential partner. Any good scientist or clinician requires a healthy dose of introspective analysis and skepticism, or what one academic calls the "irony of abnegation" [4] which we interpret to mean, a technical person cannot define success without first exploring and explaining every source of failure. Although his approach is a legitimate asset in becoming a better scientist, this type of communication with your potential partner can turn your deal into a train wreck in minutes.

It is not that you must ask your scientist to lie, merely to answer the question as it is posed and not as it might be interpreted. For example, the answer to the question, "do you have animal data showing efficacy" is "Yes, let me show you the data from our rat study." The answer *should not be* "We couldn't make work it in dogs so we did it in rats." The discussion about the failed dog experiment should and will occur later when the parties are in diligence, but on a first date, there is no need to talk about your early tentative efforts. Potential partners need to first see value in the deal before they hear the concerns; otherwise, you will never find a partner. Before each and every meeting, review with your team the goals and scope of the meeting/presentation and make sure they understand the limits of the subject matter to be discussed at any particular moment in time.

Keeping the CEO, the Board, and the Scientific Advisory Board (SAB) Updated

Even if the CEO is not on the deal team, let us not pretend for a moment that they will not be involved in your deal. The amount of CEO involvement is directly proportional to the importance of the deal to the company. If the CEO has no interest in the deal, you should probably think about working on something else. As we have previously discussed, not having the CEO involved in the day-to-day of a deal has its advantages. However, while you may be running the deal, the CEO is still running the company. If you and the CEO are not in agreement at the outset, the situation is unlikely to improve over time. It is a good idea to remind yourself that the CEO directly answers to the shareholders and those shareholders are not part of the deal team and are mainly influenced by events outside of your company. So, if the shareholders pressure the CEO, the CEO will pressure you.

Working with the CEO while still managing the deal process is a balancing act that all BD executives must accomplish. There are things that can help make this work: (1) make sure you and the CEO have regular face-to-face meetings in which you provide an accurate and honest update on the process; (2) make sure there are no surprises for the CEO, keep them up-to-date so they can inform the board effectively; and (3) avoid making predictions and try never to quantify the possibility of a getting the deal done. We suggest that all the key players, the CEO, and the board, get regular updates on the deal process. Knowing that you will be called upon to update the progress and status of a deal means that BD must keep track of all communications, meetings, personnel (both teams), and decisions (those made and the process for making new ones).

Select and Manage the Point(s) of Contact in Each Target Company

The next step in the plan will be to work out who within each company will be the initial point of contact for your proposition. Our advice on this point is to recruit as much help as you can to develop this list—it makes everyone feel involved and it actually helps. There are some fundamental questions that need to be answered, such as how will the dialog begin and who will manage it? Sometimes BD, sometimes R&D, and sometimes another person in your company will manage the initial contact. By working on an inventory of individuals who have contact with any given target partner, you give your company the best opportunity to get a deal done. Also note that the best method of approach for one target company may not be the best method for the next company. Consequently, choosing the initial contact point at a target company can have a significant impact on your deal process.

Develop a Script for Your First Communication

The first communication between you and any potential partner is perhaps the most critical and most difficult to prepare. Later in this chapter, we will describe the various pitch formats that the deal team will require in order to reach a successful conclusion. This first communication is little more than a written variation of the company's known "Elevator Pitch." There are no more than five things you should try to communicate in this first step:

1. The mission and purpose of your company.
2. What you are trying to sell?
3. What your asset is capable of achieving?
4. The stage of development of your asset.
5. How your asset will help this potential partner?

To do this effectively the initial pitch should be no more than one page of the text or approximately 10–15 PowerPoint slides. All individuals involved in delivering a pitch to any potential partner should use the same documents. It is incumbent upon the deal team leader to make sure that everyone understands the key points of the message and to ensure that team members are willing and capable of delivering the same message.

Prepare a Number of Presentations for Your Deal Campaign

Although the partnering campaign will begin with a simple, short nonconfidential introduction, such as described earlier, it requires much more than this to get the deal done. It is anticipated that you may need up to five different presentations in addition to the nonconfidential introduction. These presentations are intended to reveal increasing levels of details and confidentiality. In our experience the process more or less follows the following steps, with the required presentations highlighted in italics:

1. Nonconfidential introduction
2. *Nonconfidential presentation (more information than the intro but still not everything)*
3. Sign (first) confidential disclosure agreement (CDA)
4. *First confidential presentation (new data included)*
5. *Second confidential presentation (plans and progress)*
6. Sign second CDA (sometimes required)
7. *Intellectual property (IP) presentation*
8. *Commercial presentation that may include forecasts (if appropriate)*
9. Diligence

It is best to have these presentations prepared at the outset of the process, although they will need to be updated as time passes.

Start Planning for the Diligence Process

It may seem overly optimistic to think about the due diligence process at the beginning of the partnering campaign, but preparing the diligence documents early can positively impact the deal process in a number of ways. There are two clear benefits to considering the due diligence process at this early stage. First, the team will be forced to confront the status of the documentation required to support the transaction. If the gaps in this paper trail can be identified at this stage of the process, there is time to remedy or correct the flaws. If the flaws cannot be corrected (and there are circumstances where this might occur) the understanding of these deficiencies can at least be factored into the partnering process and the valuation exercise. The second is that it can have a significant positive impact on the actual deal itself. At some point a potential partner will want to access the diligence documents and if they are ready to go, it sends the message that your company is competent and confident. It also suggests that they might not be the first or only party to begin diligence.

Today, almost all diligence processes are conducted primarily through the use of a secure virtual data room. It is key to ensure that you closely manage access to your data room, providing access to specific folders only when appropriate and to only the appropriate individuals within the target company. Partnering companies need to demonstrate their intent in moving forward with a deal before fully opening your confidential data room.

Determine Who Will Be on the Negotiation Team

The negotiation team is not the same group of people who make up the deal team. Typically, the negotiation team is much smaller, comprising usually two or three members—we prefer the two-member team, one from BD and a transaction lawyer (many times an outside lawyer). The relationship between the lead negotiator and the transaction lawyer is the key to a successful negotiation and both individuals need to develop a clear understanding of the other's roles. On occasion, the negotiation team may also include someone from finance or some technical discipline if the deal hinges on some creative financing structure or on some complex technical element. As with the deal team, there are advantages to the CEO not being on the negotiations team, yet the CEO has an essential role in the negotiation. Using the presence and absence of the CEO in a well-organized manner can be a key element in closing the deal. In abstentia, the CEO can be both a "good cop and bad cop[5]" who can influence deal discussions at critical points but this type of role play has to be used sparingly; otherwise, eventually, the other side will insist on negotiating directly with the CEO.

Closing the Deal

There will come a point in the discussions when some kind of financial proposal will be appropriate. Assuming that your party is selling the asset, we are great believers in retaining the power of the pen, meaning that the first proposal should come from you. Once this initial offer is presented, assuming it has some basis in commercial reality, both parties tend to treat it as a benchmark. We recommend discussing your opening bid in person (face-to-face or over the phone) before submitting the formal written offer as it limits surprises and saves embarrassing misunderstanding. Once you have discussed what your opening bid will be, your second decision becomes how you want to appear to the other party, that is, a hard bargainer or moderate. Whichever you choose, the chances are that the other negotiator will respond in kind, so make sure you select a style with which you are comfortable because it is likely to be present throughout the negotiations. Your opening offer will be met, hopefully, with a counteroffer, and thus the negotiations begin. By the time the parties have exchanged two or three versions of the term sheet or contract, it should be apparent where the deal is heading and, with any good fortune, the terms and conditions agreed in those drafts will be consistent with the terms discussed in the deal preparation process.

If the terms don't meet your desired goals, there are some difficult decisions to make, but first it is helpful to understand why you are not getting what you need from this deal. There can be a number of reasons, the most likely being a lack of leverage in the negotiation. The absence of an alternative buyer always limits leverage and the other side eventually knows they are the only party at the table. Your leverage in a negotiation can also be reduced by other circumstances, including your company's financial position or the failure of a related technology or product which can undermine the perceived value of your asset. It could be that the world around your asset has changed or perhaps the strengths of your program have been undermined or devalued by new information on IP or discovery of another disease mechanism. Do you take the offered terms or walk away? There can be no universal answer to this question and each organization will need to carefully examine the original reasons for doing the deal. That is why those preparatory activities you conducted are so important to the deal process.

Mostly, negotiations fall into one of the two styles; the win/win where both sides believe in enlarging the pie before dividing it or the distributive approach where the size of the pie is fixed and one side wins as the other losses. If you have a choice, although you may not, avoid the distributive approach. Many times, the parties that adopt this method do not have interest in a relationship and inevitably these deals do not stand the test of time. We should point out that because the biotechnology/pharma world is relatively small, it is very likely that you will know someone who has done a deal with the organization with which you are about to enter into negotiations. Talk with them on the phone and ask how the other side operates—it will help you prepare for the next steps. If you find out that they don't have a track record of adopting the win/win approach, you can adjust your style accordingly.

Regardless of the approach, we recommend that during the negotiation it is best to avoid adopting direct conflict as a strategy for completing the negotiation. If you are the smaller company it is unlikely that this path will be tolerated for long. If conflict does occur the leader needs to refocus all parties on the mutual benefits of the deal, rather than the specific issue and then pursue an indirect approach to resolving the source of conflict. Your responsibility as the negotiation leader is to control any conflict that might arise and limit the amount of damage to the credibility of your side. Demonstrations of anger, no matter how much they are provoked, are usually not the best way to get your argument across. If there is a point at which the proposed position is unacceptable to you or is inconsistent with a previously agreed position, say "no"—at some point the other side needs to know that there are some things you cannot agree to.

If the discussion gets emotional, try to stop the discussion and refocus. There are a number of alternatives which can be used by themselves or together: (1) take a break (someone always needs to go to the restroom or to get some fresh air); (2) break the tension by making a joke, but not at the expense of the protagonist; and (3) table the subject for now and move on to a more resolvable topic. Keeping the dialog moving forward can significantly change the dynamic in the room.

Most conflicts in a negotiation are based on one or more of the following traits: (1) competitive personalities, (2) misperceptions and bias, (3) poor communication of the issues, and (4) rigid "policy" commitments. The basic individual personality traits cannot probably be changed, although the "flash points" can be limited by careful alterations of your message and style.

If you reach an acceptable end by narrowing the differences, you are now ready to close the deal. It is essential to close the deal as quickly as possible. The deal should never be assumed to be done until the contract agreement is signed. In order to help close the deal quickly, create some context of a ticking clock, the end of fiscal year will usually provide impetus to get it done.

At the end of the negotiation, you will have won some points and lost some points. To get the deal approved, you are going to have to match the points won and lost with the goals that were agreed upon at the outset of this process. If you have communicated effectively throughout this process and followed the rule of no surprises, the CEO and board are more likely to approve the final transaction. If you don't think the deal is good enough to sign, tell your CEO and board and let the board override you if they want. If you believe the deal is good but the CEO or board does not approve it, then somewhere along the way you have made a mistake in your process. Work out what that mistake was and don't make it again!

A Summary of the Deal Process

We refer to the process of bringing a deal to the table and closing it, as a "dance." Like dancing, it is best learned by practice. To give the readers a flavor of this dance, we conclude with a summary, but by no means all, of the steps involved.

- ***The role of BD is different in every company.*** These can include in-licensing, out-licensing, alliance management, strategy development, fund raising, product development, and many others. Understand the true needs of your business and be careful not to be distracted or sidelined by other assignments. At the end of the day the core BD needs must be taken care of, all else is secondary.
- ***Understand the environment into which you will be "selling."*** Understand what drives companies, people, competitors, suppliers, bankers, and the board. By understanding these players, it will help you plan a partnering campaign.
- ***Think first.*** BD is not a ready, fire, aim process. Thoughtful analysis, talking with contemporaries, and "reading between the lines" are all part of the preparation before you approach your targets. There is a huge amount of background information available to you, take some time to review it.
- ***Understand big pharma (or the inverse, small biotech).*** If you have not walked in their shoes, you need to learn about the pressures and constraints they operate under. Take someone in that organization to lunch and listen.
- ***Get your "elevator pitch" down cold.*** If you cannot tell your story and have interest in 30 seconds or less, you are in trouble. Don't use a computer or props, nothing but your voice. Practice it every day, in the car, to your partner, to the dog, to your coworkers. This elevator pitch will grow into an opening slide of your presentation and change over time. See it as the backbone of everything your company is.
- ***Understand what you want to buy or sell.*** If you don't, then the path is long and rough, and you may never get to complete a deal.
- ***Think through all the materials you need to line up.*** Collateral materials, slide decks, patent summaries, bibliographies, scientific champions, an internal survey of employees for industry contacts, and lots more.
- ***Prepare multiple presentations.*** The partnering meeting slide deck, the nonconfidential introduction deck, and the confidential deck I and II (hold something back for another meeting). Avoid background colors, too much animation, slides that cannot be read from the back of the room for which you always apologize. Never distribute slides to the other side in anything other than a pdf format.
- ***Always review materials before sending.*** Circumstances, data, and messages change. No excuses accepted. At the

same time avoid creating new decks for every request or there will be confusion and chaos.

- ***We have a mantra about carefully listening to others: "You have two ears and one mouth ... for a reason!"*** If you have ever been exposed to a sales technique course, you learn early to listen to your customer carefully. The more you listen, the more you will uncover needs, concerns, and get direction on moving forward.
- ***Partnering meetings.*** You can spend a lifetime and a fortune going to these meetings. They are very helpful when introducing a company or a project or after a major inflection point. Go to meetings to inform, not close. *At some point sitting in partnering booths is not appropriate!*
- ***Bluebirds and frogs.*** Even though you have your priority target list, sometimes serendipity works in your favor. *Open all your windows and sometimes a bluebird will fly in. Said another way, kiss all the frogs. There is a prince there somewhere.* Who and why deals get done is not entirely predictable, it is a mistake not to allow luck to help.
- ***Follow-up.*** Like everything else in life, follow-up is critical. Keep doors open, respond to requests, summarize meetings, send new information, build your case, and get to another meeting.
- ***Term sheets.*** Pretty standard formats. Creativity here is many times not appreciated. Mark everything draft. Never agree to a binding term sheet. If they want a deal, do the deal. Keep term sheet development low key with lots of back and forth. Keep board informed. Move to approvals once all the cats are herded and key points are settled. Generally, a term sheet is prepared by the seller.
- ***Agreement draft.*** Who writes? Emotional issue. Either side can write, but the power of the pen is real. Small companies can avoid large legal fees by letting other team write. Yes, there will be some bias but that can work in the seller's favor. Set a timeframe for completion.
- ***Negotiations.*** Yes you can take a workshop or just use common sense. Know your *musts* versus your *wants*. Have a good, experienced transaction lawyer alongside you. Work out roles and responsibilities with your attorney before you sit down. Leave egos at the door.
- ***Due diligence.*** Use electronic data rooms. Answer direct questions—directly. If you don't have a data point or know an answer, just say so. No hand waving please.
- ***After the signing.*** Have a nice social affair and a little gift token. Give good toasts. Enjoy.
- ***Alliance management.*** As important as all that has gone before, keeping a deal going is as important as getting it. BD should remain involved as they know the faces and the background. Do not distribute the contract to new players internally, only the grant, the governance clauses, and other key operating terms.

What Is the Secret to Being an Effective Business Development Executive?

As an early senior executive of Genentech once remarked, the really great BD executives possess a "secret sauce" to make things happen when others might give up and walk away. The secret sauce of BD executives includes the experience necessary to lead a company's internal team to success in completing a deal. What may appear to be a series of random events but in actuality is a very organized effort, over many months or years, to attract significant funding for company operations from partners.

BD executives are partially born and partially made. The right temperament, style, sense of humor, ability to know when to press and when not to, the ability to read people, a sense of drama, etc. are probably ingrained into a personality from their early years. This can be described as the ability to know when to talk and when to listen, process information, ask direct probing questions or indirect probing questions, engage in light conversation, and look people in the eye when addressing them. It includes the ability to write and talk precisely, avoid the "ums" and "you-knows" that one hears so often from the podium, and understanding about cultural sensitivity—these come from experience on the job and just plain common sense about your profession. Everyone can develop their own secret sauce. It's about style, timing, and momentum. Having a mentor or two somewhere along the way speeds the process. You will know you have it when you the first time a potential partner says to you "Okay, sounds good, let's do this deal...."A dedicated and effective BD executive must balance and resolve "internal" aspirations and goals with the inevitably differing external reality.

The Internet provides the BD executive with a huge amount of data to assist with our work, and it also provides everyone else with vast amounts of data. Large amounts of information, whether it be real or fake, require time to analyze and understand. Finding consensus within this mass of information has become one of the most important skills required of a BD executive. Recently, in the biotechnology industry, we have seen astounding growth in the fields of immuno-oncology and cell-based therapies that has altered both the therapeutic and deal landscapes.

New approaches to treatment and new business models have also brought a new generation of BD executives with innovative ideas and new skills. But the essential function of BD remains unchanged requiring an understanding of the commercial and clinical environment in which your company will operate going forward and to position your company to take maximum advantage of its own strengths. This chapter will not teach you clairvoyance, but we hope that it will show you some of the basic techniques necessary to both prepare and to close a deal, part art and part science. We acknowledge that when successfully managed, BD is the most fun one can have in the biotechnology industry and the satisfaction derived from a job well done is immense.

References

[1] Ulam SM, Eckhardt R. Stan Ulam, John von Neumann, and the Monte Carlo method. Los Alamos Science; 1987. p. 131−7. Special Issue (15).

[2] Desai PS, Purohit D. "Let me talk to my manager": haggling in a competitive environment. Market Sci 2004;23(2):219.

[3] Kahneman D. Think fast and slow. Penguin; 2011. ISBN-13: 9780141033570.

[4] Pappas HJ. How to be a good scientist, the irony of abnegation. Denmark: Kunkliga Tekniska Hogskolan School of Information and Communication Technology.

Endnotes

1. Validation has become a term of art often used by biotech people which has little to no substantive meaning in essence the term tries to capture the notion that if someone important cares about what I am doing, then what I am doing must be important. We can all understand the attractiveness of this idea but in truth, it is just the lack of self-esteem.
2. www.recap.com
3. www.evaluatepharma.com
4. Leading-Minds.com
5. The good cop/bad cop analogy has evolved from a stereotypic style used in TV shows and movies where it is routinely used as a psychological tactic in interrogation. The "bad cop" takes an aggressive, negative stance toward the subject, making blatant accusations, derogatory comments, threats, and in general creating antipathy between the subject and himself. This sets the stage for the "good cop" to act sympathetically: appearing supportive, understanding, in general, showing sympathy for the subject. The good cop will also defend the subject from the bad cop. The subject may feel he can cooperate with the good cop out of trust or fear of the bad cop. He may then seek protection by and trust the good cop and provide the information the interrogators are seeking. These same techniques are used regularly in the context of a negotiation.

Chapter 37

Biotech-Pharma Collaboration—A Strategic Tool: Case Study of Centocor

Lara V. Marks, D.Phil Oxon, FRSB

Honorary Research Associate, Department of Science and Technology Studies, University College London and Managing editor of www.whatisbiotechnology.org, London, United Kingdom

Chapter Outline

The estimated value of alliances signed between pharmaceutical and biotechnology companies was $160 billion per annum in 2011.[1] Underlying the vast sums being paid out for alliances is the fact that such collaboration is a lifeline for pharmaceutical companies scouting for new products to fill their dwindling portfolios in the face of expiring patents and rising generic competition. It is also vital to biotechnology companies seeking to raise funds for their research and development (R&D) and establishing a footprint on the market.

Since their inception, biotechnology companies have depended on partnerships for their survival and growth. This chapter looks at the pivotal role alliances played in the foundation and growth of Centocor, one of America's pioneering monoclonal antibody (mAb) companies. Set up in 1979, 3 years after Genentech, the world's first dedicated biotechnology company, Centocor was among the first handful of biotechnology companies started in the 1970s. Within 5 years of its founding, Centocor had become a highly competitive and profitable diagnostics company based on mAbs. As this chapter shows, much of this success rested on the collaborations its founders secured with research institutes and larger health-care companies. Through skillful networking, Centocor's executives secured the scientific and technological expertise, products, capital, and market distribution necessary to mature from a small start-up company to a major player in the global diagnostic market. In 1992, however, Centocor faced imminent collapse, brought on in part by its executives' decision to go it alone in the development and marketing of the company's first therapeutic. What saved the company from extinction and allowed it to subsequently succeed in therapeutics was a reversion to its strategy of collaboration [2].

The Birth of Centocor

In May 1979, Hilary Koprowski, a Polish virologist, immunologist, and director of the Wistar Institute[3], entered a

1. This figure is based on figures of over 800 deals signed in 2011, each of which was worth approximately $200 million. It is based on data from the EvaluatePharma Deals Database.

2. Research for this chapter is based on Centocor's company papers and the personal papers of Hubert Schoemaker (hereafter HS-PP) kindly provided by his widow Anne Faulkner Schoemaker and on oral interviews with Centocor's employees undertaken by the author in collaboration with the Chemical Heritage Foundation which houses the interview transcripts. The author conducted all interviews listed below except where specified. Interview transcripts are kept at the Chemical Heritage Foundation.

3. For Koprowski's biography see Vaughan R. Listen to the music: the life of Hilary Koprowski. Springer; 2000.

Biotechnology Entrepreneurship. DOI: https://doi.org/10.1016/B978-0-12-815585-1.00037-1

partnership with Michael Wall, an MIT-educated electrical engineer and founder of several electronics, computer, and biological start-up companies, to establish a new biotechnology company.[4] Calling the company Centocor, Koprowski and Wall aimed to create, develop, and market diagnostics and therapeutics based on mAbs. mAbs were new to the scientific and commercial world, having been devised by César Milstein and Georges Köhler at the Laboratory of Molecular Biology, Cambridge in 1975. Derived from natural antibodies (proteins produced by the immune system that are designed to attach to and inactivate foreign particles, or antigens), mAbs were produced as a result of the fusion of myeloma cells with antibodies taken from the spleen of previously immunized animals [5].

Providing for the first time a long-lasting and standardized form of antibodies that could be used for various medical applications, mAbs were quickly adopted by various academic and commercial laboratories globally. This included Koprowski and his team at the Wistar Institute. Using cells sent by Milstein, Koprowski, and his colleagues began to develop mAbs against the influenza virus and malignant cancer tumors.[6] Funded by government grants, this research formed the basis for patent applications in 1978. Granted in 1979 and 1980, these patents were the first-ever patents for mAbs.[7] In 1978 Koprowski offered to license the patents to Boehringer-Ingelheim for $500,000 annually over 10 years. The pharmaceutical company, however, had dragged out negotiations for 6 or 8 months before saying no on the basis that they saw no future for mAb products [8].

Frustrated by his experience with Boehringer-Ingelheim and other companies, Koprowski realized that the only way forward would be to establish a separate company. He decided to do this in partnership with Wall. At the time that Wall and Koprowski started discussing their plans for a company, Wall was getting itchy feet for a change of scenery, having just sold Flow Laboratories, a company he had set up to produce and sell cell cultures and related products. Wall had various business schemes in mind, including growing orchids. His idea of founding a company based on flowers, however, soon dissipated on talking to Koprowski. What captured Wall's attention was the fact that Koprowski believed he could have in hand a mAb diagnostic very quickly. This was named 19-9, a mAb developed at the Wistar Institute that Koprowski saw as having potential as a diagnostic for pancreatic cancer [9].

Setting up an office in downtown Philadelphia in May 1979, Wall started to build Centocor's executive team as the company chairman with scientific support from Koprowski and the Wistar Institute. One of the first to join the executive team was Ted Allen. Allen's background was ideal for Centocor as he had been a marketing manager at Corning Medical, a Boston-based division of Corning Glass Works. More importantly, he came from a company that had begun to establish a strong portfolio of diagnostic immunoassays. Such diagnostics were rapidly replacing the more traditional chemical-based tests that had dominated the diagnostics market since the 1940s [10].

With Allen on board, Centocor soon attracted the interest of another Corning employee who would prove pivotal in moving the company forward. This was Hubert Schoemaker, one of Allen's former Corning colleagues who had been instrumental in building up Corning's pioneering portfolio of diagnostics. Schoemaker was a biochemist by training and had completed a doctorate at MIT within a department at the cutting edge of biotechnology research. One of the factors determining Schoemaker's decision to join the Centocor start-up was his desire to find a way to improve people's lives. His inspiration came from the profound disabilities of his daughter, who was born with lissencephaly, a rare brain malformation causing severe mental disability and motor dysfunction. Schoemaker joined Centocor initially in an unofficial capacity, helping with research and planning while continuing to work at Corning. In early 1980, however, he began officially, taking over the position of chief executive officer in the wake of a sudden departure by Allen.[11] (See Fig. 37.1.)

Within months of joining Centocor's team, Schoemaker had sourced another individual who soon became vital to the company's operation. This was Vincent Zurawski. He joined Centocor in August 1979 as the company's first Chief Scientific Officer. Zurawski came well equipped for

4. HS-PP: Centocor, Centocor Oncogene Research Partners LP, June 9, 1984.

5. For the early development of monoclonal antibodies see Marks L. A healthtech revolution: the story of César Milstein and the making of monoclonal antibodies, <www.whatisbiotechnology.org>.

6. Vaughan, Listen to the music, 174–177.

7. Koprowski H, Croce C. Method of producing tumor antibodies, U.S. Patent 4,172,124 (filed April 28, 1978, issued October 23, 1979); Koprowski H, Gerhard W, Croce C. Method of producing antibodies, U.S. Patent 4,196,265 (filed June 15, 1977, issued April 1, 1980).

8. Vaughan, Listen to the music, 179.

9. Centocor, Centocor Oncogene Research Partners LP, June 9, 1984, HS-PP; Interview with Hilary Koprowski by author and Ted Everson (July 13, 2006), transcript, 16–17; Interview with David Holveck by Lara Marks and Ted Everson (July 14, 2006).

10. Wall MA, Allen EC. Investment prospectus: medical diagnostic business, HS-PP, n.d., p. 34–35.

11. For a detailed biography of Schoemaker go to his profile on <www.whatisbiotechnology.org/people/Schoemaker>.

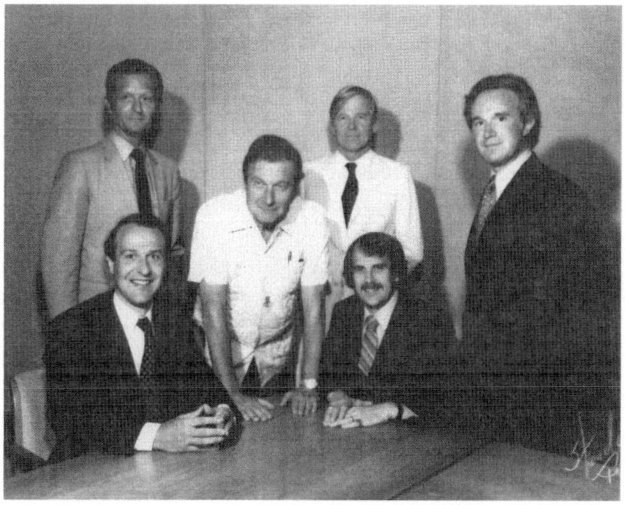

FIGURE 37.1 The earliest founders of Centocor. In the front, from left to right are: Schoemaker, Koproski, Zurawski, and Evnin. Behind from left to right are Allen and Wall. Photo credit: *Anne Schoemaker.*

the post. A chemist by training, he had been a pioneer in mAb production at Harvard Medical School and Massachusetts General Hospital (MGH), where he had held a postdoctoral research fellowship.

The Collaborative Journey Begins

The founders decided to focus their resources initially on diagnostics, predicting $17 million in revenues by 1984,[12] with therapeutics as their long-term goal. Diagnostics were easier to develop and could win regulatory approval more easily than therapeutics, thereby enabling faster revenue growth.[13] In addition to developing diagnostic products, they aimed to supply antibodies on contract to other companies for using their proprietary diagnostic kits [14].

Entering the diagnostics sector was ambitious. The $2 billion diagnostics market was highly competitive, dominated at that time by health-care giants such as Abbott Laboratories, F. Hoffman-La Roche, and Warner Lambert who had developed tests that could only be analyzed through their own proprietary instruments. In 1979 two companies were already offering mAbs on a commercial basis: Sera Lab, a British company (with which César Milstein was involved) and Hybritech, a San Diego start-up founded in 1978 by Ivor Royston, a professor at the University of California San Diego and his research assistant Howard Birndorf. Both of these companies were marketing mAbs as reagents to researchers and exploring their use as diagnostics.[15] The competitive landscape, however, quickly changed. By 1983 more than 150 companies, including large pharmaceutical companies, had mAb-based diagnostic programs, and 23 such diagnostics were being marketed and another 100 were in the pipeline [16].

From the start, Wall and Koprowski saw collaboration as key to their business model. The very name "Centocor" was derived from the words (1) "cento" that describes (in Latin) an old garment made of hundreds of patches of material or a literary or musical composition made up of parts of other works, and (2) "cor(e)" as in the center.[17] Centocor's collaborative philosophy was unusual for the time. In 1979 most start-up biotechnology companies were trying to do everything internally from the discovery process through development. Centocor's founders believed, however, that rather than depending solely on in-house research they should use internal skills to identify and fund prominent external researchers and laboratories working in areas where the company wanted to develop and where there was an appropriate license for the technology.[18] As Wall told *Forbes* magazine in May 1985, "You can have a garage full of Ph.D.s working on a project and nine times out of ten some guy across the street is going to come up with the discovery that beats them all" [19].

Central to Centocor's policy of collaboration was Wall and Schoemaker's remarkable ability to network.[20]

12. Wall and Allen, Investment prospectus, 30.

13. Interview with Tony Evnin, Venrock Associates partner and Centocor director (1981–1999) by author and Ted Everson (September 14, 2006).

14. Wall and Allen, Investment prospectus, 6.

15. Wall and Allen, Investment prospectus, 28 and 31; Author Unknown, A medical marvel goes to market, 56; Author Unknown, Biotechnologists are ready to market another trick, 87; Author Unknown, Smart bombs of biology, 59. For a history of Sera-Labs see Marks, A healthtech revolution; and Marks LV. The "Lock and Key" of medicine: monoclonal antibodies and the transformation of healthcare. Yale University Press; forthcoming [chapter 7].

16. Author Unknown, A medical marvel goes to market, 56; Hamilton MM, Competition feverish in health field: immunodiagnostics in infancy, The Washington Post, Sunday Final Edition, October 30, 1983, G1.

17. Vaughan, Listen to the music, 179; interview with Koprowski. See also interview with Michael Dougherty by author and Ted Everson (January 23, 2007), transcript. Dougherty was Centocor's assistant controller, treasurer, chief financial officer and senior vice president (1983–1993).

18. Interview with Evnin; HS-PP: Rothschild LF, et al. Centocor Inc: prospectus for public offering, July 22, 1983, 21; Teitelman R. Searching for serendipity: Centocor Combs University Labs for Technology, Forbes, May 6, 1985, 80.

19. Teitelman R. Searching for serendipity: Centocor Combs University Labs for Technology. Forbes; 1985, p. 80–81.

20. Interview with former NCI researcher and Centocor collaborator Robert Gallo (July 11, 2006). See also interview with Sarah Cabot, Centocor's technology licensing director (1986–1990), by Jennifer Dionisio (November 7, 2007).

By being well-connected and plugged into the academic world, Wall and Schoemaker realized they stood a better chance of finding promising products at a relatively early stage when they were not unduly expensive.[21] As Schoemaker later recalled, "We realized it was a lot cheaper to roam academe and pay a royalty back for what we developed than start our own research facilities. Collaboration was the best way to be competitive" [22].

One of Centocor's strongest academic collaborations was with the Wistar Institute, fueled in part by Koprowski's connection with the company. In 1979 Centocor signed three licensing deals with the institute for rights to four approved and pending patents for diagnostic and therapeutic purposes. Centocor paid $25,000 upfront and agreed to make royalty payments of 4%–6% for any resulting products [23].

Centocor's alliance with the Wistar was helped by the fact that the latter had its own charter and board. This allowed greater flexibility for an academic–company collaboration than otherwise was normally possible in the late 1970s. Although the pioneering academic–company relationship between Centocor and the Wistar raised some concern about conflict of interest for one Wistar board member, this was soon overcome[24]. The relationship set an important precedent for the partnerships Centocor-entered thereafter [25].

Centocor, like other biotechnology companies, was helped enormously by passing of the Bayh–Dole Act in late 1980, which established for the first-time uniform guidelines for the patenting and commercialization of government-funded academic research.[26] Between 1985 and 1990 Centocor's partnerships with research institutions grew from 15 to more than 80 worldwide, many involving license and license-option agreements.[27] These collaborations were vital to Centocor's business, providing materials for some of its early products.[28] Crucially, it allowed the company to keep its costs to a minimum while increasing sales: between 1984 and 1990 Centocor's R&D budget remained at the same level while its sales increased fivefold [29].

In addition to partnering with research institutions to fill its product pipeline, Centocor pursued marketing alliances. Facing a highly competitive environment, Wall and Schoemaker realized they could strengthen the company's market position by having licensing agreements with companies that had well-established market positions and distribution channels. This would eliminate the time and expense of establishing Centocor's own distribution mechanism and facilitate faster entry to the market [30].

Centocor's team deliberately secured agreements with key diagnostic companies, whereby the companies would buy and sell Centocor's antibodies in completed test kits and separate antibodies to be used in their own proprietary machines.[31] All of Centocor's diagnostic tests were designed to be compatible with existing diagnostic systems that allowed for both the testing and analysis of results, such as those marketed by Abbott and Roche, and used by the majority of clinical laboratories.[32] This arrangement not only helped Centocor gain a broad market penetration but also allowed it to leverage its technical strength without threatening competitors.[33] As David Holveck, who headed up Centocor's diagnostics department from 1983, stated, "Because of the marketing

21. Interviews with Evnin and Anne Faulkner Schoemaker (July 10, 2006). See also HS-PP: Centocor, Annual Report, 1983, 6. Hereafter all Centocor's *Annual Reports (A/R)*. The *A/R*s are contained in HS-PP.

22. Schoemaker cited in Vaughan, Listen to the music, 186; and interview with Faulkner Schoemaker.

23. HS-PP: Rothschild LF, et al. Centocor Inc: prospectus for public offering, December 14, 1982, 19 and 25. Stanley Cohen and Herbert Boyer faced similar hostility to the commercialization and patenting of their technology and founding of Genentech (see Smith Hughes S. Making dollars out of DNA: the first major patent in biotechnology and the commercialization of molecular biology, 1974–1980. ISIS 2001;92:541–575, 551).

24. Vaughan, Listen to the music, 182–186.

25. Interview with Gallo; Schoemaker, cited in Vaughan, Listen to the music, 186.

26. Before the Bayh-Dole Act, universities wishing to obtain a patent arising from federally funded research required permission from federal authorities to do so. See Hughes, Making dollars out of DNA, 551.

27. Centocor, A/R (1985), 5 and Rothschild, Centocor Inc. (1983), 22; Momich B. Building something significant at Centocor. Pennsylvania Technology, Second Quarter, 1990, p. 25–31.

28. Interview with Koprowski. Interview with Zurawski by Ted Everson, (January 4, 2007).

29. Dickinson S. Biotech's Centocor jockeys for position in drug field. The Scientist 1990;4:1–5.

30. Wall and Allen, Investment prospectus, 6.

31. Interview with Holveck by author and Ted Everson (July 14, 2006). Holveck was Centocor's head of diagnostics from 1983 and Centocor's chief executive officer from 1992.

32. Rothschild, Centocor Inc. (1982), 15; Rothschild, Centocor Inc. (1983); Centocor, A/Rs (1983), 2 and (1985), 15; Correspondence between author and David Holveck, November 2007; Interview with Holveck.

33. By 1983 the company had formed a number of marketing and manufacturing partnerships with key companies for distribution of the test in different parts in the world. This included Warner-Lambert to cover the USA, Toray/Fujizoki for Japan, and Byk-Mallinckroft for Europe. Centocor, A/Rs (1983), 2, 14, 18 and (1985), 15.

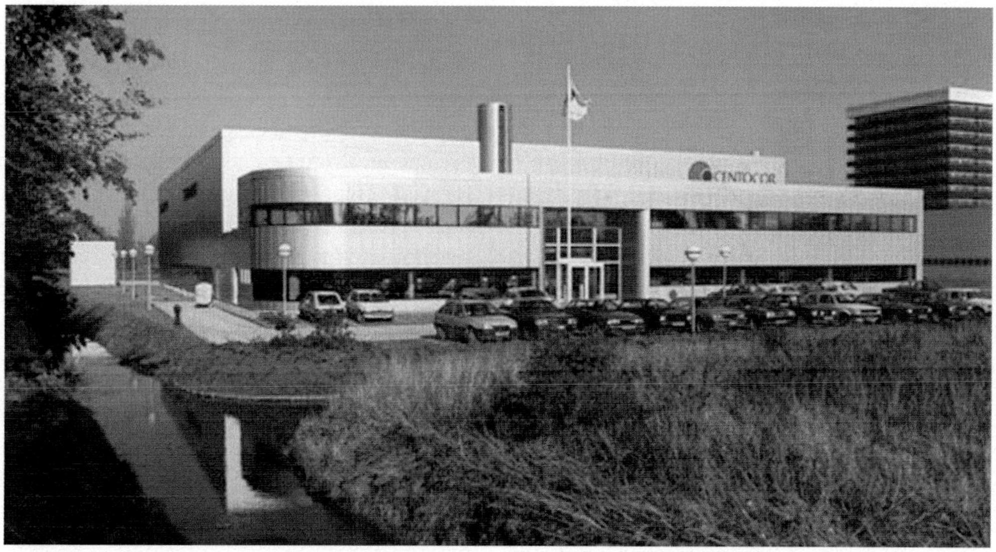

FIGURE 37.2 Centocor headquarters in Malvern, Pennsylvania.

strategy of networking with all of the major suppliers, we insulated ourselves from competition because we were the suppliers of the reagents, and they were looking for ways of adding tests to their instrumentation" [34]. In 1983 61% of Centocor's product sales were being sold by major distributors. Two years later, this had increased to 74%.[35] (See Fig. 37.2.)

An important catalyst in Centocor's early success was its swift winning of regulatory approval for two diagnostic tests: one for gastrointestinal cancer (using an antibody licensed from the Wistar) and the other for hepatitis B (developed by Zurawski and licensed from MGH). Both the tests had reached the market by 1983. The approval of the hepatitis test was significant as it was the first mAb-based test approved for this disease by the Food and Drug Administration (FDA). Centocor's hepatitis B test was in high demand because from the early 1970s many countries, including the United States, required the screening of blood intended for blood transfusion. Some idea of how popular the test was can be seen from the fact that between April and December 1983 Centocor sold 600,000 of its hepatitis tests.

Between 1983 and 1986, Centocor introduced another three tests to the market: one for diagnosing ovarian cancer (licensed from the Dana–Farber Cancer Institute), the first diagnostic tool available for the disease; a test for breast cancer (licensed from Scripps Clinic and Research Foundation); and another for colorectal cancer (licensed from the Wistar) [1]. All three tests are still used in clinical practice today. In addition to these diagnostics, Centocor also put into the market the first diagnostic test for multidrug resistance, a major problem for cancer patients. By 1990, Centocor had captured more than a quarter of the world's market for antibody-based tests for cancer [36].

Between 1979 and 1985, Centocor's team built up a profitable business with revenues of just under $50 million. It was highly lucrative because most of the bottom-line revenue came from royalties.[37] By 1987 Centocor was one of the very few mAb companies with earnings [38].

Finance: "GRAB as Many Cookies as You Can"

Just as fundamental as partnering was to Centocor's early success was Wall and Schoemaker's ability to find capital. What helped this process was the fact that soon after setting up the company, Wall, using his previous reputation in the business world, persuaded Tony Evnin, a senior partner in Venrock Associates, a venture capital firm, to become one of the company's directors. This was important as Venrock

34. Interview with Holveck by Sally Smith Hughes (1998, 1999), transcript, 43, Regional Oral History Office, Bancroft Library.

35. Centocor, A/R (1985), 27.

36. Interview with Zurawski; Author Unknown, TWST names award winners biotechnology, The Wall Street Transcript, 97/11 (December 14, 1987) HS-PP: Centocor, A/R (1990), 14.

37. HS-PP: H. Schoemaker, Wharton Talk, April 17, 2000 and interview with Holveck.

38. Bylinsky G. Coming: star wars medicine. Fortune; April 27, 1987.

had a history of investment in the diagnostics and therapeutic sector. Venrock subsequently became the first major investor in Centocor, providing $300,000. This would just be the start of raising funds. Between 1979 and 1981 Centocor raised approximately $7 million through private placement of its stocks.[39] The Centocor executives raised further cash from public offerings in 1983, 1986, 1990, and 1991, the last raising $100 million [40].

Wall and Schoemaker also secured funds through R&D limited partnerships. First used by the Delorean Car Company in 1975, R&D partnerships allowed companies to raise capital from private individual investors for specific research projects off the balance sheet, providing investors with tax benefits and potentially higher returns than equity investments.[41] In 1982 Genentech was the first biotechnology company to use the mechanism to develop human growth hormone and gamma interferon drugs.[42] Centocor was one of the most successful and aggressive users of R&D limited partnerships within the biotechnology industry, establishing at least four such partnerships between 1984 and 1987 [43].

Central to Centocor's fundraising was Schoemaker's philosophy that it should not be driven by the company's business plan. He believed that even if Centocor had a lot of money on the balance sheet, more money should be raised whenever the opportunity arose. As he explained, "In Centocor's early days, Bill Hambrecht of Hambrecht and Quist advised me: 'When the cookie jar comes around, grab as many cookies as you can because you'll never know when it comes around again'. He also advised me to discard all of the traditional business evaluations such as cash flow, price/earnings, etc. in deciding when and how much money to raise. He told me that each week he had five CEOs in his office who had insufficient capital and that he had never had a CEO come to him and tell him he had too much money" [44].

Expanding Its Market Potential

While initially funneling resources into blood-based diagnostics, Wall and Schoemaker quickly looked for ways to expand into the therapeutics sector. Therapeutics posed greater uncertainties than diagnostics. Much of the commercial attention in the nascent biotechnology therapeutics industry was focused on using recombinant DNA technology for the production of drugs for which there were existing therapeutic models and markets.[45] Therapy based on mAbs was a novel idea and remained uncharted territory.

Using mAbs for therapeutic purposes presented considerable new challenges. Unlike the blood-based diagnostics that Centocor had heretofore been developing, which involved the deployment of mAbs in tests on blood removed from the human body, therapeutics required the administration of mAbs directly into the human body. mAb drugs therefore posed greater safety concerns. Therapeutics also required far greater quantities of mAbs than needed for diagnostics, posing new manufacturing and quality-control challenges [46].

In order to gain experience in the therapeutic sector, Centocor devised a strategy to initially develop mAbs as contrast agents for diagnostic-imaging procedures. While not therapies in themselves, the use of mAbs as imaging agents tested the safety of mAbs for potential therapies and provided useful aids for the evaluation and therapeutic treatment of a patient. In 1985 Centocor established an in vivo diagnostic-imaging unit and began to develop three products directed toward imaging diseases such as cancer and conditions of the cardiovascular system. The market for mAb-imaging diagnostic products was expected to be between five and ten times larger than that of blood-based diagnostics.[47] Within the field of cancer alone, imaging

39. Centocor, A/R (1982).

40. Rothschild, Centocor Inc. (1982) and (1983); HS-PP: Paine Webber, Centocor, Common Stock, December 13, 1985, 7; Centocor, A/R (1986), (1987), 2, and (1990), 3.

41. Interviews by author and Ted Everson with PaineWebber investment bankers Stephen Evans-Freke (September 14, 2006) and Stephen Webster (July 13, 2006), and by author with Bruce Peacock, Centocor's chief financial officer 1981–1992 (July 10, 2006). See also Schiff L, Murray F. Biotechnology financing dilemmas and the role of special purpose entities. Nat Biotechnol 2004;22:271–277.

42. Interview with Fred A. Middleton, by G.E. Bugos (2001), transcript, Regional Oral History Office, Bancroft Library.

43. Interviews with Evans-Freke and Webster. See also HS-PP: Centocor, Centocor Oncogene Research Partners LP; PaineWebber, Centocor Common Stock, 22; PaineWebber, Tocor II and Centocor Prospectus, January 21, 1992, 5; Centocor, A/Rs (1985–1988) and (1989), 31.

44. Bill Hambrecht, cofounder of Hambrecht and Quist in 1968, an investment bank specializing in emerging high-growth technology companies, was one of Genentech's early investors. See Interview with Middleton, 28. Schoemaker, Wharton Talk.

45. For more on the development of recombinant insulin see Hall S. Invisible frontiers: the race to synthesize a human gene. Oxford: Oxford University Press; 1987.

46. Interview with Centocor's vice president of pharmaceutical development (1988–1993) Renato Fuchs (July 1, 2008). See also Bylinsky, Coming: star wars medicine.

47. Bylinsky, Coming: star wars medicine.

diagnostics were expected in 1985 to grow by 200% each year, reaching $200 million by 1988. The market size for cardiac imaging was also projected to increase from $70 to $130 million between 1985 and 1988 [48].

In their reports to investors, Centocor's executives predicted the company's imaging diagnostics would swiftly be on the market within a couple of years of their first testing.[49] What they hoped to do was capitalize on the mAbs, it was already deploying in the development of its in vitro blood tests. To this end, early on the team looked into developing CA 19-9 as a tool for imaging gastrointestinal cancers and CA-125 for imaging ovarian cancer.[50] Progress, however, was slow and not as straightforward as anticipated. One of the problems was that while the mAbs proved good imaging agents, they took a long time to clear from the body which delayed the reading of the images and thus obtaining the diagnostic results [51].

Centocor's difficulties in utilizing mAbs for imaging diagnostics were not unique. Indeed, many other companies would struggle to reach the market with such products, and their overall worldwide sales would remain small. In 1998, for example, the worldwide sales of diagnostic-imaging products using mAbs were worth $10 million. The sales revenue would grow over the coming years, but would continue to be small, estimated to be $15 million in revenue in 2005. Such figures were well below the projected figures Centocor, and others had forecast back in the 1980s. Back in 1987 one financial analyst had forecast the annual sales for Centocor's cardiovascular imaging tests could reach between $300 and $400 million [2].

Despite the slow progress, in August 1989, Centocor won European approval for its first imaging product called Myoscint. Licensed originally from MGH, Myoscint could locate and estimate the amount of dead heart tissue from a heart attack. The product was first marketed in France, Germany, Italy, Spain, and the United Kingdom and then in America from 1996[52]. Overall the product did not take off in a significant way. By the time the product reached the market, other methods had appeared that proved less invasive for the patient and more accurate in terms of the data they provided. In the end, Myoscint proved more useful for detecting heart transplant rejection and myocarditis (inflammation of the heart muscle). It was used for these purposes off-label in Europe, where those performing heart transplants found it an invaluable tool [53].

Therapeutics

While the experience with imaging diagnostics proved disappointing, it gave the Centocor team some expertise in the development of mAbs for use directly in humans. This was invaluable in going forward in the creation of mAb-based medicines. Importantly, it provided a starting point in terms of what was needed for the R&D for a therapeutic as well as learning the ropes for clinical trials and manufacturing. Going, forward with therapeutics, however, was by its nature a much bigger risk for the company. Nothing could fully prepare Centocor's executives, then more familiar with the business model for developing diagnostics, with what would be needed for the development of mAbs as drugs. Moreover, they had little to go on from the nascent biotechnology therapeutics industry. At the time, companies in this sector had more expertise in using the new recombinant DNA technique to develop drugs in disease areas for which there were already well-established treatment protocols and market systems. By contrast, few knew which disease areas mAbs could be successfully used therapeutically or which market they would be able to penetrate.

Early on, Wall and Schoemaker recognized that the time and cost required to bring therapeutic products to market exposed their newly emerging company to unacceptable financial risks, which could divert resources and hinder innovation. In order to minimize the risk and gain financial, scientific, and technical resources as well as credibility, they therefore devised a strategy to generate

48. Centocor, A/R (1985), 11.

49. Centocor, Investment prospectus, December 14, 1982, 17; Centocor, A/R (1983), 2.

50. Centocor, A/R (1983), 2.

51. Interview with Fuchs; Interview with Jeffrey Mattis by Lara Marks. Mattis was Centocor's vice president of pharmaceutical development (1979–1998) (February 22, 2007). Notes.

52. PaineWebber, Centocor Common Stock (1985), 4, 6, 34; PaineWebber, Tocor II; Centocor, Annual Report (1990), 7; Centocor *SEC filing Form 10-K* for the year ending, December 31, 1995; Pollack, The Next Wave of Diagnostics. Interviews with David Holveck by author and Everson (July 14, 2006 and September 9, 2009), Harlan Weisman (November 30, 2006) and Mattis. Harlan Weisman was Centocor's president of R&D and team leader for ReoPro development (1990–1999).

53. Centocor, A/R (1988), 4 and (1990), 7; Interview with Mattis; Interviews with Fuchs, notes and with Stelios Papadopolous (October 19, 2006). Papadopolous was an investment banker with Paine Webber (1987–2000). Centocor's Myoscint imaging agent backed in USA, The Pharmaletter, February 5, 1996, <http://www.thepharmaletter.com/file/25880/centocors-myoscint-imaging-agent-backed-in-usa.html>.

relationships with leading companies. By 1983 Centocor had established collaborations with two companies for this purpose: the American chemicals company FMC Corporation and the Swiss-based pharmaceutical company F. Hoffmann-La Roche [54].

Centocor's alliance with FMC began in 1980 with FMC agreeing to contribute a total of $12.4 million. Split 50/50 and managed by a committee with a representative from each company, each partner had the option to purchase all of the other's interest in the joint venture.[55] One of the aims of the collaboration was to find a way to produce mAbs from cell lines more closely resembling human antibodies. This was particularly important if Centocor was to gain leadership in the mAb therapeutics field. Most of the early mAbs developed from the time of Köhler and Milstein were derived from mouse cells. These mAbs had certain drawbacks: a short half-life, poor recognition by receptors in the human body, necessitated administration in high doses, and had greater potential to cause life-threatening allergic reactions and viral safety problems. For Centocor, human antibodies not only promised greater safety and efficacy for therapeutic products but also provided a competitive advantage in securing investment.[56] In 1986 Centocor gained exclusive rights to the human antibody technology developed through the venture. In return, FMC received 1.35 million shares of Centocor's stock.[57] The only other biotechnology company that had managed to develop human antibodies by then was Cetus [58].

Centocor Goes It Alone

In 1986 Wall and Schoemaker decided that while they would continue to develop therapeutic products through joint ventures, the profits generated from the highly successful blood test business and contract revenue from technology licensing, and selected product marketing arrangements could be used to build Centocor into a major pharmaceutical company. Their ambition was for the company to be as big as Merck, by the year 2000.[59] Transforming Centocor into a globally integrated pharmaceutical company was not an unusual goal for the time. Other executives from leading biotechnology companies were pursuing the same vision with some success. In 1985 Genentech launched Protropin to treat growth hormone deficiency in children. It was the first recombinant pharmaceutical product to be manufactured and marketed by a biotechnology company without the help of a partner [60].

By 1988 Centocor's research group had identified 30 new entities for possible drug development and had 12 Investigational New Drug Applications filed with the US FDA, many of which were mAbs, and had clinically evaluated 10 products.[61] While many of Centocor's competitors at this time were focusing on deploying mAbs for cancer treatment and Centocor had its own cancer program,[62] Centocor's preferred lead candidate was an antibody-targeting septic shock, a deadly disease usually acquired in hospitals and traditionally treated, ineffectively, with antibiotics. By 1986 Centocor had two human antibodies, one developed in-house through their collaboration with FMC, and one licensed in from the University of California San Diego, known as HA-1A [63].

At least, a third of septic shock cases are caused by Gram-negative bacteria, a class of bacteria that possesses a unique outer membrane that hinders cell penetration by antibiotics and other drugs. During the 1980s, Gram-negative sepsis was the third leading cause of death in the United States, with over 100,000 people dying from the condition each year, accounting for up to $10 billion in health-care expenditures annually. Wall and Schoemaker believed that should Centocor develop a drug to combat a critical medical problem, they would have a major blockbuster. The estimated market for products to treat septic shock in 1990 was more than $300 million [64].

In order to maximize the potential of HA-1A, trade named Centoxin, Wall and Schoemaker, in part encouraged by their Wall Street advisors, decided that rather

54. Centocor, A/R (1983), 6.
55. Centocor, A/Rs (1983), 18, 28, and (1985), 2; Rothschild, Centocor Inc. (1983), 47.
56. Interview with Evans-FrekeCentocor, A/R (1986).
57. Centocor, A/R (1986), 3.
58. Bylinsky, Coming: star wars medicine.
59. Centocor, A/Rs (1986), 17 and (1988), 5; Dickinson, Biotech's Centocor jockeys for position, 2.
60. Interview with Middleton. Interview with Fuchs.
61. Centocor, A/R (1988), 2 and 12.
62. Interview with Richard McCloskey (January 19, 2007). McClosky was Centocor's vice president of clinical research and medical research (1990–1997).
63. Centocor, A/R (1985), 29. Interviews with Denise McGinn (September 12, 2006), Zurawski and Fuchs. McGinn was Centocor's development project manager (1983–1999).
64. Momich, Building something significant at Centocor, 26–28.

than selling the rights to the drug to another company they would develop and market Centoxin internally. This they believed would give them greater control over the product and larger revenues.[65] As Tony Evnin, one of Centocor's first investors and directors, explained, "At that point in time it seemed like such an important product and it was a product in a new area. We wanted the ability to keep it all to ourselves. Perhaps we were a bit greedy, but it seemed like it was something that, by bringing in ... additional talent [from the pharmaceutical industry], we could take on ourselves" [66] (Fig. 37.3).

One of the reasons the Centocor executives decided to develop and market Centoxin internally was that it would help build the necessary infrastructure for becoming an integrated pharmaceutical company.[67] This, however, required major upscaling of the company's manufacturing capabilities and marketing that involved large sums of cash. At least, $150 million was needed to get Centoxin to market. Between 1986 and 1992, Centocor went through nine different equity, debt, and off-balance sheet financings, netting more than $500 million. By 1992 $450 million had been spent on clinical trials, building a sales force of 275 people (200 in the United States and 75 in Europe) and two new factories—one in Holland and one in the United States [68].

Heeding advice from Wall Street, the management team was also restructured to bring on board skills in pharmaceutical development, regulation, and marketing by the hiring of staff from large pharmaceutical companies. In December 1987 James Wavle, the former president of Parke-Davis, Warner–Lambert's pharmaceutical unit, became Centocor's president and chief operating officer. Working alongside Schoemaker, who retained his position as chief executive officer and replaced Wall as chairman, Wavle took on the responsibility for turning Centocor into a globally integrated pharmaceutical company [3]. The recruitment of pharmaceutical executives had a major impact on the culture within Centocor, bringing in new management styles, more aggressive marketing, and a higher cash burn [69].

Confidence was high that Centoxin would succeed. Such optimism was not unfounded. In February 1991 a leading American journal ran an article indicating Centoxin reduced Gram-negative sepsis by 39%. For those who went into septic shock, the drug reduced mortality by 47%.[70] The same month the United States Army administered the drug to soldiers fighting in the first Gulf War.[71] A month later the European drug regulatory body approved Centoxin for the treatment of Gram-negative sepsis. Six months later, in September 1991, a FDA panel

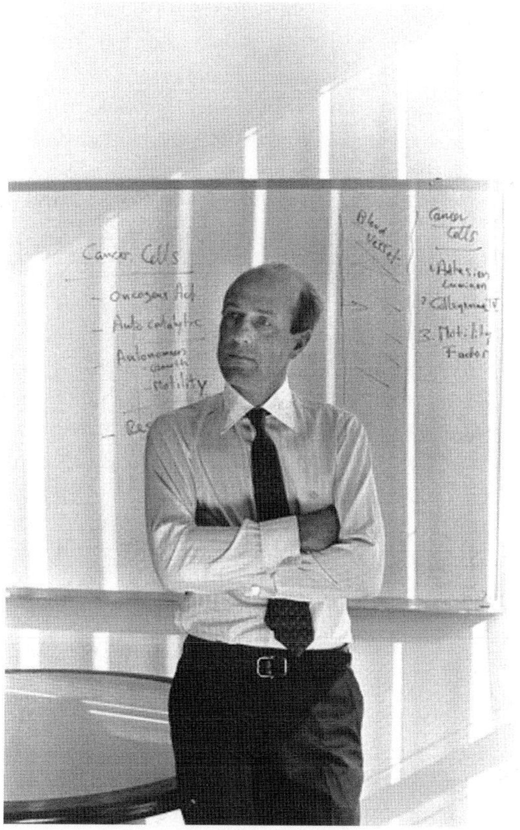

FIGURE 37.3 Hubert Schoemaker during his early years at Centocor. He was known for being able to convey very quickly a vision of the future as well as listening to those around him. Those who worked with him recall his overwhelming sense of optimism. Photo credit: *Anne Schoemaker.*

65. Interview with Bernard Schaffer. Schaffer is a Philadelphia-based market analyst.
66. Interview with Evnin.
67. Interview with Fuchs.
68. Winslow, Centocor's new drug clears FDA panel; Dickinson, Biotech's Centocor jockeys for position in drug field; and Longman R. The lessons of Centocor, in vivo: the business and medicine report, May 1992, p. 24.
69. Interviews with Holveck, Peacock, and Cabot. Joint interview with Sandra Faragalli, Patty Durachko, and Ray Heslip (September 12, 2006). All three were long-time employees of Centocor, working in the administrative, finance, warehouse, and shipping sections. Interview with Centocor's vice president of diagnostics operations (1985–1998), Paul Touhey by author and Ted Everson (September 15, 2006).
70. Ziegler EJ, Fisher CJ, Sprung CL, et al. Treatment of Gram-negative bacteremia and septic shock with HA-1A human monoclonal antibody against endotoxin. A randomized, double-blind, placebo-controlled trial. The HA-1A Sepsis Study Group. N Engl J Med 1991;324(7):429–436.
71. Author Unknown, Blasting Bacteria; Author Unknown, Centocor, Inc.

advised approval of Centoxin to treat septic shock.[72] Centocor's sales were predicted to soon be in excess of $1 billion. On this basis, Schoemaker believed Centocor would have more than 50% of the share of the antibody pharmaceuticals market in Europe, the United States, and Japan by 2000 [73].

"Centocorpse": Centocor in Crisis

The good news, however, did not last. In late October 1991 an American federal court ruled that Centocor's patent for Centoxin infringed on one held by Xoma Corporation, a competitor biotechnology company based in California developing a similar drug for septic shock in partnership with the pharmaceutical company Pfizer Inc.[74] Centocor's executives were unsure how they should handle the matter. This was the first major case of litigation they had experienced. Initially, Schoemaker wanted to settle, but Wavle persuaded him to fight based on the belief that a settlement could result in cross-licensing and thereby a loss in revenues. The hope was Centocor might strike as lucky as the biotechnology company Amgen in its patent dispute with Genetics Institute.[75] In retrospect, Schoemaker believed the decision to fight Xoma was one his biggest strategic errors.[76] Losing the patent battle to Xoma, the litigation cost Centocor dearly in terms of time and money. It also publicly aired questions about the design of Centoxin's trials and the data analysis [77].

Adding to the company's woes, from late 1991, some medical practitioners began to question the potentially high price of Centoxin (between $3000 and $4000 for each patient) and the degree to which they could predict which patients would most benefit from the drug.[78] By early 1992 initial European sales of the drug were also far below expectations. More pessimistic news was to follow when, on February 20, 1992, the FDA requested additional information about Centoxin. Triggering shock in the financial community, the tidings sent Centocor's shares tumbling 19% or $8.125 a share, closing at $33.125 a share. Only 2 weeks before, the stock had traded at $50 a share. The slide in Centocor's share represented a $675 million drop in its market value [79].

Despite the negative publicity, Schoemaker believed the problems could be resolved. Three months later, however, on a public holiday in April, he received a telephone call at home from David Kessler, head of the FDA, indicating that Centoxin would not be approved because of insufficient evidence to establish its efficacy and the necessity of more trials before it could be reconsidered for approval.[80] For Schoemaker, usually a great optimist, this news was "the worst thing that could have happened." The devastation was great for everyone in the company [81].

Hitting media headlines on April 15, 1992, the news stunned investors. Nicknamed "Centocorpse" by Wall Street, Centocor's stock dropped 41% in 1 day.[82] In the week that followed, disgruntled investors filed six lawsuits against Centocor's executives alleging violation of federal securities laws and called for damages.[83] Shareholders had seen $1.5 billion of Centocor's market capitalization disappear, its stock rate having fallen from

72. Usdin S, Wall Street vents frustration at Centocor, BioWorld Today, February 20, 1992, 1; Shaw D, FDA, Wall Street bring bad tidings to Centocor, The Philadelphia Inquirer, 1992, B11; Author Unknown, FDA Snag and Loss Hurt Centocor Stock; Valeriano LL, Centocor stock slides on news of drug snag, Wall St J, 1992; Newman A, Pettit D, Biotech Stock Lead Index 0.64% lower; Centocor plunges on worry over drug, Wall St J, 1992.

73. Author Unknown, Centocor, Inc.

74. Patent disputes were common in the industry and could be devastating for the companies concerned. See, for example, the case of CellPro which became bankrupt after failing to win a patent dispute as described in Bar-Shalom A, Cook-Deegan R. Patents and innovation in cancer: lessons from CellPro. Millbank Q 2002;80(4):637–676.

75. Interviews with Centocor's attorney (1987–1999), George Hobbs (September 30, 2006); Papadopoulos; and chief executive officer of Cephalon, Frank Baldino by author and Ted Everson (July 14, 2006). Amgen and Genetics Institute's patent dispute started in 1988 and ended in May 1993 with the Genetics Institute paying Amgen $15.9 million. Amgen SEC filing: Form: 10-Q, 8/10/1994.

76. Interviews with Faulkner Schoemaker, and Schaffer.

77. Interviews with Holveck and Papadopoulos. Centocor, A/R (1991), 38 and 39; Valeriano, Centocor stock slides on news of drug snag; Fisher LM. Centocor and Xoma settle patent fight. The New York Times; July 30, 1992.

78. Hinds CJ. Monoclonal antibodies in sepsis and septic shock. Br Med J 1992;304:132–133. Interviews with Peacock, Holveck, and Papadopoulos.

79. Usdin, Wall Street vents frustration at Centocor; Shaw, FDA, Wall Street bring bad tidings to Centocor; Author Unknown, FDA snag and loss hurt Centocor stock; Valeriano, Centocor stock slides on news of drug snag; Newman and Pettit, Biotech stock lead index 0.64% lower; Longman, The lessons of Centocor, 25.

80. Interview with Schaffer.

81. Interviews with Faulkner Schoemaker, Holveck (by author and Everson), Faragalli, Durachko, and Heslip.

82. Shaw, Centocor absorbs new blows. See also interview with Papadopoulos.

83. Author Unknown. FDA: Centoxin data insufficient. In: 74E, Shaw D, editor. Centocor absorbs new blows. The Philadelphia Inquirer. Interview with Holveck.

a high of $60 to just $6.[84] Sensitive to the calamities of one of its leading companies, the biotechnology industry suffered its own financial aftershock [85].

Collaboration—A Means of Rescue

The FDA's decision had not killed Centoxin, but Centocor desperately needed time and money to save the drug, develop its other products, and survive. With the future of the company at stake, Schoemaker and Wall immediately crafted a rescue strategy. To stop the company's cash burn they rapidly laid off hundreds of people, primarily the sales representatives hired for Centoxin's launch. Within a short period the company's employee base had shrunk by a quarter. The company's management team was also reshuffled: Wavle and other recent recruits from the pharmaceutical industry departed.

Crucial to the company's financial survival was also Schoemaker and Wall's reversion to collaboration. The income generated from the diagnostics division, which was bringing in millions of dollars, was insufficient to keep the company afloat and they could not rely on the investment community with the fall in Centocor's stock.[86] Within days of the FDA's announcement, Wall and Schoemaker plunged into a frenzy of partnership and fundraising efforts with a number of pharmaceutical companies, including SmithKline Beecham and Eli Lilly.[87] Schoemaker's dynamism and optimism were major factors in driving this forward [88].

What Wall and Schoemaker had on their side were some other promising products in Centocor's pipeline plus the fact that half the industry wanted to obtain Centoxin despite its problems. J.P Garnier, who headed SmithKline Beecham at the time, recalled, "We tried to convince Hubert [Schoemaker] to do a deal with us, and Centoxin turned into a bidding contest between several companies.... I remember a phone call coming in over the weekend saying, 'It's going to cost you $100 million in an upfront payment to get Centoxin now'. Now, it doesn't sound impressive, but it was the equivalent of saying a billion today. A $100 million was unheard of. Nobody had ever paid this kind of upfront money." As Garnier explained, "Hubert was a terrific salesman. He whipped up this asset into something that got to be very appealing. He packaged Centoxin very effectively and before you knew it, the bride looked sensational. Everybody was influenced by his sincere belief in the drug and what it could do" [89].

In July 1992 Centocor finalized a licensing agreement with Eli Lilly. Under the agreement, Centocor received $100 million upfront from Eli Lilly, an unprecedented large payment for the time. Half of this amount went toward Eli Lilly purchasing 2 million shares in Centocor, thereby giving it a 5% stake in the company. The other half went toward providing the much needed cash to continue developing and seeking clearance for Centoxin. In the event that Centoxin failed, Eli Lilly agreed to pay a further $25 million toward the development of ReoPro, a cardiovascular drug that Centocor was currently developing clinically [90].

The alliance was strategically useful for Centocor not only because of the capital Eli Lilly was to provide, but also because they had a significant presence in the antibiotics field and a strong understanding of the United States infectious disease market crucial for the further development of Centoxin. Eli Lilly was also more receptive to biotechnology than many other pharmaceutical companies, having partnered with Genentech to launch the first genetically engineered insulin and having acquired Hybritech, Centocor's main competitor in mAb diagnostics in 1986.[91] For Eli Lilly the alliance gave them a chance to enhance their knowledge in the application of mAbs for infectious disease therapeutics and access to Centocor's European sales team, thereby opening up a new avenue for selling Lilly products [92].

In the following months, Eli Lilly and Centocor worked closely together, overseen by product committees established at both companies, on a new trial for Centoxin, launched in June 1992.[93] Despite Eli Lilly's support, in January 1993, Centoxin's development was abandoned because interim trial data indicated unexpected high mortality. The poor results were attributed to a flawed trial design. Centoxin proved effective in treating

84. Schoemaker, Wharton Talk; Longman, The lessons of Centocor, 23; interview with Holveck.
85. Usdin, Wall Street vents frustration at Centocor, 1; Longman, The lessons of Centocor, 27.
86. Interview with Touhey.
87. HS-PP: Centocor, CenTropics, 1/4 (Fall 1992), 1.
88. Interview with Papadopoulos.
89. Interview with J.P Garnier by Ted Everson (July 12, 2006).
90. Author Unknown, Lilly to acquire marketing rights to Centocor drug, Centocor, Centropics.
91. Author Unknown, Lilly to acquire marketing rights to Centocor drug, Centocor, Centropics.
92. Interview with Fuchs; Centocor, CenTropics, 1.
93. Centocor, CenTropics, 2–4.

septic shock stemming from Gram-negative bacteria, but this accounts for only about a third of patients who present with sepsis. No diagnostic tool existed, however, to detect which of the patients presenting in the trials had Gram-negative sepsis. In the absence of a diagnostic tool, Centocor's clinical team had insufficient data to convince the FDA of the drug's efficacy [94].

Centocor Becomes Profitable

Despite the setback with Centoxin, by early 1993, Centocor was financially turning a corner. Its cash burn rate had fallen from $50 to $30 million between the first and last quarter of 1992. Part of this had been achieved through layoffs, but it had also been helped by the reversion back to collaboration.[95] Good results were also beginning to be reported for other products in Centocor's pipeline.

Some of the most cheering news was the positive data Centocor's clinical team was getting from the cardiovascular drug ReoPro. Licensed from the State University of New York, Stony Brook, in 1986, much of the early development and testing of ReoPro had been undertaken by Centocor with funds raised from a R&D-limited partnership set up in 1987.[96] By 1992 when Centocor signed its alliance with Eli Lilly, ReoPro was in Phase III clinical trials and Centocor had plans to file for FDA and European regulatory approval the following year [97].

In early 1993 when the first results from the drug's trial emerged positive, it was clear Centocor not only possessed a marketable drug, but its future was now secure.[98] Submitted for approval in 1993, ReoPro took just 10 months to be approved by the European regulatory authorities and 12 months by the FDA. These approvals came through in December 1994. ReoPro's approval marked a key milestone for Centocor and placed mAbs firmly on the therapeutic map, showing for the first time they could be used for acute conditions. The drug was the second mAb to win approval as a therapeutic, the first having been approved in 1986 by Johnson & Johnson's Orthoclone OKT3 (used to prevent kidney transplant rejections).[99] The first therapeutic product ever to receive simultaneous the United States and European approval, ReoPro was the only new biotechnology product sanctioned in 1994. In December 1995 the drug's marketing potential was further boosted when clinical trials showed it was effective for unstable angina, broadening its potential market to more than 1 million patients [100].

Centocor's partnership with Eli Lilly was crucial to the development of ReoPro. While Centocor had undertaken and internally financed much of its early development and clinical trials, the alliance provided the time to do further necessary work [101]. Under the alliance agreement, Eli Lilly exercised its right to market the drug in the United States and most of Western Europe. ReoPro rapidly became a success, with worldwide sales of $23 million in its first year, 1995. By 1999 worldwide sales had increased to $447.3 million. Four years later, the drug was being investigated for noncardiac indications, including sickle-cell anemia and cancer [102].

Following ReoPro's success, Centocor's team soon had another major breakthrough with a drug called Remicade. The drug, based on an antibody called cA2, originated from a collaborative R&D agreement established in January 1984 between Centocor and the laboratory of Jan Vilcek, a scientist based at the New York University School of Medicine.[103] Initially, Centocor's researchers investigated cA2 in-house alongside Centoxin to combat sepsis, but clinical studies showed it more promising for treating autoimmune disorders. In 1998 Centocor won FDA approval for Remicade, to treat Crohn's disease. A year later, Remicade was approved for rheumatoid arthritis. By 2007 the drug had received approval in 88 countries for 15 inflammatory disease indications and was being used to treat over 1 million patients worldwide, commanding 23% of the arthritis drug market. In 2006 Remicade generated the US $3.77 billion in worldwide sales. It would rise to $8 billion in 2010, making it the third medicine in history to top $8 billion in annual sales, and the best-selling biological medicine in the world for that year [4]. The approval of Remicade

94. Interviews with Holveck. Papadopoulos. Interview with Michael Melore by Ted Everson. Melore was Centocor's head of human resources (1990–1999).

95. Centocor, A/R (1992), 7.

96. Centocor, A/Rs (1987–1988).

97. Centocor, A/R (1992), 4.

98. Interview with McGinn.

99. Bylinsky, Coming: star wars medicine; Centocor, A/R (1994), 2 and 4; Cochlovius B, Braunagel M, Welschof M, Therapeutic antibodies, American Chemical Society: Modern Drug Discovery, October 2003; Farrell C, Barnathan E, Weisman HF. The evolution of ReoPro clinical development. In: Dembowsky K, Stadler P, editors. Novel therapeutic proteins: selected case studies. Weinheim: Wiley-VCH Verlag GmbH; 2003, p. 323–346.

100. New York Times (December 22, 1995).

101. Interview with Holveck.

102. Interview with Holveck.

103. Interview with Jan Vilcek (July 12, 2006). Vilcek is a microbiology professor at New York University School of Medicine.

marked a significant point in the development of mAbs as therapeutics, showing for the first time that mAbs could be deployed for chronic conditions.

The approval of ReoPro and then Remicade signaled how far Centocor had come from its humble beginnings as a company specializing in mAb diagnostics. By 1999, 20 years after its founding, Centocor had raised $1.5 billion and brought to market ten products [104]. Despite this success, Schoemaker and David Holveck, Centocor's chief executive officer from September 1992, realized their company could no longer remain independent if it was to go forward as a serious player. The cash they had secured was insufficient for maintaining and growing the company's R&D program and expanding the company's manufacturing and marketing capabilities. They also recognized that having become so successful, the company could be subject to a take-over bid. In order to prevent a hostile bid, in 1998 they began to assess the company's value and identify possible partners.[105] A year later Holveck and Schoemaker secured a deal for $5.2 billion from Johnson & Johnson. Making Centocor a subsidiary of Johnson & Johnson, the deal allowed Centocor to continue to operate independently while benefiting from the large company's infrastructure, financial resources, and credibility. Within 3 years of the deal, Centocor more than doubled its work force from 1200 people to 2800 worldwide, and more than tripled the number of new drug candidates entering late-stage testing, many in disease areas Centocor had not explored before, including diabetes, organ transplant rejection, and asthma [5].

Conclusion

This case study of Centocor is illustrative of the important role collaboration has played in the building up of the biotechnology industry. A key lesson from Centocor is how important R&D partnerships can be to a young company just beginning to create a portfolio, and how critical alliances with established companies can be to breaking into a competitive market place. Nearing bankruptcy when straying away from collaboration, the story of Centocor is a salutary reminder of the risks for newly emerging companies of going it alone.

The experiences of Centocor's executives with collaboration and the attempts to go it alone, however, are not universal in the biotechnology industry. Plenty of collaborations between biotechnology companies and large pharmaceutical companies have failed in the past and continue to do so to this day. Amgen, a biotechnology company founded just 1 year after Centocor, landed up in a costly court case over its patents and experienced huge financial losses as a result of the marketing partnership it formed in 1985 with Johnson & Johnson for its first drug erythropoietin, a treatment for anemia [106]. The company had more success when it decided to develop and market its second drug Neupogen, a treatment for neutropenia, independently.[107] The contrast between Centocor and Amgen shows how idiosyncratic the risks and outcomes can be for biotechnology companies when deciding to collaborate or go it alone. This is highly influenced by the personalities involved, market conditions, scientific and technical developments, and the cultural fit between organizations.

Acknowledgments

The author would like to thank Anne Faulkner Schoemaker for allowing generous access to Hubert Schoemaker's personal files and reading earlier drafts of this paper. Grateful thanks also go to Stelios Papadopoulos, Alison Kraft, and David Holveck for providing insightful comments on initial drafts of the paper. Much appreciation also goes to all the people who agreed to be interviewed for the research that led to this chapter which was supported by the Chemical Heritage Foundation.

References

[1] HS-PP: Centocor Press Release. Centocor receives FDA panel recommendation to Approve Ovarian Cancer Test, November 3, 1986; Thompson L. New test for ovarian cancer detects residual cells in the blood, The Washington Post, June 16, 1987.

[2] BCC Research. Antibodies for therapeutic and diagnostic imaging applications. In: Report BIO016D, February 2000; BCC Research. Dynamic antibody industry. In: Report BIO016F, August 2005; Wolf R. Centocor makes a deal on product marketing, The Inquirer, December 7, 1987.

[3] Author Unknown. Centocor Inc. Chief Hubert Schoemaker Adds Chairman's Post.

[4] Wiki Analysis. Arthritis drug market, <http://www.wikinvest.com/wiki/Arthritis_Drug_Market#_note-13>; PharmaLive. Top 500 Prescription Medicine, Special Report, October 2011.

[5] George J. Centocor now bigger than ever. Philadelphia Bus J August 16, 2002?.

104. Schoemaker, Wharton Talk.

105. Interview with Holveck; Knox A. He is building on his success. The Philadelphia Inquirer; May 7, 2000.

106. Moschol A, Leiter J. Perfect partnering, Nat Biotechnol, Supplement to Vol. 19, July, 2001, BE21–BE22. For more on Amgen's development and marketing of Epogen see Goozner M. The $800 million pill: the truth behind the cost of new drugs. Berkeley, CA: University of California Press; 2004, p. 13–34.

107. Interview with Papadopoulos.

Chapter 38

The Emergence and Transformation of China in Biotechnology

Jimmy Zhimin Zhang, PhD, MBA[1,2]

[1]*Founder, Chairman and CEO, AccuGen Therapeutics, Inc., San Francisco, CA, United States,* [2]*Venture Partner, Lilly Asia Ventures (LAV), Shanghai, P.R. China*

Chapter Outline

China has made growing the biotechnology industry one of its national top priorities. Although they are late to the party compared to other countries, China has undergone a massive transformation that is a testament to what can be accomplished when a government focuses on a key objective. China has seen a double-digit growth in its biotechnology industry since 1984 and has gone from being one of the slowest, to one of the fastest nations in the adoption of biotechnology.

Brief History of China and Its Reform

China has a history of more than 5000 years of civilization. However, its modern history only started in the early 1900s, way behind the Western civilization that started in the Renaissance during 14th–17th centuries, or Japan's Meiji Restoration (Meiji Ishin) in 1868. China opened its door and started reform in 1978. In 2010 it became the second largest economy of the world. Although the China gross domestic product (GDP) growth has slowed down to 6.6% in 2018 from the previous average double-digit growth in 1978–2010, this growth rate is still every country's envy. China has a population of 1.4 billion, therefore GDP per capita is still relatively low, only ranked 78th in 2016. China's total national healthcare expenditure was only about 6.2% of its GDP, far behind the 16.8% in the United States, and 10.9% in Japan, while China's per capital health spending was only $425.6, much less than the United States' $9535.9 and Japan's $3732.6 [1]. China's total pharmaceutical expenditure was about 39% of the total health expenditure in 2015 [2], compared to 10.1% as the percentage of retail prescription drug spending of national health expenditure in the United States in 2015 [3].

Like many other countries, China is facing the issue of an aging society. In 2018 the number of senior citizens of 65-year old or above reached 166.58 million, about 11.9% of the total population [4]; the percentage of senior citizen is expected to be over 35% by 2050 [5]. With the single-child policy implemented between 1978 and 2015, this issue is much more devastating than most other countries. In 2015 the Chinese government started allowing, and then encourages, families to give birth of a second child. However, due to many factors, such as a reduced number of women in childbearing age, high housing

Biotechnology Entrepreneurship. DOI: https://doi.org/10.1016/B978-0-12-815585-1.00038-3

price, high costs to raise a child, and being busy at work, many young families still choose to have a single child, some even choose not to have one, and some young people even choose not to get married, especially in relatively well-developed cities. The number of newly born babies in 2018 is only 15.23 million, much less than the 20 million predicted by the government in 2015.

A Long History of Interest in Medicine

Chinese traditional medicine had dominated the Chinese medicinal history prior to its modern days. The establishment of Canton Hospital (廣州博濟醫院), also known as Ophthalmic Hospital in Canton or Canton Pok Tsai Hospital, by Protestant medical missionary Peter Parker in 1835, marked the official entry of Western medicine into China. The supermajority of Chinese traditional medicine is composed of multiple herbs; only very few, for example, arsenic trioxide (As_2O_3) and artemisinin, have been identified and purified as a functional single pharmaceutical ingredient. Dr. Zhu Chen, together with his mentor Dr. Zhen-Yi Wang, demonstrated in clinical trials that combining arsenic trioxide with all-*trans* retinoic acid is effective in turning the most fatal hematological malignancy acute promyelocytic leukemia to a curable disease. Dr. Zhu Chen later became China's Minister of Health and is currently a vice chairman of the Standing Committee of the National People's Congress. Dr. Youyou Tu (aka Tu Youyou) discovered and purified artemisinin (also known as *qinghaosu*) and dihydroartemisinin to treat malaria and won 2015 Nobel Prize in Physiology or Medicine.

Evolution of China's Biotech Industry

China is a planned "market economy." Every 5 years, the central government would announce the major economic development directions, policies, and goals for the next 5 years. The current "Outline of the 13th Five-Year Plan for the National Economic and Social Development of the People's Republic of China" for years 2016–20 was announced on March 16, 2016. The biotechnology was reaffirmed as one of the six emerging strategic industries for further promotion and support. The 13th Five-Year Plan also laid out the foundation for "Healthy China 2030" planning outline, which was announced on October 25, 2016 and is the most recent comprehensive framework on the goals and plans of China healthcare reform.

Transition From a Generic Industry to Me-Too/Me-Better in 2000s

China's biotech industry had focused on generics and APIs (active pharmaceutical ingredients). Around 2000, many Chinese students who had gone to Western countries for their graduate education since the 1980s, and many of them also worked in the United States and European pharmaceutical and biotech companies, started returning to China to establish their biotech start-up companies. These Chinese oversea students are often referred to as Hai Gui ("sea turtles", returnees).

In 2000 Dr. Ge Li et al. cofounded WuXi PharmaTech and later turned it into today's hugely successful CRO (contract research organization) powerhouse WuXi AppTec.

In 2001 Drs. Xianping Lu, Zhiqiang Ning, and their friends cofounded Shenzhen Chipscreen Biosciences Co., Ltd. and later developed Chidamide [trade name Epidaza, a selective HDAC inhibitor approved by China Food and Drug Administration (CFDA) for treating relapsed or refractory peripheral T-cell lymphoma in December 2014]. Chidamide is considered as the first China-discovered new drug compound that was licensed to the United States and Europe (in 2007).

In 2002 Dr. Samantha Du founded Hutchison MediPharma and later established several research collaboration and licensing deals with multinational pharma companies, such as Merck, Eli Lilly, Johnson & Johnson, and AstraZeneca. Its internally discovered and developed Fruquintinib (trade name Elunate, an oral inhibitor of vascular endothelial growth factor receptor) was approved for metastatic colorectal cancer in September 2018 in China.

In 2003 Drs. Lieming Ding, Yinxiang Wang, and Xiaodong Zhang cofounded Zhejiang Betta Pharmaceuticals Co., Ltd. and later developed Icotinib hydrochloride (trade name Conmana, approved by China's CFDA in June 2011). Icotinib is a tyrosine kinase inhibitor against the same target, epidermal growth factor receptor (EGFR), of AstraZeneca's Gefitinib (trade name Iressa). Icotinib is considered as the first home-grown anticancer-targeted drug in China.

Even long after 2000, most Chinese companies focused on me-too and me-better strategy. Many foreign innovative new drugs entered the China market long after their initial US or European launches. Some were due to strategic reasons of these foreign sponsors; however, the majority were due to the challenges in China's regulatory process. These products were often categorized as imported drugs and had to go through a lengthy clinical trial application and approval, additional clinical trials in China, and subsequent marketing application review and approval. It typically took an additional 5 years, and in some cases more than 10 years for a new drug to go through the registration process with the CFDA, formerly the State Food and Drug Administration (SFDA). In addition, the agency had little experience in approving innovative drugs with new mechanisms of action (MOAs) or new drug targets. These gave many Chinese pharmaceutical and biotech companies a window of opportunity to pick "low-hanging fruits" and to develop new molecular entities (NMEs) against the same drug targets that already had drugs being approved by the US FDA or European Medicines Agency (EMA), or that had already been clinically validated in late stage clinical development outside of China (e.g., in phase III). These NMEs are often referred to as "me-too's" or "me-better's".

Transition to "Fast Follow-On" and Innovation in Global for China

Due to the low entry barriers of "me-too/better," many Chinese biotech companies and even large Chinese pharma companies crowded into this business model. For example, as of May 2018, there were 26 Investigational New Drug (IND) filings and clinical trials of biosimilars in China to Humira, mAb against TNFα, and 26 to Avastin, against VEGF-A [1]. There are even more small molecule "me-too/betters". Some more innovative companies tried to move earlier in the drug-development chain. Instead of developing NMEs against FDA-approved or clinically-validated drug targets, these companies quickly developed NMEs against drug targets that have compound(s) just having entered clinical phase I or phase II in the United States or Europe, as a "fast follow-on."

In 2011 Mr. John Oyler and Dr. Xiaodong Wang founded BeiGene to develop "drug candidates to be first-in-class locally and to obtain approval in China prior to ex-China developed candidates" [6]. BeiGene quickly developed BGB-283, a second-generation BRAF inhibitor, and BGB-290, an inhibitor of the enzyme poly ribose polymerase (PARP), and out-licensed the ex-China worldwide rights of both to Merck KGaA in 2013 in two separate out-licensing and collaboration deals. BeiGene also quickly developed BGB-3111, a BTK inhibitor, which is now in phase III clinical trials in the United States and under priority review for the New Drug Application (NDA) in China, and BGB-A317, a PD-1 antibody, that was out-licensed to Celgene in 2017 for its ex-China worldwide right and is now under priority review for NDA in China. BeiGene went to public at NASDAQ in February 2016 and became China's first pre-revenue biotech company that went to public in the United States.

Some of the Chinese biotech companies even jump-started their R&D pipeline by in-licensing clinical stage assets from the US and European pharma and biotech companies. They structured the deal either as a straightforward licensing deal for the China market right, or as a co-development deal to synchronize clinical trials globally and share clinical data that are generated both in China and outside of China.

In 2014 Dr. Samantha Du started her second biotech company, Zai Lab, in China, which initially filled its pipeline by in-licensing from US and European companies. In 2016 it obtained an exclusive license from Tesaro for the development and commercialization of niraparib in China, Hong Kong, and Macau. Niraparib (trade name Zejula) is an orally active small molecule PARP inhibitor developed by Tesaro and approved to treat ovarian cancer in March 2017 in the United States. Zai received the approval of niraparib for ovarian cancer in Hong Kong in October 2018 and NDA acceptance from China's NMPA (National Medical Products Administration, successor of CFDA). Zai went to public at NASDAQ in September 2017.

Transition to Indigenous Innovation in China for Global

China's CFDA (now NMPA) joined ICH (International Council for Harmonisation) in June 2017, which would allow international pharmaceutical companies to introduce their new drugs into China much more timely and efficiently, but much less costly. AstraZeneca's third-generation EGFR inhibitor osimertinib (trade name Tagrisso) received CFDA approval on March 27, 2017 under CFDA's priority review, only a couple of months after AstraZenca submitted its NDA to CFDA, and 16 months after it received US FDA's accelerated approval but 4 days before FDA's full approval. Less than one month later, Tagrisso was on China market. Roche's emicizumab (trade name Hemlibra), a humanized bispecific antibody for the treatment of hemophilia A was approved by NMPA in December 2018, about 12.5 months after it was first approved by US FDA in November 2017. In December 2018, San Francisco—based FibroGen and its commercial partner AstraZeneca secured China NMPA approval for their oral drug, roxadustat, for anemic patients. This is significant because the China approval of roxadustat was ahead of its pivotal US data and marked for the first time that a non-Chinese pharmaceutical company can sell its innovative drug in China before the United States or Europe.

Under China's CFDA (now NMPA) reform, the window for "me-too/better's," even for "fast follow-on's," is becoming narrower and narrower. Many Chinese biotech companies adjusted their strategic directions and business models and started indigenous innovation internally or increased collaboration and licensing activities with academics both inside and outside of China and with US and European pharma and biotech companies. For example, both BeiGene and Zai Lab announced that they started investing heavily in internal discovery and research of unannounced novel MOAs and targets for the global market. Other companies also collaborate with US and

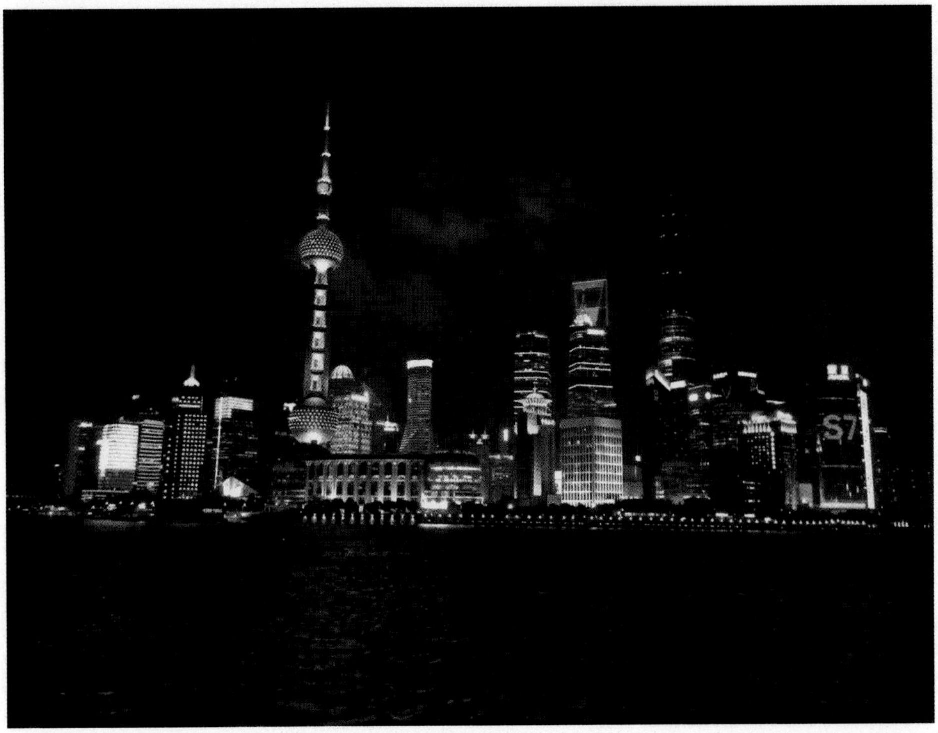

FIGURE 38.1 Shanghai in 2016.

European companies on the codevelopment of novel drugs that are even in clinical phase I or preclinical studies and carry out multicenter global or regional clinical trials aiming at simultaneous regulatory approvals in the United States, Europe, and China (Fig. 38.1).

The Current Landscape of China's Biotech Industry

The China Biotech Market

China became the second largest pharmaceutical market in 2014, from the 11th in 2000 (behind Mexico), and is expected to surpass the United States and become the largest pharmaceutical market in 5 years. However, the majority, more than 75%, of sales have been generic drugs in the last 5 years.

Traditional Chinese medicine is still a big portion of the total pharmaceutical sales in China, though it has been steadily declining from 19.1% in 2013 to 16.8% in 2017. The biologic product sales only account for 6.0%–7.4% of the Chinese pharma market but have been growing the fastest at 13.7% per year in the last 5 years. In contrast, the biologics sales take about 26.5% of the global market [1] (Fig. 38.2).

Although medical device sector is not a focus of this chapter, it is worth noting that China has also become the second largest medical device market in the world, with the average annual growth rate at 17.5% [7] (Fig. 38.3).

Government Policies and Supports

General Policies From Central Government

Recognizing the critical roles of biotechnology in "healing, fueling, and feeding" the world, the Chinese central government has enacted a series of policies to strongly support the development of biotechnology. In October 2010, Chinese government declared biotechnology as one of the seven strategic emerging industries in its "Decision of the State Council on Accelerating the Fostering and Development of Strategic Emerging Industries." Two months later, the State Council detailed its policy and support in its "Bioindustry Development Plan." Biotechnology was reaffirmed as one of the six strategic emerging industries in China's 13th Five-Year Plan (2016–20) in March 2016. Consequently, State Council issued "13th Five-Year National Plan for the development of Strategic Emerging Industries" in November 2016, National Development and Reform Commission (NDRC) issued "13th FYP Bio-Industry Development Plan" in December 2016, and Ministry of Science and Technology (MOST) issued "13th FYP Biotechnology Innovation Plan" in April 2017, and MOST, National Health and Family Planning Commission, CFDA, and other three ministries jointly issued "13th FYP Health Technology Innovation Plan" in May 2017.

As China is still primarily a "planned market economy," the favorable policies from the central government will make it easy for biotech companies to receive strong supports not only from central government and its

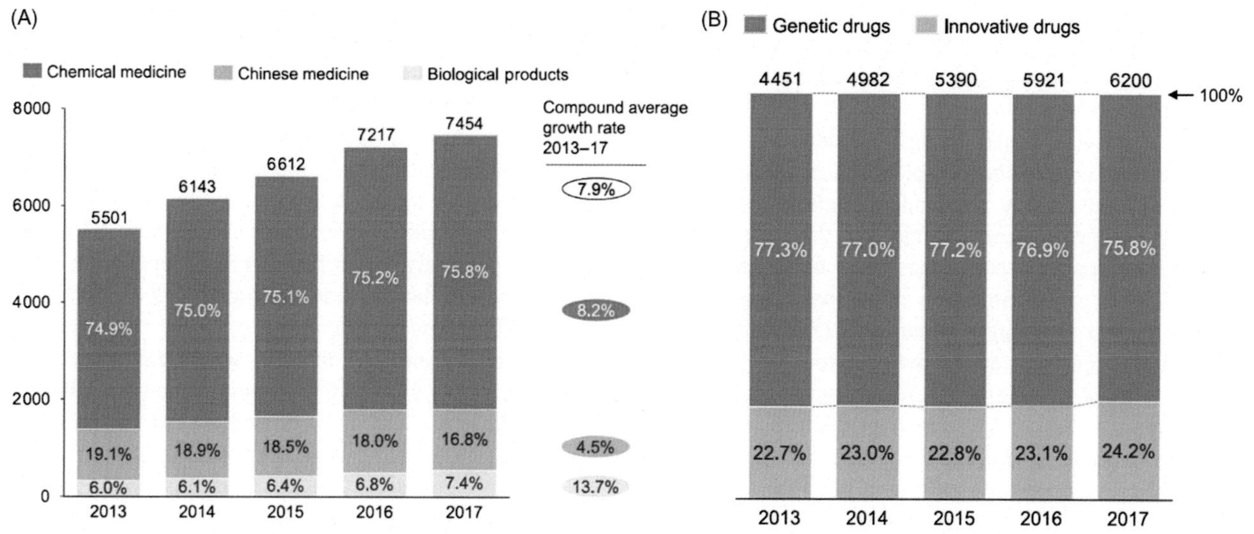

FIGURE 38.2 (A) Market size of drugs in China's hospital in 2013–17 (RMB 100 million). (B) Sorted by drug types (2013–17). *Note:* Based on data in hospitals that have over 100 beds. Source: *IPM Database, Research and Analysis by Pharmcube.*

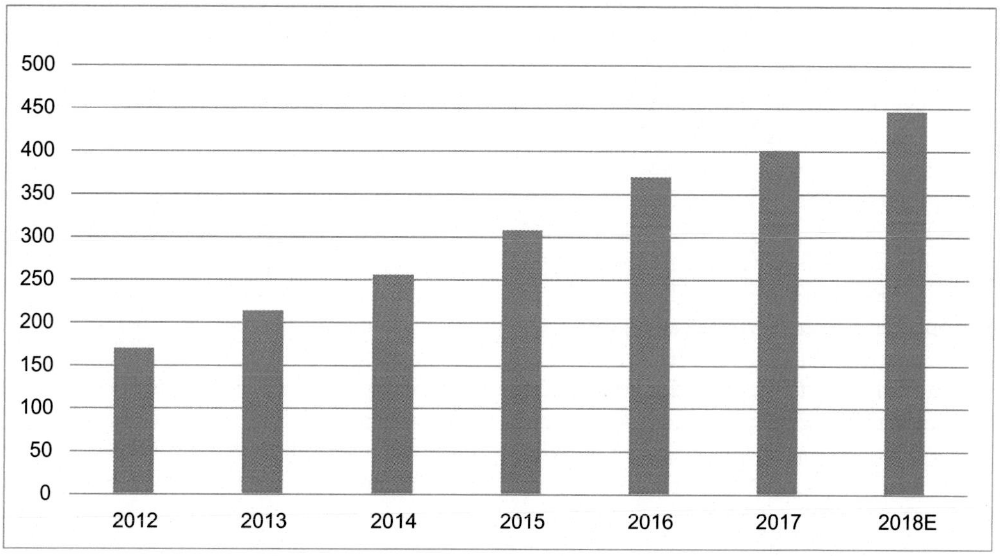

FIGURE 38.3 Total China medical device market size (in billion Chinese yuan) 1 USD = 6.8783 Chinese yuan (December 31, 2018).

agencies but also from local government at provincial, city, and high-tech park levels. These supports may include administrative support (such as easiness to set up, register and grow companies, and convenience to deal with government agencies, such as industry and commerce, tax, and custom) and monetary support (such as government grants, R&D rebates, tax incentives, and bank loans).

Clinical Trials and Regulatory Affairs

The clinical trial and approval of drugs and medical devices are mainly regulated under the authority of NMPA. It was officially established on April 11, 2018, at a vice-ministry level under the State Administration for Market Regulation. Its predecessors include CFDA (2013–18, ministry level under the State Council), SFDA [2008–13, vice-ministry level under the Ministry of Health (MOH), and 2003–08, vice-ministry level under the State Council], State Food Administration (1998–2003, under the State Economic and Trade Commission), Bureau of Medicine and Drugs (1982–98, under the State Council or State Economic and Trade Commission), General Bureau of Medicine and Drugs (1979–82, under the MOH).

Prior to 2015 CFDA reform, CFDA had very little experience in evaluating truly innovative drugs that had new MOAs or new drug targets and had never been approved anywhere else. Most of CFDA's experience had been in approving generic drugs and new drugs that had not been marketed inside China, which included imported drugs that had already received marketing approvals by US FDA or EMA. However, most of these "new drugs" from China domestic companies were either me-too/betters, isomers, or reformulation of known drugs. In 2014 China's Center for Drug Evaluation (CDE) recommended 501 drug approvals, among which were 410 domestic chemical drugs (256 generics, 26 reformulations, and 128 new chemical drugs), 68 were imported chemical drugs, 12 were biologics (10 domestic and 2 imported), and 11 were Chinese traditional medicine.

In addition, CFDA had very limited manpower. Before 2015, CDE had only 115 staff (89 technical staff), compared to its US counterpart the FDA's CDE and Research (CDER) which had more than 5000 staff members. In 2014 the CFDA CDE received 8868 NDAs and by the end of 2014, 18,597 drug registration applications had been queued waiting for approvals. In contrast, in the same year the US FDA CDER received only 1515 IND applications for drugs, biologicals, and biosimilars [8].

State Council Document (2015) No. 44 "Opinions of the State Council on the Reform of the Review & Approval System for Drugs and Medical Devices" issued on August 18, 2015 instigated the reform of CFDA. Document 44, among others, allows foreign new drugs to enter clinical trials simultaneously in China, pilots the marketing authorization holder (MAH) system, and accelerates the review and approval of innovative drugs.

On October 8, 2017 the General Office of the CPC Central Committee and the General Office of the State Council printed and issued the "Opinions on Deepening the Reform of Review and Approval System and Encouraging the Innovation of Drugs and Medical Devices" (Document 42). It reaffirms Document 44 and goes even further to reform clinical trial management and accept foreign clinical data for the approval of innovative drugs in China, to accelerate the approval of innovative drugs for urgent unmet medical needs and rare diseases, and to implement the MAH system.

Soon after the two Documents, CFDA was busy in drafting and announcing new regulations to accelerate the review and approval of innovative drugs. There was a grapevine among regulatory affair personnel that they could not sleep in the nights or enjoy the weekends, since CFDA often announced a new regulation at midnight, and frequently it would be in a Friday night. The industry, especially the biotech companies working on innovative drugs, accepted it with joys. By the end of 2017, only about 4000 drug registration applications left in queue waiting for reviews and approvals, compared to the peak of 22,000 in September 2015. In 2017 CFDA approved 394 drugs, among which were 278 domestic drugs (28 new chemical drugs, 10 biologics, 238 generics, and 2 Chinese traditional medicine), 103 imported chemical, and 13 biological drugs. Among these, 53 were accepted as priority review; the first-round review of INDs, NDAs, and ANDAs took an average of 39, 59, and 81 working days, respectively, after they were accepted for priority review, much shorter than the legal limit of 90 working days for IND review [9].

One of the notable reforms was the new regulation issued on July 31, 2018, "Announcement on Adjusting the Review & Approval Procedures of Drug Clinical Trials." Sixty working days after the acceptance of clinical trial application and receipt of corresponding payment by CDE, if CDE does not issue an opinion of rejection or questioning, the applicant can conduct the clinical trials in China per the submitted protocols. This silent approval process is now in-line with the practice at US FDA. Previously, before each phase of the clinical trials (phases I–III), applicants had to wait for CDE approval before conducting the trials; sometime the wait could be years.

On August 8, 2018, CDE proposed a "List of the First Batch of Overseas New Drugs Urgently Needed in Clinical Settings." The 48 listed drugs had been approved in the United States, Europe, or Japan. If the sponsor believes that there is no ethnic difference, the sponsor can submit clinical data obtained from overseas to directly support China registration, without the need of additional clinical trials in China before the marketing approval. Most of these 48 drugs are for cancer or rare diseases. Among these 48 drugs, 8 had already been approved or nearly approved when CDE officially released the list on November 1, 2018. Sponsors can apply to CDE to include their oversea-approved drugs into future lists.

All the reforms at NMPA seemed to have moved at full speed ahead. However, on July 15, 2018, Changchun Changsheng was put on notice by NMPA for falsifying manufacturing records of its rabies vaccine (the "Changsheng vaccine incident"); and subsequently, Mr. Jingquan Bi, NMPA Commissioner, resigned on August 16, 2018, together with some of his lieutenants. Although sadden by these developments, the general consensus of the industry is that as long as Document 42 and Document 44 are in effect, NMPA will continue its reform and implement what it has already announced.

In addition to NMPA, a parallel regulatory pathway supervises cell therapy in China as a medical technology. For investigator-sponsored noncommercial cell therapy clinical studies, the review and approval of NMPA is not necessary; instead, the clinical studies are approved by the IRB and the president of some certain hospitals that are under the authority of MOH (predecessor of National

Health Commission). Consequently, Chinese biotech companies gained significant head-start advantages in cell therapy, particularly in chimeric antigen receptor (CAR) T-cell therapy. For example, Nanjing Legend treated 35 multiple myeloma patients with its CAR T-cell drug candidate, LCAR-B38M, which specifically targets the B-cell maturation antigen, through the medical technology pathway, and won a worldwide collaboration and license deal with an upfront payment of $350 million from Johnson & Johnson's Janssen in December 2017. Although China had about the same amount of cell therapy clinical trials posted on the ClinicalTrials.gov as the United States at the end of 2017, none of those clinical trials in China had actually conducted under an IND application. Both the drug regulatory authority and the industry are pondering how to utilize those massive non-IND trial data for drug registration.

Biotech and pharma companies need to pay particular attention to the "Interim Measures for the Administration of Human Genetic Resources" published in 1998. The measures cover the gathering, collection, sales, export, and cross-border transfer of human genetic materials and information, such as those obtained in clinical trials, if participated by a foreign enterprise including its agent or subsidiary in China. Before clinical trials start, the foreign enterprise and all participating enterprises, such as clinical sites, CROs, and third-party laboratories, need to file a report to the Administration of China Human Genetic Resources ("yi-chuan-ban") of MOST.

Pricing, Drug Tender, and Reimbursement

Drug pricing and affordability have been major concerns for many governments, including the US government. This is even more entangled for the Chinese government, as China is mostly a single-payer system. The government-run medical insurance, through three major medical insurance programs, covers more than 95% of the Chinese population, while commercial health insurance remains immaterial. However, Chinese patients' out-of-pocket spending was 32.4% of the national healthcare expenditure, compared to 11.1% in the United States and 13.1% in Japan [1].

While the accessibility issue of innovative drugs is addressed by regulatory reforms at NMPA, the drug pricing and reimbursement become an imminent issue, and a bottleneck, for Chinese patients to use the most current therapies and treatment for devastating diseases. In May 2018, Chinese government created a new State Medical Insurance Administration (SMIA) to consolidate the supervision and regulation of government-run medical insurance programs, drug pricing, and drug tendering.

There are two drug reimbursement lists under the government-run insurance: one at the national level, and the other at the province level:

1. The National Reimbursement Drug List (NRDL) was first created in 2004 and revised in 2007 and 2009; however, the next revision was not until 2017. But the government promised that NRDL would be dynamic for novel and patented drugs and newly launched drugs, and a full revision would be at least once every 2 years in the future. There are two categories of drugs in the NRDL: (1) Catalog A: these drugs are medical necessary with long prescription and efficacy histories and relatively lower costs. They are reimbursed 100% by the government insurance. Only the central government can make adjustment to this catalog. (2) Catalog B: these drugs are usually newer drugs and are not fully reimbursed by the government insurance (usually at 50%–90% rate depending on the province and city).
2. The Provincial Reimbursement Drug List (PRDL): Each province has the option to make adjustment (i.e., add or subtract) on about 15% of the drugs in NRDL Catalog B, as well as its reimbursement rate. The provinces usually take consideration of the surplus of local medical insurance fund, the location of the drug manufacturers (local manufacturers usually have some advantages), and the local medical needs and prescription habits. Entering PRDL is important for new drugs, as the number of the PRDLs that a new drug has entered is one of the criteria for being included in the next round of NRDL.

In the two rounds of NRDL negotiation in 2017 and 2018, the average reduction of drug prices was about 44% in 2017 and 56.7% in 2018, and the reduction of oncology drugs ranged from 30% to 80%. For example, Roche's Bevacizumab (trade name Avastin) entered eight PRDLs since its launch in China in 2010 and entered NRDL Catalog B in July 2017. Roche reduced its price by 61.4% to ¥1998 [100 mg (4 mL)/vial, about US$295 at then exchange rate]. However, its sales more than doubled in Q3 2017 and Q4 2017, respectively, and tripled in Q1 2018.

The pricing and sales of PD-1 monoclonal antibodies in China will be interesting. BMS's Opdivo and Merck's Keytruda were approved in China on June 15, 2018 and July 25, 2018, respectively. Two domestic PD-1s from Junshi and Innovent were approved on December 17, 2018 and December 27, 2018, respectively. As of December 31, 2018, there were two domestic PD-1s, from Hengrui and BeiGene, respectively, that had filed for NDAs in China, and another nine were in clinical trials or had applied for clinical trials (Table 38.1).

TABLE 38.1 PD-1 antibodies in China.

Manufacturer	BMS	Merck/MSD	Junshi	Innovent
Product	Opdivo (nivolumab)	Keytruda (pembrolizumab)	JS001 (toripalimab)	Tyvyt (sintilimab)
Approval date	June 15, 2018	July 25, 2018	December 17, 2018	December 27, 2018
Indication	Non-small-cell lung carcinoma (NSCLC)	Melanoma	Melanoma	Hodgkin's lymphoma
Pricing	¥9260 (100 mg/10 mL, $1354 vs $2600 in the United States) ¥4591 (40 mg/4 mL, $671 vs $1100 in the United States)	¥17,918 (100 mg/4 mL, $2616 vs $4800 in the United States)	¥7200 (240 mg/6 mL, $1051)	¥7838 (240 mg/10 mL, $1168)
Dosage	3 mg/kg/2 weeks	2 mg/kg/3 weeks		
Annual list price (est.)	$84,000 (vs ~$150,00 in the United States)	$54,200	¥187,200 ($27,324)	¥266,500 ($39,732)
PAP	5 + 6 (free, undecided)	3 + 3 (free)	4 + 4 (free)	3 + 3 (free)

Talent

In the last 6 years, there have been more than 2 million "sea turtles" ("Hai Gui's," returnees) coming back to China after completing their studies overseas. Among them, more than 250,000 were in life sciences. Most of these Chinese students went to study life-sciences in the United States as graduate students, somewhat due to that American-born students had been losing interests in STEM (science, technology, engineering, and mathematics) and Chinese students seemed to be just in time to fill the gap. Many of these life sciences sea turtles had rich working experience in the pharmaceutical and biotech companies in the United States, Europe, and Japan. Some of them were senior R&D scientists and executives at these companies, including vice presidents and senior vice presidents at multinational large pharmas. Reduced federal funding to biomedical sciences and reorganizations at pharmaceutical and biotech companies in the United States seemed to have helped accelerating the tides of sea turtles. The BayHelix Group, a nonprofit organization of leaders of Chinese heritage in the global life sciences and healthcare community, was founded in the San Francisco Bay Area in 2001, but 58% of its more than 700 members, are now in China, who are the "who's who" in the China biotech industry.

The home-grown students, more than 150,000 a year in life sciences-related majors at undergraduate, master, and PhD levels, have also received strong educations. Many of the professors at top universities are sea turtles. Eighty-one percent academicians of Chinese Academy of Sciences and 54% of Chinese Academy of Engineers are sea turtles [10]; these percentages are even higher in the life sciences-related divisions.

Almost all top 20 multinational large pharma and biotech companies have established R&D centers in China since 2001. Some of the R&D centers had more than 500 staff. The multinational pharma and biotech companies brought expats, most of them Chinese nationals, from their headquarters and R&D centers into China, as well as recruited locally within China. Many of these scientists and executives left the multinational R&D centers, starting their own biotech companies or joining a start-up. Since 2015, due to strategic changes from headquarters, many multinational pharmas, such as AbbVie, Novartis, Roche, Eli Lilly, and GSK, started to close their R&D centers in China or reduce the head counts. However, these are the music to the ears of start-up companies, VCs, and CROs. Just like in the United States, even more and more senior scientists and executives are jumping ship from large pharm and biotech companies. For example, BayHelix now only has 24% of its members remaining in multinational companies at the end of 2018, compared to 30% in 2012–14.

Although there is an increasing pool of talents, yet it is still challenging to recruit top talents in China. Unlike in the United States where there is a large pool of professional managers, many top talents in China rather start their own companies due to easy access to capitals. It is particularly difficult to recruit experienced Chief Medical Officer (CMO) and business development (BD) executives. The grapevine rumored that a highly experienced and sought-after CMO in China would command almost twice the cash compensation of whom would in the United States, and an experienced BD executive with experiences in both buy and sell sides would be similar. In contrast, since most founders are CEOs themselves, CEO does not seem to be a challenging position to fill at the beginning of the start-up. However, a professional CEO is very hard to recruit, since an experienced CEO would rather start his or her own company, or the founder(s) may still want to control the company and a professional CEO would not be willing to take the task. Another alternative is to recruit talents directly from the United States. However, some of them may still like to keep their homes in the United States due to family reasons, such as spouse's work and children's education. *Nature* magazine, in 2018, featured a story how a biotech entrepreneur benefited from splitting time between China and the United States [11]. However, some misconceptions still exist in a small handful of investors and employers requiring such talents to be in China 100% of the time. This may defeat the purpose of taking advantage of the talents for their Western vision, cross-border experience, and network—killing the goose for its golden eggs.

It is challenging to keep talents in China as well. Although the turnover rate of 18.6% in biotech R&D is lower than the national average of 19.7% in 2017, according to Aon Hewitt, the salary increases of 7.4% were higher than the national average of 6.5%. Many mid and lower level managers and employees are ready to jump ship when there is a higher offer of salaries. Therefore, company's culture, mission, future prospective and working environment, employee's career-development opportunities, responsibilities, and cash and equity compensations, and CEO's personal charm, charisma, and leadership become even more important for the biotech companies in China.

Intellectual Property Protection

Recognizing that intellectual property (IP) is the fountain of innovations, Chinese government has been trying hard to strengthen the IP protection and enforcement. The patent law was first enacted in 1985 and revised in 1993, 2001, and 2009. It is in its fourth revision and expected to become effective in the second half of 2019.

China takes part in the Patent Cooperation Treaty (PCT). Therefore, a patent application originated from a PCT Contracting State can select to enter China at the national phase. Invention patents have a term of 20 years from the filing date of the patent application, and utility and design patents have a term of 10 years (the draft revision of 2019 patent law proposed to extend design patent term to 15 years). China adopts "first-to-file" system and does not accept provisional applications as in the United States. The grace period and associated activities allowed for novelty determination are also different from those in the United States. Another caveat to which biotech companies need to pay attention is the national security considerations. Like many other PCT Contracting States including the United States, China requires that for an invention made in China, the applicant(s) need to either request a preclearance from the National Intellectual Property Administration (CNIPA, successor of State Intellectual Property Office) before filing the patent application in a foreign country, or file the international patent application through CNIPA.

Two proposals in the draft revision of China's 2019 Patent Law could significantly benefit innovative drugs. (1) To compensate the time in reviewing and approving innovative drugs, for the invention patents of innovative drugs that apply for synchronized approval in China with oversea approval, the State Council may decide to extend the patent terms for up to 5 years, so long as the total valid patent life would not exceed 14 years after the innovative drug goes on sales. (2) The willful infringement of a patent could be panelized for one to five times of the damage incurred to the patent right holder, the benefit received by the infringer, or the amount of license fee.

To better resolve IP disputes, China established IP Court in Beijing, Shanghai, and Guangzhou in 2014. From January 1, 2019, a new IP Court in Supreme People's Court hears all the appeals of IP cases. This newly established IP Court is intended to function similarly to the US Court of Appeals for the Federal Circuit. It will unify and regulate law application criterion and defuse local pressure. It will likely become a preferred court for international patent litigations.

Partnering With China

Company Formation: Structure, Location, and Registration

Company Structure

Most Chinese companies adopt the following three-layer structure for flexibility:

1. An offshore company, registered in such as Cayman Island or British Virgin Island, to receive investment from investors; most of the founder shares are also in this offshore company, which is a nonoperating company.
2. An intermediary company, registered in Hong Kong, as the wholly owned subsidiary of the offshore company. This Hong Kong–based company is also a nonoperating company. Some lawyers argue that this intermediary company in Hong Kong is not necessary, especially when its China wholly foreign-owned entity (WFOE) is not profitable yet. However, some lawyers suggest to have such intermediary company regardless.
3. A local company, registered in China, which is WFOE, that is, the subsidiary of the Hong Kong company. This is usually the operating company; if not, it would have another subsidiary company in China as the operating company. For certain industry sectors,

such as human stem cell, gene testing and therapy that are prohibited from foreign investments, a VIE (variable interest entity) structure is usually adopted. The investors would own the equity of a holding company, which de facto controls over the VIE-operating company through a series of contractual arrangements. The VIE structure is widely used in telecom, e-commerce, and online-game industries, such as by SINA, Alibaba, Tencent, and Baidu.

Site Selection

Most Chinese biotech companies are clustered in so-called biotech parks, a special area that is allocated by the central or local government for biotech development. This is unlike in the United States where biotech clusters, such as the San Francisco Bay Area, the Greater Boston Area, and the San Diego Area, were usually formed by the market force and the industry itself. San Francisco Mission Bay is probably the only biotech-innovative hub designated by the State of California.

China has more than 150 biotech parks, by ChinaBio's last count in 2016. Some biotech parks are mixed with high-tech parks, while some are stand-alone. These biotech parks are mainly clustered in the following four regions:

1. The Yangtze Delta Region, which is centered in Shanghai. The most notable ones are Zhangjiang Medicine Valley in Shanghai, BioBay in Suzhou, Jiangsu, Pharma Town in Hangzhou, Zhejiang, China Medical City in Taizhou, Jiangsu, Nanjing Biotech and Pharmaceutical Valley in Nanjing, Jiangsu, and many others. This region is the most matured region in China for innovative drugs and medical devices. For example, Suzhou BioBay clusters more than 400 biotech companies, including publicly listed biotech companies such as BeiGene (NASDAQ, February 2016), Zai Lab (NASDAQ, September 2017), Innovent [Hong Kong Exchanges and Clearing Limited (HKEX, October 2018)], and many other unicorn and uprising companies. Sanofi announced in November 2018 to launch its fourth global research institute in Suzhou BioBay, after the ones in France, the United States, and Germany.
2. The BoHai Bay Region, which spans from Beijing to Tianjin. The most notable ones are Zhongguanchun Life Science Park at Changping, Beijing, which hosts many R&D-type biotech companies, and Beijing E-town, which hosts many manufacturing-type biotech companies.
3. The Pearl Delta Region, which was recently expanded to include Guangdong (including nine cities such as Guangzhou, Shenzhen, Zhuhai, Foshan, Dongguan, and Zhongshan), Hong Kong, and Macau as Greater Bay Area.
4. The Southwest region, which includes Sichuan Province (in particular its capital city Chengdu) and Chongqing.

The "Guan-Wei-Hui" (the Administrative Committee) of the biotech park is the local government that biotech start-up companies interact with the most, starting from the site selection and negotiation of administrative and financial support. Different companies have different goals and strategies; therefore, the site selection criteria would be different. For example, factors for consideration could include: location (including the maturity of the biotech park, proximity to a metro city location, convenience of short commute, and long-distance transportation), accessibility of talent (including the living conditions, such as work and education opportunities for the family, healthcare services, and living expenses), availabilities of facility and land, and government incentives and policies. The requirements on environmental impact evaluation and fire code are the two redlines that must be met during site selection. Some biotech parks do not welcome chemical drug or API manufacturing any more. Some biotech parks provide waste management, such as wastewater treatment before discharging to the municipal sewage, but some would require the company itself to manage the waste, or the mixture of two.

As in the United States for a large project, which may bring in large tax revenue and/or employment, to negotiate with state or city authority on supports such as tax incentives, in China a project as small as a biotech start-up can negotiate with biotech park Guan-Wei-Hui for administrative and financial support. Examples of such support may include start-up funding, equity investment, R&D rebates and awards, facility lease rebates, tax incentives for the company and/or its senior executives, salary supplements to senior R&D personnel, housing allowance for senior executives, and assistance to family relocation, for example, employment opportunities for spouse and education opportunities for children.

If the biotech company is going to build a R&D and/or manufacturing facility, there is a possibility to acquire the land use right from the government. In China the land is owned by the government. A private enterprise cannot own the land; it leases the land use right from the government. Therefore, the company needs to plan well how to effectively use the piece of acquired land. Unlike in the United States, after having purchased the land, a company can, at its own wish, stage the development of the land and construct buildings in several phases or even leave the land unused. In China, if a company does not fully utilize the acquired land to a certain degree by certain time as required by the government, the government has the right to reclaim the unused portion of the land.

If the company owns a piece of land (lease right), the company may have the option to take a bank loan. If approved, the company can apply to Guan-Wei-Hui for rebates on the bank loan interests. Depending on the interest rate, sometimes the rebate can fully offset the loan interests. Usually, it is challenging for a R&D company without a manufacturing facility, especially a start-up company, to obtain a meaningful amount of bank loan, as Chinese banks do not usually accept intangible assets, such as intellectual properties or equities, as collaterals. However, there are some emerging funds, some of which are supported by the government, modeling after Silicon Valley Bank to provide loans to biotech start-up companies who have received venture capital funding.

Company Registration

Company registration is usually done at the local level, either in the city or in the biotech park. One of the significant differences from the United States is the concept of registered capital. The registered capital is the number that appears on company's business license issued by the government and presumably represents the size of the company. Certain types of companies need to declare a minimal size in order to meet certain qualifications set by the government. Since 2014 the registered capital is on a subscription-basis and does not have to be paid-in within a certain period of time. However, the size of the registered capital is not "the bigger the better"; unpaid-in registered capital could become a liability later as well as incur tax consequences.

Outsourcing: Contract Research Organizations

China probably has the greatest number of CROs covering drug discovery, preclinical, clinical, and manufacturing services; some providing "end-to-end" services. Almost all global CROs have a presence in China one way or the other. This chapter introduces some "homegrown" domestic CROs that serve both Chinese and foreign companies but do not mean an exhaustive list or an endorsement of any companies.

WuXi AppTec (http://www.wuxiapptec.com/) is publicly listed in both China and Hong Kong (Stock Code: 603259.SH/2359.HK). It provides a broad and integrated portfolio of services in small molecule drug R&D and manufacturing, cell therapy and gene therapy R&D and manufacturing, and drug R&D and medical device testing. For example, in small molecule drug R&D services, it spans from assay development, library screening, and lead identification and optimization, to animal model studies and IND-enabling studies. It recently launched a new 80 billion DNA-encoded small molecule libraries and screening platform. It also recently expanded its clinical and regulatory services, encompassing all phases of clinical trials. WuXi has more than 17,000 employees, 27 R&D sites and offices in China, the United States, and Germany, and 6 million square feet of office, laboratory, and manufacturing space. Its platform is enabling more than 3000 innovative collaborators from more than 30 countries to bring innovative healthcare products to patients, and to fulfill WuXi's dream that "every drug can be made and every disease can be treated."

WuXi Biologics (https://www.wuxibiologics.com/), WuXi's sister company, is also a Hong Kong-listed company (Stock Code: 2269.HK). It provides open-access biologics technology platform offering end-to-end solutions and *one*-stop service to empower organizations to discover, develop, and manufacture biologics from concept to commercial manufacturing. The fastest timeline from DNA to IND was about 9 months. As of June 30, 2018, there were a total of 187 integrated projects, including 98 projects in preclinical development stage, 78 projects in early-phase (phases I and II) clinical development, 10 projects in late-phase (phase III) development, and 1 project in commercial manufacturing. With total estimated capacity of biopharmaceutical production planned in China, Ireland, Singapore, and the United States reaching 220,000 L by 2021, WuXi Biologics will provide its biomanufacturing partners with a robust and premier-quality global supply chain network.

GenScript Biotech Corp. (https://www.genscript.com/) is also a public company listed at HKEX in Hong Kong (Stock Code: 01548.HK). GenScript has been the world leader in biotechnology reagent service and recently expanded its business into immunotherapy, COMO, laboratory equipment, and microbial industry. GenScript has established open and innovative technology-driven platforms and GMP facilities for preclinical drug discovery and pharmaceutical product development, along with a completed industrial microbial research, development, and industrialization platform for enzyme screening, genetic engineering, synthetic biology, protein and antibody engineering, and fermentation process optimization and research application. GenScript recently launched MolecularCloud as a more intuitive way to manipulate DNA, as well as a website for researchers to share and communicate DNA components. The MolecularCloud is the capstone for GenScript's CloneArk and GenSmart platforms. CloneArk lets scientists archive cloned genetic sequences for their own subsequent use. Approximately 1 million clones already are archived in this system. It has operational sites in China and New Jersey, and business centers in Europe and Japan. GenScript has been serving more than 100 countries and 200,000 + customers around the world.

BioDuro (https://bioduro.com/), headquartered in San Diego, California with main operations in China, provides comprehensive, integrated drug-discovery services spanning from target identification through phase III, with a broad range of capabilities in chemistry, discovery biology, drug metabolism and pharmacokinetics, pharmacology, and integrated preclinical research and development services, for both small molecule discovery and large molecular development and scale-up. BioDuro's global operations include a total of about 700 employees in San Diego, Beijing, and Shanghai. It has a 100,000 ft^2 facility in Beijing, a 92,000 ft^2 state-of-the-art facility in Shanghai, and a team of highly experienced research staff and scientists, of whom 20% have PhD degrees and 15% overseas background.

Fountain Medical Development Ltd. (FMD, www.fountain-med.com) provides one-stop high-quality clinical development services for pharmaceutical and medical device companies. FMD supports client's global drug-development programs and product registration in the United States, Europe, and East Asia (including China), with more than 1700 employees located in more than 20 offices in China, the United States, Armenia, the United Kingdom, Japan, South Korea, India, and Philippines. FMD differentiates from local competition by rigorously adhering to international quality standards and focusing on innovative new drugs. It has a very strong regulatory affairs team in China and a large and experienced data management and biostatistics team with state-of-art standards and most extensive global experiences. FMD provides full-services including regulatory affairs and operations, medical affairs, clinical monitoring and management, data management and statistical analysis, SMO, pharmacovigilance, medical translation, third-party audit, safety evaluation, toxicology, and e-submissions/CDISC. FMD has vast experience conducting trials for global companies and China-specific development programs in the therapeutic areas, such as oncology, infectious disease, central nervous system, immunology GI Disorders, reproductive health, respiratory and Gastroenterology, cardiovascular, endocrine and metabolic disorders, and hematology.

There are many other high-quality CROs and Contract Development and Manufacturing Organization (CDMOs) in China, such as Pharmaron (https://www.pharmaron.com/), TigerMed (https://www.tigermed.net/en/), and Asymchem (http://www.asymchem.com.cn/en/).

Some of these CROs and CDMOs also provide equity investments in start-up companies either by themselves or through their affiliated VCs. Some of these investments are without any strings attached, while some would like the invested portfolio companies to contract their services.

Like biotech companies in China, these CROs and CDMOs treat IP very seriously and protect IP as the lifeline for themselves and their clients. As Dr. Ge Li, cofounder, Chairman, and Co-CEO of WuXi AppTec states in its IP protection credo: "IP is our shared lifeline. We guard it at WuXi with our founding principles of integrity, world-class security, zero tolerance policies, and relentless pursuit of justice against any criminal act. This is our highest priority, and we must hold ourselves accountable. We are determined to earn the trust of our partners by committing to success together" (Fig. 38.4).

Venture Capital

A total of $80 billion in VC and PE funds targeting China healthcare were raised since 2015; however, nearly $45 billion remained uninvested by October 2018, according to ChinaBio. Limited by the opportunities inside China, Chinese investors poured money into the US biotech industry and participated in investment rounds in the US biotech companies worth $5.1 billion in the first half of 2018 (about 41% of the total investment in the US biotech companies), well exceeding the $4 billion (about 23%) in 2017, according to PitchBook.

The Chinese VC funds can be generally categorized into the following four types:

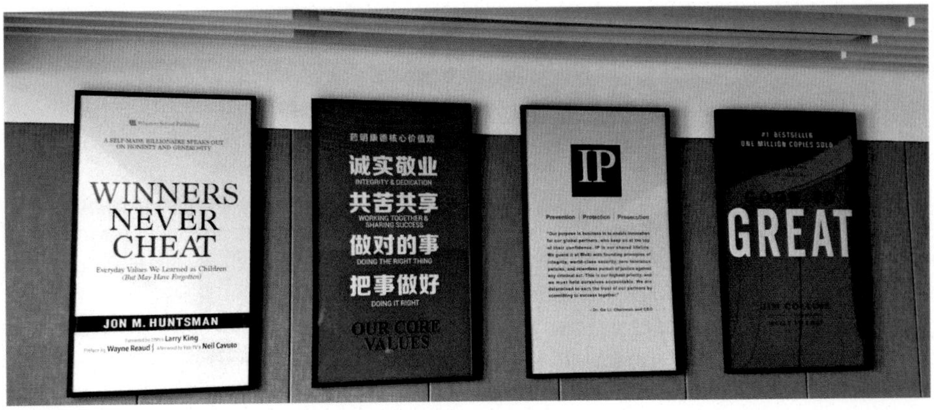

FIGURE 38.4 A picture of WuXi's IP protection credo hung on the wall of its conference rooms.

1. Government-sponsored funds: which includes those venture funds with LPs mainly from central, local, and biotech park government, and state-owned enterprises (SOE), for example, SDIC, Shenzhen Capital Group, and Suzhou Oriza Holdings. These funds are generally only allowed to invest in companies domiciled inside China.
2. Traditional VCs, which can be further roughly categorized into
   a. foreign VCs in China, such as KPCB China, Lilly Asia Ventures, Morningside, and OrbiMed Asia;
   b. VCs founded by returnees, such as 6-dimensions, CD Capital, Cenova, Decheng Capital, Qiming, and Quan Capital; and
   c. VCs founded by local Chinese investors.
3. Corporate VCs, which are mainly from Chinese pharmaceutical companies, such as Fosun, Fosun Pharma, and Hengrui. Some multinational pharmaceutical companies also have their corporate venture arms in China, such as JJDC (Johnson & Johnson Development Corp), and Merck Research Venture Fund. However, these multinational pharma's corporate VCs mostly make strategic investments in-line with their R&D strategies and apply the same investment criteria as in the United States or EU.
4. Investors converted from other industries, such as real estate, mining, IT, manufacturing, and insurance. These new biotech investors may have a different risk tolerance, time horizon, or even expectations on return on investment.

Many PE funds, such as Hillhouse, Ally Bridge, and Sequoia China, also started investing in the biotech companies that are inside and outside of China.

Many Chinese VCs and PEs tend to invest in more matured biotech companies, such as those with clinical stage assets. In the United States, they tend to coinvest with leading US investors or to lead the next round of investments in companies that have existing leading US investors or have collaboration and/or licensing deals with large multinational pharmas.

Both the central government (mostly through MOST and NDRC) and local government provide nondiluting fundings to biotech companies residing in China. Just like Small Business Innovation Research and Small Business Technology Transfer grants in the United States, these nondiluting fundings go through an application and vigorous review process.

Unfortunately, recent practical, legal, and political developments may restrict the investments from Chinese sources to the US biotech companies. If not handled appropriately, it might be devastating to the US biotech companies who are hungry for money to survive and grow.

Since 2016 the Chinese government started to control outbound investments by Chinese investors, especially in real estate, hotels, resorts, entertainments, etc. If the Chinese investors have not already had foreign currencies, for example, US dollars or Euros, outside of China, they are subject to regulatory scrutiny by the Chinese government. Although biotech investment is not currently on the list of "sensitive sectors," the tedious and time-consuming approvals sometime make Chinese investors, or even US companies, give up the investments.

The Trump Administration signaled that it would scrutinize Chinese funding of US biotech companies, as well as other US tech companies. The Foreign Investment Risk Review Modernization Act of 2018 (FIRRMA) passed in August 2018 increased the power of the Committee on Foreign Investment in the United States (CFIUS), a small government agency in the Treasury Department. CFIUS will not only, as previously, review acquisition of a US company by a foreign entity but also review any foreign investments that are even not going to take a controlling stake. These new rules apply to areas deemed to be "critical technologies," "critical infrastructure," or "sensitive personal data of US citizens."

In light of these developments both in China and the United States, US biotech companies need to plan carefully when seeking Chinese investment, for example, the timing to close an investment round, whether and when to file a report to CFIUS, and backup plans if the Chinese investment is not approved by either the Chinese or the US government.

Partner With Chinese Biotech and Pharma Companies

Chinese biotech and pharma companies are hungry for innovative technologies and assets. Though many companies prefer IND-ready and clinical stage assets, some are interested in preclinical stage assets, or even new discoveries at academic institutes. Most of these deals are US type of deals, but with much more flexible deal structures, such as research collaboration, codevelopment, risk sharing, licensing, options, joint ventures, equity investments, or the combination of two or even more. Many people have asked me, what would be a proper financial term for a China deal? As the China market is 5%–7% of the global innovative drugs for most of the multinational large pharma companies, as a simple rule of thumb, the financial terms for a rational China deal are about 5%–15% of a global deal, including the upfront, milestones, and the same or similar royalty rates. Some "hot" assets may demand higher payments. Recently, however, due to the "red-hot" biotech market and lack of good assets in China, some in-licensing deals for the China market have driven up the upfront payments by several folds.

In light of the recent regulatory reform and proposed new patent law, non-Chinese biotech and pharma companies should take particular consideration of the synchronized clinical development in China. The China market cannot be an "after-thought" any more. Due to the still popular "me-too/better" and "fast follow-on" business models, if the originator delays the development of its asset in China, the imitator would have a good chance to become the "first-in-China" and gain significant advantages, such as in pricing and reimbursement. For foreign companies with limited capabilities or capacities in China, working with a credible Chinese company would be one of the best options to capture the China market and extend the patent life in China. Otherwise missing timely China development would be a value-subtraction when out-licensing the asset to a multinational large pharma or when entering the China market.

In general, Chinese biotech and pharma companies can be divided into the following three categories:

1. SOE, such as SinoPharm, Shanghai Pharma, and CSPC Pharma. These large Chinese pharma companies are mostly controlled by the central, provincial, or city municipal government.
2. Private enterprises, such as Fosun Pharma, Hengrui, Simcere, and Lvye. These Chinese pharmas were mostly founded by private citizens who have built them into significant sizes.
3. Returnee-founded biotech companies, such as BeiGene, Zai Lab, Ascletis, Hua Medicine, Innovent, and Junshi. These Chinese biotech companies usually focus on new drug R&D, and some later have also built commercial capabilities. Most of their founders and senior executives are returnees, who have worked in multinational large pharma and biotech companies. Some global business partners commented: "discussing with them (returnees), just like having a group meeting with a bunch of colleagues (in large pharmas)."

A US biotech company may choose a potential partner based on its strategy and needs. For example, a US company with products already in the US or European market or close to the market approval may choose an SOE or a large private Chinese pharma as the partner, as they can provide not only regulatory assistance but also sales and marketing resources. In addition, some SOE own distribution channel as well. For a R&D type US company with early stage innovative asset, a returnee-founded company or a private enterprise with appetite in early stage assets may be a more appropriate partner, especially a small China biotech company would take care of an in-licensed asset as its own "baby."

Experienced BD executives are in severe shortage in China, especially those having international experiences. On a good note, some experienced BD executives from multinational large pharmas, some of them at vice president, executive, and senior director levels, are returning to China. In addition, many eager young people are interested in, and are moving into, this function. When I first coorganized with BIO (then US Biotechnology Industry Organization) a "Business Development Fundamentals Workshop" at BIO China in 2013, there were less than 20 registered students. However, in August 2016, when my multinational pharma BD friends and I coorganized a workshop "Path to Become an Excellent BD Executive" at Tongxieyi, there were more than 400 attendees. The next year when we repeated it, there were still more than 300 attendees. In the summer of 2018, when I cochaired a deep-dive workshop "Pharma Business Development and External Collaboration," spanning three long weekends, with Yeehong Business School and Pharmcube, we had to turn away a long queue of applicants to limit the class size to about 75 in order to have a close and meaningful interaction and case practices. Hopefully, many of these students would become the main BD force in interacting with US and European biotech and pharma companies, so that both sides would be speaking the same language and on the same page.

China NMPA's participation in ICH allows synchronized clinical trials in the United States, Europe, Japan, and China. Since China has a much larger population base and many patients are naïve to many treatments that have already existed in Western countries, China will provide necessary and high-quality clinical trial data, at lower per-patient cost, to support drug registration in the United States, Europe, and Japan. For example, NASDAQ-listed US biotech company BeyondSpring is using one global clinical protocol in one single global multicenter clinical trial, in the United States, China, and other Western countries, to support parallel NDA filing in China and the United States in 2019 and 2020.

The recent political development may severely hamper the US–China cross-border research collaboration and licensing activities. Under the Export Control Reform Act of 2018 (ECRA), Bureau of Industry and Security under the Department of Commerce published, on November 19, 2018, an advance notice of proposed rulemaking "Review of Controls for Certain Emerging Technologies" for public comments. Biotechnology was included in the advance notice, such as (1) nanobiology, (2) synthetic biology, (3) genomic or Genetic Engineering, or (4) neurotech. However, the exact impact would not be known until the official rule is enacted.

Exits at Public Markets in China

HKEX revised its listing rules in April 2018, allowing prerevenue biotech companies to be listed at HKEX under certain conditions, for example, a core product has completed phase I of human clinical trials and received no objection to commence phase II (or later) from NMPA, US FDA or EMA, and the market cap would be larger than HK$1.5 billion. Under the new rules, Chinese biotech companies, such as Ascletis, BeiGene (as a second listing in addition to NASDAQ), Hua Medicine, Innovent, and Junshi, were listed at HKEX in 2018. Some US biotech companies, such as GRAIL and Moderna (went to IPO at NASDAQ instead on December 6, 2018), were rumored to explore IPO opportunities at HKEX.

Stock exchange markets in mainland China do not yet permit public listing of prerevenue companies, although new rules are under consideration.

Conclusion

The China biotech industry is booming amid government's strong support owing to its recognition that biotech plays critical roles in human health, aging Chinese society and increasing level of pollution, returning of Chinese students from overseas and home-grown talents, and ever-increasing funding and investment. The IP protection is progressively strengthening. Recent regulatory reform at NMPA has been sending fresh air and excitements to the China biotech industry to advance innovative drug clinical trials and registration. The US biotech and pharma companies need to take advantage of these new progresses to accelerate the development and entry of their innovative drugs to China, to compete with potential "me-too/better's" and "fast follow-on's" and capture the full value of their products in China. However, the pricing and reimbursement of innovative drugs are still uncertain at this time. New measures from the newly established SMIA would clarify and improve the situation.

Entrepreneurs and US biotech companies should take advantage of the vast CRO resources and deep pockets of Chinese investors to advance their innovative technologies and drug candidates more rapidly and efficiently. However, CFIUS reviews under FIRRMA and export control under ECRA might significantly hinder US biotech companies to receive investments from Chinese investors and to establish collaboration and licensing deals with Chinese companies.

Case studies

Mr. Oyler Goes to China: BeiGene

In 2010 John Oyler, an American entrepreneur, and Xiaodong Wang, a Chinese native, cofounded BeiGene in China, on the premise that they could capitalize on that many global standard-of-care therapies were not timely

(Continued)

(Continued)

approved or available in China, and locally developed drug candidates would gain more rapid approval due to a separate regulatory framework at that time. They strived to discover and develop a pipeline of drug candidates with the potential to be best-in-class globally and first-in-class in China. BeiGene went to IPO at NASDAQ successfully on February 8, 2016 and was dual-listed in HKEX on August 8, 2018. Its stock had been traded as high as 220, more than nine times of its initial IPO price of $24.

BeiGene's road to IPO within 6 years from inception was not without bumps, which was described in a Harvard Business School (HBS) case coauthored by HBS Prof. Willy Shih and me [Shih, W and Zhang, JZ (2017) *BeiGene* (HBS No. 618-033), HBS Publishing, Boston, MA]. I was representing Merck/MSD on BeiGene's Board of Directors and witnessed BeiGene's ups and downs during that time. At its most difficult time, BeiGene only had a bit more than 10,000 Yuan (about US$2–3000) in its bank account, according to its cofounder Wang. After Merck/MSD offered a bridge loan in early 2013, BeiGene established two consecutive licensing and collaboration deals with Merck KGaA on BeiGene's internally discovered and developed BRAF inhibitor and PARP inhibitors in May and October 2013, respectively. BeiGene raised Series A funding of $75M in November 2014 and Series A-2 funding of $97M in May 2015, from both US and Chinese investors. By the time in February 2016 when it became the first development-stage Chinese biotech to IPO on NASDAQ, BeiGene had four assets in clinical development in the United States, Australia, New Zealand, and China.

A Tale of Two Countries: Inhibrx and Elpiscience

Inhibrx is a biotech company based in La Jolla, CA. Elpiscience is a start-up company based in Shanghai, China, cofounded in 2017 by three friends. Two of them are returnees: Dr. Darren Ji was previously Global Vice President of Roche Partnering for Asia and Emerging Markets based in Shanghai and South San Francisco, and Dr. Hongtao Lu was previously cofounder and Chief Scientific Officer (CSO) of Zai Lab based in Shanghai and had worked for GSK and Bayer. Their friend, Dr. David Shen, was still in South San Francisco and had worked for Merck and Amgen. The super management team attracted Inhibrx instantly with trust and chemistry. The undivided attention from a start-up company as its own "baby" also appealed to Inhibrx. Inhibrx and Elpiscience formed a strategic codevelopment partnership in 2018 to jointly develop Inhibrx's bispecific antibody that targets 4-1BB and PD-L1 in the United States and China. The codevelopment would accelerate the clinical trials through a large pool of naïve patients in China. In addition, Elpiscience would provide high-quality manufacturing in China. Soon after, Inhibrx filed IND with FDA in the United States, and Elpiscience

(Continued)

(Continued)

filed IND with China's NMPA. They will start phase I clinical trials in the United States and China in 2019, respectively, and multicenter global trials later.

When US Professor Met Chinese Investor: Tmunity

When Professor Carl June and Judith Li, a partner of Lilly Asia ventures (which is now independent from Eli Lilly), first met in Philadelphia in 2015, they knew a new company would be born. On January 12, 2016, Philadelphia-based Tmunity Therapeutics announced that it was raising $10 Million in equity financing from Penn Medicine and Lilly Asia Ventures. Late 2016, Tmunity recruited Usman "Oz" Azam, who was the Global Head of the Cell & Gene Therapies Unit at Novartis, as president and CEO. On January 23, 2018 a Chinese investor, Ping An Ventures, led a syndicate of $100 million Series A, including Parker Institute, Gilead, and Be The Match BioTherapies, which later joined by $35 million from Kleiner Perkins. Tmunity moved two programs into the clinic: PSMA CAR-T for prostate cancer and a CRISPR-edited NYESO-1 triple knockout T-cell receptor therapy for myeloma, melanoma, and sarcoma. On October 2, 2018, Tmunity was named as one of FierceBiotech's 2018 Fierce 15 biotech companies.

References

[1] Ye R, Chen Z. China Biotech Primer. Goldman Sachs. 2018.

[2] Sun J, et al. BMC Health Serv Res 2018;18:125.

[3] <https://www.cms.gov/Research-Statistics-Data-and-Systems/Statistics-Trends-and-Reports/NationalHealthExpendData/NationalHealthAccountsHistorical.html> [accessed December 11, 2018].

[4] <http://www.stats.gov.cn/tjsj/sjjd/201901/t20190123_1646380.html> [accessed January 23, 2019].

[5] State Information Center and China Economic Information Network. 2019 China pharmaceutical industry development report (Outlook). November 2018. <http://www.cei.gov.cn/>.

[6] BeiGene Ltd. Form-S1. February 2016. p. 140. <https://www.nasdaq.com/markets/ipos/filing.ashx?filingid = 11141700> [accessed February 22, 2019].

[7] <http://news.pharmnet.com.cn/news/2018/12/21/514538.html> [accessed December 28, 2018].

[8] CFDA. CDE: 2014 drug evaluation report. <http://www.cde.org.cn/news.do?method = viewInfoCommon&id = 313425> [accessed December 27, 2018].

[9] CFDA. CDE: 2017 drug evaluation report. <http://samr.cfda.gov.cn/WS01/CL0844/226865.html> [accessed December 27, 2018].

[10] Beijing Youth Daily. January 17, 2018.

[11] <https://www.nature.com/articles/d41586-018-00543-2> [accessed December 31, 2018].

Chapter 39

Ethical Considerations for Biotechnology Leaders

Gladys B. White, PhD

Adjunct Professor of Liberal Studies, Georgetown University, Washington, DC, United States

Chapter Outline

It may come as a surprise that the innovation and promise offered by advances in biotechnology raise any ethical issues at all. If biotechnology entrepreneurs are engaged in activities that have as their goal, improvements in the health and well-being of humankind, then why is it that these activities warrant ethical scrutiny? If good people with good ideas start, maintain, and operate companies that develop new drugs, devices, and products aimed at curing diseases and the improvement of human health, what's not to like?

The Nature of Ethical Reasoning

In order to answer these questions it is important to first have an understanding of philosophical ethics. In essence, ethics is simply concerned with the examination of important questions related to what it means to be human. Ethical considerations are tools which help us analyze the relevant strengths of arguments about what is right and wrong conduct, or what should be done in important endeavors in life. Because the activities within the biotechnology industry are vital to human health and well-being now and in the future, ethical issues, or arguments, need to be a foundational part of our understanding. What we term ethical "arguments" are simply the reasons and justifications for choosing a particular course of action. Having an understanding of ethics helps one recognize the significance of these arguments and their relative weight when major decisions need to be made. For example, such a decision could be which drug to develop and market for which disease over what period of time with the reason and justification being clearly understood and compelling to others. There is also an ethical aspect to a company's economic decisions. For instance, the strategies that entrepreneurs employ to promote short-term versus long-term profitability should be justifiable and have a rational supporting argument. Cost/benefit analysis and bottom-line viewpoints in the business world are not solely a matter of a computation involving dollars and cents, but also judgments about what constitutes the greatest good for the greatest number of people. The type of ethical analysis and the utilitarian system of justification I describe are not new but date back to the work of philosophers such as Jeremy Bentham (1748 to 1832) and John Stuart Mill (1806 to 1873) [1]. It is important to recognize that entrepreneurs are faced with significant challenges and alternatives to every rational argument and in order to support their choices they must have an understanding of

Biotechnology Entrepreneurship. DOI: https://doi.org/10.1016/B978-0-12-815585-1.00039-5

ethical tools and be familiar with ethical principles and theory.

Ethics is simply a "reason-giving" enterprise. This means that ethical arguments leading to good or right actions must be based upon supporting reasons that are both meaningful and understandable to others. Any reason-supporting argument about what should be done in any given circumstance needs to be more than a statement such as "because I said so," "because it's a rainy day," or "because this is how I feel at the moment." Subjective declarations of how an individual or group feels, or verbalization of the gut reaction of a leader should not be the primary basis for a sound ethical argument. Poor or weak ethical justifications highlight another important point—often critical decisions are made without ethical reasoning and on a basis that is not rational or objective.

Why should biotechnology entrepreneurs pay attention to the characteristics of sound ethical arguments? There are many reasons why this is relevant and two of the most important reasons are:

1. Biotechnology companies are businesses and therefore they must operate using a commonly accepted set of business ethics that include such tenets as fairness, trust, absence of conflict-of-interest, and good business practices.
2. Biotechnology companies face ethical dilemmas as do all companies and the consequences of poor decisions can be devastating. For small biotechnology companies, the costs and stakes are high. There are often competing pressures to achieve goals and accomplish results within a limited timeframe, and this creates a climate in which ethical dilemmas can arise.

Even in larger organizations, we have seen instances of pharmaceutical product development in human clinical trials revealing adverse conditions which were kept from the U.S. Food and Drug Administration (FDA), and subsequently these products were removed from the market due to deaths during commercialization [2].

A true ethical dilemma is a problem of one of two types. An ethical dilemma exists when:

1. No matter what action is taken, some harm will occur.
2. There are equally strong-reasoned arguments for taking completely different courses of action.

Accurate facts are crucial to the analysis and resolution of ethical dilemmas, but additional facts alone cannot solve or resolve a true ethical dilemma. A true ethical dilemma requires that the leader makes a wise choice. There are key features of reasoned arguments in ethics and the value of each can be assessed based upon the conceptual level or strength of each argument. There are four types of arguments ranging from weak to strong as listed in the following four levels:

Level 1: Ethical Judgments

Ethical judgments consist of simple pronouncements of right or wrong without stipulating any particular reason. When a particular action is characterized as right or wrong without an identified reason, there is no way another individual can assess its value. Also, no one can associate or compare its reasoning to similar situations because there is no information offered as to why the judgment has been made. This is why ethical judgment alone is relatively weak.

Level 2: Ethical Rules

The second level in the hierarchy of ethical reasoning is the use of ethical rules. Examples of ethical rules are statements such as thou shall not kill, lie, steal, and the like. Ethical rules are found in documents such as the Ten Commandments but also permeate codes of ethics in various professions, codes of good business practices, and corporate policy documents. A rule such as "do not lie" has more power than an ethical judgment because the rule can be used as a guide for ethical action in similar situations. Most of our everyday ethical actions are based on ethical rules. In this fashion, we readily understand the motivations of our coworkers, business partners, and customers and the use of commonsense ethical rules builds trust.

Level 3: Ethical Principles

The third level of reasoning in ethics entails ethical principles. These principles differ from ethical rules as they are guiding values by which to make decisions rather than hard and fast rules. For ethics in the life sciences, there are already well-defined principles. The Belmont Report published in 1978 was the result of a collaborative effort to determine the characteristics of ethical research when human subjects were involved, and it is generally cited as a key source for ethics in the life sciences [3]. In the Belmont report, these ethical principles are described and explained as (1) respect for autonomy, (2) beneficence, (3) nonmaleficence, and (4) justice. These are important themes for ethical action. A fifth principle is respect for persons as ends in themselves, rather than merely as means to the ends or purposes of others. When individuals are respected as ends unto themselves, their lives, interests, and well-being cannot be compromised in pursuit of the goals of others. Respect for persons carries considerable weight and importance in ethical analysis and is also an important feature of Kantian ethics (see Level 4: Ethical Theories).

Ethical principles have the advantage of conveying important concepts such as the importance of free and self-directed action (autonomy), being of benefit or good use to others (beneficence), avoiding harm to others (nonmaleficence), and acting in a way such that fair and equal treatment will result for individual human beings as well as for groups. Most ethical arguments with sufficient depth and breadth make use of ethical principles as part of their rationale.

Level 4: Ethical Theories

Ethical theories are the most powerful form of reasoning in ethics. Examples of such theories are consequentialism of which utilitarianism is one type and the duty-based theory like that of Immanual Kant which offers a justification for right action. Kant (1724 to 1804) developed a theory of ethics based on duty as perceived by human reason. Ethical analysis serves as a sorting device to unpack complicated ethical dilemmas and simultaneously offer a detailed outline of justification for the right action. Ethical theories are powerful, but can also have their weak points. The primary limitation of consequentialist-based ethical reasoning is related to a principle of justice, namely what if by securing the greatest good, or the greatest happiness for the greatest number of individuals, this results in an unacceptable level of harm for a few. For example, what if the risk of death for a few people in the clinical trial of a new drug is high but the eventual research results could benefit many? A utilitarian would regard this as an acceptable risk, whereas a Kantian ethicist would not. That is because Kant believed that the conditions of duty-based ethics should be determined in advance of the actual situation and their consequences. Kant also believed that an argument is very weak if it rests on an assessment of consequences, since we should to be able to discern what our ethical duties are in advance of taking any action.

The basis for determining our duties results from consulting our reasons. The result is what Kant identifies as the categorical imperative which has two formulations or forms of expression, namely: (1) always act in such a way that a tenet describing your action can serve as the basis for universal law; and (2) always treat human beings as ends in themselves and not merely as means to the ends of others. This theory is in stark contrast to the consequentialist, utilitarian theory of Mill in part because it is prospective and says that we need to decide on right or ethical action in advance of particular circumstances and apart from consequences [4].

In addition to duty-based ethics and consequentialism, there are other ethical theories such as virtue ethics, the ethics of care, casuistry, or case-based analysis and rights-based approaches to ethical problems that offer insights and advantages in understanding important ethical controversies. Due to the limitations of space these possibilities will not be explored in detail here but the reader is referred to other articles on these topics in the literature of philosophy and ethics. One good online source for more information is the "Stanford Encyclopedia of Philosophy" [5].

Key Issues and Practical Matters for Biotechnology Entrepreneurs

For biotech entrepreneurs, certain key ethical issues are embedded within their company's everyday practice and product development. Chief among these are informed consent, concepts of ownership of substances ranging from natural resources to human tissues and cells, and justice and intellectual property in the broad sense, to name a few. It is also important that the possible needs and interests of future generations be taken into account by the biotech industry. In ethics this concept is captured by the term "intergenerational justice" which refers to the obligations and duties we have to ensure that the Earth, for example, remains habitable for our future descendants. An even more futuristic question for biotechnology is how might the creation of synthetic forms of life impact the human race now and in the future?

The responsibilities of an industry, particularly in the for-profit world, are sometimes expressed as corporate social responsibilities. The concept of corporate social responsibility is often a matter of debate and discussion. Some argue that this responsibility is relatively narrow and consists chiefly of staying in business, making a profit, and satisfying customers and shareholders. It is implied that any broader obligations or duties to society are regarded as above and beyond company business, or as something that governments should handle. The "let government do it" notion is generally considered to be a narrow view of corporate social responsibility. This can be contrasted to the broad view of corporate social responsibility that is a more justice-based view for the entire human community in which it is unjust to leave anyone out. This view stands in stark contrast to the utilitarian bottom-line calculation of the greatest good for the greatest number irrespective of the consequences for a few. The broad view of corporate social responsibility means that individual companies should look beyond merely making money for themselves. Needless to say this may be somewhat idealistic or even unreasonable for small biotech start-up companies. Nonetheless it is important to recognize that all corporations exist within the same global social community and that there is a network of interdependencies, duties, and obligations.

The following themes are pervasive areas of ethical concern that arise in the day-to-day practices and activities of biotechnology and serve as an organizing framework for the case studies.

Informed Consent

Informed consent is required before companies can perform medical research on individuals using their specimens or tissues. Informed consent can be defined as autonomous authorization by a competent, comprehending adult who authorizes a professional to involve the subject in research, initiate a medical plan for the patient, or both [6]. The belief that human beings are entitled to give informed consent arises from the insight and conviction that each individual has the right to say what will, or what will not, be done to their own body. This pertains to all human beings and not just to those who happen to be patients or research subjects. This may appear to be self-evident, but in the biotech world problems can arise, for example, when stored biospecimens are collected for purposes other than research and informed consent was never initially sought. Obtaining informed consent is a multifaceted process involving a determination of the consenting individual's competence to decide, the provision of full and objective information, some determination of whether or not the consenting individual has actually understood the relevant information, and then the production of a signed written consent form with a copy provided to the consenting individual. No one individual or government official, for example, can give valid consent to a biotech company or biotech entrepreneur on behalf of an entire community without the knowledge of the consent of the particular individuals who are involved.

Concepts of Ownership

Generally speaking, the concept of ownership implies that an object or entity belongs to a given individual who can control its use and call it theirs. To own something has historically referred to objects or even experiences external to the person. More recently, the concept of the body as owned property has been highlighted in disputes concerning the status of human tissues and cells, particularly in cases in which something valuable can be created. Biotechnology has had a direct influence on the ability to transform a particular human cell into an immortal cell line that can be patented and then yield profits as royalties that are paid to the patent owner. In cases such as that of John Moore who was diagnosed with hairy cell leukemia in 1976 and the case of Henrietta Lacks who was diagnosed with cervical cancer in the 1950s, the patients who were the original sources of the cells were not even aware that their biological materials had been developed into something valuable (see Case Study 1 and 2).

To what extent is the human body property, and who owns human tissues and cells? Many have argued that in every case the body is property and belongs to the individual. The issue becomes more complicated when particular tissues and cells have been excised as a part of a surgical procedure, but were retrieved when they would have otherwise been abandoned.

Justice as Fair and Equal Treatment

Access to medicines domestically and globally is one issue that is of importance to biotech entrepreneurs. Justice, namely fair and equal treatment globally, is one issue that arises again and again with respect to the identification of what is important in pharmaceutical development, namely what drugs to create, which diseases to target, and what population groups to serve. The answers to these questions may pose ethical dilemmas; for example, in situations in which the populations who will purchase the individual pharmaceutical downstream are very different from those who participated in the drug development. This is an ethical dilemma that has plagued the HIV/AIDS community for some time [7]. Because the biotechnology industry exists largely in the for-profit world, the presence of consumers who can pay for pharmaceutical products is of practical importance. But if the selection of future research and development (R&D) is shaped solely by the interests and needs of those who can pay then, obviously, important priorities that serve the interests of the developing world will be proportionately overlooked or short-changed. These issues have been deliberated in the fields of philosophy and ethics for a long time, even going back to the work of Aristotle in the *Nicomachean Ethics.* Aristotle described the virtue of justice as aimed toward "another's good" [8]. In matters of distribution of resources, he defined justice as a matter of receiving what one deserves. Because of the somewhat imprecise nature of this stipulation, a fuller account of social justice is needed and one can be found in the work of the 20th century philosopher, John Rawls. In *A Theory of Justice*, Rawls identifies two principles of justice which he posits would be selected by a group of rational disinterested human beings in attempting to establish the structure and shape of a fair or ideal society. These principles are: [9]

First principle—Each person is to have an equal right to the most extensive total system of equal basic liberties compatible with a similar set of liberties for all.

Second principle—Social and economic inequalities are to be arranged so that they are both: (1) to the greatest benefit of the least advantaged; and (2) available and accessible to all.

The broad implications of this theory are that everyone in the developed world has obligations to the developing world. Is there a right to essential medicines and, correspondingly, does the human right to basic necessities override shareholder rights? Unfortunately, it is often the case that social and economic inequalities come to rest on those who are already the least advantaged. From a justice perspective, this is counterintuitive and unfair.

Intellectual Property: How Patenting Raises Ethical Issues

"A patent for an invention is the grant of an exclusive property right to the inventor for a limited amount of time" [10]. The act of patenting serves as a clear incentive for innovation and development as it establishes a structure through which scientists, product developers, and inventors of various types are motivated to engage in competition and can also be rewarded monetarily through the payment of royalties. But this incentive rests on the promise of exclusivity, which means that those other than the patent holders may have difficulty accessing the patented product or at least have to pay for the privilege. Because many biotech products are closely aligned with, or derived from, plant or human substances that exist in nature, restricting access to these products strikes many as unfair. In addition, as the cases that follow indicate, human sources of biological materials and/or their families believe that they are entitled to share in the profits generated from these products.

Traditional knowledge, for example, about the medicinal benefits of plants also seems to be a kind of commodity that has value. This knowledge may be generally available in the developing world, but cannot be legitimately borrowed by researchers of the developed world without giving credit and arguably some share of the profits to the sources and points of origin of these materials. Some researchers and policy experts have suggested that what is needed here are "models of cooperation for the benefit of global health" [11] (see Case Studies 3 and 4).

Case Studies

Ownership of Human Tissues and Cells and Patenting Cell Lines

Case 1: John Moore

In 1976, John Moore was diagnosed as having a rare form of cancer called hairy cell leukemia, a condition that affects an estimated 250 Americans yearly. The recommended treatment for Moore's condition was the removal of the spleen and surgery was performed at the University of California, Los Angeles Medical Center. As a patient, Moore had signed a standard surgical consent form (providing for the postoperative disposition of the tissue) to remove his diseased spleen, which had enlarged to approximately 40 times its normal size.

After the surgery, Moore's doctor and his technician developed a cell line (designated "Mo") from a sample of Moore's spleen obtained from the pathologist. (It also appears that some of Moore's blood cells contributed to the development of the cell line GW.) The scientists found that the cell line developed from the spleen produced high quantities of a variety of interesting and potentially interesting proteins. In 1979, the university applied for a patent on the "Mo" cell line and in 1984 a patent naming the scientists as inventors was obtained and assigned to the university. In 1981, the university, on behalf of the scientists, entered into a 4-year collaborative research program with two biotechnology and pharmaceutical companies for exclusive use of the "Mo" cell line.

In 1984, Moore filed a lawsuit claiming that his blood cells were misappropriated and that he was entitled to share in the profits derived from the commercial uses of these cells and any other products resulting from research on any of his biological materials [2]. Moore was never successful in convincing the court that he deserved a share of the profits from the patented cell line although it was clear that he had not given informed consent for this particular eventuality.

Discussion

This case is one of a number of similar cases in which a patient, through the course of medical treatment and care, unwittingly serves as the source of human tissues and cells that are later developed into a valuable product. The unimproved tissues and cells on their own do not have monetary value and also have been excised and discarded in the course of medical care. The development of a cell line that has characteristics of long life or even immortality in a laboratory setting is not something which the patient/research subject or source of the biological material could have accomplished on their own. And yet the product could not have been developed without this source material. Hours of refinement, development, and trial-and-error research have transformed this biological material into something of value that can be patented and used for a wide array of useful purposes. It is not surprising that the individual whose cells and tissues have been used in this fashion feels that he or she has been duped!

Case 2: Henrietta Lacks

Her name was Henrietta Lacks, but scientists know her as HeLa. She was a poor Southern tobacco farmer who worked the same land as her slave ancestors, yet her

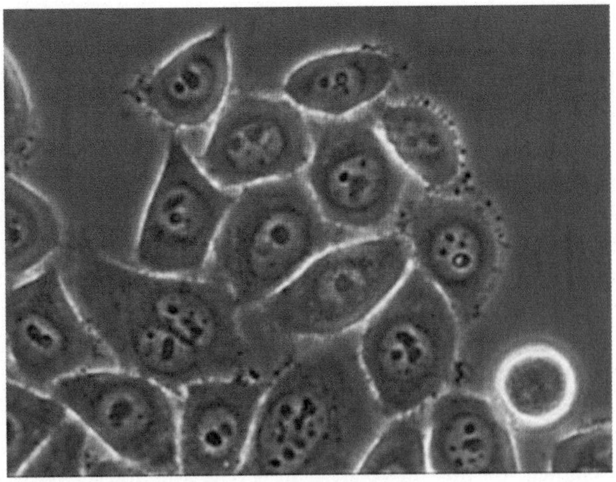

FIGURE 39.1 HeLa Cells: immortal cancer cells of Henrietta Lacks. *Source: Kristina Yu, © Exploratorium, www.exploratorium.edu, accessed February 25, 2019.*

cells—taken without her knowledge–became one of the most important tools in medicine. These were the first "immortal" human cells grown in a culture as they are still alive today although she has been dead for more than 60 years. If you could pile all the HeLa cells ever grown onto a scale, they would weigh more than 50 million metric tons—as much as a hundred Empire State Buildings. HeLa cells were vital for developing the polio vaccine; uncovering secrets of cancer, viruses, and the atom bomb's effects; helping lead to important advances like *in vitro* fertilization, cloning, and gene mapping; and have been bought and sold by the billions. (See Fig. 39.1.)

Lacks remains virtually unknown and is buried in an unmarked grave. Lacks' family did not learn of her "immortality" until more than 20 years after her death when scientists investigating HeLa began using her husband and children in research without their informed consent. And although the cells had launched a multimillion-dollar industry that sells human biological materials, her family never saw any of the profits [12]. (See Fig. 39.2.)

Discussion

In the cases of John Moore and Henrietta Lacks, the subjects were not told about the subsequent uses of their biological material even though they may have signed what was considered to be standard surgical consent at that particular point in time. They later discovered (the patient himself in the case of Moore, and the patient's family in the case of Lacks) that profits had accrued from their products and this understandably resulted in their sense of having been seriously wronged. Why couldn't these patients and/or their families have shared in this monetary value? As of this writing, neither the medical research community nor the biotech community at large has been inclined, or figured out a way, to share profits with patient sources. In the case of the family of Lacks, they have also never shared in the accrued value of the HeLa cell line. They continue to wonder why, given that their ancestor's body was the source of something so valuable, they cannot even obtain needed health insurance at this point in time. So the ethical question of what is fair in these cases remains to be answered.

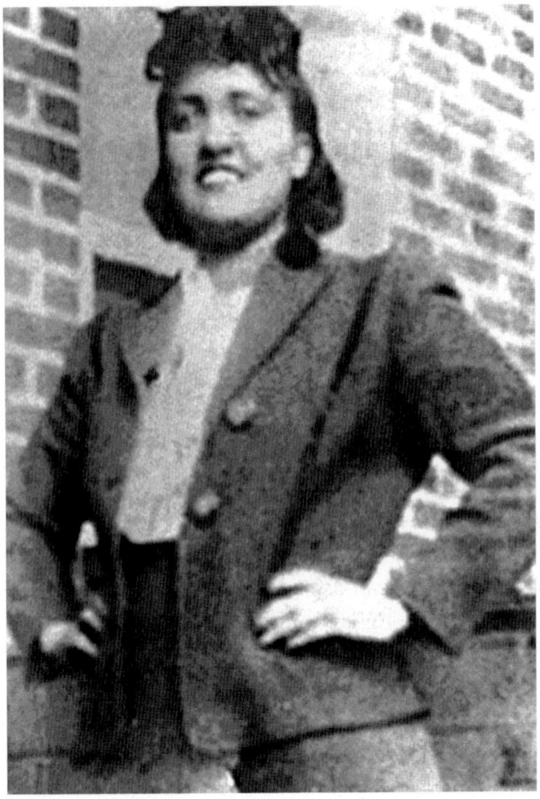

FIGURE 39.2 Henrietta Lacks died of cervical cancer at age 51. *Source: Wikipedia.*

Biopiracy

The definition of biopiracy is controversial and the legitimacy of the topic as a whole is a matter of debate. But a general definition of biopiracy is "when multinational corporations profit from the medicinal and agricultural uses of plants known to indigenous or native societies and fail to compensate these communities" [13]. One reason why this definition is controversial is that some will argue that plants belong to the global commons, that is, they belong to all of us generally and are not owned by anyone in particular. The same argument might be applied to the knowledge freely shared by indigenous or native societies, namely that if the information is freely given then there is not necessarily a legitimate expectation for compensation should this knowledge prove to be valuable in the developed world. The two case studies below, one hypothetical and one actual, illustrate what is at stake in this debate.

Case 3: Visplantia

Imagine that a Brazilian scientist visits Wyoming. On his way to the mountains, he encounters a Cheyenne shaman who joins him. The shaman is particularly talkative that day and so they engage in an entertaining conversation. The shaman tells the scientist the story of a very important and powerful plant. The Brazilian scientist learns that the shaman is visiting the mountains to gather this plant that his tribe has nurtured for many generations and that they use to cure a very aggressive disease. The scientist feels curious and decides to visit that site. Once they arrive at the site, the scientist notices that the shaman is performing a ritual ceremony, after which he picks up some plants. The shaman explains later that this plant is sacred to the Cheyenne. The scientist takes a sample of the plant back to Brazil and years later patents a medicine based on the plant compounds called Visplantia that cures HIV. Suppose that Visplantia has generated millions of dollars in profit for the Brazilian company and the scientist. The Cheyenne tribal members complain to the United States government arguing that they discovered the plant, they nurtured it for centuries, and they used the plant in important religious ceremonies. The Brazilian pharmaceutical company argues that the plant is a product of nature, that it belongs to humanity, and it is a heritage of "humankind," and that the company spent 10 years and millions of dollars of research to develop the drug [13].

Discussion

In this hypothetical case, it appears that the amount of the plant that was originally taken could not in any way have depleted the source community of this particular vegetation. The traditional community was not deprived of anything that originally existed and, in fact, the drug development that took place subsequently was not necessarily anticipated nor did it make use of traditional knowledge. No harm was done initially. The later drug development created an effective therapy for HIV. We do not know whether HIV was prevalent in the traditional society, but if it was initially or later when the drug became available, a claim for access to the drug might have some justification. The biotech company could freely provide this drug to the native population or provide it at a discount based on a broad concept of corporate social responsibility and the ethical principle of beneficence, but they would not necessarily be obliged to do so.

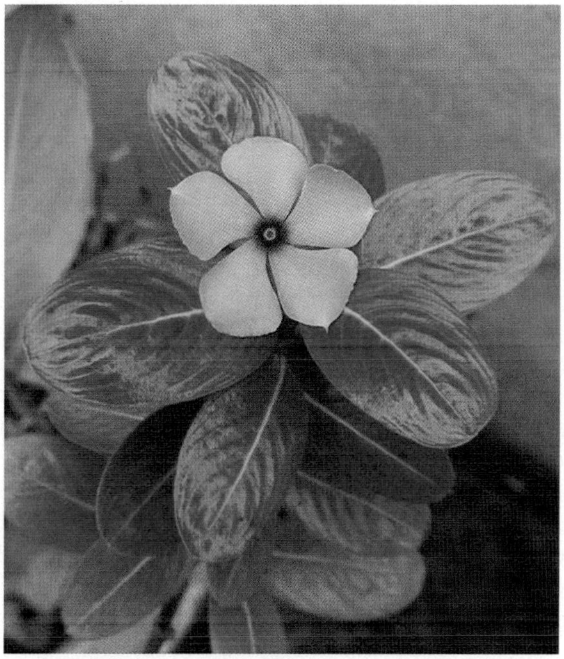

FIGURE 39.3 Rosy periwinkle (*Catharanthus roseus*).

Case 4: Rosy Periwinkle (*Catharanthus roseus*)

Scientists from developed nations engineered the cancer-fighting medicines vinblastine and vincristine from the rosy periwinkle plant found in Madagascar. Vinblastine has increased the chance of surviving childhood leukemia and is used to treat Hodgkin's disease. The U.S. pharmaceutical company Eli Lilly has patented and generated huge profits from Vincristine despite the fact that none of the financial benefits have gone to Madagascar or to the indigenous group that first made use of the plant. (See Fig. 39.3.)

The difficulty with this situation is that the pharmaceutical industry took the rosy periwinkle out of Madagascar and used it in ways other than what was initially suggested by the indigenous people. This example illustrates the difficulties inherent in the protection of traditional knowledge and biodiversity, especially when the final pharmaceutical use differs from the use suggested by indigenous communities [13].

Discussion

Once again, the test that should be applied to this case initially is whether any harm occurred to the indigenous community. Unless the quantity of rosy periwinkle plants was depleted or significantly diminished in Madagascar, it does not appear that any harm was done. In addition, there was no use made of traditional knowledge as the pharmaceutical company discovered uses that were previously unknown and they exploited this discovery. Only a much-expanded notion of corporate social responsibility extending to pure altruism would support the need for any type of in-kind compensation to the traditional community.

Summary

The dynamic world of corporate biotechnology is one of possibility, productivity, and progress. Like other endeavors that exist at the intersections of science, technology, and public policy, there are successes, failures, and hazards along the way. Ethical issues and dilemmas are serious questions about what ought to be done, often in situations of uncertainty. Ethical arguments that make use of judgments, rules, principles, and theories are the rational responses to circumstances in which it is important to decide on the best course of action. Important themes for biotech entrepreneurs are informed consent, ownership of human tissues and cells and derivative products, intellectual property, patenting, and the possibility of biopiracy. The biotechnology industry's response to these issues and others will depend, in part on whether the industry as a whole embraces a narrow or a broad concept of corporate social responsibility.

References

[1] Mill J.S. Utilitarianism. In: (editor: Crisp Roger.) Oxford University Press: New York.

[2] Congress US. Office of Technology Assessment. New Developments in Biotechnology: Ownership of Human Tissues and Cells-Special Report, OTA-BA-337, Washington, D.C. U.S. Government Printing Office; 1987.

[3] National Commission for the Protection of Human Subjects of Biomedical and Behavioral Research. The Belmont Report: Ethical Principles and Guidelines for the Protection of Human Subjects of Research. DHEW Publication OS: Washington, D.C.

[4] Kant I. Foundations of the Metaphysics of Morals. Translation by Lewis White Beck. Bobbs-Merrill: Indianapolis, Indiana.

[5] http://plato.stanford.edu/ (accessed February 25, 2019).

[6] Faden R.; Beauchamp T. A History and Theory of Informed Consent. Oxford University Press.

[7] Treating AIDS, Dilemmas of Unequal Access in Uganda. In: (editors: Petrynna A.A.; Lakaff A.; Kleinman.) Global Pharmaceuticals, Ethics, Markets, Practices. Duke University Press: Durham.

[8] Aristotle. The Basic Works of Aristotle. Random House: New York.

[9] Rawls J. A Theory of Justice. The Belnap Press of Harvard University Press: Cambridge, Massachusetts.

[10] United States Patent and Trademark Office, https://www.uspto.gov/patents-getting-started/general-information-concerning-patents#heading-2 (accessed February 25, 2019).

[11] Gupta R, Gabrielsen B, Ferguson SM. Nature's Medicines: Traditional Knowledge and Intellectual Property Management. Case Studies from the National Inst Health, Current Drug Discovery Technol 2005;2:1–17.

[12] Skloot R. The Immortal Life of Henrietta Lacks. Random House: New York.

[13] Biopiracy Dwyer L. Trade, and Sustainable Development. Colorado J Int Environ Law and Policy 2008;19:219–56.

Chapter 40

Diverse Career Opportunities in the Biotechnology and Life Sciences Industry

Toby Freedman, PhD
President, Synapsis Search Biotech Recruiting, Portola Valley, CA, United States

Chapter Outline

The biotech/biopharma industry is dynamic and continues to change and evolve with the fast speed of scientific progress. This is an exciting time to be in or to join the life sciences industry, as the industry is booming due to an influx of cash from wealthy high-tech investors, therapeutic product development successes and from initial public offerings (IPOs). As the industry continues to boom, companies are building their scientific departments and the need to hire talent has intensified.

There are many career opportunities in industry, in nonprofit organizations, and in government for individuals with science backgrounds. Whether you have an interest in laboratory work, business, sales, marketing, or clinical studies, there are hundreds of different careers in the life sciences—and as a consequence, there are numerous opportunities to find that ideal job that matches your unique personality attributes, skills, interests, and long-term goals.

A science or medical background is a valuable asset to have and will provide lifelong credibility. Whether you are writing a patent, marketing a product, conducting a clinical trial, or doing a business deal, a science background will greatly enhance your career and add credibility. The chart shown in Fig. 40.1 delineates over 100 distinct careers in the life sciences industry where you can apply your scientific or medical educational training.

For those wishing to escape bench work, there is good news: there are many nonbench roles for scientists in industry. Many PhD and MD level researchers in discovery research quickly leave the bench behind as they rise in the ranks to more strategic and higher level functions. Depending on one's ability to manage people, many PhD and MD level scientists will quickly leave the bench to supervise research associates, entry-level graduate students, and postdocs. At the same time, there are a plethora

Biotechnology Entrepreneurship. DOI: https://doi.org/10.1016/B978-0-12-815585-1.00040-1

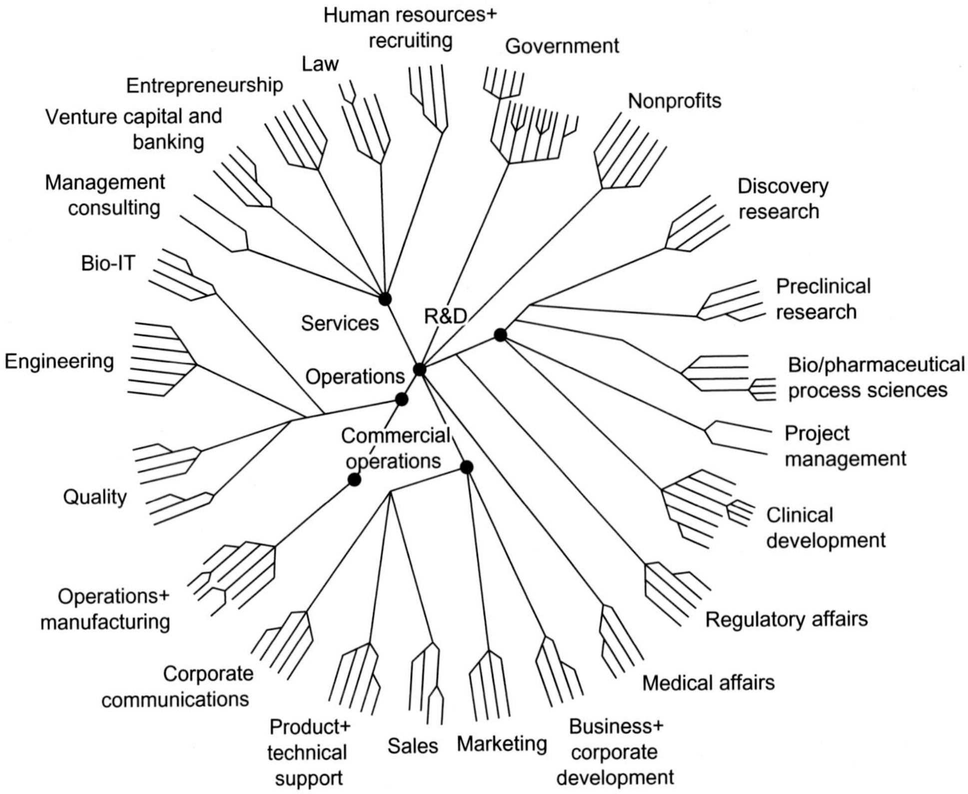

FIGURE 40.1 Career chart.

of careers for scientists to transition into nonbench roles, which are described in this chapter. These additional career areas provide an opportunity to explore other areas, such as general management, team-building, project management, creative writing, clinical development, and more.

An Overview of the Many Different Vocational Areas in the Life Sciences Industry

This chapter provides a high-level summary of 24 significant career areas in the life sciences industry, as shown in Fig. 40.1. If you identify a career that interests you, I recommend additional reading in the specific area that piques your interest. At the conclusion of this overview, there are two sections to help you move into a particular vocational area, one on steps for making a career transition and the other one describes job-finding strategies.

Entrepreneurship

Do you have a fantastic idea that has the potential of being developed into a successful business? There are few things as exciting as starting a new company and attempting something that no one else has ever done before.

Entrepreneurship can be a stimulating and rewarding career, but it is not for everyone. It helps to be financially secure and to have done it before. However, I have seen many postdoctoral fellows, graduate students, professors, and even undergraduates start and manage highly successful ventures without prior business training. If you are considering entrepreneurship, I highly recommend considering joining one of the growing number of “incubators” or “accelerators” that are cropping up worldwide. An incubator is a supportive place where a cluster of start-up companies thrive. At an incubator, start-ups can share lab equipment, office space, and gain support from fellow entrepreneurs who are working down the hall.

One highly successful example of an incubator is University of California’s QB3 (QB3 stands for California Institute for Quantitative Biosciences, which includes three institutions, University of California at San Francisco, Berkeley, and Santa Cruz). The goal of QB3 is to benefit society by commercializing university research. QB3 provides a supportive environment where new companies are being founded where professors, graduate students, and postdocs are conducting their research. Venture capital, biopharmaceutical, management consulting, and accounting firms are also actively partnering and assisting these start-up companies. This type of collaborative environment fosters communication, sharing of knowledge, and innovation. To learn more, visit https://qb3.org.

Similar incubators can be found across the United States at top universities, such as Harvard University, University of Florida, University of Washington, and SUNY in Brooklyn. Also consider off-campus incubators, such as Phoenix's TGen (Translational Genomics Research Institute), Kendall Square's incubator in Boston, and many others. Working at an incubator will provide you with first-hand experience in a start-up environment where you will be exposed to the challenges of raising capital, building teams, and developing products. Also consider attending "boot camp" programs that can help you develop your business plan, raise venture capital, and be mentored by executives who have experience in building companies.

Venture Capital

Venture capital is among the most coveted and exciting career in the life sciences industry. This career has real appeal to socially minded and team-oriented scientists because venture capitalists have opportunities to meet and work with successful entrepreneurs who are developing and commercializing ground-breaking technologies.

Most of the people think of venture capitalists as the people you go to when raising capital to fund start-ups, but these individuals also must first raise money which they then can use to invest in start-ups. Corporate venture capitalists work in large pharmaceutical or biotechnology companies and, similar to venture capitalists, they also fund private companies using money from the biopharmaceutical company that they represent. There are institutional investors (also called equity research analysts) who invest in public companies.

There are some other venture-type careers that involve working with biotech companies. These include angel investors, who are people of high net worth that financially support private companies, usually before venture capitalists invest.

Venture capitalists provide considerably more than being just a source of money. After venture capitalists invest in a company, they may assume positions on the company board of directors to monitor their investment and also to assist the company with the many challenges that are encountered in emerging businesses. Therefore an operational background and prior experience in several successful start-ups is considered an optimal background for a venture capitalist.

If you are interested in seeking a career in venture capital, consider applying for a fellowship with the Kauffman Foundation—a nonprofit organization committed to fostering entrepreneurism. Visit www.kauffman.org for more information. Many venture capital firms also hire associates and advisors (academic scientists or industry experts), consultants, and entrepreneurs-in-residence (EIRs). EIRs are experienced senior-level executives capable of running venture capital portfolio companies and managing their investments.

Investment Banking

There are three major career areas in investment banking: advisory services, sell-side equity research, and sales trading. Advisory service providers are involved in large financial transactions, such as helping their clients raise capital, complete IPOs, or mergers and acquisitions (M&As). This is a highly competitive career and can involve extensive travel, but the payoffs are large, as investment bankers are amply compensated for their hard work. If you enjoy transactional work or have an interest in finance, this is a promising career to consider.

Sell-side equity research analysts conduct and publish background research on the particular public companies that they follow. These analysts provide ratings of public companies stock, such as "buy," "sell," or "hold" and they publish informative reports for clients. It is becoming more common for investment banks to hire MDs, PhDs, and MBAs who can analyze and ascertain the chances of success for clinical trials, and by extension, they predict changes in stock value. Sales traders conduct stock sales transactions and promote stock sales.

Discovery Research

Discovery research is similar to academic research and it is the most commonly followed path for science graduates who enter industry. If you enjoy working at the scientific frontier, have an interest in benefiting human health, are an idea generator with a creative mind that can make unique connections, or if you simply enjoy lab work and would like to apply your laboratory skills to industry, this is the career to consider. There are many career levels within discovery research, such as a research associate for undergraduates and master's students as well as a scientist track for PhD graduates.

For creative scientists who do not wish to advance up the administrative path to director and vice president levels, there are the prestigious "fellow" or "staff scientist" positions that allow scientists to remain close to the research and at the same time minimize their administrative load. There are also non-bench-related positions in discovery research, including project management (see the project management section), program management, portfolio management, and many more. If your interests evolve over time, discovery research can provide you with an excellent launching pad to other careers in life sciences industry.

There is currently a shortage of talent in specific areas of discovery research, namely, protein biochemists who have antibody experience, scientists with experience using computational biology for drug discovery, flow cytometrists, and scientists focusing on specific areas, such as the neurosciences, infectious diseases, and oncology.

Some highly desirable and active areas of discovery research include new "cutting edge" technologies, such as CRISPR, gene and cell therapy, immunotherapy, combination therapy, microbiome research, and many other areas. CRISPR is a particularly exciting new area. CRISPR and genome editing are the latest breakthrough discoveries in biotechnology and companies are capitalizing on the site-specific genomic editing technologies. Some companies are providing CRISPR-related services, while others are directly applying CRISPR to edit genomes. In addition to "CRISPR babies," there are companies developing functional cures. For example, one company is using CRISPR to stop the growth of HIV by targeting HIV regulatory genes, thus preventing replication in latent, infected T cells. CRISPR is being used to edit human T cells for personalized cancer immunotherapy. One company is using CRISPR for precision-breeding strategies for plant health and to increase crop yields; and to improve microbial production strains to produce new fragrances and flavors. CRISPR might be used to engineer malaria-resistant mosquitoes to help eradicate the disease.

The biotech industry is currently witnessing a resurgence in gene therapy—a technology that in principal has been around for decades. The basic premise of gene therapy: replacing a defective gene with a working one, seems easy in concept, but the field has had many dismal clinical failures over the years. GlaxoSmithKline developed an approved gene therapy to cure adenosine deaminase deficiency, a rare pediatric disease. This was the first ex vivo stem cell gene therapy treatment approved. Thankfully, the field is seeing a comeback with new clinical successes in treatment for retinal diseases, some leukemias, Parkinson's disease, and more.

Likewise, there is a renewed interest in cell therapy and immunotherapies. Although gene therapy inserts a single gene, either on a plasmid or integrated into cells, cell therapy involves injecting live cells into patients. For allogeneic cell therapy, the donor provides cells, and companies are developing "off-the-shelf" products, whereas autologous cell therapy provides cells from self, thereby avoiding graft-versus-host disease.

The ability to manipulate the immune system has led to the field of immunotherapy. In 2010 the Food and Drug Administration (FDA) approved the first cancer vaccine for castration-resistant prostate cancer, sipuleucel-T, a dendritic cell vaccine. With new chimeric antigen receptor (CAR) T-cell therapy and adoptive cell therapies, which are types of immunotherapies, this burgeoning field is expected to grow. There will be an increased need for more cell therapy specialists skilled in manufacturing and processing of cells in a good manufacturing practice (GMP) environment. In addition, flow cytometry scientists as well as molecular biologists/geneticists and biochemists with gene or cell therapy backgrounds will be needed.

By combining two different therapies that target different mechanisms of actions or biochemical pathways, the likelihood of avoiding cancer relapse or growth is increased. Therefore drug combinations can be synergistic and thus this effective approach has become ever more popular.

Originally, chemotherapy with check point immuno-oncology and/or small molecule drug combinations was shown to be effective. However, there are other types of drugs that can synergistically be effective in combination, such as drugs that can amp up the immune system or drugs that can be used in combination that allow lower doses of chemotherapy. In addition, there are new modalities, such as bispecifics and CAR T therapies and many other types of similar modalities that can be used in combination—reflecting an endless possible array of combinations.

With the number of cancer therapeutics approved and in development increasing steadily, it would be impossible to test every combination. There is the need to determine which patients will benefit from various therapy combinations, which translates into more jobs in the growing fields of personalized medicine and molecular diagnostics.

There is a growing need to develop novel biomarkers and molecular diagnostics to identify those specific patients who are biochemically suited for therapeutic applications. This information can help one to stratify patients for selection criteria for clinical trials. This has the twofold application of helping one to obtain the approval of the therapy by virtue of selecting the patients most likely to respond, and also, developing a molecular diagnostic at the same time (called companion diagnostic), so that the diagnostic can be used to identify the appropriate patients after the drug is approved.

With next generation sequencing (NGS) and the use of artificial intelligence (AI) in predicting patient populations, molecular diagnostics is poised for growth, providing more career opportunities for computational scientists, geneticists, and genomics scientists.

Preclinical Research

Preclinical research bridges the gap between discovery research and clinical development and encompasses the areas of pharmacology, toxicology, pharmacokinetics, pathology, and chemical optimization. This is the area where prospective drug candidates are tested in animals and optimized before entering into human clinical studies. Scientists find this a rewarding area to work because while research projects are frequently terminated in discovery research, preclinical scientists have an opportunity to work on the "winners"—the most promising drug candidates that have a higher chance of clinical success. Toxicologists and pharmacologists with immunology backgrounds are in high demand.

Process Sciences

Like discovery research, process sciences offers many great entry-level industry positions for academic scientists, particularly for chemists and biochemists. This is where the steps for chemical synthesis, production of drugs, or products and scale-up processes are developed. A candidate drug might be easy to synthesize in the test tube, but during clinical trials, methods are developed to scale up production of the drug for clinical studies and eventually for large-scale manufacturing. This vocational area is a great way to apply your scientific knowledge and laboratory skills to create products and develop synthesis steps that will eventually be used for large-scale manufacturing. Scientists enjoy this field because they can be creatively involved in designing scaled-up reactions and they have the chance to see the end result of their work products.

If you have a background in process chemistry, formulation, analytical chemistry, or on the biologics side, a background in cell culture, fermentation, protein purification, or biologics scale-up, there are many jobs available in this area.

Clinical Development

There are many vocational areas and niches within clinical development—the process of testing drugs in human clinical trials. Clinical development includes areas such as medical monitoring, clinical project management, or working as a clinical research associate. There are also positions in biometrics (statistics and statistical programming), medical writing, data management, drug safety, and many more. People enjoy working in clinical development because of the rapid pace of the work environment and because there is the opportunity to work with the drug candidate "winners" developed in discovery research. In general, clinical development departments employ people with medical, pharmacological, nursing, or scientific backgrounds.

The number of careers in clinical development and clinical operations has expanded tremendously over the years as the FDA has become more demanding and there are more chemical entities to take through the clinic. Currently, contract research organizations (CROs) and biotech companies cannot staff their clinical teams quickly enough because of a shortage of talent. Over the last 20 years, there has been a tremendous increase in the processes and plans for conducting clinical studies. There are more monitoring plans for protocol deviations, for example, and many more requirements for clinical trial oversight. As a consequence, there has been a rapid growth and demand for clinical quality affairs. They are involved in documentation, planning vendor selection, providing vendor oversight, auditing, and assessing and supporting compliance of clinical development projects with good clinical practice (GCP) standards and much more.

As a consequence, MD, PhD, and MS graduates are being hired to manage clinical development. If you have an interest in clinical careers, consider taking classes or obtaining a certificate. The easiest entry is to work as a study coordinator or trial monitor at a university. For PhDs, consider medical writing, where you would be involved in writing up the clinical results for regulatory filings; or clinical scientists who write clinical protocols and are involved in clinical study design strategy. Some contract research organizations (CROs) provide excellent training programs.

Regulatory Affairs

Regulatory affairs liaisons manage the process of working with project teams and interacting with the regulatory health agencies, such as the FDA or the International Conference on Harmonization of Technical Requirements for Registration of Pharmaceuticals for Human Use. In addition to regulatory affairs liaisons positions, there are a vast array of other career opportunities, such as managing and submitting regulatory information, document management, and publishing.

There is a shortage of skilled and trained regulatory affairs professionals and as a consequence, regulatory affairs professionals are in demand. This career offers excellent job security and it pays well due to the shortage of talent. In addition, as the biopharma industry is segregating into various therapeutic areas, regulatory affairs experts must also specialize. It can take years to learn the nuances of each of the many therapeutic areas, such as small and large molecules, oncology, neurosciences, infectious diseases, cell and gene therapy, medical devices, molecular diagnostics, and new foods (i.e., lab grown meats).

Companies are currently so desperate to hire regulatory affairs personnel that they are providing internships to graduates and postdocs and are willing to train them on the job. If you are a detail-oriented scientist, possess strong writing skills, and are able to manage and influence members of the teams to write their regulatory sections, this is one of the most in-demand careers. Also consider regulatory compliance, quality assurance, and working at the FDA as a regulatory reviewer. Working as a regulatory reviewer at the FDA will provide valuable training in regulatory affairs and will make you more marketable to biotech companies, because the training will provide deep insights into the inner workings of the FDA and drug-approval process. Companies enjoy employing full time hires and consultants who were former FDA reviewers. Because of the emerging fields of gene and cell therapies and CRISPR technologies, there currently is a shortage and large demand for regulatory affairs scientists who have the appropriate experience.

Medical Affairs

After a drug has been approved, medical affairs professionals run additional clinical studies to test the drug in off-label trials for other disease indications, to study drug–drug interactions, or to test the drug in different patient populations. They are also involved in disseminating this newly discovered information to relevant parties, such as practicing medical doctors and key opinion leaders.

There are several departments within medical affairs. Clinical development professionals conduct Phase IV clinical trials, medical communications executives run medical educational events for practicing physicians, and medical science liaisons provide recently published clinical data to clinicians and doctors of various specialties. Another area of medical affairs is pharmacovigilance and drug safety. This involves monitoring the drug's performance and handling adverse drug events as individual cases after the drug has been approved. If adverse events are associated with the drug, these must be reported to the regulatory authorities. The backgrounds for these positions include medical doctors, nurses, pharmacists, and scientists.

Project Management

If you are interested in learning about the many nuances of the different steps of drug discovery and development and wish to avoid bench work, consider project management. Project managers do not actually make the critical decisions but facilitate the decision-making process and manage multidisciplinary teams. They spend their time providing vision and leadership, communicating with team members and management, running meetings, allocating resources, doing risk management, and problem-solving. Each of the areas of drug discovery and development and medical device development requires project management. Common areas include discovery research, clinical, and chemistry manufacturing and controls. Project managers are also needed in many other areas, including finance, facility management, portfolio management, and many more.

This is a wonderful area to develop your interpersonal, influencing, and leadership abilities, and to gain deeper problem-solving aptitude while moving projects forward. After working as a project manager, you will have developed the ability to enter just about any of the vocational areas in a company. If you are interested in reading more about this career, there is a free chapter on project management careers on my website at www.careersbiotech.com.

Business and Corporate Development

Professionals in business and corporate development work with the company's executive team to determine the strategic objectives of the company. For example, they determine which internal products will be funded and which will be out-licensed.

Corporate development is the department where strategic decisions are made about securing enough financial resources to ensure continued operations and to reach strategic objectives. Corporate development executives are often involved in the company's fundraising efforts, whether they are raising venture or corporate capital or doing a private investment in a public entity transaction.

Business development is the department that creates and implements the deals, which are in alignment with the company's strategic objectives. A deal can be a technology that is in-licensed (acquired) or out-licensed (sold) to another company. Small biotech companies usually do not have the financial resources to bring a drug all the way through clinical trials. Instead, most small biotech companies rely on out-licensing their initial products to larger cash-rich biopharmaceutical companies that are seeking to fill their own drug development pipelines with new products. In exchange, the large biopharmaceutical companies will pay for part, or all, of the remaining clinical development and provide the small biotech company with much-needed milestone-based cash.

There are many steps in business development, and each step involves different roles. Examples include commercial strategy consultants and advisors who provide commercial insight into finance and strategic directions; portfolio managers who determine which products have the highest probability of success; technology scouts and analysts who identify and evaluate new business opportunities; licensing officers who are involved in closing deals—they could be involved in negotiations, designing payments, or arranging the final terms of the deal; and finally, alliance managers who implement the deal and manage the partnership. Alliance managers serve as the main point of contact and ensure that deliverables are met.

With the escalating number of potential combination therapies for treating cancer and other diseases, there will be an increased need for more business development executives to be engaged in partnering deals, and also an expansion in the number of alliance managers to implement the terms of the partnerships. In addition, with more incubators and accelerators on campuses across the nation, scientists are being hired to run these facilities and start-up programs.

If you are currently a student in academia, one of the easiest ways to enter business development is to work at the Office of Technology Transfer on campus. There you will learn about patents, technology management, and be exposed to the business of biotech. Alternatively, consider working in sales or patent law—important components to business development. If you are currently working in a company, volunteer to do some business development assessments in your area of expertise. Another great way to gain entry into business development is to work at a trade association or to join an incubator.

Scientists with advanced degrees are well situated to make strategic and commercial decisions about which products to acquire or license—your science background will be well utilized in this career.

One final note for job seekers: a "business development" position on the Internet frequently means a "sales" opportunity. In fact, business development is in a way, a sales transaction—it is just that the transaction takes longer and is more complicated.

Marketing

Marketing professionals work with sales executives to determine how products are sold and advertised. They manage brands and determine how the product is perceived by the target consumers. Marketing is about communicating a message to consumers and developing a business strategy. There is a psychological component to marketing as well—how do people make purchasing decisions and how do you go about providing the right message to your target audience? Marketing is needed throughout a company's life cycle. Even at the early stages of a company, market research analyses might be conducted. Just about every CEO raising money from venture capitalists will discuss the market opportunity in a company's business plan.

Marketing careers provide excellent training in leadership. Many large pharmaceutical company CEOs started their careers in marketing. If you have ambitions of eventually becoming a CEO one day, a career in marketing is a great way to acquire some of the strategic leadership training and skills needed to run a company.

Like business development, marketing is an exciting area and a highly coveted career. Once you have gained some marketing experience, it is easier to navigate between the many careers in marketing.

Brand managers are commercially responsible for specific products. The basic areas of brand management in the life sciences include promotional, medical education, consumer, global, and managed-care marketing. New product-planning professionals help clinical teams strategize on the best market for their drug development plans. In addition, there are other branches of marketing, including commercial strategy, data analytics, and forecasting, to name a few.

One of the easiest ways for science graduates to get into marketing is through sales or market research. Market research is a career involved with gathering data about the size of a market, the target customers, and the customer's interest. Applying your science background will add a great value to a career in marketing.

Sales

Sales executives work directly with customers to develop business and conduct sales transactions. They help customers use products correctly, inform doctors about drugs and products, for example, and ensure that any questions and concerns that customers have are promptly answered. Sales can be a financially rewarding and lucrative career for those that are highly motivated and energetic. There are many perks to a career in sales, and quite possibly the best, besides the commissions, is that many sales reps work from home. This can provide an opportunity to live in areas where there are limited jobs (like Hawaii, for example). Plus, you cannot beat the commute from your kitchen to your home office! However, there can also be extensive travel in sales in order to meet customers and provide sales presentations.

Sales positions provide great entry-level opportunities for new graduates and job changers, and companies in general offer excellent training in sales. Once you have mastered sales basics, you will find a multitude of different positions within sales, including sales management, operations, and account management. There are many types of sales positions, such as selling reagents, instruments, microscopes, and preclinical and clinical trial services, for example. Specialty and primary drug sales reps visit doctors' offices frequently to promote their products and establish relations with doctors. For scientists with a driving interest in making science easier to understand for customers, consider technical sales—sales for biological and medical research products such as instruments, biotools, software, and services. You might have an opportunity to work with high-level research executives or well-known professors in academia and help them make technical decisions. Working closely with the sales reps, Field Application Specialists or Scientists provide their technical expertise to help with sales transactions. For recent graduates, this is an exciting entry-level position that will allow you to work with technical leaders in academia and industry, learn business fundamentals, and become an expert in the products that you are promoting.

Management Consulting

Management consulting is a great way to apply your analytical skills in a fast-paced, intellectually intense occupation where you can drive change and help companies become more successful. Management consultants serve as high-level strategic advisers to companies. They might conduct strategic analyses on just about any aspect of a company's business, including strategy, portfolio management, pricing, operations, productivity, finance, cost reduction, competition, and more. There are several major global management consulting firms and many small boutiques that specialize in the life sciences. Also consider the many accounting firms that have life science advisory service arms. Management consulting can involve extensive travel, and the position pays well, accordingly. Most management consulting firms offer training and some offer a mini-MBA, in which you can learn business fundamentals.

Corporate Communications

If you have a flair for writing, consider corporate communications. Corporate communications professionals are involved in managing the image of the company—how the company is perceived by investors, customers, and the general public.

There are several career areas within corporate communications. Investor relations professionals interact with the company's investors, public relations professionals manage the corporate image and news about a company, and government affairs professionals develop science policies and inform and influence the government. If you are interested in a corporate communications career, consider applying for a policy fellowship with the American Association for the Advancement of Science (AAAS).

Corporate affairs and marketing communications (marcom) are careers for scientists with an interest in business, who possess excellent writing skills. In an entry-level position, you might participate in writing press releases or creating investor packages.

Engineering

There are many opportunities for engineers in the life sciences, particularly in the biotools, biofuels, computational sciences, and medical devices industries. Some opportunities include conceiving, developing, and testing human prosthetic devices, such as bionic arms, legs, ankles, and hands. There are other opportunities in the development and production of new gene sequencing instruments. In the biofuels sector, chemical and mechanical engineers develop new methods for renewable fuel sources and the processing machinery that produces them. An engineering, bioengineering, or biochemical engineering background is needed in all sectors of the biotechnology industry including therapeutics, diagnostics, medical devices, research reagents and tools, agtech, biofuels, and industrial biotechnology products.

Operations

If you enjoy making things more efficient and improving the workplace, a career in operations might interest you. This area is focused on manufacturing and distributing products to customers at the highest level of quality for the lowest cost. People in operations enjoy making processes more efficient and are good at problem-solving and delivering on expectations. This is a fast-paced position with job variety and where you can apply your science and business acumen and directly affect the company's bottom line.

Quality

If you are one to pay meticulous attention to detail and enjoy ensuring that things are done correctly, a quality role might be for you. Quality positions tend to have good job security. Most positions require little if any travel, unless you are an auditor. Quality work ensures that products and procedures are consistent and comply with FDA regulations. For therapeutic companies, quality ensures that products are pure and safe for human or animal consumption.

Quality offers many great entry-level positions for new graduates and career-changers. Quality-control specialists test products and make sure that manufactured products meet specifications. Quality assurance professionals provide the documentation that shows that production is being done correctly. Regulatory compliance ensures that systems and procedures have accounted for quality and are compliant with the regulations. Most biotools and medical device companies have a quality-systems branch that is involved in validation of computer systems.

There will be an increased need for (and a currently tremendous demand for) clinical laboratory scientists and in particular, CLIA-certified (Clinical Laboratory Information Amendments) scientists and medical directors to oversee the development of the many molecular diagnostic tests. CLIA ensures quality laboratory testing of human samples for laboratory diagnostics.

Information Sciences—Artificial Intelligence and Bio-IT

The AI explosion and computational sciences are taking the life sciences industry by storm. The biomedical sciences industry is data rich and increasing in complexity, and the need for automation and robotics has increased. For example, NGS or SAR analyses generate large amounts of data which need to be analyzed and managed. There is an increased need for applying AI and computational analyses in just about every step of drug discovery and development, including discovery and preclinical, clinical development, risk prediction, portfolio management, patient registries, medical imaging, electronic health records, mobile health applications, medical insurance, and more. In addition, there is a need to enhance the research infrastructure, such as enotebooks, and electronic data capture.

Animal models are difficult and often not well correlated with human disease equivalents, particularly for the neurodegenerative diseases, and they can be costly. The use of in silico drug design could save millions of dollars of the companies by avoiding the use of animal models and could theoretically predict more effective therapeutics.

Computational modeling and AI are being applied to gather, manage, and intelligently use the massive amount of structured and unstructured data. Machine learning applies statistical techniques to give computer systems the ability to "learn" from the data. Using machine learning data, for example, scientists can better predict patient care by having a better understanding of each patient's unique physiology and genetic makeup. Machine learning models can help with structure–activity relationships in drug discovery, predicting toxicity and efficacy in combination therapies, and computer vision and automated tasks, for examples. The outcomes of machine learning predictions can be tested in the wet lab, more data can be obtained after each test, and the process can be reiterated until it precisely identifies what scientists are looking for—perhaps the perfect drug or drug target.

Molecular dynamics principals can be applied to predicting better protein–protein interactions and reiterative processes of machine learning and math models to identify mutations and permutations that will result in increased protein–protein interactions. This can eventually allow predictive simulations of more efficacious and possibly even new chemical entities. It can also be applied to predicting how therapeutics/antibodies react to each other and their solubility in various solutions and drug concentrations, for examples.

Big data analytics is the science of analyzing large volumes of data gathered from a wide variety of sources to uncover patterns and connections to identify new relationships and insights, which could have otherwise not been noticed. Patient data, such as from electronic health records, patient registries, and personalized genomics DNA information, represent resources of data that can be mined for potential targets for drug discovery and drug development or for patient monitoring.

There will be a growing need for people skilled in managing the large amounts of data in the cloud and in other large data repositories. Repositories that house biomedical data have grown and some have become publicly available. For example, genomics, transcriptomes, proteomics, clinical outcomes, and side effects of drugs represent large data sets that can be mined and leveraged for drug discovery and development efforts and predictive modeling and to increase the likelihood of clinical trial success.

AI technology involving self-learning machines is being developed for human augmentation and robotics. For example, AI technology can be used to tailor implanted devices or limb prosthetics that can be used to extend human sensory, physical, or cognitive abilities.

Merging high-tech applications to consumer medical products is a growing trend. For example, mobile health blood glucose monitoring for diabetics. There are numerous high-tech life science applications, such as Proteus, which developed a pill that allows doctors to monitor patient compliance.

Demand for talent is ever increasing as computational tools are being applied to the many steps of developing biomedical products and for post product approval applications, such as patient monitoring, billing, electronic health records, patient registries, and insurance.

There is a shortage of scientists with a background in both the biological sciences and computer technology—generally candidates tend to have one or the other, and there are few with a combination of both. Scientists with this combination of backgrounds are at the center of AI research and are in high demand. In addition, many trained in machine learning and AI generally tend toward the consumer tech companies, such as Google and Amazon where they can earn higher incomes.

Scientists can enter this field from either the computer or biological sciences. If you are considering making the leap and have a biological background, you can obtain computational training from Coursera classes, which generally have the nod of approval from most hiring managers. Also consider joining high-tech companies with life science arms, such as Oracle, Google/Verily, and Apple.

Technical and Product Support

If you enjoy working with customers and want to be a technical expert, you might consider careers in product and technical support. Technical support representatives manage phone calls, answer customer-related questions, and solve technical and product-related problems. They also become experts in each of the specific products, and as such, frequently these individuals later move into product development. Technical support can be a collegial and friendly working environment and most of the positions are 9–5 and involve little travel.

If you have a passion for teaching, consider a career as a technical trainer. Technical trainers teach clients how to use new products by conducting workshops. An added perk is that many trainers work from home when they are not offering a workshop.

Law

Intellectual property—patents, copyrights, and trademarks are often the most valuable assets held by a biotechnology company, especially at the early stages. Patent attorneys and agents draft and manage the patent applications. But there are other equally interesting areas of law to consider, such as transactional, corporate law, and litigation.

Transactional lawyers draft and negotiate business transactions. Corporate lawyers incorporate companies and help structure business deals, such as M&As, IPOs, and venture financings. Litigators are involved in lawsuits, typically patent infringements, which have heated up over the years as large successful biotech companies have more money worth suing for.

There are other law careers, such as regulatory law or general counsel as well as opportunities to work as a patent examiner or attorney at the US Patent and Trademark Office in Alexandria, VA. Law is a highly competitive occupation, but it also is intellectually interesting and financially rewarding.

Human Resources and Recruiting

Having the right team in an early-stage start-up is exceedingly important. It is essential that the company hires people who have the appropriate skill sets and who will also fit in with the corporate culture. The field of human resources, which is managing the corporate culture of a company, employee relations, and governance of employees, is generally occupied by people with business backgrounds; however, scientists can enter this field as well.

Recruiting can be a gratifying occupation because you are helping companies identify and hire people with the appropriate skill sets and corporate match and also helping job seekers find promising jobs. There are many different types of recruiting companies ranging from the large international executive retained search, to contingency, temp-to-hire, and staffing firms.

Careers in Government

Government and nonprofit careers generally do not pay as well as in industry, but they offer much greater job security and pension plans—so in the long term, it can balance out. This is a great way to apply your business and scientific training and contribute to society. There are many opportunities in the government sector. At the FDA, there are numerous career fields in addition to regulatory or medical affairs, such as basic research and pharmacovigilance opportunities. To find out more and to learn about student internships, visit www.usajobs.com and https://usphs.gov.

In addition to the FDA, there is a plethora of government opportunities, such as working at the departments of Agriculture, Energy, Veterans Affairs, and Defense; the CDC, NASA, NIH, Homeland Security, Department of Infectious Diseases, crime labs/forensics, the military, and many more research institutes and government labs.

Careers in Nonprofit Organizations

Nonprofit organizations can offer stimulating and altruistic work environments and are a way to apply your scientific and business acumen and work with academics, medical advocacy groups, and philanthropists. In addition to the traditional nonprofit organizations, many nonprofits are developing their own drug discovery and development or diagnostics efforts in-house, just like a biotech company. For example, the Myelin Repair Foundation, Melanoma Research Alliance, and the Michael J. Fox Foundation are actively involved in advancing treatments through the FDA. As such, the same types of positions discussed in this chapter might also be available in some nonprofit organizations.

There are nonprofit organizations for just about every known disease. Most nonprofits are philanthropic organizations that provide grants for research or patient advocacy for a specific disease, such as the Alzheimer's Association or the American Cancer Society. The Bill and Melinda Gates Foundation's mission is to improve people's health around the world. For example, grants are used for research to find cures, for vaccinations, or medical assistance for patients, for epidemiological research, or simply for raising disease awareness.

There are many different positions for business and science majors in nonprofits, including project management, social work, development (fundraising), marketing, outreach, operations, scientific affairs, finance, communications, science positions ranging from research associate or scientist to chief scientific officer, program management, patent and licensing positions, and much more.

There are also a variety of jobs at lobbying and educational nonprofit organizations, such as the Biotechnology Industry Organization, Pharmaceuticals Research and Manufacturers of America, and the Drug Information

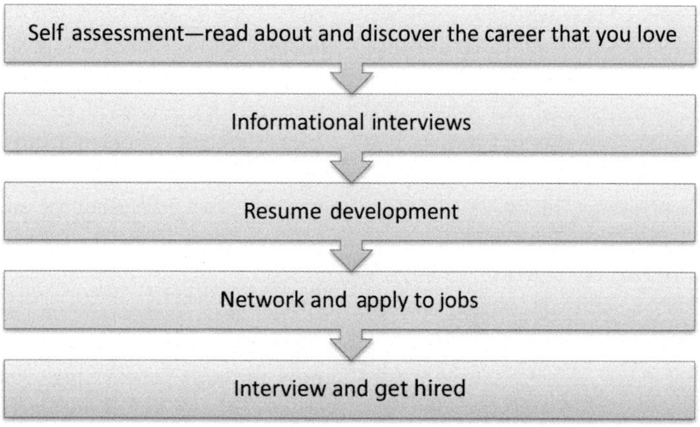

FIGURE 40.2 Basic steps for a career transition.

Association. There are many regional nonprofits that serve as lobbying and educational organizations, such as the AAAS and the Massachusetts Biotechnology Council. In addition, scientific societies, such as the American Chemical Society, provide job opportunities for business and science majors. Also consider government-run trade associations and international innovation centers that are located at biotech hubs. These opportunities would provide exposure to many start-up companies.

Making a Career Transition

Whether you wish to transition from academia to industry or from one career to another, with proper planning and some good fortune, it is possible to make a smooth career transition. As shown in Fig. 40.2, the first step includes self-assessment. Work with career counselors and take self-assessment tests in order to identify your interests, skills, personality attributes, values, and goals. If you are a student or postdoctoral fellow, most universities provide free career services on campus. Alumni are frequently provided with free career services on campus. If you are employed in a company, speak to human resources representatives, consider getting mentored or hire a personal career counselor.

The next step is to identify those vocational areas that best match your self-assessment results to find your prospective "ideal career." After researching the many careers and identifying several possibilities, conduct informational interviews. An informational interview is simply a way to interview professionals currently working in a chosen vocational field that interests you. Note that this is not a job interview—it is a way to gain more knowledge and insights about a vocational area to determine if it is right for you. To learn more about informational interviewing, visit your career services department on campus as they generally have an abundance of material on the topic. There is also extensive information available on the Internet.

There may be additional classes, degrees, or certificates that would expedite a career transition. For example, a certificate in project management would provide you with practical training using the project management tools utilized in companies.

As shown in Fig. 40.2, the third step is to prepare a resume specific for the new career and to continue networking by attending local and international conferences and events that are in line with the career area that interests you. For example, if you are interested in a career in business development, you might want to attend the Licensing Executives Society association conference; for regulatory affairs, the Regulatory Affairs Professionals Society (RAPS) society would be a good choice.

For readers who wish to make a career transition, try to obtain on-the-job training. For example, if you are a scientist working at the bench and would like a career in project management, become a team member on a project at your current job, and become familiar with the process so that you can more easily make the transition. If you are interested in business development, ask to assist with technical assessments of new technologies that the business development department is considering. If you are in academia, consider volunteering at the office of technology transfer department on campus.

Finding a Job in the Life Sciences Industry

Be sure to extensively fill out your LinkedIn profile. Recruiters and hiring managers alike are relying on LinkedIn to find and recruit talent by searching for key words. You might never know what the key words will be, so just like your resume, the more information provided in your profile (briefly though, it is not a place for your thesis, just a short summary is needed), the better. For example, list where you have worked and briefly describe your research projects. Also list your technical skills and include publication titles in your LinkedIn profile. You want to provide enough information so that someone can gleam your technical expertise and therapeutic area of study so that they can determine if you might be qualified for an opportunity. Examples of therapeutic areas are infectious diseases, neurosciences, oncology, metabolic diseases, drug delivery, biofuels, food tech, computational sciences, molecular diagnostics, etc. Technical expertise examples: molecular biology, biochemistry, antibody phage display, crystallography, mass spec, flow cytometry, cell culture, animal husbandry, etc. Also create an endorsement section with key words and technical skills for your friends to endorse—recruiters also view these sections. Broad key words, such as biotechnology and pharmaceutical companies are a good start but also provide more specific key words for endorsement, such as flow cytometry, project management, and machine learning, for examples.

Most people first apply to the well-established biopharmaceutical companies with name-recognition, such as Amgen, Vertex, Genentech/Roche, Biogen, Gilead, Pfizer, and Merck. However, these high-caliber companies are also the most competitive to get into, because everyone else is also applying to them. You should also consider the less well-known and emerging venture-backed companies and start-ups. The trick is to find companies that are working in the therapeutic area that interests you and then target those specific companies. This will increase your likelihood of success because these companies will be more interested in your technical skills and experience based on your similar interests and appropriate background. After all, companies want to hire the top experts in their technical area.

Other places to look for employment are at the service companies, such as CROs and contract manufacturing organizations. These companies will provide you with exposure to numerous different processes and products. As large and small biotech companies tend to outsource many aspects of drug discovery and development, there can be more jobs available in the service companies.

There are many nontherapeutic biotech companies to consider, for example, molecular diagnostics, personalized medicine, and next-generation sequencing companies; biotools, instruments, and reagents; consulting services; biofuels; industrial biotechnology; systems biology; nanotech; agtech; food tech; numerous large and small agencies; and the medical device industry. In addition to jobs in government and nonprofits, there are many areas of employment in academia in addition to professorships. For examples, program directorships, working at the office of technology transfer, education-related positions, laboratory management, core facility directorship, working in public relations and development (fundraising), working in an entrepreneurial start-up on campus or incubator, working in doctoral career services, and many more. A list of job posting websites and news sources is included at the end of this chapter under Resources.

I cannot stress enough how important it is to be flexible and open-minded in your job search. Consider job areas that you might not have thought about and keep an open mind while exploring your options. Also consider working as a consultant or on a contract/temporary basis.

Networking

The vast majority of people in biotechnology find their jobs through networking. The reason that networking is so effective is that hiring managers are more likely to consider candidates who are personally vouched for—perhaps a company employee has worked previously with a candidate or met him or her at a networking event and can forward their resume. Networking is also effective because company employees are frequently financially motivated to bring on hirees. The more people that you know, the more likely someone will recommend you for an opportunity.

What does "networking" actually mean? It means meeting people—whether at local and national meetings, on airplanes, at trade booths at conferences, etc. It means developing personal connections and informing your network about your job status and the types of positions that interest you. It also means being helpful and supportive of your fellow colleagues so that they can contact you for your guidance and support when they are looking for a job.

Interviewing

It is very important to apply for and interview for as many positions as possible. The more positions that you interview for, the more likely that you will find the ideal job. Likewise, companies often also interview several candidates for each position in order to hire the one with the best technical and corporate match. It is a good idea to prepare for common interview questions in advance—this is not the time to wing it. There are some excellent resources to help prepare you for interviewing, such as the book *301 Smart Answers to Tough Interview Questions*. Most of the career services on campus provide interviewing workshops that can offer valuable preparation.

Careers in the Life Sciences Industry: Job Security and Volatility

Careers in biotechnology can be as volatile as careers in other technology sectors. The reasons for volatility are due to many factors, including the dynamic nature of the life sciences industry, the ever increasing costs of developing drugs, and the difficulty of getting drugs and products approved by regulatory authorities in addition to larger economic forces, such as recessions and the political nature of drug pricing.

If job security is your major concern, some careers offer better job security than others. For example, careers in regulatory affairs or in government provide significantly better job security compared to most other areas. A particular skill set in a new or uncommon and high-demand area, such as a CLIA certification, is another way to enhance your job security.

During tough economic times, companies tend to focus on gaining revenues, which translates into a focus on products closest to sales. Therefore careers in sales, marketing, regulatory affairs, clinical development, and medical affairs tend to be more stable, whereas early drug discovery research jobs can be more volatile. By nature, early-stage biotech start-ups tend to have less job security compared to the more established biopharmaceutical companies because in the large companies, a clinical failure will likely not have as much impact as it would in a small start-up. However, even at the larger companies, frequent reorganizations and removal of redundancies after an acquisition are common.

Final Comments and Conclusion

I hope that I have provided persuasive evidence that there are a myriad of vocational areas in the life sciences industry for you to explore. It is important to find a career that you are passionate about and will enjoy. Make sure that you read about the various career options, and conduct self-assessment tests to determine which career areas best match your skills, interests, and professional and personal goals. Over the years, your interests and personal or professional goals will likely change. You should conduct periodic self-assessments, revisit your "ideal career," or change directions.

As opposed to other industries, working in the life sciences provides a unique opportunity to make a meaningful and positive impact in the world—to cure diseases, to improve the quality of people's lives, and so much more. This is your opportunity to contribute to global health.

In closing, it is my wish that you will be productive in developing drugs or products and services for unmet medical needs, that you will start companies, and be highly successful in your career.

*Toby Freedman is a recruiter, author, and career development expert. Her book, Career Opportunities in Biotechnology and Drug Development, published by Cold Spring Harbor Laboratory Press (*www.careersbiotech.com*), provides an in-depth and comprehensive overview of the many careers in the life sciences industry. This information was derived from her insights acquired from many years of working as a recruiter and based on interviews with over 200 industry executives. Each chapter describes the aspects of each career area, including descriptions of a typical day; personality attributes to be successful; pros and cons of the job; career potential; experience and educational requirements, and much more. She provides career development workshops at academic centers. Toby founded her own recruiting firm, Synapsis Search, which is focused on life science R&D and business placements. Toby previously worked at BioQuest and SLIL Biomedical (a biotech start-up). She earned a Ph.D. in biology/molecular biology from UNC Chapel Hill and her postdoctoral fellowship was at Harvard University. For more information, visit* www.amazon.com *and* www.careersbiotech.com.

Resources

Job Posting Websites

LinkedIn—www.linkedin.com is becoming the leading resource to find employment in the life sciences.

Drop Out Club—www.docjobs.com, posts jobs for MDs and PhDs who have an interest in clinical development, financial, investment banking, and venture capital opportunities.

Medical Science Liaison Society—www.themsls.org

Venture Loop—www.ventureloop.com: jobs in venture-backed companies.

Craig's List—www.craigslist.org: postings of entry-level and higher level jobs; there is a biotech section.

BioSpace—www.biospace.com: biotech and medical device job posting website and life sciences news service.

Indeed—www.indeed.com: a good place to source for jobs.

Fierce Biotech—www.fiercebiotech.com: a summary of biotech news.

Fierce Biotech Research—www.fiercebiotechresearch.com: research coverage in the life sciences.

Big 4 Bio—www.big4bio.com–biotech news in Boston, San Francisco, Philadelphia and San Diego and job postings.

Chapter 41

Common Biotechnology Entrepreneur Mistakes and How to Avoid Them

Craig Shimasaki, PhD, MBA
CEO, BioSource Consulting Group and Moleculera Labs, Oklahoma City, OK, United States

Chapter Outline

All entrepreneurs start out with boundless optimism as they perceive a visionary product or service that could revolutionize some facet of medicine, health, and life. They embark on this journey full of energy, excitement, and motivation which drives them to step out into this high-risk endeavor. However, unless they are a "seasoned entrepreneur," they are typically unaware of the "Unknown-Unknowns." The "Unknown-Unknowns" are the things entrepreneurs don't know ... that they don't know. Unknown-Unknowns are difficult, if not impossible to fix because by definition, you don't know these critical entrepreneurial problems are looming ahead. In this chapter, I'll share with you some of the most common mistakes that I have encountered myself, and also from mentoring other biotech entrepreneurs. I am a firm believer of the quote by Eleanor Roosevelt (or Groucho Marx—whomever really said this) "*Learn from the mistakes of others because you will never live long enough to make them all yourself.*" In this chapter, we will review the seven most common mistakes that biotech entrepreneurs make when starting and growing their companies. Along with each of these, I'll share ways in which to avoid them. By doing this, my desire is to help you avoid these pitfalls through careful planning and forewarning. There are certainly more than seven mistakes biotech entrepreneurs can make, but these tend to be the most common and the most impactful on the growth and development of their organization.

Biotechnology Entrepreneurship. DOI: https://doi.org/10.1016/B978-0-12-815585-1.00041-3

The Seven Most Common Biotechnology Entrepreneur Mistakes

1. ***Unclear/Undefined goals and not recognizing the difference between a method and the goal:*** Not knowing your ultimate objectives and not recognizing the difference between a method and a goal.
2. ***Misalignment of technology toward a lukewarm market: a technology solution in search of a problem to solve:*** You find yourself possessing a technology solution that is in search of a big problem to solve, but the one you have chosen does not align with the most strategic market need.
3. ***Poorly planned corporate documents with many hastily prepared agreements that have conflicting language:*** Poorly planned and piecemeal documents that have not been produced by an experienced start-up corporate attorney. These foundational legal problems impact your future ability to raise capital and grow.
4. ***Failing to recognize and leverage untapped "human capital" resources:*** There are unrecognized and untapped resources available that you need, but you are not utilizing.
5. ***Flawed capital management: fundraising is not strategically timed to a value-enhancing milestone:*** Your capital raises are not timed to occur after reaching a value-enhancing milestone, thus impacting investor interest and valuation of the company at these stages.
6. ***Not recognizing when or how to pivot or reinvent your business model. Failing to take advantage of "serendipity" and not listening to the surrounding environment:*** Missing critical external queues that lead to monumental problems and failing to take advantage of "serendipity."
7. ***Short-term commitment and wavering internal motivation leads to a self-limiting enterprise:*** Misaligned internal motivation which ultimately leads to a self-limiting enterprise. Motivation and energy wane and perseverance is short lived.

Common Mistake 1: Unclear/Undefined Goals and Not Recognizing the Difference Between a Method and the Goal

One of the most critical mistakes entrepreneurs can make is not clearly defining their goals at the outset when deciding to start a company. There are many goals that need to be defined, such as goals for a business model, goals for a value proposition and target market, product development goals, and the overall business goals that the entrepreneur is wanting to achieve. Granted, not everyone can predict what the end goal will ultimately be, but you must start out with a clear idea of your goals in order to know what direction to take in the beginning. When you begin raising money from investors, you will find that they instinctively know whether an entrepreneur really understands where they are going, or if they are just on a "fishing expedition," hoping to figure out things out along the way after they get money. All entrepreneurs need clear goals for each of these areas, and they will need to have defined them in order to have others follow.

For example:

- *Regarding your overall business goal:* If you are a full-time professor, is your overall goal to advance your technology and increase its value while staying employed at your academic institution? Do you want to license the technology to a company that will develop and commercialize your product idea, and you plan to consult and be an advisor for the company? Is your goal to advance the technology all the way through to product commercialization and marketing? Is your overall goal to develop a prototype or reach the preclinical stage, then license the project to a medical device, pharmaceutical company, or diagnostic company?
- *Regarding your business model goal:* If you have a diagnostic technology, is your business model goal to develop an in-vitro diagnostic kit that you manufacture and sell, or do you want to reach the market sooner and become a clinical lab service and offer a laboratory developed testing service?

Entrepreneurial leaders should recognize that the choice of a business goal (end goal) affects the optimal enterprise structure, the amount of capital you need, and the time required to reach an investor exit. Different goals carry differing amounts of risk and differing valuations. By defining your business goal at the outset, you and your team can use your creative ability to overcome obstacles to arrive at your desired destination. However, if your business goal is not clearly defined, often an organization will take the path of least resistance, only to later discover that their past decisions directed them *away* from their desired goal. This is why we hear the saying "*There never seems to be enough time and money to do it right the first time, however, we always seem to find time and money to do it over.*"

Recognize the Difference Between *the* Goal and a Method

There can be confusion between a *method* and the *goal* which sometimes becomes blurred by entrepreneurs who are rapidly working toward advancing their product and building their company. Because starting and building a biotech company or entrepreneurial organization is not prescriptive, often *methods* that have worked for others are followed. Although there are good methods to reach your goal, many different paths can lead to success. For instance, when raising capital, one entrepreneur may be successful by building their company using nondilutive capital in the form of grants, donations, and crowdfunding. However, for another entrepreneur if this funding "method" becomes the "goal" and they are not successful in raising nondilutive capital, they waste precious time trying to achieve a "goal" that was simply one of the many "methods" for raising capital. Because there are many methods to reach the same goal, you must be able to recognize the difference.

Here is an analogy as to why it is critical to define your goal at the outset. Suppose 10 people living in Oklahoma City have a common goal of arriving at New York City by automobile. Each one can choose from dozens of routes to reach this goal. Some choices will allow one individual to arrive sooner than others, while other choices will cause an individual to arrive later, whereas *all* 10 individuals will eventually reach the same destination goal—as long as they constantly head northeast. If a person heads south, west, or northwest, they will not arrive at their destination goal. This may seem remedial, but it is an important analogy that a goal is not the same as a method, and that there are often many methods to reach your goal. However, if you do not define your goal clearly, you will not know the difference.

Can Your Goal Change?

Absolutely. In fact, a good number of successful businesses and products are the result of a strategic business change that occurred because of an insurmountable roadblock in the original product idea or market. However, you first need to have a goal defined before you can change it. I'll share more about this principle in *Mistake 6 "Not knowing when or how to pivot or reinvent your business model or product"—missing critical external queues and failing to take advantage of "serendipity."*

For entrepreneurial success, you must clearly define your business goals, business model, and product development goals as well as other goals for your company. Well-defined goals provide a destination that team members can focus upon and help overcome obstacles and roadblocks encountered along the way. Entrepreneurs must clearly identify their goals at the outset because those who join your team are motivated by your vision, because your goal is the description of your ultimate destination. Like the reply from the Cheshire cat to Alice in Wonderland after she asked him "*which road do I take?*" he said, "*If you don't know where you are going, any road will take you there*!" Be an entrepreneur with clearly defined goals, so others can creatively help you arrive at your destination.

How to Avoid This Mistake

Every entrepreneur begins with a product idea from the technology they developed or plan to license. During the inception stage, before the company is incorporated or launched, there is no overhead cost structure or payroll to maintain. It is during this time that a variety of goals should be examined, tested, and defined—*prior* to starting the organization. This is a time when literally no one is looking at your organization and you can make as many mistakes as you want—and no one even notices. During this time, practice sharing your vision and goals with other seasoned entrepreneurs, then listen to their feedback. Share your goals with others in the industry and see if they get excited about your vision. If you have already launched your company and you are struggling, reexamine your business model and product development goals to see if they are truly aligned with an acute market need. As described in *Chapter 13: Directing Your Technology Toward a Market Problem: What You Need to Know Before Using the Business Model Canvas?*, sometimes a product application is selected but it turns out not to be the best market application. In that chapter, we review how technology can be applied to many different market applications, and a prudent entrepreneur can change or modify the market application to find a more suitable and receptive audience. Another important point that will help is to be sure to reduce your product concept and business goals into understandable terminology so that even your grandmother can understand. If you can successfully do this, and people get excited about your goal, you are on to something.

Common Mistake 2: Misalignment of Technology Toward a Lukewarm Market: A Technology Solution in Search of a Problem to Solve

Most successful products today are supported by a novel technology that provides the product's features and benefits. Entrepreneurs utilize the underlying technology and direct it toward a particular market application they have chosen. A common mistake of emerging life science and biotech entrepreneurs is that, although they have identified a great technology, their choice of market application is not ideal. This problem usually occurs when the product application was chosen because of the entrepreneur's familiarity with one particular problem—or shall we say—their lack of familiarity with a more acute problem.

As a consequence, they face lackluster investor interest and limited support for their product. Entrepreneurs should recognize two important principles at the outset.

Principle 1: Most Products Today Possess an Underlying Technology Platform

Technology-based products arise because of an underlying "technology platform" that enables the product to possess its unique features, but the technology is capable of being directed toward many other products for different market applications. Often, the underlying technology platform is not recognized because the focus has been on the product application. Also, the platform technology of a particular product is sometimes difficult to characterize at first, but with practice it becomes easier to identify and redirect. Technology transfer offices at universities and research institutions possess shelves full of unlicensed patents, not because the technology is ineffective but because the market application chosen is not appealing to potential licensees. Almost all products possess an underlying technology platform that would allow it to be redirected toward another, possibly better, market application.

Principle 2: Technology Is Agnostic to Any Single Market Application

Technology itself is not beholden to any specific market application. For example, in the biotechnology industry, a scientific technology discovery that interrupts cell-cycle control could be directed toward the development of a therapeutic for breast cancer, prostate cancer, or brain cancer (See Fig. 41.1). Many times, the choice of application is a result of the entrepreneur's familiarity with a market problem, or more often—convenience. For instance, if down the hall from the entrepreneur is a researcher who has tumor tissue available from breast or prostate cancer patients, the market application can conveniently be directed toward breast or prostate cancer therapy. However, glioblastoma, a type of brain cancer with a more acute market need, has a lower barrier for adoption in terms of effectiveness. The National Cancer Institute's website lists over 55 drugs used to treat breast cancer, whereas the FDA approved just 5 drugs for glioblastoma—none are curative. This technology applied to breast cancer or prostate cancer would have higher hurdles of efficacy than for glioblastoma due to the greater number of effective alternatives. The market application for a technology may have been selected because of convenience when it may not have been the best application for business success. Certainly, there are technical, biological, and regulatory issues that factor into the selection of a market application, but at the outset, entrepreneurs must first seek to align their technology with an acute market need in order to be successful.

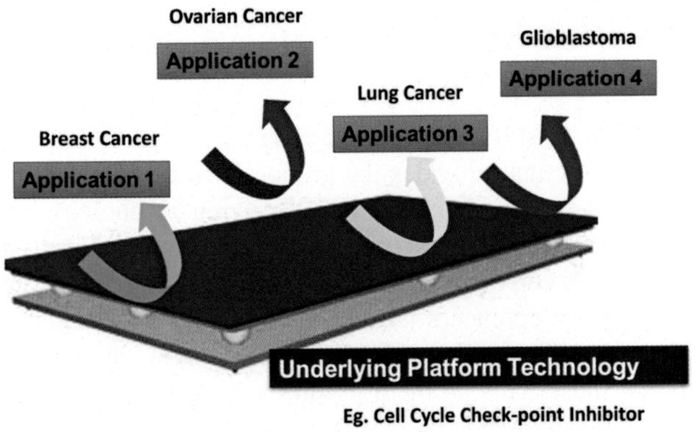

FIGURE 41.1 Your Technology Platform is Agnostic to a Market Application.

How to Avoid This Mistake

Realize that the market application of a technology is usually a choice which is often selected based upon the entrepreneur's personal awareness of a particular market need. To avoid this mistake, practice getting out of your comfort zone and force yourself to be exposed to different problems in medicine and science. Learn from experts who have different backgrounds and experiences than yours. When you become familiar with the nuances of diverse problems, you can apply an underlying technology solution to solve that particular need. Successful entrepreneurs make themselves aware of problems confronted in different sectors and markets. Unfortunately, if you are *un*aware of market problems, your options are self-limited. Like the handyman with only one tool—if it's a hammer, everything begins to look like a nail. The most successful products arise from an entrepreneur's awareness of an acute unmet market need *and* a great technology solution. In other words, successful products combine great technology directed toward a market application that has an acute unmet need with few alternative or substitute products.

There are two critical elements that underlie successful products: (1) the novelty and useful capabilities of the technology and (2) the acuteness of the market need and the lack of adequate substitutes for the product that the technology supports.

If you recognize these principles at the outset of your entrepreneurial career, you can better align technology with a critical market need, and you will have greater investor interest and market receptivity. Remember, technology is agnostic to the market application—the same technology utilized in cell phones for wireless communication can be applied to medical devices for heart rate monitoring or leveraged in the petroleum industry for real-time assessment of oil rig production.

Never forget that the bigger or more critical the problem, the greater the market need and the more important the solution. Find critical problems, even if they are in a niche market. There will be lower hurdles for acceptance in markets where few effective products exist. The height of the barrier for product acceptance is directly proportional to the number of competitive products and good substitutes available for that particular need. A market that is void of effective products or good substitutes will receive increased interest from investors and have lower hurdles for adoption. Remember to align your technology to solve the most critical need, and you will never be stuck with a great technology solution in search of an important problem to solve.

Common Mistake 3: Poorly Planned Corporate Documents With Many Hastily Prepared Agreements That Have Conflicting Language

A third common mistake of entrepreneurs is that while they grow their business, they haphazardly, although unintentionally, put together a disorderly array of foundational documents which impedes their ability to raise capital from sophisticated investors in the future. These documents are usually piecemealed together by do-it-yourself downloaded documents, blindly accepted agreements, and conflicting contracts drafted by a hodgepodge of less-experienced attorneys. Early-stage companies may move forward for a period of time, but at some point, you will find yourself with a costly mess that has to be undone by an experienced start-up corporate attorney.

In this situation, requisite documents may have simply been omitted or, if they exist, they contain conflicting language with other documents. You find that you end up with loosely assembled or completely omitted founder agreements. As a result, there may be ownership issues or ownership uncertainty because of verbal agreements made to individuals who could come back and claim rights. If multiple founders started the company, one of the founders may no longer be working to advance the business, yet they walked away with a large chunk of equity with no agreement for reacquiring those shares. You may find yourself with an inadequate technology license agreement or missing key agreements that fail to ascribe value to the organization from its founders and stakeholders. All this creates unnecessary roadblocks for raising capital in the future.

Other problems can include the following:

- A license agreement that does not allow the rights to sell the technology (business) without prior approval from the licensee.
- Missing employment agreements that assure investors that key employees will not be leaving to start a competing business after their investment.
- Inappropriately structured funding agreements with angel investors.
- Missing invention assignment agreements from key employees who are inventors of the technology.

In many cases, institutional investors may simply walk away from deals that require too much work because of uncertainties and the potential pitfalls of your deal.

Why This Frequently Occurs

This mistake happens more frequently than one may realize, simply because early-stage entrepreneurs are solely focused on the most urgent things first, such as fundraising and product development. Rightly so, but when entrepreneurs become only focused on fundraising and advancing product development, they neglect other critical aspects of the business that don't show up immediately, but disaster may be awaiting. Although it may feel like company progress is made, it is like plugging a hole in your boat to prevent it from sinking, not realizing you are headed toward a waterfall. This piecemeal, deal-with-it-when-you-need-it, and do-it-yourself approach may suffice *for a short period of time*. Unfortunately, as your business gains momentum and interest from sophisticated institutional investors, they will have grave concerns over this legal quagmire and the lack of clear ownership of the assets and legal structure of the organization. Entrepreneurs need to recognize that these corporate hindrances impact your ability to raise future capital and grow your business. Think of this as watching a building grow atop a foundation that later needs to be torn up and relaid in order for the structure to be finished.

Entrepreneurs must realize at the outset that there are four essential components of a business that must be simultaneously advanced in order for optimal chances of success. These include the following:

1. *Product development*
2. *Market development*
3. *Financing development*
4. *Corporate development*

All entrepreneurs understand the need for the product development component and they are usually deeply entrenched in this. However, the other three components are equally essential in order to build a successful business. Entrepreneurs may not be focusing on the less visible "corporate development" component of the business.

In order to have the best chance of success, entrepreneurs need to identify key milestones within each of these four development categories and manage and monitor the progress towards reaching each of them. Be sure to select milestones that demonstrate to investors a reduction in risk for each of these components.

In order to create an overall business strategy, you will need the help of an experienced and seasoned *start-up corporate attorney*. You need to find one who is experienced with development-stage companies in your sector, someone who is supportive of entrepreneurs, and one with whom you can establish a good working relationship. Realize that you will be paying for experienced business and legal advice, not for someone who fills in boilerplate documents. As a general rule, look for senior partners in small-to-mid-sized firms rather than someone in a enormous law firm that may relegate your work to junior or novice individuals. There are other attorneys you will likely need help from during your business venture, such as a patent attorney and possibly a securities attorney. For more information on finding and hiring an attorney you can review an article I wrote for *Nature Biotechnology's Bioentrepreneur titled "Why You Need a Lawyer"* [1].

A good corporate attorney is someone who will assist you with the overall impact and align each of the following (and more) to your overall business strategy:

- Choosing the right legal corporate structure and at appropriate stages
- Properly securing the rights to your company name, trademarks, and product names
- Negotiating technology license agreements with rights that are needed to sell the company in the future
- Creating founders agreement and founders stock or options with buy back rights
- Creating key employee agreements with nondisclosures and assignment of inventions to the company
- Establishment of stock option plans
- Properly constructing financing and shareholder agreements

Documents outlining the aforementioned are foundational because they define your corporate entity and its ties to licensed entities, founders, and employees, and they describe the various restrictions and rights of your organization.

How to Avoid This Mistake

If you realize that you may have created a legal document mess, in order to repair it, there must be a process of creating new documents, obtaining required signatures from past shareholders and other potential stakeholders who could possibly claim rights to some parts of the business. It is important to find a good corporate attorney and work through arrangements with them to put together a plan to fix your issues. If you do not have a large budget, some attorneys will help by deferring part of their fees to the next funding. If you find yourself in this situation, recognize that in order to secure subsequent financing, some of your agreements may need to be renegotiated or canceled which takes time and effort in order to move forward. Remember, it is not too late to begin. In order to be successful, entrepreneurs should ensure they advance each of the four essential components of a business simultaneously. Stephen Covey speaks about the "Urgent/Not Important" quadrant activities we do that displace the "Important/Not Urgent" quadrant type of activities, in his book *7 Habits of Highly Effective People* [2]. Be sure that you do not simply focus on the urgent but also the important. Allocate time and attention to the corporate development component of your business. Set value-enhancing milestones in each of these four development areas and check monthly to be sure you are engaged in activities that move each of these forward simultaneously. By consistently and progressively reaching incremental milestones in each of these areas, you will find that your business will be viewed with interest by investors. Be sure to find a good corporate attorney who has experience in your sector and at your stage of business, whom you get along with and gives you good advice. They are extremely valuable for their strategic business advice and as a trusted adviser rather than someone who provides you with just legal templates. *Focus your attention on all four areas of business for your best opportunity for success.*

Common Mistake 4: Failing to Recognize and Leverage Untapped "Human Capital" Resources

A fourth common mistake of entrepreneurs is that they actually have at their disposal untapped and unrecognized human resources that are not fully leveraged to assist in accomplishing their goals. The challenge for early-stage companies is that cash is sparse and, therefore, the company cannot hire a full team of individuals with all the requisite skills to accomplish everything they need. Early-stage companies generally have goals greater than the human resources they possess to achieve them. The irony is that these companies have a truly innovative product concept, but they don't have the abundance of resources that well-established companies do. Because of this dilemma, it is critical for early-stage companies to recognize and utilize several untapped human resources.

Without question, a critical success factor of all entrepreneurial organizations is the quality and breadth of the team who works together seamlessly toward the same goal. We typically refer to individuals who comprise the team as "human capital." Unfortunately, human capital is often thought of as *full-time employees*, whereas start-up and early-stage companies rarely can afford to hire an adequate team of full-time employees. Early-stage companies are usually challenged to raise enough capital to support their limited team and to make progress fast enough so they can raise more money to support the overhead. All too often the investment capital does not arrive in a timely manner, and these companies end up laying off team members to maintain and sustain the company. Alternatively, I encourage you to recognize that your *human capital* is much broader than simply your full-time paid employees but should include each of the following resources:

1. *Full-time company employees*
2. *Part-time company employees*
3. *Trusted consultants with a specific focus and applicable expertise*
4. *Mutually beneficial partnerships with companies and organizations*
5. *Community leaders, advocacy groups, local supporters of your mission*

Capitalizing on Your Expanded Human Capital

We can group our human capital resources into three categories: 1) Internal company employees 2) External individuals with vested interest and 3) External organizations and partner relationships. Whereas each of these groups are held together by your common core values (See Figure 41.2).

Internal Company Employees

Your "full-time company employees" is self-explanatory; but while we are discussing the subject of employees I would like to briefly share the importance of looking for three characteristics in any individual that you are considering hiring. These include (1) relevant experience, (2) ability to execute and (3) core values. The first one is what we find on a resume and what we ask questions about in an interview. The second characteristic is hard to find out unless you probe in different ways because it is easy to show experience but hard to learn if they are just good at talking. The third characteristic is the most difficult to identify but it becomes evident when a person is in different surrounding and talking with different individuals at different levels of responsibility related to the position for which they are interviewing. For instance, an interviewee who talks in a condescending manner to individuals who are in lower positions and pays careful attention to those in superior positions is one that does not have a core value that honors all individuals. As discussed in *Chapter 35: Company Growth Stages and the Value of Corporate Culture*, the cumulative core values of the employees form the culture of the company and the culture of your company will either be an asset or a liability. There are other tips on how to select these individuals for their ability to execute and their core values, described in the book *The Business of Bioscience: What Goes Into Making a Biotechnology Product* [3].

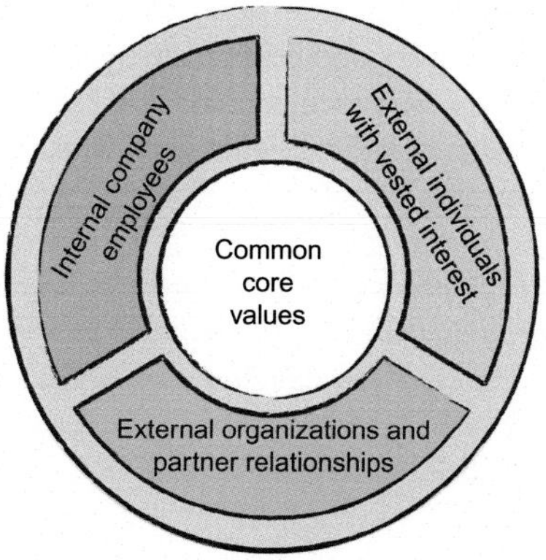

FIGURE 41.2 Your human capital assets.

External Individuals with Vested Interest

This next human capital category includes all external individuals with specialized knowledge and expertise that your full-time employees do not possess. These include more people than you initially think. They can include your corporate attorney, patent attorney, board members, scientific and clinical advisory members, business and technical advisers, mentors, technical and regulatory consultants, and angel investors. In some cases this can include the academic university professors and staff that you may be able to "lease" for a period of time. Although you will likely interact with these individuals less frequently than your full-time employees, *you should treat them, and communicate with them, as important members of your integrated team.* These relationships should be established on common goals, mutual benefit, and especially, common core values. You should keep these individuals updated on your progress and the milestones of your company, as they can better assist you if they know your company's issues. I have met many unpaid supporters of the businesses I started, who were individuals in influential positions who simply believed in me and our company's mission. Building these types of relationships also provides valuable learning and informal mentorship opportunities for you. Be willing to ask difficult questions and do not be afraid to receive candid feedback.

As another example, angel investors are typically viewed as a source of money but never forget they also have achieved success in business and can be called upon for help and advice with issues that you may not have faced before. *Leverage the knowledge of these advisers* knowing they have a vested interest in your company's success. Often, you may find that some of your investors have connections or expertise in an area that you need help, and they can advise you for free. As an entrepreneur, I have had the privilege of working with many great investors. They have provided valuable advice in sales and marketing, financial matters, regulatory and business counsel, and even moral support. Be sure to include them in your business decisions and you will find a willing group of individuals who can help advise you and introduce you to others in their network who can provide help.

Board members also fall into the category. The appointment of board members typically includes individuals who have financed your company. Therefore be sure to choose financial partners who share your company's vision and your core values. All cash from investors spends the same but recognize that when you accept equity capital, you are entering into a formal agreement with the investor's values or the institutional philosophy from which the cash comes. Board members are a key component of your human capital and, when properly selected, provide a valuable resource of expertise, contacts, and advice to help you reach your company goals. Many of my board members have provided invaluable help and advice, as their goal is the ultimate success of the organization.

External Organizations and Partner Relationships

This third category of human capital includes all the "outsourcing" organizations for activities that you do not perform internally or cannot perform as well as they do. Choose them for their expertise and experience with your specific needs in mind. Early-stage companies should be "virtual" as much as possible. In other words, keep your core expertise activities inside the company, and outsource as many noncore activities to others who can do them better, for less. For instance, most development-stage companies do not have an HR department and do not keep up with employment law requirements. Partnering with a good *professional employer organization* (PEO) leverages expertise for all the HR and payroll functions without having this burden on the entrepreneurial organization. *contract research organizations* (CRO) are utilized by development-stage biotechnology companies, and early-stage companies should outsource all activities that are not core to their expertise. This allows them to extend their time horizon to reach critical product development milestones. The key factor is to view these organizations as an integral part of your team. If you select these organizations as you would any employee, and work with them as such, you establish a trust relationship with them. Don't forget that with outsourcing, you cannot just turn over complete responsibility without constant input, rather you need to carefully manage these activities and relationships because you have less control compared to internal activities.

This human capital component also includes organizations you work with that have overlapping interests. If you have collaborations with other companies or nonprofit organizations where each receives a different benefit by working together, learn to leverage their expertise and experience. These types of mutual relationships can also provide external validation of your company's value, or they even may result in future investments in your organization, or possibly a future acquisition partner.

This component of human capital also includes supportive civic and community leaders, your legislators, and people who are supportive of your organization and its mission, especially those that may not be paid by the company. If you have a strong civic leader who believes in your mission, they are usually well connected and can introduce you to others within the community for help. Sometimes, you may need a legislator to champion a cause for you if you find the right ones that align with your mission and vision. If your product market has a patient advocacy group, these organizations can be great supporters of your organization, they can help get the word out about your fundraising and they can assist with connections to key opinion leaders.

How to Avoid This Mistake

Entrepreneurs with an early-stage company must perform many activities in which they are not experts. These activities include everything from building a website or putting out press releases to managing your financing and ensuring scientific progress of your product. However, the number of activities consuming an entrepreneur's attention increases exponentially as the company grows, making it harder for them to wear many hats successfully. As you grow, realize that there are talented individuals and partnerships outside your organization who can perform functions beyond your realm of expertise. Sometimes, they can be paid but often they can just be helping you achieve your mission. As you hire full-time employees to be a member of your team it is important to remember that these individuals should be selected based upon their expertise, ability to execute, and, more importantly, that they all share the same core values of your organization.

I often remind myself of a saying: "*At some point in your career, your success will no longer depend solely on what you accomplish alone, but by what you accomplish with and through the help of others.*" I can truly say that I have not encountered a development-stage company that claimed to have all the human resources they needed. Therefore it is critical to identify and leverage these external human capital resources your company needs. These external individuals are people whom you have chosen to rely upon for certain functional aspects of your business—or for business advice and help—who are an addition to your full-time employees.

Successful entrepreneurs *strategically leverage all their human resources* as integrated components of their human capital and overall company strategy. Carefully select these individuals and they will provide valuable advice, assistance, network contacts, and mentorship to ensure you can overcome the challenges you will face as a growing company. Recognize that your board, scientific advisers, consultants, and mentors are part of your human capital as they have a vested interest in seeing your company succeed.

Common Mistake 5: Flawed Capital Management: Fundraising Is Not Strategically Timed to a Value-Enhancing Milestone

An unintentional but common mistake of an entrepreneur is that their capital raises are not timed to occur *after* reaching the next value-enhancing milestone. Less-experienced entrepreneurs will think about raising capital as they need it. If a company attempts to raise capital because they are close to running out of money, yet they have not accomplished a value-enhancing milestone, this negatively impacts investor interest and company valuation. Determining the amount of capital to raise, and the timing in which to raise, is an important strategy for success. Although you should plan that the amount of capital you raise will allow you to reach certain milestones, it is not just the amount of money raised that is important but also the *timing* of raising money. When a company wants to raise money but has not reached the next value-enhancing milestone, it is more difficult to raise money for three reasons, (1) it is not clear what will be accomplished with the new money as the company has not increased in value from the last raise, (2) there is a perception that the company is desperate for money because they are raising money out of need rather than from strength, and (3) there is a perception that the entrepreneur leader is not capable of properly managing funds for the company. To be clear, a *value-enhancing milestone* is an accomplishment that increases the valuation of the company because by accomplishing this, *the risk of product development failure has been reduced.* To see examples of value-enhancing milestones, see *Chapter 10: Understanding Biotechnology Product Sectors.*

How to Avoid This Mistake

First you must list your value-enhancing product development milestones, then time your funding closings to be *after* completing key milestones (Fig. 41.3). This means that you must identify and estimate the amount of capital needed to reach each value-enhancing milestone. Begin

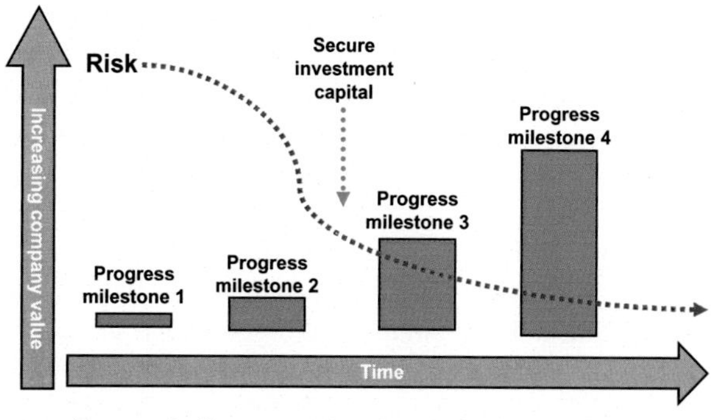

FIGURE 41.3 Company value increases as company risk is reduced.

raising capital 9 months, to as long as 18 months prior to needing the capital, depending on the size of the round, as it can take this long to close a new financing. Ample time is needed to make connections, give pitches, investor due diligence, negotiation of terms, and then the final closing. One way to help shorten the timeframe to closing is to always be "pitching to investors" even between financings. Practically speaking, you should always be in a mode of "raising money" whether you need it or not, as you can always say "no" but you cannot say "yes" without an offer. For capital raises that are $0.5MM or less, the timeframe is shorter as the investors for seed funding are usually a different investor category (see *Chapter 17: Sources of Capital and Investor Motivations*). By timing your closings to occur *after* completing key milestones, you will improve your ability to raise the needed funds. Also, remember to stay as virtual as possible and focus on your core activities and outsource the things that others can do better than you, such as noncore activities, and keep your expenses to a minimum. Consider a subleasing agreement with the university for lab space and equipment and even lease their personnel during your early stages. Consider compensating critical individuals with some equity for reduced fees. The key is to efficiently use the capital you have, and to raise money on strength to improve your likelihood of success. Without a continuous source of capital, you cannot develop your product.

Common Mistake 6: Not Recognizing When or How to Pivot or Reinvent Your Business Model. Failing to Take Advantage of "Serendipity" and Not Listening to the Surrounding Environment

There are numerous roadblocks early-stage companies will face, such as running short of cash, key experiments that did not work, the emergence of new competitors, an important patent did not issue, your key scientist joins another company, a regulatory rule changed that impacted your company, or the field of medicine you are working on is no longer of interest to investors. These are all potential roadblocks, or they can be a source of motivation to pivot or adjust your business or alter your product market focus.

If you find that investors are not interested in the field of medicine you are working in, rather than fighting over it, look for a more significant opportunity using your technology. You may stumble across information that sparks an idea that you can use to pivot or transform what you are doing into success. Train yourself to become aware of "serendipity" and learn to observe things that are presented to you in a different light. You can only take advantage of "serendipity" if you are open to it and are not dismissive of things that you don't believe pertain to you.

The discovery of penicillin was serendipitous and was a major breakthrough that changed medicine and reduced the death toll during World War II. Alexander Fleming was a brilliant researcher who studied Staphylococci but he kept an untidy laboratory (Fig. 41.4). After completing his experiments, he stacked his Petri dishes in his lab and went on vacation for a month. On September 3, 1928, he returned and found a culture contaminated with fungus and he observed that the bacterial colonies were cleared around the mold (Fig. 41.5). He recognized an opportunity and was curious enough to look into it and found a result different from what he planned.

He said:

"It arose simply from a fortunate occurrence which happened when I was working on a purely academic bacteriological problem which had nothing to do with antagonism, or moulds, or antiseptics, or antibiotics.

... penicillin started as a chance observation. My only merit is that I did not neglect the observation and that I pursued the subject as a bacteriologist. My publication in 1929 was the starting-point of the work of others who developed penicillin especially in the chemical field".

Serendipity is another word for "good fortune," or "luck," and other random circumstances. Although luck is not just chance, it requires someone to be open to new opportunities. As Louis Pasture said "*In the fields of observation, chance favors only the prepared mind.*" A good book that may help you understand ways to take advantage of serendipity is *Make Your Own Luck* [4].

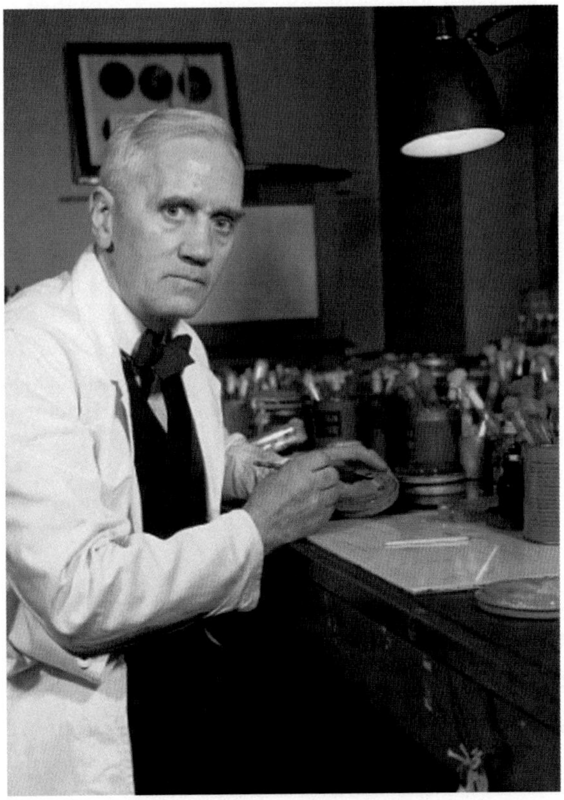

FIGURE 41.4 Alexander Fleming: an accidental discovery changed how medicine is practiced today. Source: https://upload.wikimedia.org/wikipedia/commons/b/bf/Synthetic_Production_of_Penicillin_TR1468.jpg.

How to Avoid This Mistake

Learn to see solutions rather than just problems. Be observant and train your mind to take advantage of "serendipity" when it presents itself. It is likely that as an entrepreneur, you will need to pivot (adjust/modify) your product, business model, or company at some point

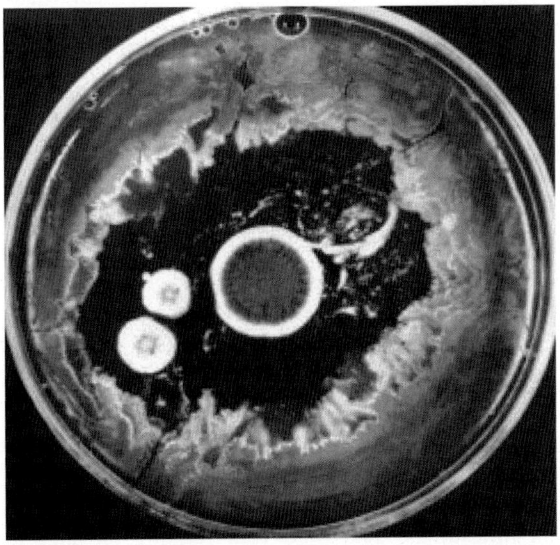

FIGURE 41.5 Penicillium mold clearing a bacterial culture of Staphylococcus. *With Permission from MSD http://www.biology-pages.info/A/Antibiotics.html.*

(and it may be multiple times). Therefore train yourself ahead of time to take advantage of chance occurrences, unexpected meetings with people, bits of information that trigger ideas, and circumstances around you. If you do this, you will never run out of ideas for solving the problems and roadblocks you face. Successful entrepreneurs instinctively see solutions while others see problems. Successful entrepreneurs see opportunities and they learn to take advantage of "serendipity."

Common Mistake 7: Short-Term Commitment and Wavering Internal Motivation Leads to a Self-Limiting Enterprise

You can be sure that sometime during your journey as an entrepreneur, things will get tough and you may even be tempted to quit. This is true of anyone in any industry who is building a company. The difference is that in the biotechnology industry, the timeframe, the costs, the regulations, are longer, higher, and more burdensome than in other industries. Many biotech entrepreneurs have quit prior to reaching their goal because they ran out of motivation, energy, or they believed that there was no way for what they were doing to become successful. I would encourage you to review the common mistake 6 and then find ways that keep yourself motivated to continue. Sometimes, discouragement comes from institutional investors who say that it is a bad idea, or it is not needed, or no one would buy that. Sometimes, those sentiments are true and you should do something to pivot. Then other times, these individuals just don't see what you see.

Bessemer Venture Partners is a 108-year-old venture fund with 120 IPO and $5 billion under management. They have 51 investment professionals and have made over 1177 investments having over 463 exits and they have seen and done so many deals that they have an "anti-portfolio" on their website [5] listing the companies they turned down for investments sometimes more than once. These include:

- Airbnb
- Apple Computer
- Google
- Cisco Systems
- PayPal
- Intel
- Ebay
- Snapchat
- FedEx
- Kayak
- Tesla
- Intuit
- Lotus
- Facebook
- Atlassian
- Okta
- Zoom

One thing you can learn from list of very successful companies that were turned down (sometimes more than once) by very smart investment professionals, is that even *they* do not know every company that will become successful.

How to Avoid This Mistake

Perseverance is the hallmark of a successful entrepreneur. Don't give up. The saying that it is only over when you quit is good advice to the biotech entrepreneur. Constantly share your vision so that others will want to follow. Many times, the difference between success and failure is that the entrepreneur did not quit. Sometimes, a breakthrough is just around the corner, and short-term perseverance is really *no* perseverance. The question was asked of Thomas Edison about his numerous unsuccessful attempts or failures to find the perfect filament for the light bulb, he responded by saying, "*I never failed once, it just happened to be a 2000-step process.*" He understood that what others call *failure* is really a lack of perseverance. If Edison would have stopped at his 1999th attempt, he would not have been credited with the discovery of the light bulb. Remember that perseverance is one of the characteristics of successful entrepreneurs and they find ways to keep themselves motivated to continue. You should also find your own ways to keep yourself motivated when you become discouraged, because it is not over unless you quit. Who knows, you may be on your 1999th experiment before your success.

References

[1] Shimasaki CD. Why you need a lawyer. Nature Publishing; 2010 <https://www.nature.com/bioent/2010/100801/pdf/bioe.2010.8.pdf> [accessed February 25, 2019].

[2] Covey SR. The 7 habits of highly effective people: powerful lessons in personal change. revised ed. New York: Free Press; 2004.

[3] Shimasaki CD. Chapter 10: Corporate culture and core values in a biotechnology company. The business of bioscience: what goes into making a biotechnology product. New York: Springer; 2009.

[4] Kash P, Monte T. Make your own luck: success tactics you'll never learn in b-school. NJ: Prentice Hall Press; 2002.

[5] Bessemer Venture Partners. The Anti-Portfolio, Honoring the Companies We Missed. <https://www.bvp.com/anti-portfolio> [accessed March 1, 2019].

Chapter 42

Summary

Craig Shimasaki, PhD, MBA

CEO, BioSource Consulting Group and Moleculera Labs, Oklahoma City, OK, United States

Chapter Outline

By now, you may have come to appreciate that the biotechnology industry is complex, multifaceted, yet tremendously exciting, with proven capabilities of delivering innovative and life-saving products previously considered impossible. This industry is immensely diverse and constantly expanding with new scientific discoveries uncovered daily. Biotechnology encompasses a breadth of products such as medical cures and treatments for severe diseases, tests that can predict recurrence of cancer, methods for improving crop yields, and unique ways of producing renewable fuels that are environment-friendly. Almost all biotechnology products originate from basic research discovered in an academic or research laboratory. However, producing commercial products from this research requires a company and a team of talented individuals to translate these research discoveries into commercial products. A seasoned and skillful entrepreneur is first required to establish and lead these companies down a chosen path that will ultimately deliver these innovative products to the marketplace. In this chapter, we will briefly review a few of the key topics covered in this book.

Biotechnology Entrepreneurship

There are vast differences between the biotechnology industry and most other industries such as the need for tremendous amounts of capital, lengthy product development cycles, and the requirement for extensive field testing, or clinical testing in animals and in humans. There is also a need for specialized expertise to overcome arduous regulatory hurdles before a biotechnology product can reach the market. Once on the market, these products must be accepted by government agencies and third-party insurers who have stringent criteria for reimbursement. Although the challenges in this industry are great, so are the opportunities for success.

A biotechnology entrepreneur is the original company builder, but they are also product developers and risk managers. These individuals are the initial source of the motivation, vision, and forward momentum of any new organization. Without them, the company and its products would not exist. Biotechnology entrepreneurship is unique in that it requires individuals who are skilled in both the technology and the business aspects of an enterprise.

Biotechnology Entrepreneurship. DOI: https://doi.org/10.1016/B978-0-12-815585-1.00042-5

Biotechnology is the melding of both scientific and business disciplines, and by integrating these activities a company can effectively develop novel products. Success in the biotechnology industry requires individuals who can effectively communicate and understand the language of business and the language of science. A key criterion for any technology leader is the ability to be a multidisciplined translator. Often, this is one of the most challenging aspects of leading and managing a biotechnology business; however, individuals who avail themselves to learning opportunities can become proficient at communicating the central issues in both these disciplines. For those who are interested in reading about additional experiences of early pioneers in the biotechnology industry, there is a wealth of information chronicled at Ref. [1]. We can learn valuable lessons from their stories, their successes, as well as their failures.

Biotechnology entrepreneurs are individuals with vision and passion that drives them to pursue their goals with the belief that their product or service will ultimately impact the well-being of multitudes. Much is riding on the shoulders of the biotechnology entrepreneur and, as a result, we have identified some characteristics that will help improve an entrepreneur's success such as:

- a driving passion for their work with an innate ability to inspire others to follow;
- the ability to communicate their vision so others can buy into that mission;
- not being afraid to take carefully calculated risks, and accepting responsibility and ownership for problems;
- viewing their environment through optimistic eyes with the desire and humility to learn from others;
- perseverance in the face of adversity, applying creativity and imagination to arrive at resourceful solutions;
- an understanding of the real purpose of negotiation;
- the ability to raise needed capital and manage it well while simultaneously multitasking critical activities;
- possessing leadership wisdom and an awareness of the unknown-unknowns;
- being a multidisciplined translator with the ability to understand and speak the language of both business and science; and
- possessing desirable core values with the ability to identify others who share similar values.

The biotechnology entrepreneur cannot accomplish this work alone but must find and motivate a creative team and build a culture of innovation in order for their product to be developed and reach commercialization. Without a dedicated and skilled team of individuals, it would be impossible for any entrepreneur to accomplish much. Therefore this team of individuals must also be talented, experienced, and able to equip and motivate others to contribute in their own unique ways to the enterprise.

Growing Biotechnology Clusters

Because of the great value generated by the biotechnology industry, there is widespread interest in developing biotechnology clusters in most all countries around the world. Biotechnology companies thrive in an ecosystem that has support services, a technically skilled workforce and access to capital. This is evidenced by the many well-established and growing concentrations of biotech activity in the United States, the United Kingdom, Canada, France, Germany, Netherlands, Switzerland, Europe, the Middle East, Japan, and Australia with emerging clusters in China, India, Indonesia, and Singapore, to name just a few.

Biotechnology clusters provide benefits to the local region and to the community they reside such as creating clean, high-technology, and high-paying jobs. In 2016 the nation's bioscience workers earned nearly $99,000, on average, which is more than $45,000 (85%) above the average for the nation's private sector. This wage premium earned by bioscience workers has grown from 64% in 2001 to 85% today. Of course, these added high-paying jobs generate personal and sales taxes for local government. Biotechnology companies also attract an innovative and skilled workforce, collateral businesses, and a host of other support services. Established biotechnology clusters have large talent pools bringing cross-creativity to the local region, and as a result, shorten product development time. As we previously discussed, there are five essential elements that must be present in any geographical region in order for a biotechnology cluster to develop. These include (1) the abundance of high quality, adequately funded academic research; (2) a ready resource of seasoned and experienced biotechnology entrepreneurs and mentors; (3) ready access to at-risk, early and development-stage capital willing to fund start-up concepts; (4) an adequate supply of technically skilled workforce, experienced in the biotechnology industry; and (5) availability of dedicated wet laboratory and specialized facilities at affordable rates.

In order to successfully create an environment with these five essential elements, both the industry and government must play a role in the development of biotechnology clusters. Traditionally, the way government has participated is through economic stimulation, financing, and incentives for companies within particular industries. Because funding is always a critical need for biotechnology companies, one of many ways government can help to stimulate private investments in biotechnology companies is by providing investment tax credits for qualified investing in life science companies.

Biotechnology Sectors and Product Diversity

As you have already learned, there is a diversity of sectors within the biotechnology industry. On the surface, this industry may appear to be complex because of the vast array of products that biotechnology is capable of producing. The "biotechnology industry" is a general reference to all of the products within sectors that include therapeutics, biologics, diagnostics, medical devices, clinical laboratory tests, instruments, agricultural, industrial, and biofuel applications.

Each sector focuses on a certain group of products and utilizes many similar tools and methods to create these products. The human health sector creates innovative medical products that decrease human suffering and improves our lives in ways that were not previously possible. New vaccines have been created to treat cancer, and others have been developed to ward off all types of infectious diseases. More accurate diagnostics have been developed to quickly identify origins of disease and determine treatment options. Many therapies have now been developed to treat orphan diseases, which are debilitating diseases that afflict fewer than 200,000 people, all of whom previously had limited treatments for their conditions. With the aid of biotechnology, as of 2020, there are over 770 orphan drugs approved by the FDA and more then 550 are in the development pipeline.

Advances in personalized medicine are accelerating as practical applications of the human genome research are being developed and used. Breakthroughs in sequencing technology are astounding. To sequence the first human genome, it required 13 years and approximately $3 billion, now, within a decade and a half, we have the ability to sequence an entire genome within days for about $1000. Sequencing technology is advancing so rapidly that it soon will be possible to sequence an individual's entire genome within an hour for about $100. Greater medical advances are realized because of an increased understanding of our genetics and our environment, which will continue to result in novel treatments to enhance our longevity and provide us with a better quality of life. Revolutionary biotechnology research tools continue to be created from innovative discoveries such as polymerase chain reaction. This technique expanded the field of diagnostic medicine and forensic science by providing us the ability to amplify minute quantities of genetic material from a human specimen and to determine if an individual will respond appropriately to a particular drug.

Major advances are also being made in the food and agriculture biotechnology sector. These include unique ways to more efficiently grow crops, novel ways to increase product yields, and to significantly increase nutritional benefits of the foods we consume. Agricultural biotechnology has delivered insect-resistant crops that greatly reduce the need to use pesticides on our food sources, herbicide tolerance crops that allow farmers to use weed killers without damaging crops and to produce crops that have increased resistance to harsh environmental conditions such as drought, floods, and extreme cold and heat. Biofuel development and production have significantly advanced because of biotechnology with the use of corn, switchgrass, and cellulosic feedstocks that decrease our dependence on foreign oil and to reduce greenhouse gas emissions. All these advances have been made possible because of the creative ideas of individuals who utilized biotechnology tools and techniques to solve some of the greatest problems of our day.

From the birth of biotechnology in the mid-1970s with the discovery of genetic engineering tools that can transplant a desirable human gene into the genome of bacteria to express this needed protein, the biotechnology industry was begun. Originating from only a handful of start-ups, now there are more than 10,000 biotechnology companies worldwide, which are creating novel products to solve some of our most challenging problems. These companies forged the way and ushered in the development of additional tools needed to advance research discoveries that, in turn, led to more innovative products. The biotechnology industry is constantly expanding as new scientific and technical discoveries are uncovered and new applications are identified. The overarching goal of this industry is to create unique products and processes that improve life, health, and well-being of individuals and society as a whole.

Technology Opportunities

Biotechnology companies are birthed from novel product ideas that are conceived to provide value for a specific group of individuals. If you examine the original source of most successful biotechnology products, you will find that the vast majority of them originated from basic research conducted by a scientist, professor, physician, or engineer at an academic or research institution. Basic research has a fundamental goal of acquisition and discovery of new knowledge by exploring new ideas, testing new concepts, and better understanding previously unknown processes in biology, science, and engineering. Unfortunately for the commercially minded, academic research goals rarely include product development or commercialization. Technology transfer offices (TTOs) at universities are increasing efforts to advance basic research ideas further along to early stages of product development. However, academic and research institutions are not typically well equipped or experienced in assessing the potential of technology concepts destined to be blockbuster products, nor do they possess depth of expertise in biotechnology product development. As a result, very few products have been fully developed within academic and research institutions because this is not one of their major goals. Because the most advanced product development work is performed in companies, it is critical for a functional avenue of exchange to be created between research institutions and biotechnology industry enterprises.

For biotechnology entrepreneurs who are considering licensing a basic research technology application from an institution, be sure to first conduct a technology evaluation because that decision has long-term impact on the potential success of your future company. After you select a technology and product application, a team of individuals will be committing an enormous amount of time and resources to the development of this future product. Therefore technology concepts and product ideas should be selected based upon certain criteria, and some ideas should be avoided because of shortcomings that may limit their likelihood of success. Several criteria have been elaborated upon in this book to assist in evaluating new product technology ideas, and to assess those with the likelihood of future commercial success.

Company Formation, Ownership Structure and Security Issues

Upon deciding to start a biotech company, it is essential to secure the support of a good corporate attorney with experience in start-ups in the biotechnology industry. There are many legal issues that can negatively impact a company as it grows if they are not handled properly in the beginning. Choosing the right legal structure, properly issuing founders stock and stock options to employees, intellectual property (IP) ownership agreements and employment agreements and securities agreements when raising capital; these are just some of the issues that you need to contend with when starting a company. Therefore is it essential to have selected an experienced biotech start-up attorney to help you from the very beginning to have consistency throughout your company development.

Licensing the Technology

During the early stages, one of the most valuable assets a company has is its IP. The rights given to the company allow it to raise capital so it can make product development progress. Most of the technologies that form the basis of biotechnology products originate in academic and research institutions. Knowing how to work with these entities, understanding what terms are conventional to agree to, is critical to the long-term value of the company. When licensing technology from academic institutions, you will be interfacing and negotiating with someone in the TTO. Public and private research institutions have legal obligations to fulfill. Knowing how to help them fulfill their obligations, while finding a compromise such that you are not committing large amounts of capital in the beginning, allows your company to fund product development milestones that increase the value of the organization for future fundraising. With the help of your corporate attorney, they can guide you through this process and help you understand the terms you are agreeing to, and how these may impact the future obligations of the company.

Intellectual Property Protection Strategies

Prior to, and during product development at a biotechnology company, a major asset the company must secure is the IP rights to the technology. This initially occurs through a negotiated license from the owning institution, but the entrepreneur must pursue additional IP as the product is developed by their company. Much of the early value that investors attribute to a development-stage biotechnology company is the "ownership" of these technological concepts and new product ideas as embodied in the company's IP. In order for a company's product or service to be successful, it must have a technological and beneficial advantage over other products in the market. To gain a competitive advantage, your company must provide something unique. Legal protection of these assets is essential. As improvements, new product concepts and ideas are implemented, it is likely that others will desire to copy them. We previously reviewed a number of legal tools for protecting your assets and for achieving exclusivity or at least a head start over your competition. A good patent counsel is essential in helping you devise a strategy to properly protect these assets through a variety of protective barriers such as general patents, design patents or industrial designs, utility model patents or petty patents, and plant patents, as well as trademarks, service marks, and layout designs of integrated circuits, commercial names and designations, geographical indications, protection against unfair competition, and trade secrets.

Company Business Models

Products are developed and marketed by companies, and every commercial enterprise must operate through an underlying business model. Business models are simply the way in which a company makes money and the manner in which all these functions are interrelated internally and externally. Choosing the right business model is essential to ensure that a company has the best opportunity for success. The selection of a business model should be made during the inception of the company, and chosen to give the future organization a strategic competitive advantage. Selecting the optimal business model is the first step to building business success and reducing the risk of failure. This is because the entrepreneur and leadership team are the "risk managers" of the company, and in order to manage risks, they must know what they are. We reviewed some business model examples used in the biotechnology industry and described the components that make up a business model. We then discussed five segments of business risk that entrepreneurial leaders must manage in order to optimize success. The purpose was to give the entrepreneur a better understanding of how a business model helps manage and reduce the risks of their company.

The Virtual Company

Start-up biotechnology companies rarely have enough money to accomplish everything they would like because of limited capital. This is why I am a strong proponent of operating as a "virtual company" during the start-up phase of a company. Operating as a virtual company simply means that the company does not perform all the necessary functions internally but still accomplishes all the necessary activities as if it did. The way this is accomplished is by carefully selecting outsourcing partners. For most early-stage companies the extent of outsourcing can be significant where almost all development functions are performed under contract through specialty organizations. Sometimes, the types of R&D activities required by some early-stage biotechnology companies are so unique and specialized that their only option is to perform these functions in-house; however, the more common functions can still be outsourced to keep overhead costs down. During start-up stages, capital is usually quite limited and a company cannot hire many full-time employees, but substantial progress must still be made in order to gain interest from investors. Operating as a virtual company during the formative stages allows entrepreneurs to extend the time horizon of their operations, and it requires much less capital to maintain and sustain the company while their product is initially being developed.

Sources of Capital for Product Development

A company cannot survive without continued access to capital, no matter how great the technology or product is. Fortunately, there are many sources of capital available to biotechnology companies. However, each source has limitations as to the amount of capital they can invest, and the time frame in which they can invest. The most common sources of capital that are available to biotechnology companies at various stages of development include:

1. Personal Capital
2. Friends and Family
3. Grants: Local and Federal
4. State Financing/Funding Programs
5. Angel Investors/Family Fund Offices
6. Nonprofit Foundations
7. Venture Capital (VC)
8. Corporate Sponsors or Partnerships
9. Private Equity/Institutional Debt/Mezzanine Financing

It is important to remember that each capital source has different investing limitations, different expectations for returns, and different motivations that drive their investing decisions. Most investor groups have well defined expectations for returns on their investment, and these expectations are commensurate with the level of risk they are taking. Investors typically describe their expectations as a multiple of their investment, a return on investment (ROI), and also by the number of years in which to exit. Also, remember that there are "dilution effects" on shareholders, founders, and management with each new round of capital raised. Therefore it is advantageous for existing shareholders to ensure that the company valuation is constantly increasing as each new round of capital is raised.

We described what we called funding alignment principles. These will improve the likelihood of success in raising the needed amount of capital from the right source at the optimal time of company development. Finding the ideal funding partner is not easy but the likelihood increases by following these funding alignment principles that include the following:

1. Identify the target capital source that has the greatest interest in the development stage of your company and product.
2. Make sure there is alignment with your company's financial needs and the funding source criteria for investing such as dollar amount, type of equity, and length of investment time.
3. Make sure that your opportunity provides the necessary return expected by your target funding source in terms of ROI and multiple-of-investment.
4. Make sure there is alignment in the motivations and core values of your organization with those of the target funding source.

Each of the capital sources we described have a preferred stage at which they like to invest. As companies transition through distinct product development and capital financing stages, these different funding sources become more interested or less interested depending on their investing criteria. Entrepreneurs can save themselves time and energy by focusing only on the funding sources most likely to invest at their particular development stage.

Financing stage terminology may vary but listed early are some of the terms most commonly used. For those that are more familiar with product development stages rather than financing stages, a particular product development stage can be implied by the stage of financing.

1. ***Start-up or preseed capital***: Also known as formation capital and is typically the smallest amount of money the company raises at any one time. These funds are usually used to establish corporate operating and employment agreements, file and prosecute IP and to incrementally advance the technology. Often these are the funds that allow the company to fully develop their business plan and marketing strategy.
2. ***Seed capital***: Is sometimes called proof-of-concept capital and is the next larger round of capital after start-up capital. The money raised in this round can range between $100,000 to more than $1,000,000 and is typically used to advance the technology or product to a stage that increases the value of the company by reaching a key development milestone. Other uses of this capital may go toward expanding the target market research, hiring consultants, subcontracting to contract research organizations and to hire part-time or temporary employees.
3. ***Early-stage capital: series A/B preferred rounds***: These are the next significant funding rounds for the organization and may come from a syndicate of Angels or a group of Angels and local funding programs. Early-stage capital can also come from institutional investors such as early-stage investing venture capital firms. These rounds can range from $3 to $25 million or more, depending on the product sector.
4. ***Mid-stage or development-stage capital: series C/D preferred round***: These follow-on rounds usually involve some or all of the investors in the previous preferred rounds plus new investors that typically come from institutions such as venture capital and corporate partners. Greater numbers of VCs invest in mid-stage development companies than in early-stage development companies. The number and size of these subsequent rounds vary and the letter designation increases with each round.
5. ***Later stage and expansion capital: series E/F preferred rounds***: Therapeutics and biologics typically require more funding rounds and larger capital investments as compared to diagnostics, medical devices, and molecular testing products. The good news is that there are greater numbers of VC firms that invest in these later-stage rounds.
6. ***Mezzanine capital***: For companies that need it, this is usually the last round of capital before an exit for investors such as an acquisition or initial public offering (IPO) of the company. Venture capital funds are plentiful at this stage when product development risks have been greatly reduced. Investors at this stage enjoy a shorter time from investment to exit than for those who invested at early or development stages.
7. ***Acquisition or IPO***: These are exit events where the investors and shareholders can reap a financial reward for their work and perseverance. However, for drug development and biologics companies the requirement for capital is so high that usually an IPO really becomes another later-stage financing round.

Cash is a precious and limited commodity to a start-up company. The hard fact is that there is just not enough investment capital to fund all the good ideas for every biotechnology company. Securing biotech funding requires perseverance, and the ability to learn from each investor presentation to improve the chances of funding the company at subsequent junctures. The greatest idea imagined, the most powerful drug concept ever conceived, or the grandest life-saving medical device dreamed, is of no consequence if one cannot finance its development to commercialization. Someone once said, "a vision without execution is a hallucination." To have a vision without funds to execute it is an exercise in frustration and futility. Perseverance, flexibility, creativity, and finding a team of exceptional people are key ingredients for successful fundraising.

Financial Ramifications of Funding a Biotechnology Venture: What You Need to Know About Valuation and Term Sheets

Understanding what premoney and postmoney values are and how they can be determined are important factors in negotiating funding rounds. Even more important are the terms that are set such as liquidation preferences, dividends, antidilution or price protections, drag-along and tag-along provisions, piggy-back rights, board composition, and voting rights. These terms greatly impact the rights of shareholders and the rights of management and the board and determine how payouts are shared at an exit. Entrepreneurial leaders need to understand the impact of these terms on their company and their potential impact on raising the next round of capital.

Investor Presentations: What Do You Need in an Investor Pitch Deck

One of the key tools that a biotech leadership team will use when raising capital is an investor pitch deck. This is a set of PowerPoint slides that succinctly convey the fundamental facets of your company to potential investors. What you put in them will tell investors a lot about your company and about the management. In the past, a formal business plan was used to communicate to prospective investors, but the pitch deck has become the preferred communication tool by most investors today. There are a number of topical subjects that need to be covered in an investor pitch deck to tell the story of your company and to expound on the key aspects of your business. These 18 topical subjects in slides are the key ones you need in a Biotech Investor Pitch Deck:

- **Title slide**
- **Topic 1:** Company purpose, history, and mission
- **Topic 2:** The problem or "pain," unmet medical need, and "why" there is a problem
- **Topic 3:** Technology and product "solution"
- **Topic 4:** Target market opportunity
- **Topic 5:** Competition and/or substitutes
- **Topic 6:** Describe your business model
- **Topic 7:** Product development and regulatory pathway
- **Topic 8:** Intellectual property and/or secret sauce, and partnerships
- **Topic 9:** Insurance reimbursement strategy
- **Topic 10:** Go-to-market strategy
- **Topic 11:** Proforma projections and financing "ask"
- **Topic 12:** Use of proceeds
- **Topic 13:** Likely exits and estimated time frame
- **Topic 14:** Leadership team
- **Topic 15:** Reasons to Invest Summary
- **Topic 16:** Thank you Q&A
- **Topic 17:** Potential risks and how they will be mitigated
- **Topic 18:** Support and appendix slides

However, there is one pitfall that occurs in that transition toward the pitch deck as the preferred communication tool for investors; it allows the entrepreneurial team to bypass the requirement to carefully think through the entire business and product development strategy as you would if preparing a complete business plan. For that reason, I recommend that you complete a business plan for your company as an internal tool for your direction and strategic planning. This process will help you think through the assumptions to see if they are correct and identify the hurdles you need to overcome as you build your business.

Development of a Company Culture With Core Values

A company's culture is a good predictor of the future success of the organization and their likelihood of achieving their product development and commercialization goals. For a biotech start-up company, developing a corporate culture may not seem like a high priority compared to other pressing needs such as raising capital, hiring a team, and quickly making product development progress. One can even temporarily ignore the development of a company culture without much consequence; however, at some point, the culture will affect a company's ability to get work done effectively.

Each company should develop a culture suitable for their needs and their particular objectives. It is best to purposefully build a culture that adds strength, rather than a divisive one that occurs by default. At some point the company reaches a critical mass, and the culture of the organization becomes set. Fortunately, most start-up biotechnology companies begin with an entrepreneurial culture. An entrepreneurial culture is one where there is excitement and anticipation about the company's work and mission. Employees have aspirations of contributing to a greater good along with opportunities of professional advancement and expectations about working in an organization with a great future. A one-size-fits-all corporate culture does not work, but there are certain qualities and values that are always advantageous to have.

Just as an organization's strength is the sum total of the strengths of the individuals, the culture of a company is the sum total of the individual core values of its employees. Each one of us possess a set of core values whether we recognize it or not. These are the guiding principles upon which we operate and make decisions. Sometimes, these core values are clearly defined, and other times these guiding principles are simply understood. Successful companies have been built upon strong core values. An employee having a core value of "*mutual respect for others*" will make a different decision about leaving a job unfinished for another employee, and an individual with the core value of "*acceptance of responsibility for one's actions*" will readily admit a mistake rather than cover it up or blame someone else. These instances may seem inconsequential by themselves, but when you add these up amongst 20, 50, 100, or 1000 employees, this becomes the culture of the company. A fundamental error of business is to focus only on product development and marketing without consideration to the core values of the people that produce these products.

Company Growth Stages

All companies transition through growth stages along their pathway to commercialization and maturity. This transition is a real process that occurs subtly over time. As this transition takes place, there is a corporate culture that becomes established and it originates from the core values of the leaders and the sum total of the core values of the new hires. There are distinct growth stages of every company, and during these stages, there are transition phases in which a company moves to the next growth stage successfully or unsuccessfully. The ability of an organization to make this transition is dependent upon the leadership and their ability to make management style changes as the company grows. For individuals who work daily within an organization, these transition stages and changes are not obvious, whereas for those coming into the organization from the outside, it is very obvious.

As a company works to accomplish its objective of creating a valuable product or service, it adds staff, expands activities, and establishes corporate relationships and its business practices evolve. Changes will also occur in the process of how a company makes decisions. A company that comprises 10,000 employees, and manufactures and distributes products worldwide, typically makes decisions differently than a start-up organization with a handful of employees and one product in development. The optimal methods and processes of decision-making for an early-stage company do not necessarily work well for a mature company and vice versa; however, even though the methods and processes may change, the culture should not, nor does it need to change with growth.

Biologics Manufacturing

Once a biotechnology product has been fully developed, it must be manufactured in large enough quantities to meet the market demand for the product. In the case of biologics manufacturing (or biomanufacturing, for short), it is quite different from traditional small molecule pharmaceutical manufacturing. Biomanufacturing is a complex process using recombinant DNA technology to develop procedures and analytics to manufacture these biologic products. These biologic product processes are developed using several platforms such as whole *multicellular* systems encompassing transgenic plants, animals, and *unicellular* microbial (bacteria and yeast), insect and mammalian cell culture. The discovery and "proof of concept" from the research bench is transferred to a process development group that will use science and engineering as well as regulatory expertise to scale-up the product efficiently. The process for different biologics platforms are complex, and unlike traditional chemical synthesis, the biologic product resulting from a living system is not an exact science. Because of this biologic complexity, it is important to remember that "*the process is the product,*" and any variation in the process could impart a change in the product's safety and efficacy, and ultimately regulatory approval.

Regulatory Approval for Biotechnology Products

The entrepreneurial team must develop a clear regulatory strategy during the early stages of product development that can later be presented to national regulatory authorities (NRAs) such as the FDA. NRAs regulate products developed for treating and diagnosing patients to facilitate access to high quality, safe, and effective products and restrict access to those products that are unsafe or have limited clinical use. Regulatory procedures have an impact on all stages of biomedical product development. Biotechnology companies must have well thought-out plans for safety review during development stages, regulatory approval, and legal registration which are all required before product commercialization. When appropriately implemented, this type of regulation and oversight ensures public health benefits and safety for patients, health-care workers and the broader medical community. Therefore it is essential that developers of biomedical products (drugs, biologics, devices, in vitro diagnostics, or some combination) possess the knowledge and awareness of the regulatory challenges and opportunities to expedite the development of safe and effective products in a cost-effective manner.

Biotechnology Products Have Three Customers

Compounding these challenges that have been described, the biotechnology entrepreneur and management team must be sure that their product meets the needs of three different "customers" rather than just one. These three include the *patient*, the *physician* (or provider), and the *payer*, all of whom need to realize value from your product in order for it to be successful. In the biotechnology industry, one customer is the decision-maker who decides *which* product should be used, another customer makes an independent decision whether or not to *pay* for the product (and how *much* to pay for the product) and a totally different customer *uses* the product. In other industries the customer is the same individual who makes the decision to purchase, and he or she is the same one who uses the product. This is *not* how product decisions, purchasing, and utilization occur for biomedical products. This partitioning of customer decisions is an aspect that can hamper the success of many biotechnology companies. It is vital to have a clear understanding of the three independent customers of biotechnology products and to provide a compelling value proposition to each. This can be accomplished if you understand each of their motivations and responsibilities which will then improve your product marketing success.

Business Development and Partnering

For biotechnology companies, it seems like the need for cash is constant. Very few, if any, biotech companies have been able to raise enough capital to cover all their research, development, clinical, regulatory, and manufacturing costs through to commercialization. Venture capital has provided a significant portion of the later-stage funding for many companies, but there are still requirements for larger amounts of capital at final stages of human clinical trials, and a need for a commercialization partner. For therapeutic, biologic and many medical devices, forming partnerships with large pharmaceutical companies or medical device companies, can provide the needed capital and a valuable marketing partner. Therefore it is important for the entrepreneurial team to assess who these likely future partners may be, and to keep them apprised of your product development progress along the way. The benefits of having a strategic partner are many. In a typical partnership the biotech company may receive up-front, milestone, fee-for-service payments and, eventually, royalties on sales. In exchange the partner receives ownership or exclusive license and marketing rights to the biotechnology company's product. Also, this partnership event may also ultimately become the exit event for your investors. Having a strategic commercial partner is almost essential, but keep in mind that successful deals can take at least 12 months to conclude so be sure to plan and prepare early.

Public Relations for Biotechnology Companies

Finding the right partner can be difficult especially when the management team usually has more priorities than it has resources. One great tool to help future partners to find you is through public relations (PR), which is the art of creating, broadcasting, and maintaining your message and company image with your targeted audiences.

PR is often overlooked by many early-stage biotechnology companies, but it is an excellent tool for supporting your company objectives such as finding funding, partnerships, customers or employees, or just carrying out various business activities. One critical step in reaching a particular audience is to determine the story you want to tell about your company and products in terms of your target audience's needs and interests. Once you have defined your positioning and key messages, these can then be tailored to specific objectives for specific audiences and used as part of a strategic communications program that supports your corporate goals. Entrepreneurs should consider the various PR methods, including building a steady stream of news and media coverage, contributed articles, speaking platforms, and strategic use of social media. Strategically incorporating these tools will help you reach your desired audience and will help potential partners find you, along with providing visibility and credibility for your company over time.

Ethics in Biotechnology

All companies are faced with challenges, and some challenges are greater than others. Biotechnology companies may also face ethical dilemmas at some time, even in an industry where life-saving products are developed for the good of others. For small biotechnology companies, consequences can be devastating for poor decisions, and the cost and stakes are high. Challenges can arise because of competing pressures to achieve goals and accomplish results within a limited time frame, and this could set up a climate in which a bad choice could be made and, as a consequence, ethical dilemmas can arise. We have seen the setbacks of ImClone, the developers of the chemotherapeutic Erbitux, in 2002 when Sam Waksal, their CEO, was convicted of securities fraud, bank fraud, obstruction of justice, and perjury. Even in larger organizations, we have also seen instances of pharmaceutical products such as Vioxx, where the product was subsequently removed from the market due to heart attack deaths during commercialization. It has been stated that there were indications in human studies supporting the drug's association with increased risk of heart attack much earlier, but not made public. All companies must strive to operate in a manner that would not give reason for the public to be skeptical about its motives or its mission and purpose. Biotechnology companies also need to operate using a commonly accepted set of business ethics that include such tenets as fairness, trust, absence of conflict-of-interest, and good business practices.

In rare cases, companies may find themselves in a dilemma when no matter what action is taken, some harm will occur, and there are equally strong reasons for taking either course of action. In these cases, accurate facts are vital to resolving ethical dilemmas, but these facts alone will not solve the problem. Ethical dilemmas require that the leader make wise choices. The choices individuals make are based upon core values. Fortunately, these instances described are rare, and the examples of dilemmas most likely arise because of a series of unethical or at best, poor decisions made over time, rather than one solitary decision. For a biotechnology company to have success, it is vital that the leader and the entrepreneurial team possess similar core values, and that they lead and manage using these values to inspire their team to follow. By doing this, your company will improve its decision-making skills, and this will exceedingly reduce the number of ethical issues they may face in the future.

Career Opportunities in the Life Sciences Industry

Individuals with a life science education and background are essential to the biotechnology industry and a company's success. You should realize that having this background does not limit your career to just laboratory research and benchwork. We described a number of sectors within the biotechnology industry, and within each of these sectors, having diverse career opportunities. Life science careers are not limited to biotechnology sectors either, as there are a multitude of opportunities in other industries such as those that support the biotechnology industry. A sample of career opportunities for individuals with life science background include discovery and preclinical research, process sciences, clinical development, regulatory or medical affairs, scientific project management, business and corporate development, marketing, sales, technical and product support, management consulting, corporate communications, operations, manufacturing, quality control, bio-IT, law, human resources and recruiting, venture capital and investment banking, and careers in nonprofit organizations and in government. Whether or not you have an interest in laboratory work, business, sales, marketing or clinical studies, there are hundreds of different career options. Some of the different career paths can lead you to writing a patent, marketing a product, conducting a clinical trial or doing a business deal. It is important to realize that there are numerous opportunities for you to find that ideal job that matches your unique personality attributes, skills, interests, and long-term goals.

For individuals with a scientific or technology background who are conducting laboratory benchwork and want to transition from bench research to other vocational areas, the good news is that many scientists do transition to other careers and bring with them the depth of experience and knowledge from their field of science. Be sure to pursue your interests and explore the various opportunities available. As I tell students, be sure to find the career opportunity that inspires you and the one that you would do even if you did not get paid, for that is the place where you will excel and fulfill your vocational destiny.

Conclusion

The information and guidance in this book will help you start, manage, and lead a life science company or give you an understanding of how to operate as an "entrepreneur" or team member within this remarkable industry. The two goals of this work have been (1) to train future biotechnology leaders and managers to become more successful by learning from the previous generations of entrepreneurs and biotech leaders sharing their experiences, knowledge, and life lessons (2) to educate and expand the working knowledge about this industry to the vital service providers and partners who are essential to the success of biotechnology companies.

It would be impossible to cover in enough detail all the topical information relevant to the needs of this expanding industry. However, it is our desire to have conveyed enough information to better equip you to operate, manage, lead within, or support companies in this biotechnology industry. I hope that these experiences and teachings have provided you with greater knowledge and inspiration to pioneer new product opportunities, to lead and manage more effectively, to overcome technical, financing, and regulatory challenges as you journey alongside the multitudes of individuals within this vast and growing industry. A familiar saying is "*There is no trying, only doing.*" All biotechnology entrepreneurs must begin with a foundational belief that their technology and product possess great value to those in need of their treatment, test, or service. And it is through the continual "*doing*" rather than "*trying*" you will create an opportunity to make a difference in this world. Keep "*doing*" and don't quit.

I wish you the best of success in all your entrepreneurial endeavors!

Reference

[1] Program in BioScience and Biotechnology Studies, Regional Oral History Office, The Bancroft Library. Berkeley, CA: University of California, 2014. <http://bancroft.berkeley.edu/ROHO/projects/biosci/oh_list.html> [accessed March 9, 2019].

Index

Note: Page numbers followed by "*f*," "*t*," and "*b*" denote figures, tables, and boxes, respectively.

B

C

D

J

K

L

M

O

P

Q

R

S

T

U

V